This is the first comprehensive work of reference to survey in depth the wide-ranging variability in the response of individuals to drugs. Such variability may result from differences in bio-transformation of drugs or in receptor responses: it has profound implications in terms of drug therapy, understanding mechanisms of drug metabolism and action, and awareness of genetic polymorphism and its links with disease. New human genes have been discovered by studying these phenomena. Adverse reactions occur more commonly on standard drug dose regimens in some phenotypes. Similarly the response of disorders to standard treatments is affected by genetic constitution. Also, the possession of certain pharmacogenetic phenotypes renders some individuals more prone to develop spontaneous disorders.

Advances in molecular genetics are revolutionizing the whole field – for which this authoritative book forms the invaluable reference base.

GENETIC FACTORS IN DRUG THERAPY
Clinical and molecular pharmacogenetics

GENETIC FACTORS IN DRUG THERAPY
Clinical and molecular pharmacogenetics

David A. Price Evans, MD, DSc, PhD, FRCP
Director of Medicine, Riyadh Armed Forces Hospital, Saudi Arabia

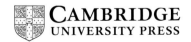
CAMBRIDGE
UNIVERSITY PRESS

Published by the Press Syndicate of the University of Cambridge
The Pitt Building, Trumpington Street, Cambridge CB2 1RP
40 West 20th Street, New York, NY 10011-4211, USA
10 Stamford Road, Oakleigh, Melbourne 3166, Australia

First published 1993

Printed in Great Britain at the University Press, Cambridge

A catalogue record for this book is available from the British Library

Library of Congress cataloguing in publication data

Price Evans, David A.
Genetic factors in drug therapy: clinical and molecular pharmacogenetics/David A. Price
Evans.
p.   cm.
Includes index.
ISBN 0 521 41296 X (hc)
1. Pharmacogenetics.   I. Title.
[DNLM: 1. Pharmacogenetics. 2. Drug Therapy. 3. Genetics,
Medical. 4. Variation (Genetics)–drug effects. QV 38 P945g 1993]
RM301.3.G45P75 1993
615'.7–dc20
DNLM/DLC
for Library of Congress   93-17041   CIP

ISBN 0 521 41296 X

Cyflwynedig i'm rhieni

CONTENTS

Preface

The purpose of writing this book was to make available in a convenient and illustrated form a general overview of pharmacogenetics. The time was judged opportune because the newer techniques of genetics are now beginning to demonstrate clearly the molecular mechanisms involved. It must be emphasized that this is neither a textbook of pharmacology nor a treatise on therapeutics. Readers are expected to have a working knowledge of these topics.

The author's interest in drug metabolism was first aroused when as a science undergraduate he was taught by Professor R. Tecwyn Williams, FRS. His interest in genetics came into being by working with Professor Lord Cohen of Birkenhead, Professor Sir Cyril A. Clarke, FRS and Dr Richard B. McConnell who greatly influenced his thinking as a medical undergraduate and subsequently. These two themes came together when the author became a Fellow in Professor Victor A. McKusick's department at Johns Hopkins Hospital where he worked on the genetics of isoniazid metabolism.

An opportunity further to study genetic factors in drug metabolism and effect came about by joining the staff of the Department of Medicine at the University of Liverpool which was headed first by Lord Cohen and later by Sir Cyril Clarke, both of whom were generous in their support, interest and encouragement.

During the production of this book the author has been fortunate in receiving an enormous amount of help from friends and colleagues. Many, who are world authorities in their particular fields, have read individual chapters and offered criticism and advice. Acknowledgements to them appear at the ends of the appropriate chapters.

Professor H. F. Woods and Professor G. T. Tucker of the Department of Medicine and Pharmacology of the University of Sheffield have been through the whole book and gave advice which led to extensive improvements.

Many of the good points that appear in the book are due to the efforts of the persons listed above. However, the sole responsibility for any errors, omissions and misrepresentations lies with the author.

The production of the book would not have been possible were it not for the active participation of the staffs of the Medical Library and Medical Illustration departments of the Riyadh Armed Forces Hospital and to them the author owes a debt of gratitude. Very special thanks are due to Mrs Tracey Atkinson, Personal Assistant to the author, who in addition to her demanding ordinary duties took an especial interest in the production of this book and was responsible for all the correspondence involved, and for typing many successive drafts.

Mr I. P. Silver, of the Cambridge University Press, and Mrs J. K. Bulleid have been most helpful in providing advice and in guiding the book through its various stages of production.

PART I   Introduction

1   The arrangement of the information in this volume

PROGRESS has been faster in the study of the genetics of drug metabolism than in the study of the genetic phenomena of drug receptors. It is not clear why this should be, but some possibilities are:

1 That there is more genetic variability in the drug biotransforming mechanisms than in the receptor mechanisms.
2 That more effort has been put into investigating drug metabolism than drug response. This is understandable because the same expertise, technology and apparatus can be used to study various biotransformation phenomena whereas the study of receptors tends to be more individualized.

However, the difference is currently being redressed as progressively more receptor genes are being cloned (Barnes 1992).

Within the field of drug metabolism it is customary to describe the chemical reactions as either Phase I or Phase II. The former are primary changes in the molecule, which typically consist of the addition of polar groups such as $-OH$, $-NH_2$, $-COOH$ and $-SH$, or hydrolyses. The latter are various types of conjugations in which higher polar entities are added, e.g. glucuronide, acetyl, methyl, sulphate and amino acid groups.

Hence the first section of this book deals with cytochrome P450 based phenomena since these constitute the most important Phase I reactions. Following a general introduction, individual chapters are devoted to categories of cytochrome P450 which are of especial clinical importance.

The plasma cholinesterase, alcohol-metabolizing enzymes and some other polymorphisms take up the next Phase I sections.

Turning to Phase II reactions the *N*-acetyltransferase polymorphism has been studied for over 30 years and so a large amount of information about it is available, which occupies one section.

Miscellaneous Phase II drug biotransformations are then gathered together.

The remainder of the book consists of sections devoted to items which can be considered to show genetic variability in drug response and these include glucose-6-phosphate dehydrogenase, the hepatic porphyrias, phenylthiocarbamide (PTC) tasting, chlorpropamide–alcohol flushing, etc.

Finally, short sections are devoted to gathering together ideas which are common to a number of the different systems discussed in the book and drawing some conclusions.

Barnes, P. J. (1992). Molecular biology of receptors. *Quarterly Journal of Medicine, New Series*, **83**, 339–53.

2   General introduction

VARIABILITY of response to drug medications between patients is a commonplace observation, and often there is no satisfactory explanation. This book aims to describe how genetic factors can explain why people differ in the way they react to ordinary drug medications.

ADVERSE REACTIONS

An adverse reaction has been defined as 'one which is noxious and unintended and which occurs at doses used in man for prophylaxis diagnosis or therapy' (WHO 1969).

Adverse reactions to drugs are common events in all branches of medical practice and at all ages but are particularly highlighted in the elderly, who because they have more chronic illness receive more drug therapy than persons of other age groups (Lancet 1988; Tanner & Baum 1988).

An item in the BMA News Review (1984) announced that in the UK 75% of persons over the age of 75 years were taking some kind of drug. Of these two thirds were taking up to three different drugs at the same time and one third were receiving four or five drugs. Apparently 30% of women aged over 70 years were taking sedatives or tranquillizers continuously and 15% of patients admitted to geriatric hospitals were suffering from side effects of drugs.

However, in the paediatric population also analogous data have been revealed. Mitchell *et al.* (1988) found that among 6546 non-neonatal children without cancer monitored on general medical and speciality wards at two teaching hospitals and

three community hospitals, 2% of admissions were prompted by adverse drug reactions. Two patients died because of their drug reactions.

A table (Venulet 1975) gathered together eleven hospital series and indicated an adverse reaction frequency of 1.5 to 25%. Other studies revealed that 3.7% of 7017 (Miller 1974) and 6.2% of 481 patients (Black & Somers 1984) were admitted to hospital because of adverse drug reactions. Out of 177 patients admitted because of adverse reactions 6.2% died (Caranasos *et al.* 1974).

Since the thalidomide disaster focused the attention of governments and doctors on adverse reactions to drug treatment an enormous amount of research has been carried out on the epidemiology and on the mechanisms involved in producing adverse reactions to various medications. Nevertheless hundreds of deaths continue to be attributed to suspected adverse reactions (Bem *et al.* 1988). Adverse reactions can result from both environmental and genetic influences and their interaction. It is not the purpose of the book to deal with the environmental aspects. In the chapters that follow it will be shown how genetic factors can explain the predisposition of certain individuals to develop adverse reactions to drugs, especially the non-allergic variety.

LACK OF EFFICACY

The study of adverse reactions is an area of clinical investigation in which it is difficult to obtain reliable data. It is even more difficult to get accurate data on what may be regarded as 'the other side of the coin', namely, ineffectiveness of drug therapy. Obviously, many factors could contribute to produce ineffectiveness in an individual patient, in particular the nature of his disease. For example, an infective microorganism might not be sensitive to an antibiotic prescribed. Even after excluding such patients there remain an unquantified but substantial number in whom there is no clear reason why conventional doses of appropriate medications are ineffective. It is true that many environmental influences can contribute to an unsatisfactory outcome, but many instances arise where such an explanation is untenable. This is another grey area on which pharmacogenetics can shed some light.

VARIATION: THE RAW MATERIAL OF GENETICS

For many practical people such as industrial producers and animal breeders, variation in their product is a great nuisance. Medicine too is a practical art and on a superficial level it could be considered that variation in the response of patients to standard drug therapy is a great nuisance. Variation, however, is the very stuff out of which the study of genetics has arisen. (It will be recalled that the historic compilation of Bateson in 1894 was entitled *Materials for the Study of Variation.*)

In this book it is hoped to show three benefits derived from the study of variation in response to drug treatment: first, something of the manner in which adverse reactions are produced, so that they may then more readily be avoided; secondly, improvement in the efficacy of drug treatment; thirdly, that the genetic phenomena discovered as a result of studying variability in response to drugs may explain the mechanism of production of common spontaneous disorders.

Where possible the clinical relevance of each pharmacogenetic system has been emphasized. Animal studies have not been discussed in detail except where they are especially important to the understanding of human phenomena.

Throughout this book the author has used the historical approach in the belief that it enables the reader to perceive how the present state of knowledge has evolved, and more clearly to discern areas that merit further research.

The book deals with genetic phenomena which have been discovered or brought into prominence by the investigation of the variability in the effects or metabolism of drugs or drug-like chemicals. It does not deal with spontaneous conditions which are genetically determined but which vary in their response to drug medications (such as vitamin D resistant rickets).

The chapters are mainly named after the relevant enzyme. In some cases, however, this would not be appropriate even though the relevant enzymes are known (e.g. the porphyrias). In other examples it would not be possible because the enzymic basis is unknown (e.g. the phenylthiocarbamide tasting polymorphism).

HISTORICAL PERSPECTIVE

The two divisions of pharmacogenetics – drug biotransformation and responses of cells or tissues to drugs – have different antecedents. The most clearly definable is the former.

That part of pharmacogenetics which deals with the biotransformation of drugs has as its starting point the discovery of the first 'detoxication mechanism' which was the synthesis in the mammalian organism of hippuric acid from ingested benzoic acid. The first unequivocal proof of the occurrence of the synthesis was provided in 1842 by Keller (cited by Williams 1959). Many more mammalian detoxication mechanisms involving the chemical biotransformations of foreign compounds were discovered during the remainder of the nineteenth century.

In 1902 Garrod published his paper on alkaptonuria, which provided the first proof of Mendelian genetics in man. The disease was attributed to a block or interruption at some point in a metabolic reaction sequence and it was thought likely that the block was due to the congenital deficiency of a specific enzyme (Dunn 1965). Though this study laid the basis for the development of biochemical genetics it was only many years later that this field really developed and along with it biochemical pharmacology and the idea of genetically controlled interindividual variation (see Scriver & Childs 1989).

The next relevant step which was unrelated to the foregoing was the discovery of the inheritance of the ability to taste phenylthiocarbamide (PTC). This compound had been synthesized by Fox who noted that some persons were able to detect a bitter taste easily when the crystals were placed on the tongue whereas other persons could detect only a very slight taste or none at all. The heritable basis of this variation was independently reported in 1931 by Blakeslee & Salmon and by Snyder and the validity of the genetic hypothesis was established on the gene frequency basis by Snyder in 1932. This was the first described genetic variation of the response of a tissue to a chemical compound.

The ability to taste or not taste PTC (which is chemically closely related to the drugs methyl thiouracil and propyl thiouracil) was a clear example of what subsequently became known as genetic polymorphism. The biological importance of this concept was established by Ford in 1940 and was clearly expounded by him in his book (Ford 1965).

The first example of a biotransformation of a drug in a mammal shown to be under genetic control was provided by Sawin & Glick (1943) who studied the fact that serum from some rabbits can destroy atropine whereas the sera from other rabbits lack this ability.

A new branch of biochemistry called 'Detoxication Mechanisms' was established in 1947 when R. Tecwyn Williams published his book thus entitled. This book gave numerous examples of differences between species in the biotransformation of foreign compounds. From then on a tremendous increase occurred in activity in this field of science (Williams 1959).

Another book which aroused considerable interest was that of Roger J. Williams published in 1956. It was entitled *Biochemical Individuality* (mirroring the title of Garrod's 1902 paper) and emphasized the differences between individuals. It included a section on variability in pharmacological manifestations, but did not distinguish between continuous and discontinuous variability.

The 1950s was the decade when pharmacogenetics as a definite separate branch of science came into being. The term was introduced into the medical literature by Motulsky (1957) and Vogel (1959) and was defined as the study in animal species of genetically determined variations that are revealed by the effects of drugs.

During the 1950s the human genetic polymorphisms for glucose-6-phosphate dehydrogenase deficiency and isoniazid metabolism together with the rare genetic variants of plasma pseudocholinesterase (explaining succinylcholine apnoea) and acatalasia were described.

Subsequently progress was made in diverse directions. It was well established in the 1960s that one of the most common primary biotransformations which happen to drugs (and other foreign compounds) in the mammalian body is the addition of oxygen i.e. hydroxylation. This process was found to vary greatly between individuals and twin studies indicated that it was under genetic control.

In the 1970s the genetic polymorphisms of the hydroxylation of sparteine and debrisoquine were described and later were found to be due to the same genes. Subsequently a similar but independent polymorphism for the hydroxylation of (S)-mephenytoin was discovered.

The 1980s saw a surge of new knowledge and understanding of the cytochromes P450 which are the enzymes responsible for carrying out oxidation reactions.

Currently the immensely powerful techniques of molecular genetics, including 'reverse genetics' and the use of expression vectors are being deployed to solve pharmacogenetic mysteries (see, for example, Gonzales 1989 and Meyer 1990). It seems an opportune time to review the subject, in the belief that we are at the start of an era of rapid progress.

Many genes which are responsible for the variability in responses between patients have been mapped and cloned. In some instances, for example the acetylation polymorphism, a single base difference leading to a single amino acid difference is responsible for the variability. This situation is reminiscent of haemoglobins A and S. In other examples, e.g. the debrisoquine polymorphism, more complex differences based on splicing variants exist which bear some similarity to the well established models of some types of thalassaemia.

A point of difficulty has now arisen. In some instances knowledge of the molecular genetics has run on ahead, independent of knowledge of the related phenotypic characteristics.

Painstaking work will be required to match up the phenomena of molecular genetics, e.g. restriction fragment length polymorphisms (RFLPs), with the effects of drugs on cells, tissues and whole human beings. However, the accessibility of DNA from circulating leucocytes, the possibility of making much more of it with the polymerase chain reaction and the relative ease of the laboratory techniques involved, should make it possible to dissect phenotypic variability much more easily in the future than has been possible in the past.

As a result of such work it may prove possible to provide predictive information as to how an individual person will respond to a drug without having first to expose him to that medication.

At a clinical level there have been only a few good clinical studies designed to assess the therapeutic benefits of knowing the phenotypes of patients being treated with the drugs described in this book and this is an aspect which needs more attention.

Bateson, W. (1984) *Materials for the Study of Variation.* London: MacMillan.

Bem, J. L., Mann, R. D. & Rawlins, M. D. (1988) CSM Update. Review of yellow cards 1986 and 1987. *British Medical Journal*, **296**, 1319.

Black, A. J. & Somers, K. (1984). Drug-related illness resulting in hospital admission. *Journal of the Royal College of Physicians (London)*, **18**, 40–1.

BMA (1984). News Review, **9** (9), 3.

Caranasos, G. H., Stewart, R. B. & Cluff, L. E. (1974). Drug-induced illness leading to hospitalisation. *Journal of the American Medical Association*, **228**, 713–17.

Dunn, L. C. (1965) *A Short History of Genetics.* New York: McGraw-Hill.

Ford, E. B. (1965) *Genetic Polymorphism.* London: Faber & Faber.

Fox, A. L. (1932). The relationship between chemical constitution and tastes. *Proceedings of the National Academy of Sciences (USA)*, **18**, 115–20.

Garrod, A. E. (1902). The incidence of alkaptonuria: a study in chemical individuality. *Lancet*, **2**, 1616–20.

Gonzalez, F. J. (1989). The molecular biology of cytochrome P450s. *Pharmacological Review*, **40**, 243–88.

Lancet editorial (1988). Need we poison the elderly so often? *Lancet*, **2**, 20–2.

Meyer, U. A. (1990) Molecular genetics and the future of pharmacogenetics. *Pharmacology and Therapeutics*, **46**, 349–55.

Miller, R. R. (1974) Hospital admissions due to adverse drug reactions. A report from the Boston Collaborative drug Surveillance Program. *Archives of Internal Medicine*, **134**, 219–23.

Mitchell, A. A., LaCouture, P. G., Sheehan, J. E., Kauffman, R. E. & Shapiro, S. (1988). Adverse drug reactions in children leading to hospital admission. *Pediatrics*, **2**, 24–9.

Motulsky, A. G. (1957). Drug reactions, enzymes and biochemical genetics. *Journal of the American Medical Association*, **165**, 835–7.

Sawin, P. B. & Glick, D. (1943). Atropine esterase – a genetically determined enzyme in the rabbit. *Proceedings of the National Academy of Sciences (USA)*, **29**, 55–9.

Scriver, C. R. Childs, B. (1989) *Garrod's Inborn Factors in Disease. Oxford Monographs on Medical Genetics* 16. New York: Oxford University Press.

Snyder, L. H. (1932). Studies in human inheritance IX. The inheritance of taste deficiency in man. *Ohio Journal of Science*, **32**, 436–40.

Tanner, L. A. & Baum, C. (1988). Spontaneous adverse reactions reporting in the elderly. *Lancet*, **2**, 580 (letter).

Venulet, J. (1975). Increasing threat to man as a result of frequently uncontrolled and widespread use of various drugs. *International Journal of Clinical Pharmacology*, **12**, 387–94.

Vogel, F. (1959). Moderne probleme der humangenetik. *Ergebnisse der Innere Medizinische und Kinderheilkunde*, **12**, 52–62.

WHO (1969). International Drug Monitoring: The role of the hospital technician. Report Series No. 425, 6.

Williams, R. J. (1956) *Biochemical Individuality. The basis of the genetotrophic concept.* New York: University of Texas Press.

Williams, R. T. (1959) *Detoxication Mechanisms.* London: Chapman & Hall.

3   Classification of pharmacogenetic phenomena

INTRODUCTION

PHARMACOGENETIC phenomena can be classified by combining two criteria: pharmacological and genetic. From a genetic point of view the big subdivision is into single gene effects (including polymorphisms), and polygenic effects which are phenomena described in terms of quantitative (or biometrical) genetics. From a pharmacological viewpoint subdivision can be made into the time course of drug action (pharmacokinetics) which includes the influence of biotransformation, and the effects of drugs on cells tissues and organs (pharmacodynamics) (see Table 3.1).

Table 3.1. *Pharmacogenetic phenomena*

Single gene effect
Pharmacokinetic
All phenotypes common (polymorphisms)
One phenotype rare ('idiosyncrasy')
Pharmacodynamic
All phenotypes common (polymorphisms)
One phenotype rare ('idiosyncrasy')
Polygenic effects (quantitative genetics)
Pharmacokinetic
Pharmacodynamic

DISCOVERY OF SINGLE GENE EFFECTS

Single gene effects in pharmacogenetics have mainly been discovered as discontinuous variability. Ima-

gine an experiment involving a population of healthy people. Each person is given a standard dose of a drug. Then a pharmacokinetic parameter, such as plasma half-life or metabolite production, is measured in a standard manner. The results would

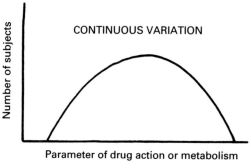

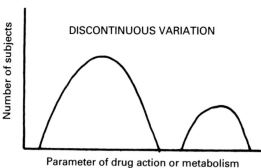

Fig. 3.1. The types of variability of frequency distributions which may be observed when large numbers of persons are given a standard dose of a drug in exactly the same manner. (From Evans 1963.)

6

enable a frequency distribution to be constructed. This frequency distribution could be unimodal or contain two or more modes (Fig 3.1). Provided artefact and stratification had been avoided the finding of, say, a bimodal distribution would strongly suggest the possibility that the population consisted of two types of individual with regard to the property measured. In fact these would be two phenotypes. Such a finding would need to be followed up with family studies to see whether or not the phenotypes were genetically determined.

Exactly similar considerations would appertain for pharmacodynamic measurements, e.g. fall in blood pressure on a standard drug dosage.

The most powerful biological systems of single gene effects are polymorphisms.

THE CONCEPT OF POLYMORPHISM

Polymorphism is defined as the occurrence together in the same locality of two or more discontinuous forms of a species in such proportions that the rarest of them cannot be maintained merely by recurrent mutation (Ford 1971).

As pointed out by Ford (who has been largely responsible for defining the biological importance of the phenomenon) polymorphism does not include certain important types of variation. Different human races (where intermarriage gives offspring with intermediate properties), continuous variation controlled by a number of genes, and the occurrence of rare genetically determined phenotypes are not covered by the concept of polymorphism.

The great advantage in a medical context of dealing with a genetic polymorphism is that associations can be defined in terms of frequency. Thus, in a well known example there has been found to be a much higher frequency of HLA B27 in a population of patients with ankylosing spondylitis than in control populations. Similar associations have been found between pharmacogenetic polymorphic phenotypes and clinical events.

According to one school of thought, one of the central biological ideas derived from the study of genetic polymorphisms runs as follows:

The population has built within it genetically determined variation, so that a swift response can be made to an environmental change. One phenotype will survive better than another to propagate the species whatever the direction of the environmental change.

In some situations one phenotype has the advantage, but in another set of circumstances that same phenotype is at a disadvantage.

This fundamental strategy of nature is mirrored in the case of some pharmacogenetic polymorphisms in different clinical situations.

However, this neat and attractive concept is difficult to reconcile with the enormous number of polymorphisms which have been found by the study of enzymes and other proteins and especially of DNA. Many of these polymorphisms appear to be quite neutral, i.e. to confer no selective advantage.

POLYGENIC EFFECTS

In the introduction to the discussion of single gene effects an imaginary experiment was described. A population of healthy people was given a standard dose of a drug, following which standard metric observations were made. When such an experiment yields a unimodal frequency distribution curve (Fig. 3.1) an entirely different philosophy has to be deployed to that concerned in the elucidation of single gene effects.

In this case (which is by far the most common) it is not possible to discuss the results in terms of different 'types' of individuals; and consequently it is not possible to recognise the influences of single alleles. That being so, the observed phenomenon must be analysed by means of a completely different technique.

The manipulation of observed frequencies of different types of individuals is replaced by the manipulation of variances. The variance of an observation in a population (the square of the standard deviation) is very easily computed. This is the phenotypic variance. Variance has the useful mathematical property of additivity. It can be therefore considered that different components have been added together to make up the phenotypic variance. The most obvious components are the variance due to genetic factors and the variance due to environmental factors. This branch of science is called quantitative or biometrical genetics since it deals with measured properties (Falconer 1964; Cavalli-Sforza & Bodmer 1971). A chapter dealing with quantitative genetic aspects of pharmacogenetics follows later.

INTER-ETHNIC VARIABILITY

Another aspect of pharmacogenetics, not made apparent by the classification of Table 3.1, is the difference between racial groups. This aspect is of great medical importance, and will also be discussed in a later chapter.

Cavalli-Sforza, L. L. & Bodmer, W. F. (1971) *The Genetics of Human Populations.* San Francisco: Freeman.

Evans, D. A. P. (1963). Pharmacogenetics. *American Journal of Medicine,* **34**, 639–62.

Falconer, D. S. (1964). *Introduction to Quantitative Genetics.* (Reprinted with amendments.) Edinburgh: Oliver & Boyd.

Ford, E. B. (1971). *Ecological Genetics,* 3rd edition. London: Chapman & Hall.

Part II   Cytochrome P450 based phenomena

4   Cytochromes P450 – general features

INTRODUCTION

P450 is the name given to a class of cytochromes whose nomenclature has now been rationalized and which are controlled by genes called *CYP* (Nebert *et al.* 1991). The name is derived from the fact that these compounds are demonstrable spectroscopically by reduction with excess TPNH and then gassing two portions of the solution, one with nitrogen and the other with carbon monoxide (CO). The difference spectrum (reduced/nitrogen minus

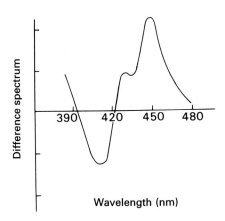

Fig. 4.1. Difference spectrum of cytochrome P450. Samples of reduced cytochrome P450 and reduced cytochrome P450 treated with carbon monoxide are placed in the path of a double-beam spectrometer, and a difference spectrum is plotted. (From Thomas & Gillham 1989.)

reduced/CO) gives a broad absorption band (hence the term 'pigment' which gives the P) with its peak at 450 nm (Omura & Sato 1964; Remmer & Merker 1965) (see Fig. 4.1). The CO complex gives this absorption peak due to the configuration of a cysteine thiolate in the protein (Guengerich 1991).

A similar class of compounds was termed P448 because the absorption spectra of their reduced CO forms gave peaks at 448 nm. They are now called P450 1A2 (Ioannides & Parke 1987).

Cytochrome P450 was first discovered in the 1950s and was recognized to be a haemoprotein by Omura & Sato (1964). Personal accounts of early history of P450 research have been given by Cooper (1973), Levin (1990) and Sato (1991). This group of compounds is extremely widespread in nature, occurring in all living organisms. In mammals there are particularly large amounts in the liver where they constitute the major haem protein. A cytochrome P450 molecule catalyses the insertion of one O_2 derived oxygen atom into an aliphatic or aromatic molecule. An enormous amount of research work has taken place on P450 activities in the last 30 years. Since they are concerned both with the metabolism of drugs and also exhibit genetic variability in their action, they are of great pharmacogenetic importance. The purpose of this section is to present some relevant background information before considering individual pharmacogenetic *CYP* gene product polymorphisms in greater detail.

9

MOLECULAR STRUCTURE

The basic structure is a single polypeptide chain consisting of 500 ± 60 amino acids and containing a single non-covalently bound haem (the same as in haemoglobin, myoglobin, cytochrome *c*, etc.). The crystalline structure of the camphor mono-oxygenase P450 (P450$_{cam}$) from *Pseudomonas putida* has been determined and this is currently the only known crystal structure of a cytochrome P450. It is thought likely that all other cytochrome P450 proteins are similar in general construction.

The haem group is completely buried within the protein. There is a cysteine at position 357 (Cys 357) and the sulphur atom of this cysteine coordinates with the iron atom of the haem. This accounts for one of the six valencies of the iron atom, another four being taken up by bonds to the nitrogen atoms of the pyrrole rings of the haem molecule. The sixth valency is unoccupied when the substrate is bound to the cytochrome P450. When the substrate is removed this valency is taken up with either a water molecule or a hydroxyl group. There is a 'pocket' in the protein molecule into which the substrate fits. The cysteine forms part of this pocket. The structure of the pocket seems to have been highly conserved during evolution. For example, phenylalanine at position 350, glycine at 353 and a branched aliphatic side chain at 359 are invariant (the actual numbering is that of P450$_{cam}$ and may differ in other forms) (see Fig. 4.2).

A second pocket, spatially close to the substrate pocket, accepts the oxygen molecule. This again is formed from a sequence of amino acids which has been highly conserved in evolution. For example, –gly 248–gly 249–X 250–Y 251–thr 252, or ala 248–gly 249–X 250–Y 251–thr 252– seems invariable. The numbering is that of P450$_{cam}$ and may differ in other forms. X and Y represent a variety of other amino acids but X is commonly threonine and Y is commonly glutamic acid.

The overall three-dimensional structure of the cytochrome P450 molecule seems very similar in prokaryotic and eukaryotic organisms, except that in the latter P450s are membrane-bound whereas they are not in the former (P450$_{cam}$ being an example). Eukaryotic microsomal P450 contain a hydrophobic N-terminal tail which probably serves as a membrane anchor leaving the rest of the enzyme external to the membrane (Poulos 1988).

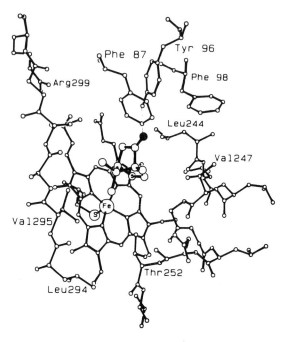

Fig. 4.2. The P450$_{cam}$ active site. Notice that the camphor and O_2 binding pocket are surrounded by aliphatic and aromatic residues. Unlike peroxidase and catalase there are no acid–base or polar catalytic residues (His, Arg, etc.) capable of directly assisting in fission of the O–O bond. (From Poulos 1988.)

A PROTEIN IN EVOLUTION

As a result of examining the amino acid composition of cytochromes P450 mainly as deduced from cDNA sequences of different organisms it has been possible to work out an evolutionary tree (Fig. 4.3).

The way in which the phylogenetic tree was constructed was explained by Nelson & Strobel (1987). Pairs of cytochromes P450 were compared for their amino acid sequences and a percentage difference determined for each pair. From this percentage difference the evolutionary distance in 'accepted point mutations' was estimated using the atlas of protein sequence and structure of Dayhoff (1979). A phylogenetic tree produced by an unweighted-pair-group method of analysis was constructed using the evolutionary distance. The calibration of the time scale was determined as follows. The divergence of bacterial and eukaryotic cytochromes P450 was set at 1400 million years before the present (My BP); the bird–mammal divergence time ($d = 0.71$) at 300 My

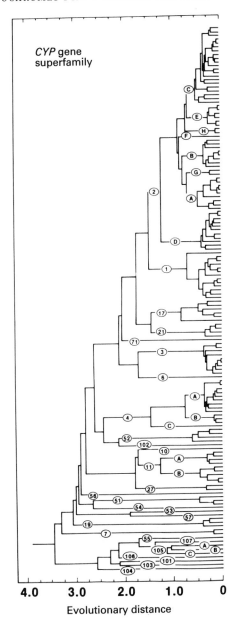

CYP gene
superfamily

4.0   3.0   2.0   1.0   0

Evolutionary distance

Fig. 4.3. The P450 superfamily. The genes within each subfamily represent all those that have been characterized in various species. This tree was calculated using amino acid sequences deduced from 147 of the 154 cDNA sequences available. (From Nebert *et al.* 1991.)

BP and the rat–mouse divergence ($d = 0.27$) at *c.* 20 My BP (Nelson & Strobel 1987; Dayhoff 1979).

The amino acid sequence of a cytochrome P450 from one family is $< 36\%$ similar to P450s from other families.

On the other hand cytochromes P450 within the same subfamily have $> 68\%$ similarity.

A list of 154 *CYP* genes and seven putative pseudogenes has been provided by Nebert *et al.* (1991). Twenty-seven gene families have been described; 10 of them exist in all mammals and comprise 18 subfamilies (16 mapped in man). Each subfamily appears to represent a cluster of tightly linked genes some of which have arisen by gene duplication.

FUNCTION

In mammals P450 proteins are usually located in the endoplasmic reticulum (which *in vitro* becomes the microsomal preparation of the biochemist), but some are mitochondrial.

The generally accepted scheme by which a cytochrome P450 molecule functions at the end of an electron-transport chain is shown in Fig. 4.4. It seems likely that one P450 reductase molecule services a number of cytochrome P450 molecules.

The cytochrome P450 catalyses the reaction whereby one oxygen atom from molecular oxygen is incorporated in the drug substrate molecule to form a hydroxyl group. The exact way in which this happens is not understood. It is likely that a peroxy O–O bond is cleaved heterolytically with the transient formation of an hypothetical ferryl-oxy Fe^{4+}-O intermediate (see Guengerich 1990a, b, 1991 for detailed discussions).

The threonine at position 252 in P450$_{cam}$ has been replaced by serine (which also has a hydroxyl group) and by alanine and valine (which do not possess hydroxyl groups) by Imai *et al.*(1989). The catalytic activity of the enzyme to oxidize camphor was 90% reduced when alanine or valine was substituted but was much the same when serine was substituted. On the other hand, oxygen consumption was unimpaired by the loss of the hydroxyl group and most of the oxygen formed hydrogen peroxide. So, the conclusion was that possessing a hydroxyl group bearing amino acid at position 252 is essential for the proper functioning of the enzyme.

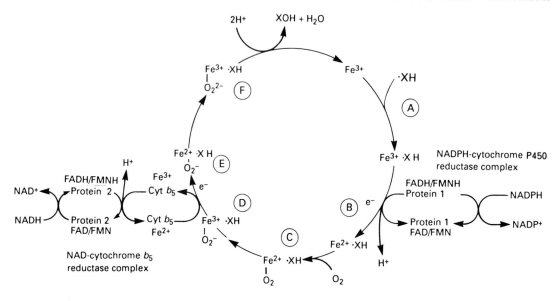

Fig. 4.4. Mode of action of cytochrome P450. Fe^{3+} and Fe^{2+} represent the haem iron of cytochromes P450 and b_5 in the oxidized and reduced form respectively. Proteins 1 and 2 (FAD/FMN) represent flavoproteins. (From Thomas & Gillham 1989.)

The types of oxygenation which occur under the influence of P450 enzymes are shown in Fig. 4.5 and Table 4.1. Many endogenous compounds such as steroids, fatty acids and prostaglandins are substrates for some of these reactions. A huge number of foreign compounds including drugs, carcinogens and pesticides are metabolized in the body by cytochromes P450. Generally speaking the introduction of an oxygen atom into a molecule makes the compound more polar, i.e. water-soluble, by producing a hydroxyl group. This is the most important example of Phase I detoxification reactions. Phase II reactions which follow later generally involve conjugating the oxygenated compound with some other moiety creating an even more water soluble molecule. Examples are glucuronic acid, sulphuric acid, mercapturic acid and amino acid conjugations.

Multiple forms of cytochrome P450 are active in all tissues of all living things; for example, 38 distinct P450 genes have been cloned from rat liver. A single type of cytochrome P450 can have very specific or relatively non-specific affinity for various substrates. A single substrate (e.g. propranolol) can be oxidized at more than one position in its molecule by different cytochromes P450, giving several metabolites. Also, one substrate can be oxidized at the same position by more than one cytochrome P450 having different degrees of affinity.

Since there are many cytochromes P450 with widely different specificities the whole overlapping system is able to deal effectively with a large number and variety of substrates.

We are mainly concerned in pharmacogenetics with the membrane-bound cytochromes P450 of liver. The P450 enzymes of other organs such as the adrenals and lungs will not be discussed in detail. We will be particularly concerned with allozymes which are different P450 enzymes produced by variant genes at the same locus (sometimes called isozymes, but this term should really refer to very similar molecules which are produced by genes at different loci).

Although there is now considerable unanimity about the nomenclature, recognition and actions of different types of P450 cytochromes, there are still some difficulties.

For example different groups give different subfamily designations to the enzyme oxidising mephenytoin. Because of this some workers refer to P450 2C8/9/10 and others to 2C18. Another example is in the subfamily P450 3A. Some workers regard this a major form in the human liver, but

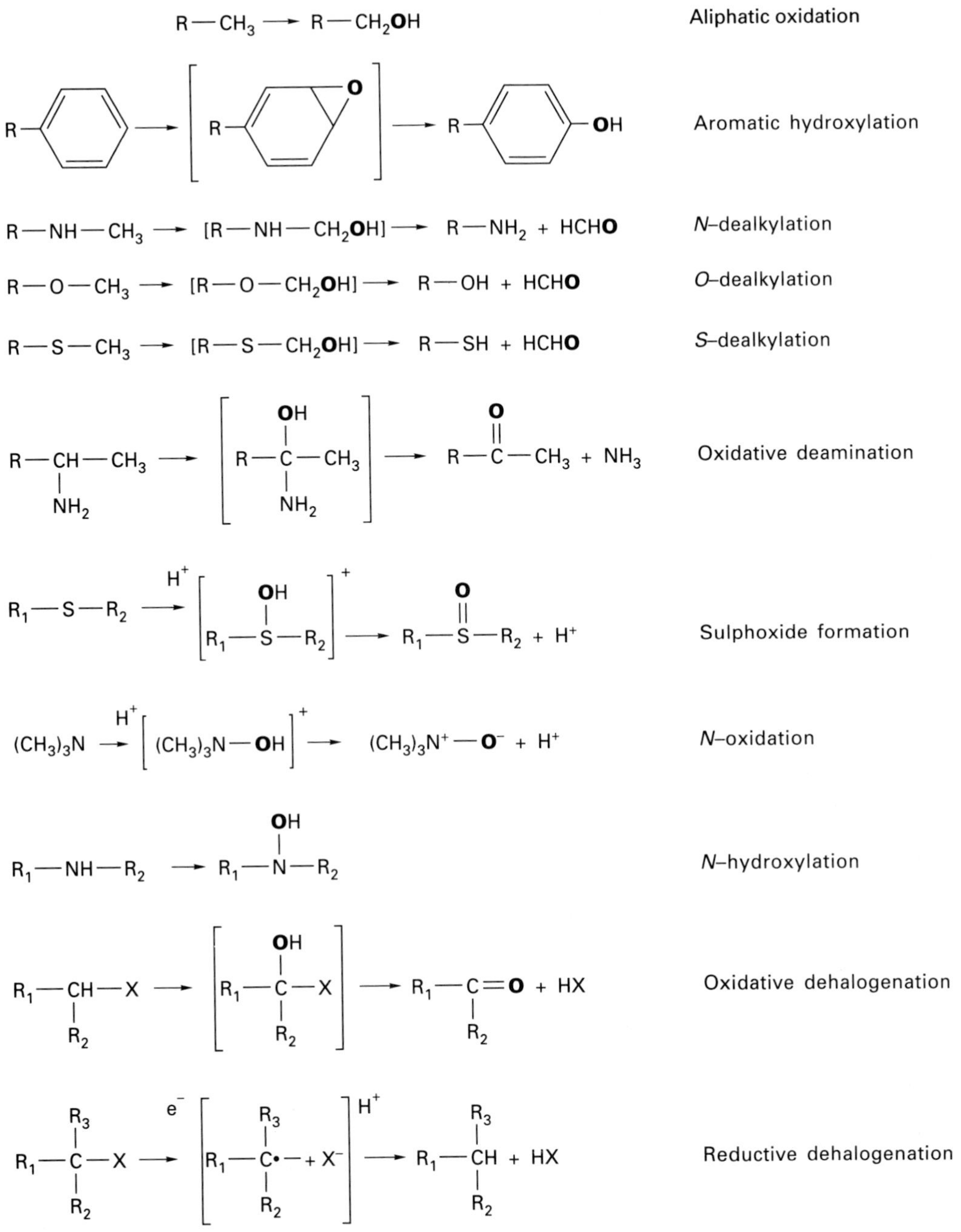

$$R—CH_3 \longrightarrow R—CH_2OH \qquad \text{Aliphatic oxidation}$$

Aromatic hydroxylation

$$R—NH—CH_3 \longrightarrow [R—NH—CH_2OH] \longrightarrow R—NH_2 + HCHO \qquad \textit{N}\text{–dealkylation}$$

$$R—O—CH_3 \longrightarrow [R—O—CH_2OH] \longrightarrow R—OH + HCHO \qquad \textit{O}\text{–dealkylation}$$

$$R—S—CH_3 \longrightarrow [R—S—CH_2OH] \longrightarrow R—SH + HCHO \qquad \textit{S}\text{–dealkylation}$$

Oxidative deamination

Sulphoxide formation

N–oxidation

N–hydroxylation

Oxidative dehalogenation

Reductive dehalogenation

Fig. 4.5. Examples of the many diverse mono-oxygenase activities of the P450 enzymes. The oxygen derived from atmospheric oxygen is denoted by bold print. (From Nebert & Gonzalez 1987.)

Table 4.1. *Some CYP genes in man and their clinical significance*

CYP family			Inducing agents				Medical interest and/or drug substrates
1	A	1	PO	IS			Procarcinogen polycyclic hydrocarbons, 17β-oestradiol
		2	PO	IS	OM	3MC	Acetanilide, phenacetin, caffeine, theophylline, N-hydroxylation of aromatic amines and amides
2	A		PO	IS			Coumarin
	B		PH				
	C	8	PH	RI			Tolbutamide
		9	PH	RI			Diazepam, N-desmethyldiazepam, tolbutamide, mephenytoin, hexobarbital, methylphenobarbital, alprenolol[a]
	D	6					Debrisoquine/sparteine, etc.[a]
	E		ET				Oestradiol, ethanol, paracetamol, chlorzoxazone
3	A	3	PH	ST	RI		Benzo[a]pyrene, 6β-OH cortisol, tamoxifen
		4	CL	RI	DPH	DX	EE quinidine, cortisol, midzolam, lidocaine, cyclosporin A, nifedipine, erythromycin
		5					Overlaps with 3A4[c]
		6					Testosterone[d]
4			CL				
11	A						Cholesterol side chain cleavage
	B	1					Steroid 11β hydroxylase (congenital adrenal hyperplasia)
17							Steroid 17α hydroxylase (adrenal hyperplasia)
19							Aromatization of androgens (? gynaecomastia)
21							Steroid 21-hydroxylase (congenital adrenal hyperplasia)

(Note: rows for 3A3 and 3A4 are joined by a brace labelled [b])

PO, polycyclic aromatic compounds; IS, isosafrole; PH, phenobarbital; ET, ethanol; ST, steroids; CL, clofibrate; OM, omeprazole; RI, rifampicin; DPH, phenytoin; DX, dexamethasone; EE, 17α ethynyl oestradiol; 3MC, 3-methyl cholanthrene. (The condition resulting from a deficiency of an enzyme is indicated in parentheses.)
[a]Polymorphic.
[b]One of the major forms of cytochrome P450 in the adult liver.
[c]Polymorphic, in that it is present in only about 10 to 20% of human adult livers (with cytochrome P450 3A4) and one liver described with cytochrome P450 3A5 only (Aoyama *et al.* 1989). Present in 1 of 10 human fetal livers (Wrighton *et al.* 1990).
[d]The major form of cytochrome P450 in the fetal liver.
Information from: Aoyama *et al.* 1989; Bargetzi *et al.* 1989; Brosen 1990; Gonzalez 1990, 1992; Hunt *et al.* 1992; Liu *et al.* 1991; McManus *et al.* 1990; Morel *et al.* 1990a, b; Pichard *et al.* 1990; Relling *et al.* 1990; Wolf *et al.* 1990; Wrighton *et al.* 1990; Gonzalez 1992.

Jacolot *et al.* (1991) refer to it as 'only a very minor form in human liver'. Wrighton *et al.* (1990) point out that it is not possible to separate P450 3A3 from P450 3A4. Park & Kitteringham (1990) refer to P450 3A3 as being responsible for 80% of cyclosporin oxidation activity as well as for the metabolism of nifedipine, erythromycin, etc. Others refer to this category of function as cytochrome P450 3A4.

These difficulties most probably arise because the cytochrome P450 molecules within a subfamily are very closely similar with regard to their structure and so possess overlapping specificity. Gradually, by means of multiple correlative experiments, the important and major substrate for each subtype will be established.

CATEGORIES OF HUMAN CYTOCHROMES P450

Some of the human cytochromes P450 have a bulk of interesting information so as to warrant their own independent sections in this book. These include P450 1A1 and 1A2, P450 2C8, 9 and 10, P450 2D6, and P450 3A4 and 5.

The essential molecular specificities which differentiate the last named three major varieties of human drug metabolizing cytochrome P450 (CYP) enzyme can be summarized as follows. (Smith 1991).

CYP 2D6

Polar or non-polar basic drugs with the chargeable

nitrogen atom 5 to 7Å from the site of oxidation, the favourite pathway being hydroxylation, an essential activity, non-inducible, stereoselective, saturable, with a rat model.

CYP 3A

An open substrate site which takes large lipophilic molecules, less selective than 2D6, with a slow turnover. Substrates manoeuvre in the substrate pocket. Less specific and inducible by various drug compounds.

CYP 2C 8/9/10

Acts on molecules with areas of hydrophilicity and strong hydrogen bond forming potential, e.g. the carbonyl groups of the hydantoin ring and the sulphonylurea of tolbutamide.

There remain four other categories concerning which the information in man is very much more limited and they will be discussed at this point.

P450 2A

This enzyme is encoded by *CYP 2A* (localized at 19q13.1–13.2), is capable of oxidising coumarin and activating aflatoxin B1 and is induced by phenobarbitone and phenytoin (Wolf 1990).

P450 2B

The function of this enzyme in the human is unknown. The localisation of the gene *(CYP 2B)* is the same as for *CYP 2A*, and this enzyme is also induced by phenobarbitone and phenytoin (Wolf 1990).

P450 2E1

The encoding gene *CYP 2E* is on chromosome 10. The enzyme cytochrome P450 2E is responsible for nitrosamine activation, paracetamol and oestradiol oxidation and ethynyloestradiol 2-hydroxylation, and the metabolism of ethanol and enflurane (Wolf 1990; Hunt *et al.* 1990). It can be induced by ethanol consumption, fasting and diabetes. The activity of P450 2E in hepatocyte cultures was not affected by 3-methylcholanthrene, phenobarbital or rifampicin and was not present in fetal liver (Morel *et al.* 1990b).

The amount of P450 2E1 protein may be increased following exposure to ethanol, fasting or isoniazid, does not diminish with age and may be reduced by cimetidine (Hunt *et al.* 1990).

The clinically most important aspects of this enzyme as known at present are: (1) it is the major catalyst of microsomal paracetamol metabolism to its hepatotoxic electrophilic metabolite; (2) the amount of the protein in the liver is increased in chronic alcoholism (Hunt *et al.* 1990), and (3) the activity is moderately inhibited by cimetidine (Knodell *et al.* 1991). This cytochrome is also considered to be of importance in carcinogen activation (Paolini *et al.* 1989).

Two genetic polymorphisms, each having two alleles, were detected in the *CYP 2E* gene by Watanabe *et al.* (1990) using *Pst*I and *Rsa*I. These two polymorphisms were in complete linkage disequilibrium with each other.

Another restriction fragment length polymorphism (RPLF) in the second intron of *CYP 2E1* was detected using *Dra*I and a 1.0 kb DNA probe from the 3′-end of the cDNA by Uematsu *et al.* (1991). They were able to detect three genotypes CC, CD and DD, which they investigated in normal control subjects and patients with cancers of the lung and other organs. Their claim that the distribution of the genotypes among the lung cancer patients was different from that among controls is not statistically valid.

The idea was put forward that Parkinson's disease may be due to the accumulation of neurotoxins, and that this occurs in persons who by reasons of genetic endowment are unable properly to detoxify and eliminate these unknown toxins. Because of this reasoning the metabolism of paracetamol (as a test drug for P450 cytochromes) was investigated by Factor *et al.* (1989) in 26 patients with Parkinson's disease and 18 control subjects. Both paracetamol (P) and 3-hydroxyparacetamol (3HP) were measured in the urine following the ingestion of a single 1000 mg dose. No significant difference was observed between patients and controls in the excretion of either compound or in the ratio 3HP/P. . Also there was no difference between patients who contracted Parkinson's disease before and after 40 years of age or those receiving or not receiving anti-Parkinsonian medications. Hence there was no support for the hypothesis.

Cytochrome P450$_9$

Beaune *et al.* (1985) purified this enzyme which is capable of oxidizing 4-nitroanisole, aniline, benzo[a]pyrene and 7-ethoxycoumarin. There were very considerable intra-individual variations in the amount of this cytochrome in the nine microsomal liver preparations studied. The exact role of P450$_9$ in xeno- or endobiotic metabolism in the human liver and any genetically determined variation remains to be worked out.

INDUCIBILITY

An important property of the cytochromes P450 is that many of them are inducible. The observation which first aroused interest was an increase in the amount of liver protein which followed the administration of foreign compounds. This increase in liver protein was soon shown to be correlated with the enhanced elimination of test drugs and was found to be due to increased amounts of liver enzymes. Later, specific forms of cytochrome P450 were shown to be involved. The idea that the administration of a foreign compound could result in the enhanced detoxification and elimination of the same compound captured the scientific imagination and analogies were drawn with the immune system.

At first two classes of inducers were recognized, namely, the phenobarbital and 3-methylcholanthrene classes. Now more inducibility groups are known and some are shown in Table 4.1.

The actual induction mechanisms are now known in detail for some categories of cytochrome P450. Porter & Coon (1991) give five mechanisms for the regulation of *CYP* expressions: (1) gene transcription, (2) processing, (3) mRNA stabilization, (4) translation, (5) enzyme stabilization. Examples of induction involving all these mechanisms are known in animal systems (Goldfarb 1990), but some human induction phenomena are not well understood at the molecular level.

The topic of enzyme induction of P450 cytochromes in man has recently been reviewed by Breckenridge (1987) and by Park & Kitteringham (1990). The common inducing drugs in man are the antiepileptics phenobarbitone, carbamazepine and phenytoin, and rifampicin. There is an almost infinite variety of non-drug environmental chemicals which can cause induction. Cigarette smoke, various constituents of diet, alcohol and pesticides are individual factors which have been studied.

The effects of induction vary widely with the nature of the inducing compound, the effect which is being observed, and between the individuals being studied.

The existence of varying dosages of inducing drugs and environmental chemicals and varying degrees of induction produced between individuals in response to a standardized stimulus make this a difficult area in which to measure the influence of individual factors. Relatively few studies have addressed the objective of disentangling genetic and environmental influences. Where the individual genes could not be recognized the techniques used have been those of quantitative (i.e. multifactorial) genetics. They were basically the study of twins and the study of families (see later section on polygenic effects).

Following the discovery of pharmacogenetic polymorphisms it turns out that phenotypes within a polymorphism can be affected differently by inducing agents.

CHROMOSOMAL LOCALIZATION

A number of *CYP* genes have recently been assigned (or 'mapped') to chromosomal locations. These are shown in Appendix IV. Details of the evidence for the chromosomal 'mapping' of some individual pharmacogenetically important genes will be provided in the ensuing sections.

The chromosomal distribution of the *CYP* genes provides a further illustration of the peculiar functional anatomy of the human genome pointed out by McKusick (1986) in that *CYP* genes which control similar functions are located on different chromosomes.

The author would like to express his gratitude to Professor Barry Helliwell, Department of Medical Biochemistry, King's College, University of London, UK who made many helpful suggestions about the contents of this chapter.

Aoyama, T., Yamano, S., Waxman, D. J., Lapenson, D. P., Meyer, U. A., Fischer, V., Tyndale, R., Inaba, T., Kalow, W., Gelboin, H. V. & Gonzalez, F. J. (1989). Cytochrome P450 hPCN³, a novel cytochrome P450 IIIA gene product that is differentially expressed in the adult human liver. *Journal of Biological Chemistry*, **264**, 10388–95.

Bargetzi, M. J., Aoyama, T., Gonzalez, F. J. & Meyer, U. A. (1989). Lidocaine metabolism in human liver microsomes by cytochrome P450 III A4. *Clinical Pharmacology and Therapeutics*, **46**, 521–7.

Beaune, P., Flinois, J. P., Kiffel, L., Kremers, P. & Leroux, J. P. (1985). Purification of a new cytochrome P-450 from human liver microsomes. *Biochimica et Biophysica Acta*, **840**, 364–70.

Breckenridge, A. (1987). Enzyme induction in humans. Clinical aspects – an overview. *Pharmacology and Therapeutics*, **33**, 95–9.

Brøsen K. (1990). Recent developments in hepatic drug oxidation. Implications for clinical pharmacokinetics. *Clinical Pharmacokinetics*, **18**, 220–39.

Cooper, D. Y. (1973). Discovery of the function of the heme protein P-450: a systematic approach to scientific research. *Life Sciences*, **13**, 1151–61.

Dayhoff, M. O. (1979). *Atlas of protein sequence and structure*. Silver Spring, MD: National Biomedical Research Foundation, **5**, Suppl. 3.

Factor, S. A., Weiner, W. J., & Hefti, F. (1989). Acetaminophen metabolism by cytochrome P450 monoxygenases in Parkinson's disease. *Annals of Neurology*, **26**, 286–28.

Goldfarb, P. (1990). Molecular mechanisms of cytochrome P450 gene regulation. *Biochemical Society Transactions*, **18**, 30–2.

Gonzalez, F. J. (1990). Molecular genetics of the P450 super-family. *Pharmacology and Therapeutics*, **45**, 1–38.

Gonzalez, F. J. (1992). Human cytochromes P450: problems and prospects. *Trends in Pharmacological Sciences*, **13**, 346–52.

Guengerich, F. P. (1990a). Enzymatic oxidation of xenobiotic chemicals. *Critical Reviews of Biochemistry and Molecular Biology*, **25**, 97–153.

Guengerich, F. P. (1990b). Chemical mechanisms of cytochrome P-450 catalysis. *Asia Pacific Journal of Pharmacology*, **5**, 253–68.

Guengerich, F. P. (1991). Reactions and significance of cytochrome P450 enzymes. *Journal of Biological Chemistry*, **266**, 10019–22.

Hunt, C. M., Strater, S. & Stave, G. M. (1990). Effect of normal aging on the activity of human hepatic cytochrome P450 II E1. *Biochemical Pharmacology*, **40**, 1666–9.

Hunt, C. M., Watkins, P. B., Saenger, P., Stave, G. M., Barlascini, N., Watlington, C. O., Wright, J. J. Jr & Guzelian, P. S. (1992). Heterogeneity of CYP3A isoforms metabolizing erythromycin and cortisol. *Clinical Pharmacology and Therapeutics*, **51**, 18–23.

Imai, M., Shimada, H., Watanabe, Y., Matsushima-Hibiya, Y., Makino, R., Koga, H., Horiuchi, T. & Ishimura, Y. (1989). Uncoupling of the cytochrome P-450 cam monoxygenase reaction by a single mutation, threonine-252 to alanine or valine; A possible role of the hydroxyl amino acid in oxygen activation. *Proceedings of the National Academy of Sciences (USA)*, **86**, 7823-7.

Ioannides, C. & Parke, D. V. (1987). The cytochromes P-448 – a unique family of enzymes involved in chemical toxicity and carcinogenesis. *Biochemical Pharmacology*, **36**, 4197-207.

Jacolot, F., Simon, I., Dreano, Y., Beaune, P., Riche, C. & Berthou, F. (1991). Identification of the cytochrome P450

IIIA family as the enzymes involved in the *N*-demethylation of tamoxifen in human liver microsomes. *Biochemical Pharmacology*, **41**, 1911–9.

Knodell, R. G., Browne, D. G., Gwozdz, G. P., Brian, W. B. & Guengerich, F. P. (1991). Differential inhibition of individual human liver cytochromes P450 by cimetidine. *Gastroenterology*, **101**, 1680–91.

Levin, W. (1990). Functional diversity of hepatic cytochromes P-450. *Drug Metabolism and Disposition*, **18**, 824–30.

Liu, G., Gelboin, H. V. & Myers, M. J. (1991). Role of cytochrome P450 1A2 in acetanilide 4-hydroxylation as determined with cDNA expression and monoclonal antibodies. *Archives of Biochemistry and Biophysics*, **284**, 400–6.

McKusick, V. A. (1986). The morbid anatomy of the human genome. A review of gene mapping in clinical medicine (first of four parts). *Medicine*, **65**, 1-33.

McManus, M. E., Burgess, W. M., Veronese, M. E., Huggett, A., Quattrochi, L. C. & Tukey, R. H. (1990). Metabolism of 2-acetylaminofluorene and benzo(a)pyrene and activation of food derived heterocyclic amine mutagens by human cytochromes P-450. *Cancer Research*, **50**, 3367–76.

Morel, F., Beaune, P. H., Ratanasavanh, D., Flinois, J. P., Yang, C. S., Guengerich, F. P. & Guillouzo, A. (1990a). Expression of cytochrome P450 enzymes in cultured human hepatocytes. *European Journal of Biochemistry*, **191**, 437–44.

Morel, F., Beaune, P., Ratanasavanh, D., Flinois, J. P., Guengerich, F. B. & Guillouzo A. (1990b). Effects of various inducers on the expression of cytochromes P-450 IIC8, 9, 10 and IIIA in cultured adult human hepatocytes. *Toxicology in vitro*, **4**, 458–60.

Nebert, D. W. & Gonzalez, F. J. (1987). P450 genes: structure, evolution and regulation. *Annual Review of Biochemistry*, **56**, 945–93.

Nebert, D. W., Nelson, D. R., Coom, M. J., Estabrook, R. W., Feyereisen, R., Fuji-Kuriyama, Y., Gonzalez, F. J., Guengerich, F. P., Gunsalus, I. C., Johnson, E. F., Loper, J. C., Sato, R., Waterman, M. R. & Waxman, D. J. (1991). The P450 superfamily: update on new sequences, gene mapping, and recommended nomenclature. *DNA and Cell Biology*, **10**, 1–14.

Nelson, D. R. & Strobel, H. J. (1987). Evolution of cytochrome P450 proteins. *Molecular and Biological Evolution*, **4**, 572–93.

Omura, T. & Sato, R. (1964). The carbon monoxide-binding pigment of liver microsomes I: evidence for its hemoprotein nature. *Journal of Biological Chemistry*, **239**, 2370–8.

Paolini, M., Bauer, C., Biagi, G. L. & Cantelli-Forti, G. (1989). Do cytochromes P-448 and P-450 have different functions? *Biochemical Pharmacology*, **38**, 2223–5.

Park, B. K. & Kitteringham, N. R. (1990). Assessment of enzyme induction and enzyme inhibition in humans: toxicological implications. *Xenobiotica*, **20**, 1171–85.

Pichard, P., Fabre, I., Fabre, G., Domergue, J., Aubert, B. S., Mourad, G. & Maurel, P. (1990). Cyclosporin A drug interactions: screening for inducers and inhibitors of cytochrome P450 (cyclosporin A oxidase) in primary cultures of hepatocytes and in liver microsomes. *Drug Metabolism and Disposition*, **18**, 595–606.

Porter, T. D. & Coon, M. J. (1991). Cytochrome P450.

Multiplicity of isoforms, substrates, and catalytic and regulatory mechanisms. *Journal of Biological Chemistry*, **266**, 13469–72.

Poulos, T. L. (1988). Cytochrome P450: Molecular architecture, mechanism and prospects for rational inhibitor design. *Pharmaceutical Research*, **5**, 67-75.

Relling, M. V., Aoyama, T., Gonzalez, F. J. & Meyer, U. A. (1990). Tolbutamide and mephenytoin hydroxylation by human cytochrome P450s in the *CYP2C* subfamily. *Journal of Pharmacology and Experimental Therapeutics*, **252**, 442–7.

Remmer, H. & Merker, H. J. (1965). Effect of drugs on the formation of smooth endoplasmic reticulum and drug metabolizing enzymes. *Annals of the New York Academy of Sciences*, **123**, 79-97.

Sato, R. (1991). Cytochrome P450: An inconspicuous start. *Current Contents, Life Sciences*, **34** (8), 9.

Smith, D. A. (1991). Species differences in metabolism and pharmacokinetics: are we close to an understanding? *Drug Metabolism Reviews*, **23**, 355–73.

Thomas, J. H., Gillham, B. (1989). *Wills' Biochemical Basis of Medicine*, 2nd edition, p. 465. London: Wright.

Uematsu, F., Kikuchi, H., Motomiya, M., Abe, T., Sagami, I., Ohmachi, T., Wakui, A., Kanamaru, R. & Watanabe, M. (1991). Association between restriction fragment length polymorphism of the human cytochrome P450 II E1 gene and susceptibility to lung cancer. *Japanese Journal of Cancer Research*, **82**, 254–6.

Watanabe, J., Hayashi, S. I., Nakachi, K., Imai, K., Suda, Y., Sekine, T. & Kawajiri. K. (1990). Pst 1 and Rsa 1 RFLP's in complete linkage disequilibrium at the CYP 2E gene. *Nucleic Acids Research*, **18**, 7194.

Wolf, C. R., Miles, J. S., Gough, A, & Spurr, N. K. (1990). Molecular genetics of the human cytochrome P-450 system. *Biochemical Society Transactions*, **18**, 21–4.

Wrighton, S. A., Brian, W. R., Sari, M. A., Iwasaki, M., Guengerich, F. P., Raucy, J. L., Molowa, D. T. & Vandenbranden, M. (1990). Studies on the expression and metabolic capabilities of human liver cytochrome P450 III A5 (HLp3). *Molecular Pharmacology*, **38**, 207–13.

5 Arylhydrocarbon hydroxylase (cytochrome P450 1A1 and 1A2)

INTRODUCTION

A SHORT chapter is included on this topic because it represents an important application of knowledge gained about cytochrome P450 (CYP) enzymes to medical problems which arise from exposure to drugs and other chemical compounds.

Most of the basic work on this topic has been carried out in mice and largely in the laboratories of Dr Daniel W. Nebert from whose numerous contributions the following account is derived. It is necessary to summarize the advances in knowledge made in mice because there are some important human implications which will be described later.

A comprehensive review of the animal data on the cytochrome P450 1 gene family and its role in the metabolic activation of chemicals was published by Ioannides & Parke (1990).

THE *Ah* LOCUS IN THE MOUSE

The initial observation was that liver benzo[a]pyrene metabolism could be induced in B6 mice (b/b) but not in D2 mice (d/d) by 3-methylcholanthrene (3-MC). In fact subsequent studies on over 30 inbred mouse strains showed that about 2/3 were responsive like B6 and about 1/3 were non-responsive like D2. The property of 3-MC responsiveness was found to be an autosomal dominant in some of the strains examined and the lack of responsiveness was an autosomal recessive character. This could be proved by examining the progeny of appropriate crosses and back crosses (Thorgeirsson & Nebert 1977). The same genetically determined 3-MC inducibility of benzo[a]pyrene hydroxylation was also found to be present in other tissues. The results were confirmed by Thomas *et al.*(1972).

Other enzymic activities were also shown to be induced by 3-MC under the same genetic control, including phenacetin *O*-deethylase, acetanilide-4-hydroxylase, NAD(P)H:menadione oxidoreductase, UDP-glucuronosyl transferase and glutathione transferase. It is interesting to note that both phase I and phase II detoxification reactions are included in this list (Nebert 1988).

The term Ah was derived from *a*romatic *h*ydrocarbon responsiveness.

A non-invasive test

A useful advance was the development of a non-invasive test based on zoxazolamine paralysis. This test was as follows. Weanlings of either sex were treated with intraperitoneal β-naphthoflavone for 36 hours at which time induction was maximal in b/b and b/d mice but negligible induction occurred in d/d mice. Zoxazolamine was then given intraperitoneally. Because of the enhanced metabolism which had been induced b/b and b/d mice were paralysed for only a few minutes whereas d/d mice were paralysed for 30 to 120 minutes. This test did not influence the outcome of later toxicological and other studies on the animals thus phenotyped.

The responsible cytochromes P450

Two cytochromes P450 were isolated from B6 mouse liver and were identified as the enzymes whose production was induced by 3-MC. Cytochrome P450 1A1 was specific for the metabolism of benzo[a]pyrene whilst cytochrome P450 1A2 was specific for the oxidation of acetanilide and other arylamines. Similar results were obtained in rat and rabbit (Nebert 1989).

The degree of induction of cytochrome P450 1A1 is huge. Due to the low constitutive level the amount of mRNA and transcription rises by 5 to 100-fold. For cytochrome P450 1A2 the constitutive level is high and the transcription only rises by 4 to 5-fold. The former induction occurs early in embryogenesis whereas the latter only arises in the postnatal period.

The Ah receptor

The compound 2,3,7,8-tetrachlorodibenzo-*p*-dioxin (TCDD, 'dioxin') was found to be 30 000 times more powerful an inducer than 3-MC (Poland & Glover 1974). TCDD at a higher dose was capable of inducing cytochrome P450 1A1 activity in D2 mice to almost the same degree as B6 mice, a finding which showed that the D2 (d/d) mouse had a functioning structural gene encoding for cytochrome P450 1A1.

The idea thus came into being that the lack of inducibility was due to a defective regulatory gene. Assays and purification techniques have been developed for a cytosolic Ah receptor (Nebert 1989). The exact molecular mechanism of how the inducer hydrocarbon changes the receptor in order to become active is not yet understood; it is possible that it may be conformational or chemical. Somehow TCDD is able to produce an effective hydrocarbon-inducer complex in D2 mice whereas 3-MC cannot.

A special protein moves the hydrocarbon Ah receptor complex from the cytoplasm into the nucleus. The gene for this protein has been localized to mouse chromosome 3 (Brooks *et al.* 1989).

Following the translocation of the hydrocarbon–receptor complex into the nucleus or the acquisition of chromatin-binding properties, the expression of several genes is augmented (Nebert 1988).

The *Ah* locus is the gene which encodes the Ah receptor(s) and is located on the proximal portion of mouse chromosome 12 (Nebert 1989).

The relationship of the *Ah* gene to the *cyp 1a1* gene

A complicated *Ah* regulatory region was identified between 880 and 1090 bases upstream from the cyp 1a1 mRNA cap site and this has been characterized. It seems likely that there are several functional regions within the upstream sequence: a promoter region, a region that is negatively autoregulated, possible repressor binding and inducer–receptor complex-binding sites and an upstream activation element that is required for transcriptional activation by TCDD (Gonzalez & Nebert 1985).

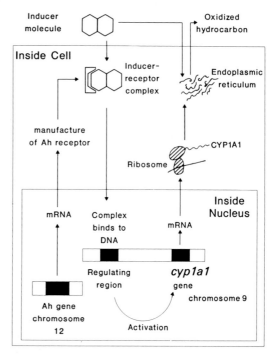

Fig. 5.1. Diagram of the action of a polycyclic hydrocarbon inducing the aryl hydrocarbon hydroxylase system in the mouse. The hydrocarbon combines with the cytosolic Ah receptor. The complex enters the nucleus and binds to a regulatory region of DNA. As a result the structural gene produces mRNA molecules at a faster rate. This results in the existence of more cytochrome P450 (CYP 1A1) molecules which increase the hydrocarbon oxidizing activity (adapted from Nebert 1989, with permission). In man the *CYP 1A1* gene is on chromosome 15.

When the inducer–receptor complex gains chromatin-binding properties and moves into the nucleus to bind with its target, the *cyp 1a1* gene is activated by an increase in transcription. Post-transcriptional activation of the *cyp 1a2* gene also occurs. Increases in the respective mRNA levels are followed by increases in the amounts of the cytochrome P450 proteins and enzymic activities (Fig. 5.1).

Recently two nuclear factors have been described in addition to the Ah receptor which also interact with the response elements of the *cyp 1a1* gene in cultured rat hepatocytes. XF1 and XF2 are nuclear factors which bind to three DNA elements with five invariant nucleotides. Induced Ah receptor complex also binds to three DNA elements, and two DNA elements are common to both sets (Saatcioglu *et al.* 1990).

The effects of Ah responsiveness in mice

The main phenotypic effects of the differences in Ah responsiveness between mouse strains are summarized in Table 5.1. Most of the information has been derived from the excellent review article of Nebert (1989).

In view of the widespread effects of this single gene interstrain difference in mice it was natural for a search to have been made for an analogous genetic polymorphism in humans.

STUDIES OF ARYLHYDROCARBON HYDROXYLASE IN HUMANS

Human lymphocyte preparations

A paper by Busbee *et al.* (1972) introduced a new method of studying the metabolism of drugs and other foreign compounds in humans. Leucocytes were harvested from sedimented dextran-treated heparinized blood. These leucocytes were incubated with phytohaemagglutinin (PHA) and then 'induced' with 3-methylcholanthrene (3-MC) for 24 hours. A homogenate of the leucocytes was then incubated with NADPH and benzo[a]pyrene (BP). The 3-hydroxy BP which was produced was measured spectrofluorimetrically, and this was the index of arylhydrocarbon hydroxylase (AHH) activity.

[The AHH activity is correlated with cytochrome P450 1A1 levels ($r = 0.68$) but 7-ethoxyresorufin *O*-deethylase is more highly correlated ($r = 0.92$); see Wheeler & Guenthner 1991.]

A similar paper was also published by Whitlock *et al.* (1972) who employed a nylon column and Ficoll–Hypaque purification of the leucocytes after which they were treated with either PHA or poke-weed mitogen (PWM) followed by BP. The leucocytes so prepared were shown to be able to hydroxylate BP.

Then Kellermann *et al.* (1973a) published work which at the time seemed an amazing new break-through but which subsequently turned out to be difficult to corroborate in other laboratories. Sixty-seven families with 165 children were studied by a technique very similar to those described above, 3-MC being used as the inducing agent. The repeatability of the test within individuals over months was claimed to be high. The distribution histogram of the inducibility levels was trimodal (Fig. 5.2) and a genetic analysis of the pedigrees indicated that there were three Mendelian autosomal genotypes (Table 5.2).

By incorporating a number of technical refinements such as assessing AHH activity when the lymphocytes were maximally stimulated, using cryopreserved lymphocytes so that many samples could be run simultaneously and relating the activity to cytochrome *c* reduction, Kouri *et al.* (1984) were able to re-examine the topic. Nine pairs of monozygous and 10 pairs of dizygous twins were studied and the results indicated a small but real genetic component of the variability of AHH activity among these twins (Table 5.3).

Using the same technique there was an important side-product from the survey of Levine *et al.* (1984) of the primary relatives of patients with leukaemia, solid tumours and controls. By comparing variances within families (0.36) and within comparable groups of unrelated subjects (0.61) for the value of AHH activity/cyt *c* reductase activity the heritability was computed to be 0.41, indicating a small genetic component. This ratio described by Kouri *et al.* (1984) was shown to correlate closely in six individuals with the cytochrome P450 1 mRNA/actin mRNA ratio (Jaiswal *et al.* 1985), indicating the likelihood that it gives a measure of the activity of the *CYP 1A1* gene (Fig 5.3).

However, despite these advances in technique

Table 5.1. *Effects of Ah responsiveness in mice*

Polycyclic hydroxcarbon-induced carcinogenesis	b/b and b/d are at higher risk than d/d of developing cancer when polycyclic hydrocarbons are administered topically or by injection.
Mutagenesis	In the Ames test 3-MC was metabolized more effectively to a potent mutagen by mice with a high affinity Ah receptor. The ultimate mutagen *in vitro* and carcinogen *in vivo*, the trans-7,8-diol-9,10-epoxide of benzo[a]pyrene, is formed to a much greater extent in b/b and b/d mice than in d/d mice.
Toxicity	
1. Bone marrow toxicity	d/d mice develop fatal marrow toxicity whereas b/b and b/d mice do not when benzo[a]pyrene and other polycyclic hydrocarbons are fed orally. This is due to the latter two genotypes detoxifying the chemicals by a first-pass effect whereas d/d is ineffective in this regard.
2. Hepatic toxicity	Activity of the CYP 1A2 enzyme produces toxic metabolites from many organic molecules including paracetamol (acetaminophen). Increased levels of covalently bound metabolites of paracetamol occurred in 3-MC pretreated b/b and b/d but not in d/d mice.
3. Ocular toxicity	Intraperitoneal and oral paracetamol following 3-MC pretreatment caused cataracts in b/b and b/d mice but never in d/d mice. The Ah^b containing (B6) mice exhibited 2 to 5 times greater uptake of paracetamol into the eye. Concomitantly administered phenobarbital protects b/b and b/d from developing cataracts.
4. Ovarian toxicity	Oocyte toxicity is much more prevalent in b/b and b/d than in d/d mice following i.p. hydrocarbons. Inducible *cyp 1a1* mRNA is present in mouse ovarian cells. These phenomena are not seen in the testis of the mouse.
5. Immunotoxicity	Immunotoxicity induced by i.p. hydrocarbons and TCDD is more pronounced in b/b and b/d mice than in d/d mice. Both B cell suppression and T cell toxicity are involved.
6. Atherosclerosis	3-MC enhanced atherosclerosis was shown to be more prevalent in b/b and b/d mice than in d/d mice. The mechanism is unknown but the following two possibilities are suggested: (1) 3-MC induces CYP 1A1 in the arterial wall which then produces toxic products from endogenous compounds or 3-MC itself; (2) the production in the liver, lung, etc. of stable reactive compounds which then circulate in the blood and enter the arterial endothelium.
7. Ethanol resistance	Mice selected for short sleeping time following i.p. ethanol were found to have high liver content of Ah receptor and in them hepatic CYP 1A2 could be induced by 3-MC. On the other hand mice selected for long sleeping time had negligible amounts of liver Ah receptor and their hepatic CYP 1A2 could not be induced by 3-MC.
8. Fertility fitness and longevity	Recombinant inbred lines were studied and phenotyped with the β-naphthoflavone and zoxazolamine procedure. Those with high Ah activity produced 4 times as many offspring as those without and also had significantly longer life spans.
Teratogenesis	i.p. benzo[a]pyrene administered to pregnant mice on gestational days 7 to 10 produced more malformations in the b/d fetus than in the d/d fetus in the same uterus. Oral benzo[a]pyrene produced exactly the opposite result.

b/b, b/d, d/d homozygotes and heterozygotes were derived from B6 and D2 lines of inbred mice.
3-MC, 3-methylcholanthrene; i.p., intraperitoneal; TCDD 2,3,7,8-tetrachlorodibenzo-*p*-dioxin; CYP 1A2, cytochrome P450 1A2. *From:* Nebert 1989.

and the establishment of quantitative genetic control of AHH activity in lymphocytes the monogenic model advanced by Kellermann *et al.* (1973a) remained unconfirmed.

Human peripheral blood monocytes

One of the difficulties with the lymphocyte test referred to above was that it was not possible to differentiate between the influences of the mitogen (PHA or PWM) and the hydrocarbon (e.g. 3-MC). This difficulty was not present when monocytes were used because they already have cytoplasm and so stimulation by a mitogen was not necessary.

A twin study was reported by Okuda *et al.* (1977) in which the AHH inducibility in monocytes from

Table 5.2. *Family studies*

Mating type	N	Total number of children	Phenotypes		
			AA	AB	BB
AA × AA	17	39	39	–	–
AA × AB	28	63	31	32	–
AA × BB	4	10	–	10	–
AB × AB	10	35	9	17	9
AB × BB	6	13	–	9	4
BB × BB	2	5	–	–	5
Total	67	165	79	68	18

From: Kellerman *et al.* 1973a.

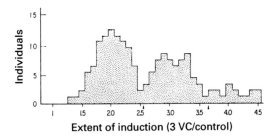

Fig. 5.2. Distribution of inducibility levels. Extent of induction expressed as the ratio of AHH activity after induction with 3-methylcholanthrene to activity before induction. (From Kellermann *et al.* 1973a.)

10 pairs of monozygous and 17 pairs of dizygous twins was examined. The heritability was computed as 0.57 ± SE 0.19 (p = 0.03). It was noted that the intrapair differences of more than 30% in inducibility were only seen in two of 17 sets of dizygous twins, which suggested the possibility that only a small number of genes might be involved.

Human blood monocytes from 86 members of 15 families were assayed by Nowak *et al.* (1988) for (1) water-soluble [³H]-benzo[a]pyrene metabolite production estimated by liquid scintillation counting (LSC) and (2) DNA adducts from BP also estimated by LSC. The two measurements were correlated and for both the intrafamilial variance was less than the interfamilial variance, indicating a measure of genetic control.

So for monocytes the evidence was similar to that for lymphocytes, indicating a measure of quantitative genetic (i.e. 'polygenic') control of AHH activity.

Bronchogenic carcinoma

The well-known causation of bronchial carcinoma by cigarette smoke, which contains many polycyclic hydrocarbons as well as other carcinogens, stimulated a lot of research to see if lymphocyte or monocyte AHH inducibility was related to this disorder.

(1) Estimations of AHH inducibility in peripheral blood lymphocytes only

The relationship between the inducibility of AHH in blood lymphocytes and bronchial carcinoma was investigated by Kellermann *et al.* (1973b) in 50 patients who were typed into the three alleged groups of low, intermediate and high inducibility. The results are shown in Table 5.4, indicating that generally the patients had higher inducibilities.

This interesting finding, which might mean that either the higher inducibility phenotypes were more prone to develop lung cancer or alternatively that the presence of lung cancer might give rise to a

Table 5.3. *Data suggesting genetic basis for observed differences in AHH levels among humans: twin study*[a]

Cases[b]	Pairs	x̄ AHH[c]	σ^2b	σ^2w	r	σ^2w-DZ/σ^2w-MZ
MZ	9	0.40	0.49	0.06	0.81	2.33
DZ	10	0.44	0.50	0.14	0.58	p = 0.055

[a]σ^2b, between twin variance; σ^2w, within twin variance; σ^2w-DZ, within twin variance of dizygotic twins; σ^2w-MZ, within twin variance of monozygotic twins; r, correlation coefficient.
[b]MZ, Monozygotic twins; DZ, UCL Dizygotic twins.
[c]Mean (x̄) AHH values in units AHH per unit cytochrome *c* activity.
From: Kouri *et al.* 1984.

Table 5.4. *Comparison of healthy control group, tumour control group and lung cancer group for arylhydrocarbon hydroxylase (AHH) inducibility*

Group	Number in group	AHH inducibility %			Gene frequencies*	
		AA	AB	BB	AHH^a	AHH^b
Healthy control	85	44.7	45.9	9.4	0.676	0.324
Tumour control	46	43.5	45.6	10.9	0.663	0.337
Lung cancer	50	4.0	66.0	30.0	0.370	0.630

AA, Low; AB, intermediate; BB, high.
* Superscripts refer to the 2 alleles.
From: Kellermann *et al.* 1973b.

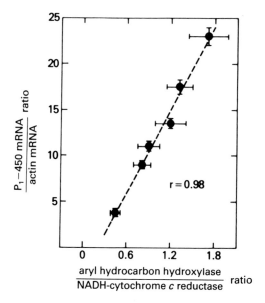

Fig. 5.3. Comparison of P$_1$450 mRNA levels with AHH inducibility among six patients. Closed circles and brackets denote the means ± standard deviations (*n* = 3) for both mRNA and enzyme determinations. (From Jaiswal *et al.* 1985.)

then subject them all to exactly the same *in vitro* procedures at the same time and (4) measure DNA synthesis by means of radioactive thymidine uptake and measure NADH-dependent cytochrome *c* reductase activity.

The mean AHH/cytochrome *c* reductase activity ratio for 21 lung cancer patients was 0.89 and for 30 non-lung cancer pulmonary disease patients was 0.47 (p > 0.001). There was no difference between the two sets of patients as regards thymidine incorporation per unit of cytochrome *c* reductase activity.

Similar results were obtained by Kouri *et al.* (1984). A shift to higher values was found in lung cancer patients as compared with normal persons and hospitalized non-lung cancer patients (Fig 5.4).

As the authors point out, the question whether the higher AHH activities in the cancer patients were the cause or the result of the lung cancer remained to be determined. On this point the study of Ward *et al.* (1978) is relevant. They studied 32 patients who had their lung carcinomas successfully resected 1 to 10 years before the survey was carried out and were apparently disease-free. Their lymphocyte AHH inducibility was not significantly different to that of 57 normal controls. However, it is true that Ward *et al.* (1978) did not incorporate in their assay procedure the requirements subsequently developed by Kouri *et al.* (1984).

(2) Estimations of AHH inducibility in monocytes

The work of Nowak *et al.* (1988) who studied benzo(a)pyrene metabolism to water-soluble meta-

higher inducibility state, was further examined by many other research groups with indifferent success.

Real progress in this field had to await the study of Kouri *et al.* (1982). Their innovations were to (1) place patients on a standard diet before the lymphocytes were obtained, (2) select carefully matched controls, (3) use cryopreserved lymphocytes and

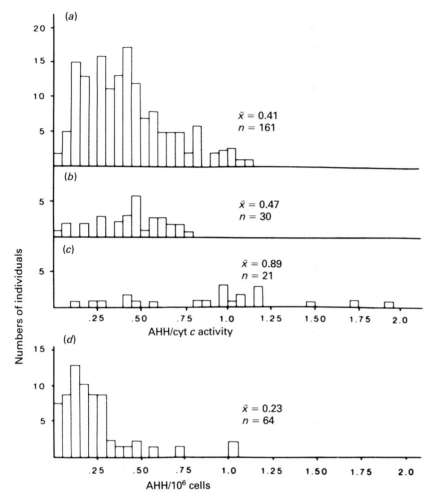

Fig. 5.4. AHH/cyt *c* activities in mitogen-activated lymphocytes from (a) normal individuals, (b) hospitalized individuals without lung cancer, (c) hospitalized patients with lung cancer, (d) AHH activities in 64 healthy baboons from different families. (From Kouri *et al.* 1984.)

bolites and DNA adduct formation by monocytes, has been referred to earlier. Using the same technique Rudiger *et al.* (1985) observed enhanced metabolism and formation of DNA adducts in the monocytes of lung cancer patients compared with normal subjects. The difference from normal subjects was larger in subgroups of lung cancer patients who were non-smokers or who had a particularly early onset of the disease and who could therefore be considered to be genetically cancer-prone.

(3) Estimations of AHH inducibility in pulmonary alveolar macrophages and lung tissue

The AHH activity of pulmonary alveolar macrophages (PAM) was assayed and compared with the activity which could be induced in blood lymphocytes *in vitro* as described above. It was found by Cantrell *et al.* (1973) that the AHH activity per 10^6 PAM was much higher in smokers than in non-smokers and in both groups it correlated with the inducibility generated by 3-MC in blood lymphocytes. A similar effect in both cell types was shown to be produced by cigarette tars by McLemore *et al.* (1977a). The same group (McLemore *et al.* 1977b) extended their observations to include benzo[a]-pyrene induction of PAMs as well as lymphocytes

Table 5.5. *Comparison of AHH activities in PAMs and blood lymphocytes*

AHH activity	PAMs			Lymphocytes		
	Non-smoker (n=8)	Smoker (n=15)	p value[a]	Non-smoker (n=8)	Smoker (n=15)	p value
Non-induced[b]	24 ± 2[c]	45 ± 5	<0.002	20 ± 2	57 ± 6	<0.001
BA-induced[d]	104 ± 22	166 ± 30	>0.1	99 ± 22	168 ± 23	<0.04
Delta-induction[e]	78 ± 19	122 ± 26	>0.1	79 ± 21	112 ± 20	>0.2
Fold-induction[f]	3.11 ± 60	2.46 ± 0.37	>0.3	3.66 ± 0.83	2.07 ± 37	>0.1

[a] t test for non-paired data with degrees of freedom adjusted for unequal variances. Values considered significant if $p < 0.05$.
[b] Cells cultured without the inducer BA. Value expressed as milliunits/10^6 cells.
[c] Means $\pm$ SEM.
[d] Cells cultured with BA. Values represent milliunits/10^6 cells.
[e] Represents the BA-induced − non-induced AHH activity expressed as milliunits/10^6 cells.
[f] Represents the [(BA-induced AHH/non-induced AHH) − 1].
From: McLemore *et al.* 1973b.

in smokers and non-smokers. The smokers had much higher non-induced AHH activities in both cell types, otherwise the responses were similar (Table 5.5). Both the increment in AHH and the fold-induction of AHH showed correlations between PAM and induced lymphocytes.

When the same research group (McLemore *et al.* 1978) investigated lung cancer patients with the same techniques, the correlation between PAM and peripheral blood lymphocytes was not present. This non-correlation in the cancer patients was found with both fresh and cultured PAMs. The conclusion was that the use of a single tissue such as lymphocytes for evaluation of the relationship between AHH activity and cancer susceptibility was questionable. However, in a later paper (McLemore *et al.* 1981) the authors point out that when the PAM and lymphocyte AHH levels were considered simultaneously the cancer group contained a significantly higher percentage of persons with high results compared with an age-matched group of non-cancer patients.

Arylhydrocarbon hydroxylase (assayed using the same technique as that of Kellermann *et al.* 1973a) was found to be present in 41 human lung tissue samples from carcinoma of bronchus and other patients, by Karki *et al.* (1987). There was a 67-fold inter-individual variation. There were significant correlations between the lung AHH activity and the inducibility ratio with ($r = 0.618$) and without ($r = 0.442$) correction by thymidine incorporation deter-

mined in lymphocytes by AHH assay. The AHH activities in lymphocytes from smokers were much higher than in those from non-smokers.

A strong positive association was observed between active cigarette smoking and the presence of the mRNA for *CYP 1A1* in normal lung tissue by McLemore *et al.* (1990). The *CYP 1A1* gene expression was closely associated with CYP 1A1 (cytochrome P450 1A1) enzyme activity as monitored by ethoxy-resorufin O-deethylation. These findings provided support for the idea that the *CYP 1A1* gene might have a role in the causation of bronchial carcinoma bearing in mind the capability of the relevant enzyme to biotransform polycyclic hydrocarbons to carcinogenic metabolites.

(4) Molecular genetic studies

Using DNA derived from peripheral blood leucocytes an *Msp* I restriction fragment length polymorphism (RFLP) was detected with a 3′-specific cDNA probe for *CYP 1A1* by Petersen *et al.* (1991). The 2.5 and 1.9 kb fragments had allelic frequencies of 88% and 12% respectively in a mixed-race sample of 47 unrelated volunteers. It was found that a high CYP 1A1/cytochrome *c* reductase activity ratio segregated with the 1.9 kb *Msp*I allele in one three-generation family. Kawajiri *et al.* (1990) reported the 1.9 kb allele to have a frequency of 31% in Japanese and they found the 1.9/1.9 homozygote to be about twice as common amongst lung cancer patients as in non-cancer subjects. Unfortunately Tefre *et al.* (1991), who studied the same RFLP in 221 Norwegian lung cancer patients and 212 controls found no significant difference in the frequencies of the genotypes between the two populations.

Another genetic polymorphism in the coding region of *CYP 1A1* has been found. A mutation from adenine to guanine causes a replacement of isoleucine (Ile) to valine (Val) in the haem-binding region of the cytochrome. When expressed *in vitro* in yeast cells the Val/Val enzyme had a higher catalytic and mutagenic activity towards benzo[a]-pyrene than the Ile/Ile form. The percentage frequencies of the genotypes as determined using the polymerase chain reaction on DNA from blood lymphocytes in 358 healthy controls were Ile/Ile 65.1, Ile/Val 30.2 and Val/Val 4.7 (Hayashi *et al.* 1992). In 116 patients with lung carcinomas of histological types known to be associated with smoking, the corresponding figures were 56.9, 29.3 and 13.8 ($\chi^2 = 10.1$, $p < 0.01$). This was accompanied by an increased frequency of the null genotype for glutathione-S-transferase 1 [GST 1(−)] as described in Chapter 19.

These observations will require independent corroboration. Nevertheless it is an exciting possibility that predisposition (or resistance) to lung cancer may be determinable by means of a single blood test.

Leukaemia and solid tumours

In a large study of 248 lymphocyte samples from the primary relatives of 38 patients with leukaemia, 32 with solid tumours and 45 controls (friends and neighbours), Levine *et al.* (1984) found no difference between the groups with regard to median units of maximally induced AHH activity per unit of NADH-dependent cytochrome *c* reductase activity.

The Ile/Val genotypes referred to above were found in frequencies not significantly different from controls in cancers of stomach, colon and breast by Hayashi *et al.* (1992).

Smoking appears to protect against aflatoxin hepatoma

At a time when the evidence concerning the many harmful effects of cigarette smoking is overwhelming it is interesting to note that Nebert (1989) mentions that the primary hepatoma which is common in the aflatoxin-endemic region of China appears to be less common in cigarette smokers than among non-smokers. This is paralleled by experimental evidence in ducks where exposure to cigarette smoke is protective against aflatoxin B_1-induced hepatoma formation.

Aflatoxin B_1 is known to be metabolized by one or more forms of phenobarbital-inducible cytochrome P450 activity to the 2,3 oxide that is believed responsible for DNA adducts and aflatoxin B_1-induced hepatomas. Cytochrome P450 1A2 catalyses the 4-hydroxylation of aflatoxin B_1 which is actually a detoxification pathway because less of the 2,3 oxide is formed (Nebert 1989).

It is possible therefore that the protective effect of smoking in humans consuming aflatoxin may be the result of AHH induction by the inhaled polycyclic hydrocarbons.

Earlier menopause in smoking women

Oocyte toxicity is much more prevalent after intra-peritoneal 3-MC or BP in b/b and b/d in mice than in d/d mice, whereas a similar effect is not seen in the testis (Mattison & Thorgeirsson 1978a, 1979). By means of *in situ* hybridization Dey *et al.* (cited by Nebert 1989) were able to find inducible *cyp 1a1* mRNA in particular ovarian cell types but not in any cells of the mouse testis. These observations may provide the explanation for the clinical observation that women who smoke cigarettes have their menopause at a significantly younger age than women who do not smoke (Mattison & Thorgeirsson 1978b).

Arylhydrocarbon hydroxylase activity and drug metabolism

In an attempt to find common patterns of drug oxidation the plasma half lives and metabolic clearance rates of several drugs given by mouth were determined in subjects who also had their lymphocyte inducibility of AHH determined. The results are condensed in Table 5.6. Many high correlations were observed. The 4-hydroxylation of acetanilide shows considerable inter-individual variability in man (Cunningham *et al.* 1974) and cytochrome P450 1A2 mRNA was seen to vary more than 15-fold between 12 human liver samples (Ikeya *et*

Table 5.6. *The correlations of plasma half lives and metabolic clearance ratios of various drugs with lymphocyte inducibility*

Reference	Number and sex of experimental subjects	Antipyrine	Phenylbutazone	Phenobarbital	Acetanilide	Theophylline	Phenacetin
Kellermann *et al.* 1975	23 (17 F, 6 M)	Correlation of $T^{1/2}$ with AHH $r = 0.84$ Also correlation between single dose AP $T^{1/2}$ with multiple dose $T^{1/2}$ of PBZ $r = 0.82$	Correlation of $T^{1/2}$ with AHH $r = 0.86$				
Kellermann *et al.* 1976	57 'selected subjects' (41 M, 16 F)	Correlation of $T^{1/2}$ with AHH ratio $r = 0.923$					
	'Unselected subjects' (46 M, 34 F)	Correlation of $T^{1/2}$ with AHH ratio -0.425 (-0.751 when the females excluded)					
Kellermann *et al.* 1977	28 M + 3 F in correlation study	Half lives correlated with AHH $r = 0.94$		Half lives correlated with AP $r = +0.88$ and with AHH inducibility $r = 0.88$			
	20 M + 2 F in induction study (one week's phenobarbital pretreatment)	Reduced $T^{1/2}$ 13.3 to 30.6%. No correlation between initial $T^{1/2}$ and the reduction after phenobarbital					
Kellermann *et al.* 1978	30 M + 4 F				Half lives correlated with AHH $r = 0.721$; clearance rate correlated with AHH $r = 0.644$	Both half lives and clearance rates correlated with AHH $r = 0.850$ and $r = 0.753$ respectively	Half lives correlated with AHH $r = 0.787$ but clearance rate did not $r = 0.041$
					The half lives of the three drugs correlated with each other and with antipyrine. Antipyrine, theophylline and acetanilide clearance rates all correlated with each other but phenacetin clearance rates did not correlate with any of the others		

$T^{1/2}$, Plasma half life; AHH, aryl hydrocarbon hydroxylase induction ratio; AP, antipyrine; PBZ, phenylbutazone; M, male; F, female; r, correlation coefficient.

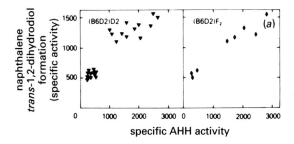

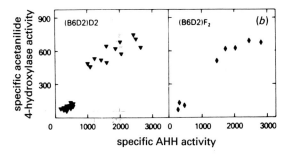

Fig. 5.5. Relationship between AHH activity and (a) rate of naphthalene *trans*-1,2-dihydrodiol formation or (b) acetanilide 4-hydroxylase activities in MC-treated (B6D2)D2 and (B6D2)F$_2$ progeny. (From Atlas & Nebert 1976.)

al. 1989). Acetanilide 4-hydroxylation is controlled by the *Ah* system in mice and segregates into two clear groups in 3-MC-treated (B6 D2) F$_1$ × D2 backcross and in 3-MC treated (B6 D2) F$_2$ progeny (Atlas & Nebert 1976) (Fig 5.5).

Kalow & Tang (1991) described the use of caffeine as a way of measuring cytochrome P450 1A2 activity in man. This is possible because cytochrome P450 1A2 catalyses the 7 demethylation of the compound. Hence the ratio of urinary concentrations [AAMU + 1X + 1U]/17U gives an estimate of the enzymic activity (AAMU = 5-acetylamino-6-amino-3-methyl uracil; 1X = 1-methyl xanthine; 1U = 1-methyl urate; 17U = 1,7-dimethyl urate). The frequency distribution of the ratio in 178 healthy subjects was unimodal, and there was no significant difference between the sub-distributions of Chinese subjects and those of European extraction.

A different ratio was investigated by Butler *et al*. (1992). Urinary [17X + 17U]/137X following caffeine ingestion indicated the presence of different phenotypes. Family studies will be required to see if

these phenotypes are genetically determined (17X = paraxanthine, 137X = caffeine).

The same ratio was found to be raised in smokers by Sherson *et al*. (1992), indicating induction of cytochrome P450 1A2 activity.

Recently it has been shown that human phenacetin deethylation is mediated by cytochrome P450 1A2 which is also responsible for the 3-demethylation of caffeine and the *N*-oxidation of carcinogenic arylamines like 4-aminobiphenyl (Butler *et al*. 1989). This observation regarding phenacetin O-deethylation may well tie up with previous reports on the subject. It is mentioned elsewhere that phenacetin is metabolized by the cytochrome P450 2D6 which is responsible for the debrisoquine polymorphism. The observation of Butler *et al*. (1989) may well match that of Distlerath *et al*. (1985) who identified a cytochrome P450 different from that involved in the debrisoquine polymorphism as having the ability to oxidize phenacetin. So this drug is an example of one whose metabolism by the same biotransformation is mediated by two different enzymes.

It had previously been shown by Grygiel & Birkett (1981) that theophylline metabolism was greatly enhanced in smokers. The basis for this observation has now been revealed by more modern methods.

The demethylation of theophylline was studied with microsomes from 22 different human livers by Sarkar *et al*. (1992). The formation of 3-methylxanthine and 1-methylxanthine correlated best with an immunoreactive protein representing cytochrome P450 1A2.

The influence of omeprazole (OM) on cytochrome P450 1A1 (as indicated by ethoxyresorufin deethylase and benzopyrene hydroxylase) and P450 1A2 (as indicated by phenacetin deethylase and acetanilide hydroxylase), plus their respective mRNAs by Northern blot analysis was investigated by Diaz *et al*. (1990). They found that human microsomal mono-oxygenase activities specifically associated with these two cytochromes P450 (e.g. phenacetin deethylase and acetanilide hydroxylase) were induced several-fold by OM. This was related to an increase in specific mRNAs and an increase in *de novo* synthesis of the protein.

The authors made the suggestion that, since OM is an inducer of phenacetin deethylation to acetaminophen (paracetamol), patients being treated with OM have an increased risk of acetaminophen hepatotoxicity. Also since cytochromes P450 1A1 and 1A2 activate carcinogenic compounds these patients may have an increased risk of developing malignant neoplasms. However, some objections were raised by Wrighton & Watkins (1991) to the methodology used by Diaz et al. (1990), based on the facts that cytochrome P450 1A2 is not uniformly distributed in the liver and that the samples of liver taken by Diaz et al. (1990) were taken from different sites before and after omeprazole administration. These objections were not considered justified by Farrell (1992) and Golor et al. (1992), but Humphries (1991), remarks that the interactions of omeprazole with other drugs are not likely to be clinically significant.

This forecast turned out to be correct in the case of theophylline, as studied by Taburet et al. (1992) who found that the oral clearance and urinary excretion of various metabolites were not significantly different with or without omeprazole in eight volunteers. However, the possibility arises that they may all have been extensive metabolizers in the mephytoin polymorphism (cytochrome P450 2C 18), because Rost et al. (1992) found that only in poor metabolizers of S-mephytoin were large increases in the exhalation of $^{13}CO_2$ observed after consumption of ^{13}C-[N-3-methyl]-caffeine, indicating induction of cytochrome P450 1A2. So there is a possibility that a small proportion of Caucasians (and a larger proportion of Orientals) may be adversely affected by omeprazole via this mechanism (see p. 45).

Using human liver microsomes furafylline was found to be a potent non-competitive inhibitor of high-affinity phenacetin deethylase (a reaction catalysed by cytochrome P450 1A2) and also of the 3-demethylation of caffeine (Sesardic et al. 1990). The drug had very little or no effect on enzymic activities mediated by various other cytochromes P450. Similarly, Fuhr et al. (1990) showed that quinoline antibiotics, e.g. ciprofloxacin, selectively inhibited the 3-demethylation of caffeine.

The molecular genetics of cytochromes P450 1A1 and 1A2 in man

The existence of the Ah receptor (AhR) in human tissues has been shown in a squamous cell carcinoma cell line, and placenta (Harper et al. 1988), colon adenocarcinoma cell line (Harper et al. 1991), lymphoblastoid cell line (Waither et al. 1991),

human liver cell line M2-Hep-1 (Roberts et al. 1991) and Hep-G2 (Wang et al. 1991).

The gene for the human arylhydrocarbon receptor nuclear transporter (ARNMT protein 'C' MIM 126110) has been isolated and localized to chromosome 1pter–1q12. A potentially useful RFLP has been detected using the restriction endonuclease MspI (Brooks et al. 1989).

The human CYP 1A1 gene (6311 base pairs, bp) as well as the 5' (1604 bases) and 3' (113 bases) flanking regions were completely sequenced by Jaiswal et al. (1985). The gene contains seven exons (Fig. 5.6) and the cDNA is 2596 bp long and has a continuous reading frame from 117 to 1656 (so giving 512 amino acids plus a stop codon). The exon–intron pattern and total gene size of human CYP 1A1 and mouse cyp 1a1 genes are strikingly similar though the encoded proteins are 20% divergent. It seems likely that this similarity of structure is paralleled by a similarity of control and function. The human CYP 1A1 gene is located on chromosome 15 at 15q22–qter.

The cDNA and complete amino acid sequence of human CYP 1A2 has also been worked out (Jaiswal et al. 1986); it has 515 residues compared with 512 in CYP 1A1. No RFLPs or variants have hitherto been described for CYP 1A2.

The cDNA of human CYP 1A1 has been expressed in the yeast Saccharomyces cerevisiae by Eugster et al. (1990) and Ching et al. (1991). The enzyme kinetics were studied by the former authors using the deethylation of 7-ethoxyresorufin. Ketoconazole and α-naphthoflavone were found to be strong inhibitors.

A human hepatoma cell line devoid of significant basal levels of cytochrome P450 was used by Aoyama et al. (1989) to carry a vaccinia virus cDNA expression system for human cytochrome P450 1A2. It was shown that the enzyme could hydroxylate aniline, O-deethylate ethoxyresorufin and 7-ethoxycoumarin. Also, an ability to activate various aromatic amines, heterocyclic amines and polycyclic hydrocarbons was demonstrated.

Similarly, Wölfel et al. (1992) expressed human cytochrome P450 1A2 in genetically engineered V79 Chinese hamster cells. They found that methoxyresorufin was metabolized by cytochrome P450 1A2 but not by 1A1. In addition, they pointed out that expressing P450 1A2 in V79 cells already having N-acetyltransferase activity may be particularly useful for assessing the production of mutagens from aro-

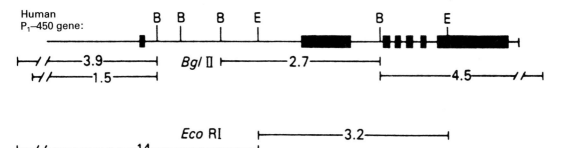

Fig. 5.6. Diagram of the human P$_1$450 gene, having seven exons (black boxes). Because about 9 kb of the gene and 5'- and 3'-flanking regions have been sequenced, it is relatively easy to assign RFLP patterns within and near the gene – shown here with *Bgl*II (3.9 and 1.5 kb pattern) and *Eco*RI (14 and 7.5 kb pattern). (From Nebert & Jaiswal 1987.)

matic amines.

McManus *et al.* (1990) expressed human *CYP 1A1* and *CYP 1A2* in Cos-1 cells. The products of these genes were shown to be able to *N*-hydroxylate the carcinogen 2-acetylaminofluorene, and were inhibited by α-naphthoflavone. Various other carcinogenic aromatic amides and amines were similarly 'activated' by human liver microsomal preparations (which lack cytochrome P450 1A1) and this process was inhibited by α-naphthoflavone. It was therefore considered that the gene *CYP 1A2* may be of importance in carcinogenesis.

The level of cytochrome P450 1A2 and of 7-ethoxyresorufin *O*-deethylase activity was shown to be increased in cultured human hepatocytes by 3-methylcholanthrene but not by various other compounds (Morel *et al.* 1990).

These discoveries should open the way to a greater understanding of the role of these enzymes in drug metabolism and in the aetiology of disease.

Aoyama *et al.* (1989) point out that assembling a large library of cDNAs coding for unique human cytochromes P450 will enable a catalogue of substrates for each cytochrome to be defined. This may be particularly valuable for the study of carcinogens.

CONCLUSIONS

A single gene interspecies difference has been found in mice which profoundly influences the activities of a number of enzymes. The phenotypic consequences in terms of carcinogenesis and toxicity from various drugs and chemicals are widely divergent between animals which do and do not carry the allele for Ah responsiveness.

Studies to find a human counterpart have on the whole been disappointing. As studied hitherto in blood lymphocytes and monocytes, arylhydrocarbon hydroxylase appears to be a biometrical trait with a relatively weak heredity probably under polygenic control. The *CYP 1A1* and *CYP 1A2* genes have had their chromosomal localizations and structures determined. Restriction length polymorphisms have been described in the former and the different genotypes may have clinically relevant contrasting phenotypic features. When the structure of the *Ah* gene has been determined in humans then variants may be found which can be correlated with different clinical events.

The author would like to express his gratitude to Dr Daniel W. Nebert, Centre for Environmental Genetics, Department of Environmental Health, University of Cincinnati Medical Centre, USA who made many helpful suggestions about the contents of this chapter.

Aoyama, T., Gonzalez, F. J. & Gelboin H. V. (1989). Human cDNA-expressed cytochrome P450 1A2: mutagen activation and substrate specificity. *Molecular Carcinogenesis*, **2**, 192–8.

Atlas, S. A. & Nebert D. W. (1976). Genetic association of increases in naphthalene acetanilide and biphenyl hydroxylations with inducible arylhydrocarbon hydroxylase in mice. *Archives of Biochemistry and Biophysics*, **175**, 495–506.

Brooks, B., Johnson, B., Heinzmann, C., Mohandas, T., Sparkes, R., Jones, S., Bennett, P., Balacs, T., Moore, G., Conley, L., & Hankinson, O. (1989). Localization of a gene required for the nuclear translocation of the dioxin receptor to human chromosome 1 and mouse chromosome 3 and a human RFLP with Msp 1. *American Journal of Human Genetics*, **45**, Suppl A 132 (0513).

Busbee, D. L., Shaw, C. R. & Cantrell, E. T. (1972). Aryl hydrocarbon hydroxylase induction in human leucocytes. *Science*, **178**, 315–16.

Butler, M. A., Iwasaki, M., Guengerich, F. P. & Kadlubar, F. F. (1989). Human cytochrome P-450$_{PA}$(P-450IA2) the phenacetin O-deethylase, is primarily responsible for the hepatic 3-demethylation of caffeine and N -oxidation of carcinogenic arylamines. *Proceedings of the National Academy of Sciences (USA)*, **86**, 7696–700.

Butler, M. A., Lang, N. P., Young, J. F., Caporaso, N. E., Vineis, P., Hayes, R. B., Teitel, C. H., Messengrill, J. P., Lawsen, M. F. & Kadlubar, F. F. (1992). Determination of CYP 1A2 and NAT 2 phenotypes in human propulations by analyses of caffeine urinary metabolites. *Pharmacogenetics*, **2**, 116–27.

Cantrell, E., Busbee, D., Warr, G. & Martin, R. (1973). Induction of arylhydrocarbon hydroxylase in human lymphocytes and pulmonary alveolar macrophages – a comparison. *Life Sciences*, **13**, 1649–54.

Ching, M. S., Lennard, M. S., Tucker, G. T., Woods. H. F., Kelly, D. E. & Kelly, S. L. (1991). The expression of hyman cytochrome P450 1A1 in the yeast *Saccharomyces cerevisiae* . *Biochemical Pharmacology*, **42**, 753–8.

Cunningham, J. L., Bullen, M. F. & Evans, D. A. P. (1974). The pharmacokinetics of acetanilide and diphenylhydantoin sodium. *European Journal of Clinical Pharmacology*, **7**, 461–6.

Dey, A., Westphal, H., Jones, J. E. & Nebert, D. W. (Cited by Nerbert 1989). Cell specific Cyp1a1 and Cyp1a2 induction by 3 methylcholanthrene in mouse tissues.

Diaz, D., Fabre, I., Daujat, M., Aubert, B. S., Bories, P., Michel, H. & Maurel, P. (1990). Omeprazole is an aryl-hydrocarbon-like inducer of human hepatic cytochrome P450. *Gastroenterology*, **99**, 737–47.

Distlerath, L. M., Reilly, P. E. B., Martin, M. V., Davis, G. G., Wilkinson, G. R. & Guengerich, F. P. (1985). Purification and characterization of the human liver cytochromes P-450 involved in debrisoquine 4-hydroxylation and phenacetin O-deethylation, two prototypes for genetic polymorphism in oxidative drug metabolism. *Journal of Biological Chemistry*, **260**, 9057–67.

Eugster, H. P., Sengstag, C., Meyer, U. A., Hinnen, A., & Würgler, F. E. (1990). Constitutive and inducible expression of human cytochrome P450IA1 in yeast *Saccharomyces cerevisiae*: an alternative enzyme source for *in vitro* studies. *Biochemical and Biophysical Research Communications*, **172**, 737–44.

Farrell, G. (1992). P450 1A2 and omeprazole. *Gastroenterology*, **102**, 1822–3.

Fuhr, U., Wolff, T., Harder, S., Sghymanski, P. & Staib, A. H. (1990). Quinolone inhibition of cytochrome P-450-dependent caffeine metabolism in human liver microsomes. *Drug Metabolism and Disposition*, **18**, 1005–10.

Golor, J., Neubert, D., Krüger, N. & Helge, H. (1992). Omeprazole and hepatic mono-oxygenase. *Gastroenterology*, **102**, 1443–4.

Gonzalez, F. J. & Nebert, D. W. (1985). Autoregulation plus upstream positive and negative control regions associated with transcriptional activation of the mouse P₁-450 gene. *Nucleic Acids Research*, **13**, 7269–88.

Grygiel, J. J. & Birkett, D. J. (1981). Cigarette smoking and theophylline clearance and metabolism. *Clinical Pharmacology and Therapeutics*, **30**, 491–6.

Harper, P. A., Golas, C. L. & Okey, A. B. (1988). Characterization of the Ah receptor and arylhydrocarbon hydroxylase induction by 2, 3, 7, 8-tetrachlorodibenzo-p-dioxin and benz(a)anthracene in the human A431 squamous cell carcinoma line. *Cancer Research*, **48**, 2388–95.

Harper, P. A., Golas, C. L. & Okey, A. B. (1988). Characterization of the Ah receptor and arylhydrocarbon hydroxylase induction by 2, 3, 7, 8-tetrachlorodibenzo-p-dioxin and benz(a)anthracene in the human A431 squamous cell carcinoma line. *Cancer Research*, **48**, 2388–95.

Hayashi, S.-I., Watanabe, J. & Kawajiri, K. (1992). High susceptibility to lung cancer analyzed in terms of combined genotypes of P450 IA1 and Mu-class glutathione S-transferase genes. *Japan Journal of Cancer Research*, **83**, 866–70.

Humphries, T. J. (1990). Clinical implications of drug interactions with the cytochrome P450 enzyme system associated with omeprazole. *Digestive Diseases and Sciences*, **36**, 1665–9.

Ikeya, K., Jaiswal, A. K., Owens, R. A., Jones, J. E., Nebert, D. W. & Kimura, S. (1989). Human CYP1A2: sequence, gene structure, comparison with the mouse and rat orthologous gene, and differences in liver 1A2 mRNA expression. *Molecular Endocrinology*, **3**, 1399–1408.

Ioannides, C. & Parke, D. V. (1990). The cytochrome P450 1 gene family of microsomal hemoproteins and their role in the metabolic activation of chemicals. *Drug Metabolism Reviews*, **22**, 1–85.

Jaiswal, A. K., Gonzalez, F. J. & Nebert, D. W. (1985). Human P₁-450 gene sequence and correlation of mRNA with genetic differences in benzo[a]pyrene metabolism. *Nucleic Acids Research*, **13**, 4503–20.

Jaiswal, A. K., Nebert, D. W. & Gonzalez, F. J. (1986). Human P₃-450: d DNA and complete amino acid sequence. *Nucleic Acids Research*, **14**, 6773–4.

Kalow, W. & Tang, B. K. (1991). Use of caffeine metabolite ratios to explore CYP1A2 and xanthine oxidase activities. *Clinical Pharmacology and Therapeutics*, **50**, 508–19.

Karki, N. T., Pokela, R., Nuutinen, L. & Pelkonen, O. (1987). Arylhydrocarbon hydroxylase in lymphocytes and lung tissue from lung cancer patients and controls. *International Journal of Cancer*, **39**, 565–70.

Kawajiri, K., Nakachi, K., Imai, K., Yoshi, A., Shinoda, N. & Watanabe, J. (1990). Identification of genetically high risk individuals to lung cancer by DNA polymorphisms of the cytochrome P450 1A1 gene. *FEBS Letters*, **263**, 131–3.

Kellermann, G. & Luyten-Kellermann, M. (1977). Phenobarbital-induced drug metabolism in man. *Toxicology and Applied Pharmacology*, **39**, 97–104.

Kellermann, G. & Luyten-Kellermann, M. (1978). Benzo[a]pyrene metabolism and plasma elimination rates of phenacetin acetanilide and theophylline in man. *Pharmacology*, **17**, 191–200.

Kellermann, G., Luyten-Kellermann, M., Horning, M. G. & Stafford, M. (1975). Correlation of arylhydrocarbon hydroxylase activity of human lymphocyte cultures and plasma elimination rates for antipyrine and phenyl-butazone. *Drug Metabolism and Disposition*, **3**, 47–50.

Kellermann, G., Luyten-Kellermann, M., Horning, M. G. &

Stafford, M. (1976). Elimination of antipyrine and benzo[a]pyrene metabolism in cultured human lymphocytes. *Clinical Pharmacology and Therapeutics*, **20**, 72–80.

Kellermann, G., Luyten-Kellermann, M. & Shaw, C. R. (1973a). Genetic variation of arylhydrocarbon hydroxylase in human lymphocytes. *American Journal of Human Genetics*, **25**, 327–31.

Kellermann, G., Shaw, C. R. & Luyten-Kellermann, M. (1973b). Arylhydrocarbon hydroxylase inducibility and bronchogenic carcinoma. *New England Journal of Medicine*, **289**, 934–37.

Kouri, R. E., McKinney, C. E., Levine, A. S., Edwards, B. K., Vessell, E. S., Nebert, D. W. & McLemore, T. L. (1984). Variations in arylhydrocarbon hydroxylase activities in mitogen-activated human and non-human primate lymphocytes. *Toxicologic Pathology*, **12**, 44–8.

Kouri, R. E., McKinney, C. E., Slomiany, D. J., Snodgrass, D. R., Wray, N. P. & McLemore, T. L. (1982). Positive correlation between arylhydrocarbon hydroxylase activity and primary lung cancer as analysed in cryopreserved lymphocytes. *Cancer Research*, **42**, 5030–37.

Levine, A. S., McKinney, C. E., Echelberger, C. K., Kouri, R. E., Edwards, B. K. & Nebert, D. W. (1984). Arylhydrocarbon hydroxylase inducibility among primary relatives of children with leukaemia or solid tumours. *Cancer Research*, **44**, 358–62.

McLemore, T. L., Adelberg, S., Liu, M., McMahon, N. A., Yu, S. J., Hubbard, W. C., Czerwinski, M., Wood, T. G., Storeng, R., Lubet, R. A., Eggleston, J. C., Boyd, M. R. & Hines, R. N. (1990). Expression of CYP1A1 gene in patients with lung cancer: Evidence for cigarette smoke-induced gene expression in normal lung tissue and for altered gene regulation in primary pulmonary carcinomas. *Journal of the National Cancer Institute*, **82**, 1333–9.

McLemore, T. L., Martin, R., Toppell, K. L., Busbee, D. L. & Cantrell, E. T. (1977b). Comparison of arylhydrocarbon hydroxylase induction in cultured blood lymphocytes and pulmonary macrophages. *Journal of Clinical Investigation*, **60**, 1017–24.

McLemore, T. L., Martin, R. R., Wray, N. P., Cantrell, E. T., & Busbee, D. L. (1978). Dissociation between arylhydrocarbon hydroxylase activity in cultured pulmonary macrophages and blood lymphocytes from lung cancer patients. *Cancer Research*, **38**, 3805–11.

McLemore, T. L., Martin, R. R., Wray, N. P., Cantrell, E. T. & Busbee, D. L. (1981). Reassessment of the relationship between arylhydrocarbon hydroxylase and lung cancer. *Cancer*, **48**, 1438–43.

McLemore, T. L., Warr, G. A. & Martin, R. R. (1977a). Induction of arylhydrocarbon hydroxylase in human pulmonary alveolar macrophages and peripheral lymphocytes by cigarette tars. *Cancer Letters*, **2**, 161–8.

McManus, M. E., Burgess, W. M., Veronese, M. E., Huggett, A., Quattrochi, L. C. & Tukey, R. H. (1990). Metabolism of 2-acetylaminofluorene and benzo(a)pyrene and activation of food derived heterocyclic amine mutagens by human cytochromes P-450. *Cancer Research*, **50**, 3367–76.

Mattison, D. R. & Thorgeirsson, S. S. (1978a). Gonadal arylhydrocarbon hydroxylase in rats and mice. *Cancer Research*, **38**, 1368–73.

Mattison, D. R. & Thorgeirsson, S. S. (1978b). Smoking and industrial pollution and their effects of menopause and ovarian cancer. *Lancet*, **1**, 187–8.

Mattison, D. R. & Thorgeirsson, S. S. (1979). Ovarian arylhydrocarbon hydroxylase activity and primordial oocyte toxicity of polycyclic hydrocarbons in mice. *Cancer Research*, **39**, 3471–5.

Morel, F., Beaune, P. H., Ratanasavanh, D., Flinois, J. P., Yang, C. S., Guengerich, F. P. & Guillouzo, A. (1990). Expression of cytochrome P-450 enzymes in cultured human hepatocytes. *European Journal of Biochemistry*, **191**, 437–44.

Nebert, D. W. (1988). Genes encoding drug-metabolizing enzymes: possible role in human disease. In *Phenotypic Variations in Populations*, ed. A. D. Woodhead, M. A. Bender, R. C. Leonard, pp. 45–64. New York: Plenum.

Nebert, D. W. (1989). The Ah locus: genetic differences in toxicity, cancer, mutation and birth defects. *Critical Reviews in Toxicology*, **20**, 153–74.

Nebert, D. W. & Jaiswal, A. K. (1987). Human drug metabolism polymorphisms: use of recombinant DNA techniques. *Pharmacology and Therapeutics*, **33**, 11–17.

Nowak, D., Schmidt-Preuss, U., Jorres, R., Liebke, F. & Rudiger, H. W. (1988). Formation of DNA adducts and water-soluble metabolites of benzo[a]pyrene in human monocytes is genetically controlled. *International Journal of Cancer*, **41**, 169–73.

Okuda, T., Vessell, E. S., Plotkin, E., Tarone, R., Bast, R. C. & Gelboin, H. V. (1977). Interindividual and intraindividual variations in arylhydrocarbon hydroxylase in monocytes from monozygous and dizygous twins. *Cancer Research*, **37**, 3904–11.

Petersen, D. D., McKinney, C. E., Ikeya, K., Smith, H. H., Bale, A. E., McBride, O. W. & Nebert, D. W. (1991). Human CYP1A1 gene: cosegregation of the enzyme inducibility phenotype and an RFLP. *American Journal of Human Genetics*, **48**, 720–5.

Poland, A. & Glover, E. (1974). Comparison of 2,3,7,8 tetrachlorodibenzo-p-dioxin, a potent inducer of arylhydrocarbon hydroxylase with 3-methylcholanthrene. *Molecular Pharmacology*, **10**, 349–59.

Roberts, E. A., Johnson, K. C. & Dippold, W. G. (1991). Ah receptor mediating induction of cytochrome P450 1A1 in a novel continuous human liver cell line (Mz-Hep-1). *Biochemical Pharmacology*, **42**, 521–8.

Rost, K. L., Brösicke, H., Brockmöller, J., Scheffler, M., Helge, H. & Roots, I. (1992). Increase of cytochrome P450 1A2 activity by omeprazole: evidence by the ^{13}C-[N-3-methyl]-caffeine breath test in poor and extensive metabolizers of S-mephenytoin. *Clinical Pharmacology and Therapeutics*, **52**, 170–80.

Rudiger, H. W., Nowak, D., Hartmann, K. & Cerutti, P. (1985). Enhanced formation of benzo(a)pyrene: DNA adducts in monocytes of patients with a presumed predisposition to lung cancer. *Cancer Research*, **45**, 5890–94.

Saatcioglu, F., Perry, D. J., Pasco, D. S. & Fagan, J. B. (1990). Multiple DNA-binding factors interact with overlapping specificities at the arylhydrocarbon response element of the cytochrome P450IA1 gene. *Molecular and Cellular Biology*, **10**, 6408–16.

Sarkar, M. A., Hunt, C., Guzelian, P. S. & Karnes, H. T. (1992). Characterization of human liver cytochromes P-450 involved in theophylline metabolism. *Drug Metabolism and Disposition*, **20**, 31–7.

Sesardic, D., Boobis, A. R., Murray, B. P., Murray, S., Segura, J., de la Torre, R. & Davies, D. S. (1990). Furafylline is a potent and selective inhibitor of cytochrome P450 1A2 in man. *British Journal of Clinical Pharmacology*, **29**, 651–63.

Sherson, D., Sigsgaard, T., Overgaard, E., Loft, S., Pulsen, H. E. & Jongeneelen, F. J. (1992). Interaction of smoking, uptake of polycyclic aromatic hydrocarbons, and cytochrome P450 1A2 activity among foundry workers. *British Journal of Industrial Medicine*, **49**, 197–202.

Taburet, A. M., Geneve, J., Bocquentin, M., Simoneau, G., Caulin, C. & Singlas, E. (1992). Theophylline steady state pharmacokinetics is not altered by omeprazole. *European Journal of Clinical Pharmacology*, **42**, 343–5.

Tefre, T., Ryberg, D., Haugen, A., Nebert, D. W., Skang, V., Brøgger, A. & Børresen, A. L. (1991). Human *CYP1A1* (cytochrome P_1 450) gene: lack of association between the Msp 1 restriction fragment length polymorphism and incidence of lung cancer in a Norwegian population. *Pharmacogenetics*, **1**, 20–5.

Thomas, P. E., Kouri, R. E. & Hutton, J. J. (1972). The genetics of arylhydrocarbon hydroxylase induction in mice: a single gene difference between C57 BL/6J and DBA/2J. *Biochemical Genetics*, **6**, 157–68.

Thorgeirsson, S. S. & Nebert, D. W. (1977). The Ah locus and the metabolism of chemical carcinogens and other foreign compounds. *Advances in Cancer Research*, **25**, 149–93.

Waither, W. I., Michaud, M., Harper, P. A., Okey, A. B. & Anderson, A. (1991). The Ah receptor, cytochrome P450 1A1 mRNA induction, and arylhydrocarbon hydroxylase in a human lymphoblastoid cell line. *Biochemical Pharmacology*, **41**, 85–92.

Wang, X., Narasimhan, T. R., Morrison, V. & Safe, S. (1991). In situ and in vitro photoaffinity labelling of the nuclear arylhydrocarbon receptor from transformed rodent and human cell lines. *Archives of Biochemistry and Biophysics*, **287**, 186–94.

Ward, E., Paigen, B., Steenland, K., Vincent, R., Minowada, J., Gurtoo, H. L., Satori, P. & Havens, M. B. (1978). Arylhydrocarbon hydroxylase in persons with lung or laryngeal cancer. *International Journal of Cancer*, **22**, 384–9.

Wheeler, C. W. & Guenthner, T. M. (1991). Cytochrome P-450-dependent metabolism of xenobiotics in human lung. *Journal of Biochemical Toxicology*, **6**, 163–9.

Whitlock, J. P., Jr, Cooper, H. L. & Gelboin, H. Y. (1972). Aryl hydrocarbon (benzopyrene) hydroxylase is stimulated in human lymphocytes by mitogens and benz[a]-anthracene. *Science*, **177**, 618–19.

Wölfel, C., Heinrich-Hirsch, B., Schulz-Schalge, T., Seidel, A., Frank, H., Ramp, U., Wächter, F., Wiebel, F. J., Gonzalez, F., Greim, H. & Doehmer, J. (1992). Genetically engineered V79 Chinese hamster cells for stable expression of human cytochrome P450 IA2. *European Journal of Pharmacology – Environmental Toxicology and Pharmacology Section*, **228**, 95–102.

Wrighton, S. A. & Watkins, P. (1991). Non-uniform distribution of cytochrome P450 1A2 in liver. *Gastroenterology*, **100**, 1487–8.

6 The mephenytoin hydroxylation polymorphism (cytochrome P450 2C18)

THE DISCOVERY OF THE POLYMORPHISM

MEPHENYTOIN (3-methyl-5-phenyl-5-ethyl-hydantoin) has been in use for the treatment of epilepsy for over 40 years. It has been known for a long time that the drug is partially metabolized in man by demethylation to 5-phenyl-5-ethyl-hydantoin (nirvanol). Alternatively, mephenytoin is metabolized by aromatic hydroxylation to 3-methyl-5- (4-hydroxyphenyl) -5-ethylhydantoin (4'-OH-M).

Mephenytoin has a centre of asymmetry at the 5-position of the hydantoin ring (Fig. 6.1) and undergoes substrate-stereoselective metabolism. It has been found that there is marked stereoselectivity of the alternate metabolic pathway of metabolism to 4'-OH-M so that S-mephenytoin is rapidly and almost quantitatively eliminated in urine as the phenolglucuronide. The R-enantiomer which undergoes less aromatic hydroxylation is demethyl-

ated to R-nirvanol which is much more slowly excreted than S4'-OH-M (Fig. 6.2).

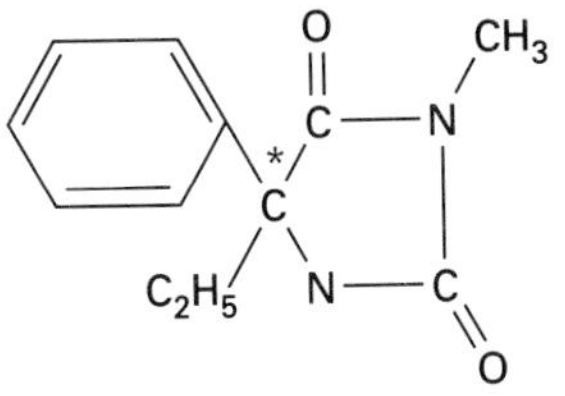

Kupfer and his associates, in studies to investigate the kinetic consequences of stereoselective S-mephenytoin hydroxylation during long-term racemic mephenytoin dosing in normal subjects, found one subject who had a defect in the aromatic hydroxylation of S-mephenytoin (Kupfer *et al.* 1979). Consequently 221 healthy unrelated Caucasian Swiss subjects were each given 100 mg racemic mephenytoin orally (Kupfer & Preisig 1984). Urine was collected for 8 hours after drug ingestion and the following 'hydroxylation index' determined:

$$\frac{\mu mol \ mephenytoin \ dose \ (S\text{-}enantiomer)}{\mu mol \ 4'\text{-}OH\text{-}mephenytoin \ in \ urine \ 0 \ to \ 8 \ hours}$$

This ratio was discontinuously distributed in the population (Fig. 6.3) so that 12 individuals were classified as poor metabolizers (PM_M) and 209 individuals were classified as extensive metabolizers (EM_M).

On another occasion a panel of 10 extensive and 10 poor metabolizers of mephenytoin were also given 50 mg of S-nirvanol only and the urine collected for 8 hours thereafter. Unlike mephenytoin, S-nirvanol is excreted in the urine and this compound and 4'-OH-nirvanol were assayed so yielding the urinary metabolic ratio:

$$MR_N = \frac{\mu mol \ S \ nirvanol}{\mu mol \ 4'\text{-}OH\text{-}S \ nirvanol} \quad over \ 8 \ hours$$

The results showed an unexceptional concordance

Fig. 6.1. The structural formula of mephenytoin (3-methyl-5-phenyl-5-ethylhydantoin).
* Indicates the centre of asymmetry.

35

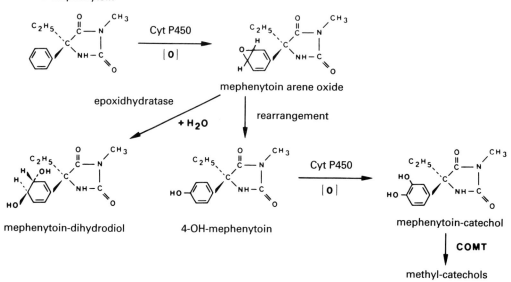

Fig. 6.2. Metabolic pathways of *R*- and *S*-mephenytoin in man. Cyt, cytochrome; PEH, 5-phenyl-5-ethylhydantoin; COMT, catechol-*O*-methyltransferase. (From Kupfer *et al.* 1984a.)

with the mephenytoin results (Kupfer & Preisig 1984).

GENETIC NATURE OF THE POLYMORPHISM

The same 221 subjects were also investigated with a debrisoquine test (Fig 6.3). The population fell into four classes (Table 6.1) showing that the two polymorphisms were independent. Similar results were obtained in Caucasians by other groups of experimenters (Table 6.1 and Fig. 6.4).

Five families each ascertained via a poor metabolizer of mephenytoin were investigated by

Kupfer & Preisig (1984) using nirvanol as the test compound. The poor metabolizers of nirvanol (PM$_N$) appeared to be homozygous recessives for deficient aromatic hydroxylation of nirvanol and mephenytoin (Fig. 6.5). Extensive metabolizers (EM$_N$) were dominants. Within the 23 related subjects studied in five families seven heterozygotes could be recognized. The metabolic ratio for nirvanol (MR$_N$) values (4.7 ± 3.2, range 1.2–8.5) were intermediate between PM$_N$ (17.1 ± 7.6, range 9–34) and EM$_N$ phenotypes (1.2 ± 0.6, range 0.6–2.4) but did not form a separate recognizable group. This is in keeping with the bimodal distribution obtained in the population study. In one family the proposita was PM$_N$ PM$_D$ but the remainder of the persons in the pedigree showed results compatible with independent assortment of the responsible alleles.

Similar results were obtained by Inaba *et al.* (1986) who studied 33 individuals in five families ascertained via PM$_M$ probands. Three of the families

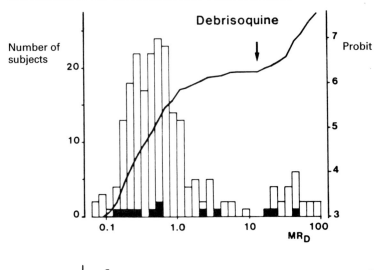

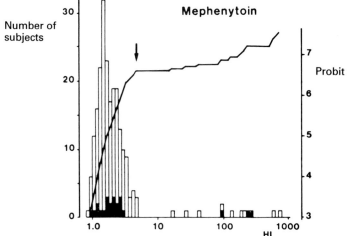

Fig. 6.3. Frequency histograms of the debrisoquine metabolic ratios (*upper panel*) and the mephenytoin hydroxylation indices (*lower panel*) on a logarithmic scale. The closed bars indicate the PM_M in the debrisoquine and the PM_D phenotypes in the mephenytoin histograms, respectively. The solid line indicates the results of the probit analysis by which the antimodes (*black arrows*) were determined. (From Kupfer & Preisig 1984.)

were Japanese and two Caucasian. Ward *et al.* (1987) investigated four Japanese extended families. Their findings also were in keeping with PM individuals being autosomal recessives (Fig. 6.6). In their families six PM × PM matings produced only

PM offspring; and the numbers of offspring of different phenotypes produced from other matings did not differ significantly from those predicted by the Hardy–Weinberg equilibrium. (Table 6.2).

Another five pedigrees published by Drøhse *et al.* (1989) indicated that poor metabolizers of mephenytoin were autosomal recessives, and an individual was identified who was a poor metabolizer of both sparteine and mephenytoin.

COMPARISONS OF VARIOUS POPULATIONS

The available data for inter-ethnic comparisons are shown in Table 6.3. (The series of Britto *et al.* 1991

Table 6.1. *Distribution of debrisoquine/sparteine and mephenytoin phenotypes in Caucasians*

Reference	Location	Total number	Comparison drug	Phenotype			
				$EM_M EM_X$	$EM_M PM_X$	$PM_M EM_X$	$PM_M PM_X$
Kupfer & Preisig 1984	Switzerland	221	Debrisoquine (Deb)	189	20	9	3
Wedlund et al. 1984	Tennessee, USA	156	Debrisoquine (Deb)	141	11	4	0
Inaba et al. 1984	Canada	83	Sparteine (S)	78	3	2	0
Jacqz et al. 1988a	France	132	Dextromethorphan (Dex)	121	3	7	1
Drøhse et al. 1989	Denmark	358	Sparteine (S)	317	32	8	1
Sanz et al. 1989	Sweden	253	Debrisoquine (Deb)	224	22	7	0
Guttendorf et al. 1990	Kentucky, USA	519	Dextromethorphan (Dex)	468	32	16	3

M, mephenytoin; X, S or Deb or Dex; EM, extensive metabolizer; PM, poor metabolizer.

Table 6.2. *Observed and predicted frequency of PMs of mephenytoin in Japanese families*

Phenotype	N	Total number of offspring	Number of PM offspring		χ^2
			Expected	Observed	
PM × PM	3	6	6	6	–
PM × EM	6	11	3.3	3	0.027*
EM × EM	4	13	1.3	3	2.220*

*$p > 0.05$

From: Ward *et al.* 1987.

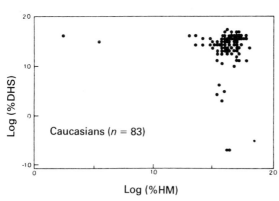

Fig. 6.4. Scatter plot of $p(4')$-hydroxymephenytoin (HM) against 2- and 5-dehydrosparteine (DHS) in 83 unrelated subjects. Spearman rank correlation coefficient $r_s = 0.10$ (NS). (From Inaba *et al.* 1984.)

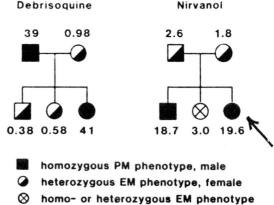

Fig. 6.5. Pedigrees and metabolic ratios of debrisoquine and nirvanol hydroxylation in the same family (Family S). The numbers indicate the metabolic ratios of debrisoquine and nirvanol. (From Kupfer & Preisig 1984.)

Table 6.3. *Inter-ethnic variability of the mephenytoin hydroxylation polymorphism*

Reference	Location studied	Ethnic group	Total number of subjects studied	Number of poor metabolizers	q	SE (q)
Kupfer & Preisig 1984	Berne	Caucasians	221	12	0.233	0.0327
Wedlund et al. 1984	Nashville	Caucasians	156	4	0.1601	0.0395
Jurima et al. 1985a	Toronto	Caucasians	118	5	0.2058	0.0450
Jaczq et al. 1988a	Le Vesinet, France	Caucasians	132	8	0.2462	0.0422
Breimer et al. 1988	Leiden	Caucasians	172	4	0.1525	0.0377
Sanz et al. 1989	Huddinge, Sweden	Caucasians	253	7	0.1663	0.0310
Bertilsson et al. 1992	Huddinge, Sweden	Caucasians	488[a]	16	0.1811	0.0223
Drøhse et al. 1989	Odense, Denmark	Caucasians	358	9	0.1586	0.0261
Baumann et al. 1992	Prilly-Lausanne	Caucasians	58	3	0.2274	0.0639
Pollock et al. 1991	Pittsburgh	White elderly Americans	123	5	0.2016	0.0442
		Black elderly Americans	27	5	0.4303	0.0869
Jurima et al. 1985a	Toronto	Chinese	39	2	0.2264	0.0780
Horai et al. 1989	Changsha Hunan	Chinese	98	17	0.4165	0.0459
Bertilsson et al. 1989	Beijing	Chinese	99	16	0.4020	0.0460
Bertilsson et al. 1992	Beijing	Chinese (Han)	137[b]	20	0.3821	0.0336
Sohn et al. 1992	Chinju, Seoul & Pusan	Koreans	208	26	0.3535	0.0324
Jurima et al. 1985a	Toronto	Japanese	31	7	0.4752	0.0790
Nakamura et al. 1985	Tsukuba Japan	Japanese	100	18	0.4243	0.0453
Horai et al. 1989	Tokyo & Osaka	Japanese	200	45	0.4743	0.0311
Setiabudy et al. 1992	Jakarta	Indonesians	10	3	0.5477	0.1323
Clasen et al. 1991	East Greenland	East Greenlanders (mongoloid 'Dorset' people)	300	28	0.3055	0.0275
	West Greenland (Nuuk)	West Greenlanders (Inuit/Caucasian)	171	5	0.1710	0.0377
Inaba et al. 1988	Panama	Cuna Amerindians	90	0	0.0000	0.0000
Doshi et al. 1990	Bombay	Indians	48	10	0.4564	0.0642

q, Frequency of the allele controlling poor hydroxylation.
[a] Includes the 253 subjects of the Sanz et al. (1989).
[b] Includes the 99 subjects of Bertilsson et al. (1989).

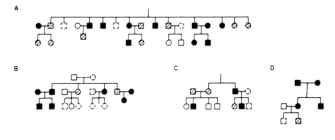

A

B C D

○ = ♀ EM   ■ = PM   ⚏ = Unknown phenotype
□ = ♂ EM   ▨ = Obligate heterozygote

Fig. 6.6. Family pedigrees from four extended Japanese families for the mephenytoin 4-hydroxylation polymorphism. The hatched symbols represent subjects who have an obligate heterozygous genotype. (From Ward et al. 1987.)

was not included because it does not give the number of poor metabolizers in each racial group.) Eight Caucasian samples amongst whom PMs are 3.52% can be compared with six Japanese and Chinese samples amongst whom PMs are 18.52%. Pooling the estimates for these two ethnic groups yields the hugely significant $\chi_1^2 = 133$. The absence of PMs amongst the Cuna Amerindian sample could be interpreted as an example of genetic drift. If the single Indian sample can be taken as representative of the Indian subcontinent then the change in gene frequency must occur between Bombay and Berne. There is a deficiency of gene frequency estimates in Africans.

METABOLIC DIFFERENCES BETWEEN PHENOTYPES

The kinetic implications of the mephenytoin polymorphism were studied in one poor metabolizer (PM) and four extensive metabolizers (EM) by Kupfer *et al.* (1984b). They gave these subjects a single oral dose of differentially radiolabelled enantiomers. A pseudo-racemic mixture of ^{14}C-labelled S-mephenytoin with the ^{14}C in the 4-position of the hydantoin ring, and ^{3}H-labelled R-mephenytoin with the ^{3}H in the 4'-position of the phenyl ring, was employed. This was followed by single daily doses of unlabelled racemic mephenytoin for the next few days.

In EM subjects there was substrate stereoselective

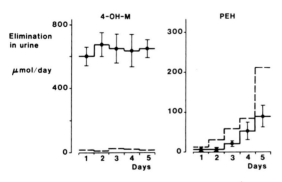

Fig. 6.7. Daily urinary excretion of 4-OH-M (*left*) and PEH (*right*) in four normal subjects (● with mean ± SD) and in one mephenytoin hydroxylation-deficient subject (– – –) after oral racemic mephenytoin (1.4 mmol/day for 5 days). (From Kupfer *et al.* 1984b.)

metabolism with the S-enantiomer rapidly excreted as 4'-OH-M (Fig. 6.7) and the R-enantiomer slowly excreted as 5-phenyl-5-ethylhydantoin (nirvanol) (PEH). Stereoselective metabolism persisted during repeated dosing.

In the PM individual there was no evidence of stereoselective metabolism, recovery of 4'-OH-M was low and both enantiomers were slowly excreted predominantly as PEH (Fig. 6.7). The plasma PEH concentrations and urinary PEH excretion rates were approximately twice those in normal subjects. So the genetically determined inability to 4'-hydroxylate S-mephenytoin resulted in the S-enantiomer being metabolized by demethylation to PEH which was more slowly excreted than 4'-OH-M. Consequently, S-PEH as well as R-PEH accumulated in the body eventually, effectively doubling the body content of hydantoin (Fig. 6.8). This was demonstrated in terms of plasma concentration in the above survey and carries the implication that a PM individual, if recognized before treatment with mephenytoin was started, would require only half the conventional dose to achieve the same total plasma hydantoin concentration as an EM individual.

Similar results were obtained by Wedlund *et al.* (1985) who showed that following a single oral dose of racemic mephenytoin the consequences were very different for the two enantiomers in the two phenotypes.

In EM subjects the plasma concentration of the R-enantiomer increased rapidly to a peak value within 2 to 4 hours and then declined exponentially with a mean half life of 76 hours. The peak concentration of the S-enantiomer was also achieved rapidly but the value was only about 25% of that of the R-enantiomer. The rate of elimination was 30 to 40-fold faster with a mean half life of 2.13 hours. The metabolite R-PEH accumulated slowly reaching a peak at about 5 days and declining slowly thereafter. A small amount of S-PEH was detected and rapidly eliminated.

In contrast, the stereoselective elimination of mephenytoin was reduced markedly in subjects of the PM phenotype, with the disposition of the S-enantiomer being the same as that for R-mephenytoin, which in turn was similar to that observed for this enantiomer in EM individuals. Comparable plasma levels of S- and R-PEH were also present in PM subjects.

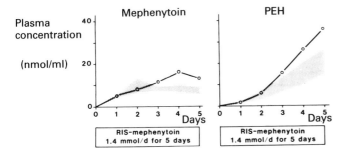

Fig. 6.8. Plasma concentration of mephenytoin (*left*) and PEH (*right*) in four normal subjects (hatched areas represent mean ± SD) and in one mephenytoin hydroxylation-deficient subject (o) after oral racemic mephenytoin. (From Kupfer *et al.* 1984b.)

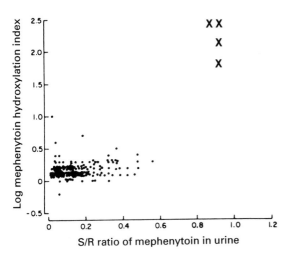

Fig. 6.9. Comparison of the hydroxylation index and the *S/R* ratio of mephenytoin in an 8 h urine sample from 156 unrelated Caucasians after 100 mg mephenytoin. (From Wedlund *et al.* 1984.)

In the urine, EM individuals excreted almost 50% of the dose over 4 days as 4'-hydroxymephenytoin with only 5 to 15% being eliminated as PEH over 14 days. On the other hand, PM persons eliminated negligible amounts of the 4-hydroxymetabolite and PEH excretion accounted for 30 to 40% of the administered dose.

Wedlund *et al.* (1985) also made the observation that the S/R enantiomeric ratio of mephenytoin could be determined in an 8 hour urine sample. Even though less than 2% of the dose was excreted unchanged by both phenotypes the urinary concentrations were high enough to allow determination of the enantiomeric ratio with stereoselective capillary gas chromatography. In 156 unrelated Caucasians a high S/R urinary enantiomeric ratio (of unity) clearly separated four individuals who had a high hydroxylation index categorizing them as poor hydroxylators (Fig. 6.9). Consequently, the S/R enantiomeric ratio can be used as a phenotyping test. The S/R ratio is of course low (> 0.6) in extensive metabolizers because a high proportion of the S-enantiomer they consume is 4'-hydroxylated, a fate which does not befall either the S-enantiomer in poor metabolizers or the R-enantiomer in either of the two phenotypes.

A chiral high-performance liquid chromatographic method employing β-cyclodextrin as a mobile phase additive has been introduced by Rona & Szabo (1992) which achieved enantiomeric separation.

An *in vitro* change in urines from the mephenytoin phenotyping test was described by Zhang *et al.* (1991). If the urines were kept at −20° C there was a change in the S/R enantiomeric ratio, which was quite large enough to alter the apparent phenotype in some instances. This change was attributed to the decomposition of an acid-labile urinary metabolite of S-mephenytoin. Three possible ways of ensuring correct phenotyping were described: (1) measure the enantiomeric ratio within at least 1 month of collection: (2) store a dichloromethane extract rather than the urine: (3) treat a sample of the urine with 12 N hydrochloric acid; in the true poor metabolizer urine the S/R ratio never increased above 1.2 whereas the extensive metabolizer urine exhibited a several-fold change in the ratio.

ENZYMIC BASIS OF THE POLYMORPHISM

The rate of 4′-hydroxylation and of N-demethylation of S- and R-mephenytoin was determined in liver microsomes of 13 EM and 2 PM metabolizers of mephenytoin by Meier *et al.* (1985). Microsomal mephenytoin metabolism in PMs was characterized by an increased K_m (150.6 and 180.6 vs a mean $\pm$ SD of 37.8 $\pm$ 9.6 µmol/l S-mephenytoin in 8 EMs) a decreased rate of metabolism for S-mephenytoin hydroxylation (0.76 and 0.69 vs 4.85 $\pm$ 1.65 nmol 4′-hydroxy-mephenytoin per mg protein per hour) and loss of stereoselectivity for the hydroxylation of the R- and S-enantiomers of mephenytoin (R/S ratio 1.10 and 0.76 vs 0.11 $\pm$ 0.04 in 13 EMs). The formation of 4′-OH-mephenytoin from R-mephenytoin and the demethylation reaction remained unaffected. These results strongly suggested that the mephenytoin polymorphism was caused by a partial or complete absence or inactivity of a cytochrome P450 isozyme with high affinity for S-mephenytoin.

The same group (Gut *et al.* 1986) monitored the activities of the two major oxidative pathways of mephenytoin metabolism in column eluates of human liver preparations. They purified a cytochrome P450 isozyme 'P450$_{meph}$' which exclusively and stereoselectively catalysed the 4′-hydroxylation of S-mephenytoin. This cytochrome P450 had an apparent molecular weight of 55 000 and a λ_{max} in the reduced CO-binding spectrum of 450 nm. Polyclonal rabbit antibodies against purified P450$_{meph}$ almost completely inhibited the 4-hydroxylation of mephenytoin in human liver microsomes. In microsomes of liver biopsies of two subjects characterized *in vivo* as PMs of mephenytoin, immunocrossreactive and immunoinhibitable material was observed with similar or identical properties to P450$_{meph}$. There was no difference in the extent of the immunochemical reaction between microsomes of *in vivo* phenotyped PMs and EMs of mephenytoin. These data suggest that P450$_{meph}$ is the site of the genetic variation and support the concept that a functionally altered variant form of P450$_{meph}$ is the cause of this polymorphism.

A human autoimmune antibody has been found in patients suffering from tienilic acid (ticrynafen, a diuretic: Fig. 6.10) -induced hepatitis which specifically inhibits human mephenytoin hydroxylation because it 'recognizes' cytochrome P450$_{meph}$. The

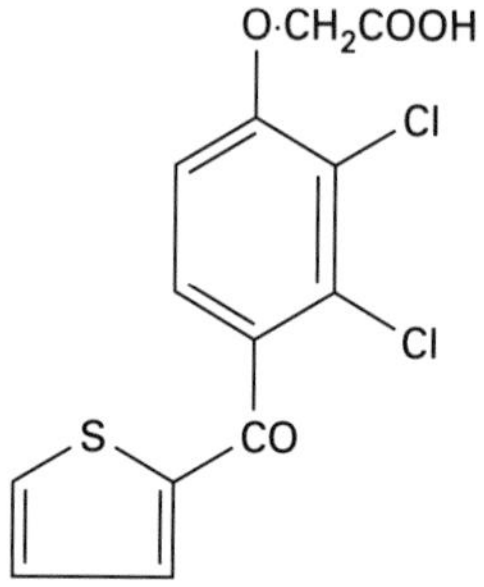

Fig. 6.10. Structural formula of tienilic acid (ticrynafen).

cytochrome P450 so recognized was immunopurified from microsomes of EM$_M$ and PM$_M$ subjects. No difference could be found with regard to immuno-crossreactivity, molecular weight, isoelectric point, relative content in microsomes, two-dimensional tryptic peptide maps, one-dimensional peptide maps with three proteases, amino acid composition and amino-terminal protein sequence. These data strongly suggest that the mephenytoin deficiency is caused by a minor structural change leading to a functionally altered cytochrome P450 isozyme (Meier & Meyer 1987). Somewhat similar results (but lacking the *in vivo/in vitro* correlations) were found by Shimada *et al.* (1986).

CHEMICAL INHIBITION STUDIES

The underlying idea of these studies was to see whether cytochrome P450$_{meph}$ was inhibited from metabolizing mephenytoin by a given chemical. If this occurs then it is likely that the cytochrome 'recognizes' the chemical in question presumably because of a molecular fit. This suggests the possibility that the new chemical *may* be a substrate for the enzyme activity of P450$_{meph}$.

An experiment based on this reasoning was carried out by Jurima *et al.* (1984) who showed that mephenytoin did not inhibit sparteine oxidation by human liver. This was evidence suggesting that the sparteine/debrisoquine and the mephenytoin polymorphisms are separate, a finding confirmed by both population studies and the physical separation of the two responsible P450s by Gut *et al.* (1986).

It is known that large quantities of steroids are metabolized daily by humans and that they are

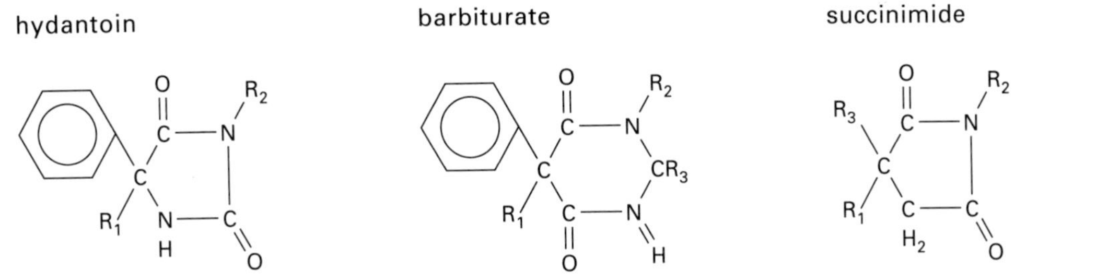

	R$_1$	R$_2$			R$_1$	R$_2$	R$_3$			R$_1$	R$_2$	R$_3$
MEPHENYTOIN	C$_2$H$_5$	CH$_3$		MEPHOBARBITAL	C$_2$H$_5$	CH$_3$	=0		METHSUXIMIDE	C$_6$H$_5$	CH$_3$	CH$_3$
ETHOTOIN	H	C$_2$H$_5$		N^4-ETHYLPHENOBARBITAL	C$_2$H$_5$	C$_2$H$_5$	=0		PHENSUXIMIDE	C$_6$H$_5$	CH$_3$	H
PEH	C$_2$H$_5$	H		N^1-METHYLPRIMIDONE	C$_2$H$_5$	CH$_3$	H		ETHOSUXIMIDE	C$_2$H$_5$	H	CH$_3$
PHENYTOIN	C$_6$H$_5$	H		N^1-ETHYLPRIMIDONE	C$_2$H$_5$	C$_2$H$_5$	H					
N^3-METHYLPHENYTOIN	C$_4$H$_5$	CH$_3$		PHENOBARBITAL	C$_2$H$_5$	H	=0					
				PRIMIDONE	C$_2$H$_5$	H	H					

Fig. 6.11. Chemical structures of related anticonvulsants studied for their ability to inhibit competitively the
formation of 4-OH-M from racemic mephenytoin by
human liver microsomes. Solid underline indicates that
the K_i/K_m value is low (0.2–1.2), a dashed underline identifies less potent inhibitors (K_i/K_m >2.0) and compounds
that exhibit no inhibition are not underlined. (From Hall
et al. 1987.)

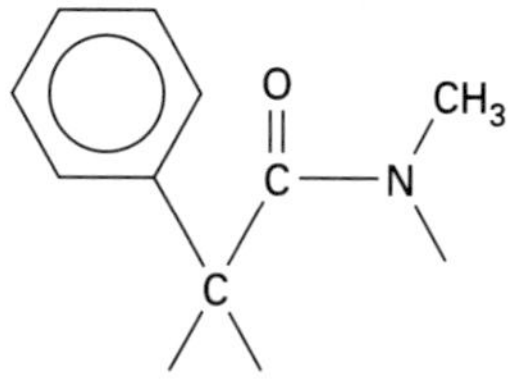

Fig. 6.12. A compound containing the group –CO–NH–
which forms part of a cyclic structure is called a lactam.
This diagram shows an aryl residue α to the carbonyl
carbon of an N-alkyl lactam.

oxidised by P450 enzymes. Jurima et al. (1985b)
therefore investigated which steroids inhibited
mephenytoin hydroxylation by human liver preparations in vitro. Cortisone and ethynyloestradiol
gave fairly strong inhibition. Cortisol, oestradiol,
adrenosterone and testosterone demonstrated weak
but distinct inhibition. It is conceivable that P450$_{meph}$
may be a steroid-metabolizing enzyme which happens to metabolize a man-made foreign compound.
This concept has considerable clinical implications.

An in vitro study involving various anticonvulsants was conducted by Hall et al. (1987).
Competitive inhibition of 4-hydroxylation of
mephenytoin was observed with ethotoin, mephobarbital, methsuximide and phensuximide but not
with other commonly used anticonvulsants such as
ethosuximide, phenobarbital, phenytoin and primidone (Fig. 6.11). However, synthetic N-alkyl analogues of the latter compounds were found to be
inhibitory. An aryl residue α to the carbonyl carbon
of an N-alkyl lactam in a 5- or 6-membered ring
(Fig. 6.12), therefore, appears to be a minimal

requirement for strong interaction with P450$_{meph}$.

Relling et al. (1989) demonstrated that teniposide
competitively inhibited the 4-hydroxylation of
S-mephenytoin and that etoposide and flavone
acetic acid were weak inhibitors of this reaction.

Nilutamide is a non-steroidal anti-androgen
derivative behaving as a competitive inhibitor of the
androgen receptor. This drug is used in the treatment of metastatic prostatic carcinoma. It was
shown by Horsmans et al. (1991) that nilutamide
at the concentrations expected during therapeutic
usage is a powerful inhibitor of the human liver
microsomal 4-hydroxylation of mephenytoin. The
inhibition was not specific because hydroxylations
mediated by cytochromes P450 which do not oxidize mephenytoin were also inhibited.

A summary of in vitro inhibition studies is shown
in Tables 6.4 and 6.5.

Table 6.4. *Drugs which have been shown to inhibit mephenytoin 4'-hydroxylation* in vitro

Cimetidine	Mephobarbital
Cortisone	Methsuximide
21-Deoxycortisone	Malamide
Diazepam	Nilutamide
Ethinyl oestradiol	Papavarine
Ethotoin (racemic)	Progesterone
Etoposide	Propanolol
Flavone acetic acid	Temazepam
Flurazepam	Teniposide
Hexobarbital	Tolbutamide
Ketoconazole	Tranylcypromine

From: Hall *et al.* 1987; Horsmans *et al.* 1991; Jurima *et al.* 1985b; Relling *et al.* 1989; Wilkinson *et al.* 1989.

Table 6.5. *Drugs which have been shown not to inhibit mephenytoin 4'-hydroxylation* in vitro

Iodochlorohydroxyquin
PEH
Phenytoin
Primidone

PEH, 5-phenyl-5-ethylhydantoin; Nirvanol.
From: Wilkinson *et al.* 1989.

STUDIES ON MOLECULAR STRUCTURE AND GENE LOCALIZATION

Shimada *et al.* (1986) and Umbenhauer *et al.* (1987) have both purified the cytochrome P450 responsible for mephenytoin 4'-hydroxylase activity.

The former authors purified two forms designated $P450_{MP-1}$ and $P450_{MP-2}$ from human liver microsomes. *In vitro* translation of liver RNA yielded polypeptides migrating on polyacrylamide gel electrophoresis with either $P450_{MP-1}$ or with $P450_{MP-2}$ activities depending upon which form was in each liver sample, indicating that the two cytochromes P450 are translated from different mRNAs. The molecular weights were 48 000 and 50 000 and they were capable of catalysing S-mephenytoin 4'-hydroxylation, S-nirvanol 4'-hydroxylation, S-mephenytoin N-demethylation and diphenylhydantoin 4'-hydroxylation. Some liver samples contained only $P450_{MP-1}$, others contained only $P450_{MP-2}$ and some contained a mixture. Unfortunately, the *in vitro* performance was not correlated with the *in vivo* phenotypes of the individual from whom the liver tissue was obtained.

Umbenhauer *et al.* (1987) isolated human cDNA clones related to cytochrome P450 S-mephenytoin 4'-hydroxylase using specific isolating antibodies. The predicted *N*-terminal sequence matched that determined for $P450_{MP-1}$ and $P450_{MP-2}$ at all unambiguous positions. The genomic DNA blot analysis and the existence of multiple mRNAs indicated that at least several genes were present. It is to be noted that the human library studied was obtained from a single human liver and so this work represented only one step towards elucidating the complex genetic polymorphism in human liver S-mephenytoin 4-hydroxylase activity.

Later, Meehan *et al.* (1988) utilized the fact that there is a measure of homology between human liver $P450_{MP-1}$ and $P450_{MP-2}$ on the one hand and rat liver P450 molecules in the PB-1 group on the other (P450 2C8, according to the nomenclature of Nebert *et al.* 1991). Radiolabelled cDNA probes prepared from a rat PB-1 clone were hybridized to rodent–human hybrid cells' chromosomal complements. It was found that the maximal signal occurred in the region 10q24.1 to 10q24.3 which may therefore be taken as the tentative localization of the gene controlling $P450_{MP}$ (*CYP 2C8* according to Nebert *et al.* 1991).

The complexity of the genes controlling mephenytoin oxidation in man was illustrated by the results of Brian *et al.* (1989). A probe was derived from a human liver cDNA library which was believed to encode a *CYP* related to S-mephenytoin 4'-hydroxylase. This clone was termed MP-8, and it was used to probe genomic DNA isolated from several human livers. Different patterns were obtained indicating at least seven related genes.

Studies of the amounts of specific mRNA isolated from human livers also indicate individual differences in the transcription of the relevant genes.

There is substantial evidence that tolbutamide and mephenytoin hydroxylations are largely independent. Relling *et al.* (1990) showed that there was no correlation between the two activities in a population of 38 human livers. However, both these workers and Veronese *et al.* (1991) showed that cytochrome P450 2C9 was able to hydroxylate both drugs and that this activity was inhibited by sulphaphenazole. On the other hand Srivastava *et al.* (1991) found that cytochromes P450 2C8, 2C9 and

2C10 all catalysed the oxidation of tolbutamide but not of mephenytoin, and that the two activities could be separated chromatographically. As a result of studying a number of clones from human livers Romkes et al. (1991) found a range of cytochromes P450. When these were expressed in Cos-1 cells their cytochrome P450 2C9 did not hydroxylate mephenytoin but another cytochrome P450, tentatively designated 2C18, was able to catalyse this activity. A cytochrome P450 called 'human-2' was described by Yasumori et al. (1991) which was able to hydroxylate S-mephenytoin five times faster than R-mephenytoin.

So it can be said at the time of writing that it is known that there are a number of cytochromes P450 in the 2C subfamily. The differences between many of them consist of one or two amino acids. Some of these cytochromes have the ability to hydroxylate S-mephenytoin, but the exact basis of the metabolic polymorphism of S-mephenytoin hydroxylation is not yet determined.

OTHER DRUGS METABOLIZED POLYMORPHICALLY BY THE MEPHENYTOIN POLYMORPHISM

It has already been mentioned that phenylethyl hydantoin (nirvanol) (PEH) is subject to the same polymorphic oxidation as mephenytoin (Kupfer & Preisig 1984).

Mephobarbital hydroxylation has been shown by Kupfer & Branch (1985) to co-segregate with mephenytoin hydroxylation. Also Jacqz et al. (1986) showed that the ingestion of mephobarbital prior to a dose of racemic mephenytoin resulted in increased peak levels of S-mephenytoin but not of R-mephenytoin (as compared with control observations made when racemic mephenytoin was ingested alone).

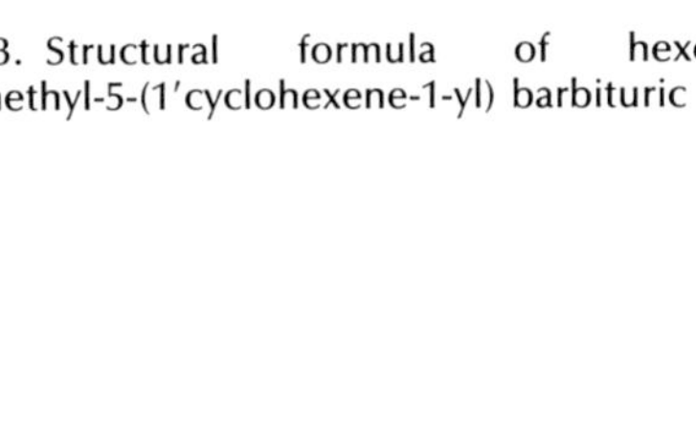

Fig. 6.13. Structural formula of hexobarbital [1,5-dimethyl-5-(1'cyclohexene-1-yl) barbituric acid].

Both in vitro and in vivo observations by Knodell et al. (1988) indicated that hexobarbital, which fulfils the specifications for molecular structure suggested by Hall et al. (1987) (and which is hydroxylated at the 3'-position in humans) (Fig. 6.13) was also metabolized by the polymorphic cytochrome $P450_{meph}$ responsible for the aromatic hydroxylation of S-mephenytoin.

An observation was made by Fritz et al. (1987) concerning the chiral metabolites of phenytoin, namely, the S- and R-enantiomers of 5-(4-hydroxyphenyl)-5-phenyl-hydantoin (HPPH). The S-enantiomer of HPPH was the major urinary phenytoin metabolite irrespective of the hydroxylation phenotype. However, R-HPPH was significantly decreased in poor metabolizers of mephenytoin leading to a bimodal distribution of HPPH S/R ratio which was closely correlated with the mephenytoin hydroxylation index. Since only a small fraction of the phenytoin consumed is metabolized to R-HPPH in either phenotype this polymorphic step is unlikely to be of clinical significance.

A somewhat clinically more interesting finding was that of Ward et al. (1989a) who looked at the metabolism of propanolol (which is racemic and has long been known to exhibit great inter-subject variability) in relation to both the debrisoquine and the mephenytoin hydroxylation polymorphisms. They found that the partial metabolic clearance to naphthoxylactic acid (NLA) was 55% less in the PM_M group than in the EM and PM_D groups indicating that the enzyme S-mephenytoin 4-hydroxylase contributes to the metabolic conversion of propanolol to NLA (Table 6.6). An individual who was a double recessive, i.e. $PM_D PM_M$ was the only one observed to have a reduced total propanolol clearance and prolonged elimination half-life.

Other correlations are shown in Table 6.7. With regard to diazepam and desmethyl diazepam Zhang et al. (1990) demonstrated that there was a significant difference between Chinese and Caucasian subjects. The metabolism of diazepam was slow in both extensive and poor metabolizers of mephenytoin amongst the Chinese so that they both resembled Caucasian poor metabolizers. This may be due to the possession of an S-mephenytoin hydroxylase with different specificities in the two races (Zhang et al. 1990). Strangely, the metabolism of both diazepam and desmethyldiazepam (the major metabolite) correlated exactly (and polymorphically) with that of

Table 6.6. *Partial metabolic clearance of individual routes of each enantiomer of propanolol in a panel of normal subjects of known debrisoquine and mephenytoin phenotypes*

Route of metabolism (ml/min)	Enantiomer	EM	PM_D	PM_M	$PM_{D/M}$
PG	R	259 ± 75	264 ± 140	207 ± 153	293
	S	292 ± 104	254 ± 107	240 ± 162	278
NLA	R	379 ± 190	408 ± 224	$174 \pm 99^*$	183
	S	393 ± 199	278 ± 227	$181 \pm 79^*$	181
Total 4-OH-P	R	1155 ± 566	$309 \pm 269^*$	1157 ± 904	117
	S	483 ± 283	$119 \pm 84^*$	477 ± 356	67
4-OH-P sulphate	R	854 ± 392	$233 \pm 200^*$	935 ± 751	91
	S	165 ± 100	$40 \pm 25^*$	196 ± 151	41
4-OH-P glucuronide	R	302 ± 200	$77 \pm 63^*$	203 ± 127	27
	S	318 ± 192	$87 \pm 73^*$	281 ± 207	27

P, propanolol; PG, propanolol glucuronide; NLA, naphthoxylactic acid; EM, extensive metabolizer of debrisoquine and mephenytoin; PM_D, poor metabolizer of debrisoquine; PM_M, poor metabolizer of mephenytoin; $PM_{D/M}$, poor metabolizer of both compounds; $^*p < 0.05$ in comparison with EM group for the same route of metabolism.
From: Ward *et al.* 1989a.

Table 6.7. *Drugs whose metabolism has been shown to be controlled by the mephenytoin-hydroxylation polymorphism by means of* in vivo *observations*

Drug	Reference
Nirvanol	Kupfer & Preisig 1984
Mephobarbital	Kupfer & Branch 1985; Jacqz *et al.* 1986
Hexobarbital	Knodell *et al.* 1988
HPPH → R-HPPH	Fritz *et al.* 1987
Propanolol → NLA	Ward *et al.* 1989a
Methylphenytoin	Schellens *et al.* 1990
Omeprazole	Andersson *et al.* 1990
Diazepam	Bertilsson *et al.* 1989; Sohn *et al.* 1992
Desmethyl diazepam	Bertilsson *et al.* 1989; Sohn *et al.* 1992
Imipramine (demethylation)	Skjelbo *et al.* 1991
Warfarin	
Proguanil → cycloguanil	Ward *et al.* 1989b

R-HPPH – Only the production of this R-enantiomer of para hydroxy diphenyl hydantoin is influenced by the polymorphism.
NLA, naphthoxylactic acid.

mephenytoin in Koreans (Sohn *et al.* 1992). This raises the possibility that there may be genetic heterogeneity in drug metabolizing enzymes between Oriental populations.

The polymorphic hydroxylation of omeprazole correlated closely that of mephenytoin in Caucasians and Chinese (Andersson *et al.* 1992). A consequence of this was demonstrated by Rost *et al.* (1992) in that a study using the ^{13}C-[*N*-3-methyl]-caffeine breath test suggested that omeprazole induced cytochrome P450 1A2 in poor metabolizers

of S-mephenytoin. The polymorphic hydroxylation of omeprazole, however, was almost exactly similar to mephenytoin in both phenotypes in both races (Andersson *et al.* 1992).

The spread of chloroquine resistant malaria has led to a great deal of interest in other antimalarial compounds both new and old. These alternative drugs have included the biguanide drug proguanil (Fig. 6.14) which has been available for nearly 50 years. It is known to require metabolism to the dihydrotriazine metabolite cycloguanil (Fig. 6.14) in

Proguanil (paludrine)
(*N'*-*p*-chlorphenyl-
N^5-isopropyldiguanide)

Cycloguanil
(4,6-diamino-1-p-chlorphenyl-
1,2-dihydro-2,2-dimethyl-1,3,5-triazine)

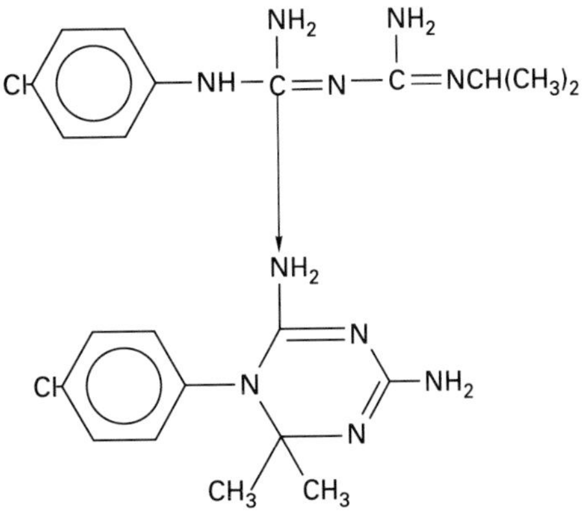

Fig. 6.14. The metabolism of proguanil.

order to become active. Cycloguanil (CG) is a powerful inhibitor of difolate reductase which is an enzyme vital to the parasite and has activity against the erythrocytic forms of *Plasmodium falciparum*.

When sensitive and specific analytical methods – particularly high performance liquid chromatographic (HPLC) methods – became available it was possible to study cycloguanil concentrations in blood and urine. Interest in this topic was generated by the fact that prophylactic failures had been observed even in patients receiving carefully monitored daily dosages. There followed a series of studies in which the variability in the biotransformation of proguanil (PG) became apparent.

Sixty-five healthy black Kenyan adult volunteers took 200 mg proguanil orally and their urine 6 hours afterwards revealed a frequency distribution of the PG/CG ratio which contained a main mode and was highly skewed to the right (Watkins *et al.* 1990). The results of tests performed on two occasions on 30 individuals were highly correlated. Concentration/time profiles for CG were very much lower in poor metabolizers (urinary PG/CG ratio <10) than in extensive metabolizers.

A similar study was carried out in Kenya on 108 British soldiers and the results showed a similar pattern. The urinary PG/CG ratio showed 10% of the population to be poor metabolizers. Twenty-seven Gurkhas formed a discrete mode in the lower half

of the main mode of extensive metabolizers (Ward *et al.* 1989b).

The 0 to 8 hour urinary PG/CG ratio following the ingestion of 200 mg proguanil showed a clear separation between three poor metabolizers and 134 extensive metabolizers from the Liverpool population. The former had much lower peak CG concentrations (Helsby *et al.* 1990a).

An experiment to find out the metabolic basis for this polymorphism (Helsby 1990b) involved the use of microsomal preparations from three human livers, which could effect the biotransformation of PG to CG. It was found that this oxidation could be competitively inhibited by mephenytoin but not by either sparteine or tolbutamide. This finding suggested that the same cytochrome P450 might be responsible for the oxidation of both PG and S-mephenytoin.

This idea was put to the test using the 'typed panel' approach by Ward *et al.* (1991). Eighteen Danish subjects had been previously characterized as mephenytoin poor (PM_m) or extensive metabolizers (EM_m) and sparteine poor (PM_s) or extensive metabolizers (EM_s). Five subjects had the phenotype PM_m EM_s, one was PM_m PM_s, six were EM_m PM_s and six were EM_m EM_s. It was found the PM_m individuals had significantly higher PG/CG ratios than EM_m individuals. There was no significant difference between PM_s and EM_s subjects. These findings provided strong evidence that proguanil and mephenytoin oxidations are controlled by the same genes in the *CYP 2C* subfamily.

The co-segregation of urinary proguanil/cycloguanil metabolic ratio and the mephenytoin hydroxylation index was independently corroborated in 21 extensive and three poor metabolizers of mephenytoin by Funck-Brentano *et al.* (1992).

The practical therapeutic implications of this polymorphism of proguanil metabolism are: (1) poor metabolizers are deprived of protection when given proguanil prophylactically, (2) resistant strains of plasmodia may develop because of low-level exposure to cycloguanil in poor metabolizers, (3) it is possible that the intrahepatocyte phase of plasmodial development may also be subject to lack of control in poor metabolizers.

DRUGS WHICH ARE NOT INFLUENCED BY THE MEPHENYTOIN POLYMORPHISM

The results obtained with reconstituted preparations and antibody inhibitions enabled Shimada *et al.* (1986) to conclude that P450$_{MP}$ is the major P450 involved in the 4'-hydroxylation and *N*-demethylation of S-mephenytoin, the 4'-hydroxylation of S-nirvanol and the 4'-hydroxylation of diphenylhydantoin.

The immunochemical inhibition studies suggest that P450$_{MP}$ does not contribute extensively to:
total *N*-methyldiphenylhydantoin 4'-hydroxylation and *N*-demethylation
R-mephenytoin 4'-hydroxylation and *N*-demethylation
R-nirvanol 4-hydroxylation
p-nitroanisole *O*-demethylation
D-benzphetamine *N*-demethylation
benzo[a]pyrene hydroxylation
diazepam *N*-demethylation
phenacetin *O*-deethylation
nifedipine oxidation
± bufuralol 1'-hydroxylation

The last three results are particularly interesting because these three compounds are thought to be metabolized by cytochromes P450 belonging to other subfamilies. Antibodies raised to P450$_{MP}$ did not react with isolated purified cytochromes P450 specific for these three compounds, and antibodies raised against the other cytochromes P450 did not react with P450$_{MP}$.

Other compounds unlikely to be candidates for P450$_{MP}$ mediated metabolism are mentioned under

'Chemical Inhibition Studies' above.

Glibenclamide pharmacokinetics were not significantly different in the two mephenytoin phenotypes (Dahl-Puustinen *et al.* 1990). *In vitro* studies indicated that the hydroxylations of tienilic acid and mephenytoin were carried out by different members of the cytochrome P450 2C subfamily (Dansette *et al.* 1991). *In vivo* studies indicated that PMs of MP appear to hydroxylate tolbutamide at normal rates (Knodell *et al.* 1987).

In vitro studies, however, reveal a complex, and at present rather confused picture; some cytochromes P450 appear to metabolize both tolbutamide and mephenytoin but it seems that the major enzyme responsible for mephenytoin hydroxylation does not have activity for tolbutamide (see the subsection on molecular genetics).

The results of inhibition studies conducted *in vivo* are shown in Table 6.8.

Table 6.8. *The results of inhibition studies in vivo*

Inhibition produced	No inhibition produced
Ethotoin	Ethosuximide
Mephobarbital	Phenytoin
Methsuximide	D-Propoxyphene

From: Sanz J, Bertilsson 1990; Wilkinson *et al.* 1989.

INDUCTION

Rifampicin was shown to induce S-mephenytoin hydroxylation *in vivo* in extensive metabolizers only (Zhou *et al.* 1990). Pentobarbital is also an inducer. The hydroxylase activity is reduced by ketoconazole and liver disease (Wilkinson *et al.* 1989).

PHENOTYPING PROCEDURES

The phenotyping procedures of Kupfer & Preisig (1984) and Wedlund *et al.* (1985) have been described earlier. The latter method is now the most popular and gives excellent separation of phenotypes (see Drøhse *et al.* 1989; Spina *et al.* 1989; Sanz *et al.* 1989; Doshi *et al.* 1990; Guttendorf *et al.* 1990). It has become popular to test simultaneously for both the debrisoquine/sparteine polymorphism and the mephenytoin polymorphism. The co-administration of the following compounds was demonstrated not to interfere with mephenytoin phenotyping: sparteine (Drøhse *et al.* 1989), metoprolol (Horai *et al.* 1989), debrisoquine (Sanz *et al.* 1989), dextromethorphan (Guttendorf *et al.* 1990). The mephenytoin phenotype was not disturbed when subjects were taking diazepam (Spina *et al.* 1989).

Bertilsson *et al.* (1992) point out that a wider separation of S/R urinary ratios was found in the 8–24 or 24–38 hour urines than in the 0–8 hour urine collection after a 100 mg dose of racemic mephenytoin. Their Fig. 4 is reminiscent of Fig. 2 of Evans *et al.* (1965), which shows the results of an isoniazid phenotyping test on a population, where the separation of phenotypes is much greater at 6 hours than at 2 hours. The reason is the same in both cases, namely that allowing more time allows the more powerful enzyme to show itself to greater advantage.

Significant adverse effects were observed by Setiabudy *et al.* (1992) in two out of 10 Indonesians given the standard 100 mg racemic mephenytoin phenotyping dose. These consisted of dizziness, drowsiness, intellectual impairment and inability to stand up. The two affected individuals were poor metabolizers. Seven extensive and one poor metabolizers were unaffected. These authors advocate the use of a 50 mg phenotyping dose in Orientals. Sleepiness was found to occur significantly more frequently in poor metabolizers during phenotyping by Sohn *et al* (1992): see below. Urinary enantiomeric S/R ratios (used as a phenotyping test) were not related to age or creatinine clearance in the study of Pollock *et al.* (1991).

In contrast to its effect on cytochrome P450 2D6 phenotyping with dextromethorphan, thioridazine had no effect on mephenytoin phenotyping. Amitriptyline was also shown not to influence the phenotying test (Baumann *et al.* 1992).

DIRECT CLINICAL EFFECTS

According to Di Palma (1965), 'the hydantoin structure was introduced into therapy in 1916 in the form of phenylethyl hydantoin (nirvanol) a sedative drug. After a brief trial this drug was withdrawn because it caused blood dyscrasias. It is probable that had it enjoyed a longer clinical life its value in epilepsy would have been empirically discovered.'

Serious toxicity to mephenytoin is common and includes 'morbilliform rash (in 10% of patients),

fever, lymphadenopathy, pancytopenia, agranulocytosis, hepatotoxicity, periarteritis nodosa and lupus erythematosus. Death attributed to aplastic anaemia has occurred. Acute overdosage results in coma' (Woodbury & Fingl 1975).

It is to be noted that S-mephenytoin, R-mephenytoin, S-PEH and R-PEH (nirvanol) are all active compounds in that they have an effect on the central nervous system. As has been seen the total of their plasma concentrations is much higher especially after repeated dosages in the poor metabolizer as compared with the extensive metabolizer. Kupfer *et al.* (1984b) noted mild sedation in poor a metabolizer experimental volunteer after only 5 days dosing with 1.4 mmol racemic mephenytoin daily (M_r mephenytoin = 218). These symptoms did not occur in extensive metabolizers.

Similarly, Sohn *et al.* (1992), whilst testing Korean subjects with a single dose of 100 mg racemic mephenytoin, noticed sleepiness in eight out of 26 poor metabolizers but only in five out of 180 extensive metabolizers ($p > 0.001$).

Whilst deficient epoxide hydrolase may be involved in the production of the marrow toxicity, lymphadenopathy, hepatotoxicity, etc. (Spielberg 1986), it is also possible that poor metabolizers of mephenytoin may be more prone than extensive metabolizers to adverse effects, especially those involving an action on the central nervous system.

ASSOCIATION OF PHENOTYPES WITH SPONTANEOUS DISORDERS

An investigation of multiple factors associated with bladder cancer was carried out by Kaisary *et al.* (1987). Different results were obtained when aggressive (Stage III) and non-aggressive (Stages I and II) neoplasms were considered. Normit plots of the distribution of the R/S mephenytoin ratio showed that patients with non-aggressive tumours were slightly more likely to be faster metabolizers than were the controls. Logistic regression analysis confirmed a weak but significant association ($p = 0.04$). In contrast, after controlling for sex, age, smoking habit, alcohol intake, acetylator phenotype and debrisoquine recovery ratio there was no difference in the cumulative frequency distribution of the mephenytoin phenotype (R/S ratio) between the patients with aggressive tumours and normal subjects and this parameter was not associated with increased relative risk.

The idea that Parkinson's disease might be due to a chemical agent in the environment, and that this agent might be detoxified well by most people, leaving a few people vulnerable has been referred to elsewhere in this book. An investigation into both the sparteine/debrisoquine and the mephenytoin polymorphisms in Parkinsonism was carried out by Gudjonsson *et al.* (1990) who phenotyped 34 patients. Of these patients 2.94% were poor hydroxylators of debrisoquine and 3.28% were poor hydroxylators of mephenytoin. This study lends no support to the basic idea but is of course open to a type II error of interpretation (i.e. erroneously believing the null hypothesis to be true: Wulf 1981).

A more exciting study was that of May *et al.* (1990) who, based on a similar philosophy, examined the mephenytoin polymorphism in 84 patients with scleroderma. They also tested for dapsone acetylation, dapsone hydroxylation and debrisoquine hydroxylation. The phenotype frequencies for acetylation and debrisoquine oxidation did not differ between patients and controls. When the results for dapsone hydroxylation and mephenytoin hydroxylation were combined the relative risk of developing the disease was as follows:

$$EM_{dap} \, EM_{meph} = 1$$
$$PM_{dap} \, EM_{meph} = 2.5$$
$$PM_{dap} \, PM_{meph} = 10$$

The nine individuals in the last group were mainly women who developed the disorder at a relatively young age. So this study constitutes a *prima facie* case for scleroderma possibly being a disorder due to poor oxidation of some environmental chemical.

The relationship of the S-mephenytoin hydroxylation polymorphism to food preferences was investigated by Britto *et al.* (1991). A population of 178 drug-free non-smoking males (almost all white) were asked to rate their preferences for 150 foodstuffs. The 18 poor metabolizers of mephenytoin showed a diminished stated preference for spinach and cabbage.

SIMILAR POLYMORPHISM IN NON-HUMAN PRIMATE

Investigations into the mephenytoin polymorphism may be very substantially helped by the discovery of Jacqz *et al.* (1988b) who determined the mephenytoin metabolic index in 64 adult 'crab-eater' monkeys. Two of the animals gave very convincing results indicating that they were poor metabolizers widely separated from the 62 extensive metabolizers.

The author would like to express his gratitude to Dr Dominick A. Minotti, Pacific Health Associates, Seattle, USA and Dr Immaneni Viswanath, Barking Hospital, Barking, Essex, UK who made many helpful suggestions about the contents of this chapter.

Andersson, T, Regårdh, C. G., Dahl-Puustinen, M. L. & Bertilsson, L. (1990). Slow omeprazole metabolizers are also poor S-mephenytoin hydroxylators. *Therapeutic Drug Monitoring*, **12**, 415–6.

Andersson, T., Regårdh, C. G., Lou, Y. C., Zhang, Y., Dahl, M. L. & Bertilsson, L. (1992). Polymorphic hydroxylation of S-mephenytoin and omeprazole metabolism in Caucasian and Chinese subjects. *Pharmacogenetics*, **2**, 25–31.

Baumann, P., Meyer, J. W., Amey, M. Baettig, D., Bryois, C., Jonzier-Perey, M., Koeb, L., Mommey, C. & Woggon, B. (1992). Dextromethorphan and mephenytoin phenotyping of patients treated with thioridazine or amitriptyline. *Therapeutic Drug Monitoring*, **14**, 1–8.

Bertilsson, L., Henthorn, T. K., Sanz, E., Tybring, G., Säwe, J. & Villeen, T. (1989). Importance of genetic factors in the regulation of diazepam metabolism, relationship to S-mephenytoin but not to debrisoquine, hydroxylation phenotype. *Clinical Pharmacology and Therapeutics*, **45**, 348–55.

Bertilsson, L., Lou, Y. Q., Du, Y. L., Liu, Y., Kuang, T. Y., Liao, X. M., Wang, K. Y., Reviriego, J, Iselius, L. & Sjöqvist, F. (1992). Pronounced differences between native Chinese and Swedish populations in the polymorphic hydroxylations of debrisoquine and S-mephenytoin. *Clinical Pharmacology and Therapeutics*, **51**, 388–97.

Breimer, D. D, Schellens, J. H. M. & Soons, P. A. (1988). Assessment of *in vivo* oxidative drug metabolizing enzyme activity in man by applying a cocktail approach. In *Proceedings of the VIIth International Symposium on microsomes and drug oxidations (Adelaide 17 to 21 August 1987)*, ed. J. Miners, D. J. Birkett, R. Drew & M. McManus, pp. 232–40. London, Taylor and Francis. Cited by Alvan, G., Bechtel, P., Iselius, L. & Gundert-Remy, U. (1990). Hydroxylation polymorphisms of debrisoquine and mephenytoin in European populations. *European Journal of Clinical Pharmacology*, **39**, 533–7.

Brian, W. R., Ged, C., Bellew, T. M., Srivastava, P. K., Bork, R. W., Umbenhauer, D. R., Lloyd, R. S. & Guengerich, F. P. (1989). Human liver mephenytoin 4'hydroxylase cytochrome P-450 proteins and genes. *Drug Metabolism Reviews*, **20**, 449–65.

Britto, M. R, McKean, H. E., Bruckner, G. G. & Wedlund, P. J. (1991). Polymorphisms in oxidative drug metabolism, relationship to food preference. *British Journal of Clinical Pharmacology*, **32**, 235–7.

Clasen, K., Madsen, L., Brøsen, K., Alboge, K., Misfelt, S. & Gram, L. F. (1991). Sparteine and mephenytoin oxidation – genetic polymorphisms in east and west Greenland. *Clinical Pharmacology and Therapeutics*, **49**, 624–31.

Dahl-Puustinen, M. L., Alm, C., Bertilsson, L., Christenson, I., Östman, J., Thunberg, E. & Wikström, I. (1990). Lack of relationship between glibenclamide metabolism and debrisoquine or mephenytoin hydroxylation phenotypes. *British Journal of Clinical Pharmacology*, **30**, 476–80.

Dansette, P. M., Amar, C., Valadon, P., Pons, C. . Beaune, P. H. & Mansuy, D. (1991). Hydroxylation and formation of electrophilic metabolites of tienilic acid and its isomer by human liver microsomes. Catalysis by a cytochrome P450 II C different from that responsible for mephenytoin hydroxylation. *Biochemical Pharmacology*, **41**, 553–60.

DiPalma, J. R. (1965) Drugs in epilepsy and hyperkinetic states. In *Drill's Pharmacology in Medicine*, 3rd edition, ed. J. R. Di Palma, p. 235. New York: McGraw-Hill.

Doshi, B. S., Kulkarni, R. D., Chauhan, B. L. & Wilkinson, G. R. (1990). Frequency of impaired mephenytoin 4'hydroxylation in an Indian population. *British Journal of Clinical Pharmacology*, **30**, 779–80.

Drøhse, A., Bathum, L., Brøsen, K. & Gram, L. F. (1989). Mephenytoin and sparteine oxidation, genetic polymorphisms in Denmark. *British Journal of Clinical Pharmacology*, **27**, 620–5.

Evans, D. A. P., Davison, K. & Pratt, R. T. C. (1965). The influence of acetylator phenotype on the side effects of treating depression with phenelzine. *Clinical Pharmacology and Therapeutics*, **6**, 430–5.

Fritz, S., Lindner, W., Roots, I., Frey, B. M. & Kupfer, A. (1987). Stereochemistry of aromatic phenytoin hydroxylation in various drug hydroxylation phenotypes in humans. *Journal of Pharmacology and Experimental Therapeutics*, **241**, 615–22.

Funck-Brentano, C., Bosco, O., Jacqz-Agrain, E., Keundijian, A. & Jaillon, P. (1992). Relation between chloroguanide bioactivation to cycloguanil and the genetically determined metabolism of mephenytoin in humans. *Clinical Pharmacology and Therapeutics*, **51**, 507–12.

Gudjonsson, O., Sanz, E., Alvan, G., Aquilonius, S. M. & Reviriego, J. (1990). Poor hydroxylator phenotypes of debrisoquine and S-mephenytoin are not over-represented in a group of patients with Parkinson's disease. *British Journal of Clinical Pharmacology*, **30**, 301–2.

Gut, J., Meier, U. T., Catin, T. & Meyer, U. A. (1986). Mephenytoin-type polymorphism of drug oxidation; purification and characterisation of a human liver cytochrome P-450 isozyme catalysing microsomal mephenytoin hydroxylation. *Biochimica et Biophysica Acta*, **884**, 435–47.

Guttendorf, R. J., Britto, M., Blouin, R. A., Foster, T. S., John, W., Pittman, K. A. & Wedlund, P. J. (1990). Rapid screening for polymorphisms in dextromethorphan and mephenytoin metabolism. *British Journal of Clinical Pharmacology*, **29**, 373–80.

Hall, S. D., Guengerich, F. P., Branch, R. A. & Wilkinson, G. R. (1987). Characterisation and inhibition of mephenytoin 4-hydroxylase activity in human liver microsomes. *Journal of Pharmacology and Experimental Therapeutics*, **240**, 216–22.

Helsby, N. A., Ward, S. A., Edwards, G., Howells, R. E. & Breckenridge, A. M. (1990a). The pharmacokinetics and activation of proguanil in man, consequences of variability in drug metabolism. *British Journal of Clinical Pharmacology*, **30**, 593–8.

Helsby, N. A., Ward, S. A., Howells, R. E. & Breckenridge, A. M. (1990b). *In vitro* metabolism of the biguanide

antimalarials in human liver microsomes, evidence for a role of the mephenytoin hydroxylase (P450 MP) enzyme. *British Journal of Clinical Pharmacology*, **30**, 287–91.

Horai, Y., Nakano, M., Ishizaki, T., Ishikawa, K., Zhou, H. H., Zhou, B. J., Liao, C. L. & Zhang, L. M. (1989). Metoprolol and mephenytoin oxidation polymorphisms in Far East Oriental subjects, Japanese versus mainland Chinese. *Clinical Pharmacology and Therapeutics*, **46**, 198–207.

Horsmans, Y., Lannes, D., Larrey, D., Tinel, M., Letteron, P., Loeper, J. & Pessayre, D. (1991). Nilutamide inhibits mephenytoin 4-hydroxylation in untreated male rats and in human liver microsomes. *Xenobiotica*, **12**, 1559–70.

Inaba, T., Jorge, L. F. & Arias, T. D. (1988). Mephenytoin hydroxylation in the Cuna Amerindians of Panama. *British Journal of Clinical Pharmacology*, **25**, 75–9.

Inaba, T., Jurima, M. & Kalow, W. (1986). Family studies of mephenytoin hydroxylation deficiency. *American Journal of Human Genetics*, **38**, 768–72.

Inaba, T., Jurima, M., Nakano, M. & Kalow, W. (1984). Mephenytoin and sparteine pharmacogenetics in Canadian Caucasians. *Clinical Pharmacology and Therapeutics*, **36**, 670–6.

Jacqz, E., Billante, C., Moysan, F. & Mathieu, H. (1988b). The non-human primate; a possible model for human genetically determined polymorphisms in oxidative drug metabolism. *Molecular Pharmacology*, **34**, 215–7.

Jacqz, E., Dulac, H. & Mathieu, H. (1988a). Phenotyping polymorphic drug metabolism in the French Caucasian population. *European Journal of Clinical Pharmacology*, **35**, 167–71.

Jacqz, E,, Hall, S. D., Branch, R. A. & Wilkinson, G. R. (1986). Polymorphic metabolism of mephenytoin in man, Pharmacokinetic interaction with a co-regulated substrate, mephobarbital. *Clinical Pharmacology and Therapeutics*, **39**, 646–53.

Jurima, M., Inaba, T., Kadar, D. & Kalow, W. (1985a). Genetic polymorphism of mephenytoin p(4')-hydroxylation, difference between Orientals and Caucasians. *British Journal of Clinical Pharmacology*, **19**, 483–7.

Jurima, M., Inaba, T. & Kalow, W. (1984). Sparteine oxidation by human liver; absence of inhibition by mephenytoin. *Clinical Pharmacology and Therapeutics*, **35**, 426–8.

Jurima, M., Inaba, T. & Kalow, W. (1985b). Mephenytoin hydroxylase activity in human liver; inhibition by steroids. *Drug Metabolism and Disposition*, **13**, 746–9.

Kaisary, A., Smith, P., Jacqz, E., McAllister, C. B., Wilkinson, G. R., Ray, W. A. & Branch, R. A. (1987). Genetic predisposition to bladder cancer; ability to hydroxylate debrisoquine and mephenytoin as risk factors. *Cancer Research*, **47**, 5488–93.

Knodell, R. G., Dubey, R. K., Wilkinson, G. R. & Guengerich, F. P. (1988). Oxidative metabolism of hexobarbital in human liver; Relationship to polymorphic S-mephenytoin 4-hydroxylation. *Journal of Pharmacology and Experimental Therapeutics*, **245**, 845–9.

Knodell, R. G., Hall, S. D., Wilkinson, G. R. & Guengerich, F. P. (1987). Hepatic metabolism of tolbutamide, characterization of the form of P-450 involved in methyl hydroxylation and relationship to *in vivo* disposition. *Journal of Pharmacology and Experimental Therapeutics*, **241**, 1112–19.

Kupfer, A. & Branch, R. A. (1985). Stereoselective mephobarbital hydroxylation cosegretes with mephenytoin hydroxylation. *Clinical Pharmacology and Therapeutics*, **38**, 414–18.

Kupfer, A., Desmond, P., Patwardhan, R., Schenker, S. & Branch, R. A. (1984b). Mephenytoin hydroxylation deficiency, kinetics after repeated doses. *Clinical Pharmacology and Therapeutics*, **35**, 33–9.

Kupfer, A., Desmond, P., Schenker, S. & Branch, R. (1979). Family study of a genetically determined deficiency of mephenytoin hydroxylation in man. *Pharmacologist*, **21**, 173.

Kupfer, A., Lawson, J. & Branch, R. A. (1984a). Stereoselectivity of the arene epoxide pathway of mephenytoin hydroxlation in man. *Epilepsia*, **25**, 1–7.

Kupfer, A. & Preisig, R. (1984). Pharmacogenetics of Mephenytoin, A new drug hydroxylation polymorphism in man. *European Journal of Clinical Pharmacology*, **26**, 753–9.

May, D. G., Black, C. M., Olsen, N. J., Csuka, M. E., Tanner, S. B., Bellino, L., Porter, J. A., Wilkinson, G. R. & Branch, R. A. (1990). Scleroderma is associated with differences in individual routes of drug metabolism, A study with dapsone, debrisoquine, and mephenytoin. *Clinical Pharmacology and Therapeutics*, **48**, 286–95.

Meehan, R. R., Gosden, J. R., Rout, D., Hastie, N. D., Friedberg, T., Adesnik, M., Buckland, R., Van Heyningen, V., Fletcher, J., Spurr, N. K., Sweeney, J. & Wolf, C. R. (1988). Human cytochrome P-450 PB-1; A multigene family involved in mephenytoin and steroid oxidations that maps to chromosome 10. *American Journal of Human Genetics*, **42**, 26–37.

Meier, U. T., Dayer, P., Mule, P. J., Kronback, T. & Meyer, U. A. (1985). Mephenytoin hydroxylation polymorphism; characterisation of the enzymatic deficiency in liver microsomes of poor metabolizers phenotyped in vivo. *Clinical Pharmacology and Therapeutics*, **38**, 488–94.

Meier, U. T. & Meyer, U. A. (1987). Genetic polymorphism of human cytochrome P-450 (S)-mephenytoin 4-hydroxylase. Studies with human autoantibodies suggest a functionally altered cytochrome P-450 isozyme as cause of the genetic deficiency. *Biochemistry*, **26**, 8466–74.

Nakamura, K., Goto, F., Ray, W. A., McAllister, C. B., Jacqz, E., Wilkinson, G. R. & Branch, R. A. (1985). Interethnic differences in genetic polymorphism of debrisoquine and mephenytoin hydroxylation between Japanese and Caucasian populations. *Clinical Pharmacology and Therapeutics*, **38**, 402–8.

Nebert, D. W., Nelson, D. R., Coon, M. J., Estabrook, R. W., Feyereisen, R., Fujii-Kuriyama, Y., Gonzalez, F. J., Guengerich, F. P., Gunsalus, I. C., Johnson, E. F., Loper, J. C., Sato, R., Waterman, M. R. & Waxman, D. J. (1991). The P450 superfamily, update on new sequences, gene mapping and recommended nomenclature. *DNA and Cell Biology*, **10**, 1–14.

Pollock, B. G., Perel, J. M., Kirshner, M., Altieri, L. P., Yeager, A. L. & Reynolds, C. F., III. (1991). S-mephenytoin 4-hydroxylation in older Americans. *European Journal of Clinical Pharmacology*, **40**, 609–11.

Relling, M. V., Aoyama, T., Gonzalez, F. J. & Meyer, U. A. (1990). Tolbutamide and mephenytoin hydroxylation by human cytochrome P450s in the *CYP2C* subfamily. *Journal of Pharmacology and Experimental Therapeutics*, **252**, 442–7.

Relling, M. V., Evans, W. E, Fonne-Pfister, R. & Meyer, U. A. (1989). Anticancer drugs as inhibitors of two polymorphic cytochrome P-450 enzymes, debrisoquine and mephenytoin hydroxylase in human liver microsomes. *Cancer Research*, **49**, 68–71.

Romkes, M., Faletto, M. B., Blaidell, J. A., Raucy, J. L. & Goldstein, J. A. (1991). Cloning and expression of complementary DNAs for multiple members of the human P450 IIC subfamily. *Biochemistry*, **30**, 3247–55.

Rona, K. & Szabo, I. (1992). Determination of mephenytoin stereoselective oxidative metabolism in urine by chiral liquid chromatography employing β-cyclodextrin as a mobile phase additive. *Journal of Chromatography*, **573**, 173–7.

Rost, K. L. Brösicke, H., Brockmöller, J., Scheffler, M., Helge, H. & Roots, I. (1992). Increase of cytochrome P-450 1A2 activity by omeprazole: evidence by the ^{13}C[*N*-3-methyl]-caffeine breath test in poor and extensive metabolizers of S-mephenytoin. *Clinical Pharmacology and Therapeutics*, **52**, 170–80.

Sanz, J. & Bertilsson, L. . (1990). d-Propoxyphene is a potent inhibitor of debrisoquine but not S-mephenytoin 4-hydroxylation *in vivo*. *Therapeutic Drug Monitoring*, **12**, 297–9.

Sanz, E. J., Villen, T., Alm, C. & Bertilsson, L. (1989). S-mephenytoin hydroxylation phenotypes in a Swedish population determined after co-administration with debrisoquine. *Clinical Pharmacology and Therapeutics*, **45**, 495–9.

Schellens, J. H. M., Van der Wart, J. H. F. & Breimer, D. D. (1990). Relationship between mephenytoin oxidation polymorphism and phenytoin, methylphenytoin and phenobarbitone hydroxylation assessed in a phenotyped panel of healthy subjects. *British Journal of Clinical Pharmacology*, **29**, 665–71.

Setiabudy, R., Chiba, K., Kusaka, M. & Ishizaki, T. (1992). Caution in the use of a 100 mg dose of racemic mephenytoin for phenotyping South Eastern Oriental subjects *British Journal of Clinical Pharmacology*, **33**, 665–6.

Shimada, T., Misono, K. S. & Guengerich, F. P. (1986). Human liver microsomal cytochrome P-450 mephenytoin 4-hydroxylase, a prototype of genetic polymorphism in oxidative drug metabolism. *Journal of Biological Chemistry*, **261**, 909–21.

Skjelbo, E., Brøsen, K., Hallas, J. & Gram, L. F. (1991). The mephenytoin oxidation polymorphism is partially responsible for the N-demethylation of imipramine. *Clinical Pharmacology and Therapeutics*, **49**, 18–23.

Sohn, D. R., Kusaka, M., Ishizaki, T., Shin, S. G., Jang, I. J., Shin, J. G. & Chiba, K. (1992). Incidence of S-mephenytoin hydroxylation deficiency in a Korean population and the interphenotypic differences in diazepam pharmacokinetics. *Clinical Pharmacology and Therapeutics*, **52**, 160–9.

Spielberg, S. P. (1986). *In vitro* analysis of idiosyncratic drug reactions. *Clinical Biochemistry*, **19**, 142–4.

Spina, E, Buemi, A. L., Sanz, E. & Bertilsson, L. (1989). Diazepam treatment does not influence the debrisoquine or mephenytoin hydroxylation phenotyping tests. *Therapeutic Drug Monitoring*, **11**, 721–3.

Srivastava, P. K., Yun, C. H., Beaune, P. H., Ged, C. & Guengerich, F. P. (1991). Separation of human liver tolbutamide hydroxylase and (S)-mephenytoin 4'-hydroxylase cytochrome P-450 enzymes. *Molecular Pharmacology*, **40**, 69–79.

Umbenhauer, D. R., Martin, V. M., Lloyd, R. S. & Guengerich, F. P. (1987). Cloning and sequence determination of a complementary DNA related to human liver microsomal cytochrome P-450 S-mephenytoin 4-hydroxylase. *Biochemistry*, **26**, 1094–9.

Veronese, M. E., Mackenzie, P. I., Doecke, C. J., McManus, M. E., Miners, J. O. & Birkett, D. J. (1991) Tolbutamide and phenytoin hydroxylations by cDNA-expressed human liver cytochrome P450 2C9. *Biochemical and Biophysical Research Communications*, **175**, 1112–18.

Ward, S. A., Goto, F., Nakamura, K., Jaqz, E., Wilkinson, G. R. & Branch, R. A. (1987). S-mephenytoin 4-hydroxylase is inherited as an autosomal-recessive trait in Japanese families. *Clinical Pharmacology and Therapeutics*, **47**, 96–9.

Ward, S. A., Helsby, N. A., Skjelbo, E., Brøsen, K,. Gram, L. F. & Breckenridge, A. M. (1991). The activation of the biguanide antimalarial proguanil co-segregates with the mephenytoin oxidation polymorphism - a panel study. *British Journal of Clinical Pharmacology*, **31**, 689–92.

Ward, S. A., Walle, T., Walle, U. K., Wilkinson, G. T. & Branch, R. A. (1989a). Propranolol's metabolism is determined by both mephenytoin and debrisoquine hydroxylase activities. *Clinical Pharmacology and Therapeutics*, **45**, 72–9.

Ward, S. A., Watkins, W. M., Mberu, E., Saunders, J. E., Koech, D. H., Gilles, H. M., Howells, R. E. & Breckenridge, A. M. (1989b). Inter-subject variability in the metabolism of proguanil to the active metabolite cycloguanil in man. *British Journal of Clinical Pharmacology*, **27**, 781–7.

Watkins, W. M., Mberu, E. K., Nevill, C. G., Ward, S. A., Breckenridge, A. M. & Koech, D. K. (1990). Variability in the metabolism of proguanil to the active metabolite in healthy Kenyan adults. *Transactions of the Royal Society of Tropical Medicine and Hygiene*, **84**, 492–5.

Wedlund, P. J., Aslanian, W. S., Jacqz, E., McAllister, C. B., Branch, R. A. & Wilkinson, G. R. (1985). Phenotypic differences in mephenytoin pharmacokinetics in normal subjects. *Journal of Pharmacology and Experimental Therapeutics*, **234**, 662–9.

Wedlund, P. J., Aslanian, W. S., McAllister, C. B., Wilkinson, G. R. & Branch, R. A. (1984). Mephenytoin hydroxylation deficiency in Caucasians. Frequency of a new oxidative drug metabolism polymorphism. *Clinical Pharmacology and Therapeutics*, **36**, 773–80.

Wilkinson, G. R., Guengerich, F. P. & Branch, R. A. (1989). Genetic polymorphism of S-mephenytoin hydroxylation. *Pharmacology and Therapeutics*, **43**, 53–76.

Woodbury, D. M. & Fingl, E. (1975). Drugs effective in the therapy of the epilepsies. In *The Pharmacological basis of therapeutics*, 5th edition, ed. L. S. Goodman & A. Gilman, New York: Macmillan p. 208.

Wulf, H. R. (1981) *Rational Diagnosis and Treatment*, p. 147. Oxford: Blackwell.

Yasumori, T., Yamazoe, Y. & Kato, R. (1991). Cytochrome P450 human-2 (P450 II C9) in mephenytoin hydroxylation polymorphism in human livers, differences in substrate and stereoselectivities among microheterogenous P-450 II C species expressed in yeasts. *Journal of Biochemistry*, **109**, 711–17.

Zhang, Y., Blouin, R. A., McNamara, P. J., Steinmetz, J. & Wedlund, P. J. (1991). Limitation to the use of the urinary S-/R-mephenytoin ratio in pharmacogenetic studies. *British Journal of Clinical Pharmacology*, **31**, 350–2.

Zhang, Y., Reviriego, J., Lou, Y. Q., Sjoqvist, F. & Bertilsson, L. (1990). Diazepam metabolism in native Chinese poor and extensive hydroxylators of S-mephenytoin, inter-ethnic differences in comparison with white subjects. *Clinical Pharmacology and Therapeutics*, **48**, 496–502.

Zhou, H. H., Anthony, L. B., Wood, A. J. J. & Wilkinson, G. R. (1990). Induction of polymorphic 4'hydroxylation of S-mephenytoin by rifampicin. *British Journal of Clinical Pharmacology*, **30**, 471–5.

7 The debrisoquine/sparteine polymorphism (cytochrome P450 2D6)

THE METABOLISM OF DEBRISOQUINE AND THE DEFINITION OF PHENOTYPES

DEBRISOQUINE (3,4-dihydro-2-(1-H)-isoquino-linecarboxamide) lowers blood pressure by blocking the transmission of sympathetic nerve impulses at the nerve terminals, thus diminishing peripheral resistance. The reduction in post-ganglionic sympathetic transmission is achieved by interfering with the physiological release of norepinephrine.

There was found to be a wide inter-individual variation in the blood pressure response of patients (Silas *et al.* 1977) and normal subjects to standard dosages. It was also found that the hypotensive response correlated with the plasma concentration and urinary excretion of unchanged drug.

It was some years after the introduction of the drug that detailed studies were made in individuals and populations of its pharmacokinetics and meta-bolism. Debrisoquine was found to be promptly absorbed after oral doses (Idle *et al.* 1979a).

The major metabolite in man was found to be the aliphatic 4-hydroxydebrisoquine (Fig. 7.1). Small amounts of phenolic metabolites 5-, 6-, 7- and 8-hydroxydebrisoquine were also formed (Idle *et al.* 1979a).

Smith (1986) describes how, in 1975, he sustained a severe attack of hypotension after ingesting 32 mg of debrisoquine base for experimental purposes. Other volunteers had only trivial effects and their urine samples showed that they excreted the drug mainly as 4-hydroxydebrisoquine. Smith (1986) himself excreted the drug almost entirely unchanged. It had previously been noticed that he was a poor oxidizer of amphetamine and poor oxidative demethylator of 4-methoxyamphetamine. These observations led to a systematic search for a genetic polymorphism in debrisoquine hyd-roxylation.

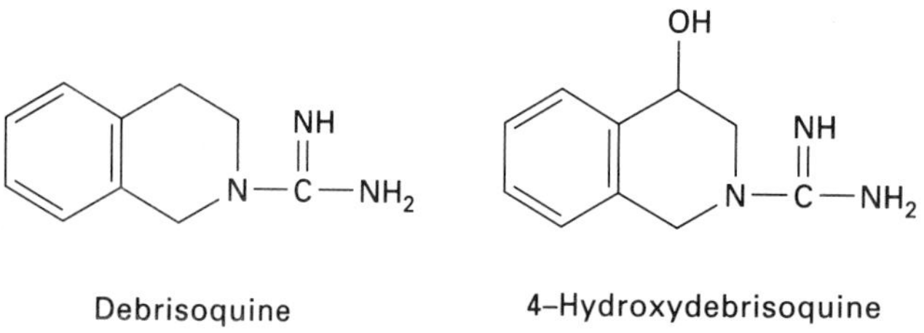

Debrisoquine   4–Hydroxydebrisoquine

Fig. 7.1. Chemical structure of debrisoquine and its major metabolite, 4-hydroxydebrisoquine. (From Mahgoub *et al.* 1977.)

54

As a result of the study of 94 human volunteers it was found that 91 individuals excreted considerable amounts of 4-hydroxydebrisoquine relative to the unchanged debrisoquine. In three individuals, however, only a very small amount of this main metabolite was excreted in the urine, and a relatively large amount of the unchanged drug compound (Mahgoub *et al.* 1977). It was most convenient to express the result as a metabolic ratio = debrisoquine concentration/4-hydroxydebrisoquine concentration, determined in the urine excreted during 8 hours following the oral ingestion of 10 mg debrisoquine. Values of this ratio greater than 20 defined 'poor metabolizers' which were clearly separated from 'extensive metabolizers' in a bimodal frequency distribution histogram (Fig. 7.2).

THE SPARTEINE POLYMORPHISM

A parallel line of research in Germany had meanwhile revealed that the drug sparteine exhibited wide variability in its metabolism to dehydrosparteines (Fig. 7.3) in the population. The ratio, Concentration of sparteine/Concentration of dehydrosparteines, in urine excreted during 12 hours following ingestion of 100 mg sparteine sulphate, showed a definite bimodal distribution (Fig. 7.4). Of the 360 persons tested, 18 had a high ratio and constituted one of the modes. (Eichelbaum *et al.* 1978; Eichelbaum *et al.* 1979a). These persons could be termed 'poor metabolizers' of sparteine, a terminology substantiated by meticulous pharmacokinetic investigations (Eichelbaum *et al.* 1979b).

Subsequently, it was established in selected volunteers (Inaba *et al.* 1980; Eichelbaum *et al.*

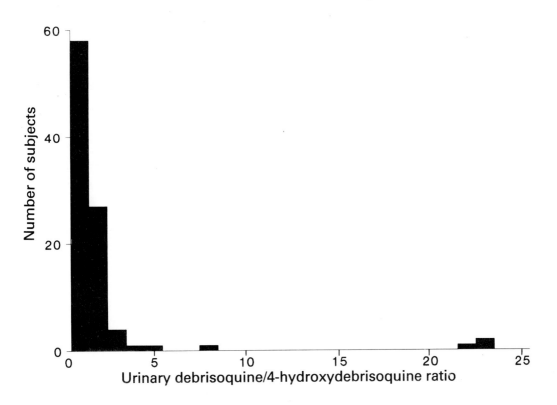

Fig. 7.2. Frequency distribution of the ratio, urinary debrisoquine/4-hydroxydebrisoquine, in 94 human volunteers. (From Mahgoub *et al.* 1977.)

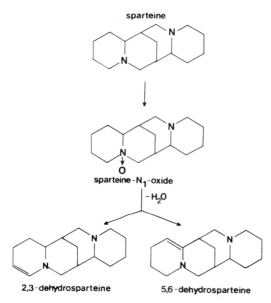

Fig. 7.3. Metabolic pathway of sparteine in man. (From Eichelbaum *et al.* 1978.)

1982; Inaba *et al.* 1983), in random individuals from the population and in families ascertained via poor hydroxylator probands (Evans *et al.* 1983), that in European subjects debrisoquine and sparteine are under common genetic control.

FAMILY STUDIES OF DEBRISOQUINE METABOLISM

Twenty-three poor metabolizers (PMs) were found in a new population survey of unrelated subjects carried out by Evans *et al.* (1980). The families of nine of these PMs were studied and the results are shown in Table 7.1. Metabolic ratios greater than 12.6 ($\log_{10}$ MR > 1.10) were taken to indicate PMs. In pedigrees 1 to 5 all PM offspring had a PM parent (either sex) but for pedigrees 6 to 9 both parents of PM offspring were extensive metabolizers. This clearly shows that PM is an autosomal recessive character. Similar results were obtained by Dick *et al.* (1982). Separate modes indicating homozygous and heterozygous dominants could not be recog-

Fig. 7.4. Distribution of $\log_{10}$ sparteine/dehydrosparteines in urine. (From Eichelbaum *et al.* 1978.)

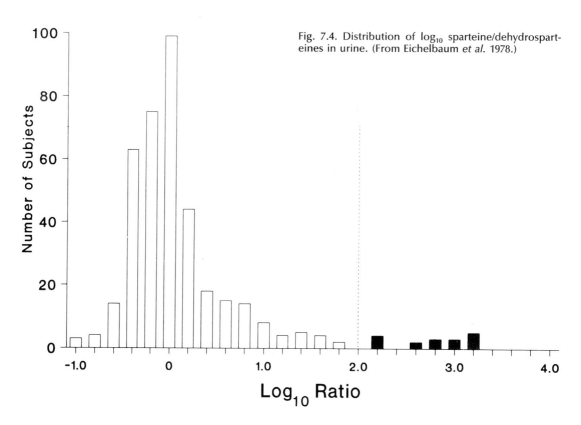

Table 7.1. Log_{10} urinary metabolic ratios in 9 pedigrees ascertained through probands who are poor metabolizers

Pedigree no.	Parents		Offspring				
	Father	Mother	1	2	3	4	5
1	1̄.48	→ 1.52	0̱.15 M	0.18 M	0̱.42 M	0.11 M	0.15 M
2	→ 1.29	1̄.78	1̄.78 M	0.58 M	1̄.95 M	–	–
3	1.32	0.23	1.43 M	→ 1̱.33 M	0.40 M	–	–
4	1.40	Not available	→ 1̱.32	1̄.90 M	–	–	–
5	2.29	0.04	→ 1.48 M	1.88 M	–	–	–
6	0.28	0.48	→ 1.41	1.32 M	0.32 M	1.84 M	–
7	0.48	0.34	→ 1.59	1.26	–	–	–
8	0.63	1.00	→ 1.30 M	–	–	–	–
9	0.72	0.04	→ 1.32 M	0.77 M	0.64 M	–	–

→, proband; M, male offspring. *From:* Evans *et al.* 1980.

nized. However, heterozygotes could be identified in the pedigrees and by utilizing the information provided by them the means of the two genotypes responsible for the dominant phenotype could be computed by the method explained in Appendix 1. In the debrisoquine studies the dominance was computed by this method to be approximately 30% (Evans *et al.* 1980).

Using a much more sophisticated computer methodology a similar figure was obtained by Steiner *et al.* (1985).

The results of phenotyping the members of two Chinese Han families, ascertained by means of PM probands, gave results consistent with them being Mendelian autosomal recessives (Du & Lou 1990).

FAMILY STUDIES OF OTHER DRUGS

A family study of sparteine metabolic ratio (see below) by Evans *et al.* (1983) showed poor metabolizers of sparteine to be poor metabolizers of debrisoquine as well, and to be autosomal recessives. Dominance was computed as 66.7%. Brøsen *et al.* (1986a) also conducted a family study and reached the same conclusion, computing dominance at 77%.

A study of 12 persons in a Japanese family with sparteine (Chiba *et al.* 1988) gave results in keeping with the PM phenotype being a Mendelian recessive character in this racial group.

The genetics of phenformin oxidation was studied in families by Shah *et al.* (1985), who showed that poor metabolizers were autosomal recessives and who computed dominance to be 63%. Finally, McGourty *et al.* (1985) investigated metoprolol and debrisoquine metabolism in families and found that the poor metabolizers of both drugs were autosomal recessives.

DRUGS WHOSE METABOLISM IS CONTROLLED BY THE ALLELES CONTROLLING THE DEBRISOQUINE AND SPARTEINE HYDROXYLATION POLYMORPHISM

Oxidation is such a common fate for drug molecules that from the outset it seemed likely that other drugs might have their biotransformations influenced by the same alleles. Since debrisoquine is a strongly basic guanidine (pK_a 12.5), other basic drugs seemed probable candidates for the same polymorphic oxidation.

Whilst this theoretical prediction proved to be correct, it also turned out that a large number of drug compounds of very different molecular constitutions and pharmacological actions are substrates for this polymorphic oxidation process. A list of drugs is presented in Table 7.2 and their molecular structures in Fig. 7.5. The information has been gathered, mainly in healthy individuals by using either a 'typed panel' approach (Idle *et al.* 1979c) or by studying a random population sample. In either case each individual has been tested with both the test drug and a reference compound.

Table 7.2. *Drugs whose metabolism* in vivo *is polymorphic under the control of the same alleles as debrisoquine and sparteine in Caucasians*

Drug	Reference
Analgesics	
Phenacetin[a]	Kong *et al.* 1982; Devonshire *et al.* 1983
Codeine	Chen *et al.* 1988, 1991; Mortimer *et al.* 1990; Yue *et al.* 1989a
Antianginal	
Perhexilene	Wagner *et al.* 1987
Diltiazem	Cooper *et al.* 1984
Antiarrhythmics	
Encainide	Woosley *et al.* 1981, 1986; Wang *et al.* 1984; Roden & Woosley 1988
Flecainide	Beckmann *et al.* 1988 (especially R-flecainide: Gross *et al.* 1989)
Propafenone	Siddoway *et al.* 1983, 1987; Latini *et al.* 1992
Mexiletine	Broly *et al.* 1991a
N-Propylajmaline	Zekorn *et al.* 1985
Quinidine	Brøsen *et al.* 1990 (minor pathway)
Antidepressives	
Amitriptyline	Mellstrom *et al.* 1986; Zhang *et al.* 1992
Imipramine	Brosen *et al.* 1986b, c; Brosen & Gram 1988; Brosen 1988; Spina *et al.* 1987
Nortriptyline	Mellstrom *et al.* 1981; Nordin *et al.* 1985; Gram *et al.* 1989
Perphenazine	Dahl-Puustinen *et al.* 1989
Clopromazine	Balant-Gorgia *et al.* 1986
Desipramine	Dahl *et al.* 1992
Minaprine	Davi *et al.* 1992; Marre *et al.* 1992
Paroxetine	Bloomer *et al.* 1992; Sindrup *et al.* 1992a, b
Clomipramine	Nielsen *et al.* 1992
Antipsychotics	
Zuclopenthixol	Dahl *et al.* 1991
Thioridazine	von Bahr *et al.* 1991
Haloperidol	Llerena *et al.* 1992a, b
Antihypertensive	
Guanoxan	Sloan *et al.* 1978
Indoramin	Pierce *et al.* 1987
Beta blockers	
Alprenolol	Alvan *et al.* 1982
Bufuralol	Dayer *et al.* 1982a, b, 1983, 1985
Metoprolol	Alvan *et al.* 1982; Lennard *et al.* 1982a, b; Jack & Kendall 1982[b]; Jack *et al.* 1983a,[b] b[b]
Propanolol (4-hydroxylation)	Raghuram *et al.* 1984; Lennard *et al.* 1984; Shaheen *et al.* 1989
Propanolol (5-hydroxylation)	Otton *et al.* 1990
Timolol	Shah *et al.* 1982a; Alvan *et al.* 1982; McGourty *et al.* 1985; Lennard *et al.* 1986
Bronchodilator	
Methoxyphenamine	Roy *et al.* 1984, 1985
Cough suppressant	
Dextromethorphan	Kupfer *et al.* 1984; Schmid *et al.* 1985; Henthorne *et al.* 1989; Mortimer *et al.* 1989
H_2 inhibitor	
Metiamide	Idle *et al.* 1979b
Hallucinogen	
4-methoxyamphetamine	Kitchen *et al.* 1979
5-HT uptake inhibitor	
CGP15210 G	Gleiter *et al.* 1985

Table 7.2. (*cont.*)

Drug	Reference
Monoamine uptake inhibitor	
Amiflamine	Alvan *et al.* 1983, 1984
Oral hypoglycaemic	
Phenformin	Oates *et al.* 1982a, 1983; Shah *et al.* 1985; Fletcher *et al.* 1986
Chlorpropamide	Kallio *et al.* 1990

[a] Subsequent studies have shown that phenacetin is metabolized by two enzymes and is much more complex than was at first realized (see pages 29 and 133).
[b] These authors were sceptical that the metabolism of metoprolol was controlled by the debrisoquine/sparteine polymorphism.

Similar information has emerged from studying patients. For example, Tacke *et al.* (1992) showed that amongst 16 patients with exceptionally high concentrations of antidepressants (amitriptyline, doxepin, trimipramine, imipramine and clomipramine), there were eight poor metabolizers. On the other hand, amongst 16 patients with low or normal levels of the same antidepressants there were only two poor metabolizers ($p = 0.03$).

PHENOTYPING TESTS

Debrisoquine has been the favourite reference compound and sparteine has also been used. However, these two compounds are relatively unobtainable in many places, and sparteine in the 100 mg oral dose which has been used may cause cramping abdominal pains and premature menstruation in some women. For these reasons the harmless, freely available 'over the counter' cough remedy dextromethorphan (Fig. 7.6) which was first recognized as having wide inter-individual variation in its metabolism by Pfaff *et al.* (1983), is now becoming established as a favourite phenotyping agent (see, eg, Guttendorf *et al.* 1988; Chen *et al.* 1990; Wenk *et al.* 1991; Perault *et al.* 1991) by virtue of its oxidative demethylation (Fig. 7.6). Codeine which is also oxidatively demethylated was used as a phenotyping drug by Yue *et al.* (1989a), whereas Ishizaki (1991) advocates the use of metoprolol because it is widely available and harmless.

High performance liquid chromatographic techniques are now replacing the previously used gaschromatographic analytical methods both for debrisoquine (e.g. Johnson *et al.* 1990) and for dextromethorphan (e.g. Jacqz-Aigrain *et al.* 1989; Chen *et al.* 1990). A gas chromatography–mass spectrometry method for debrisoquine was reported by Daumas *et al.* (1991). An ELISA method has been introduced for dextromethorphan phenotyping by Freche *et al.* (1990). Simple thin-layer chromatography methods have been published by Ebner *et al.* (1989) for sparteine and by Guttendorf *et al.* (1988) for dextromethorphan (Fig. 7.7).

The daytime performance of the debrisoquine phenotyping test appeared to give better phenotypic separation than a night-time test (Shaw *et al.* 1990) whilst age (Siegmund *et al.* 1990; Pollock *et al.* 1992) and urinary pH (Kallio 1990) did not influence the metabolic ratio obtained. Paar *et al.* (1989) favoured a 90 minute blood sample rather than a 6 hour urine collection to determine the metabolic ratio for sparteine after studying 121 healthy students, 12 of whom were discovered to be PM.

No attention has been paid to the information provided by Cooper *et al.* (1984), who administered one oral 300 mg dose of perhexiline maleate and collected one urine sample 12 to 24 hours later and one blood sample at 24 hours. In both plasma and urine the concentration of the M1 hydroxylated metabolite, determined by gas liquid chromatography, showed a huge gap between the phenotypes making this the most unequivocal phenotyping method.

The study of Latini *et al.* (1992) indicates that the urinary metabolic ratio of propafenone might be used as a phenotyping procedure.

Cirrhosis of the liver was shown by Debruyne *et al.* (1989) to impair the debrisoquine phenotyping test by increasing the metabolic ratio.

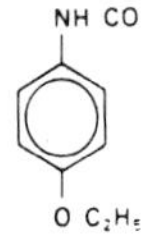

Phenacetin 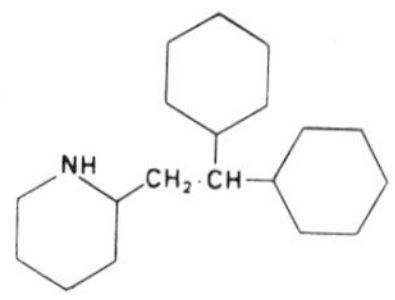   **Perhexiline** 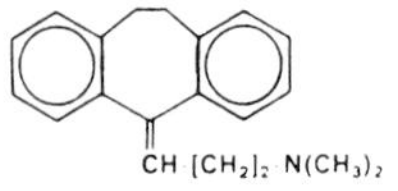   **Amitriptyline**

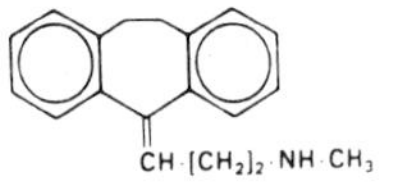

Nortriptyline 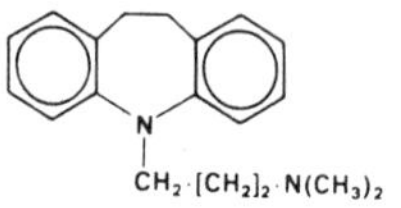   **Imipramine** 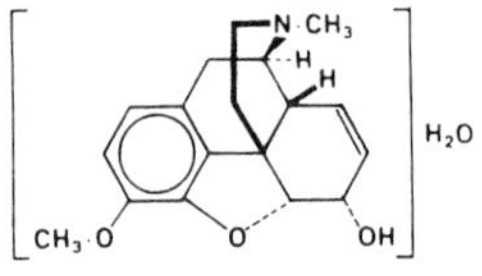   **Codeine**

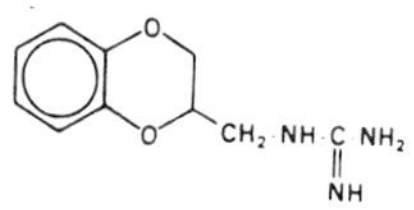

Guanoxan 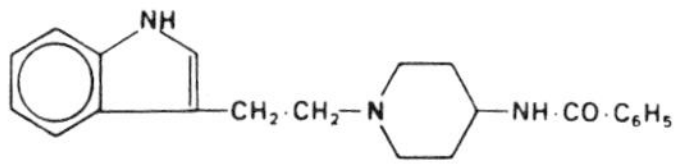   **Indoramin**

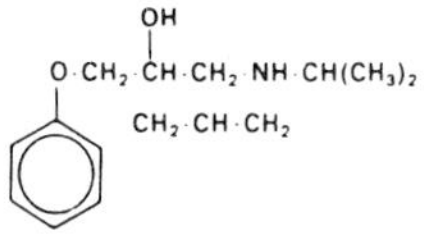

Alprenolol 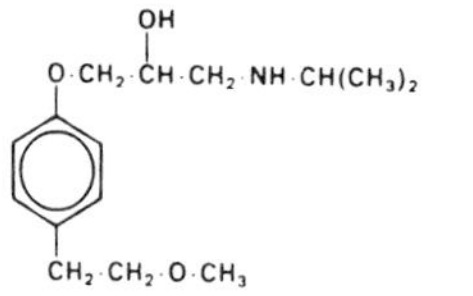   **Metoprolol**

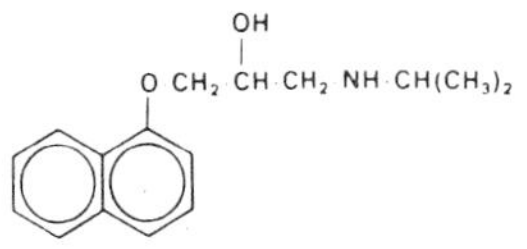

Propranolol 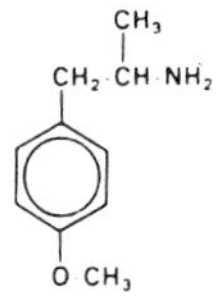   **Methoxyamphetamine**

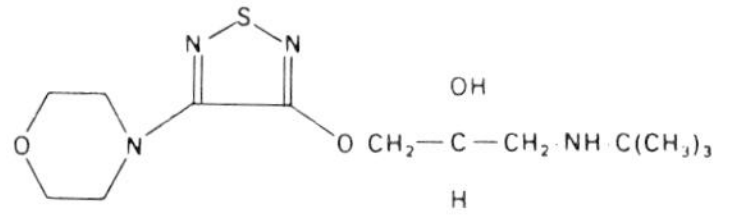

Timolol 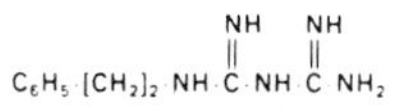   **Phenformin**

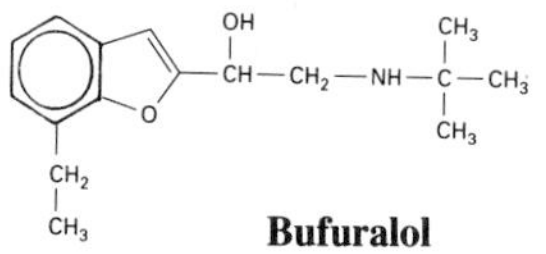

Bufuralol

Fig. 7.5. The molecular structures of some drugs which are polymorphically oxidized by the debrisoquine/ sparteine system. (From *Clarke's Isolation and Identification of Drugs*, 1986.)

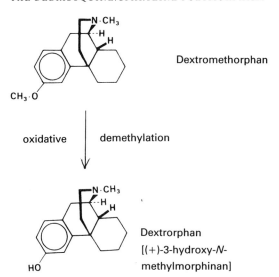

Dextromethorphan

oxidative | demethylation

Dextrorphan
[(+)-3-hydroxy-*N*-
methylmorphinan]

Fig. 7.6. The polymorphic metabolism of dextro-methorphan. Dextromethorphan is the non-opioid dextrorotatory stereoisomer of the levorotatory narcotic methorphan (*N*-methyl-methoxymorphinan). (Structural formulae from *Clarke's Isolation and Identification of Drugs, 1986*.)

The newer DNA-based genotyping methods described in a later section may render obsolete *in vivo* phenotyping methods where the subject being investigated has to ingest a drug compound.

DRUGS WHOSE METABOLISM IS NOT CONTROLLED BY THE DEBRISOQUINE/SPARTEINE POLYMORPHISM

These drugs are listed in Table 7.3.

INTERACTIONS *IN VIVO* BETWEEN DRUGS KNOWN TO BE SUBSTRATES FOR DEBRISOQUINE/SPARTEINE POLYMORPHIC OXIDATION

A startling clinical example of the importance of this topic was provided by Wagner *et al.* (1987). A 47 year old man with coronary arterial disease was admitted to a coronary care unit with third degree heart block and seriously impaired ventricular function.

Fig. 7.7. Semilogarithmic frequency distribution histogram of dextromethorphan metabolic rates in 8 hour urine samples of 65 subjects. Extensive metabolizers = metabolic ratio < 0.3; poor metabolizers = metabolic ratio > 0.3. (From Guttendorf *et al.* 1988.)

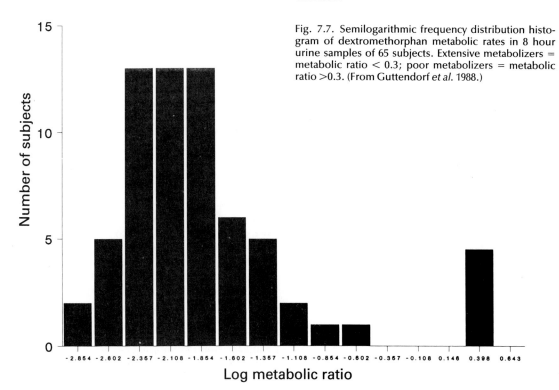

Log metabolic ratio

Table 7.3. *Drugs and chemicals whose oxidations have been shown* in vivo *not to be controlled in Caucasians by the debrisoquine/sparteine polymorphism*

Drug	Reference
Almitrine	Herchuelz *et al.* 1990
Amylobarbitone	Inaba *et al.* 1980; Kalow 1982
Antipyrine	Bertilsson *et al.* 1981; Danhof *et al.* 1981; Eichelbaum *et al.* 1983
Atenolol	Lennard *et al.* 1986
Carbamazepine	Eichelbaum *et al.* 1985
Carbocysteine	Mitchell 1984
Clothiapine	Spina *et al.* 1991
Glibenclamide	Dahl-Puustinen *et al.* 1990
Mephenytoin	Kupfer & Preisig 1984; Inaba *et al.* 1984a
Methaqualone	Oram *et al.* 1982; Dayer *et al.* 1984a
Midazolam	Kasai *et al.* 1988
Paracetamol	Veronese & McLean 1991a
Phenacetin	Veronese & McLean 1991a[a]
Pinacidil	Shaheen 1986
Phenytoin	Steiner *et al.* 1987
Prazosin	Lennard *et al.* 1988a
Quinidine	Mikus *et al.* 1989[b]
Quinine	Wanwimolruk & Chalcroft 1991
Theophylline	Dahlqvist *et al.* 1984
Tolbutamide	Miners *et al.* 1985; Peart *et al.* 1987
Toluene	Löf *et al.* 1990

[a] See also Table 7.2.
[b] But also see Brøsen *et al.* (1990) who detected a minor influence of the polymorphism on 3-hydroxylation.

One week prior to this admission metoprolol therapy had been commenced and 2 days prior to admission diltiazem had been added. He was found to have very high plasma levels of both drugs. The liver and kidney functions were normal.

It was also noted that earlier in his history he had sustained many syncopal attacks whilst on treatment with metoprolol and propafenone together. After he had recovered from his toxic episode he was tested with all three drugs plus sparteine and was shown to be a poor metabolizer for them all.

All the drugs listed in Table 7.2 have the potential to interact with each other *in vivo*. However, this theoretical possibility may not actually occur in practice. For example, the effect of a variety of β-blockers on the debrisoquine metabolic ratio was shown to be only marginal by Kallio *et al.* (1990).

OTHER INTERACTIONS

Some drugs which are not themselves substrates for the polymorphic debrisoquine/sparteine oxidation can have a considerable effect on drugs which are.

The most notable example is quinidine (Fig. 7.8) which has been extensively studied both *in vitro* on liver microsomal oxidation of substrates for the debrisoquine/sparteine polymorphic oxidation and also for its effect *in vivo*.

Six research groups have investigated the effect of a dose of quinidine taken just before a standard debrisoquine or sparteine phenotyping test. Thirty-eight out of 46 EM became apparent PM and this effect lasted about 3 days (Inaba *et al.* 1986; Speirs *et al.* 1986; Brinn *et al.* 1986; Brøsen *et al.* 1987; Nielsen *et al.* 1990; Ayesh *et al.* 1991).

The effect of quinidine has also been investigated on the metabolism and clinical effects of drugs which are under the control of the debrisoquine/sparteine polymorphism. Quinidine was shown by Zhou *et al.* (1990) greatly to diminish the 4-hydroxylation of propanolol, especially (+)propanolol with the effect of raising the plasma concentration and producing an enhanced β-blockade. In this context the EM is likely to be more deleteriously affected than the PM patient.

Similarly imipramine and desipramine (Brøsen & Gram 1989), nortriptyline and desipramine (Ayesh *et al.* 1991), mexiletine (Broly *et al.* 1991a) and R(−) flecainide (Birgersdotter *et al.* 1992) plasma

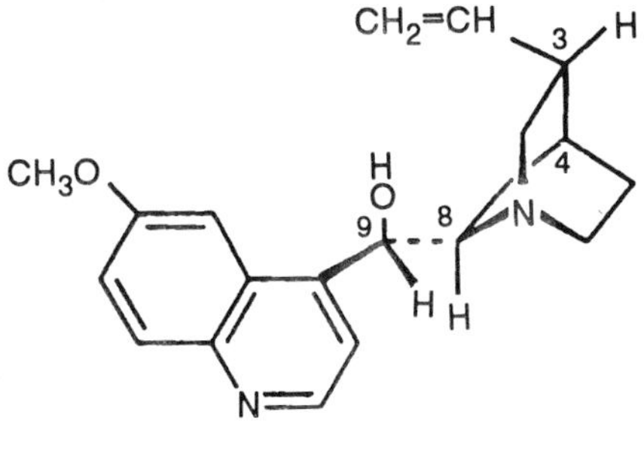

Quinidine (8R, 9S)

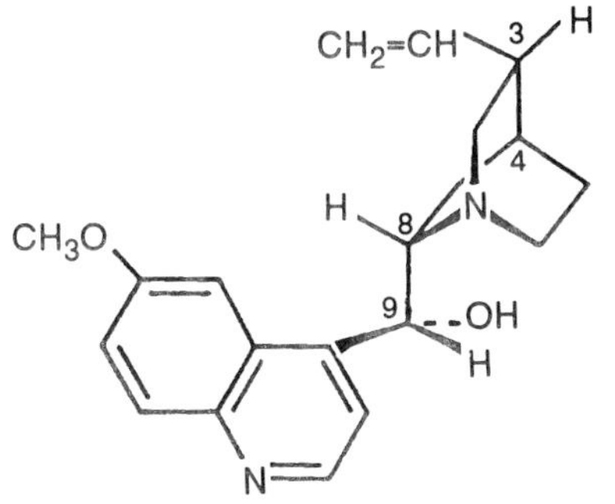

Quinine (8S, 9R)

Fig. 7.8. Chemical structures of quinidine and quinine. They are related to each other as diastereoisomers having the configurations around carbons 8 and 9 of (8R, 9S) and (8S, 9R), respectively. (From Ayesh et al. 1991.)

concentrations were all higher after a dose of quinidine.

Where a drug undergoes oxidation by more than one pathway, only certain routes may be inhibited by quinidine. This may indicate that these specific biotransformations are governed by the debrisoquine/sparteine genetic polymorphism. Thus Turgeon et al. (1991) showed that quinidine decreased the partial metabolic clearances of mexiletine (me) to the three metabolites hydroxymethyl-me, m-hydroxy-me and p-hydroxy-me but not the partial metabolic clearance to N-hydroxy-me in EM. There was no effect in PM individuals. Similarly the O-demethylation and 5-hydroxylation of methoxyphenamine but not the N-demethylation were inhibited by quinidine sufficiently to change the apparent phenotype in 11 out of 12 EM (Muralidharan et al. 1991).

It was thought that quinidine is not metabolized at all by the cytochrome P450 responsible for the debrisoquine/sparteine polymorphism since Mikus et al. (1986) found that the pharmacokinetics of quinidine and its metabolites were the same in 3 EM as in 3 PM. A different conclusion was reached by Brøsen et al. (1990) who found in 4 EM and 4 PM that the formation of 3-hydroxyquinidine (as expressed by its clearance from quinidine) was slightly but significantly higher in the EM then in the PM phenotype. So it would appear that the vast bulk of quinidine is metabolized by a cytochrome P450 other than the CYP 2D6 gene product which only deals with a small fraction.

Dextropropoxyphenene was shown to cause an apparent change of phenotype by inhibiting debrisoquine metabolism (Sanz & Bertilsson 1990).

Flecainide administration caused an increase in the dextromethorphan/dextrorphan urinary ratio causing an apparent change of phenotype EM → PM in one individual (Haefeli et al. 1990). Similarly, the sparteine metabolic ratio was increased during paroxetine treatment causing an apparent change in phenotype EM → PM in two persons (Sindrup et al. 1992a).

The psychotropic drugs are of great importance in this context. Thioridazine and levopromazine elevated debrisoquine metabolic ratios probably causing an apparent change of phenotype (Syvalahti et al. 1986). Haloperidol appeared to increase the urinary metabolic ratio of sparteine but not sufficiently to cause an apparent change of an EM into a PM (Gram et al. 1989a). Levopromazine was shown to increase the debrisoquine metabolic ratio markedly by Kallio et al. (1990); in one patient this produced an apparent change of phenotype (EM → PM). The frequency of PM as assessed by a debrisoquine test was shown to be 46.2% amongst 91 schizophrenics surveyed by Spina et al. (1991). The explanation was that various patients were receiving chlorpromazine, levopromazine, thioridazine and haloperidol, all of which were inhibiting the oxidation of debrisoquine.

Similarly, Gram et al. (1989b) observed that plasma nortriptyline concentrations were elevated by concurrent perphenazine administration.

THE EFFECTS OF INDUCER AND INHIBITOR COMPOUNDS *IN VIVO* ON DRUG METABOLISM MEDIATED BY THE DEBRISOQUINE/SPARTEINE POLYMORPHISM

The metabolism of many drugs which are oxidized by a cytochrome P450 mechanism is known to be influenced by the preceding or simultaneous administration of other compounds. Probably the best known examples in the clinical setting are phenobarbitone and cimetidine. Phenobarbitone causes, over a few days, an increase in the protein endoplasmic reticulum and total cytochrome P450 contents of the liver. Now that it is known that there are different cytochromes P450 with their own specific array of substrates, the influence of phenobarbitone induction must be assessed on each cytochrome P450 separately. Another drug which is used clinically more than phenobarbitone and which is known to be an inducer is rifampicin. Cimetidine is a compound well known to inhibit liver drug metabolism.

According to Schellens *et al.* (1989) phenobarbitone appears to be without effect on sparteine metabolism. Rifampicin, however, caused changes in both the elimination half-life and the metabolic clearance of sparteine in extensive metabolizers (Eichelbaum *et al.* 1986). It seems likely that the further metabolism of dihydrosparteines may be induced. Renal clearance was not altered. The urinary metabolic ratio was not significantly changed. There were no significant changes in poor metabolizers.

Rifampicin treatment was found to lower the debrisoquine metabolic ratio in PM by Leclercq *et al.* (1989) to the extent that two out of six individuals became apparent EM subjects. No change of apparent phenotype was detected under the influence of phenobarbitone or cimetidine.

Cimetidine has been shown to influence the kinetics of desmethyl-imipramine (DMI) by increasing the plasma half-life and area under the concentration/time curve and by decreasing the total plasma clearance and urinary 2-hydroxy DMI production in extensive metabolizers (Steiner & Spina 1987). There was no significant effect in poor metabolizers. Another group (Philip *et al.* 1989) investigated the effect of cimetidine treatment for the three preceding days on a standard debrisoquine phenotyping test. The metabolic ratio was raised in extensive metabolizers but not sufficient to cause an apparent change of phenotype.

ENZYMOLOGICAL STUDIES

During the 1980s steady progress was made in elucidating the enzymological basis for the debrisoquine/sparteine polymorphism.

An important preliminary step was the development of methods to determine mixed function oxidase activity in microsomal fractions from percutaneous needle biopsies of human liver (Boobis *et al.* 1980). These methods were subsequently available to be deployed in the investigation of the debrisoquine/sparteine polymorphism and Davies *et al.* (1981) duly reported the results of investigating five persons. These individuals were phenotyped with a debrisoquine test subsequent to their liver biopsies being obtained for diagnostic purposes; four were shown to be extensive metabolizers (EM) and one was a poor metabolizer (PM). Incubations were prepared with liver microsomal protein and the ability to oxidize debrisoquine was confirmed to be dependent on NADPH. Their livers showed that the total cytochrome P450 content was not different in the EM and PM phenotypes but the microsomal oxidative capacity as shown by the ability to form 4-hydroxydebrisoquine from debrisoquine was zero in the PM compared with 25 to 50 pmol/mg protein per minute in the EM phenotype.

The results were confirmed by Meier *et al.* (1983) who showed an exact correlation of *in vivo* and *in vitro* debrisoquine hydroxylation in 14 EM and two PM individuals.

The next step was to purify the cytochrome P450 from the microsomal preparations of EM and PM subjects and this was performed by Gut *et al.* (1984) and by Dayer *et al.* (1984b). Bufuralol was used as the substrate for these investigations. This β-adrenergic blocker was known to be polymorphically 1'-hydroxylated *in vivo* and furthermore is enantiomeric. In extensive metabolizer microsomes the enzymatic reaction displayed apparent Michaelis–Menten kinetics and the (+) enantiomer was preferentially metabolized. By contrast the enzyme reaction in poor metabolizer microsomes was characterized by a 4 to 5-fold greater K_m and by absence of stereoselectivity.

[The Michaelis–Menten expression

$$V_i = V_{max}[S]/\{K_m + [S]\}$$

where V_i = initial velocity of the reaction, V_{max} = maximal velocity of the reaction, $[S]$ = substrate concentration, K_m = Michaelis constant (substrate concentration that produces half-maximal velocity), describes the behaviour of many enzymes as the substrate concentration is varied. See Martin *et al.* 1985 for a full explanation.]

After cholate solubilization the microsomal supernatant was subjected to column fractionation and each of the fractions was assayed for bufuralol 1'-hydroxylation activity. A cytochrome P450 fraction with high activity and which displayed a single homogenous band on SDS polyacrylamide gel electrophoresis was used for further studies and called cytochrome P450$_{buf}$.

In a non-membranous reconstituted system containing NADPH, cytochrome P450 reductase, a NADPH regenerating system and phospholipids, P450$_{buf}$ exhibited an almost complete substrate stereoselectivity for bufuralol (+) isomer 1'-hydroxylation. It was concluded that the purified cytochrome P450$_{buf}$ was the enzymic site for the debrisoquine/sparteine type oxidation polymorphism and that poor metabolizers had a quantitative or qualitative deficiency of the isozyme.

Somewhat analogous results were obtained by Distlerath *et al.* (1985) who made considerable use of specific anti-cytochrome P450 antibodies but did not correlate biochemical findings with *in vivo* phenotyping, and also by Birgersson *et al.* (1986). These studies indicated that only about 1% of the total cytochrome P450 content of the liver was involved in the debrisoquine/sparteine/bufuralol/desmethyl imipramine oxidizing activity.

Zanger *et al.* (1988) utilized purified cytochrome P450 liver preparations from persons of known phenotypes in a more extensive analysis. Two cytochromes P450 oxidizing bufuralol were obtained by column purification as above and termed cytochrome P450$_{buf I}$ and cytochrome P450$_{buf II}$. By using a peroxide system instead of the usual NADPH and O_2 supported system it was shown that cytochrome P450$_{buf I}$ mediated the 1'-hydroxylation of bufuralol whereas cytochrome P450$_{buf II}$ did not. Using the peroxide system microsomes from poor metabolizers (PM) were shown to have a higher K_m and very low V_{max} compared with microsomes from extensive metabolizers. Furthermore, the PM microsomes showed no stereoselectivity in bufuralol metabolism.

An anti-rat cytochrome P450$_{db1}$ IgG antibody (db stands for debrisoquine) reacted with purified cytochrome P450$_{buf I}$ from the microsomes of extensive metabolizers. No such immunoreactive material of the same molecular weight (50 000) could be detected in microsomes from PM individuals.

These findings further confirmed the basis of the polymorphism to be in one specific type of human cytochrome P450. The thrust of research then took a different direction based upon the application of molecular genetic techniques; this will be described in a later section.

The studies of Ladona *et al.* (1991) and Treluyer *et al.* (1991) reveal that cytochrome P450 2D6 is virtually absent before birth.

IN VITRO INHIBITION STUDIES OF THE CYTOCHROME P450 RESPONSIBLE FOR THE DEBRISOQUINE/SPARTEINE POLYMORPHISM

The idea behind these studies is as follows.

If a substrate has been found which is metabolized well by an enzyme, then other potential substrates can be investigated to see if their presence in the incubate will inhibit the metabolism of the original substrate. Inhibitions can be competitive or noncompetitive. In the Dixon plot method of expressing rates of catalysis, regression lines of the reciprocal of the velocity of the reaction against the concentration of the inhibitor are constructed using varying concentrations of the original substrate. If they meet at one point competitive inhibition is demonstrated. The strength of the inhibition is expressed as K_i which is the concentration (stated as the positive) of the inhibitor corresponding to the point of intersection. When no inhibition occurs horizontal lines are produced, rising up the ordinate as the concentration of the substrate diminishes. Fig. 7.9 shows examples of the two processes. It is to be noted that competitive inhibition can be overcome at a sufficiently high substrate concentration, whereas noncompetitive inhibition *cannot* be overcome by increasing the substrate concentration.

Most of the work in this area has been carried out using sparteine, debrisoquine and bufuralol as the

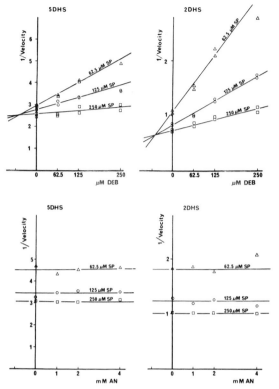

Fig. 7.9. Dixon plots showing (above) competitive inhibition by debrisoquine (DEB) of 5-dehydrosparteine (5DHS) and 2-dehydrosparteine (2DHS) formation by a human liver preparation: $K_i = 60$ μM; (below) antipyrine (AN) produced no inhibition. The velocity is expressed as nanomoles per mg protein per 30 min. (From Otton et al. 1982a.)

substrates being oxidized by human liver microsomal preparations.

Bufuralol 1'-hydroxylation has been shown to be a highly active and specific biotransformation mediated by the cytochrome P450 responsible for the polymorphic oxidations of debrisoquine and sparteine. For this reason it has been used, particularly by Swiss investigators, as a research tool to see if other compounds cause inhibition.

When a compound has been shown to cause inhibition of the polymorphic debrisoquine/sparteine polymorphic cytochrome P450 in vitro it means that it may (1) cause similar inhibition in vivo, (2) fit into the active site of the cytochrome P450 and (3) be polymorphically metabolized in vivo . The most striking exception to (3) is quinidine

which is an extremely powerful inhibitor of the oxidation of the relevant drugs by extensive metabolizers in vivo and in vitro (Otton et al. 1984) but is not itself a substrate for polymorphic oxidation in vitro. (Otton et al. 1988b). In vivo evidence, however, as already mentioned suggests a minor role for the polymorphic enzyme in the 3-oxidation of quinidine (Brøsen et al. 1990).

The results obtained by a number of research groups investigating a large number of compounds are shown in Tables 7.4 and 7.5. Some of these results are worthy of comment.

The many plant alkaloids which are competitive antagonists for the polymorphic debrisoquine/sparteine cytochrome P450 with low K_i values suggest the possibility that this cytochrome may have evolved to deal with toxic food constituents (Fonne-Pfister & Meyer 1988).

An antibody called LKMI occurs in patients with chronic active hepatitis and is directed against the specific cytochrome P450 now called CYP 2D6 and so can be used as an investigative tool. If the metabolism of a compound by a liver preparation is inhibited by this antibody then it is likely that it is metabolized by this specific cytochrome P450 (Kroemer et al. 1989).

Some compounds are metabolized in the body by more than one biotransformation. The in vitro technique gives an opportunity to examine the reactions separately. For example, metoprolol is metabolized by α-hydroxylation and O-demethylation (Fig. 7.10). Otton et al. (1988a) showed that in the case of the former process complete and stereoselective inhibition occurred in the presence of quinine and quinidine. Also, poor metabolizers in the debrisoquine/sparteine polymorphism do not perform α-hydroxylation. On the other hand, O-demethylation was only partly inhibited by quinine and quinidine. This suggests that the activity is catalysed by two different cytochrome P450 systems (1) partly by the debrisoquine/sparteine cytochrome P450 in extensive metabolizers and (2) partly by another route responsible for the quinidine-resistant low activity.

These illustrative examples make the point that competitive inhibition studies in vitro are potentially quick and easy ways of finding out whether new substrates are likely to be polymorphically metabolized in vivo. Many drugs can be screened with a few liver samples and these in vitro tech-

Table 7.4. *Compounds inhibiting the activity of the debrisoquine/sparteine P450 in human liver* in vitro

Drugs	Parkinson's disease producers[a]
Ajmaline	MPDP+
Alprenolol	MPTP
Amitriptyline	MPP+
Apomorphine	PTP
Budipine	
Bufuralol	*Alkaloids*
1-t-Butyl-4-hydroxyphenyl-4-phenyl piperidine	Ajmalicine
Chloroquine	Ajmaline
Chlorpromazine	Berberine
Cimetidine	Cinchonidine
Desipramine	Cinchonine
Dextroproproxyphene	Corynanthine
Diphenylhydramine	Harmaline
4,4-Diphenylpiperidine	Ibogaine
Flecainide	Laudanosine
Fluoxetine	α-Lobeline
Fluphenazine	Tetrahydropapaverine
Guanoxon	Yohimbine
Haloperidol (and reduced metabolite)	
Imipramine	*Endogenous substances and steroids*
Levomepromazine	Androstene-3,17-dione
Lidocaine	Norethindrone acetate
Medipine	Progesterone
Mefloquine	Tryptamine
Metoclopramide	
Metoprolol	Very weak inhibition shown by Amobarbital
Mexiletine	Guanethidine and Tolazoline
Nicardipine	
Nortriptyline	
Norfluoxetine	
Oxyprenolol	
Paroxetine	
Phenylcyclopropylamine	
Pilocarpine	
Pindolol	
Primaquine	
Priscoline	
Prodipine	
Propafenone (R- and S-)	
Propanolol	
Quinine	
Quinidine	
Timolol	
Trifluperidol	

[a] MPDP+ 1-methyl-4-phenyl-2,3-dihydropyridinium perchlorate
MPTP *N*-methyl-4-phenyl-1,2,3,6-tetrahydropyridine hydrochloride
MPP+ 1-methyl-4-phenylpyridinium iodide
PTP 4-phenyl-1,2,3,6-tetrahydropyridine hydrochloride
From: Bloomer *et al.* 1992; Boobis *et al.* 1985; Broly *et al.* 1990; Brøsen & Skjelbo 1991; Brøsen *et al.* 1991a, b; Dayer *et al.* 1987; Fonne-Pfister *et al.* 1987; Fonne-Pfister & Meyer 1988; Haefeli *et al.* 1990; Inaba *et al.* 1984b; Knodell *et al.* 1991; Kroemer *et al.* 1989, 1991; Lancaster *et al.* 1990; Otton *et al.* 1982, 1983, 1984; Sanz & Bertilsson 1990; Spina *et al.* 1984; Tyndale *et al.* 1991; Von Bahr *et al.* 1983, 1985.

Table 7.5. *Compounds which do not inhibit the activity of the debrisoquine/sparteine cytochrome P450 2D6 in human liver* in vitro

Amobarbital	Isoproterenol
Antipyrine	Oubain
Caffeine	Phenytoin
Disopyramide	Theophylline
Ethosuximide	Tolbutamide
Hexamethonium	Valproic acid
Various anti-cancer drugs (Relling *et al.* 1989)	

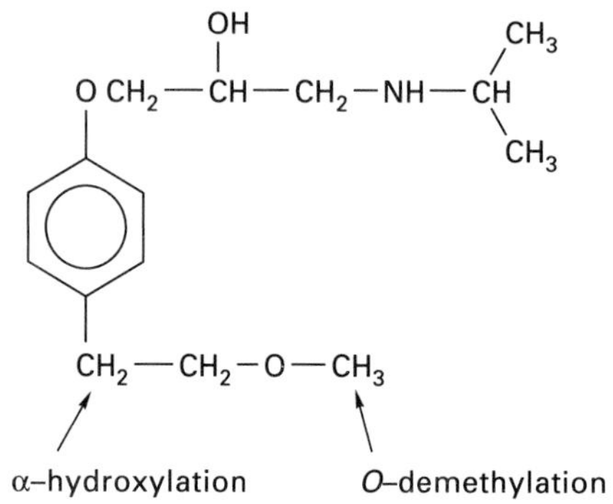

Fig. 7.10. The sites of α-hydroxylation and O-demethylation of metoprolol.

niques are obviously easier and cheaper to carry out than large population studies of pharmacokinetic behaviour *in vivo*.

The heterologous expression of *CYP 2D6* in a functional form in the yeast *Saccharomyces cerevisiae* reported by Ellis *et al.* (1992) is another interesting development. There is already a large body of information available about the yeast and it is easy to maintain in culture, so it may well turn out to provide a more convenient test mechanism than liver cells.

These studies also make one wonder about the structure of the relevant cytochrome P450. It must have a very special construction because (a) on the one hand, it can deal with such a huge variety of substrate molecules and (b) on the other hand, the performance of the cytochrome P450 is exquisitely sensitive to the tiny difference between quinine and quinidine (Fig. 7.8). The latter is much more potent an inhibitor than the former (Otton *et al.* 1988b).

The suggestion has been made (Wolff *et al.* 1985)

that a common feature of substrates is that they have a spatial distance of about 5 Å between the basic nitrogen atom carrying the positive charge and the lipophilic region where oxidation recurs. Similarly, Meyer *et al.* (1986) proposed a distance of 7 Å between the basic nitrogen and the oxygen of the reaction site of the enzyme for dextromethorphan and bufuralol. It can be deduced from this that the positively charged position of the substrate requires a corresponding negatively charged site in the protein for binding – possibly the carboxylate anion group of aspartate or glutamate and a 'pocket' formed by lipophilic parts of aminoacids close to the iron atom of the haem group (cf. cytochrome P450$_{cam}$, p. 10).

Koymans *et al.* (1992) reconcile the two distances by pointing out that the distance between the two oxygen atoms of a carboxylic group is 2 Å, hence it depends which one is used to measure the distance to the basic nitrogen of the substrate.

A large number of molecules known to be substrates for the polymorphism were used to produce a molecular template by means of a computer-based interactive molecular graphics technique combined with energy calculations (Islam *et al.* 1991). The template was then used to determine the likelihood that new compounds were substrates for cytochrome P450 2D6. Tamoxifen was shown not to fit the template, and subsequently this prediction was verified by *in vitro* enzymological observations using human liver microsomes which showed that it was not a substrate for this cytochrome.

Despite the ability of the relevant cytochrome P450 to deal with many diverse structures (as illustrated in Fig. 7.5) there is at the same time a very precise stereospecificity. The stereoselectivity for bufuralol-1′-hydroxylation and metoprolol α-hydroxylation have already been mentioned.

Debrisoquine itself is achiral but 4-hydroxylation gives the possibility of producing two enantiomers R (rectus) and S (sinister). [The R and S notation sometimes referred to as the 'sequence rule' (Cahn–Ingold–Prelog convention) enables configuration to be assigned directly from the three-dimensional structure. For a full explanation see *The Pharmaceutical Handbook*, ed. A. Wade (1980) and Seymour 1990.]

It has been found that 98% of the 4-hydroxy debrisoquine (4OHD) produced in EM is in the S form whereas 5 to 36% of the R form is present in the small amount of 4OHD produced by the PM pheno-type (Meese *et al.* 1988; Eichelbaum 1988; Lennard *et al.* 1988b).

Nortriptyline 10-hydroxylation introduces chiral-ity since E and Z enantiomers are produced as metabolic products. The E and Z notation defines stereoisomers in relation to ethylene double bonds and replaces the terms *cis* and *trans* . The terms Z (*zusammen*: together) and E (*entgegen*: opposite) refer in the case of nortriptyline to the orientation of the hydroxyl group of the metabolite to the methyl propylamine side chain (see Fig. 7.11, and also *The Pharmaceutical Handbook*, ed. A. Wade (1980)). Only E hydroxylation was found to be subject to the deb-risoquine polymorphism by Mellstrom *et al.* (1981).

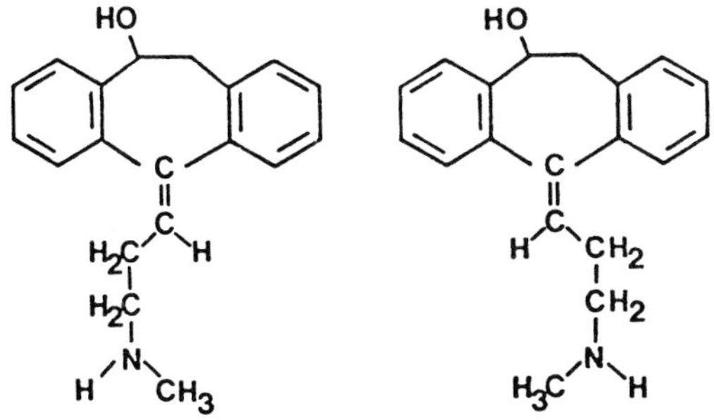

Z-10-OH-NT   E-10-OH-NT

Fig. 7.11. E- and Z-enantiomers of 10-hydroxy-nortriptyline. (From Mellstrom *et al.* 1981.)

MOLECULAR GENETICS

In this section only the work carried out on the cytochrome P450 enzymes controlling the debrisoquine/sparteine polymorphism in humans will be described. This work in humans was per-formed against a huge background experience of work in many other species. There are extensive and authoritative reviews covering the whole topic (e.g. Nebert & Gonzalez 1987; Gonzalez 1989). The place of the debrisoquine/sparteine polymorphism as per-ceived in the general evolutionary scheme can be appreciated by reference to the general section on cytochromes P450. Some confusion has arisen from

the nomenclature in that individual workers have tended to coin their own. Now, however, there is general acceptance of the scheme portrayed in Table 4.1 in the cytochromes P450 chapter. The opera-tional terms cytochrome $P450_{buf}$ and cytochrome $P450_{db}$ have been replaced by the term cytochrome P450 2D6 (Nebert *et al.* 1991).

There are significant advantages in the molecular biological approach to the study of cytochromes P450 and this is why it has been making all the running in the last few years. Some of these advant-ages are worth noting because this knowledge is widely applicable.

Cytochromes P450 which are membrane bound can prove difficult to purify especially from human tissue which may only be available in small amounts. The detection of tiny changes (which may be very important functionally) between cyto-chromes P450 from different individuals constitutes another problem. Molecules with very small differ-ences can have the same mobility on electrophoretic gels and may not be differentially recognized by antibodies.

Recombinant DNA technology overcomes many of these obstacles to progress. Individual cytochrome P450 molecules can be purified and made available in useful amounts by means of molecular cloning and the functional expression of an individual cytochrome P450 can be examined by introducing its genome into a suitable cell.

Returning to the specific subject of the debriso-quine/sparteine polymorphism, there are some important publications which will now be briefly reviewed.

The first study on the structure of the deb-risoquine gene variants was that of Gonzalez *et al.* (1988a), who isolated the relevant cDNA in liver samples using an anti-rat db1 antibody. Then, using a human expression library from the liver of an extensive metabolizer (EM), a 1568 base pair cDNA was obtained. This cDNA was inserted into the SV40 and adenovirus expression vector p91023 (B) and this construct was transfected into COS cells in cul-ture. This procedure enabled these cells to produce an enzyme with high bufuralol 1'-hydroxylase activity which had the same electrophoretic mobility as the enzyme purified from liver microsomes and recognized by the anti-rat db1 antibody.

From seven livers (4 EM 3 PM) phenotyped using the *in vitro* bufuralol 1'-hydroxylase assay the mRNA was subjected to electrophoresis and a ^{32}P-labelled db1 cDNA probe. Four variant RNAs were identified in PM livers and compared with the 'wild type' (wt) RNA of about 1.8 kb size found in EM individuals. The sizes and putative structures of the corresponding cDNA molecules of these variants were as follows:-

a	larger than wt	– retained intron 5
b	larger than wt	– retained intron 6
c	about the same size as wt	– loss of the 3' half of exon 6 in combination with the removal of intron 6
b'	considerably smaller than wt	– a similar structure to the wt but possessed several amino acid substitutions

The next step was taken by Skoda *et al.* (1988) who investigated blood leucocyte DNA from 53 unrelated Caucasians (29 EM 24 PM) and 29 phenotyped members of six families each ascertained via a PM. The DNA was digested with restriction endonucleases (RE) subjected to electrophoresis and probed with ^{32}P-labelled db1 cDNA. Restriction fragment length polymorphisms (RFLP) were demonstrated using 13 of the 20 RE indicating that the gene is highly polymorphic. The pattern obtained with the RE *Xba*I was informative and will suffice to illustrate the results (Fig. 7.12). It is to be noted, however, that RFLP analysis with any RE tested so far can predict only 20 to 25% of PM phenotypes.

The complete cDNA of the debrisoquine hydroxylase gene (now known as *CYP 2D6*) was published by Gonzalez *et al.* (1988b). It had nine exons. Kimura *et al.* (1989) constructed a genomic library from the lymphocytic DNA of an EM identified by pedigree analysis to be homozygous. There followed the discovery of two genes closely resembling but different from *CYP 2D6*. Three genes aligned in a row were designated *CYP 2D6*, *CYP 2D7* and *CYP 2D8*. The complete DNA sequences of all three genes are shown in the paper of Kimura *et al.* (1989). Due to the insertion of an extra T in the first exon at position +226 the reading frame of *CYP 2D7* is disrupted leading to a termination codon in exon 5. Probably the mRNA is unstable and incapable of producing a functional enzyme. The *CYP 2D8* gene as compared with *CYP 2D6* has multiple deletions and insertions in its exonic sequences so that it can be regarded as a pseudogene.

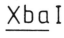

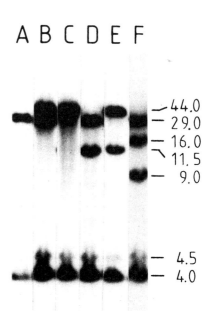

Fig. 7.12. Southern blot analysis of human leucocyte DNA after digestion with the restriction nuclease *Xba*I and hybridization with the ^{32}P-labelled full-length human cytochrome P450 db1 cDNA probe. One example of each observed restriction pattern is shown. Numbers indicate fragment size in kb. (From Skoda *et al.* 1988.)

It was suggested that the *CYP 2D6* gene may be beginning to vanish due to the lack of selection pressure from plant toxins (Heim & Meyer 1992) and the occurrence of gene conversion between the pseudogene and the *CYP 2D6* gene might hasten the introduction of mutations into *CYP 2D6* (Kimura *et al.* 1989).

Eight mutant *CYP 2D6* alleles are described in Table 7.6.

The variant **b** described by Gonzalez *et al.* (1988a) is considered now not to arise from *CYP 2D6* (Kimura *et al.* 1989; Gough *et al.* 1990).

The variant **a** of Gough *et al.* (1990) is the same as the variant 29B of Kagimoto *et al.* (1990). The main transition is at base No. 1934 in Kagimoto *et al.* (1990) but the change is shown at base No. 506 in Gough *et al.* (1990) because the latter do not include intronic bases in their enumeration. Gonza-

Table 7.6. CYP2D6 *alleles in Europeans*

XbaI alleles (kb) [a]	Bam HI alleles (kb) [b]	Structural characteristics	Designation according to Broly *et al.* 1991[c]	Functional capability of the gene product	Estimated population frequency[c]
29	Wt (7 + 4.4) present	29N wild type (wt)	D6	Normal conferring the EM phenotype	0.66 ± 0.02
44	No information	wt complex gene rearrangement (see text)[c]	D6(E)	Normal conferring the EM phenotype	0.03 ± 0.01
29	Mutant (7 + 4.4) present	29A. Deletion of nucleotide 2637A in exon 5 leading to a frameshift [d]	D6(A)	Nil	0.02 ± 0.01
29	Mutant (7 + 4.4) absent	29B. The most important change is one nucleotide deletion 1934 G → A at the 3' end of intron 3 leading to the formation of a premature stop codon and the production of a truncated gene produce [d,e]	D6(B)	Nil	0.13 ± 0.01
29	Mutant presumably (7 + 4.4) absent	29B' same as 29B plus a silent 1749 G → C mutation in exon 3d	D6(B)	Nil	Incorporated in above
44	No information	Same as 29B with additional intronic mutations deletions and insertions plus a 15 kb insertion of D7' [a,c,f,g,h]	D6(B)	Nil	0.08 ± 0.01
(16 + 9)	No information	Contains the splice-site mutation 29B [c,i]	D6(B)	Nil	0.01 ± 0.01
11.5	No information	Deletion of the entire functional gene [g,e]	D6(D)	Nil	0.05 ± 0.01
29	No information	Three base pair deletion at the 3' end of exon 5 leads to loss of lys 281[j]	D6(C)	K_m same as wt but low V_{max} and diminished quantity of immuno-reactive protein	0.02 ± 0.01

[a] Skoda *et al.* 1988a.
[b] Evans & Relling 1990.
[c] Broly *et al.* 1991b.
[d] Kagimoto *et al.* 1990.
[e] Gough *et al.* 1990.
[f] Hanioka *et al.* 1990.
[g] Gaedigk *et al.* 1991.
[h] Gonzalez & Meyer 1991.
[i] Daly *et al.* 1990.
[j] Tyndale *et al.* 1991a.

lez *et al.* (1988a) also marked base 506 but no comment was made about it.

The most important single base change is considered to be 1934 G → A because it should cause the formation of an incorrectly spliced primary transcript and result in an mRNA having a single base deletion. This change would lead to a stop codon 40 bases further on giving a non-functional truncated gene product (Fig. 7.13). The production of such a molecule has not, however, as yet been directly demonstrated.

The other mutations in the 29B alleles were found by Kagimoto *et al.* (1990) to be:

Silent mutation   1085 C → G   (exon 2)
Silent mutation   1749 G → C   (exon 3)
Silent mutation   2185 A → G   (intron 4)
Mutation 188 C → T giving   34 Pro → Ser (exon 1)
Mutation 1062 C → A giving   91 Leu → Met (exon 2)
Mutation 1072 A → G giving   94 His → Arg (exon 2)
Mutation 4268 G → C giving   486 Ser → Thr (exon 9)

The paper of Hanioka *et al.* (1990) dealt with the 44 kb mutant allele. This had the same base changes as the 29B allele of Kagimoto *et al.* (1990) with the following additions:

398 G → T   (intron 1)
688 C deleted   (intron 1)
834 C → G   (intron 1)
931 T → G   (intron 1)
P1413/1414 G inserted (intron 2)
G1520 C1521 → CA   (intron 2)
A1524 G1525 → GC   (intron 2)
3472 A → C   (intron 7)
3670 A → G   (intron 7)

So the effective mRNA and protein production is the same as 29B.

An interesting family study (Evans & Relling 1990) demonstrated that the *Xba*I (16 + 9) allele conferred a non-functional enzyme. The same family also showed the existence of three types of

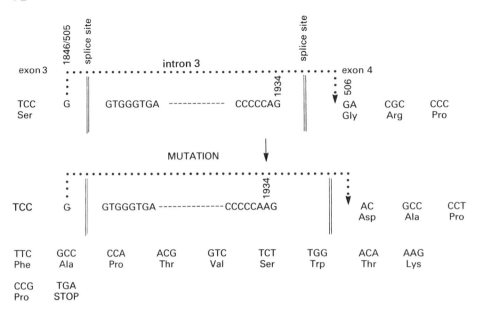

Fig. 7.13. The proposed mechanism for the B variants. When 1934G is mutated to A, the end of intron 3 is then signalled by an AG base pair which is one base further on. The G from the end of exon 3 was formerly part of a triplet GGA coding for glycine, but in the mutant is part of the triplet GAC coding for aspartic acid. Due to the frameshift, new triplets code for a new series of amino acids and at 1974 1975 and 1976 the triplet TGA is a STOP codon. The numbers 505 and 506 relate to the cDNA. Alternatively if intron 3 is not spliced out the message reads GGT (Gly) GGG (Gly) TGA (STOP). [Explanation provided by Professor Urs A. Meyer.]

*Xba*I 29 kb alleles, one (29N) giving a functional enzyme and the other two governing non-functional enzymes. The mother in the family who was a PM transmitted different 29 kb alleles encoding non-functional enzymes to her two PM daughters as shown by different *Bam*HI RFLP patterns.

A new mutant was found in the liver of a poor metabolizer by Tyndale *et al.* (1991a). This mutant had a three base pair deletion at the 3'-end of *CYP* 2D6 exon 5 leading to a loss of a lysine. The interesting thing about this mutant is that the gene product retains some degree of enzymic activity.

The gene now designated D6(E) needs some explanation. At first it was thought that a 44 kb fragment on *Xba*I digestion represented an allele which did not produce an active enzyme since it contained a 29B mutation. However, it was found

that in Chinese it was associated with an almost normal functioning enzyme; the same is true for about 9% of European 44 kb fragments. It is suggested that it arose as a result of a crossing over giving a 44 kb allele containing a normal *CYP 2D6* gene and a 11.5 kb allele with a deleted *CYP 2D6* gene (Broly *et al.* 1991b).

The polymerase chain reaction (PCR) was used by Heim & Meyer (1990) to identify the 3 different types of 29 kb alleles produced by *Xba*I digestion of lymphocytic DNA. These alleles were additional to the 44 and 11.5 kb alleles also revealed by *Xba*I digestion. Applying these two techniques to 38 individuals demonstrated the ability to identify over 95% of PM individuals and heterozygous dominants even though the study did not include the rare (16 + 9) kb allele revealed by *Xba*I digestion and the Tyndale *et al.* (1991a) variant.

It was further pointed out by Gonzalez & Meyer (1991) that using both PCR and RFLP analyses the genotypes of the vast majority of phenotypes can be detected. An impressive demonstration of this capability was provided in the paper of Broly *et al.* (1991b). These authors studied a total of 410 healthy European volunteers including 35 members of five families. Of these, 333 individuals including 27 family members had a phenotyping test, PCR and *Xba*I RFLP determined. Of 318 unrelated phenotyped volunteers 77 were PM which is a frequency more than three times higher than in the general population and this selection was deliberate to study as many mutants as possible. Using the figure of 7.40% given by Alvan *et al.* (1990) the population frequencies of the alleles were computed as shown in Table 7.6. A few rare mutant alleles may still remain to be discovered in Europeans.

With the 9 alleles in Table 7.6 45 genotypes are possible and some of them will be excessively rare. For practical purposes all the D6(B) mutations can be combined to given an allele frequency of 0.22, and reduces the number of combinations to 21. The combinations estimated to represent more than 1% of the population are as follows with their percentages:-

EM	D6/D6	43.56
	D6/D6(E)	3.96
	D6/D6(A)	2.64
	D6/D6(B)	29.04
	D6/D6(D)	6.60
	D6/D6(C)	2.64
	D6(E)/D6(B)	1.32
PM	D6(B)/D6(B)	4.84
	D6(B)/D6(D)	2.20

leaving less than 5% to be accounted for by the other 12 combinations. Three genotypes stand out, namely, the homozygous D6/D6 and heterozygous D6/D6(B) amongst the extensive metabolizers, whilst the homozygous D6(B)/D6(B) account for a majority of poor metabolizers.

A Swedish study of 223 individuals (Dahl *et al.* 1992) which included RFLP analysis and *CYP 2D6*-specific PCR amplification for the *wt*, *29A* and *29B* alleles, and a British study of 72 individuals (Armstrong *et al.* 1992) which included RFLP analysis for *CYP 2D6 D* and *E* with PCR amplification for *CYP 2D6 A* and *B*, gave similar results. There was a suggestion that *CYP 2D6 B* may be commoner in the Swedish than in the British population.

Previously it was possible (Evans *et al.* 1980, Steiner *et al.* 1985) to (1) observe heterozygotes in pedigrees and show that they were widely distributed in the EM mode in a histogram of $\log_{10}$ debrisoquine MR values, (2) compute the mean value for EM homozygotes and (3) compute the degree of dominance. In the papers of Broly *et al.* (1991) and Dahl *et al.* (1992) the frequency distributions of homozygous and heterozygous EM individuals were

demonstrated as a result of direct genotyping, in histograms of debrisoquine/sparteine and desipramine $\log_{10}$ MR values.

Chimeric genes were constructed by Kagimoto *et al.* (1990), each containing a 5'-end, a middle portion and a 3'-end, derived variously from wt and 29B genes. These chimeric genes were expressed in COS-1 cells in culture. Mutations in exon 1 resulted in a functionally deficient protein and the mutation at the intron 3/exon 4 splice site in an absent protein. Mutations in exons 2 and 9 were of no consequence for function. This work emphasizes the functional significance of the D6(B) mutations.

The debrisoquine polymorphism is probably the mechanistically best understood variation in drug metabolism. The molecular genetics has been dealt with in some detail because of this and to illustrate the future potential of genetic analysis in pharmacogenetics.

CHROMOSOMAL LOCALIZATION

In order to discover the chromosomal assignment of the gene controlling cytochrome P450 2D Eichelbaum *et al.* (1987) carried out a linkage study of 29 polymorphic markers with the debrisoquine phenotype.

After phenotyping 990 unselected subjects of German origin 64 poor metabolizers were identified. The metabolism of sparteine was then studied in the families of 21 of them.

Linkage analysis to the marker systems yielded negative or non-informative results for all polymorphisms with the exception of the P_1 blood group. A computer calculation based on 15 informative families gave a maximal LOD (logarithm of the odds ratio) score of 3.35 for both paternal and maternal recombination fractions $\Theta m = \Theta f = 0.0$. This result proved tight linkage since recombination is less than 2%. (For an explanation of LOD scores and linkage calculations see Emery 1976.)

It was already known that P_1 was located on the long arm of chromosome 22 and so this is the chromosome which carries the gene for the debrisoquine/sparteine polymorphism. Gonzalez *et al.* (1988b) reached the same conclusion, localizing the gene *CYP 2D* at 22q11.2–q12.2.

INTER-ETHNIC VARIABILITY

A large number of population studies have been performed and a representative selection is shown in Table 7.7.

An important point was emphasized by Idle (1989), Caporaso & Pickle (1989), Yue *et al.* (1989a), Lee *et al.* (1988) and Arias & Jorge (1989), namely, that the antimodal dividing point for metabolic ratio to define phenotypes needs to be determined from the frequency distribution of each ethnic group and not transposed from one ethnic group to another.

Considering the debrisoquine tests alone, it is clear that there is a profound difference between Europeans and Orientals. Pooling the series gives a frequency of the PM phenotype in Europeans of $596/7577 = 7.87\%$ (Alvan *et al.* (1990) performed a meta-analysis incorporating many personal communications and gave a figure of $7.65 \pm \text{SD } 2.17$), and in the Orientals $12/1287 = 1.12\%$ ($\chi_i^2 = 82.78$, $p > 0.001$).

Tests performed with sparteine and other compounds have given very similar results.

The African results are variable and native American series few in number. It is possible that results like those found in the San Bushmen and the two Amerindian series could have arisen by means of genetic drift.

When two compounds have been tested on the same population then some interesting results have been found. In Europeans there is ample evidence that debrisoquine and sparteine are detecting the same genetically determined phenotypes (e.g. Evans *et al.* 1983; Inaba *et al.* 1983).

The results of debrisoquine and dextromethorphan phenotyping tests have been shown to correlate well by, for example, Jacq *et al.* (1988) and Henthorne *et al.* (1989); likewise, debrisoquine and metoprolol (McGourty *et al.* 1985). Debrisoquine 4-hydroxylation and codeine oxidative demethylation (Fig. 7.14) have also been shown to correlate in Caucasians by Yue *et al.* (1989a) but no poor metabolizers were demonstrable using codeine in Chinese (Yue *et al.* 1989b). The frequency distribution histograms for codeine *O*-demethylation metabolic ratio published by Yue *et al.* (1989b) show a bimodality in Europeans similar to that found with debrisoquine. In 133 Chinese, however, there was no bimodality and the whole histogram was at a

higher level than that of the Europeans. This is unlike the result obtained using debrisoquine in Chinese by Xu & Jiang (1990), where three poor metabolizers were discerned separate from the mode of the 217 extensive metabolizers.

The comparison of Chinese and Caucasian populations with respect to *CYP 2D6* alleles has yielded interesting results. A low frequency of poor metabolizers of debrisoquine was found in Oriental populations, but the matter on closer examination turns out to be more complex than a simple difference in the frequency of the same alleles. When codeine *O*-demethylation was studied in 115 Chinese only one PM by Caucasian criteria was found whilst the other 114 were distributed in a single mode (Johansson *et al.* 1991b). A detailed pharmacokinetic study of eight Caucasian EM and eight Chinese showed no significant difference in their partial metabolic clearance of codeine by *O*-demethylation (Yue *et al.* 1991). Examination of *CYP 2D6* by *Xba*I RFLP analysis showed the presence of heterozygotes and homozygotes for the 44 kb allele in the EM mode (Yue *et al.* 1989c) though the latter did lie at the high MR end. The techniques employed in this study were not able to differentiate different 29 kb fragments, a situation which was remedied by Johansson *et al.* (1991), who used in addition PCR specific amplification of the wild type gene and *CYP 2D6A* (29A) and *CYP 26B* (29B). Neither 29A nor 29B was discovered amongst the 115 subjects. One individual with an 11.5/11.5 kb genotype was the only PM. It was clear that the Chinese 44 kb fragment did not contain the 29B mutation and did possess considerable enzymic activity. This is the D6(E) mutant of Broly *et al.* (1991b), which was noted by them to occur in a Korean and an Egyptian and in a small minority of Europeans with the 44 kb allelic fragment. By changing the electrophoretic conditions on agarose gel Mura *et al.* (1991) were able to show that the apparent size of the Chinese fragment was 40 kb. The Caucasian fragment continued to exhibit a 44 kb size with the changed electrophoretic technique.

In Japanese subjects Horai *et al.* (1989) studied 55 individuals out of 292 who had previously been tested with metoprolol. The 55 included the 1 PM of metoprolol found on the previous survey (Horai *et al.* 1988). When the 55 subjects were tested with debrisoquine and sparteine this one individual was shown to be the only PM for both drugs. So the

Table 7.7. *Inter-ethnic variability in the debrisoquine/sparteine polymorphism*

Reference	Ethnic group	Total number examined	Number of poor metabolizers	q
Debrisoquine tests				
Europeans				
Alvan *et al.* 1982	Swedish	155	5	0.180
Arvela *et al.* 1988	Finns	155	5	0.180
Arvela *et al.* 1988	Lapps	70	6	0.293
Bechtel *et al.* 1986	French	116	11	0.308
Benitez *et al.* 1988	Spanish	185	25	0.368
Clark *et al.* 1985	Presumed British Whites	104	6	0.240
Dick *et al.* 1982	Swiss	222	22	0.315
Evans *et al.* 1980	British white	258	23	0.299
Evans *et al.* 1983	British white	215	14	0.255
Henthorn *et al.* 1989	Spanish	124	13	0.324
Inaba *et al.* 1983	Canadian Caucasians	32	4	0.353
Kallio *et al.* 1988	Finns	211	11	0.228
McGourty *et al.* 1985	British white	143	12	0.290
Mahgoub *et al.* 1977	Presumed British	94	3	0.179
Meier *et al.* 1983	Swiss	61	2	0.181
Peart *et al.* 1986	Caucasian Australians	100	6	0.245
Roots *et al.* 1988	German	270	30	0.333
Zschiesche *et al.* 1990	German	145	17	0.342
Sylvalahti *et al.* 1986	Finns	107	6	0.237
Szorady & Santa 1987	Hungarians	100	8	0.283
Veronese & McLean 1991b	Tasmanians	152	13	0.292
Vincent-Viry *et al.* 1991b	French	3065	250	0.286
Spina *et al.* 1991	Italians	67	5	0.273
Horsmans *et al.* 1991	Belgians	167	12	0.268
Spina *et al.* 1992a	Italians	137	10	0.270
Bertilsson *et al.* 1992	Swedish[a]	1011	69	0.261
Wanwimolruk *et al.* 1992	New Zealand Caucasians	111	8	0.268
Middle Eastern populations				
Islam & Idle 1980	Saudis	102	1	0.099
Idle & Smith 1984	Egyptians	72	1	0.118
Idle & Smith 1984	Iraqis	260	9	0.186
Sardas *et al.* 1991	Turks	93	1	0.104
Asiatics				
Idle & Smith 1984	Indians	147	3	0.143
Africans				
Iyun *et al.* 1986	Nigerians (Ibadan)	138	0	0.000
Mbanefo *et al.* 1980	Nigerians (Ibadan)	123	10	0.285
Sommers *et al.* 1988	San Bushmen	96	18	0.433
Woolhouse *et al.* 1985	Ghanaians	141	10	0.266
Sommers *et al.* 1989b	Venda (South Africa)	98	4	0.202
Lennard *et al.* 1992	Nigerians	102	5	0.221
Americans				
Arias & Jorge 1989	Ngawbé Guaymi Amerindians (Panama)	84	5	0.244
Jorge *et al.* 1990	Cuna Amerindians (Panama)	89	0	0.000
Orientals				
Lee *et al.* 1988	Chinese	97	0	0.000
Nakamura *et al.* 1985	Japanese	100	0	0.000
Lou *et al.* 1987	Chinese	269	2	0.086

Table 7.7 (*cont.*)

Reference	Ethnic group	Total number examined	Number of poor metabolizers	q
Xu & Jiang 1990	Chinese	220	3	0.117
Du & Lou 1990	Chinese	140	2	0.119
Wanwimolruk *et al.* 1990	Thai	173	2	0.107
Bertilsson *et al.* 1992	Chinese: Han[b]	279	3	0.104
Bertilsson *et al.* 1992	Mongolian[b]	128	1	0.088
Bertilsson *et al.* 1992	Wei	153	1	0.080
Bertilsson *et al.* 1992	Zang	135	2	0.122
Polynesians				
Wanwimolruk *et al.* 1992	New Zealand Polynesians	55	4	0.270
Sparteine tests				
Arias *et al.* 1988a	Cuna Indians (Panama)	142	0	0.000
Arias *et al.* 1998b	Ngawbe Guaymi Amerindians (Panama)	95	5	0.227
Brosen 1986	Greenlanders	185	6	0.227
Clasen *et al.* 1991	East Greenlanders[c]	300	10	0.183
Clasen *et al.* 1991	West Greenlanders[c]	171	4	0.153
Brosen *et al.* 1985	Danes	301	22	0.270
Ebner *et al.* 1989	German	121	9	0.273
Eichelbaum *et al.* 1978	German	380	18	0.218
Eichelbaum & Woodhouse 1985	Ghanaians	154	0	0.000
Evans *et al.* 1983	British white	215	12	0.236
Ishizaki *et al.* 1987	Japanese	84	2	0.154
Vinks *et al.* 1982	Canadian Caucasians	48	4	0.289
Somers *et al.* 1990	Barakwena	97	3	0.176
Somers *et al.* 1991	Venda (South Africa)	97	0	0.000
Lennard *et al.* 1992	Nigerians	106	4	0.194
Tests using other compounds				
Bufarol				
Dayer *et al.* 1982a	Swiss	154	12	0.279
Codeine				
Yue *et al.* (1989b)	Swedes	132	18	0.369
Dextromethorphan				
Guttendorf *et al.* 1988	?Caucasian Americans	65	4	0.248
Henthorne *et al.* 1989	Spanish (with debris)	124	13	0.324
Hildebrand *et al.* 1989	?Germans	450	46	0.320
Jacq *et al.* 1988	French	132	4	0.174
Larrey *et al.* 1987	French	103	4	0.197
Faccini *et al.* 1990	Italian	146	12	0.287
Freche *et al.* 1990	French	216	11	0.226
Schmid *et al.* 1985	Swiss	268	23	0.293
Vetticaden *et al.* 1989	Dutch	44	4	0.302
Nsabiyumva *et al.* 1991	Burundis	100	5	0.224
Metoprolol				
Horai *et al.* 1989	Japanese	292	1	0.058
Iyun *et al.* 1986	Nigerian (Ibadan) (with debris)	138	0	0.000
Lennard *et al.* 1983	British white	119	8	0.259
McGourty *et al.* 1985	British white (with debris)	143	12	0.290
Sommers *et al.* 1989a	San Bushmen	98	4	0.202
Sommers *et al.* 1989b	Venda (South Africa)	94	7	0.2730
Sohn *et al.* 1991	Chinese	107	0	0.000

Table 7.7 (*cont.*)

Reference	Ethnic group	Total number examined	Number of poor metabolizers	q
Sohn *et al.* 1991	Koreans	218	1	0.068
Sohn *et al.* 1991	Japanese	295	2	0.082
Lennard *et al.* 1992	Nigerians	141	0	0.000
Phenformin				
Oates *et al.* 1982a	?British white	195	18	0.304
Woolhouse *et al.* 1985	Ghanaians (with debris)	143	11	0.277

[a]757 previously reported (Steiner *et al.* 1988)
[b]145 Han and 124 Mongolians previously reported (Lou *et al.* 1987).
[c]Antimode not distinct.
'(with debris)' indicates that the same subjects were also investigated with debrisoquine.

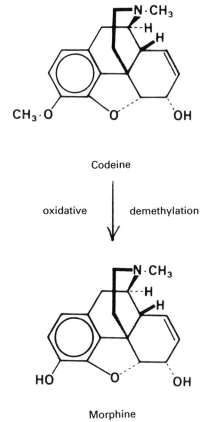

Codeine

oxidative demethylation

Morphine

Fig. 7.14. The metabolism of codeine which is controlled by the debrisoquine/sparteine polymorphism. (Structural formulae from *Clarke's Isolation and Identification of Drugs, 1986*.)

oxidation of these three compounds would appear to be under common genetic control in Japanese (see also Horai *et al.* 1990).

An inter-ethnic difference was found by Lennard *et al.* (1989) in the case of metoprolol α-hydroxylation in that amongst EMs the S/R ratios were higher in Caucasians than Nigerians. This suggests the possibility that there may be a subtle difference in the structure and/or function of the cytochrome P450 in EMs of the two ethnic groups.

Anomalies arise in studies of African populations. Iyun *et al.* (1986) found no PMs of either debrisoquine or metoprolol among 138 Nigerians in Ibadan, which was contrary to the experience of Mbanefo *et al.* (1980) who found 10 PMs among 123 Nigerians in Ibadan. Lancaster *et al.* (1990) raise the possibility that some anomalous results in Africans may be attributed to the presence of antimalarials in the livers of the individuals tested.

In a further study of Nigerians by Lennard *et al.* (1992), 141 individuals took metoprolol (M), 106 took sparteine (S) and 102 took debrisoquine (D). Of these 86 took M & S, 38 D & S, 33 M & D and 24 M, S & D on different occasions. A weak correlation ($r = 0.51$) was observed between the MR values of M & S and nil significance for the other two comparisons. Five subjects with high MR values for D indicated the presence of the polymorphism (unlike the results of Iyun *et al.* (1986)). Two out of four individuals with high MR values for S were tested with D and one was a PM and also had the highest MR for M. The frequency distribution histogram of MR values for M showed no bimodality. This study indicates a dissociation of controls of M, D and S oxidation at a phenotypic level in Nigerians. Possibly direct genotyping may clarify the situation.

Amongst Ghanaians, Woolhouse *et al.* (1985) found bimodal distributions of the metabolic ratios of debrisoquine (with 10 PMs out of 141 subjects) and phenformin (with 11 PMs out of 143 subjects). All the 10 PMs of debrisoquine were also PMs of phenformin and all the 131 EMs of debrisoquine were also EMs of phenformin. However, not a single PM for sparteine was found on testing 154 subjects (including the 143 tested for phenformin). This finding needs to be confirmed as it may indicate a difference in the genetic control of the relevant cytochromes P450 in Ghanaians compared with Europeans. At present, one can only speculate about the molecular basis of this inter-ethnic difference.

Sommers *et al.* (1988) found a relatively high frequency of PM of debrisoquine (18 PM 78 EM) amongst San Bushmen but this was not paralleled by metoprolol testing (4 PM 94 EM). Another anomaly but in a reverse direction was found by Sommers *et al.* (1989b) amongst the Venda where debrisoquine typing gave 94 EM 4 PM but metoprolol typing gave 87 EM 7 PM and none of the poor metabolizers of metoprolol were poor metabolizers of debrisoquine.

So it appears possible, from these relatively few results, that compounds which appear to be oxidized by the same mechanism in Caucasians and Orientals are oxidized by different mechanisms in Africans. These anomalous observations on African populations might be explained by a mechanism similar to that reported by Matsunaga *et al.* (1990). They found in a rat enzyme designated cytochrome P450 2D1 that a single amino acid change at position 380 from isoleucine to phenylalanine markedly lowered the catalytic activity for bufuralol, whilst debrisoquine hydroxylation was different in the two enzymes in the reverse direction. This observation suggests the possibility that a lot more is yet to be discovered about human inter-ethnic variability.

CLINICAL CONSEQUENCES

The clinical consequences of having two phenotypes in the debrisoquine/sparteine polymorphism depend upon which particular drug is being considered. In general the poor metabolizer has a much smaller 'first pass' effect than the extensive metabolizer. This means that a much larger proportion of the drug molecules which are absorbed from the alimentary tract are bio-transformed in the liver in an unit time in extensive metabolizers. The kinetics of the original molecule and of the metabolites in the plasma will depend also on other factors, particularly liver blood flow and renal excretion.

The same effects will eventually become apparent after an intravenous dose but will not be as immediate because the drug is not being passed directly into the liver from its site of entry into the body.

Repeated dosages by either route will lead to a steady state plasma concentration which will depend amongst other things on the elimination rate constant k_e and that constant will be influenced by the liver metabolism. $\bar{C}p = fD/Vd\ k_e\ T$ where $\bar{C}p$ =average concentration in the plasma at the plateau state, f = fractional absorption, D = dose, Vd = apparent volume of distribution, k_e = elimination rate constant (time^{-1}) = $0.69315/t\frac{1}{2}$, T = dosage interval (time), $t\frac{1}{2}$ = elimination half-time (Fingl & Woodbury 1973). (For an explanation of the source of 0.69315, which is $\log_e 2$: see Appendix II.)

So where the metabolism is less active or absent in the poor metabolizer the half-time will be longer and k_e smaller and $\bar{C}p$ higher than in the extensive metabolizer.

The debrisoquine polymorphism was originally discovered because a single small oral dose produced a hypotensive episode in a poor metabolizer – who was also the prinicipal investigator (Smith 1986). Subsequently, a planned study showed that blood pressure is consistently lower in poor metabolizers than in extensive metabolizers after standard doses (Idle *et al.* 1978).

As more and more drugs have been proven to be substrates for the polymorphism, it has become apparent that the clinical consequences are numerous and diverse (see Brøsen & Gram 1989; Lennard 1990; Eichelbaum & Gross 1990; Alvan 1991, for recent reviews). Usually, the drug itself as administered is the active principle. So, in most instances the poor metabolizer suffers an exaggerated degree of the desired action, as was the case with the debrisoquine/blood pressure example. This is because the standard dose is tailored for the average extensive metabolizer and, since the poor metabolizer has a much higher blood level, he ends up with an overdose and displays toxic symptoms.

Less frequently, other mechanisms operate to the detriment of the poor metabolizer, such as the formation of toxic metabolites because a higher proportion of the ingested molecules traverse what are usually very minor pathways. The most striking example concerned phenacetin, which in extensive metabolizers is mainly converted to paracetamol. Only a little is metabolized along other routes. In poor metabolizers, however, these minor routes become important and a lot of 2-hydroxyphenacetin and 2-hydroxyphenetidine are produced. The latter is responsible for causing methaemoglobinaemia (Shahidi *et al.* 1968; Kong *et al.* 1982).

With encainide the poor metabolizer is disadvantaged because of another mechanism. The compound as administered is a pro-drug, since it requires oxidative *O*-demethylation to produce the active metabolite and so the poor metabolizer fails to benefit from the anti-arrythmic effect. (This view has been disputed by Quart *et al.* 1988.)

In the case of propafenone neurological adverse effects (visual blurring, dizziness, parasthesiae) were associated with high plasma concentrations. The plasma concentrations in patients on regular treatment before dosing were 42 to 1356 ng/ml in EM and 1408 to 1801 ng/ml in PM. Of 22 EMs with chronic ventricular arrhythmia 14% had neurologic symptoms compared with 4 out of 6 PM (Siddoway *et al.* 1987).

The adverse effects suffered by poor metabolizers may occur after just one dose (as was the case with debrisoquine) or may develop after chronic dosing. An extreme example of the latter kind is seen with the anti-anginal drug perhexilene. This drug undergoes oxidation which has been shown to be controlled by the debrisoquine/sparteine polymorphism (Cooper *et al.*, 1984). Perhexilene is a racemic mixture and both enantiomers have very long plasma half-lives even in extensive metabolizers (280 hours in the D-form and 66 hours in the L-form). In poor metabolizers these half-lives are 427 and 157 hours respectively (Idle & Smith 1984). By some means elevated plasma levels lead to a severe peripheral neuropathy and liver damage which has features similar to that caused by ethanol. These two adverse reactions are overwhelmingly exhibited by poor metabolizers (Shah *et al.* 1982b).

Propanolol is subject to an interesting dual oxidation. It had previously been demonstrated that 4'-hydroxylation of propanolol was impaired in poor metabolizers but they did not have diminished oral clearance or enhanced β-blockade (Lennard *et al.*

1984, Raghuram *et al.* 1984). The drug is oxidized by two routes, namely to 4-hydroxypropanolol and to naphthoxy-lactic acid (Fig. 7.15). Now it has been shown that whilst the first pathway is impaired in poor metabolizers of debrisoquine, the second pathway is impaired in poor metabolizers of mephenytoin (qv.). So the compound is oxidized at two different sites in its molecule by two different cytochromes P450. Only in persons who were poor metabolizers of both debrisoquine and mephenytoin were the metabolism and pharmacokinetics greatly disturbed (Ward *et al.*, 1989). A similar mechanism has also been demonstrated for imipramine by Skjelbo *et al.* (1991). In a population of 22 individuals studied, one who was a poor metabolizer of sparteine and a poor metabolizer of mephenytoin had the lowest oral clearance and longest plasma half-life for both imipramine and desmethyl imipramine.

So, in Europeans, if both types of poor metabolizers (debrisoquine and mephenytoin) had a frequency, of say, 5% in the population then this double recessive would represent 1 in 400 of the population. In a general practice list of 2000 there would be about five such persons and it is probable that there might be one or two in any large hospital at any one time.

It is quite likely that other drugs which are oxidized at two molecular sites may be dealt with by two different cytochromes P450 and so an individual would be disadvantaged only if he was a double recessive. The historic phenylbutazone (anti-inflammatory antipyretic uricosuric) may be a case in point since it was oxidized by hepatic microsomes to yield two metabolites, namely, oxyphenbutazone with a hydroxyl group in the para position on a benzene ring, and γ-hydroxy-phenylbutazone with an alcoholic hydroxyl group in the ω-1 position of the η-butyl side chain.

Table 7.8 gives examples of clinical effects in poor metabolizers which have actually been authenticated, i.e. do not rely on extrapolation. There are dangers in extrapolation which are shown by the story of metoprolol. There is no doubt that metoprolol is polymorphically oxidized and that the clearance of the drug is slower in poor metabolizers who also have more long-lasting β-blockade following a single oral dose. Clark *et al.* (1984) have shown that adverse effects in patients treated for hypertension with metoprolol are not generally associated with

Propanolol

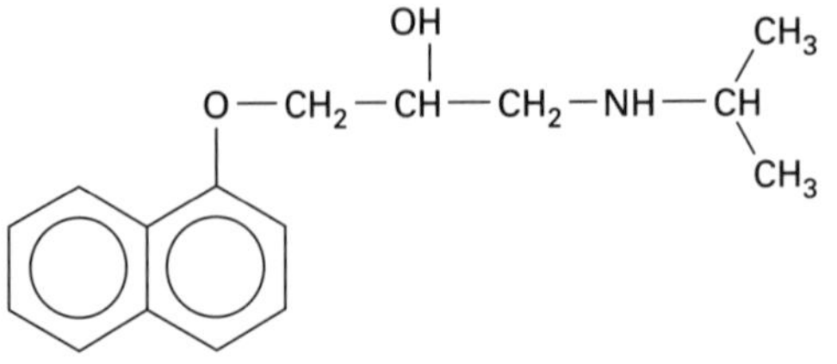

$O-CH_2-CH-CH_2-NH-CH$ with OH and CH_3, CH_3

Side chain oxidation
(mephenytoin polymorphism)

Ring oxidation
(debrisoquine polymorphism)

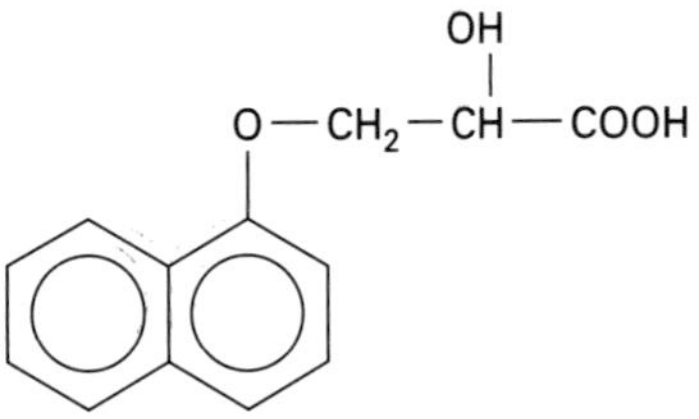

$O-CH_2-CH-COOH$ with OH

$O-CH_2-CH-CH_2-NH-CH$ with OH and CH_3, CH_3; ring OH

Naphthoxylactic acid

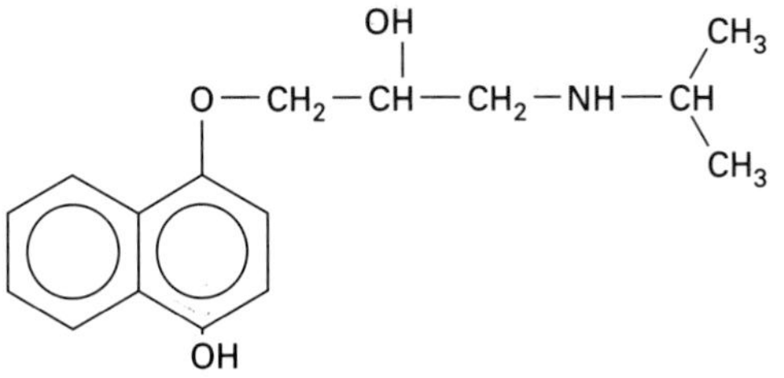

4–hydroxypropanolol

Fig. 7.15. The two routes of oxidation of propanolol, which are controlled by two different cytochrome P450 polymorphisms.

oxidation status. Also Lewis et al. (1991) found in healthy volunteers that fatigue produced by single doses of 100 mg metoprolol was not more pronounced in PM individuals. However, they caution that results obtained in healthy volunteers should not be uncritically extrapolated to patients where the dosage used is often 100 mg twice daily for long periods. Under these circumstances PM patients may be adversely affected more than EM patients. It follows from all this that individual PM patients who feel fatigue or other symptoms on metoprolol may be greatly benefited by a change to atenolol.

In the case of indoramin (an α_1-adrenoceptor antagonist) five poor metabolizer subjects experienced sedation, nausea, dizziness and headache whereas seven extensive metabolizers did not. The difference did not quite reach statistical significance but this is most likely because the numbers were small (Pierce et al. 1987).

There is ample evidence that tricyclic antidepressants are oxidized polymorphically by the debrisoquine/sparteine system, e.g. amitriptyline (Mellstrom et al. 1986), imipramine and its metabolites (Brøsen et al. 1986b,) and desmethyl impra-

mine (Spina et al. 1987). Nortriptyline E-10 hydroxylation has been referred to previously.

Now Dahl-Puustinen et al. (1989) have shown that the pharmacokinetics of the neuroleptic perphenazine are related to the debrisoquine/sparteine polymorphism. Serum concentrations of the compound were significantly higher over more than 24 hours in poor compared with extensive hydroxylators after a single oral dose of 6 mg.

This development adds weight to the previous suggestion by Balant-Gorgia et al. (1986) that interaction between tricyclic antidepressants and some neuroleptics may give more toxic effects in poor metabolizers. Some additional emphasis is provided by the observations of Derenne et al. (1989) who showed that debrisoquine metabolic ratios were moved to higher levels in persons receiving combinations of tricyclics and neuroleptics.

The observations of Llerena et al. (1992a) and Spina et al. (1992a) indicate that haloperidol is another compound which produces side effects more in poor than in extensive metabolizers. This finding matches the correlation of plasma levels with phenotyping information and the inhibition of cytochrome P450 2D6 in vitro by haloperidol. [The subject was made more complicated by the demonstration that cytochrome P450 2D6 is responsible for the oxidation of the reduced metabolite of halop-

Table 7.8. *Proven clinical consequences of the debrisoquine/sparteine polymorphism*

Drug	Clinical effect in poor metabolizer	Reference
Bufuralol	Pallor, sweating, nausea, vomiting, bradycardia, hypotension	Dayer *et al.* 1982b
Captopril	Agranulocytosis occurred as a side effect in two patients both found to be PM	Oates *et al.* 1982b
Codeine	Lack of increase in pain threshold	Sindrup *et al.* 1991
Debrisoquine	Orthostatic hypotension	Idle *et al.* 1978; Lennard *et al.* 1983
Encainide	Lack of anti-arrhythmic effect. Requires high dose. Disputed by Quart *et al.* 1988 but supported by Karalis *et al.* 1990	Carey *et al.* 1981; Roden *et al.* 1981
Flecainide	High plasma concentrations can be anticipated in PM with renal impairment. Sudden deaths in people on drug are associated with high plasma levels and are attributed to pro-arrhythmic effects (precipitation of arrhythmia by anti-arrhythmic drugs)	Mikus *et al.* 1989
Haloperidol	Stiffness, paresthesias, restlessness in 3 PM individuals	Llerena *et al.* 1992a
Haloperidol, thioridazine levopromazine & chlorpromazine	Oversedation, drowsiness, postural hypotension, diplopia, dry mouth	Spina *et al.* 1992b
Phenacetin	More methaemoglobinaemia and more 2 hydroxy-phenacetin and 2 hydroxy-phenetidine	Kong *et al.* 1982
Phenformin	Healthy subjects with genetically impaired debrisoquine oxidation also have an impaired ability to hydroxylate phenformin. After a single oral dose of 50 mg phenformin to normal healthy persons of known debrisoquine oxidation phenotype PM develop higher plasma levels of phenformin and lactate. Several patients who had developed lactic acidosis whilst on treatment with phenformin had an impaired ability to oxidize phenformin	Shah *et al.* 1985
Propafenone	Central nervous system effects (visual blurring, dizziness and paresthesia) associated with higher trough plasma concentrations. β-blockade greater	Siddoway *et al.* 1987 Lee *et al.* 1990
Propanolol	Tiredness, dizziness and syncope in a single patient. Phenotyped later as a PM	Shah *et al.* 1982a
Sparteine	Excessive uterine contraction	Filler *et al.* 1964; Newton *et al.* 1966; Eichelbaum *et al.* 1988

eridol back to haloperidol as shown by Tyndale *et al.* (1991b).

Hence, it would appear that the debrisoquine/sparteine polymorphism is of great importance in psychiatric patients with the poor metabolizers being especially at risk. Pollock *et al.* (1992) discuss the point, particularly from the geriatric aspect. Age-induced changes in physiological functions (e.g. renal function as shown by creatinine clearance) may alter the metabolism of some drugs which interact with subtrates for the debrisoquine polymorphism even though the metabolism of debrisoquine itself is not affected. Routine pretreatment phenotyping (or genotyping) was advocated in elderly psychiatric patients.

The problems of genetically determined ultra-rapid hydroxylators have largely been ignored. Their treatment with the appropriate drug may be abandoned because conventional doses fail to produce the desired effect. Bertilsson *et al.* (1993) described two depressed patients of this type who responded to high doses of tricyclic antidepressants.

There are obviously a large number of possibilities for clinically significant effects of co-administration of drugs which are listed in Table 7.2. Some combinations which occur in clinical practice (e.g. cardiovascular drugs and psychiatric drugs) have already been mentioned. Other combinations remain unexplored.

Quinidine inhibition of drug metabolism by EM patients has already been mentioned. The clinical implications were extensively reviewed by Caporaso & Shaw (1991). They point to the following possible consequences of the administration of quinidine with drugs listed in Table 7.2: toxic effects, diminished effect (in the case of codeine) and interference with phenotyping data in surveys to see if there is an association between the polymorphism and stated disorders.

In a huge screening survey of a French population (Vincent-Viry *et al.* 1991) 22 blood constituents, 6 morphologic variables, 13 types of pathology and 3 environmental variables were assessed in the two phenotypes. Statistically significant differences were found in mean red cell volume, mean corpuscular haemoglobin concentration, serum albumin concentration and ponderal index (PMs weighed more).

ASSOCIATIONS BETWEEN DEBRISOQUINE/SPARTEINE PHENOTYPES AND SPONTANEOUS DISORDERS

Cancers

The most interesting topic is undoubtedly cancer. There is a possibility that procarcinogens may be converted into carcinogens by oxidation. Consequently, cancer patient populations have been investigated for the distribution of the debrisoquine/sparteine phenotype within them.

The first account of Hetzel *et al.* (1980) was amplified by Law *et al.* (1989), who investigated 104 patients with bronchial carcinoma and found they included two poor metabolizers. This population was compared with 104 smoking controls who included nine poor metabolizers. Later the same group (Ayesh *et al.* 1984) reported a new series of patients. They found 21 poor metabolizers out of 234 smoking controls as compared with only four poor metabolizers amongst 245 patients with bronchogenic carcinoma. Furthermore, the whole distribution curve of metabolic ratios was shifted towards lower values in the cancer population, suggesting that it may have had within it a higher proportion of homozygous dominants. Roots *et al.* (1988) demonstrated that the debrisoquine metabolic ratio remained constant in 14 EM and four PM patients following tumour resection and other treatments.

More data have been gathered by other groups (Table 7.9) and when analysed together the available information indicates a significant association of the extensive metabolizer with lung cancer. How-

ever, there is also significant heterogeneity mainly due to the series of Speirs *et al.* (1990). The possible reasons why Speirs's group's results were different is extensively discussed in their paper and no explanation has been found after considering geographic location, selection of patients, histological type of tumour and the way in which the phenotyping test was conducted. Further implications of the data of Ayesh *et al.* (1984) were examined by Caporaso *et al.* (1989a, b), the latter paper exploring the EM-cancer of the lung association in relation to the synergism between smoking and occupational exposure, for example to asbestos.

Both Roots *et al.* (1989) and Horsmans *et al.* (1991) make the point that their series of bronchial carcinoma patients contained no PM individuals under 50 years of age. Obviously this could be an important observation.

Unfortunately the data given by Gough *et al.* (1990) are so sparse that it is not possible to incorporate their data into any more general analysis, but they report a significant reduction in the number of poor metabolizers.

An attempt was made by Sugimura *et al.* (1990) to genotype patients with lung cancer and controls using the *Xba*I RFLP method referred to earlier. Unfortunately, this method by itself was not very informative. Much better information would be obtained by applying the combined *Xba*I and PCR techniques of Broly *et al.* (1991b). Bronchial carcinoma is well known to produce many metabolic sequelae. Direct genotyping would eliminate such processes which have an effect on the phenotyping procedure and thus affect the observed association. If it were proved that extensive metabolizer genotypes were associated with bronchial carcinoma, then two possible interpretations might be (1) activation of procarcinogens by oxidation under the influence of *CYP 2D6* gene products, (2) linkage of *CYP 2D6* to some other gene important in cancer production.

Molecular genetic techniques were also applied to the problem by Wolf *et al.* (1992). In 361 lung cancer patients the genotype frequencies were not significantly different from those in 720 controls. These authors also make the suggestion that the presence of the disease may interfere with the phenotyping process.

Five series of bladder cancer patients have been studied (Table 7.10). Although the Japanese series

Table 7.9. *The association between extensive metabolizer phenotype and bronchial carcinoma*

Reference	Location of study	Number of Subjects Lung cancer EM	PM	Controls EM	PM	Approximate relative risk (x)	$\log_e x$ (y)	Sampling variance (V)	Weight $\left(\frac{1}{V} = w\right)$	Significance of difference from zero (wy^2)	wy
Ayesh *et al.* 1984	London	241	4	213	21	5.4044	1.6872	0.2543	3.9330	11.1959	6.6358
Roots *et al.* 1989	Berlin	280	21	328	40	1.6085	0.4753	0.0764	13.0818	2.9551	6.2176
Law *et al.* 1989	London	102	2	95	9	4.0785	1.4057	0.4535	2.2053	4.3578	3.1000
Faccini *et al.* 1990	Verona	20	0	132	12	3.8679	1.3527	1.1321	0.8833	1.6164	1.1949
Speirs *et al.* 1990	London	74	8	235	23	0.8746	−0.1340	0.1703	5.8703	0.1054	−0.7865
Caporaso *et al.* 1990	Baltimore	95	1	80	2	9.8861	2.2911	0.5997	1.6675	8.7534	3.8205
Benitez *et al.* 1991	Madrid	80	4	133	10	1.4070	0.3414	0.3107	3.2183	0.3752	1.0989
Duche *et al.* 1991	Besançon & Creteil	143	10	123	12	1.3833	0.3244	0.0914	10.9386	1.1515	3.5490
Horsmans et al. 1991	Brussels	86	51	155	2	1.2642	0.2345	0.2615	3.8242	0.2102	0.8967
								Totals	45.6225	30.7210	25.7270

Mean value of $y = Y = \frac{\Sigma wy}{\Sigma w} = 0.6734$; antilog of $Y = X = 1.9608$.

$\text{SE }(Y) = \sqrt{\frac{1}{\Sigma w}} = 0.1480$.

95% of fiducial limits of $Y = Y \pm t_{8, 0.05}\sqrt{\frac{1}{\Sigma w}} = 1.0148$ and 0.3320.

The equivalent X values to the 95% fiducial limits of $Y = 2.7588$ and 1.3937.

Significance of difference of X from unity $= \chi_1^2 = \frac{(\Sigma wy)^2}{\Sigma w} = 14.5078$ $(p < 0.001)$.

Heterogeneity estimate $\chi_8^2 = \Sigma wy^2 - \frac{(\Sigma wy)^2}{\Sigma w} = 16.2133$ $(p < 0.05)$.

The calculations were made to six places of decimals. The figures shown here have been rounded off to four places of decimals.
Source: Method of Woolf (1954) modified by Haldane (1955).

Table 7.10. *The association between the extensive metabolizer phenotype and bladder cancer*

Reference	Location of study	Number of Subjects Bladder cancer EM	PM	Controls EM	PM	Approximate relative risk (x)	$\log_e x$ (y)	Sampling variance (V)	Weight $\left(\frac{1}{V} = w\right)$	Significance of difference from zero (wy^2)	wy
Cartwright et al. 1984	Yorkshire	120	2	92	2	1.3027	0.2644	0.6857	1.4584	0.1020	0.3857
Kaisary et al. 1987	Bristol	88	4	82	10	2.5030	0.9183	0.3142	3.1828	2.6839	2.9227
Horai et al. 1989	Tokyo	51	0	202	1	0.7630	−0.2705	1.5242	0.6572	0.0369	−0.1778
Benitez et al. 1990[a]	Madrid	122	3	522	34	2.3110	0.8377	0.2886	3.4648	2.4313	2.9024
Branch 1992[a]	Pittsburgh	102	4	77	8	2.4982	0.9156	0.3336	2.9972	2.5125	2.7442
								Totals	11.7605	7.7667	8.7772

Mean value of $y = Y = \frac{\Sigma wy}{\Sigma w} = 0.7463$; antilog of $Y = X = 2.1092$.

$\text{SE}\,(Y) = \sqrt{\frac{1}{\Sigma w}} = 0.2916.$

95% of fiducial limits of $Y = 1.5558$ and $-0.0631.$

The equivalent X values to the 95% fiducial limits of $Y = 4.738947$ and $0.9387.$

Significance of difference of X from unity $= \chi^1 = \frac{(\Sigma wy)^2}{\Sigma w} = 6.55078$ ($p < 0.01$).

Heterogeneity estimate $\chi^2_8 = \Sigma wy^2 - \frac{(\Sigma wy)^2}{\Sigma w} = 1.2159$ ($p > 0.80$).

The calculations were made to six places of decimals. The figures shown here have been rounded off to four places of decimals.
Source: Method of Woolf (1954) modified by Haldane (1955).
[a] Personal communication.
Unfortunately Roots et al. (1989) provide insufficient detail for analysis. Their Figure 2 indicates that for their 82 patients compared with controls there was a deficiency of individuals of PM phenotype ($p < 0.01$).

does not match the others the overall results show a significant association of the extensive metabolizer phenotype with bladder cancer. The association is even more marked when aggressive bladder cancers only are studied.

An increase of the number of heterozygotes was found by Wolf *et al.* (1992) who genotyped 184 bladder cancer patients and compared them with 720 controls. However, the percentage of poor metabolizers in the two groups was almost identical.

Somewhat analogous findings resulted from a survey of 59 Nigerians with cancer of various abdominal viscera (Idle *et al.* 1981). There was only one PM compared with 10 out of 123 controls. Again the frequency distribution curve of metabolic ratios was shifted towards lower values.

A series of 184 gastric cancer patients was studied by Roots *et al.* (1989). They found an under-representation of the PM phenotype particularly in the histological 'intestinal' type of neoplasm.

A 'significant trend towards lower numbers of PMs' was found in a series of laryngeal cancer by Roots *et al.* (1989).

On the other hand, in cancer of the breast the association goes the other way, with three series indicating that the poor metabolizer phenotype is associated with the disease (Table 7.11). However, Wolf *et al.* (1992) found that the genotype frequencies were almost exactly the same in 313 breast cancer patients as in 720 controls.

A highly significantly greater frequency of poor metabolizers was found in both acute and chronic myelocytic leukaemias, compared with controls, by Wolf *et al.* (1992). This could be due to allele loss in the blood cells which were used for the genotyping process. Alternatively, extensive metabolizers may be more able to detoxify leukaemogenic chemicals.

Single series of colorectal cancer (Ladero *et al.* 1991), pharyngeal cancer (Roots 1989) and lymphoma (Philip *et al.* 1987) do not show any association of either phenotype with the disease. Cancers of the prostate, colon and malignant melanoma showed genotype frequencies not significantly different from normal controls (Wolf *et al.* 1992).

It seems clear that further series of genotyped patients with very carefully selected controls will be needed to sort out the disparities which exist at present in this field of knowledge.

Systemic lupus erythematosus

Systemic lupus erythematosus patients were investigated by Baer *et al.* (1986). Nine out of 42 patients were poor metabolizers compared with 12 out of 147 healthy volunteer controls. The difference in frequency was significant ($p < 0.04$). The poor metabolizer patients could not be accounted for by interference with the phenotyping test by the disease or by concomitant drug therapy. It will be interesting to see if this finding is substantiated in other series.

Parkinson's disease

The compounds MPTP, MPDP+, MPP+ and PTP (see Table 7.4) are capable of causing Parkinson's disease. They can also inhibit the activity of cytochrome P450 2D6 in human liver microsomes *in vitro*. It has been shown by Fonne-Pfister *et al.* (1987) that bufuralol hydroxylase activity is present in brain; and Tyndale *et al.* (1991c) demonstrated the gene *CYP 2D6* in the caudate nucleus of the human brain.

These considerations gave rise to the ideas (1) that compounds such as MPTP, etc. may be absorbed into the body from the environment, (2) compounds of this type may be more effectively detoxified in the liver and brain of extensive than of poor metabolizers, (3) poor metabolizers may be more prone to develop Parkinson's disease if they absorb them because they are relatively unable to detoxify them.

An initial report by Barbeau *et al.* (1985), that there was a shift of the distribution curve of metabolic ratios towards higher values in patients with Parkinson's disease compared with controls, had later to be qualified. The same group (Poirier *et al.* 1987) showed that this effect was due to diphenhydramine and similar antihistaminics which the patients were concurrently receiving.

Other groups have now examined the problem and their results are summarized in Table 7.12. It is to be noted that the studies of Armstrong *et al.* (1992) and Smith *et al.* (1992) differ from the others in that they examined DNA directly. Armstrong *et al.* (1992) used a PCR test for *CYP 2D6A* and *CYP 2D6B*, and an RFLP test for *CYP 2D6D* and *CYP 2D6E*. Smith *et al.* (1992) used PCR amplification with analysis of the G → A transition at the intron 3/

Table 7.11. *The association between poor metabolizer phenotype and carcinoma of the breast*

| Reference | Location of study | Number of Subjects | | | | Approximate relative risk (x) | $\text{Log}_e x$ (y) | Sampling variance (V) | Weight $\left(\dfrac{1}{V} = w\right)$ | Significance of difference from zero (wy^2) | wy |
| | | Breast cancer | | Controls | | | | | | | |
		EM	PM	EM	PM						
Pontin *et al.* 1990	London	16	13	121	8	1.6564	0.5046	0.1993	5.0180	1.2779	2.5323
Ladero *et al.* 1991	Madrid	88	10	423	23	2.1846	0.7814	0.1462	6.8413	4.1776	5.3460
Huober *et al.* 1991	Heidelberg	95	13	114	9	1.7038	0.5328	0.1905	5.2482	1.4901	2.7965
								Totals	17.1075	6.9456	10.6748

Mean value of $y = Y = \dfrac{\Sigma wy}{\Sigma w} = 0.6240$; antilog of $Y = X = 1.8663$.

$\text{SE}\,(Y) = \sqrt{\dfrac{1}{\Sigma w}} = 0.3060.$

95% of fiducial limits of $Y = Y \pm t_{2,\,0.05}\sqrt{\dfrac{1}{\Sigma w}} = 1.9401$ and -0.6921.

The equivalent X values to the 95% fiducial limits of $Y = 6.9593$ and 0.5005.

Significance of difference of X from unity $= \chi_1^2 = \dfrac{(\Sigma wy)^2}{\Sigma w} = 6.6609$ ($p < 0.001$).

Heterogeneity estimate $\chi_2^2 = \Sigma wy^2 - \dfrac{(\Sigma wy)^2}{\Sigma w} = 0.2846$ ($p < 0.90$).

The calculations were made to six places of decimals. The figures shown here have been rounded off to four places of decimals.
Source: Method of Woolf (1954) modified by Haldane (1955).

Table 7.12. *Test of the association between poor metabolizer phenotype and Parkinson's disease*

Reference	Location of study	Ethnic Group	Number of individuals				Approximate relative risk (x)	$\log_e x$ (y)	Sampling variance (V)	Weight $\left(\frac{1}{V} = w\right)$	Significance of difference from zero (wy^2)	wy
			Parkinson's disease		Controls							
			EM	PM	EM	PM						
Steventon et al. 1989	Birmingham, UK	Not stated	60	6	16	2	0.7091	−0.3438	0.5514	1.8135	0.2143	−0.6234
Benitez et al. 1990b	Madrid & Badajoz	Not stated	44	1	522	34	0.5105	−0.6724	0.5527	1.8093	0.8197	−1.2165
Gudjonsson et al. 1990	Uppsala & Huddinge	Unrelated Swedish Caucasians	33	1	945	69	0.6091	−0.4957	0.5447	1.8357	0.4510	−0.9099
Meillard et al. 1990	Rennes	French Caucasians	16	4	11	2	1.2545	0.2268	0.6755	1.4804	0.0761	0.3357
Chiba et al. 1991	Tokyo	Not stated	72	0	82	2	0.2276	−1.4802	1.3591	0.7358	1.6122	−1.0891
Kallio et al. 1991	Turku, Finland	Not stated for patients. Controls stated to be Finnish Caucasians	93	4	167	9	0.8486	−0.1642	0.3166	3.1587	0.0851	−0.5186
Armstarong et al. 1992	Newcastle upon Tyne	Not stated	51	2	70	2	1.3689	0.3140	0.7000	1.4286	0.1409	0.4486
Smith et al. 1992	London & Birmingham	Caucasians	202	27	684	36	2.5468	0.9348	0.0691	14.4661	12.6418	13.5232
Steiger et al. 1992	London	Not stated	45	9	130	13	2.0183	0.7023	0.2008	4.9800	2.4560	3.4973
									Totals	31.7081	18.4955	13.4463

Mean value of $y = Y = \frac{\Sigma wy}{\Sigma w} = 0.4241$; antilog of $Y = X = 1.5282$.

$\text{SE}\,(Y) = \sqrt{\frac{1}{\Sigma w}} = 0.1776$.

95% of fiducial limits of $Y = Y \pm t_{8,0.05}\,\text{SE}\,(Y) = 0.8343$ and 0.0138.

The equivalent X values to the 95% fiducial limits of $Y = 2.3032$ and 1.0139.

Significance of difference of X from unity $= \chi_1^2 = \frac{(\Sigma wy)^2}{\Sigma w} = 5.7021$ $(p < 0.02)$.

Heterogeneity estimate $\chi_8^2 = \Sigma wy^2 - \frac{(\Sigma wy)^2}{\Sigma w} = 12.7934$ $(p > 0.10)$.

The calculations were made to six places of decimals.
Source: Method of Woolf (1954) modified by Haldane (1955).

Table 7.13. *Studies which did not reveal any association with cytochrome P450 2D6 phenotypes*

Reference	Disorder
Lanthier *et al.* 1984	Alcoholic liver disease
Saner *et al.* 1986	Pulmonary hypertension of vascular origin possibly due to aminorex fumarate
Jacz-Aigrain *et al.* 1990	Autoimmune hepatitis in children
Bechtel *et al.* 1986	Epilepsy
Sabuinen *et al.* 1989	Glaucoma
Amery *et al.* 1988	Migraine
Chapman *et al.* 1981	Discoid psoriasis
Dayer *et al.* 1984c	Plasma cholesterol concentrations
Fletcher *et al.* 1986	Non-insulin-dependent diabetes mellitus
Spina *et al.* 1992a; Vallada *et al.* 1992	Schizophrenia (drug-free)
Smith *et al.* 1992; Wolf *et al.* 1992	Emphysema
Steventon *et al.* 1989	Motor neurone disease

exon 4 junction and the base pair delection in exon 5. Amongst 229 Parkinson's disease patients the frequencies of both the mutant alleles and PM phenotypes were higher than among 72 controls. The other series performed by standard phenotyping techniques (mostly using debrisoquine) might have been subject to the influence of factors such as drug consumption and age. Some involved relatively small numbers of patients. The report of Comella *et al.* (1987) does not give sufficient information to be included in Table 7.12. Despite the fact that some studies did not support the hypothesis, the analysis in Table 7.12 shows a significant association overall, which receives a large contribution from the study of Smith *et al.* (1992)

An alternative to the 'toxic chemical' hypothesis is that there may be linkage of the *CYP 2D6* locus to another gene involved in the pathogenesis of Parkinson's disease.

Other conditions

No association of either phenotype has been demonstrated in single series of a variety of conditions (Table 7.13).

CONCLUSION

In this chapter it has been shown that a major polymorphism exists in man based upon structural changes in the specific cytochrome P450 2D6 enzyme molecule. As a result there are important clinical consequences in therapeutics. For a substantial range of drugs conventional doses produce toxicity due to accumulation of excessive amounts in poor metabolizers. Considerable inter-ethnic variability in phenotype frequencies have been identified. The molecular bases of the polymorphism have been determined in Europeans. Associations have been demonstrated of the extensive metabolizers with carcinomas of the bronchus (though this is disputed) and bladder, and of the poor metabolizers with carcinoma of the breast (though this is disputed) and leukaemias. Although the natural substrates of the relevant cytochrome P450 are as yet unidentified this polymorphism may be of considerable ecological significance. One of the research groups who first identified the polymorphism hit on a true and felicitous phrase when they entitled their review paper 'The debrisoquine hydroxylation gene; a gene of multiple consquence' (Idle & Smith 1984).

The author would like to express his gratitude to Professor Urs A. Meyer, Department of Pharmacology, Biozentrum University of Basel, Switzerland who made many helpful suggestions about the contents of this chapter.

Alvan, G. (1991). Clinical consequences of polymorphic drug oxidation. *Fundamental and Clinical Pharmacology*, **5**, 209–28.

Alvan, G., Bechtel, P., Iselius, L. & Gundert-Remy, U. (1990). Hydroxylation polymorphisms of debrisoquine and mephenytoin in European populations. *European Journal of Clinical Pharmacology*, **39**, 533–7.

Alvan, G., Graffner, C., Grind, M., Gustafsson, L. L., Lindgren, J. E., Nordin, C., Ross, S., Selander, H. & Siwers, B. (1983). Pharmacokinetics metabolism and tolerance of amiflamine – a new selective and reversible MAO inhibitor. In II World Conference on Clinical Pharmacology and Therapeutics, Washington DC. *Drug Metabolism and Disposition*. Abstract 493, p. 84.

Alvan, G., Grind, M., Graffner, C. & Sjöqvist, F. (1984). Relationship to N-demethylation of amiflamine and its metabolite to debrisoquine hydroxylation polymorphism. *Clinical Pharmacology and Therapeutics*, **36**, 515–19.

Alvan, G., von Bahr, C., Seidman, P. & Sjöqvist, F. (1982). High plasma concentrations of β-receptor blocking drugs and deficient debrisoquine hydroxylation. *Lancet*, **1**, 333.

Amery, W. K., Davies, P. T. G., Caers, L. I., Heykants, J., Steiner, T. J., Woestenborghs, R. & Rose, F. C. (1988). Hepatic cytochrome P_{450}-mediated oxidation function in migraine. *Cephalalgia*, **8**, 71–4.

Arias, T. D., Inaba, T., Cooke, R. G. &, Jorge, L. F. (1988b). A preliminary note on the transient polymorphic oxidation of sparteine in the Ngawbe Guaymi Amerindians. A case of genetic divergence with tentative phylogenetic time frame for the pathway. *Clinical Pharmacology and Therapeutics*, **44**, 343–52.

Arias, T. D. & Jorge, L. F. (1989). An observation on the ethnic uniqueness of the debrisoquine and sparteine antimodes, a study in the Ngawbé Guaymi Amerindians of Panamá. *British Journal of Clinical Pharmacology*, **28**, 493–4.

Arias, T. D., Jorge, L. F., Lee, D., Barrantes, R. & Inaba, T. (1988a). The oxidative metabolism of sparteine in the Cuna Amerindians of Panama, Absence of evidence of deficient metabolizers. *Clinical Pharmacology and Therapeutics*, **43**, 456–65.

Armstrong, M., Daly, A. K., Cholerton, S., Bateman, D. N. & Idle, J. R. (1992). Mutant debrisoquine hydroxylation genes in Parkinson's disease. *Lancet*, **339**, 1017–18.

Arvela, P., Kirjarinta, M. A., Kirjarinta, M., Karki, N. & Pelkonen, O. (1988). Polymorphism of debrisoquine hydroxylation among Finns and Lapps. *British Journal of Clinical Pharmacology*, **26**, 601–3.

Ayesh, R., Dawling, S., Hayler, A., Oates, N. S., Cholerton, S., Widdop, B., Idle, J. R. & Smith, R. L. (1991). Comparative effects of the diastereoisomers quinine and quinidine in producing phenocopy debrisoquine poor metabolisers in healthy volunteers. *Chirality*, **3**, 14–18.

Ayesh, R., Idle, J. R., Ritchie, J. C., Crothers, M. J. & Hetzel, M. R. (1984). Metabolic oxidation phenotypes as markers for susceptibility to lung cancer. *Nature*, **312**, 169–70.

Baer, A. N., McAllister, C. B., Wilkinson, G. R., Woosley, R. L. & Pincus, T. (1986). Altered distribution of debrisoquine phenotypes in patients with systemic lupus erythematosus. *Arthritis and Rheumatism*, **29**, 843–50.

Balant-Gorgia, A. E., Balant, L. P., Genet, Ch., Dayer, P., Aeschlimann, J. M. & Garrone, G. (1986). Importance of oxidative polymorphism and levomepromazine treatment on the steady-state blood concentrations of clomipramine and its major metabolites. *European Journal of Clinical Pharmacology*, **31**, 449–55.

Barbeau, A., Roy, M., Paris, S., Cloutier, T., Plasse, L. & Poirier, J. (1985). Ecogenetics of Parkinson's disease, 4 hydroxylation of debrisoquine. *Lancet*, **2**, 1213–15.

Bechtel, P., Joanne, C., Bechtel, Y., Grand mottet, M. & Jounet, J. M. (1986). Stabilité et/ou variabilité de l'expression du polymorphisme génétique d'hydroxylation et d'acétylation chez des malades présentant des pathologies et soumes a des therapeutiques varieés. *Annales de Biologie Clinique*, **44**, 361–7.

Beckmann, J., Hertrampf, R., Gundert-Remy, U., Mikus, G., Gross, A. S. & Eichelbaum, M. (1988). Is there a genetic factor in flecainide toxicity? *British Medical Journal*, **297**, 1316.

Benitez, J., Ladero, J. M., Fernandez-Gundin, M. J., Llerena, A., Cobaleda, J., Martinez, C., Munoz, J. J., Vargas, E., Prados, J., Gonzalez-Rozas, F., Rodriguez-Molina, J. & Uson, A. C. (1990a). Polymorphic oxidation of debrisoquine in bladder cancer. *Annals of Medicine*, **22**, 157–60.

Benitez, J., Ladero, J. M., Jara, C., Carillo, J. A., Cobaledo, J., Llerena, A., Vargas, E. & Munoz, J. J. (1991). Polymorphic oxidation of debrisoquine in lung cancer patients. *European Journal of Cancer*, **27**, 158–61

Benitez, J., Ladero, J. M., Jimenez-Jimenez, F. J., Martinez, C., Puerto, A. M., Valdivielso, M. J., Llerena, A., Cobaleda, J. & Munoz, J. J. (1990b). Oxidative polymorphism of debrisoquine in Parkinson's disease. *Journal of Neurology, Neurosurgery and Psychiatry*, **53**, 289–93.

Benitez, J., Llerena, A. & Cobaleda, J. (1988). Debrisoquine oxidation polymorphism in a Spanish population. *Clinical Pharmacology and Therapeutics*, **44**, 74–7.

Bertilsson, L., Dahl, M.-L., Sjöqvist, F., Åberg-Wistedt, A, Humble, M., Johansson, J., Lundqvist, E. & Ingleman-Sundberg, M. (1993). Molecular basis for rational megaprescribing in ultrarapid hydroxylators of debrisoquine. *Lancet*, **341**, 63.

Bertilsson, L., Lou, Y. Q., Du, Y. L., Liu, Y., Kuang, T. Y., Liao, X. M., Wang, K. Y., Riviriego, J., Iselius, L. & Sjöqvist, F. (1992). Pronounced differences between native Chinese and Swedish populations in the polymorphic hydroxylations of debrisoquine and S-mephenytoin. *Clinical Pharmacology and Therapeutics*, **51**, 388–97.

Bertilsson, L., Mellström, B., Sjöqvist, F. & Martensson, B. & Åsberg, M. (1981). Slow hydroxylation of nortriptyline and concomitant poor debrisoquine hydroxylation, clinical implications. *Lancet*, **1**, 560–1.

Birgersdotter, U. M., Wong, W., Jurgeon, J. & Roden, D. M. (1992). Stereoselective genetically determined interaction between chronic flecainide and quinidine in patients with arrhythmias. *British Journal of Clinical Pharmacology*, **33**, 275–80.

Birgersson, C., Morgan, E. T., Jornvall, H. & von Bahr, C. (1986). Purification of a desmethylimipramine and debrisoquine hydroxylating cytochrome P450 from human liver. *Biochemical Pharmacology*, **35**, 3165–6.

Bloomer, J. C., Woods, F. R., Haddock, R. E., Lennard, M. S. & Tucker, G. T. (1992). The role of cytochrome P450 2D6 in the metabolism of paroxetine by human liver microsomes. *British Journal of Clinical Pharmacology*, **33**, 521–3.

Boobis, A. R., Brodie, M. J., Kahn, G. C., Fletcher, D. R., Saunders, J. H. & Davies, D. S. (1980). Mono-oxygenase activity of human liver in microsomal fractions of needle biopsy specimens. *British Journal of Clinical Pharmacology*, **9**, 11–19.

Boobis, A. R., Murray, S., Hampden, C. E. & Davies, D. S. (1985). Genetic polymorphism in drug oxidation, *in vitro* studies of human debrisoquine 4-hydroxylase and bufuralol 1'-hydroxylase activities. *Biochemical Pharmacology*, **34**, 65–71.

Branch, R. A., Wilkinson, G. R., McAllister, C. B., Ray, W., Kaisary, A. & Smith, P. (1985). Association of polymorphic oxidative drug metabolism cigarette smoking and alcohol consumption with bladder cancer (abstract). *Clinical Research*, **33**, 527A.

Brinn, R., Brøsen, K., Gram, L. F., Haghfelt, T. & Otton, V. (1986). Sparteine oxidation is practically abolished in quinidine-treated patients. *British Journal of Clinical Pharmacology*, **22**, 194–7.

Broly, F., Gaedigk, A., Heim, M., Eichelbaum, M., Morike, K. & Meyer, U. A. (1991b). Debrisoquine/sparteine hydroxylation genotype and phenotype, analysis of common mutations and alleles of CYP2D6 in a European population. *DNA and Cell Biology*, **10**, 545–58.

Broly, F., Libersa, C., Lhermitte, M. & Dupuis, B. (1990). Inhibitory studies of mexiletine and dextromethorphan oxidation in human liver microsomes. *Biochemical Pharmacology*, **39**, 1045–53.

Broly, F., Vandamme, N., Libersa, C. & Lhermitte, M. (1991a). The metabolism of mexiletine in relation to the debrisoquine/sparteine-type polymorphism of drug oxidation. *British Journal of Clinical Pharmacology*, **32**, 459–66.

Brøsen, K. (1986). Sparteine oxidation polymorphism in Greenlanders living in Denmark. *British Journal of Clinical Pharmacology*, **22**, 415–19.

Brøsen, K. (1988). The relationship between imipramine metabolism and the sparteine oxidation polymorphism. *Danish Medical Bulletin*, **35**, 460–8.

Brøsen, K., Davidsen, F. & Gram, L. F. (1990). Quinidine kinetics after a single oral dose in relation to the sparteine oxidation polymorphism in man. *British Journal of Clinical Pharmacology*, **29**, 248–53.

Brøsen, K. & Gram, L. F. (1988). First-pass metabolism of imipramine and desipramine, impact of the sparteine oxidation phenotype. *Clinical Pharmacology and Therapeutics*, **43**, 400–6.

Brøsen, K. & Gram, L. F. (1989a). Clinical significance of the sparteine/debrisoquine oxidation polymorphism. *European Journal of Clinical Pharmacology*, **36**, 537–47.

Brøsen, K. & Gram, L. F. (1989a). Quinidine inhibits the 2-hydroxylation of imipramine and desipramine but not the demethylation of imipramine. *European Journal of Clinical Pharmacology*, **37**, 155–60.

Brøsen, K., Gram, L. F. & Kragh-Søorensen, P. (1991a). Extremely slow metabolism of amitriptyline but normal metabolism of imipramine and desipramine in an extensive metabolizer of sparteine debrisoquine and mephenytoin. *Therapeutic Drug Monitoring*, **13**, 177–82.

Brøsen, K., Gram, L. F., Haghfelt, T. & Bertilsson, L. (1987). Extensive metabolizers of debrisoquine become poor metabolizers during quinidine treatment. *Pharmacology and Toxicology*, **60**, 312–14.

Brøsen, K., Klysner, R., Gram, L. F., Otton, S. V., Bech, O. & Bertilsson, L. (1986c). Steady state concentrations of imipramine and its metabolites in relation to the sparteine/debrisoquine polymorphism. *European Journal of Clinical Pharmacology*, **30**, 679–84.

Brøsen, K., Otton, S. V. & Gram, L. F. (1985). Sparteine oxidation polymorphism in Denmark. *Acta Pharmacologica et Toxicologica*, **57**, 357–60.

Brøsen, K., Otton, S. V. & Gram, L. F. (1986a). Sparteine

oxidation polymorphism, a family study. *British Journal of Clinical Pharmacology*, **21**, 661–7.

Brøsen, K., Otton, S. V. & Gram, L. F. (1986b). Imipramine demethylation and hydroxylation, impact of the sparteine oxidation phenotype. *Clinical Pharmacology and Therapeutics*, **40**, 543–9.

Brøsen, K. & Skjelbo, E. (1991). Fluoxetine and norfluoxetine are potent inhibitors of P450IID6–the source of the sparteine/debrisoquine oxidation polymorphism. *British Journal of Clinical Pharmacology*, **32**, 136–7.

Brøsen, K., Zeugin, T. & Meyer, U. A. (1991b). Role of P450IID6 the target of the sparteine – debrisoquine oxidation polymorphism in the metabolism of imipramine. *Clinical Pharmacology and Therapeutics*, **49**, 609–17.

Caporaso, N., Hayes, R. B., Dosemeci, M., Hoover, R., Ayesh, R., Hetzel, M. & Idle, J. R. (1989b). Lung cancer risk occupational exposure and the debrisoquine metabolic phenotype. *Cancer Research*, **49**, 3675–9.

Caporaso, N. & Pickle, L. (1989). Debrisoquine phenotype and genotype in Chinese. *Lancet*, **2**, 1534–5.

Caporaso, N., Pickle, L. W., Bale, S., Ayesh, R., Hetzel, M. & Idle, J. R. (1989a). The distribution of debrisoquine metabolic phenotypes and implications for the suggested association with lung cancer risk. *Genetic Epidemiology*, **6**, 517–24.

Caporaso, N. E. & Shaw, G. L. (1991). Clinical implications of the competitive inhibition of the debrisoquine-metabolizing isozyme by quinidine. *Archives of Internal Medicine*, **151**, 1985–92.

Caporaso, N. E., Tucker, M. A., Hoover, R. N., Hayes, R. B., Pickle, L. W., Issaq, H. J., Muschik, G. M., Green-Gallo, L., Buivys, D., Aisner, S., Resau, J. H., Trump, B. F., Tollerud, D., Weston, A. & Harris, C. C. (1990). Lung cancer and the debrisoquine metabolic phenotype. *Journal of the National Cancer Institute*, **82**, 1264–72.

Carey, E. L ,. Duff, H. J., Roden, D. M., Primm, J. A., Oates, J. A. & Woosley, R. L. (1981). Relative electrocardiographic and antiarrhythmic effects of encainide and its metabolites in man. *Circulation*, **64**, SIV–264.

Cartwright, R. A., Philip, P. A., Rogers, J. H. & Glashan, R. W. (1984). Genetically determined debrisoquine oxidation capacity in bladder cancer. *Carcinogenesis (London)*, **5**, 1191–2.

Chapman, P. H., Rawlins, M. D., Shuster, S., Idle, J. R., Ritchie, J. C. & Smith, R. L. (1981). Polymorphic 4-hydroxylation of debrisoquine in chronic discoid psoriasis. *European Journal of Clinical Pharmacology*, **21**, 257–8.

Chen, Z. R., Somogyi, A. A. & Bochner, F. (1988). Polymorphic O-demethylation of codeine. *Lancet*, **2**, 914–15.

Chen, Z. R,. Somogyi, A. A. & Bochner, F. (1990). Simultaneous determination of dextromethorphan and three metabolites in plasma and urine using high-performance liquid chromatography with application to their disposition in man. *Therapeutic Drug Monitoring*, **12**, 97–104.

Chen, Z. R., Somogyi, A. A., Reynolds, G. & Bochner, F. (1991). Disposition and metabolism of codeine after single and chronic doses in one poor and seven extensive metabolisers. *British Journal of Clinical Pharmacology*, **31**, 381–90.

Chiba, K., Imai, H., Yoshino, H., Kato, J., Ishizaki, T. &

Narabayashi, H. (1991). Sparteine oxidation in patients with early- and late-onset Parkinson's disease. In *Parkinson's disease, From clinical aspects to molecular basis*, ed. T. Nagatso, H. Narabayashi, M. Yoshida, Vol. 10, pp. 103–9. New York: Springer-Verlag.

Chiba, K., Kato, J., Hashimoto, K. & Ishizaki, T. (1988). Apparent Mendelian recessive inheritance of sparteine metabolism in an extended Japanese family. *European Journal of Clinical Pharmacology*, **34**, 661–2.

Clark, D. W. J. (1985). Genetically determined variability in acetylation and oxidation – therapeutic implications. *Drugs*, **29**, 342–75.

Clark, D. W. J., Morgan, A. K. W. & Waal-Manning, H. (1984). Adverse effects from metoprolol are not generally associated with oxidation status. *British Journal of Clinical Pharmacology*, **18**, 965–7.

Clarke's Isolation and Identification of Drugs, 2nd edn, ed. A. C. Moffat, J. V. Jackson, M. S. Moss, & B. Widdop (1986). London: The Pharmaceutical Press.

Clasen, K., Madsen, L., Brøsen, K., Albøge, K., Misfeldt, S. & Gram, L. F. (1991). Sparteine and mephenytoin oxidation, genetic polymorphisms in East and West Greenland. *Clinical Pharmacology and Therapeutics*, **49**, 624–31.

Comella, C. I., Tanner, C. M., Goetz, C. G., Gans, S., Rapp, D. & Fischer, J. (1987). Debrisoquine metabolism in Parkinson's disease. *Neurology*, **37**(Suppl.1), 261–2.

Cooper, R. G., Evans, D. A. P. & Whibley, E. J. (1984). Polymorphic hydroxylation of perhexilene maleate in man. *Journal of Medical Genetics*, **21**, 27–33.

Dahl, M. L., Ekqvist, B., Widen, J. & Bertilsson, L. (1991). Disposition of the neuroleptic zuclopenthixol cosegregates with the polymorphic hydroxylation of debrisoquine in humans. *Acta Psychiatrica Scandinavica*, **84**, 99–100.

Dahl, M. L., Johansson, I., Palmertz, M. P., Ingelman-Sundberg, M. & Sjöqvist, F. (1992). Analysis of the CYP2D6 gene in relation to debrisoquine and desipramine hydroxylation in a Swedish population. *Clinical Pharmacology and Therapeutics*, **51**, 12–17.

Dahl-Puustinen, M. L., Alm,C., Bertilsson, L., Christenson, I., Östman, J., Thunberg, E. & Wikström, I. (1990). Lack of relationship between glibenclamide metabolism and debrisoquine or mephenytoin hydroxylation phenotypes. *British Journal of Clinical Pharmacology*, **30**, 476–80.

Dahl-Puustinen, M. L., Liden, A., Alm, C., Nordin, C. & Bertilsson, L. (1989). Disposition of perphenazine is related to polymorphic debrisoquine hydroxylation in human beings. *Clinical Pharmacology and Therapeutics*, **46**, 78–81.

Dahlqvist, R., Bertilsson, L., Birkett, D. J., Eichelbaum, M., Sawe, J. & Sjöqvist, F. (1984). Theophylline metabolism in relation to antipyrine debrisoquine and sparteine metabolism. *Clinical Pharmacology and Therapeutics*, **35**, 815–21.

Daly, A. K., Armstrong, M. & Idle, J. R. (1990). Molecular genotyping to predict debrisoquine hydroxylation phenotype. *Lancet*, **336**, 889–90

Danhof, M., Idle, J. R., Teunissen, M. W. E., Sloan, T. P., Breimer, D. D. & Smith, R. L. (1981). Influence of the genetically controlled deficiency in debrisoquine hydroxylation on antipyrine metabolite formation. *Pharmacology*, **22**, 349–58.

Daumas, L., Sabot, J. F., Vermeulen, E., Clapot, P., Allegre, F., Pinatel, H., Boucherat, M. & Francois, B. (1991). Determination of debrisoquine and metabolites in human urine by gas chromatography – mass spectrometry. *Journal of Chromatography*, **570**, 89–97.

Davi, H., Bonnet, J. M. & Berger, Y. (1992). Disposition of minoprine in animals and in human extensive and limited debrisquoine hydroxylators. *Xenobiotica*, **22**, 171–84.

Davies, D. S., Kahn, G. C., Murray, S., Brodie, M. J. & Boobis, A. R. (1981). Evidence for an enzymatic defect in the 4-hydroxylation of debrisoquine by human liver. *British Journal of Clinical Pharmacology*, **11**, 89–91.

Dayer, P., Balant, L. & Fabre, J. (1984a). The genetic control of drug oxidation in the liver. *International Journal of Clinical Pharmacology*, **3**, 421–5.

Dayer, P., Balant, L., Kupfer, A., Courvoisier, F. & Fabre, J. (1983). Contribution of the genetic status of oxidative metabolism to variability in the plasma concentration of Beta-adrenergic blocking agents. *European Journal of Clinical Pharmacology*, **24**, 787–99.

Dayer, P., Balant, L., Kupfer, A., Striberni, R. & Leeman, T. (1985). Effect of oxidative polymorphism (debrisoquine/sparteine type) on hepatic first-pass metabolism of bufuralol. *European Journal of Clinical Pharmacology*, **28**, 317–20.

Dayer, P., Courvoisier, F., Balant, L. & Fabre, J. (1982a). Beta-blockers and drug oxidation status. *Lancet*, **1**, 509.

Dayer, P., Gasser, R., Gut, J., Kronbach, T., Robertz, G. M., Eichelbaum, M. & Meyer, U. A. (1984b). Characterization of a common genetic defect of cytochrome P450 function (debrisoquine-sparteine type polymorphism). *Biochemical and Biophysical Research Communications*, **125**, 374–80.

Dayer, P., Kronbach, T., Eichelbaum, M. & Meyer, U. A. (1987). Enzymatic basis of the debrisoquine/sparteine-type genetic polymorphism of drug oxidation. *Biochemical Pharmacology*, **36**, 4145–52.

Dayer, P., Kubli, A., Kupfer, A., Courvoisier, F., Balant, L. & Fabre, J. (1982b). Defective hydroxylation of bufuralol associated with side effects of the drug in poor metabolisers. *British Journal of Clinical Pharmacology*, **13**, 750–2.

Dayer, P., Suenram, A., Pometta, D. & Fabre, J. (1984c). Apparent lack of influence of the genetic drug oxidation status on plasma cholesterol concentration in man. *Pharmacological Research Communications*, **16**, 129–34.

Debruyne, D., Gram, L. F., Grollier, G., Camsonne, R., Agron, L., Dao, M. T., Lacotte, J., Bigot, M. C. & Moulin, M. (1989). Quinidine disposition in relation to antipyrine elimination and debrisoquine phenotype in alcoholic patients with and without cirrhosis. *International Journal of Clinical Pharmacology Research*, **9**, 319–25.

Derenne, F., Joanne, C., Vandel, S., Bertschy, G., Volmat, R. & Bechtel, P. (1989). Debrisoquine oxidative phenotyping and psychiatric drug treatment. *European Journal of Clinical Pharmacology*, **36**, 53–8.

Devonshire, H. W., Kong, I., Cooper, M., Sloan, T. P., Idle, J. R. & Smith, R. L. (1983). The contribution of genetically determined oxidation status to inter-individual variation in phenacetin disposition. *British Journal of Clinical Pharmacology*, **16**, 157–66.

Dick, B., Kupfer, A., Molnar, J., Braunschweig, S. & Preisig, R. (1982). Hydroxylierungsdefekt fur Medikamente (Typus Debrisoquin) in einer Stichprobe der Schweizer Bevölkerung. *Schweizerische Medizinische Wochenschrift*, **112**, 1061–7.

Distlerath, L. M., Reilly, P. E. B., Martin, M. V., Davis, G.

G., Wilkinson, G. T. & Guengerich, F. P. (1985). Purification and characterization of the human liver cytochromes P450 involved in debrisoquine 4-hydroxylation and phenacetin O-de-ethylation: two prototypes for genetic polymorphism in oxidative drug metabolism. *Journal of Biological Chemistry*, **260**, 9657–67.

Du, Y. L. & Lou, Y. Q. (1990). Polymorphism of debrisoquine 4-hydroxylation and family studies of poor metabolizers in Chinese population. *Acta Pharmacologica Sinica*, **11**, 7–10.

Duche, J. C., Joanne, C., Barre, J., de Cremoux, H., Dalphin, J. C., Depierre, A., Brochard, P., Tillement, J. P. & Bechtel, P. (1991). Lack of a relationship between the polymorphism of debrisoquine oxidation and lung cancer. *British Journal of Clinical Pharmacology*, **31**, 533–6.

Ebner, T., Meese, C. O. & Eichelbaum, M. (1989). Thin-layer chromatographic screening test for polymorphic sparteine oxidation. *Therapeutic Drug Monitoring*, **11**, 214–16.

Eichelbaum, M. (1988). *Genetic polymorphism of sparteine/debrisoquine oxidation*. ISI Atlas of Science, Pharmacology, pp. 243–51.

Eichelbaum, M., Baur, M. P., Dengler, H. J., Osikowska-Evers, B. O., Tieves, G., Zekorn, C. & Rittner, C. (1987). Chromosomal assignment of human cytochrome P450 (debrisoquine/sparteine type) to chromosome 22. *British Journal of Clinical Pharmacology*, **23**, 455–8.

Eichelbaum, M., Bertilsson, L., Kupfer, A., Steiner, E. & Messe, C. O. (1988). Enantioselectivity of 4-hydroxylation in extensive and poor metabolizers of debrisoquine. *British Journal of Clinical Pharmacology*, **25**, 505–8.

Eichelbaum, M., Bertilsson, L. & Sawe, J. (1983). Antipyrine metabolism in relation to polymorphic oxidations of sparteine and debrisoquine. *British Journal of Clinical Pharmacology*, **15**, 317–21.

Eichelbaum, M., Bertilsson, L., Sawe, J. & Zekorn, C. (1982). Polymorphic oxidation of sparteine and debrisoquine; related pharmacogenetic entitites. *Clinical Pharmacology and Therapeutics*, **31**, 184–6.

Eichelbaum, M. & Gross, A. S. (1990). The genetic polymorphism of debrisoquine/sparteine metabolism – clinical aspects. *Pharmacology and Therapeutics*, **46**, 377–94.

Eichelbaum, M., Mineshita, S., Ohnhaus, E. E. & Zekorn, C. (1986). The influence of enzyme induction on polymorphic sparteine oxidation. *British Journal of Clinical Pharmacology*, **22**, 49–53.

Eichelbaum, M., Spannbrucker, N. & Dengler, H. J. (1978). A probably genetic defect of the metabolism of sparteine. In *Biological oxidation of Nitrogen*.ed. J. W. Gorrod, pp. 113–18. Amsterdam: Elsevier, North Holland.

Eichelbaum, M., Spannbrucker, N. & Dengler, H. J. (1979b). Influence of the defective metabolism of sparteine on its pharmacokinetics. *European Journal of Clinical Pharmacology*, **16**, 189–94.

Eichelbaum, M., Spannbrucker, N., Steincke, B. & Dengler, H. J. (1979a). Defective N-oxidation of sparteine in man, a new pharmacogenetic defect. *European Journal of Clinical Pharmacology*, **16**, 183–7.

Eichelbaum, M., Tomson, T., Tybring, G. & Bertilsson, M. (1985a). Carbamazepine metabolism in man. Induction and pharmacogenetic aspects. *Clinical Pharmacokinetics*, **10**, 80–90.

Eichelbaum, M. & Woolhouse, N. M. (1985). Inter-ethnic difference in sparteine oxidation among Ghanaians and Germans. *European Journal of Clinical Pharmacology*, **28**, 79–83.

Ellis, S. W., Ching, M. S., Watson, P. F., Henderson, C. J., Simula, A. P., Lennard, M. S., Tucker, G. T. & Woods, H. F. (1992). Catalytic activities of human debrisoquine 4-hydroxylase cytochrome P450 (CYP2D6) expressed in yeast. *Biochemical Pharmacology*, **4**, 617–20.

Emery, A. E. H. (1976). *Methodology in Medical Genetics. An Introduction to Statistical Methods*, pp. 63–75. Edinburgh: Churchill Livingstone.

Evans, D. A. P., Harmer, D., Downham, D. Y., Whibley, E. J., Idle, J. R., Ritchie, J. & Smith, R. L. (1983). The genetic control of sparteine and debrisoquine metabolism in man with new methods of analysing bimodal distributions. *Journal of Medical Genetics*, **20**, 321–9.

Evans, D. A. P., Mahgoub, A., Sloan, T. P., Idle, J. R. & Smith, R. L. (1980). A family and population study of the genetic polymorphism of debrisoquine oxidation in a British white population. *Journal of Medical Genetics*, **17**, 102–5.

Evans, W. E. & Relling, M. V. (1990). XbaI 16-plus 9-kilobase DNA restriction fragments identify a mutant allele for debrisoquin hydroxylase, report of a family study. *Molecular Pharmacology*, **37**, 639–42.

Faccini, G. B., Puchetti, V. & Zatti, N. (1990). Dextromethorphan oxidation phenotypes as markers for susceptibility to lung cancer. *Clinical Chemistry*, **36**, 387.

Filler, W. W., Jr. Filler, N. & Zinberg, S. (1964). Sparteine sulphate in labour. *American Journal of Obstetrics and Gynaecology*, **88**, 737–46.

Fingl, E. & Woodbury, D. M. (1975). General principles. In *The Pharmacological Basis of Therapeutics*, 5th edition, ed. L. S. Goodman & A. Gilman, p. 22. New York, Macmillan.

Fletcher, P., Hirji, M. R., Kuhn, S., Alexander, L. & Mucklow, J. C. (1986). The effects of diabetes mellitus, exercise and single doses of biguanides upon lactate metabolism in man. *British Journal of Clinical Pharmacology*, **21**, 691–99

Fonne-Pfister, R., Bargetzi, M. J. & Meyer, U. A. (1987). MPTP, the neurotoxin inducing Parkinson's disease, is a potent competitive inhibitor of human rat cytochrome P450 isozymes (P450 buf I, P450 db I) catalyzing debrisoquine 4 hydroxylation. *Biochemical and Biophysical Research Communications*, **148**, 1144–50.

Fonne-Pfister, R. & Meyer, U. A. (1988). Xenobiotic and endobiotic inhibitors of cytochrome P450 db1 function the target of the debrisoquine/sparteine type polymorphism. *Biochemical Pharmacology*, **37**, 3829–35.

Frèche, J. P., Dragacci, S., Petit, A. M., Siest, J. P., Galteau, M. M. & Siest, G. (1990). Development of an ELISA to study the polymorphism of dextromethorphan oxidation in a French population. *European Journal of Clinical Pharmacology*, **39**, 481–5.

Gaedigk, A., Blum, M., Gaedigk, R., Eichelbaum, M. & Meyer, U. A. (1991). Deletion of the entire cytochrome P450 *CYP2D6* gene as a cause of impaired drug metabolism in poor metabolizers of the debrisoquine/sparteine polymorphism. *American Journal of Human Genetics*, **48**, 943–50.

Gleiter, C. H., Aichele, G., Nilsson, E., Hengen, N., Antonin, K. H. & Bieck, P. R. (1985). Discovery of altered pharmacokinetics of CGP 15210 G in poor hydroxylators of debrisoquine during early drug development. *British Journal of Clinical Pharmacology*, **20**, 81–4.

Gonzalez, F. J. (1989). The molecular biology of cytochrome P450s. *Pharmacological Reviews*, **40**, 243–88.

Gonzalez, F. J. & Meyer, U. A. (1991). Molecular genetics of the debrisoquine-sparteine polymorphism. *Clinical Pharmacology and Therapeutics*, **50**, 233–8.

Gonzalez, F. J., Skoda, R. C., Kimura, S., Umeno, M., Zanger, U. M., Nebert, D. W., Gelboin, H. V., Hardwick, J. P. & Meyer, U. A. (1988a) Characterization of the common genetic defect in humans deficient in debrisoquine metabolism. *Nature*, **331**, 442–6.

Gonzalez, F. J., Vilbois, F., Hardwick, J. P., McBride, O. W., Nebert, D. W., Gelboin, H. V. & Meyer, U. A. (1988b). Human debrisoquine 4-hydroxylase (P450 II D I); cDNA and deduced amino acid sequence and assignment of the CYP2D locus to chromosome 22. *Genomics*, **2**, 174–9.

Gough, A. C., Miles, J. S., Spurr, N. K., Moss, J. E., Gaedigk, A., Eichelbaum, M. & Wolf, C. R. (1990). Identification of the primary gene defect at the cytochrome P_{450} CYP2D locus. *Nature*, **347**, 773–6.

Gram, L. F., Brøsen, K., Kragh-Sørensen, P. & Christensen, P. (1989b). Steady-state plasma levels of E- and Z-10-OH-nortriptyline in nortriptyline-treated patients, significance of concurrent medication and the sparteine oxidation phenotype. *Therapeutic Drug Monitoring*, **11**, 508–14.

Gram, L. F., Debruyne, D., Caillard, V., Boulenger, J. P., Lacotte, J., Moulin, M. & Zarifan, E. (1989a). Substantial rise in sparteine metabolic ratio during haloperidol treatment. *British Journal of Clinical Pharmacology*, **27**, 272–5.

Gross, A. S., Mikus, G., Fischer, C., Hertrampf, R., Gundert-Remy, U. & Eichelbaum, M. (1989). Stereoselective disposition of flecainide in relation to the sparteine/debrisoquine metabolizer phenotype. *British Journal of Clinical Pharmacology*, **28**, 555–66.

Gudjonsson, O., Sanz, E., Alvan, G., Aquilonius, S. M. & Reviriego, J. (1990). Poor hydroxylator phentoypes of debrisoquine and S-mephenytoin are not over-represented in a group of patients with Parkinson's disease. *British Journal of Clinical Pharmacology*, **30**, 301–2.

Gut, J., Gasser, R., Dayer, P., Kronback, T., Catin, T. & Meyer, U. A. (1984). Debrisoquine-type polymorphism of drug oxidation: purification from human liver of a cytochrome P450 isozyme with high activity for bufuralol hydroxylation. *FEBS Letters*, **173**, 287–90.

Guttendorf, R. J., Wedlund, P. J., Blake, J. & Chang, S. L. (1988). Simplified phenotyping with dextromethorphan by thin-layer chromatography; application to clinical laboratory screening for deficiencies in oxidative drug metabolism. *Therapeutic Drug Monitoring*, **10**, 490–8.

Haefeli, W. E., Bargetz, M. J., Follath, F. & Meyer, U. A. (1990). Potent inhibition of cytochrome P450 II D6 (Debrisoquine 4-Hydroxylase) by Flecainide in vitro and in vivo. *Journal of Cardiovascular Pharmacology*, **15**, 776–9.

Haldane, J. B. S. (1955). The estimation and significance of the logarithm of a ratio of frequency. *Annals of Human Genetics (London)*, **20**, 309–11.

Hanioka, N., Kimura, S., Meyer, U. A. & Gonzalez, F. J. (1990). The human CYP2D locus associated with a common genetic defect in drug oxidation, a $G_{1934} \rightarrow$ A base change in intron 3 of a mutant CYP 2D6 allele results in an aberrant 3′ splice recognition site. *American Journal of Human Genetics*, **47**, 994–1001.

Heim, M. & Meyer, U. A. (1990). Genotyping of poor metabolizers of debrisoquine by allele-specific PCR amplification. *Lancet*, **2**, 529–32.

Heim, M. H. & Meyer, U. A. (1992). Evolution of a highly polymorphic human cytochrome P450 gene cluster: CYP2D6 . *Genomics*, **14**, 49–58.

Henthorne, T. K., Benitez, J., Avram, M. J., Martinez, C., Llerena, A., Cobaleda, J., Krejcie, T. C. & Gibbons, R. D. (1989). Assessment of the debrisoquine and dextromethorphan phenotyping tests by gaussian mixture distributions analysis. *Clinical Pharmacology and Therapeutics*, **45**, 328–33.

Herchuelz, A., Gangji, D., Derenne, F., Jeanniot, J. P. H. & Douchamps, J. (1991). Metabolism of almitrine in extensive and poor metabolisers of debrisoquine/sparteine. *British Journal of Clinical Pharmacology*, **31**, 73–6.

Hetzel, M. R., Law, M., Keal, E. E., Sloan, T. P., Idle, J. R. & Smith, R. L. (1980). Is there a genetic component in bronchial carcinoma in smokers? *Thorax*, **35**, 709 (Abstract).

Hildebrand, M., Seifert, W. & Reichenberger, A. (1989). Determination of dextromethorphan metabolizer phenotype in healthy volunteers. *European Journal of Clinical Pharmacology*, **36**, 315–18.

Horai, Y., Fujita, K. & Ishizaki, T. (1989). Genetically determined N-acetylation and oxidation capacities in Japanese patients with non-occupational urinary bladder cancer. *European Journal of Clinical Pharmacology*, **37**, 581–7.

Horai, Y., Ishizaki, T. & Ishikawa, K. (1988). Metoprolol oxidation in a Japanese population, evidence for one poor metabolizer among 262 subjects. *British Journal of Clinical Pharmacology*, **26**, 807–8.

Horai, Y., Taga, J,. Ishizaki, T. & Ishikawa, K. (1990). Correlations among the metabolic ratios of three test probes (metoprolol, debrisoquine and sparteine) for genetically determined oxidation polymorphism in a Japanese population. *British Journal of Clinical Pharmacology*, **29**, 111–15.

Horsmans, Y., Desager, J. P. & Hervengt, C. (1991). Is there a link between debrisoquine oxidation phenotype and lung cancer susceptibility? *Biomedicine and Pharmacotherapy*, **45**, 359–62.

Huober, J., Bertram, B., Petru, E., Kaufmann, M. & Schmahl, D. (1991). Metabolism of debrisoquine and susceptibility to breast cancer. *Breast Cancer Research and Treatment*, **18**, 43–8.

Idle, J. R. (1989). Poor metabolisers of debrisoquine reveal their true colours. *Lancet*, **2**, 1097.

Idle, J. R., Mahgoub, A., Angelo, M. M., Dring, L. G., Lancaster, R. & Smith, R. L. (1979a). The metabolism of [^{14}C] debrisoquine in man. *British Journal of Clinical Pharmacology*, **7**, 257–66.

Idle, J. R., Mahgoub, A., Lancaster, R. & Smith, R. L. (1978). Hypotensive response to debrisoquine and hydroxylation phenotype. *Life Sciences*, **22**, 979–84.

Idle, J. R., Mahgoub, A., Sloan, T. P., Smith, R. L., Mbanefo, C. O. & Bababunmi, E. A. (1981). Some observations on the oxidation phenotype status of Nigerian patients presenting with cancer. *Cancer Letters*, **11**, 331–8.

Idle, J. R., Ritchie, J. C. & Smith, R. L. (1979b). Oxidation phenotype and metiamide metabolism. Proceedings of the British Pharmacological Society, 4–6 April 1979. *British*

Journal of Pharmacology, **66**, 432P.

Idle, J. R., Sloan, T. P., Smith, R. L. & Wakile, L. A. (1979c). Application of the phenotyped panel approach to the detection of polymorphism of drug oxidation in man. *British Journal of Pharmacology*, **66**, 430P–1P

P. Idle, J. R. & Smith, R. L. (1984). The debrisoquine hydroxylation gene; a gene of multiple consequence. In *Proceedings of the Second World Conference on Clinical Pharmacology and Therapeutics*, ed. L. Lemberger & M. M. Reidenberg, pp. 148–64. Bethesda, MD: American Society for Experimental Therapentics.

Inaba, T., Jurima, M., Nakano, M. & Kalow, W. (1984a). Mephenytoin and sparteine pharmacogenetics in Canadian Caucasians. *Clinical Pharmacology and Therapeutics*, **36**, 670–6.

Inaba, T., Nakano, M., Otton, S. V., Mahon, W. A. & Kalow, W. (1984b). A human cytochrome P-450 characterized by inhibition studies as the sparteine-debrisoquine mono-oxygenase. *Canadian Journal of Physiology and Pharmacology*, **62**, 860–2.

Inaba, T., Otton, S. V. & Kalow, W. (1980). Deficient metabolism of debrisoquine and sparteine. *Clinical Pharmacology and Therapeutics*, **27**, 547–9.

Inaba, T., Tyndale, R. E. & Malion, W. A. (1986). Quinidine, potent inhibition of sparteine and debrisoquine oxidation in vivo. *British Journal of Clinical Pharmacology*, **22**, 199–200.

Inaba, T., Vinks, A., Otton, S. V. & Kalow, W. (1983). Comparative pharmacogenetics of sparteine and debrisoquine. *Clinical Pharmacology and Therapeutics*, **33**, 394–9.

Ishizaki, T. (1991). Genetically determined N-acetylation and oxidation polymorphisms, their clinical implications in Far Eastern Oriental populations. *Asia Pacific Journal of Pharmacology*, **6**, 187–99.

Ishizaki, T., Eichelbaum, M., Horai, Y., Hashimoto, K., Chiba, K. & Dengler, H. J. (1987). Evidence for polymorphic oxidation of sparteine in Japanese subjects. *British Journal of Clinical Pharmacology*, **23**, 482–5.

Islam, S. A., Wolf, C. R., Lennard, M. S. & Sternberg, M. J. E. (1991). A three-dimensional molecular template for substrates of human cytochrome P-450 involved in debrisoquine 4-hydroxylation. *Carcinogenesis*, **12**, 2211–19.

Islam, S. I. & Idle, J. R. (1980). Polymorphic drug oxidation among Saudis. *Proceedings of the 5th Saudi Medical Meeting, Riyadh*, 481–6.

Iyun, A. O., Lennard, M. S., Tucker, G. T. & Woods, H. F. (1986). Metoprolol and debrisoquin metabolism in Nigerians, Lack of evidence for polymorphic oxidation. *Clinical Pharmacology and Therapeutics*, **40**, 387–94.

Jack, D. B. & Kendall, M. J. (1982). Beta blockers and debrisoquine metaboliser status. *Lancet*, **1**, 741.

Jack, D. B., Kendall, M. J., Wilkins, M. & Quarterman, C. P. (1983a). Oxidation phenotype and Beta-blockers. *New England Journal of Medicine*, **308**, 964.

Jack, D. B., Wilkins, M. & Quarterman, C. P. (1983b). Lack of evidence for polymorphism in metoprolol metabolism. *British Journal of Clinical Pharmacology*, **16**, 188–90.

Jacqz, E., Dulac, H. & Mathieu, H. (1988). Phenotyping polymorphic drug metabolism in the French Caucasian population. *European Journal of Clinical Pharmacology*, **35**, 167–71.

Jacqz-Aigrain, E., Laurent, J. & Alvarez, F. (1990). Dextromethorphan pehnotypes in paediatric patients with autoimmune hepatitis. *British Journal of Clinical Pharmacology*, **30**, 153–4.

Jacqz-Aigrain, E., Menard, Y., Popon, M. & Mathieu, H. (1989). Dextromethorphan phenotypes determined by high-performance liquid chromatography and fluorescence detection. *Journal of Chromatography*, **495**, 361–3.

Johansson, I., Yue, Q. Y., Dahl, M. L., Heim, M., Sawe, J., Bertilsson, L., Meyer, U. A., Sjöqvist, F. & Ingelman-Sundberg, M. (1991). Genetic analysis of the interethnic difference between Chinese and Caucasians in the polymorphic metabolism of debrisoquine and codeine. *European Journal of Clinical Pharmacology*, **40**, 553–6.

Johnson, K. A., Kolatkar, V. & Straka, R. J. (1990). Improved selectivity of a high performance liquid chromatography assay for debrisoquine and its 4-hydroxymetabolite from urine. *Therapeutic Drug Monitoring*, **12**, 478–80.

Jorge, L. F., Arias, T. D., Inaba, T. & Jackson, P. R. (1990). Unimodal distribution of the metabolic ratio for debrisoquine in Cuna Amerindians of Panama. *British Journal of Clinical Pharmacology*, **30**, 281–6.

Kagimoto, M., Heim, M., Kagimoto, K., Zeugin, T. & Meyer, U. A. (1990). Multiple mutations of the human cytochrome P450 II D6 gene (*CYP2D6*) in poor metabolizers of debrisoquine. *Journal of Biological Chemistry*, **265**, 17209–14.

Kaisary, A., Smith, P., Jaczq, E., McAllister, C. B., Wilkinson, G. R., Ray, W. A. & Branch, R. A. (1987). Genetic predisposition to bladder cancer, ability to hydroxylate debrisoquine and mephenytoin as risk factors. *Cancer Research*, **47**, 5488–93.

Kallio, J. (1990). The effect of urine pH on debrisoquine phenotyping, application of an HPLC-method. *International Journal of Clinical Pharmacology, Therapy and Toxicology*, **28**, 223–6.

Kallio, J., Huupponen, R. & Pyykkö, K. (1990a). The relationship between debrisoquine oxidation phenotype and the pharmacokinetics of chlorpropamide. *European Journal of Clinical Pharmacology*, **39**, 93–5.

Kallio, J., Huupponen, R., Seppäla, M., Šakö, E. & Iisalo, E. (1990b). The effects of β-adrenoceptor antagonists and levomepromazine on the metabolic ratio of debrisoquine. *British Journal of Clinical Pharmacology*, **30**, 638–43.

Kallio, J., Lindberg, R., Huupponen, R. & Iisalo, E. (1988). Debrisoquine oxidation in a Finnish population; the effect of oral contraceptives on the metabolic ratio. *British Journal of Clinical Pharmacology*, **26**, 791–5.

Kallio, J. Martilla, R. J., Rinne, U. K., Sonninen, V. & Syvälahti, E. (1991). Debrisoquine oxidation in Parkinson's disease. *Acta Neurologica Scandinavica*, **83**, 194–7.

Kalow, W. (1982). The metabolism of xenobiotics in different populations. *Canadian Journal of Physiology and Pharmacology*, **60**, 1–12.

Karalis, D. G., Nydegger, C., Porter, S., Carver, J., Pina, I. L., Kutalek, S. P. & Michelson, E. L. (1990). Effects of encainide and metabolizer phenotype on ventricular conduction during exercise. *The American Journal of Cardiology*, **66**, 1393–6.

Kassai, A., Toth, G., Eichelbaum, M. & Klotz, U. (1988). No evidence of a genetic polymorphism in the oxidative metabolism of midazolam. *Clinical Pharmacokinetics*, **15**, 319–25.

Kimura, S., Umeno, M., Skoda, R. C., Meyer, U. A. &

Gonzalez, F. J. (1989). The human debrisoquine 4-hydroxylase (CYP2D) locus, sequence and identification of the polymorphic *CYPO2D6* gene a related gene and a pseudogene. *American Journal of Human Genetics*, **45**, 889–904.

Kitchen, I., Tremblay, J., Andre, J., Dring, L. G., Idle, J. R., Smith, R. L. & Williams, R. T. (1979). Interindividual and interspecies variation in the metabolism of the hallucinogen 4-methoxyamphetamine. *Xenobiotica*, **9**, 397–404.

Knodell, R. G., Browne, D. G., Gwozdz, G. P., Brian, W. R. & Guengerich, F. P. (1991). Differential inhibition of individual human liver cytochromes P-450 by cimetidine. *Gastroenterology*, **101**, 1680–91.

Kong, I., Devonshire, H. W., Cooper, M., Sloan, T. P., Idle, J. R. & Smith, R. L. (1982). The influence of oxidation phenotype on phenacetin metabolism and haemotoxicity. *British Journal of Clinical Pharmacology*, **13**, 275P – 276P.

Koymans, L., Vermeulen, N. P .E., van Acker, S. A. B. E., te Koppele, J. M., Heykants, J. J. P., Lavrijsen, K., Meuldermans, W. & den Kelder, G. M. D. O. (1992). A predictive model for substrates of cytochrome P-450-debrisoquine (2D6). *Chemical Research in Toxicology*, **5**, 211–19.

Kroemer, H. K., Fischer, C., Meese, C. O. & Eichelbaum, M. (1991). Enantiomer-enantiomer interaction of (S)- and (R)-propafenone for cytochrome P450IID6 - catalyzed 5-hydroxylation, in vitro evaluation of the mechanism. *Molecular Pharmacology*, **40**, 135–42.

Kroemer, H. K., Mikus, G., Kronbach, T., Meyer, U. A. & Eichelbaum, M. (1989). *In vitro* characterization of the human cytochrome P450 involved in polymorphic oxidation of propafenone. *Clinical Pharmacology and Therapeutics*, **45**, 28–33.

Kupfer, A. & Preisig, R. (1984). Pharmacogenetics of mephenytoin. A new drug hydroxylation polymorphism in man. *European Journal of Clinical Pharmacology*, **26**, 753–9.

Kupfer, A., Schmid, B., Preisig, R. & Pfaff, G. (1984). Dextromethorphan as a safe probe for debrisoquine hydroxylation polymorphism. *Lancet*, **2**, 517–18.

Ladero, J. M., Benitez, J., Gonzalez, J. F., Vargas, E. & Diaz-Rubio, M. (1991a). Oxidative polymorphism of debrisoquine is not related to human colo-rectal cancer. *European Journal of Clinical Pharmacology*, **40**, 525–7.

Ladero, J. M., Benitez, J., Jara, C., Llerena, A., Valdivielso, M. J., Munoz, J. J. & Vargas, E. (1991b). Polymorphic oxidation of debrisoquine in women with breast cancer. *Oncology*, **48**, 107–10.

Ladona, M. G., Lindström, B., Thyr, C., Dun-Ren, P. & Rane, A. (1991). Differential foetal development of the O- and N-demethylation of dextromethorphan in man. *British Journal of Clinical Pharmacology*, **32**, 295–302.

Lancaster, D. L., Adio, R. A., Tai, K. K., Simooya, O. O., Broadhead, G. D., Tucker, G. T. & Leonard, M. S. (1990). Inhibition of metoprolol metabolism by chloroquine and other antimalarial drugs. *Journal of Pharmacy and Pharmacology*, **42**, 267–271.

Lanthier, P. L., Reshef, R., Shah, R. R., Oates, N. S., Smith, R. L. & Morgan, M. Y. (1984). Oxidation phenotyping in alcoholics with liver disease of varying severity. *Alcoholism, Clinical and Experimental Research*, **8**, 435–41.

Larrey, D., Amouyal, G., Tinel, M., Letteron, P., Berson, A., Labbe, G. & Pessayre, D. (1987). Polymorphism of

dextromethorphan oxidation in a French population. *British Journal of Clinical Pharmacology*, **24**, 676–9.

Latini, R., Belloni, M., Bernasconi, R., Cappiello, E., Giani, P., Landolina, M., Leopaldi, D. & Castel, J. M. (1992). Identification of propafenone metaboliser phenotype from plasma and urine excretion data. *European Journal of Clinical Pharmacology*, **42**, 111–14.

Law, M. R., Hetzel, M. R. & Idle, J. R. (1989). Debrisoquine metabolism and genetic predisposition to lung cancer. *British Journal of Cancer*, **59**, 686–8.

Leclerq, V., Desager, J. P, Horsman, Y., van Nieuwenhuyze, Y. & Harvengt, C. (1989). Influence of rifampicin, phenobarbital and cimetidine on mixed function monooxygenase in extensive and poor metabolizers of debrisoquine. *International Journal of Clinical Pharmacology, Therapy and Toxicology*, **27**, 593–8.

Lee, E. J. D., Nam, Y. P. & Hee, G. N. (1988). Oxidation phenotyping in Chinese and Malay populations. *Clinical and Experimental Pharmacology and Physiology*, **15**, 889–91.

Lee, J. T., Kroemer, H. K., Silberstein, D. J., Funck-Brentano, C., Lineberry, M. D., Wood, A. J. J., Roben, D. M. & Woosley, R. L. (1990). The role of genetically determined polymorphic drug metabolism in the beta-blockade produced by propafenone. *The New England Journal of Medicine*, **322**, 1764–8.

Lennard, M. S. (1990). Genetic polymorphism of sparteine/debrisoquine oxidation, a reappraisal. *Pharmacology and Toxicology*, **67**, 273–93.

Lennard, J. M., Benitez, J., Jara, C., Llerena, A., Valdivielso, M. J., Munoz, J. J. & Vargas, E. (1991). Polymorphic oxidation of debrisoquine in women with breast cancer. *Oncology*, **48**, 107–10.

Lennard, M. S., Iyun, A. O., Jackson, P. R., Tucker, G. T. & Woods, H. F. (1992). Evidence for a dissociation in the control of sparteine, debrisoquine and metoprolol metabolism in Nigerians. *Pharmacogenetics*, **2**, 89–92.

Lennard, M. S., Jackson, P. R., Freestone, S., Tucker, G. T., Ramsay, L. E. & Woods, H. F. (1984). The relationship between debrisoquine oxidation phenotype and the pharmacokinetics and pharmacodynamics of propanolol. *British Journal of Clinical Pharmacology*, **17**, 679–85.

Lennard, M. S., McGourty, J. C. & Silas, J. H. (1988a). Lack of relationship between debrisoquine oxidation phenotype and the pharmacokinetics and first dose effect of prazosin. *British Journal of Clinical Pharmacology*, **25**, 276–8.

Lennard, M. S., Ramsay, L. E., Silas, J. H., Tucker, G. T. & Woods, H. F. (1983). Protecting the poor metabolizer, clinical consequences of genetic polymorphism of drug oxidation. *Pharmacy International*, **4**, 53–7.

Lennard, M. S., Silas, J. H., Freestone, S., Ramsay, L. E., Tucker, G. T. & Woods, H. F. (1982a). Oxidation phenotype - a major determinant of metoprolol metabolism and response. *New England Journal of Medicine*, **307**, 1558–60.

Lennard, M. S., Silas, J. H., Freestone, S. & Trevethick, J. (1982b). Defective metabolism of metoprolol in poor hydroxylators of debrisoquine. *British Journal of Clinical Pharmacology*, **14**, 301–3.

Lennard, M. S., Tucker, G. T., Silas, J. H. & Woods, H. F. (1986). Debrisoquine polymorphism and the metabolism and action of metoprolol timolol propanolol and atenolol. *Xenobiotica*, **16**, 435–47.

Lennard, M. S., Tucker, G. T., Woods, H. F., Iyun, A. O. & Eichelbaum, M. (1988b). Stereoselective 4-hydroxylation of debrisoquine in Nigerians. *Biochemical Pharmacology*, **37**, 97–8.

Lennard, M. S., Tucker, G. T., Woods, H. F., Silas, J. H. & Iyun, A. O. (1989). Stereoselective metabolism of metoprolol in Caucasians and Nigerians – relationship to debrisoquine oxidation phenotype. *British Journal of Clinical Pharmacology*, **27**, 613–16.

Lewis, R. V., Ramsay, L. E., Jackson, P. R., Yeo, W. W., Lennard, M. S. & Tucker, G. T. (1991). Influence of debrisoquine oxidation phenotype on exercise tolerance and subjective fatigue after metoprolol and atenolol in healthy subjects. *British Journal of Clinical Pharmacology*, **31**, 391–8.

Llerena, A., Alm, C., Dahl, M. L., Ekqvist, B. & Bertilsson, L. (1992a). Haloperidol disposition is dependent on debrisoquine hydroxylation phenotype. *Therapeutic Drug Monitoring*, **14**, 92–7.

Llerena, A., Dahl, M. L., Ekqvist, B. & Bertilsson, L. (1992b). Haloperidol disposition is dependent on the debrisoquine hydroxylation phenotype: increased plasma levels of the reduced metabolite in poor metabolizers. *Therapeutic Drug Monitoring*, **14**, 261–4.

Löf, A., Hansen, S. H., Naslund, P., Steiner, E., Wallen, M. & Hjelm, E. W. (1990). Relationship between uptake and elimination of toluene and debrisoquine hydroxylation polymorphism. *Clinical Pharmacology and Therapeutics*, **47**, 412–17.

Lou, Y. C., Ying, L., Bertilsson, L. & Sjoqvist, F. (1987). Low frequency of slow debrisoquine hydroxylation in a native chinese population. *Lancet*, **2**, 852–3.

McGourty, J. C., Silas, J. H., Lennard, M. S., Tucker, G. T. & Woods, H. F. (1985). Metoprolol metabolism and debrisoquine oxidation polymorphism - population and family studies. *British Journal of Clinical Pharmacology*, **20**, 555–66.

Mahgoub, A., Dring, L. G., Idle, J. R., Lancaster, R. & Smith, R. L. (1977). Polymorphic hydroxylation of debrisoquine in man. *Lancet*, **2**, 584–6.

Marre, F., Fabre, G., Lacarelle, B., Bourrie, M., Catalin, J., Berger, Y., Rahmani, R. & Cano, J. P. (1992). Involvement of the cytochrome P-450 II D sub-family in minoprine 4-hydroxylation by human hepatic microsomes. *Drug Metabolism and Disposition*, **20**, 316–21.

Martin, D. W., Mayes, P. A., Rodwell, V. W. & Grauner, D. K. (1985). *Harper's Review of Biochemistry* . p. 83. Los Altos CA: Lange Medical Publications.

Matsunaga, E., Zeugin, T., Zanger, U. M., Aoyama, T., Meyer, U. A. & Gonzalez, F. J. (1990). Sequence requirements for cytochrome P-450IID1 catalytic activity. A single amino acid change (ILE^{380} PHE) specifically decreases V_{max} of the enzyme for bufuralol but not debrisoquine hydroxylation. *Journal of Biological Chemistry*, **265**, 17197–201.

Mbanefo, C., Bababunmi, E. A., Mahgoub, A., Sloan, T. P., Idle, J. R. & Smith, R. L. (1980). A study of the debrisoquine hydroxylation polymorphism in a Nigerian population. *Xenobiotica*, **10**, 811–18.

Meese, C. O., Fisher, C. & Eichelbaum, M. (1988). Stereoselectivity of the 4-hydroxylation of debrisoquine in man detected by gas chromatography/mass spectrometry. *Biomedical and Environmental Mass Spectrometry*, **15**, 63–6.

Meier, P. J., Mueller, H. K., Dick, B. & Meyer, U. A. (1983). Hepatic mono-oxygenase activities in subjects with a genetic defect in drug oxidation. *Gastroenterology*, **85**, 682–92.

Meillard, M. N., Beutue-Ferrer, D., Brunet-Bourgin, F., Morel, G. & Allain, H. (1990). Etude de l'hydroxylation de la débrisoquine dans la maladie de Parkinson. *Presse Medicale*, **19**, 947–9.

Mellstrom, B., Bertilsson, L., Sawe, J., Schulz, H. U. & Sjoqvist, F. (1981). E- and Z-10-hydroxylation of nortriptyline, relationship to polymorphic debrisoquine hydroxylation. *Clinical Pharmacology and Therapeutics*, **30**, 189–93.

Mellstrom, B., Sawe, J., Bertilsson, L. & Sjöqvist, F. (1986). Amitriptyline metabolism; association with debrisoquine hydroxylation in non-smokers. *Clinical Pharmacology and Therapeutics*, **39**, 369–71.

Meyer, U. A., Gut, J., Kronbach, T., Skoda, C., Meier, U. T. Catin, T. & Dayer, P. (1986). The molecular mechanisms of two common polymorphisms of drug oxidation – evidence for functional changes in cytochrome P-450 isozymes catalysing bufuralol and mephenytoin oxidation. *Xenobiotica*, **16**, 449–64.

Mikus, G., Gross, A. S., Beckmann, J., Hertrampf, R., Gundert-Remy, U. & Eichelbaum, M. (1989). The influence of the sparteine/debrisoquine phenotype on the disposition of flecainide. *Clinical Pharmacology and Therapeutics*, **45**, 562–7.

Mikus, G., Ha, H. R., Vozeh, S., Zekorn, C., Follath, F. & Eichelbaum, M. (1986). Pharmacokinetics and metabolism of quinidine in extensive and poor metabolisers of sparteine. *European Journal of Clinical Pharmacology*, **31**, 69–72.

Miners, J. O., Wing, L. M. H. & Birkett, D. J. (1985). Normal metabolism of debrisoquine and theophylline in a slow tolbutamide metaboliser. *Australian and New Zealand Journal of Medicine*, **15**, 348–9.

Mitchell, S. C., Waring, R. H., Haley, C. S., Idle, J. R. & Smith, R. L. (1984). Genetic aspects of the polymorphically distributed suphoxidation of S-carboxymethyl-L-cysteine in man. *British Journal of Clinical Pharmacology*, **18**, 507–21.

Morgan, M. Y., Reshef, R., Shah, R. R., Oates, N. S., Smith, R. L. & Sherlock, S. (1984). Impaired oxidation of debrisoquine in patients with perhexilene liver injury. *Gut*, **25**, 1057–64.

Mortimer, O., Lindrom, B., Laurell, H., Bergman, U. & Rane, A. (1989). Dextromethorphan, polymorphic serum pattern of the O-demethylated and didemethylated metabolites in man. *British Journal of Clinical Pharmacology*, **27**, 223–7.

Mortimer, O., Persson, K., Ladona, M. G., Spalding, D., Zanger, U. M., Meyer, U. A. & Rane, A. (1990). Polymorphic formation of morphine from codeine in poor and extensive metabolizers of dextromethorphan, relationship to the presence of immunoidentified cytochrome P-450IID1. *Clinical Pharmacology and Therapeutics*, **47**, 27–35.

Mura, C., Broyard, J. P., Jacqz-Aigrain, E. & Krishnamoorthy, R. (1991). Distinct phenotypes and genotypes of debrisoquine hydroxylation among Europeans and Chinese. *British Journal of Clinical Pharmacology*, **32**, 135–6.

Muralidharan, G., Hawes, E. M., McKay, G., Korchinski, E. D. & Midha, K. K. (1991). Quinidine but not quinine inhibits in man the oxidative metabolic routes of methoxyphenamine which involve debrisoquine 4-hydroxylase. *European Journal of Clinical Pharmacology*, **41**, 471–4.

Nakamura, K., Goto, F., Ray, W. A., McAllister, C. B., Jacqz, E., Wilkinson, G. R. & Branch, R. A. (1985). Interethnic differences in genetic polymorphism of debrisoquine and mephenytoin hydroxylation between Japanese and Caucasian populations. *Clinical Pharmacology and Therapeutics*, **38**, 402–8.

Nebert, D. W. & Gonzalez, F. J. (1987). P450 genes, structure, evolution and regulation. *Annual Review of Biochemistry*, **56**, 945–93.

Nebert, D. W., Nelson, D. R., Coon, M. J., Estabrook, R. W., Feyereisen, R., Fujii-Kuriyama, Y., Gonzalez, F. J., Guengerich, F. P., Gunsalus, I. C., Johnson, E. F., Loper, J. C., Sato, R., Waterman, M. R. & Waxman, D. J. (1991). The P450 superfamily, update on new sequences, gene mapping and recommended nomenclature. *DNA and Cell Biology*, **10**, 1–14

Newton, B. W., Benson, R. C. & McCarriston, C. C. (1966). Sparteine sulfate, A potent capricious oxytocic. *American Journal of Obstetrics and Gynecology*, **94**, 234–41.

Nielsen, M. D., Brøsen, K. & Gram, L. F. (1990). A dose-effect study of the *in vivo* inhibitory effect of quinidine on sparteine oxidation in man. *British Journal of Clinical Pharmacology*, **29**, 299–304.

Nielsen, K. K., Brøsen, K., Gram, L. F. and the Danish University Antidepressant Group (1992). Steady-state plasma levels of clomipramine and its metabolites: impact of the sparteine/debrisoquine oxidation polymorphism. *European Journal of Clinical Pharmacology*, **43**, 405–11.

Nordin, C., Siwers, B., Benitez, J. & Bertilsson, L. (1985). Plasma concentrations of nortriptyline and its 10-hydroxy metabolite in depressed patients – relationship to the debrisoquine hydroxylation metabolic ratio. *British Journal of Clinical Pharmacology*, **19**, 832–5.

Nsabiyumva, F., Furet, Y., Autret, E., Jonville, A. P. & Breteau, M. (1991). Oxidative polymorphism of dextromethorphan in a Burundi population. *European Journal of Clinical Pharmacology*, **41**, 75–7.

Oates, N. S., Shah, R. R., Drury, P. L., Idle, J. E. & Smith, R. L. (1982b). Captopril-induced agranulocytosis associated with an impairment of debrisoquine hydroxylation. *British Journal of Clinical Pharmacology*, **14**, 601P.

Oates, N. S., Shah, R. R., Idle, J. R. & Smith, R. L. (1982a). Genetic polymorphism of phenformin 4-hydroxylation. *Clinical Pharmacology and Therapeutics*, **32**, 81–9.

Oates, N. S., Shah, R. R., Idle, J. R. & Smith, R. L. (1983). Influence of oxidation polymorphism on phenformin kinetics and dynamics. *Clinical Pharmacology and Therapeutics*, **34**, 827–34. Oram, M., Wilson, K., Burnett,

Oates, N. S., Shah, R. R., Idle, J. R. & Smith, R. L. (1983). Influence of oxidation polymorphism on phenformin kinetics and dynamics. *Clinical Pharmacology and Therapeutics*, **34**, 827–34.

Oram, M., Wilson, K., Burnett, D., Al-Dabbagh, S. G., Idle, J. R. & Smith, R. L. (1982). Metabolic oxidation of methaqualone in extensive and poor metabolisers of debrisoquine. *European Journal of Clinical Pharmacology*, **23**, 147–50.

Otton, S. V., Brinn, R. V. & Gram, L. F. (1988b). *In vitro* evidence against the oxidation of quinidine by the sparteine/debrisoquine mono-oxygenase of human liver. *Drug Metabolism and Disposition*, **16**, 15–17.

Otton, S. V., Crewe, H. K., Lennard, M. S., Tucker, G. T. & Woods, H. F. (1988a). Use of quinidine inhibition to define the role of the sparteine/debrisoquine cytochrome

P450 in metoprolol oxidation by human liver microsomes. *Journal of Pharmacology and Experimental Therapeutics*, **247**, 242–7.

Otton, S. V., Gillam, E. M. J., Lennard, M. S., Tucker, G. T. & Woods, H. F. (1990). Propanolol oxidation by human liver microsomes – the use of cumene hydroperoxide to probe isoenzyme specificity and regioselectivity and stereoselectivity. *British Journal of Clinical Pharmacology*, **30**, 751–60.

Otton, S. V., Inaba, T. & Kalow, W. (1983). Inhibition of sparteine oxidation in human liver by tricyclic antidepressants and other drugs. *Life Sciences*, **32**, 795–800.

Otton, S. V., Inaba, T. & Kalow, W. (1984). Competitive inhibition of sparteine oxidation in human liver by β-adrenoceptor antagonists and other cardiovascular drugs. *Life Sciences*, **34**, 73–80.

Otton, S. V., Inaba, T., Mahon, W. A. & Kalow, W. (1982a). *In vitro* metabolism of sparteine by human liver; competitive inhibition by debrisoquine. *Canadian Journal of Physiology and Pharmacology*, **60**, 102–5.

Paar, W. D., Schuhler, H., Fimmers, R. & Dengler, H. J. (1989). Sparteine oxidation polymorphism, phenotyping by measurement of sparteine and its dehydrometabolites in plasma. *European Journal of Clinical Pharmacology*, **36**, 555–60.

Peart, G. F., Boutagy, J. & Shenfield, G. M. (1986). Debrisoquine oxidation in an Australian population. *British Journal of Clinical Pharmacology*, **21**, 465–71.

Peart, G. F., Boutagy, J. & Shenfield, G. M. (1987). Lack of relationship between tolbutamide metabolism and debrisoquine oxidation phenotype. *European Journal of Clinical Pharmacology*, **33**, 397–402.

Perault, M. C., Bouquet, S., Bertschy, G., Vandel, S., Chakroun, R., Guibert, S. & Vandel, B. (1991). Debrisoquine and dextromethorphan phenotyping and antidepressant treatment. *Therapie*, **46**, 1–3.

Pfaff, G., Briegel, P. & Lamprecht, I. (1983). Inter-individual variation in the metabolism of dextromethorphan. *International Journal of Pharmaceutics*, **14**, 173–89.

Philip, P. A., James, C. A. & Rogers, H. J. (1989). The influence of cimetidine on debrisoquine 4-hydroxylation in extensive metabolizers. *European Journal of Clinical Pharmacology*, **36**, 319–21.

Philip, P. A., Rogers, H. J. & Harper, P. G. (1987). Acetylation and oxidation phenotypes in malignant lymphoma. *Cancer Chemotherapy and Pharmacology*, **20**, 235–8.

Pierce, D. M., Smith, S. E. & Franklin, R. A. (1987). The pharmacokinetics of indoramin and 6-hydroxyindoramin in poor and extensive hydroxylators of debrisoquine. *European Journal of Clinical Pharmacology*, **33**, 59–65.

Poirier, J., Roy, M., Campanella, G., Cloutier, T. & Paris, S. (1987). Debrisoquine metabolism in Parkinsonian patients treated with antihistamine drugs. *Lancet*, **2**, 386.

Pollock, B. G., Perel, J. M., Altieri, L. P., Krishner, M., Fasiczka, A. L., Houck, P. R. & Reynolds III CF. (1992). Debrisoquine hydroxylation phenotyping in geriatric psychopharmacology. *Psychopharmacology Bulletin*, **28**, 163–8.

Pontin, J. E., Hamed, H., Fentiman, I. S. & Idle, J. R. (1990). Cytochrome P450dbI phenotypes in malignant and benign breast disease. *European Journal of Cancer*, **26**, 790–2.

Quart, B., Durkee, J. & Soyka, L. (1986). Polymorphic encainide oxidation; what is the clinical significance? *Acta Pharmacologica Toxicologica*, 59, Suppl V 116 (Abstr 333) cited by Roden DM, Woosley RL. (1988). Clinical pharmacokinetics of encainide. *Clinical Pharmacokinetics*, **14**, 141–7.

Raghuram, T. C., Koshakji, R. P., Wilkinson, G. R. & Wood, A. J. J. (1984). Polymorphic ability to metabolise propanolol alters 4-hydroxy propanolol levels but not beta-blockade. *Clinical Pharmacology and Therapeutics*, **36**, 51–6.

Relling, M. V., Evans, W. E., Fonne-Pfister, R. & Meyer, U. A. (1989). Anticancer drugs as inhibitors of two polymorphic cytochrome P-450 enzymes, debrisoquine and mephenytoin hydroxylase in human liver microsomes. *Cancer Research*, **49**, 68–71.

Ritter, J., Somasundaram, R., Heinemeyer, G. & Roots, J. (1986). The debrisoquine hydroxylation phenotype and the acetylator phenotype as genetic risk factors in the occurrence of larynx and pharynx carcinoma. *Acta Pharmacologica et Toxicologica*, Suppl. IX, p. 221.

Roden, D. M., Duff, H. J., Primm, R. K., Kronenberg, M. W. & Woosley, R. L. (1981). Control of ventricular pre-excitation and associated arrhythmias by encainide. *American Heart Journal*, **102**, 794–7.

Roden, D. M. & Woosley, R. L. (1988). Clinical pharmacokinetics of encainide. *Clinical Pharmacokinetics*, **14**, 141–7.

Roots, I., Drakoulis, N., Brockmoller, J., Janicke, I., Cuprunov, M. & Ritter, J. (1989). Hydroxylation and acetylation phenotypes as genetic risk factors in certain malignancies. In *Xenobiotic Metabolism and Disposition*, ed. R. Kato, R. W. Estabrook & M. N. Cayen, pp. 499–506. London: Taylor & Francis.

Roots, I., Drakoulis, N., Ploch, M., Heinemeyer, G., Loddenkemper, R., Minks, T., Nitz, M., Otte, F. & Koch, M. (1988). Debrisoquine hydroxylation phenotype, acetylation phenotype and ABO blood groups as genetic host factors of lung cancer risk. *Klinische Wochenschrift*, 66 Suppl. XI; 87–97.

Roots, I., Heinemyer, G., Drakoulis, N. & Kampf, D. (1987). The role of pharmacogenetics in drug epidemiology. In *Epidemiological concepts in Clinical Pharmacology*, ed. H. Kemtz, I. Roots & K. Voigt. Berlin: Springer-Verlag.

Roy, S. D., Hawes, E. M., Hubbard, J. W., McKay, G. & Midha, K. K. (1984). Methoxyphenamine and dextromethorphan as safe probes for debrisoquine hydroxylation polymorphism. *Lancet*, **2**, 1393.

Roy, S. D., Hawes, E. M., McKay, G., Korchinski, E. D. & Midha, K. K., (1985). Metabolism of methoxyphenamine in extensive and poor metabolizers of debrisoquin. *Clinical Pharmacology and Therapeutics*, **38**, 128–33.

Salminen, L., Lindberg, R., Toivari, H. R., Huupponen, R., Kaila, T. & Iisalo, E. (1989). Prevalence of debrisoquine oxidation phenotypes in glaucoma patients. *International Ophthalmology*, **13**, 91–3.

Saner, H., Gurtner, H. P., Preisig, R. & Kupfer, A. (1986). Polymorphic debrisoquine and mephenytoin hydroxylation in patients with pulmonary hypertension of vascular origin after aminorex fumarate. *European Journal of Clinical Pharmacology*, **31**, 437–42.

Sanz, E. J. & Bertilsson, L. (1990).D -Propoxyphene is a potent inhibitor of debrisoquine but not S-mephenytoin 4-hydroxylation in vivo. *Therapeutic Drug Monitoring*, **12**, 297–99.

Sardas, S., Pontin, J. & Idle, J. R. (1991). Polymorphic 4-hydroxylation of debrisoquine in a Turkish population. *Pharmacogenetics*, **1**, 123–4.

Schellens, J. H. M., van der Wart, J. H. F., Brugman, M. & Breimer, D. D. (1989). Influence of enzyme induction and inhibition on the oxidation of nifedipine sparteine mephenytoin and antipyrine in humans as assessed by a 'cocktail' study design. *Journal of Pharmacology and Experimental Therapeutics*, **249**, 638–45.

Schmid, B., Bircher, J., Preisig, R. & Kupfer, A. (1985). Polymorphic dextromethorphan metabolism, cosegregation of oxidative O-demethylation with debrisoquine hydroxylation. *Clinical Pharmacology and Therapeutics*, **38**, 618–24.

Seymour, M. (1990). Stereoisomerism in pharmaceuticals. *The Pharmaceutical Journal*, **244**, 25–8.

Shah, R. R., Evans, D. A., Oates, N. S., Idle, J. R. & Smith, R. L. (1985). The genetic control of phenformin 4-hydroxylation. *Journal of Medical Genetics*, **22**, 361–6.

Shah, R. R., Oates, N. S., Idle, J. R. & Smith, R. L. (1982a). Beta blockers and drug oxidation status. *Lancet*, **1**, 508–9.

Shah, R. R., Oates, N. S., Idle, J. R., Smith, R. L. & Lockhart, J. D. F. (1982b). Impaired oxidation of debrisoquine in patients with perhexilene neuropathy. *British Medical Journal*, **284**, 295–9.

Shaheen, O., Biollaz, J., Koshakji, R. P., Wilkinson, G. R. & Wood, A. J. J. (1989). Influence of debrisoquin phenotype on the inducibility of propanolol metabolism. *Clinical Pharmacology and Therapeutics*, **45**, 439–43.

Shaheen, O., Patel, J., Avant, G. R., Hamilton, M. & Wood, A. J. J. (1986). Effect of cirrhosis and debrisoquin phenotype on the disposition and effects of pinacidil. *Clinical Pharmacology and Therapeutics*, **40**, 650–5.

Shahidi, N. T. (1968). Acetophenetidin-induced methemoglobinemia. *Annals of the New York Academy of Sciences*, **151**, 822–32.

Shaw, G. L., Falk, R. T., Caporaso, N. E., Issaq, H. J., Fox, S. D. & Tucker, M. A. (1990). Effect of diurnal variation on debrisoquine metabolic phenotyping. *Journal of the National Cancer Institute*, **82**, 1573–4.

Siddoway, L. A., McAllister, B,. Wang, T., Bergstrand, R. H., Roden, D. M., Wilkinson, G. R. & Woosley, R. L. (1983). Polymorphic oxidative metabolism of propafenone in man. *Circulation*, **68**, Suppl. III, Abstract 253, p. III–64.

Siddoway, L. A., Thompson, K. A., McAllister, C. B., Wang, T., Wilkinson, G. R., Roden, D. M. & Woosley, R. L. (1987). Polymorphism of propafenone metabolism and disposition in man, clinical and pharmacokinetic consequences. *Circulation*, **75**, 785–91.

Siegmund, W., Hanke, W., Zschiesche, M., Franke, G., Biebler, K. E. & Wilke, A. (1990). N-acetylation and debrisoquine type oxidation polymorphism in Caucasians {en} with reference to age and sex. *International Journal of Clinical Pharmacology, Therapy and Toxicology*, **28**, 504–9.

Silas, J. H., Lennard, M. S., Tucker, G. T., Smith, A. J., Malcolm, S. L. & Marten, T. R. (1977). Why hypertensive patients vary in their response to oral debrisoquine. *British Medical Journal*, **1**, 422-425.

Sindrup, S. H., Brøsen, K., Bjerring, P., Arendt-Nielsen, L., Larsen, V., Angelo, H. R. & Gram, L. F. (1991). Codeine increases pain thresholds to copper vapor laser stimuli in extensive but not poor metabolizers of sparteine. *Clinical Pharmacology and Therapeutics*, **49**, 686–93.

Sindrup, S. H., Brøsen, K. & Gram, L. F. (1992b). Pharmacokinetics of the selective serotonin reuptake inhibitor paroxetine, Nonlinearity and relation to the sparteine oxidation polymorphism. *Clinical Pharmacology and Therapeutics*, **51**, 288–95.

Sindrup, S. H., Brøsen, K., Gram, L. F., Hallas, J., Skjelbo, E., Allen, A., Allen, G. D., Cooper, S. M., Mellows, G., Tasker, T. C. G. & Zussman, B. D. (1992a). The relationship between paroxetine and the sparteine oxidation polymorphism. *Clinical Pharmacology and Therapeutics*, **51**, 278–87.

Skjelbo, E., Brøsen, K., Hallas, J. & Gram, L. F. (1991). The mephenytoin oxidation polymorphism is partially responsible for the N-demethylation of imipramine. *Clinical Pharmacology and Therapeutics*, **49**, 18–23.

Skoda, R. C., Gonzalez, F. J., Demierre, A. & Meyer, U. A. (1988). Two mutant alleles of the human cytochrome P-450 db1 gene (P450C2D1) associated with genetically deficient metabolism of debrisoquine and other drugs. *Proceedings of the National Academy of Sciences (USA)*, **85**, 5240–3.

Sloan, T. P., Mahgoub, A., Lancaster, R., Idle, J. R. & Smith, R. L. (1978). Polymorphism of carbon oxidation of drugs and clinical implications. *British Medical Journal*, **2**, 655–7.

Smith, R. L. (1986). Human genetic variations in oxidative drug metabolism. *Xenobiotica*, **16**, 361–5.

Smith, A. D., Gough, A. C., Leigh, P. N., Summers, B. A., Harding, A. E., Maranganore, D. M., Sturman, S. G., Schapira, A. H. V., Williams, A. C., Spurr, N. K. & Wolf, C. R. (1992). Debrisoquine hydroxylase gene polymorphism and susceptibility to Parkinson's disease. *Lancet*, **339**, 1375–7.

Sohn, D. R., Shin, S. G., Park, C. W., Kusaka, M., Chiba, K. & Ishizaki, T. (1991). Metoprolol oxidation polymorphism in a Korean population, comparison with native Japanese and Chinese populations. *British Journal of Clinical Pharmacology*, **32**, 504–7.

Sommers, De K., Moncrieff, J. & Avenant, J. (1988). Polymorphism of the 4-hydroxylation of debrisoquine in the San Bushmen of Southern Africa. *Human Toxicology*, **7**, 273–6.

Sommers, De K, Moncrieff, J. & Avenant, J. (1989a). Metoprolol α-hydroxylation polymorphism in the San Bushmen of Southern Africa. *Human Toxicology*, **8**, 39–43.

Sommers, De K., Moncrieff, J. & Avenant, J. (1989b). Non-correlation between debrisoquine and metoprolol polymorphisms in the Venda. *Human Toxicology*, **8**, 365–8.

Sommers, De K., Moncrieff, J. & Avenant, J. (1990). Polymorphism in sparteine oxidation in the Barakwena (Kwengo) of Southern Africa. *South African Journal of Science*, **86**, 28–9.

Sommers, De K., Moncrieff, J. & Avenant, J. C. (1991). Absence of polymorphism of sparteine oxidation in the South African Venda. *Human and Experimental Toxicology*, **10**, 175–8.

Speirs, C. J., Murray, S., Boobis, A. R., Seddon, C. E. & Davies, D. S. (1986). Quinidine and the identification of drugs whose elimination is impaired in subjects classified as poor metabolizers of debrisoquine. *British Journal of Clinical Pharmacology*, B22, 739–43.

Speirs, C. J., Murray, S., Davies, D. S., Biola Mabadeje, A. F. & Boobis, A. R. (1990). Debrisoquine oxidation phenotype and susceptibility to lung cancer. *British Journal of Clinical Pharmacology*, **29**, 101–9.

Spina, E., Ancione, M., DiRosa, A. E., Meduri, M. & Capute, A. P. (1992b). Polymorphic debrisoquine oxidation and actue neuroleptic-induced adverse effects. *European Journal of Clinical Pharmacology*, **42**, 347–8.

Spina, E., Birgersson, C., von Bahr, C., Ericsson, O., Mellstrom, B., Steiner, E. & Sjöqvist, I. (1984). Phenotypic consistency in hydroxylation of desmethylimipramine and debrisoquine in healthy subjects and in human liver microsomes. *Clinical Pharmacology and Therapeutics*, **36**, 677–82.

Spina, E., Campo, G. M., Calandra, S., Capute, A. P., Carrillo, J. A. & Benitez, J. (1992a). Debrisoquine oxidation in an Italian population, A study in healthy subjects and in schizophrenic patients. *Pharmacological Research*, **25**, 43–50.

Spina, E., Martines, C., Caputi, A. P., Copaleda, J., Pinas, B., Carrillo, J. A. & Benitez, J. (1991). Debrisoquine oxidation phenotype during neuroleptic monotherapy. *European Journal of Clinical Pharmacology*, **41**, 467–70.

Spina, E., Steiner, E,. Ericsson, O. & Sjöqvist, F. (1987). Hydroxylation of desmethylimipramine, dependence on the debrisoquin hydroxylation phenotype. *Clinical Pharmacology and Therapeutics*, **41**, 314–19.

Steiger, M. J., Lledo, P., Quinn, N. P., Marsden, C. D., Turner, P. & Jenner, P. G. (1992). Debrisoquine hydroxylation in Parkinson's disease. *Acta Neurologica Scandinavica* **86**, 159–64.

Steiner, E., Alvan, G., Garle, M., Maguire, J. H., Lind, M., Nilson, S. O., Tomson, T., McClanahan, J. S. & Sjöqvist, F. (1987). The debrisoquine hydroxylation phenotype does not predict the metabolism of phenytoin. *Clinical Pharmacology and Therapeutics*, **42**, 326–33.

Steiner, E., Bertilsson, L. Šawe, J. Bertling, I. & Sjöqvist, F. (1988). Polymorphic debrisoquin hydroxylation in 757 Swedish subjects. *Clinical Pharmacology and Therapeutics*, **44**, 431–5.

Steiner, E., Iselius, L., Alvan, G., Lindsten, J. & Sjöqvist, F. (1985). A family study of genetic and environmental factors determining polymorphic hydroxylation of debrisoquine. *Clinical Pharmacology and Therapeutics*, **38**, 394–401.

Steiner, E. & Spina, E. (1987). Differences in the inhibitory effect of cimetidine on desipramine metabolism between rapid and slow debrisoquine hydroxylators. *Clinical Pharmacology and Therapeutics*, **42**, 278–82.

Steventon, G. B., Heafield, M. T. E., Sturman, S. G., Waring, R. H., Williams, A. C. & Ellington, J. (1989). Degenerative neurological disease and debrisoquine-4-hydroxylation phenotype. *Medical Science Research*, **17**, 163–4.

Sugimura, H., Caporaso, N. E., Shaw, G. L., Modali, R. V., Gonzalez, F. J., Hoover, R. N., Resau, J. H., Trump, B. F., Weston, A. & Harris, C. C. (1990). Human debrisoquine hydroxylase gene polymorphisms in cancer patients and controls. *Carcinogenesis*, **11**, 1527–30.

Syvalahti, E. K. G., Lindberg, R., Kallio, J. & de Vocht, M. (1986). Inhibitory effects of neuroleptics on debrisoquine oxidation in man. *British Journal of Clinical Pharmacology*, **22**, 89–92.

Szorady, I. & Santa, A. (1987). Drug hydroxylator phenotype in Hungary. *European Journal of Clinical Pharmacology*, **32**, 325.

Tacke, U., Leinonen, E., Lillsunde, P., Seppala, T., Arvela, P., Pelkonen, O. & Ylitalo, P. (1992). Debrisoquine hydroxylation phenotypes of patients with high versus low to normal serum antidepressant concentrations. *Journal of Clinical Psychopharmacology*, **12**, 262–7.

Treluyer, J. M., Jacqz-Aigrain, E., Alvarez, F. & Cresteil, T. (1991). Expression of CYP2D6 in developing human liver. *European Journal of Biochemistry*, **202**, 583–8.

Turgeon, J., Fiset, C., Giguère, R., Gilbert, M., Moerike, K., Rouleau, J. R., Kroemer H. K., Eichelbaum, M., Grech-Bélanger, O. & Bélanger, P. M. (1991). Influence of debrisoquine phenotype and of quinidine on mexiletine disposition in man. *Journal of Pharmacology and Experimental Therapeutics*, **259**, 789–98.

Tyndale, R., Aoyama, T., Broly, F., Matsunaga, T., Inaba, T., Kalow W., Gelboin, H. V., Meyer, U. A. &, Gonzalez, F. J. (1991a). Identification of a new variant CYP2D6 allele lacking the codon encoding lys-281, possible association with the poor metabolizer phenotype. *Pharmacogenetics*, **1**, 26–32.

Tyndale, R., Kalow, W. & Inaba, T. (1991b). Oxidation of reduced haloperidol to haloperidol: involvement of human P450IID6 (sparteine/debrisoquine monooxygenase). *British Journal of Clinical Pharmacology*, **31**, 655–60.

Tyndale, R. F., Sunahara, R., Inaba, T., Kalow, W., Gonzalez, F. J. & Niznik, H. B. (1991c). Neuronal cytochrome P450 II D1 (debrisoquine/sparteine-type). Potent inhibition by (−) cocaine and nucleotide sequence identity to human hepatic P450 gene CYP2D6 . *Molecular Pharmacology*, **40**, 63–8.

Vallada, H., Collier, D., Dawson, E., Own, M., Nanko, S., Murray, R. & Gill, M. (1992). Debrisoquine 4-hydroxylase (CYP2D) locus and possible susceptibility to schizophrenia. *Lancet*, **340**, 181–2.

Veronese, M. E. & McLean, S. (1991b). Debrisoquine oxidation polymorphism in a Tasmanian population. *European Journal of Clinical Pharmacology*, **40**, 529–32.

Veronese, M. E. & McLean, S. (1991a). Metabolism of paracetamol and phenacetin in relation to debrisoquine oxidation phenotype. *European Journal of Clinical Pharmacology*, **40**, 547–52.

Vetticaden, S. J., Cabana, B. E., Prasad, V. K., Purich, E. D., Jonkman, J. H. J., de Zeeuw, R., Ball, L., Leeson, L. J. & Braun, R. L. (1989). Phenotypic differences in dextromethorphan metabolism. *Pharmaceutical Research*, **6**, 13–19.

Vincent-Viry, M., Muller, J., Fournier, B., Galteau, M. M. & Siest, G. (1991). Relation between debrisoquine oxidation phenotype and morphological biological and pathological variables in a large population. *Clinical Chemistry*, **37**, 327–32.

Vinks, A., Inaba, T., Otton, S. V. & Kalow, W. (1982). Sparteine metabolism in Canadian Caucasians. *Clinical Pharmacology and Therapeutics*, **31**, 23–9.

Von Bahr, C., Birgersson, C., Blanck, A., Goransson, M., Mellstrom, B. & Nilsell, K. (1983). Correlation between nortriptyline and debrisoquine hydroxylation in the human liver. *Life Sciences*, **33**, 631–6.

Von Bahr, C., Movin, G., Nordin, C., Liden, A., Hammarlund-Udenaes, M., Hedberg, A., Ring, H. & Sjöqvist, F. (1991). Plasma levels of thoridazine and metabolites are influenced by the debrisoquine hydroxylation phenotype. *Clinical Pharmacology*, **49**, 234–40.

Von Bahr, C., Spina, E., Birgersson, O., Ericsson, Ö., Goransson, M., Henthorn, T. & Sjöqvist, F. (1985). Inhibition of desmethylimipramine-2-hydroxylation by drugs in human liver microsomes. *Biochemical Pharmacology*, **34**, 2501–5.

Wade, A. (ed.) (1980). *Pharmaceutical Handbook*. 19th edition (reprinted 1985), pp. 535–49. London: The Pharmaceutical Press.

Wagner, F., Jahnchen, E., Trenk, D., Eichelbaum, M., Harnasch, P., Hauf, G. & Roskamm, H. (1987). Severe complications of antianginal drug therapy in a patient identified as a poor metabolizer of metoprolol propafenone diltiazem and sparteine. *Klinische Wochenschrift*, **65**, 1164–8.

Wang, T., Roden, D. M., Wolfenden, H. T., Woosley, R. L., Wood, A. J. J. & Wilkinson, G. R. (1984). Influence of genetic polymorphism on the metabolism and disposition of encainide in man. *Journal of Pharmacology and Experimental Therapeutics*, **228**, 605–11.

Wanwimolruk, S. & Chalcroft, S. (1991). Lack of relationship between debrisoquine oxidation phenotype and the pharmacokinetics of quinine. *British Journal of Clinical Pharmacology*, **32**, 617–20.

Wanwimolruk, S., Denton, J. R., Ferry, D. G., Beasley, M. & Broughton, J. R. (1992). Polymorphism of debrisoquine oxidation in New Zealand Caucasians. *European Journal of Clinical Pharmacology*, **42**, 349–50.

Wanwimolruk, S., Patamasucon, P. & Lee, E. J. D. (1990). Evidence for the polymorphic oxidation of debrisoquine in the Thai population. *British Journal of Clinical Pharmacology*, **29**, 244–7.

Ward, S. A., Walle, T., Walle, K., Wilkinson, G. R. & Branch, R. A. (1989). Propanolol's metabolism is determined by both mephenytoin and debrisoquine hydroxylase activities. *Clinical Pharmacology and Therapeutics*, **45**, 72–9.

Wenk, M., Todesco, L., Keller, B. & Follath, F. (1991). Determination of dextromethorphan and dextrorphan in urine by high-performance liquid chromatography after solid-phase extraction. *Journal of Pharmaceutical and Biomedical Analysis*, **9**, 341–4.

Wolf, C. R., Smith, C. A. D., Gough, A. C., Moss, J. E., Vallis, K. A., Howard, G., Carey, F. J., Mills, K., McNee, W., Carmichael, J. & Spurr, N. K. (1992). Relationship between the debrisoquine hydroxylase polymorphism and cancer susceptibility. *Carcinogenesis*, **13**, 1035–8.

Wolff, T., Distlerath, L. M., Worthington, M. T., Groopman, J. D., Hammons, G. J., Kadlubar, F. F., Prough, R. A., Martin, M. V. & Guengerich, F. P. (1985). Substrate specificity of human liver cytochrome P450 debrisoquine 4-hydroxylase probed using immunochemical inhibition and chemical modelling. *Cancer Research*, **45**, 2116–22.

Woolf, B. (1954). On estimating the relation between blood group and disease. *Annals of Human Genetics (London)*, **19**, 251–3.

Woolhouse, N. M., Eichelbaum, M., Oates, N. S., Idle, J. R. & Smith, R. L. (1985). Dissociation of co-regulatory control of debrisoquine/phenformin and sparteine oxidation in Ghanaians. *Clinical Pharmacology and Therapeutics*, **37**, 512–21.

Woosley, R. L., Roden, D. M., Dai, G., Wang, T., Altenbern, D., Oates, J. & Wilkinson, G. R. (1986). Co-inheritance of the polymorphic metabolism of encainide and debrisoquine. *Clinical Pharmacology and Therapeutics*, **39**, 282–7.

Woosley, R. L., Roden, D. M., Duff, H. J., Carey, E. L., Wood, A. J. J., & Wilkinson, G. R. (1981). Co-inheritance of deficient oxidative metabolism of encainide and debrisoquine. *Clinical Research*, **29**, 501A.

Xu, X. M. & Jiang, W. D. (1990). Debrisoquine hydroxylation and sulfamethazine acetylation in a Chinese population. *Acta Pharmacologica Sinica*, **11**, 385–8.

Yue, Q. Y., Bertilsson, L,. Dahl-Puustinen, M. L., Säwe, J., Sjöqvist, F., Johansson, I. & Ingelman-Sundberg, M. (1989c). Disassociation between debrisoquine hydroxylation phenotype and genotype among Chinese. *Lancet*, **2**, 870.

Yue, Q. Y., Hasselström, J., Svensson, J. O. & Säwe, J. (1991a). Pharmacokinetics of codeine and its metabolites in Caucasian healthy volunteers; comparisons between extensive and poor hydroxylators of debrisoquine. *British Journal of Clinical Pharmacology*, **31**, 635–42.

Yue, Q. Y., Svensson, J. O., Alm, C., Sjöqvist, F. & Säwe, J. (1989b). Interindividual and interethnic differences in the demethylation and glucuronidation of codeine. *British Journal of Clinical Pharmacology*, **28**, 629–37.

Yue, Q. Y., Svensson, J. O., Alm, C., Sjöqvist, F. & Säwe, J. (1989a). Codeine O-demethylation co-segregates with polymorphic debrisoquine hydroxylation. *British Journal of Clinical Pharmacology*, **28**, 639–45.

Yue, Q. Y., Svensson, J. O., Sjöqvist, F. & Säwe, J. (1991b). A comparison of the pharmacokinetics of codeine and its

metabolites in healthy Chinese and Caucasian extensive hydroxylators of debrisoquine. *British Journal of Clinical Pharmacology*, **31**, 643–7.

Zanger, U. M., Vilbois, F., Hardwick, J. P. & Meyer, U. A. (1988). Absence of hepatic cytochrome P450$_{buf I}$ causes genetically deficient debrisoquine oxidation in man. *Biochemistry*, **27**, 5447–54.

Zekorn, C., Achtert, G., Hausleiter, H. J., Moon, C. H. & Eichelbaum, M. (1985). Pharmacokinetics of N-propylajmaline in relation to polymorphic sparteine oxidation. *Klinische Wochenschrift*, **63**, 1180–6.

Zhang, X. H., Gu, N. F., Xu, X. M., Zia, Z. Y. & Jiang, W. D. (1992). Amitriptyline metabolism and debrisoquine hydroxylation in native Chinese subject. *Asia Pacific Journal of Pharmacology*, **7**, 21–25.

Zhou, H. H., Anthony, L. B., Roden, D. M. & Wood, A. J. J. (1990). Quinidine reduces clearance of (+) propanolol more than (−) propanolol through marked reduction in 4-hydroxylation. *Clinical Pharmacology and Therapeutics*, **47**, 686–93.

Zschiesche, M., Hanke, W., Siegmund, W., Franke, G. & Wilke, A. (1990). Oxidation phenotyping with debrisoquine in Germany (East). *Pharmazie*, **45**, 920–1.

8 The cytochrome P450 3A subfamily

INTRODUCTION

THIS subfamily of cytochromes P450 has been found to be of great importance because the isoforms metabolize many exogenous compounds especially drugs and endogenous compounds, particularly steroids.

For an individual compound such as a drug the evidence that it is metabolized by a specific cytochrome P450 is usually obtained along the following lines:

1 it competitively inhibits the catalytic activity of human liver microsomes for a previously known substrate for the cytochrome P450 in question;
2 its metabolism in human liver microsomes is selectively inhibited by a specific anti-cytochrome P450 antibody;
3 its rate of metabolism by a number of human liver microsomes correlates with the concentration of the specific cytochrome P450 in those microsomes;
4 it is metabolized by a purified and reconstituted cytochrome P450 enzyme preparation;
5 it is metabolized by tissue culture cells or yeasts or bacteria which have been transfected with the appropriate cDNA.

Hints may also be provided by clinical observations such as reduction of the rate of metabolism of one drug when another is given concomitantly, but this can be due to other mechanisms than competitive inhibition at the enzymic level.

By applying the techniques described above a picture has now been built up of the cytochrome P450 3A subfamily. Cytochrome P450 3A1 is said to metabolize the probe drug benzyloxyphenazone (Park & Kitter-

ingham 1990). Information about the other members of the cytochrome P450 3A subfamily is shown in Table 8.1. The new nomenclature is used in this account, but it must be pointed out that there is still some confusion between different workers as to the numbering of the different subclasses and which numbered subclass caries out a specific activity.

Following this brief general introduction, the metabolism of a few drug substrates which are of importance in clinical practice will be considered in more detail.

NIFEDIPINE

The frequency distributions of pharmacokinetic parameters

A study to analyse the frequency distributions of kinetic and dynamic parameters of nifedipine in 53 healthy persons was performed by Kleinbloesem et al. (1984). It was already known that the drug was metabolized into pharmacologically inactive metabolites by a number of routes, namely, oxidation of the dihydropyridine nucleus to a pyridine moiety followed by hydrolysis of the ester moiety (to give the metabolite dehydronifedipinic acid MI) and hydroxylation of the 3-methyl group (to give the metabolite hydroxydehydronifedipinic acid MII) (Fig. 8.1) and that wide inter-individual variability in drug disposition existed. The authors found a bimodal distribution of the two parameters (1) area

Table 8.1. *Cytochromes P450 3A subfamily*

Category (previous designation)	Compounds metabolized	Inhibitors	Inducers	Comments
3A3 (HLp)	As below			Minor form in human liver and is polymorphic
3A4 (NF) (hPLN1)	alfentanil erythromycin (*N*-demethylase) cyclosporine[a] aflatoxins quinidine (3-hydroxylation and *N*-oxidation) nifedipine testosterone 6β-hydroxylation androstenedione progesterone cortisol 17β-oestradiol 17α-ethynyloestradiol midozalam benzphetamine aldrin lidocaine (lignocaine, xylocaine) diltiazem dapsone hydroxylation tamoxifen troleandomycin cotrimazole benzo[a]pyrene-7,8-diol	cimetidine 3-methyl-cholanthrene erythromycin gestodene troleandomycin	dexamethasone macrolide antibiotics phenobarbital rifampicin	Most important member
3A5 (hPLN3) (HLp3)	nifedipine (but not erythromycin and quinidine)			Expressed in about 15% of the population and 1 in 10 fetal livers (i.e. polymorphic)
3A6 (HFL33) (HFLa) (HLp2)	benzo[a]pyrene 7-ethoxycoumarin testosterone dihydroepiandrosterone			Expressed in the fetus but has been found in a few adult livers.

[a]further details with regard to cyclosporine appear on p. 107 and in Table 8.4.
The information in this table has been condensed from the following sources: Aoyama *et al.* 1989; Bargetzi *et al.* 1989; Gonzalez 1990; Gonzalez *et al.* 1988; Hunt *et al.* 1992a; Jacolot *et al.* 1991; Knodell *et al.* 1991; Kronbach *et al.* 1988; May *et al.* 1990; Morel *et al.* 1990a, b; Nebert & Jaiswal 1987; Pichard *et al.* 1990; Renaud *et al.* 1990; Shimada *et al.* 1989; Watkins 1990; Wrighton *et al.* 1989, 1990; Yun *et al.* 1992.

under the plasma concentration/time curve (AUC) and (2) urinary excretion of MI during the 8 hours following the ingestion of 20 mg of nifedipine. Nine individuals in a separate mode had high AUC values and excreted little MI. Also, these nine individuals had a greater change in heart rate and drop in blood pressure than the 44 individuals in the main mode.

Subsequently, other groups evaluated this result (Table 8.2). The study of Renwick *et al.* (1988) was very carefully carried out on young male volunteers. A large study by Schellens *et al.* (1988) came from the same centre as the original report of Kleinbloesem *et al.* (1984). On the parameters studied there was no evidence for bimodality to support the idea that there might be a polymorphism in the metabolism of nifedipine.

Twelve healthy young individuals (9 male) were studied by Soons *et al.* (1992) with a single oral dose of 10 mg nifedipine on three occasions. They found that the intra-individual variability was greater than inter-individual variability for maximal plasma concentration and timing and for plasma half-life but considerably less for area under the plasma nifedipine concentration curve. The correlations between pharmacokinetic and pharmacodynamic measurements such as blood pressure were poor.

Additional information

The interesting observation was made by Snedden *et al.* (1986), that in hypertensive patients being

Table 8.2. *Population studies evaluating the existence of polymorphic metabolism of nifedipine*

Reference	Number of subjects studied	Dose of nifedipine ingested	Parameters investigated	Conclusion(s)
Lobo *et al.* 1986	12	20 mg nifedipine retard	Plasma nifedipine AUC[a] $T50\%$[b], AUC, C_{max}[c]	No evidence for bimodality
Renwick *et al.* 1988	59	10 mg nifedipine	Terminal $T^{\frac{1}{2}}$[d], AUC of nifedipine Terminal $T^{\frac{1}{2}}$ of acid metabolite[e]	No confirmation of existence of a polymorphism
Schellens *et al.* 1988	130	20 mg slow release nifedipine*	AUC, C_{max} nifedipine AUC, C_{max} pyridine metabolite[f]	No bimodality and no evidence for the existence of a polymorphism
Porchet *et al.* 1988	80	10 mg nifedipine	Blood pressure pharmacodynamics	No evidence for polymorphism

[a] Area under plasma concentration–time curve.
[b] Time taken to achieve 50% of the AUC.
[c] Maximal plasma concentration achieved.
[d] Terminal half-life.
[e] Dehydronifedipinic acid.
[f] Dehydronifedipine.
*Together with 50 mg sparteine (as sulphate) and 100 mg phenytoin.

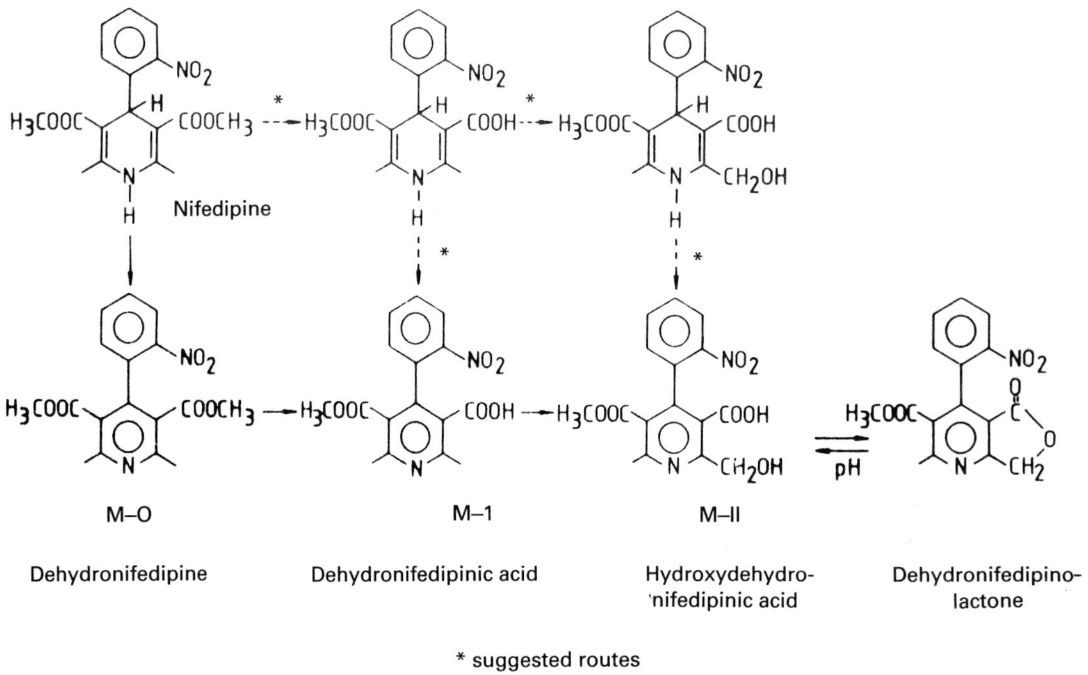

M–O	M–1	M–II	
Dehydronifedipine	Dehydronifedipinic acid	Hydroxydehydro-nifedipinic acid	Dehydronifedipino-lactone

* suggested routes

Fig. 8.1. Scheme of metabolism of nifedipine. (Supplied through the kindness of Professor D. D. Breimer, Center for Bio-Pharmaceutical Sciences, Leiden, The Netherlands.)

concomitantly treated with a variety of other cardio-vascular drugs the serum levels of nifedipine (N) and dehydronifedipine (DHN) were much higher and the ratio of DHN/N much lower than in patients receiving nifedipine alone. These observations suggested that the metabolism of the compound was prone to be influenced by environmental factors.

Similarly, Renwick *et al.* (1987) showed in 14 healthy volunteers that plasma concentrations were significantly higher after cimetidine which is known to bind to the active site of cytochrome P450, inhibiting interaction with other substrates.

The influence of oral contraceptive steroids in raising plasma nifedipine levels was emphasized by Soons *et al.* (1992a).

The major effect of pretreatment with quinidine on the disposition of nifedipine and its metabolites was a reduction of about 40% in the mean plasma concentration of the M-O metabolite (see Fig. 8.1) with a prolongation of the nifedipine plasma half-life. This inhibitory effect is to be ascribed to the fact that the 3-hydroxylation and *N*-oxidation of quinidine (which are the major routes of metabolism) are catalysed by cytochrome P450 3A4, which also metabolizes nifedipine (Schellens *et al.* 1991).

Omeprazole administration was found not to influence nifedipine pharmacokinetics by Soons *et al.* (1992b), but they did not ascertain the mephytoin phenotypes of their 10 subjects. The probability is that they were all extensive metabolizers. A different result might be obtained in poor metabolizers.

Biochemical aspects

The current state of knowledge was summarized by Guengerich (1989).

Cytochrome P450 3A4 molecules have been isolated by virtue of their ability to catalyse the oxidation of nifedipine. One difficulty in this work has been the fact that the proteins appear to lose catalytic activity on purification. The amino acid constitutions of different preparations of cytochrome P450 3A4 have been determined by various groups of researchers. Minor differences in structure have been described, possibly indicating the existence of different forms which may be allelic.

Molecular genetics

Genomic analysis suggests that four or more *CYP 3A* genes exist and that several similar cytochromes

P450 may be formed. Various cDNA clones have been isolated which were of different lengths.

An important series of discoveries was made by Gonzalez *et al.* (1988). The basis for this work lies in the following facts: (1) in rodents, studies of the enzymology, structure and regulation of cytochromes P450 are more advanced than in humans, (2) cDNA clones from human liver λ gt11 libraries can be isolated by using antibodies against rat enzymes and rat cytochrome P450 cDNA probes.

In order to characterize the cytochrome P450 that metabolizes nifedipine in man a human cytochrome P450 PCN1 cDNA (hPCN1, now known as *CYP 3A4*) was isolated from a human liver λ gt11 library using rat cytochrome P450 PCN1 DNA as a probe (PCN stands for pregnenolone 16α-carbonitrile which has been shown to induce this type of cytochrome P450 in the rat: Gonzalez 1990). The full-length cDNA was sequenced. It contained 2058 base pairs and an open-reading frame of 503 amino acids. The gene was cloned into the ECO RI site of the SV40-adenovirus-based expression vector p91023(B). Nifedipine was readily converted to its major metabolite M-O (dehydronifedipine: see Fig. 8.1) by COS cells containing *CYP 3A4* (but not by COS cells transfected with the vector alone or by COS cells containing other human cDNAs). This is the metabolite formed *in vitro* from nifedipine by human liver microsomes. It is interesting to note that this microsomal activity varied considerably among the 12 liver samples investigated by Gonzalez *et al.* (1988).

Similarly, Renaud *et al.* (1990) introduced the same or a very similar gene into the yeast *Saccharomyces cerevisiae* . They showed that this *CYP 3A* gene product had a high affinity for macrolide antibiotics, dihydroergotamine and miconazole. Oxidations of nifedipine, quinidine and erythromycin were also observed. An improved yeast-expressed human liver *CYP 3A4* system was described by Peyronneau *et al.* (1992).

With regard to cytochrome P450 3A5 the full-length cDNA has been isolated and it encodes for 502 amino acid residues with 84% similarity to cytochrome P450 3A4 (Aoyama *et al.* 1989).

Gene mapping

Using DNA from various rodent human hybrid cells and an *Eco*RI-digested fragment from the *CYP 3A4* sequences as a probe in Southern blot analysis, Gonzalez *et al.* (1988) demonstrated that this gene

(*CYP 3A4*) is localized on human chromosome 7. Later, Inoue *et al.* (1992) assigned *CYP 3A4* to 7q22.1 by fluorescence *in situ* hybridization.

Inducibility of cytochrome P450 3A4

In vivo studies suggest that the enzyme is inducible by compounds such as rifampicin, barbiturates, dexamethasone and other steroids and by macrolide antibiotics such as erythromycin. Induced persons have higher levels of immunologically detectable cytochrome P450 3A4 or related proteins (Guengerich 1989). (Reference has been made earlier to the probable inhibiting influence of cimetidine: Breimer *et al.* 1989.) The level of activity of this P450 *in vivo* can be estimated by the amount of 6β-hydroxycortisol present in urine.

Likely substrates for cytochrome P450 3A4 as suggested by immuno-inhibition studies

A list of the relevant compounds is shown in Table 8.3. It will be seen that both endogenous substances and drugs are represented.

Inter-subject variability

As yet no genetically determined variability has been described in metabolic reactions controlled by cytochrome P450 3A4. This is perhaps not surprising, for the following reasons: relatively few individuals (or livers) have been investigated by the elegant tools of molecular genetics. On the other hand *in vivo* investigations such as studying half-lives and area under the curve are probably too crude in view of the facts that (1) cytochrome P450 3A4 is inducible and inhibitable and so is likely to be at different levels of activity in different persons and (2) the metabolic fate of nifedipine as shown in Fig. 8.1 is complex. Clearly, the way is open to try and design more refined ways to look for inter-individual differences in nifedipine oxidation.

It is relevant in this context to point out that Wrighton *et al.* (1989) have discovered a new polymorphism of a human cytochrome P450 that hydroxylates testosterone at several molecular sites. The human P450 3 family contains not only cytochrome P450 3A4 but also cytochrome P450

Table 8.3. *Likely substrates for cytochrome P450 3A4 (as determined by immunoinhibition)*

1,4-Dihydropyridines
Quinidine (*N*-oxygenation and 3-hydroxylation)
Testosterone
Androstenedione
Progesterone
Cortisol (6β-hydroxylation)
17β-Oestradiol (2- and 4-hydroxylation)
17α-Ethynyloestradiol (2-hydroxylation)
Dehydroepiandrosterone 3-sulphate (16α-hydroxylation)
Erythromycin *N*-demethylation
Cyclosporine hydroxylation

Adapted from: Guengerich 1989.

3A3. Two forms of the latter were previously known. Cytochrome P450 3A6 is the major P450 present in human fetal liver and confers on it the ability to metabolize a large number of compounds. Whilst investigating liver microsomal preparations with a monoclonal anti-cytochrome P450 3A3, Wrighton *et al.* (1989) discovered another form of the enzyme with slightly faster mobility in SDS-polyacrylamide gel. This new enzyme was termed cytochrome P450 3A5. A survey of 46 liver samples revealed that 11 of them contained cytochrome P450 3A5 and the others did not, and these findings did not correlate with the drug or smoking history. Following these observations Wrighton *et al.* (1990) using highly purified cytochrome P450 preparations showed that the cytochrome 3A4 was the major enzyme catalysing nifedipine oxidation. Cytochrome P450 3A5 also catalysed nifedipine oxidation but unlike 3A4 it did not catalyse the *N*-demethylation of erythromycin and *N*-oxidation of quinidine.

Furthermore, cytochrome P450 3A5 was confirmed to be polymorphically expressed, being detectable in only 19 out of 66 livers; it accounted for 6 to 60% (and in one instance 100%) of the total cytochrome P450 3 family in the livers in which it was expressed.

In another paper Aoyama *et al.* (1989) state that a survey of 40 human livers revealed cytochrome P450 3A4 in all but one. In about 10 to 20% of the livers there was a closely similar molecule designated cytochrome P450 3A5. One liver expressed only the latter. Using the same technique as described above the cDNA coding for this protein was isolated and transfected into living cells. It was found to confer the ability to metabolize nifedipine to dehydronifedipine, the same as cytochrome P450 3A4. The two proteins are 84% similar in amino acid composition. They vary in their substrate specificities to steroids.

In view of the fact that nifedipine is oxidized by two cytochromes P450, one of which is polymorphic, and both subject to induction and inhibition, it is not surprising that a simple genetic pattern was not found by studying its metabolism and pharmacokinetics *in vivo*.

Inter-ethnic variability

Healthy individuals from the Indian sub-continent were found by Ahsan *et al.* (1991) to have a higher area under the nifedipine concentration/time curve and a longer half-life than Caucasians. The authors put forward the following possible explanations for their observations:

1 a genetically determined difference in cytochromes P450 3A;
2 increased plasma protein binding in the Asiatics;
3 the presence of an environmental factor in the Asiatics which inhibited cytochromes P450 3A;
4 the presence of an environmental factor in the Caucasians which induced cytochromes P450 3A.

The Asiatics all complained of marked palpitations, which might be an indicator of an ethnic difference in pharmacodynamic response.

CYCLOSPORINE

Cyclosporine, the widely used immunosuppressive compound (Fig. 8.2), undergoes a large number of oxidations, 28 being listed by Kahan *et al.* (1990), so that very many metabolites are produced.

Cytochrome P450 3A4 was found by Kronbach *et al.* (1988) to be the main enzyme responsible for these biotransformations.

The pattern of production of the three main metabolites was similar in all 15 livers investigated but

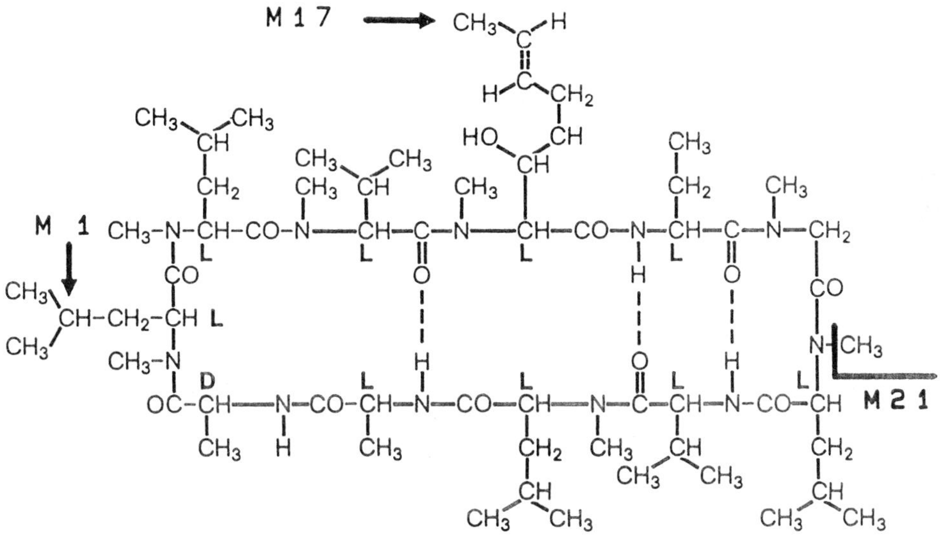

Fig. 8.2. Structure and sites of metabolism of cyclosporine (arrows indicate sites of hydroxylation; angle refers to the site of *N*-demethylation). (From Kronbach *et al.* 1988.)

In the new nomenclature M17 is AMI, M21 is AM4N and MI AM9 (see Kahan *et al.* 1990).

Table 8.4. *List of molecules that should or should not interfere with the hepatic metabolism of cyclosporin A*

Drugs that affect the rate of CsA metabolism as		Drugs that do not affect the rate of CsA metabolism
Inducers	Inhibitors (K_1 µM)	
Rifampicin	Triacetyloleandomycin[a]	Cefoperazone
Sulfadimidine	Erythromycin[a]	Cefotaxime
Phenobarbital	Josamycin	Ceftazidime
Phenytoin	Midecamycin	Isoniazid
Phenylbutazone	Ketoconazole	Doxycycline
Dexamethasone	Miconazole	Spiramycin
Sulfinpyrazone	Midazolam[a]	Sulfadiazine
Carbamazepine	Nifedipine[a]	Sulfamethoxazole
	Diltiazem[a]	Norfloxacin
	Verapamil	Pefloxacin
	Nicardipine	Vancocin
	Ergotamine	Trimethoprim
	Dihydroergotamine	Amphotericin B
	Glibenclamide	Valproic acid
	Ethynylestradiol[a]	Quinidine
	Progesterone[a]	Cimetidine
	Bromocriptine	Ranitidine
	Cortisol[a]	Omeprazole
	Prednisone	Diclofenac
	Prednisolone	Aspirin
	Methylprednisolone	Paracetamol
		Debrisoquine
		Guanoxan
		Captopril
		Frusemide
		Acetazolamide
		Sparteine
		Gliclazide
		Imipramine

[a]Molecules which have been characterized as specific P450 3A substrates.
From: Pichard *et al.* 1990.

the level of activity varied 25-fold. The authors point out that the activity of this particular cytochrome P450 is particularly susceptible to the influence of other chemicals.

Aoyama *et al.* (1989) found that whereas cytochrome P450 3A4 was able to metabolize cyclosporine to two hydroxylated metabolites (M1 and M17) and one demethylated metabolite (M21), only one metabolite (M1) was formed by cytochrome P450 3A5.

Using primary human hepatocyte cultures and human liver microsomes Pichard *et al.* (1990) surveyed 59 compounds, representing 17 different therapeutic classes, for their ability to induce and inhibit cytochrome P450 3A level and cyclosporine (CsA) oxidation. The most important items of information gleaned from this survey are shown in Table 8.4. This information is of great practical importance in clinical medicine, for the following reasons. Inducers will lower CsA levels and inhibitors will raise them. Chronic immunosuppression with CsA is required for recipients to retain transplanted organs, and on the other hand CsA is nephrotoxic. So giving an inducer may cause rejection, whilst giving an inhibitor may cause nephrotoxicity.

LIDOCAINE

Another important compound which is metabolized by cytochrome P450 3A4 is the popular anaesthetic agent lidocaine (*syn* lignocaine, xylocaine).

Bargetzi *et al.* (1989) used the biotransformation of lidocaine (Fig. 8.3) to monoethyl glycinexylidide (MEGX) as the indicator reaction to survey the microsomal activity in livers from 13 kidney transplant donors and one patient with cirrhosis. The activity in terms of mmoles MEGX/mg protein per hour varied between 100 and 850. Midazolam (512

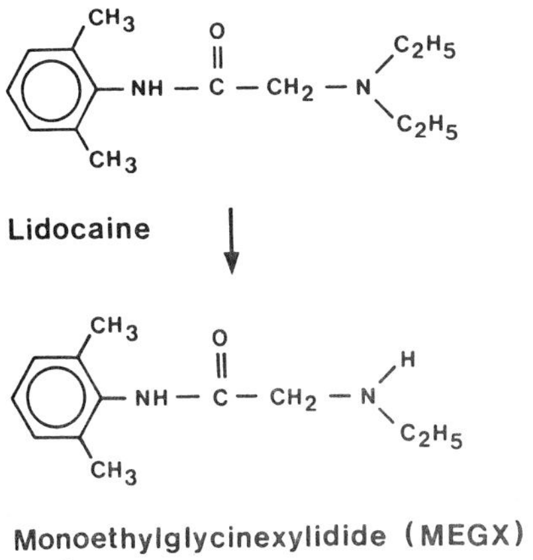

Lidocaine

Monoethylglycinexylidide (MEGX)

Fig. 8.3. Structures of lidocaine and monoethyl-glycinexylidide (MEGX). (From Bargetzi *et al.* 1989.)

μmol/l) inhibited lidocaine-deethylase activity by 87% at 10 μM and by 65% at 5 mM substrate concentration, respectively. A panel of polyclonal antibodies raised against various cytochromes P450 of man and rat was tested for inhibition of lidocaine deethylation. The antiserum directed against cytochrome P450 3A4 was strongly inhibitory, varying between individual livers. There was significant correlation between biotransforming activity and amount of immunologically detectable protein. Homogenates of Hep-G2 cells transfected with human cytochrome P450 3A4 and the related cytochrome P450 3A5 cDNAs showed specific activity for lidocaine deethylation (which the non-transfected cells did not confer).

Human cytochrome P450 3A4 seems to be responsible for the low-affinity enzyme which performs the major part of lidocaine-deethylase activity. Hitherto, no genetic variability has been demonstrated and no *in vivo/in vitro* correlations, but the subject is of intense interest because of the use of MEGX formation in liver donors as an indicator of the functional performance of the organ to be transplanted. Ollerich *et al.* (1990) reported that the capacity of the liver to biotransform lidocaine to MEGX was significantly related to the 120 day survival in a population of 58 adult cirrhotic patients.

TAMOXIFEN

The anti-oestrogen non-steroidal compound tamoxifen (TAM: Fig. 8.4) is widely used in the treatment of metastatic breast cancer.

It was thought that its use was limited to those breast cancers which possessed cytoplasmic oestrogen receptors since it was thought to act by competing with these receptors especially by means of its 4-hydroxy metabolite. However, it has recently been found to be effective even when an oestrogen mechanism is not involved. It may also be used protectively for selected cases after treatment of the primary tumour. Hence a very large number of women are, and will be, taking this compound for a long time.

The major metabolites are shown in Fig. 8.4, and they may all be biologically active as well as the unchanged original molecule.

An *in vitro* investigation was conducted by Jacolot *et al.* (1991) to find out the mechanism(s) of metabolism of TAM by human liver microsomes.

The metabolism of TAM was shown to be P450 dependent and correlated with testosterone-6β-hydroxylation and erythromycin N-demethylation. The N-oxidative demethylation of TAM was shown to correlate with the amount of cytochrome P450 3A immunodetected. Erythromycin, cyclosporine, nifedipine and diltiazem competitively inhibited TAM N-demethylase activity but oestradiol did not. All this points to TAM being N-demethylated by cytochrome P450 3A (probably 3A4 but this is not certain).

On the other hand Blankson *et al.* (1991) conducted very similar experiments with human liver microsomes one of which was from a cytochrome P450 2D6 poor metabolizer. N-dimethyl tamoxifen was the most prominent metabolite and was formed

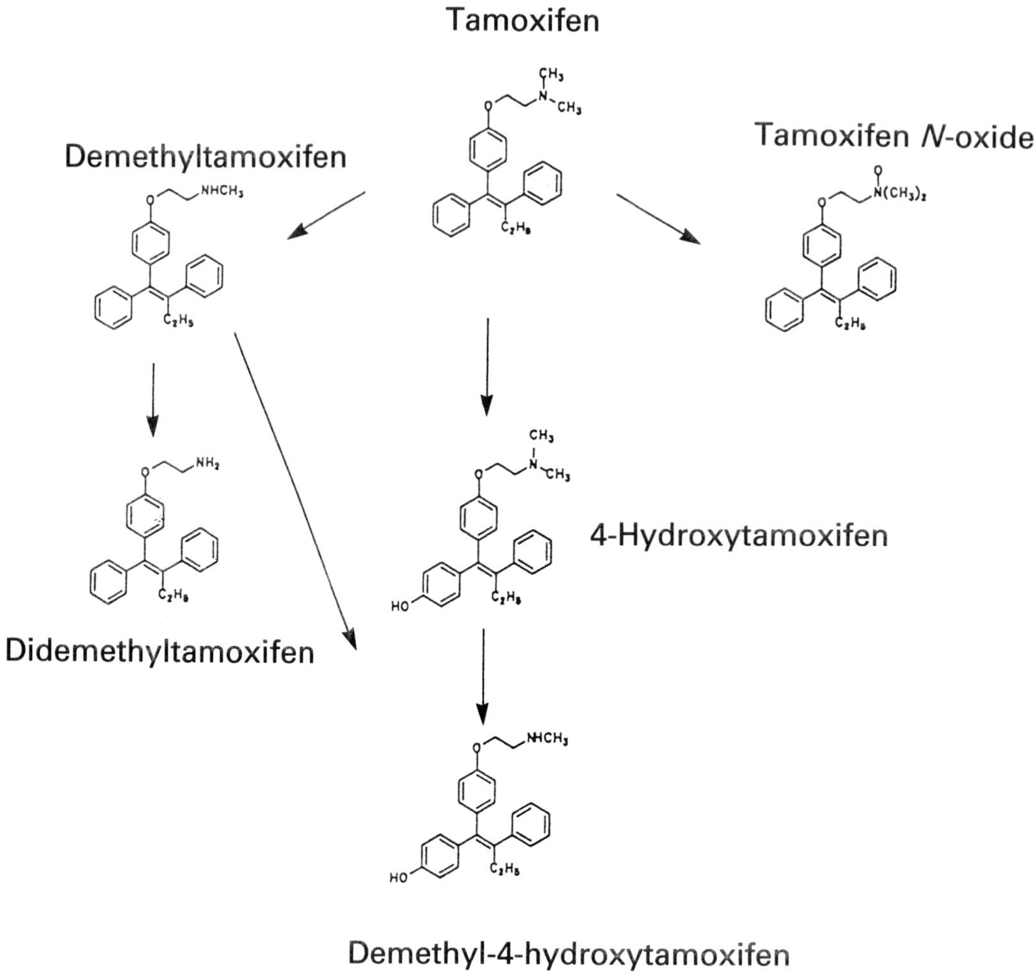

Tamoxifen

Demethyltamoxifen

Tamoxifen *N*-oxide

Didemethyltamoxifen

4-Hydroxytamoxifen

Demethyl-4-hydroxytamoxifen

Fig. 8.4. The major routes of tamoxifen metabolism in humans. (From Blankson *et al.* 1991.)

in similar amounts by both extensive and poor cytochrome P450 2D6 preparations. Quinidine did not inhibit this reaction.

It is of interest that TAM compares poorly with the molecular template for cytochrome P450 2D6 substrates generated using interactive molecular graphics by Islam *et al.* (1991).

It is possible that cytochromes P450 from subfamilies other than 3A may contribute to TAM metabolism. Meantime other 3A substrates have the potential to interact with TAM *in vivo*, either to diminish the antineoplastic effect of TAM or to increase the

chances of an adverse effect of the other compound. Examples of the latter type have been recorded in the case of warfarin and nicoumalone (British National Formulary 1992; see also p. 132).

CONCLUSION

The *CYP 3A* family contains a number of closely related genes. The gene products have overlapping specificities. The importance of these cytochrome P450 molecules in practical therapeutics would seem to be very considerable.

As pointed out by Nebert & Jaiswal (1987), it would be a great step forward if the P450 genes could be screened in patients by investigating the

DNA obtained from a sample of venous blood. This would enable large numbers of individuals to be categorized without the need to obtain liver microsomal preparations or exposing the individual to the drug under consideration.

It must be pointed out, however, that if genotypic variability could be identified in this way it would still be necessary to correlate the findings with *in vivo* events and clinical settings.

A useful clinical test for cytochrome P450 3A activity is the [*N*-methyl-^{14}C] erythromycin breath test in which the extent of desmethylation is indicated by the amount of $^{14}CO_2$ exhaled. By means of this test Hunt *et al.* (1992b) showed a higher activity in females than in males, without any significant diminution with age.

Formal clinical experiments to examine interactions between drugs which have been found by laboratory methods to be substrates of the subfamily of cytochromes P450 3A have yielded results which have varied. Sometimes the expected result was obtained and sometimes it was not.

Quinidine was found by Schellens *et al.* (1991) to inhibit nifedipine metabolism and prolong its elimination half-life by about 40%. This was an anticipated result. Similarly, Tortorice *et al.* (1990) found that verapamil caused a 45% increase in the area under the curve, maximal concentration and trough level of cyclosporine. This effect may have been due to altered bioavailability rather than inhibited metabolism.

The results of the *in vivo* [^{14}C]-erythromycin breath test performed by Hunt *et al.* (1992b) did not correlate with urinary 6β-hydroxycortisol/cortisol ratio, and this unexpected result may have indicated the fact that these two compounds are metabolized by different isoforms of cytochrome P450 3A.

The clinical importance of the polymorphisms of cytochromes P450 3A3 and 3A5 has not yet been determined.

Ahsan, C. H., Renwick, A. G., Macklin, B., Challenor, V. F., Waller, D. G. & George, C. F. (1991). Ethnic differences in the pharmacokinetics of oral nifedipine. *British Journal of Clinical Pharmacology*, **31**, 399–403.

Aoyama, T., Yamano, S., Waxman, D. J., Lapenson, D. P., Meyer, U. A,. Fisher, V., Tyndale, R., Inaba, T., Kalow, W., Gelboin, H. V. & Gonzalez, F. J. (1989). Cytochrome P450 hPCN3 a novel cytochrome P-450IIIA gene product that is differentially expressed in adult human liver. *Journal of Biological Chemistry*, **264**, 10388–395.

Bargetzi, M. J., Aoyama, T., Gonzalez, F. J. & Meyer, U. A.

(1989). Lidocaine metabolism in human liver microsomes by cytochrome P450 III A4. *Clinical Pharmacology and Therapeutics*, **46**, 521–7.

Blankson, E. A., Ellis, S. W., Lennard, M. S., Tucker, G. T. & Rogers, K. (1991). The metabolism of tamoxifen by human liver microsomes is not mediated by cytochrome P-450 II D6. *Biochemical Pharmacology*, **42**(Suppl.), S209–12.

Breimer, D. D., Schellens, J. H. M. & Soons, P. A. (1989). Nifedipine, variability in its kinetics and metabolism in man. *Pharmacology and Therapeutics*, **44**, 445–54.

British National Formulary. London. (1992). *British Medical Association and Royal Pharmaceutical Society of Great Britain*, **23**, 485.

Gonzalez, F. J. (1990). Molecular genetics of the P-450 superfamily. *Pharmacology and Therapeutics*, **45**, 1–38.

Gonzalez, F. J., Schmid, B. J., Umeno, M., McBride, O. W., Hardwick, J. P., Meyer, U. A., Gelboin, H. V. & Idle, J. R. (1988). Human P450-PCN1, sequence, chromosomal localization and direct evidence through cDNA expression that P450-PCN1 is nifedipine oxidase. *DNA*, **7**, 79–86.

Guengerich, F. P. (1989). Characterization of human microsomal cytochrome P-450 enzymes. *Annual Review of Pharmacology and Toxicology*, **29**, 241–264.

Hunt, C. M., Watkins, P. B., Saenger, P., Stave, G. M., Barlascini, N., Watlington, C. O., Wright Jr, J. T. & Guzelian, P. S. (1992a). Heterogeneity of CYP3A isoforms metabolizing erythromycin and cortisol. *Clinical Pharmacology and Therapeutics*, **51**, 18–23.

Hunt, C. M., Westerkam, W. R., Stave, G. M. & Wilson, J. A. P. (1992b). Hepatic cytochrome P-4503A (CYP3A) activity in the elderly. *Mechanisms of Ageing and Development*, **64**, 189–99.

Inoue, K., Inazawa, J., Nakagawa, H., Shimada, T., Yamazaki, H., Guengerich, F. P. & Abe, T. (1992). Assignment of the human cytochrome P-450 nifedipine oxidase gene (CYP3A4) to chromosome 7 at band q 22.1 by fluorescence *in situ* hybridization. *Japanese Journal of Human Genetics*, **37**, 133–8.

Islam, S. A., Wolf, C. R ., Lennard, M. S. & Sternberg, M. J. E. (1991). A three-dimensional molecular template for substrates of human cytochrome P-450 involved in debrisoquine 4-hydroxylation. *Carcinogenesis*, **12**, 2211–19.

Jacolot, F., Simon, I., Dreano, Y., Beaune, P., Riche, C. & Berthou, F. (1991). Identification of the cytochrome P-450 III A family as the enzymes involved in the N-demethylation of tamoxifen in human liver microsomes. *Biochemical Pharmacology*, **41**, 1911–19.

Kahan, B. D., Shaw, L. M., Holt, D., Grevel, J. & Johnston, A. (1990). Consensus document, Hawk's Cay meeting on therapeutic drug monitoring of cyclosporine. *Clinical Chemistry*, **36**, 1510–16.

Kleinbloesem, C. H., van Brummelen, P., Faber, H., Danhof, M., Vermeulen, N. P. E. & Breimer, D. D. (1984). Variability in nifedipine pharmacokinetics and dynamics; a new oxidation polymorphism in man. *Biochemical Pharmacology*, **33**, 3721–24.

Knodell, R. G., Browne, D. G., Gwozdz, G. P., Brian, W. R. & Guengerich, F. P. (1991). Differential inhibition of individual human liver cytochromes P-450 by cimetidine. *Gastroenterology*, **101**, 1680–91.

Kronbach, T., Fischer, V. & Meyer, U. A. (1988). Cyclosporine metabolism in human liver; Identification of a cytochrome P-450 III gene family as the major cyclosporine - metabolizing enzyme explains interactions of cyclosporine with other drugs. *Clinical Pharmacology and Therapeutics*, **43**, 630–5.

Lobo, J., Jack, D. B. & Kendall, M. J. (1986). The intra- and inter-subject variability of nifedipine pharmacokinetics in young volunteers. *European Journal of Clinical Pharmacology*, **30**, 57–60.

May, D. G., Porter, J. A., Uetrecht, J. P., Wilkinson, G. R. & Branch, R. A. (1990). The contribution of N-hydroxylation and acetylation to dapsone pharmacokinetics in normal subjects. *Clinical Pharmacology and Therapeutics*, **48**, 619–27.

Morel, F., Beaune, P., Ratanasavanh, D., Flinois, J. P., Guengerich, F. P. & Guillouzo, A. (1990b). Effects of various inducers on the expression of cytochromes P-450 II C 8, 9, 10 and III A in cultured adult human hepatocytes. *Toxicology in vitro*, **4**, 458–60.

Morel, F., Beaune, P. H., Ratanasavanh, D., Flinois, J. P., Yang, C. S., Guengerich, F. P. & Guillouzo, A. (1990a). Expression of cytochrome P-450 enzymes in cultivated human hepatocytes. *European Journal of Biochemistry*, **191**, 437–44.

Nebert, D. W. & Jaiswal, A. K. (1987). Human drug metabolism polymorphisms, use of recombinant DNA techniques. *Pharmacology and Therapeutics*, **33**, 11-17.

Oellerich, M., Burdelski, M., Lautz, H. U., Schulz, M., Schmidt, F. W. & Herrmann, H. (1990). Lidocaine metabolite formation as a measure of liver function in patients with cirrhosis. *Therapeutic Drug Monitoring*, **12**, 219–26.

Park, B. K. & Kitteringham, N. R. (1990). Assessment of enzyme induction and enzyme inhibition in humans, toxicological implications. *Xenobiotica*, **20**, 1171–1185.

Peyronneau, M. A., Renaud, J. P., Truan, G., Urban, P. Pompon, D. & Mansuy, D. (1992). Optimization of yeast-expressed liver cytochrome P450 3A4 catalytic activities by coexpressing NADPH-cytochrome P450 reductase and cytochrome b₅ . *European Journal of Biochemistry*, **207**, 109–16.

Pichard, L., Fabre, I., Fabre, G., Domergue, J., Aubert, B. S., Mourad, G. & Maurel, P. (1990). Cyclosporine A drug interactions, screening for inducers and inhibitors of cytochrome P-450 (cyclosporine A oxidase) in primary cultures of human hepatocytes and in liver microsomes. *Drug Metabolism and Disposition*, **18**, 595–606.

Porchet, H. C., Benveniste, C., Adler, D. & Dayer, P. (1988). Absence de polymorphisme dans la reponse individuelle aux dihydropyridines nifedipine et (±)-nicradipine. *Schweizerische Medizinische Wochenschrift*, **118**, 1918–20.

Renaud, J. P., Cullin, C., Pompon, D., Beaune, P. & Mansuy, D. (1990). Expression of human liver cytochrome P450 III A4 in yeast – a functional model for the hepatic enzyme. *European Journal of Biochemistry*, **194**, 889–96.

Renwick, A. G., Le Vie, J., Challenor, V. F., Waller, D. G., Gruchy, B. & George, C. F. (1987). Factors affecting the pharmacokinetics of nifedipine. *European Journal of Clinical Pharmacology*, **32**, 351–55.

Renwick, A. G., Robertson, D. R. C., Macklin, B., Challenor, V., Waller, D. G. & George, C. F. (1988). The pharmacokinetics of oral nifedipine – a population study. *British Journal of Clinical Pharmacology*, **25**, 701–08.

Schellens, J. H. M., Ghabrial, H., van der Wart, H. H. F., Bakker, E. N., Eilkinson, G. R. & Breimer, D. D. (1991). Differential effects of quinidine on the disposition of nifedipine, sparteine and mephenytoin in humans. *Clinical Pharmacology and Therapeutics*, **50**, 520–8.

Schellens, J. H. M., Soons, P. A. & Breimer, D. D. (1988). Lack of bimodality in nifedipine plasma kinetics in a large population of healthy subjects. *Biochemical Pharmacology*, **37**, 2507–10.

Shimada, T., Martin, M. V., Pruess-Schwartz, D., Marnelt, L. J. & Guengerich, F. P. (1989). Roles of individual human cytochrome P- 450 enzymes in the bioactivation of benzo(a)pyrene, 7,8-dihydroxy-7,8-dihydrobenzo(a)pyrene and other dihydrodiol derivatives of polycyclic aromatic hydrocarbons. *Cancer Research*, **49**, 6304–12.

Snedden, W., Fernandez, P. G. & Nath, C. (1986). The metabolism of nifedipine during long-term therapy. *Clinical and Investigative Medicine*, **9**, 244–9.

Soons, P. A., Schoemaker, H. C., Cohen, A. F. & Breimer, D. D. (1992a). Intraindividual variability in nifedipine pharmacokinetics and effects in healthy subjects. *Journal of Clinical Pharmacology*, **32**, 324–31.

Soons, P. A. van den Berg, G., Danhof, M. van Brummelen, P., Jansen, J. B. M. J., Lamers, C. B. H. W. & Briemer, D. D. (1992b). Influence of single- and multiple-dose omeprazole treatment on nifedipine pharmacokinetics and effects in helathy subjects. *European Journal of Clinical Pharmacology*, **42**, 319–24.

Tortorice, K. L., Heim-Duthoy, K. L., Awni, W. M., Venkateswara, Rao, K. & Kasiske, B. L. (1990). The effects of calcium channel blockers on cyclosporine and its metabolites in renal transplant recipients. *Therapeutic Drug Monitoring*, **12**, 321–8.

Watkins, P. B. (1990). The role of cytochromes P-450 in cyclosporine metabolism. *Journal of the American Academy of Dermatology*, **23**, 1301–11.

Wrighton, S. A., Brian, W. R., Sari, M. A., Iwasaki, M., Guengerich, F. P., Rancy, J. L., Molowa, D. T. & Vandenbranden, M. (1990). Studies on the expression and metabolic capabilities of human liver cytochrome P450 III A5 (HLp³). *Molecular Pharmacology*, **38**, 207–13.

Wrighton, S. A., Ring, B. J., Watkins, P. B. & Vandenbranden, M. (1989). Identification of a polymorphically expressed member of the human cytochrome P-450 III family. *Molecular Pharmacology*, **36**, 97–105.

Yun, C. H., Wood, M., Wood, A. J. J. & Guengerich, F. P. (1992). Identification of the pharmacogenetic determinants of alfentanil metabolism: cytochrome P-450 3A4. *Anesthesiology*, **77**, 467–74.

9 Tolbutamide

INTRODUCTION, AND A GENETIC HYPOTHESIS

TOLBUTAMIDE has been used to treat diabetes since 1956 and the hypoglycaemic action is related to the plasma concentration. This drug was found to be metabolized in man to hydroxytolbutamide and then to carboxytolbutamide (Fig. 9.1). These two metabolites together accounted in the urine for 85% of an orally administered dose of tolbutamide. About $\frac{2}{3}$ of the urinary metabolites were in the form of the carboxy compound and the remaining $\frac{1}{3}$ in the form of the hydroxy compound (Thomas & Ikeda 1966).

Isolated case reports were published of individual patients who had hypoglycaemia associated with exceptionally long plasma half-lives of tolbutamide (Kreeger 1962; Bird & Schwabbe 1965).

Considerable interest in the genetic aspects of tolbutamide metabolism was generated by the paper of Scott & Poffenbarger (1979a), who administered tolbutamide intravenously to 42 unrelated non-diabetics. The time course of plasma tolbutamide concentration was studied. The authors claimed to show a trimodal distribution of the disappearance rate constant K_d. Small numbers of families and twinships were studied. The suggestion was made that there might be a genetic polymorphism of tolbutamide oxidation to form hydroxytolbutamide.

This suggestion was further extrapolated by reference to the UGDP (University Group Diabetes Program) study, which published data indicating increased mortality in a group of diabetics treated with a fixed dose of tolbutamide compared with a group on a fixed dose of insulin and another on a variable dose of insulin. Scott & Poffenbarger (1979b) offered as an explanation that 'slow hydroxylators' might accumulate high levels of tolbutamide in the plasma, which then might have deleterious cardiovascular consequences such as ventricular fibrillation or increase the extent of ischaemic myocardial damage.

Unfortunately, there has been no confirmation of the suggestion of Scott and Poffenbarger that there is a genetic polymorphism of tolbutamide elimination kinetics. It appears from studying pharmacokinetic parameters that 'poor metabolizers' with, for example, long plasma half-lives well separated from the general mass of subjects, are quite rare. Back & Orme (1989) assembled a total of 45 subjects who had their half-lives determined in five separate studies and only two individuals with half-lives of about 14 hours seemed to be separate from the other 43. Another eight values published by Kostelnik & Iber (1973) would fit into the main mode. In a survey of 42 healthy individuals one was found with a half-life of 31.5 hours by Harmer et al. (unpublished observation). Thirteen healthy non-diabetics were given 500 mg tolbutamide orally by Peart et al. (1987). The plasma half-life and urinary excretion of OH–TOL and COOH–TOL were determined and the half lives showed a range of 2.7 to 9.0 hours with no evidence of a polymodal distribution. The authors state that of 60 subjects whose plasma tolbutamide kinetics had been studied in Australia only one was an unequivocal 'slow metabolizer'

113

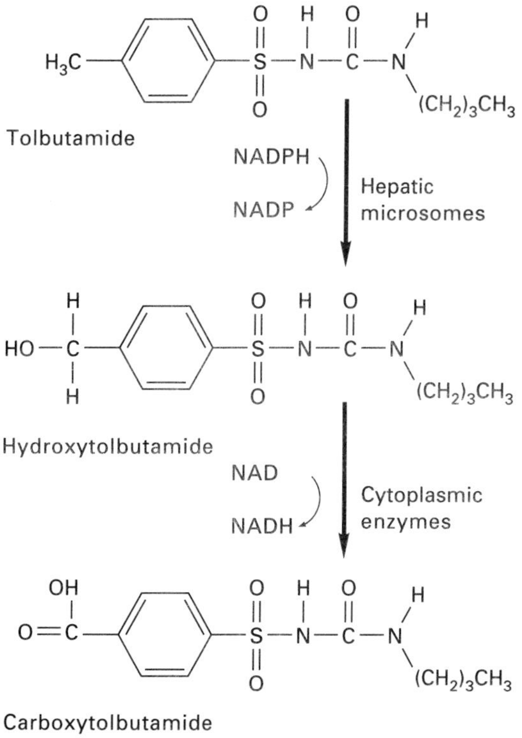

Fig. 9.1. Metabolic pathways for tolbutamide. Tolbutamide = 1-butyl-3-*p*-tolyl sulphonylurea; hydroxytolbutamide = 1-butyl-3(*p*-hydroxymethyl)phenyl sulphonylurea; carboxytolbutamide = 1-butyl-3(*p*-carboxy)phenyl
sulphonylurea. (From Peart *et al.* 1987.)

with a half-life of 37 hours (Miners *et al.* 1985).
Page *et al.* (1991) designed a simple screening test
for tolbutamide metabolism; it consisted of collecting the 4 to 8 hour urine, and blood at 8 and 24
hours, after ingesting a 500 mg dose. This test was
applied to 63 'non-diabetic volunteers of mixed
racial groups with normal renal and hepatic function'. Two subjects' results stood apart from the
remainder, with plasma half-lives of 21.6 and 16.1
hours. The urinary excretion values of hydroxy- and
carboxy-metabolites in these two individuals were
low.

So the prevalence of slow metabolizers could be
a few per cent of the population in Caucasians. This
would not be surprising in view of what we now
know about the debrisoquine/sparteine and
mephenytoin polymorphisms in Europeans. If Scott
and Poffenbarger's figures were correct, between 10

and 24% of the population would be classed as poor
metabolizers and such a figure seems far too high.

The metabolism of tolbutamide has been shown
by Miller *et al.* (1990) to diminish significantly with
age and this factor should be taken into account
when evaluating population surveys.

IN VIVO ASSESSMENTS OF INTERACTIONS OF OTHER DRUGS WITH TOLBUTAMIDE METABOLISM

A considerable number of drugs have been assessed
to see if their administration, immediately before or
together with tolbutamide, alters the metabolism of
the latter. The main results are shown in Table 9.1.
Some of the items of information are worthy of further comment.

From the work of Peart *et al.* (1987), who investigated tolbutamide pharmacokinetics in 10
extensive and three poor metabolizers of debrisoquine, it is clear that the debrisoquine/sparteine
polymorphism does not influence the metabolism of
the compound. The *in vitro* evidence points the same
way.

With regard to mephenytoin, Knodell *et al.*
(1987) found that the pharmacokinetics of tolbutamide were very similar in six extensive and four
poor metabolizers of mephenytoin.

The results found with cimetidine were perplexing. Whilst the higher doses of 1200 and 1600
mg daily used in pretreatment presumably in Caucasians produced inhibition of tolbutamide kinetics,
the smaller dose of 800 mg daily pretreatment, also
presumably in Caucasians, did not. On the other
hand 1200 mg cimetidine daily pretreatment in the
presumably Nigerian subjects of Adebaya & Coker
(1988) produced no inhibition. It is possible there
may be an ethnic difference in this effect (see Table
9.1).

IN VITRO OBSERVATIONS USING HUMAN LIVER PREPARATIONS

A large number of compounds has been examined
to see if they cause inhibition of tolbutamide
hydroxylation by human liver microsomal preparation. The results are condensed in Table 9.2. It must
be pointed out that the occurrence of inhibition does
not necessarily mean the inhibitor is metabolized by

Table 9.1. In vivo *assessments of interactions of other drugs with tolbutamide metabolism*

Reference	Effect
Christensen *et al.* 1963	Two patients presented with clinical hypoglycaemia and one patient was observed to have low blood glucose levels whilst taking tolbutamide and sulphaphenazole concurrently as therapy. Three diabetics being treated with tolbutamide were given sulphaphenazole experimentally and their blood glucose concentrations were found to be lowered.
Schulz & Schmidt 1970	Sulphaphenazole prolonged tolbutamide half-life.
Kostelnik & Iber 1973	Tolbutamide pharmacokinetics improved at the same rate as ethanol pharmaco-kinetics and NADP-dependent ethanol oxidizing activity in liver biopsies in alcoholics who became abstinent.
Rowland & Matin 1973	Sulphaphenazole inhibits the metabolism and markedly prolongs tolbutamide plasma levels.
Lumholtz *et al.* 1975	Sulphamethizole potent inhibitor of tolbutamide metabolism *in vivo*.
Pond *et al.* 1977	Tolbutamide half-life was prolonged by sulphaphenazole and this effect occurred within 2 hours. Phenylbutazone and oxyphenbutazone also prolonged tolbutamide half-life but after a 20 hour delay.
Miners *et al.* 1982	Sulphinpyrazone inhibited plasma clearance and half-life by inhibition of oxidative metabolism (the effect persisted after sulphinpyrazone had disappeared from the plasma and was much more powerful than the effect caused by the inhibition of binding to plasma proteins).
Dey *et al.* 1983	Pretreatment with 7 days 800 mg daily cimetidine did not inhibit tolbutamide elimination. (Test dose 500 mg p.o.)
Cate *et al.* 1986	Elimination kinetics of 1 gm tolbutamide p.o. markedly inhibited by 1200 mg o.d. cimetidine for 2 days before the test. No inhibiton produced by ranitidine.
Stockley *et al.* 1986	Cimetidine 400 mg BD for the preceding 4 days had no effect on the disposition of 250 mg tolbutamide p.o.
Peart *et al.* 1987	Tolbutamide pharmacokinetics same in EM and PM of debrisoquine.
Robson *et al.* 1987	Dextropropoxyphene caused no change in tolbutamide hydroxylation (it did inhibit 8 hydroxylation of theophylline by 17% but not theophylline 1-demethylation or 3-demethylation).
Adebayo & Coker 1988	Ranitidine and cimetidine (1200 mg/day for 4 days) did not affect the pharmacokinetics of 1 g tolbutamide p.o.
Back *et al.* 1988a	Effects of sulphaphenazole (A) cimetidine (B) and primaquine (C) on the disposition of antipyrine (I) and 500 mg IV tolbutamide (II) in human volunteers. A increased the $T^{\frac{1}{2}}$ of I and clearance to metabolite decreased, no effect on II. B high dose (1 g o.d. 4 days and 600 mg one hour before the test) increased $T^{\frac{1}{2}}$ of I and II. C no effect in I, half-life of II increased and clearance to metabolites decreased.
Veronese *et al.* 1990a	Urinary metabolic ratio hydroxytolbutamide + carboxytolbutamide/tolbutamide decreased after sulphaphenazole as did the plasma clearance of tolbutamide whilst the $T^{\frac{1}{2}}$ became longer.

the same cytochrome P450 as tolbutamide, but it does make it a possibility. The absence of inhibition makes it extremely unlikely that the inhibitor is metabolized by the same cytochrome P450 as tolbutamide.

In vitro evidence summarized by Knodell *et al.* (1987) was at variance with their *in vivo* evidence mentioned above. Their results indicated the possibility that tolbutamide hydroxylation and S-mephenytoin hydroxylation might be catalysed by the same cytochrome P450, as follows.

1 The addition of anti-$P450_{MP}$ to incubates strongly inhibited both tolbutamide hydroxylase and S-mephenytoin 4-hydroxylase activities.

2 Tolbutamide hydroxylase activity correlated with S-mephenytoin 4-hydroxylase activity in a population of liver samples.

3 Tolbutamide hydroxylase activity co-purified with $P450_{MP}$ and both tolbutamide and S-mephenytoin 4-hydroxylation were mediated by one electrophoretically homogenous protein.

4 S-mephenytoin and tolbutamide acted as competitive inhibitors of hydroxylation of each other (this

Table 9.2. In vitro *assessment of the inhibition of tolbutamide oxidation by P450 in human liver*

Compounds causing potent inhibition	Compounds which cause weak inhibition or no inhibition
aniline	methylimidazole
cimetidine	dimethylimidazole
dextropropoxyphene	methimazole
sulphinpyrazone	histamine
verapamil	metronidazole
chlordiazepoxide	sparteine
diazepam	chloroquine
lorazepam	aminopyrine
nordiazepam	benzo[a]pyrene
phenylbutazone	caffeine
sulphamethizole	debrisoquine
sulphamethoxazole	erythromycin
ketoconazole	norgestel
clotrimazole	sulphanilamide
miconazole	sulphamethoxazole
sulphaphenazole	dapsone
primaquine	quinidine
diethylstilboestrol	pyrimethamine
ethnyl oestradiol	cholesterol
progesterone	cortisol
nifedipine	7-ethoxycoumarin
oestradiol	paraxanthine
	phenacetin
	propanolol
	theobromine
	theophylline
	mephenytoin
	antipyrine

Data derived from: Back *et al.* 1988b; Miners *et al.* 1988; Purba & Back 1988; Purba *et al.* 1987.

is at variance with the observation of Purba *et al.* 1987).

None of this *in vitro* work provided unambiguous evidence that the two compounds are oxidized by a single protein.

Two possible explanations were discussed by Knodell *et al.* (1987): first that tolbutamide hydroxylation was catalysed by a cytochrome P450 other than P450$_{MP}$-S-mephenytoin hydroxylase; secondly, that structural alterations in a mutant P450$_{MP}$ prevent S-mephenytoin 4-hydroxylation but did not hinder the enzyme from hydroxylating tolbutamide.

The importance of studying human liver preparations and not assuming that the inferences derived from results in animal tissues can apply to humans is emphasized by the study of Veronese *et al.* (1990b). They found that cytochrome P450 3A6

tolbutamide hydroxylation in rats and rabbits was different from that found in humans. For example, sulphaphenazole inhibition was more pronounced in the human preparations.

MOLECULAR GENETICS

The understanding of tolbutamide metabolism has been greatly advanced by the study of Relling *et al.* (1990). They found that there was a large variability in both tolbutamide and mephenytoin metabolism by 38 human liver preparations *in vitro* but there was no correlation between the two activities. Both reactions shared common inhibitors.

These workers then took the cDNAs for two cytochromes P450 which had previously been isolated. These were P450 2C8 and P450 2C9. Each cDNA was inserted into a recombinant vaccinia virus and the virus then was made to infect hepatoma cells growing in culture. Both whole cell homogenates and microsomal preparations were examined for enzymic activity and cytochrome P450 content.

It was found that both cytochrome P450 2C8 and cytochrome P450 2C9 expressed significant tolbutamide hydroxylase activity. In contrast only cytochrome P450 2C9 exhibited a lower level of hydroxylase activity with mephenytoin and only with the (R)-enantiomer (Table 9.3).

Similarly, Brian *et al.* (1989) have described a clone in the CYP 2C subfamily of cytochromes P450 which when expressed in yeast can hydroxylate tolbutamide but not (S)-mephenytoin.

The two chemical reactions were also shown to be mediated by different proteins by Srivastava *et al.* (1991). Cytochromes P450 2C9 and 10 were expressed in yeast and shown to be excellent tolbutamide hydroxylases but poor (S)-mephenytoin 4'-hydroxylases. The same group had previously shown cytochrome P450 2C8 to have low tolbutamide hydroxylation ability and no (S)-mephenytoin 4'-hydroxylase activity.

However, a human *CYP 2C9* cDNA clone expressed in COS cells by Veronese *et al.* (1991) was able to oxidize both tolbutamide and phenytoin.

Furthermore, a *CYP 2C9* type clone has been isolated from an adult liver cDNA library by Ohgiya *et al.* (1992), which had a six-base deletion leading to the loss of two amino acids in the encoded protein. This clone and others lacking the deletion were expressed in yeast. The clone with the deletion con-

Table 9.3. *Enzyme activity (nanomoles per milligram of protein per hour) of expressed P450 2C8 and P450 2C9 cDNAs in homogenates of HepG2 cells*

	TB	Racemic MEPH		(R)-MEPH		(S)-MEPH	
	OH-TB	4-OH	Nirv	4-OH	Nirv	4-OH	Nirv
2C9	0.501	0.155	0.026	0.095	0.058	n.d.	n.d.
2C8	0.149	n.d.	n.d.	n.d.	n.d.	n.d.	0.016
Control	n.d.	n.d.	n.d.	n.d.	n.d.	n.d.	n.d.

OH-TB, hydroxytolbutamide; 4-OH, 4-hydroxymephenytoin; Nirv, nirvanol; n.d., not detectable. TB concentration was 2 mM; (R)-, (S)- and racemic MEPH concentrations were 1 mM.
From: Relling *et al.* 1990.

ferred only half the tolbutamide hydroxylating ability of clones lacking the deletion. This observation raises the possibility that there may be a polymorphism in the population.

Cytochromes P450 2C8, 9 and 10 have been found to be related. The two latter appear to differ by two amino acids in that 2C9 has Tyr instead of Cys at 358 and Gly instead of Asp at 417. Cytochrome P450 2C8, however, differs greatly from 2C10 (Srivastava *et al.* 1991).

So with this knowledge of the molecular genetics now available it is easy to see why the studies of the genetics of tolbutamide metabolism in human beings have been perplexing. The drug is hydroxylated by more than one type of cytochrome P450 and it is possible there may be genetic variants and/or different degrees of inducibility of each type. So the absence of a monogenic pattern of inheritance of the metabolism is understandable, as is the comparative rarity of an individual with a profound inability to hydroxylate the drug.

Also, the relationship of tolbutamide metabolism to mephenytoin metabolism is clarified in that some agents are able to inhibit more than one type of cytochrome P450 *in vitro* but the functional performance of these same cytochromes P450 *in vivo* can be very different. The tremendous value of separating individual cytochromes P450 and expressing them in cultured cells is clearly demonstrated.

Adebayo, G. I. & Coker, H. A. B. (1988). Lack of efficacy of cimetidine and ranitidine as inhibitors of tolbutamide metabolism. *European Journal of Clinical Pharmacology*, **34**, 653–6.

Back, D. J. & Orme, M. L'E. (1989). Genetic factors influencing the metabolism of tolbutamide. *Pharmacology and Therapeutics*, **44**, 147–55.

Back, D. J., Tjia, J. F., Karbwang, J. & Colbert, J. (1988b). *In vitro* inhibition studies of tolbutamide hydroxylase activity of human liver microsomes by azoles sulphonamides and quinolines. *British Journal of Clinical Pharmacology*, **26**, 23–9.

Back, D. J., Tjia, J., Monig, H., Ohnhaus, E. E. & Park, B. K. (1988a). Selective inhibition of drug oxidation after simultaneous administration of two probe drugs antipyrine and tolbutamide. *European Journal of Clinical Pharmacology*, **34**, 157–63.

Bird, E. D. & Schwalbe, F. C. (1965). Prolonged hypoglycaemia secondary to tolbutamide. *Annals of Internal Medicine*, **62**, 110–12.

Brian, W. R., Srivastava, P. K., Umbenhauer, D. R., Lloyd, R. S. & Guengerich, F. P. (1989). Expression of a human liver cytochrome P-450 protein with tolbutamide hydroxylase activity in *Saccharomyces cerevisiae*. *Biochemistry*, **28**, 4993–9.

Cate, E. W., Rogers, J. F. & Powell, J. R. (1986). Inhibition of tolbutamide elimination by cimetidine but not ranitidine. *Journal of Clinical Pharmacology*, **26**, 372–7.

Christensen, L. K., Hansen, J. M. & Kristensen, M. (1963). Sulphaphenazole-induced hypoglycaemic attacks in tolbutamide-treated diabetics. *Lancet*, **2**, 1298–1301.

Dey, N. G., Castleden, C. M., Ward, J. & Cornhill, J., McBurney, A. (1983). The effect of cimetidine on tolbutamide kinetics. *British Journal of Clinical Pharmacology*, **16**, 438–40.

Knodell, R. G., Hall, S. D., Wilkinson, G. R. & Guengerich, F. P. (1987). Hepatic metabolism of tolbutamide, Characterization of the form of cytochrome P-450 involved in methyl hydroxylation and relationship to in vivo disposition. *Journal of Pharmacology and Experimental Therapeutics*, **241**, 1112–19.

Kostelnik, M. E. & Iber, F. L. (1973). Correlation of alcohol and tolbutamide blood clearance rates with microsomal alcohol-metabolizing enzyme activity. *American Journal of Clinical Nutrition*, **26**, 161–4.

Kreeger, N. (1962). Tolbutamide-induced hypoglycaemia. *New England Journal of Medicine*, **266**, 218–20.

Lumholtz, B., Siersbaek-Nielson, K., Skovsted, L., Kampmann, J. & Hansen, J. M. (1975). Sulfamethiozole-induced inhibition of diphenyl hydantoin, tolbutamide and warfarin metabolism. *Clinical Pharmacology and Therapeutics*, **17**, 731–4.

Miller, A. K., Adir, J. & Vestal, R. E. (1990). Excretion of tolbutamide metabolites in young and old subjects. *European Journal of Clinical Pharmacology*, **38**, 523–4.

Miners, J. O, Foenander, T. K., Wanwimolruk, S., Gallus, A. S. & Birkett, D. J. (1982). The effect of sulphinpyrazone on oxidative drug metabolism in man, inhibition of tolbutamide elimination. *European Journal of Clinical Pharmacology*, **22**, 321–6.

Miners, J. O., Smith, K. J., Robson, R. A., McManus, M. E., Veronese, M. E. & Birkett, D. J. (1988). Tolbutamide hydroxylation by human liver microsomes. *Biochemical Pharmacology*, **37**, 1137–44.

Miners, J. O., Wing, L. M. H. & Birkett, D. J. (1985). Normal metabolism of debrisoquine and theophylline in a slow tolbutamide metabolizer. *Australian and New Zealand Journal of Medicine*, **15**, 348–9.

Ohgiya, S., Komori, M., Ohi, H., Shiamatsu, K., Shinriki, N. & Kamataki, T. (1992). Six-base deletion occurring in messages of human cytochrome P-450 in the CYP 2C sub-family results in reduction of tolbutamide hydroxyglase activity. *Biochemistry International*, **27**, 1073–81.

Page, M. A., Boutagy, J. S. & Shenfield, G. M. (1991). A screening test for slow metabolisers of tolbutamide. *British Journal of Clinical Pharmacology*, **31**, 649–54

Peart, G. F., Boutagy, J. & Shenfield, G. M. (1987). Lack of relationship between tolbutamide metabolism and debrisoquine oxidation phenotype. *European Journal of Clinical Pharmacology*, **33**, 397–402.

Pond, S. M., Birkett, D. J. & Wade, D. N. (1977). Mechanisms of inhibition of tolbutamide metabolism, phenylbutazone, oxyphenbutazone, sulfaphenazole. *Clinical Pharmacology and Therapeutics*, **22**, 573–9.

Purba, H. S. & Back, D. J. (1988). Inhibition of tolbutamide 4-hydroxylase activity in human liver microsomes by benzodiazepines. *British Journal of Clinical Pharmacology*, **26**, 227P.

Purba, H. S., Back, D. J. & Orme, M. L'E. (1987). Tolbutamide 4-hydroxlase activity of human liver microsomes, effect of inhibitors. *British Journal of Clinical Pharmacology*, **24**, 230–4.

Relling, M. V., Aoyama, T., Gonzalez, F. J. & Meyer, U. A. (1990). Tolbutamide and mephenytoin hydroxylation by human cytochrome P450s in the CYP 2C subfamily. *Journal of Pharmacology and Experimental Therapeutics*, **252**, 442–7.

Robson, R. A., Miners, J. O., Whitehead, A. G. & Birkett, D. J. (1987). Specificity of the inhibitory effect of dextro-propoxyphene on oxidative drug metabolism in man, effects on theophylline and tolbutamide disposition. *British Journal of Clinical Pharmacology*, **23**, 772–5.

Rowland, M. & Matin, S. B. (1973). Kinetics of drug-drug interactions. *Journal of Pharmacokinetics and Biopharmaceutics*, **1**, 553–67.

Schulz, E. & Schmidt, F. H. (1970). Abbauhemmung von tolbutamid durch sulfaphenazol beim menschen. *Pharmacologia Clinica*, **2**, 150–4.

Scott, J. & Poffenbarger, P. L. (1979a). Pharmacogenetics of tolbutamide metabolism in humans. *Diabetes*, **28**, 41–51.

Scott, J. & Poffenbarger, P. L. (1979b). Tolbutamide pharmacogenetics and the UDGP controversy. *Journal of the American Medical Association*, **242**, 45–8.

Srivastava, P. K., Yun, C. H., Beaune, P. H., Ged, C. & Guengerich, F. P. (1991). Separation of human liver microsomal tolbutamide hydroxylase and (S)-mephenytoin 4'-hydroxylase cytochrome P450 enzymes. *Molecular Pharmacology*, **40**, 69–79.

Stockley, C., Keal, J., Rolan, P., Bochner, F. & Somogyi, A. (1986). Lack of inhibition of tolbutamide hydroxylation by cimetidine in man. *European Journal of Clinical Pharmacology*, **31**, 235–7.

Thomas, R. C. & Ikeda, G. J. (1966). The metabolic fate of tolbutamide in man and in the rat. *Journal of Medicinal Chemistry*, **9**, 507–10.

Veronese, M. E., Mackenzie, P. I., Doeke, J., McManus, M. E., Miners, J. O. & Birkett, D. J. (1991). Tolbutamide and phenytoin hydroxylations by cDNA-expressed human liver cytochrome P450 2C9. *Biochemical and Biophysical Research Communications*, **175**, 1112–18.

Veronese, M. E., McManus, M. E., Laupattarakasem, P., Miners, J. O. & Birkett, D. J. (1990b). Tolbutamide hydroxylation by human, rabbit and rat liver microsomes and by purified forms of cytochrome P-450. *Drug Metabolism and Disposition*, **18**, 356–61.

Veronese, M. E., Miners, J. O., Randles, D., Gregov, D. & Birkett, D. J. (1990a). Validation of the tolbutamide metabolic ratio for population screening with use of sulfaphenazole to produce model phenotypic poor metabolizers. *Clinical Pharmacology and Therapeutics*, **47**, 403–11.

10 Phenytoin

INTRODUCTION

PHENYTOIN (diphenylhydantoin: Fig. 10.1) was introduced into clinical practice by Merritt & Putnam (1938) and is still a very useful anti-epileptic drug. Its action is considered to be the stabilization of the cell membranes of neurones and myocardial and other cells. This action is thought to be the result of phenytoin's influence on ionic fluxes across the cell membrane.

Despite its obvious clinical usefulness a lot of troubles arose in practice due to toxic manifestations in patients taking conventional doses, e.g. anorexia, nausea, drowsiness, mental dullness, confusion, hallucinations, blurred vision, ataxia, dysarthria, tremor, diplopia, vertigo and nystagmus, on the one hand, and also ineffective control of fits, on the other.

When methods to measure the concentrations of phenytoin in the serum (e.g. that of Dill *et al.* 1956) became available it was shown that superior clinical results could be obtained by keeping the plasma phenytoin concentration within a fairly narrow therapeutic range. Indeed, this observation with phenytoin was a powerful stimulus to the establishment of the now standard practice of therapeutic drug monitoring (Lund *et al.* 1972).

Some other facets were also revealed when drug levels became measurable. First, the rather atypical pharmacokinetics of phenytoin: the steady-state plasma concentration is not directly proportional to the dose ('non-linear kinetics', see Atkinson & Shaw 1973, Gugler *et al.* 1976; Levine *et al.* 1987).

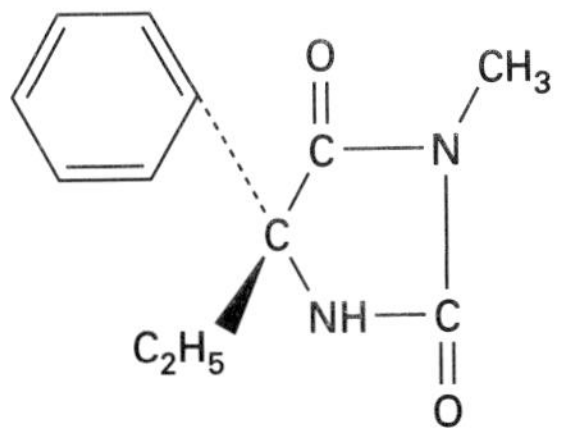

R–mephenytoin

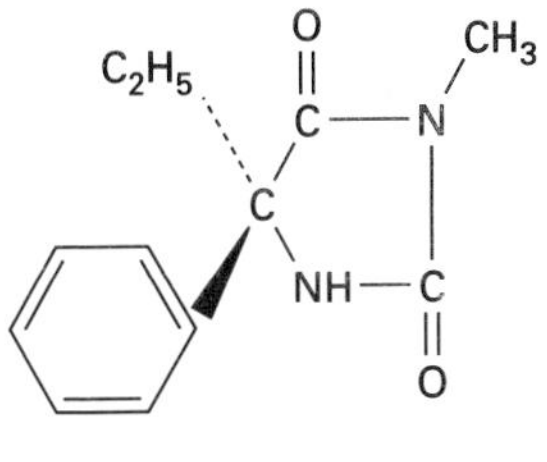

S–mephenytoin

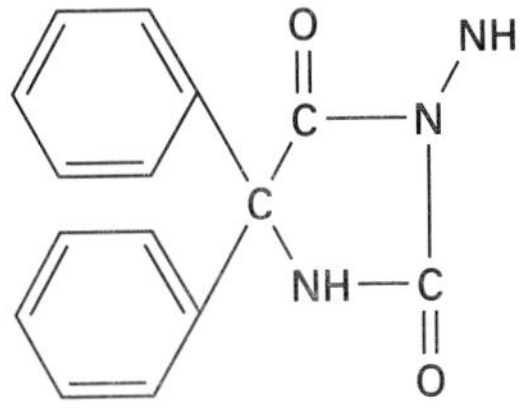

Diphenylhydantoin (phenytoin)

Fig. 10.1. Structural formulae of phenytoin and the enantiomers of mephenytoin.

Secondly, interactions between phenytoin and other drugs were shown to be clinically important and these interactions included alterations in phenytoin pharmacokinetics. Thirdly, the very large inter-individual variability in the kinetics, e.g. the steady-state plasma concentration attained on a standard dosage schedule, for example, Loeser (1961) showed blood levels ranging from 2.5 to over 40 µg/ml in 29 patients treated for fits with an average dose of 5.4 mg/kg (range 3.3 to 8.8 mg/kg).

There are four principal areas in which genetic studies on phenytoin have been revealing and they will be discussed below.

INTERACTION BETWEEN DIPHENYLHYDANTOIN METABOLISM AND THE POLYMORPHIC ACETYLATION OF ISONIAZID

It had been observed clinically that some patients who received diphenylhydantoin (DPH) in the usual dosage of 4 to 5 mg per kg body weight simultaneously with anti-tuberculosis therapy developed nystagmus, ataxia and drowsiness. A series of 24 such patients was studied by Kutt *et al.* (1966). Some of these patients had been taking DPH for years without any previous difficulties. However, some time after treatment for tuberculosis with isoniazid (INH) and para-aminosalicylic acid (PAS) was started they developed symptoms and signs of DPH toxicity whilst taking their regular phenytoin dosage. Non-epileptic tuberculous patients without any liver disease were also given DPH experimentally to study its metabolism in this setting.

Abnormally high blood levels of DPH were found in the patients who developed toxic symptoms whilst taking INH and PAS, although they previously had taken the same doses of DPH without side effects. Reduction of the DPH dosage enabled these patients to maintain seizure control without evidence of intoxication, and with a therapeutic blood DPH level. The urinary 5-phenyl-5'-para-hydroxyphenylhydantoin (HPPH) excretion revealed interesting findings. For example, one woman on 300 mg DPH daily received in addition INH plus PAS therapy. When she developed lethargy, ataxia and nystagmus the blood DPH level was 38 µg/ml and her HPPH excretion was 52% of the ingested dose. When the daily dose of DPH was

reduced to 100 mg the blood DPH level became 5 µg/ml and the HPPH output was 72% of the ingested dose.

Similar results were obtained when non-epileptic patients being treated for tuberculosis were experimentally commenced on DPH therapy at a dose of 300 mg daily. The blood DPH level rose to toxic levels over about 4 weeks and symptoms such as ataxia, lethargy, blurred vision, etc. developed.

It was observed that the addition of folic acid to the therapeutic regime for such a patient caused the blood DPH concentration to fall, and the HPPH urinary excretion to rise.

However, the authors mention in their article that not all patients were prone to this interactive adverse effect. The influence of INH and PAS separately was not assessed.

The same group (Kutt *et al.* 1968) investigated the hydroxylation of phenytoin in rats and showed that its inhibition increased with increasing doses of isoniazid. Rat liver microsomal preparations were investigated and isoniazid was shown to produce a non-competitive inhibition of phenytoin hydroxylation (Fig. 10.2). Combinations of isoniazid and PAS resulted in a greater degree of non-competitive inhibition than would be expected from the sum of inhibitions caused by either drug alone at the same concentrations. The performance of these *in vitro* studies gave rise to the idea that only patients with sufficiently high blood INH concentra-

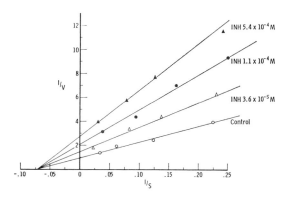

Fig. 10.2. Lineweaver–Burk plot (1/*v* vs 1/*s*; *v* = velocity, *s* = substrate) of inhibition of diphenylhydantoin parahydroxylation by INH. Note the change of slope and shift of the intercepts by increasing amounts of INH consistent with noncompetitive inhibition. (From Kutt *et al.* 1968.)

tions developed enough inhibition of DPH hydroxylation to produce DPH intoxication. The authors then speculated that polymorphic INH acetylation might influence the clinical outcome.

The hypothesis that slow acetylators were more prone than rapid acetylators to develop DPH toxicity, when simultaneously treated with isoniazid, was evaluated by Brennan *et al.* (1968) and Kutt *et al.* (1970). They investigated 36 patients, 6 of whom had developed DPH toxicity whilst on combined therapy. Acetylator phenotyping was carried out by the ingestion of 10 mg INH per kg body weight and the plasma level determined 3 hours later. A bimodal distribution curve was obtained (Fig. 10.3).

● Fast INH inactivators
▲ Slow INH inactivators, without DPH intoxication
△ Slow INH inactivators, with DPH intoxication

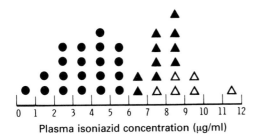

Fig. 10.3. Isoniazid plasma concentrations of 36 patients 3 hours after a test dose of 10 mg of isoniazid per kg body weight. All patients in whom diphenylhydantoin intoxication developed had high isoniazid plasma concentrations (△). (By permission of the publishers of the American Review of Respiratory Diseases.) (From Kutt *et al.* 1970.)

All six individuals who had developed DPH toxicity had values towards the upper end of the slow acetylator mode. Similarly, when blood DPH concentrations were followed sequentially in patients receiving 300 mg DPH, 300 mg INH and 1500 mg PAS daily the rise in plasma DPH levels over 21 days in rapid acetylators was similar to that obtained in persons taking the same dosage of DPH but no INH or PAS (Fig. 10.4). Amongst the slow acetylators there was a gradation with slight elevation amongst those nearer the antimode and a sharp rise to toxic levels in the slowest (Kutt 1971).

This is a classical example of a genetic polymorphism influencing the outcome of a drug interaction.

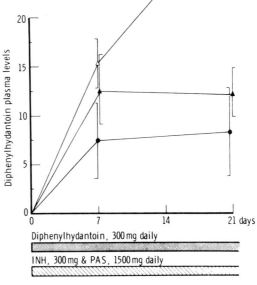

△ Slow INH inactivators, with DPH intoxication
▲ Slow INH inactivators, without DPH intoxication
● Fast INH inactivators

Fig. 10.4. Diphenylhydantoin blood concentrations of patients who were fast, moderately slow, and very slow isoniazid inactivators. There was a rapid rise to the toxic range without stabilization in the very slow inactivators, and the average level in the moderately slow inactivators was higher than in the fast inactivators. (By permission of the publishers of the American Review of Respiratory Diseases.) (From Kutt *et al.* 1970.)

GENETIC CONTROL OF PHENYTOIN METABOLISM

As has been mentioned earlier there is a very wide inter-individual variability in the metabolism of DPH which in man occurs principally by para-hydroxylation to HPPH. Soon after the phenomenon of induction was discovered to occur in human drug metabolism, it was found that phenytoin blood levels were altered by environmental influences. For example, Burns *et al.* (1965) showed that plasma phenytoin concentrations were lowered in patients receiving either phenobarbital or griseofulvin (but the phenobarbital effect was later shown not to be a sustained phenomenon: Kutt *et al.* 1969; Booker *et al.* 1971).

Nevertheless, convincing evidence has also been forthcoming of genetic control of DPH metabolism, and has been derived (as for many other drugs) from

Table 10.1. *Details of poor diphenylhydantoin hydroxylator probands*

Reference	Dose of DPH	Number of days of drug therapy to develop toxic signs	Plasma concentration of DPH when toxic signs developed	Urinary HPPH excretion when toxic signs developed	Plasma DPH half-life (hours)	Urinary HPPH excretion in 24 hours	Serum DPH/HPPH concentration ratio
Kutt *et al.* 1964	3.8 mg/kg BW/day	17	87 μg/ml (normal 3 to 5)	140 mg daily i.e. 48% of DPH dose (normal 60 to 70%)	–	–	–
Vasko *et al.* 1980	4.6 mg/kg BW/day	10	52 μg/ml approx (therapeutic range 10 to 20)	50% of DPH dose daily	–	–	–
	3.0 mg/kg BW/day	?	26	?	–	–	–
	3.0 mg/kg BW as single dose intravenously	–	–	–	30.6 hours (control 14.4 ± SEM 1.6)	27% of dose (normal 47 to 71%)	–
Vermeij *et al.* 1988	Single oral dose of 300 mg	–	–	–	–	–	about 20 (controls 37.7 ± SD 1.8)

DPH, diphenylhydantoin; HPPH, 5-(*p*-hydroxyphenyl)-5-phenylhydantoin; BW, body weight; SEM, standard error of the mean; SD, standard deviation.

twin studies and family studies. The first step in the metabolism is parahydroxylation of one of the phenyl rings to give HPPH. This is followed by glucuronidation and excretion. It is considered that there is so much capacity in the latter step that the former is rate-limiting.

Seven pairs of identical (IT) and seven pairs of fraternal (FT) twins were studied by means of their diphenylhydantoin serum half-life by Andreasen *et al.* (1973). The mean intra-pair variance of the two groups of twins was calculated as the total intra-pair variance divided by twice the number of twins. The values were, for FT = 16.49 and for IT = 2.49. An *F* test showed these variances to differ significantly (p< 0.05). The heritability index, calculated as:

$$\frac{\text{variance within pairs of FT} - \text{variance within pairs of IT}}{\text{variance within pairs of FT}}$$

was 0.85, indicating a strong genetic influence.

Family studies have been carried out following the identification of three probands who developed DPH toxicity on conventional dosage therapy. The characteristics of the probands are shown in Table 10.1.

The patient of Kutt *et al.* (1964) was treated with 1.4 mg DPH per kg daily and on this dosage maintained a blood level of about 9 μg DPH per ml without toxic symptoms. On this dosage the output of HPPH was about 70% of the drug intake. Out of the six family members investigated three handled DPH in a similar manner to the proband and three were normal. The genetic nature of the metabolic deficiency for the hydroxylation was unclear from this pedigree.

The pedigree ascertained by means of the proband of Vasko *et al.* (1980) contained four 'hypometabolizers' and seven normal metabolizers. The criteria for classification were not clear cut and the manner of inheritance was doubtful.

Much more satisfactory information was provided by Vermeij *et al.* (1988). The serum DPH/HPPH ratio 6 hours after a 300 mg DPH dose showed that the proband and two siblings formed a mode widely separated from all other subjects. The 22 offspring of these three persons constituted a mode at higher ratio levels than random healthy control subjects (Fig. 10.5). The interpretation offered by the authors is that the hydroxylation of DPH is controlled by two alleles at an autosomal locus and that the three individuals in the first generation were homozygous

recessives. Their four spouses were presumably dominant homozygotes and their 22 offspring heterozygotes. It was, however, also pointed out that more complicated genetic models could not be excluded.

Vasko *et al.* (1980) suggested that slow metabolism may not be very rare. Glazko *et al.* (1969) described one volunteer out of six who had a prolonged half-life at 28.7 hours and who excreted only 29% of a 250 mg DPH dose as HPPH over 5 days. Vermeij *et al.* (1988) state that they studied other families with high DPH/HPPH ratios. Nevertheless, at present there are no population data on the incidence of the slow metabolism character, and further genetic information has not been published. The possibility also exists of abnormally powerful hydroxylators of phenytoin (in the absence of any concomitant drug therapy). Three such patients were described by Kutt *et al.* (1966). In one of these patients an oral daily dose of 600 mg DPH produced a blood level of 7 μg/ml and 60% of the ingested dose appeared in the urine as HPPH.

In view of what we now know about the hydroxylation of many compounds in the body it seems more than likely that there are genetic variants of the cytochrome P450 which are involved in the oxidation of DPH. These variants probably have a diminished enzymic ability to parahydroxylate the DPH molecule.

Specific antibodies against purified rabbit cytochromes P450 were produced by Doecke *et al.* (1990). Only cytochrome P450 2C3 was capable of 4-hydroxylating phenytoin and this activity was inhibited by anti-P450 2C3 IgG. This same antibody inhibited the 4-hydroxylation of phenytoin by human liver microsomes by 66%. The authors suggest that an ortholog to rabbit cytochrome P450 2C3 is in part responsible for this activity in man.

CORRELATION OF DIPHENYLHYDANTOIN HYDROXYLATION WITH THE HYDROXYLATION OF OTHER COMPOUNDS

With the knowledge of the genetic polymorphism of the hydroxylation of debrisoquine/sparteine and S-mephenytoin it was attractive to see whether phenytoin metabolism was governed by the same alleles.

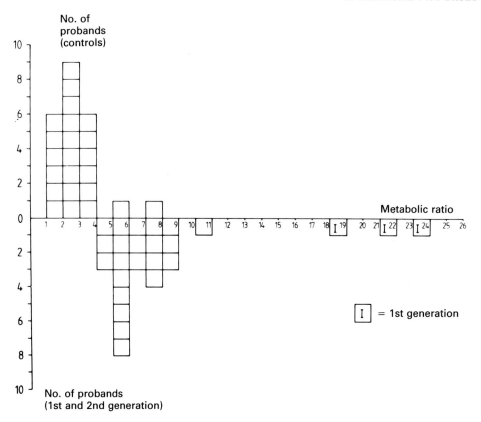

Fig. 10.5. Histogram of the metabolic ratios of serum phenytoin/hydroxyphenytoin concentrations found in subjects studied of 30 years and older. (From Vermeij et al. 1988.)

In view of the structural similarity between phenytoin and mephenytoin it is strange that the genetical relationship between the metabolism of the two compounds should have received so little attention. This defect was handsomely rectified by the study of Fritz et al. (1987). They made use of information on phenytoin metabolism previously discovered by Butler et al. (1976), namely, that when the drug was para-hydroxylated (the overwhelmingly important biotransformation) then, in man, a mixture of two isomers of HPPH was produced with a 10 to 1 preponderance of the laevorotatory form (now called S-HPPH).

Fritz et al. (1987), using chiral ligand exchange chromatography, were able to estimate the S- and R-enantiomers of HPPH independently. There was no evidence of any difference in total HPPH produc-

tion or in the production of either of the two enantiomers between the two debrisoquine/sparteine phenotypes. Both mephenytoin phenotypes produced much more S-HPPH than R-HPPH so that the overall metabolism of DPH was not different in the two phenotypes. However, R-HPPH production was deficient in poor hydroxylators of S-mephenytoin, with the result that the urinary S-HPPH/R-HPPH ratio was significantly higher in that phenotype as compared with extensive S-mephenytoin hydroxylators (Table 10.2).

Butler et al. (1976) discussed the two possibilities that one enzyme may be able to hydroxylate both phenyl rings of DPH, or there may be two separate enzymes, one for each ring. The latter view was supported by Fritz et al. (1987), principally on the grounds that the HPPH S/R ratio decreased markedly after autoinduction with DPH indicating independent control of the two catalytic activities.

The relationship of the debrisoquine/sparteine hydroxylation to phenytoin para-hydroxylation has

Table 10.2. *Enantiomeric ratio of 4-hydroxyphenytoin in different hydroxylation phenotypes*

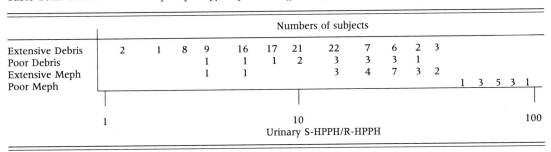

Debris, hydroxylator of debrisoquine; Meph, hydroxylator of mephenytoin.
From: Fritz *et al.* 1987.

Table 10.3. *Phenytoin metabolism in extensive and poor metabolizers of debrisoquine/sparteine*

Reference	Subjects investigated	Parameters of phenytoin metabolism studied	Result
Sloan *et al.* 1981	5 EM 6 PM	Apparent first-order rate constant for the formation of HPPH.	EM 0.030 ± 0.007 h^{-1} PM 0.016 ± 0.003 h^{-1} $p < 0.001$
		Half time for the elimination of the oral dose of DPH (200 mg) in the urine as HPPH	EM 44.3 ± 12.1 h PM 81.5 ± 23.3 h $p < 0.005$
de Wolff *et al.* 1983	1 EM	300 mg DPH daily produced severe toxicity after 11 days	HPPH/DPH in urine = 9.2 when serum concentration was 20 mg/l (normal = $33.0 \pm$ SD 12.8)
Kadar *et al.* 1983)	1 PM	Single 200 mg oral dose of DPM containing some [4–^{14}C]phenytoin	Apparent $K_{\text{formation pHPPH}}$ 0.125 mg/h and DPH serum half-life 15.2 h
	1 EM	Single 200 mg oral dose of DPM containing some [4–^{14}C]phenytoin	Apparent $K_{\text{formation pHPPH}}$ 0.133 mg/h and DPH serum half-life 15.9 h
Steiner *et al.* 1987	7 EM 5 PM	5 mg DPH per kg i.v. CL $t_{\frac{1}{2}}$ V_{area} AUC estimated by first-order kinetics C_0 K_m V_{max} V_{area} estimated by Michaelis–Menten kinetics	No significant difference between phenotypes and similarly for urinary metabolite recovery
Fritz *et al.* 1987	25 EM 7 PM	Single oral dose of 100 mg phenytoin 12 hour urinary HPPH	$14 \pm 7\%$ of dose excreted in EM 18% of dose excreted in PM
		Log urinary S-HPPH/R-HPPH	Range the same in both phenotypes (see Table 10.2)

EM, Extensive metabolizers; PM, poor metabolizers; CL, plasma clearance; $t_{\frac{1}{2}}$, plasma half-life; V_{area}, apparent volume of distribution; AUC, area under the curve; C_0, concentration extrapolated at zero time; K_m, Michaelis constant; V_{max}, maximum velocity.

been studied both *in vivo* and *in vitro*. The *in vivo* evidence is summarized in Table 10.3. It is not clear why Sloan *et al.* (1981) obtained what was subsequently shown to be an erroneous result. The *in vitro* evidence consists of the demonstration by Inaba *et al.* (1985) that phenytoin failed competitively to inhibit sparteine metabolism by human liver microsomes.

It was demonstrated by Kutt *et al.* (1964) that an individual who had insufficient capacity to parahydroxylate DPH, was able normally to hydroxylate the phenyl rings of phenobarbital, mephobarbital and phenylalanine (the last as shown by the normal decline of phenylalanine blood level).

Correlations have also been sought between the hydroxylation of phenytoin and the hydroxylation of other drugs in which no clear genetic polymorphism has as yet been delineated. Schellens *et al.* (1991) administered a cocktail of nifedipine, sparteine and phenytoin to eight healthy subjects (all extensive metabolizers of sparteine). No significant correlations were found between the three drugs when various pharmacokinetic parameters were examined.

A highly significant correlation was demonstrated between microsomal phenytoin 4-hydroxylation and tolbutamide methylhydroxylation by Doecke *et al.* (1991) using 18 human livers. In addition, competitive inhibition of each activity was demonstrated by the other drug. It is also relevant that sulphaphenazole was a powerful inhibitor of both oxidations whereas mephenytoin did not have this ability. Veronese *et al.* (1991) isolated a cytochrome P450 2C9 cDNA cloned from human liver, inserted into a plasmid which was transfected into COS-7 cells. These cells were then shown to produce a 55 kDa protein which was able to hydroxylate tolbutamide and phenytoin. Phenytoin was a competitive inhibitor of tolbutamide hydroxylation and sulphaphenazole was a potent inhibitor of both compounds.

So the conclusions at present are (1) that the S-mephenytoin hydroxylation polymorphism influences R-HPPH formation; and since the production of R-HPPH is a minor metabolic pathway the inter-individual variability in it is unlikely to have clinical significance; (2) that a cytochrome P450 2C9 type enzyme hydroxylates both tolbutamide and phenytoin, but it will have to be determined whether other cytochromes P450 in this category are involved in the metabolism of these two compounds.

POOR PARAHYDROXYLATION OF PHENYTOIN AND PARKINSON'S DISEASE

A patient with Parkinson's disease was fortuitously found to have very slow hydroxylation of phenytoin by Ferrari *et al.* (1986) during the course of a family investigation.

Prompted by this finding, Ferrari *et al.* (1990) studied the parahydroxylation of phenytoin in 17 normal controls and 24 patients with Parkinsonism. The rate of DPH metabolism was indicated by the ratio DPH/HPPH in the serum 6 hours after an oral test dose of 300 mg DPH (this was the technique

used by Vermeij *et al.* (1988) in their family study). In the normal controls the ratios varied between 1 and 3.6. In the Parkinsonian patients the patients the ratios varied between 1.4 and 23.2. Five Parkinsonian patients gave ratios between 4 and 12 corresponding to the heterozygotes in Fig. 10.5. One patient had a value of 23.2 indicating the slow hydroxylator phenotype but it is not clear if this was the patient referred to by Ferrari *et al.* (1986). The hypothesis that slow DPH parahydroxylation is associated with Parkinson's disease attained statistical significance.

It is an interesting idea, that deficient hydroxylation of a chemical substance (endogenous or xenobiotic) might be somehow responsible for Parkinson's disease. As yet, however, there is no solid supporting evidence as to its nature.

IDIOSYNCRATIC ADVERSE REACTIONS AND EPOXIDE HYDROLASES

An apparently idiosyncratic adverse reaction occurs in a very few people who are treated with phenytoin. The features of the reaction are fever, skin rash, hepatotoxicity, lymphadenopathy (pseudolymphoma) and various bone marrow responses including leucocytosis, eosinophilia, haemolytic anaemia and rarely pancytopenia. Not all these features are present in every patient.

A novel approach to the study of such adverse reactions was made by Spielberg (1984) and the essentials were as follows. It was known that a variety of drug molecules (and other xenobiotics), which are not themselves toxic, can be metabolized to produce highly reactive compounds. The latter in their turn are metabolized and rendered non-toxic. The possibility was considered that this 'defence mechanism' may be defective or inadequate in some individuals because of genetically determined variability.

In the case of phenytoin the toxic intermediary metabolite is an arene oxide produced by oxidation via a cytochrome P450 enzyme. This compound is highly reactive and capable of binding to macromolecules within the cell. The result of this process is not only a direct cytotoxicity but also the production of endogenous neo-antigens which are thought capable of producing auto-immune responses (Fig. 10.6). Normally this process is prevented by the

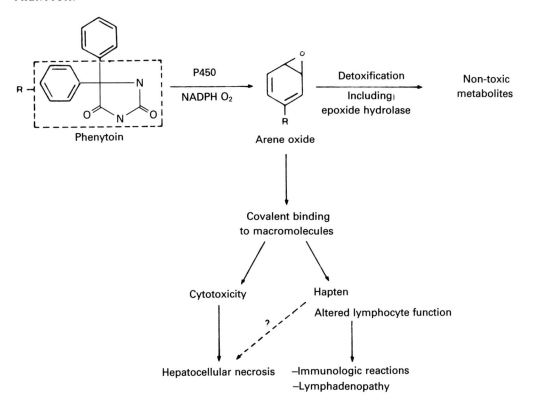

Fig. 10.6. Pathway of phenytoin metabolism and proposed role of arene oxide metabolites in the pathogenesis of hepatotoxicity. (From Spielberg *et al.* 1981.)

prompt destruction of the arene oxide by intracellular mechanisms which include epoxide hydrolase (EC 3.3.2.3) which catalyses the enzymatic hydration of alkene and arene oxides to dihydrodiols (Fig. 10.7).

Spielberg *et al.* (1981) were able to design a semi-*in vitro* system to assess this possibility (Fig. 10.8). The two principal components of the system were first liver microsomes from a mouse and secondly,

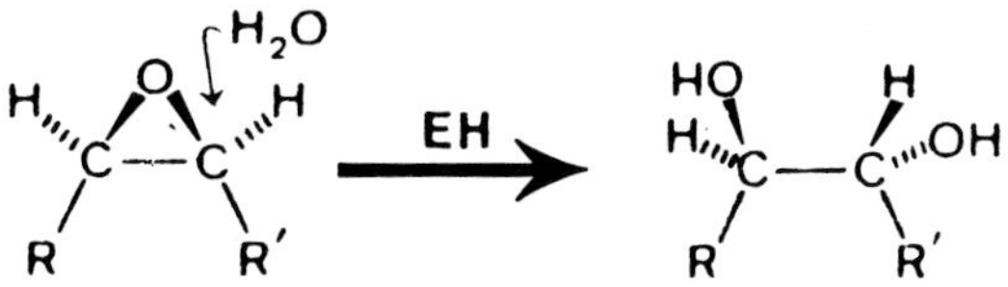

Fig. 10.7. Reaction catalysed by microsomal epoxide hydrolase. (From Seidegård & DePierre 1983.)

peripheral blood lymphocytes from the human subject being investigated. The mouse was treated with phenobarbital before being sacrificed, in order to induce a high level of liver cell enzymic activity. The microsomes were incubated with the drug being tested and the necessary NADPH-generating cofactors to facilitate oxygenation. By this means the arene oxide metabolite was produced. Lymphocytes are known to contain epoxide hydrolase, and this enzyme by its action on arene oxide enables the lymphocyte to survive. On the other hand, reduced activity or absence of epoxide hydrolase would render the lymphocyte liable to be killed. Lymphocyte viability was assessed by means of dye exclusion. The absence of epoxide hydrolase can be mimicked by the addition of 1,1,1-trichloro-2-propene oxide (TCPO) to the system because this compound is a potent non-competitive inhibitor of epoxide hydrolase.

Three patients with clinical evidence of reactions to phenytoin were investigated by Spielberg *et al.* (1981) and 10 to 20% of their lymphocytes were

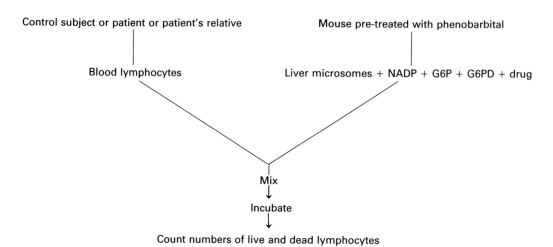

Control subject or patient or patient's relative   Mouse pre-treated with phenobarbital

Blood lymphocytes   Liver microsomes + NADP + G6P + G6PD + drug

Mix

Incubate

Count numbers of live and dead lymphocytes

Fig. 10.8. The assessment of drug toxicity *in vitro*. (Adapted from Spielberg 1984.)

found to die in the presence of up to 125 μM phenytoin in the microsomal system. No such cell death occurred in healthy control subjects in the absence of TCPO but a similar result was produced in them in the presence of TCPO (Fig. 10.9).

The same system was also used to assess mephenytoin and acetaminophen (paracetamol) toxicity. The patients' lymphocytes showed more toxicity to the former than did cells from control subjects (including patients who had been treated with phenytoin without untoward reactions). Dose-dependent paracetamol toxicity was the same for patients' and controls' cells (this compound is detoxified by a different mechanism involving glutathione).

Lymphocytes from relatives of two of the probands produced dose−response curves of three types: (a) like the proband, (b) like the controls, (c) intermediate between the proband and controls. The two small pedigrees published were compatible with the possibility of control of the epoxide hydrolase by two autosomal alleles (Table 10.4).

It is to be noted that phenytoin itself (i.e. not metabolized by a microsomal system) was not toxic to the lymphocytes. Also, in a similar animal system lymphocytotoxicity could be prevented by the addition of purified epoxide hydrolase.

The general principle (i.e. that genetic deficiency of epoxide hydrolase can lead to drug toxicity) was extended by the observations of Gerson *et al.* (1983) on a patient who had developed drug-induced hypoplastic anaemia first on phenytoin and later on carbamazepine (but not on primidone) given for post-traumatic epilepsy. His blood lymphocytes when examined by the technique explained above exhibited *in vitro* toxicity to phenytoin and carbamazepine metabolites (but not to phenobarbital metabolites), and these results were reproduced 18 months after cessation of drug therapy and recovery from the anaemia. The patient's mother showed results intermediate between the patient and normals with both drugs.

An extension of the same technique to study birth defects was made by Strickler *et al.* (1985). An investigation was made of 24 children borne of women who had taken phenytoin throughout the relevant pregnancy. The lymphocytes of 14 children and 13 out of 31 parents gave abnormal results in the *in vitro* test explained above. The abnormal lymphocytic responses fell in the range of those given by the presumed heterozygotes in the hepatotoxicity survey described above.

The children were examined for major and minor birth defects (major = those requiring medical or surgical intervention and causing major functional disturbance, e.g. cardiac malformations, cleft lip/palate and microcephaly). Twelve out of 14 children with positive assays versus two out of 10 with negative assays had one or more major birth defects ($p = 0.002$, Fisher's exact test) and five of 14 positive versus 0 of 10 negative had at least three major

Table 10.4. *Pedigree data on diphenylhydantoin-produced lymphocyte toxicity dose–response curves*

Proband	Father	Mother	Brother	Sister
1	I	I	–	P
2	I	I	C	P

C, like control; P, like proband; I, intermediate.
Constructed from data in Spielberg *et al.* 1981.

birth defects (*p* = 0.047). There was no correlation of minor birth defects with lymphocyte responses (Strickler *et al.* 1985). It was known that fetal epoxide hydrolase activity was low, and so the suggested mechanism was that the fetus was subjected to toxic metabolites when the mother (being a heterozygote) was not fully able to metabolize them. Obviously such a proposition demands much more rigorous proof.

A wealth of information exists on mammalian epoxide hydrolases which hitherto has not been applied very much to clinical situations. The subject was thoroughly reviewed by Seidegård & DePierre (1983) and Thomas & Oesch (1988).

These enzymes take part in the metabolism of many xenobiotics (including drugs) and also endogenous compounds such as leukotrienes and squalene (the cyclization of squalene epoxide is a key step in cholesterol biosynthesis). They exist in a variety of organs with the highest activities in liver, testis, kidney, ovary and lung. Within the liver cell enzymic activity is demonstrable both in the endoplasmic reticulum (microsomes) and in the cytosol.

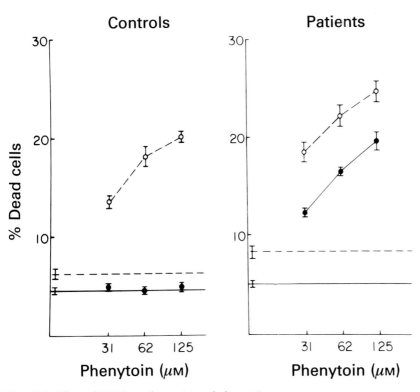

Fig. 10.9. Effect of TCPO on the toxicity of phenytoin. Values represent the mean ±1 SEM for TCPO-treated cell samples (○) and untreated samples (●). Horizontal lines indicate baseline toxicity in treated samples (– – –) and untreated samples (—). Duplicate determinations were performed in each of seven normal controls and the three patients. (From Spielberg *et al.* 1981.)

Different substrates are required to demonstrate epoxide hydrolase activity in the two locations. The microsomal enzyme is inducible by phenobarbital. Purification procedures have revealed multiple molecular forms of the enzyme. Simple spectrophotometric assays are now available for the liver cytosolic epoxide hydrolase (Wixtrom & Hammock 1988), and both membrane-bound and soluble activities can be assayed in human white blood cells using radioactive *cis-* and *trans*-stilbene oxides respectively as substrates (Seidegård *et al.* 1984). Where molecular weights have been determined they were in the range 50 000 to 58 000 Da. The cDNA for human microsomal epoxide hydrolase has been sequenced and the enzyme expressed in COS-1 cells (Skoda *et al.* 1988). The elucidation of the genetic organization of the multiple forms, and their variants, seems likely to prove important in understanding the variability in drug-produced clinical phenomena.

INTER-ETHNIC VARIABILITY IN PHENYTOIN METABOLISM

This topic was reviewed by Huidgberg (1986). He points out the difficulties in making inter-ethnic comparisons of drug metabolism. Essentially these difficulties are due to the near impossibility of completely dissociating genetic from environmental influences. In many studies the ethnic groups have differed in location, diet, weight, etc. the influence of which are difficult to assess. Different studies have employed varying methodologies and computed different metabolic parameters. Nevertheless, Huidberg (1986) was able to compile a table of seven studies which compared ethnic groups with respect to DPH half-life, total body clearance, HPPH excretion, plasma steady-state concentration and K_m.

The evidence is convincing that Eskimos have a more powerful metabolism of DPH than Caucasians as indicated by higher total clearance, greater HPPH excretion and lower steady-state plasma concentration on repeated dosing.

The studies on Africans give a confused picture.

Japanese have been reported to have a lower K_m than Caucasians, and a similar result was obtained in Chinese by Chan *et al.* (1990) though they also emphasize that there was greater inter-individual variability in the population that they studied.

The subject is one which invites *in vitro* enzymol-

ogic assessment, and eventually a molecular biological approach to the relevant cytochrome P450 enzyme.

Andreasen, P. B., Frøland, A., Skovsted, L., Andersen, S. A. & Hauge, M. (1973). Diphenylhydantoin half-life in man and its inhibition by phenylbutazone, the role of genetic factors. *Acta Medica Scandinavica*, **193**, 561–4.

Booker, H. E., Tormey, A. & Toussaint, J. (1971). Concurrent administration of phenobarbital and diphenylhydantoin: Lack of an interference effect. *Neurology*, **21**, 383–5.

Brennan, R. W., Dehejia, H., Kutt, H. & McDowell, F. (1968). Diphenylhydantoin intoxication attendant to slow inactivation of isoniazid. *Neurology*, **18**, 283.

Burns, J. J., Cucinell, S. A., Koster, R. & Conney, A. H. (1965). Application of drug metabolism to drug toxicity studies. *Annals of the New York Academy of Sciences*, **123**, 273–86.

Butler, T. C. Dudley, K. H., Johnson, D. & Roberts, S. B. (1976). Studies of the metabolism of 5,5-diphenylhydantoin relating principally to the stereoselectivity of the hydroxylation reactions in man and dog. *Journal of Pharmacology and Experimental Therapeutics*, **199**, 82–92.

Chan, E., Ti, T. Y. & Lee, H. S. (1990). Population pharmacokinetics of phenytoin in Singapore Chinese. *European Journal of Clinical Pharmacology*, **39**, 177–81.

deWolff, F. A., Vermeij, P., Ferrari, M. D., Buruma, O. J. S. & Breimer, D. D. (1983). Impairment of phenytoin parahydroxylation as a cause of severe intoxication. *Therapeutic Drug Monitoring*, **5**, 213–15.

Dill, W. A., Kazenko, A., Wolf, L. M. & Glazko, A. J. (1956). Studies on 5,5'diphenyl-hydantoin (Dilantin) in animals and man. *Journal of Pharmacology and Experimental Therapeutics*, **118**, 270–9.

Doecke, C. J., Sansom, L. N. & McManus, M. E. (1990). Phenytoin 4-hydroxylation by rabbit liver P450 II C3 and identification of orthologs in human liver microsomes. *Biochemical and Biophysical Research Communications*, **166**, 860–6.

Doecke, C. J., Veronese, M. E., Pond, S. M., Miners, J. O., Birkett, D. J., Sansom, L. N. & McManus, M. E. (1991). Relationship between phenytoin and tolbutamide hydroxylations in human liver microsomes. *British Journal of Clinical Pharmacology*, **31**, 125–30.

Ferrari, M. D., deWolff, F. A., Vermey, P., Veenema, H. & Buruma, O. J. S. (1986). Hepatic cytochrome P450 malfunction and Parkinson's disease. *Lancet*, **1**, 324.

Ferrari, M. D., Peeters, E. A. J., Haan, J., Roos, R. A. C., Vermey, P., deWolff, F. A. & Buruma, O. J. S. (1990). Cytochrome P450 and Parkinson's disease. Poor parahydroxylation of phenytoin. *Journal of the Neurological Sciences*, **96**, 153–7.

Fritz, S., Lindner, W. E., Roots, I., Frey, B. M. & Küpfer, A. (1987). Stereochemistry of aromatic phenytoin hydroxylation in various drug hydroxylation phenotypes in humans. *Journal of Pharmacology and Experimental Therapeutics*, **241**, 615–22.

Gerson, W. T., Fine, D. G., Spielberg, S. P. & Sensenbrenner, L. L. (1983). Anticonvulsant-induced aplastic anaemia: increased susceptibility to toxic drug metabolites *in vitro*. *Blood*, **61**, 889–93.

Glazko, A. J., Chang, T., Baukema, J., Bill, W. A., Goulet, J. R. & Buchanan, R. A. (1969). Metabolic disposition of diphenylhydantoin in normal subjects following intravenous administration. *Clinical Pharmacology Therapeutics*, **10**, 498–504.

Gugler, R., Manion, C. V. & Azarnoff, D. L. (1976). Phenytoin: pharmacokinetics and bioavailabitity. *Clinical Pharmacology and Therapeutics*, **19**, 135–42.

Hvidberg, E. F. (1986). Ethnic differences in phenytoin kinetics. In:*Ethnic differences in Reactions to Drugs and Xenobiotics*, ed. W. Kalow, H. W. Goedde & D. P. Agarwal. Progress in Clinical and Biological Research, **214**, 279–87. New York: Alan R. Liss.

Inaba, T., Jurima, M., Mahon, W. H. & Kalow, W. (1985). *In vitro* inhibition studies of two isozymes of human liver cytochrome P450. Mephenytoin p-hydroxylase and sparteine monoxygenase. *Drug Metabolism and Disposition*, **13**, 443–8.

Kadar, D., Fecycz, T. D. & Kalow, W. (1983). The fate of orally administered[14]C-phenytoin in two healthy male volunteers. *Canadian Journal of Physiology and Pharmacology*, **61**, 403–7.

Kutt, H. (1971). Biochemical and genetic factors regulating Dilantin metabolism in man. *Annals of the New York Academy of Sciences*, **179**, 704–22.

Kutt, H., Brennan, R., Hehejia, H. & McDowell, F. (1970). Diphenylhydantin intoxication: a complication of isoniazid therapy. *American Review of Respiratory Disease*, **101**, 377–84.

Kutt, H., Haynes, J. & McDowell, F. (1966). Some causes of ineffectiveness of diphenylhydantoin. *Archives of Neurology*, **14**, 489–92.

Kutt, H., Haynes, J., Verebely, K. & McDowell, F. (1969). The effect of phenobarbital on plasma diphenylhydantoin level and metabolism in man and in rat liver microsomes. *Neurology*, **19**, 611–16.

Kutt, H., Verebely, K. & McDowell, F. (1968). Inhibition of diphenylhydantoin metabolism in rats and in rat liver microsomes by anti-tubercular drugs. *Neurology*, **18**, 706–10.

Kutt, H., Winters, W. & McDowell, F. H. (1966). Depression of parahydroxylation of diphenylhydantoin by antituberculosis chemotherapy. *Neurology*, **16**, 594–602.

Kutt, H., Wolk, M., Scherman, R. & McDowell, F. (1964). Insufficient parahydroxylation as a cause of diphenylhydantoin toxicity. *Neurology*, **14**, 542–8.

Levine, M., Orr, J. & Chang, T. (1987). Inter-individual variation in the extent and rate of phenytoin accumulation. *Therapeutic Drug Monitoring*, **9**, 171–6.

Loeser, E. W., Jr (1961). Studies on the metabolism of diphenylhydantoin (Dilantin). *Neurology*, **11**, 424–9.

Lund, L., Lunde, P. K, Rane, A., Borga, O. & Sjöqvist, F. (1972). Plasma protein binding, plasma concentrations and effects of diphenylhydantoin in man. *Annals of the New York Academy of Sciences*, **179**, 723–8.

Merritt, H. & Putnam, T. J. (1938). Sodium diphenyl hydantoinate in treatment of convulsive disorders. *Journal of the American Medical Association*, **111**, 1068–73.

Schellens, J. H. M., Soons, P. A., van der Wart, J. H. F., Hoevers, J. W. & Breimer, D. D. (1991). Lack of pharmacokinetic interaction between nifedipine, sparteine and phenytoin in man. *British Journal of Clinical Pharmacology*, **31**, 175–8.

Seidegård, J. & DePierre, J. W. (1983). Microsomal epoxide hydrolase: properties regulation and function. *Biochimica et Biophysica Acta*, **695**, 251–70.

Seidegård, J., DePierre, J. W. & Pero, R. W. (1984). Measurement and characterization of membrane-bound and soluble epoxide hydrolase activities in resting mononuclear leucocytes from human blood. *Cancer Research*, **44**, 3654–60.

Skoda, R. C., Demierre, A., McBride, O. W., Gonzalez, F. J. & Meyer, U. A. (1988). Human microsomal xenobiotic epoxide hydrolase. Complementary DNA sequence, complementary DNA- directed expression in COS-1 cells and chromosomal localization. *Journal of Biological Chemistry*, **263**, 1549–54.

Sloan, T. P., Idle, J. R. & Smith, R. L. (1981). Influence of D^H/D^L alleles regulating debrisoquine oxidation on phenytoin hydroxylation. *Clinical Pharmacology and Therapeutics*, **29**, 493–7.

Spielberg, S. P. (1984). *In vitro* assessment of pharmacogenetic susceptibility to toxic drug metabolites in humans. *Federation Proceedings*, **43**, 2308–13.

Spielberg, S. P., Gordon, G. B., Blake, D. A., Goldstein, D. A. & Herlong, H. F. (1981). Predisposition to phenytoin hepatotoxicity assessed *in vitro*. *New England Journal of Medicine*, **305**, 722–7.

Steiner, E., Alvan, G., Garle, M., Maguire, J. H., Lind, M., Nilson, S. O., Tomson, T., McClanahan, J. S. & Sjöqvist, F. (1987). The debrisoquine hydroxylation phenotype does not predict the metabolism of phenytoin. *Clinical Pharmacology and Therapeutics*, **42**, 326–33.

Strickler, S. M., Miller, M. A., Andermann, E., Dansky, L. V., Seni, M. H. & Spielberg, S. P. (1985). Genetic predisposition to phenytoin-induced birth defects. *Lancet*, **2**, 746–9.

Thomas, H. & Oesch, F. (1988). Functions of epoxide hydrolases. *ISI Atlas of Science: Biochemistry*, 287–91.

Vasko, M. R., Bell, R. D., Daly, D. D. & Pippenger, C. E. (1980). Inheritance of phenytoin hypometabolism: a kinetic study of one family. *Clinical Pharmacology and Therapeutics*, **27**, 96–103.

Vermeij, P., Ferrari, M. D., Buruma, J. S., Veenema, H. & deWolff, F.A. (1988). Inheritance of poor phenytoin parahydroxylation capacity in a Dutch family. *Clinical Pharmacology and Therapeutics*, **44**, 588–93.

Veronese, M. E., Mackenzie, P. I., Doecke, C. J., McManus, M. E., Miners, J. O. & Birkett, D. J. (1991). Tolbutamide and phenytoin hydroxylations by cDNA-expressed human liver cytochrome P450 2C9. *Biochemical and Biophysical Research Communications*, **175**, 1112–18.

Wixtrom, R. N. & Hammock, B. D. (1988). Continuous spectrophotometric assays for cytosolic epoxide hydrolase. *Analytical Biochemistry*, **174**, 291–9.

11 Some other drugs of special interest

WARFARIN

THE ASSESSMENT of enzyme induction and enzyme inhibition by therapeutic drugs in clinical practice is a matter of great interest and in some instances of practical importance. Amongst a number of indicator drugs discussed by Park & Kitteringham (1990) is racemic warfarin, both R and S forms of which are extensively biotransformed to both oxidised and reduced metabolites. Clinically important drug interactions have been reported with the inducers rifampicin, phenytoin and phenobarbitone, and a stereoselective inhibition of the metabolism of the R form by cimetidine.

It is of considerable interest that Rettie *et al.* (1992) have shown that three cytochromes P450, i.e. 1A2, 2C9 and 3A4, catalyse highly stereoselective and regioselective oxidations of warfarin. Form 1A2 produces (R)-6-hydroxy, and 3A4 produces (R)-10-hydroxy whereas 2C9 produces (S)-7-hydroxy and (S)-6-hydroxy warfarin in the ratio of about 3.5 to 1. Since (S)-warfarin is the most biologically active enantiomer P450 2C9 mediates the most important biotransformation of this drug.

METRONIDAZOLE

The widely used antimicrobial metronidazole is extensively biotransformed by hydroxylation of its methyl group. This compound is potentially of considerable pharmacogenetic interest because the occasional patient reports the production of dark coloured urine following the ingestion of just a single tablet, in the absence of any other symptom or sign (Rollo *et al.* 1975).

This event could indicate the existence of a phenotype in which an unusual biotransformation occurs. In an investigation of the kinetics of metronidazole metabolism by microsomes prepared from the livers of kidney transplant donors, Loft *et al.* (1991) studied the inhibitory effects of selected substrates and inhibitors of specific cytochromes P450. These were: caffeine, theophylline, phenacetin and α-naphthoflavone (P450 1A2), mephenytoin (P450 2C8/9/10), tolbutamide (P450 2C10), quinidine (P450 2D6), acetone (P450 2E1) and nifedipine (P450 3A3 according to the authors, but P450 3A4/5 in this account). None of these compounds caused significant inhibition of metronidazole metabolism.

In addition, (1) microsomes from the liver of a poor metabolizer of debrisoquine metabolized metronidazole the same as those from other livers, (2) metronidazole hydroxylation *in vivo* was not inhibited by cimetidine and only very weakly by phenacetin, and it was not induced by smoking, (3) metronidazole did not inhibit phenacetin deethylation *in vitro* and did not affect the clearance of co-administered theophylline *in vivo*, (4) metronidazole clearance was increased by pretreatment with phenobarbitone, but inhibited by propanolol.

The biphasic *in vitro* kinetics indicate that metronidazole is hydroxylated by two types of P450 cytochromes. It would be of considerable interest to know which they are.

PHENACETIN

A genetic deficiency in the *O*-deethylation of phenacetin was described by Shahidi (1968). This was clinically significant since it led to methaemoglobinaemia in the affected individuals after they had taken the drug. After the debrisoquine/sparteine polymorphism was discovered Sloan *et al.* (1978) showed that poor metabolizers had an impairment of phenacetin *O*-deethylation.

The subject was reinvestigated by Kahn *et al.* (1985) who made both *in vivo* and *in vitro* observations. An impairment of phenacetin deethylation was confirmed *in vivo* in poor metabolizers of debrisoquine. *O*-deethylation of phenacetin was observed to be a biphasic process deduced to be mediated by two components, namely, high affinity–low capacity and low affinity–high capacity. There was a correlation ($r = 0.84$) between the high affinity component of phenacetin *O*-deethylation and debrisoquine 4-hydroxylase activity (P450 2D6). There was no such correlation for the low-affinity component. Debrisoquine was a competitor of the high-affinity component but phenacetin did not inhibit debrisoquine 4-hydroxylation. The conclusion was that the high affinity component of phenacetin *O*-deethylase and debrisoquine 4-hydroxylase activities are catalysed by different isozymes of cytochrome P450 but that they are most probably regulated by closely linked genes.

More recently the high affinity phase of phenacetin *O*-deethylation was found to be catalysed by 'P450$_{PA}$' which was purified by Distlerath *et al.* (1985). Studies of orthologs in animals have been used to develop probes for the human gene which is a *CYP 1A2* (see page 29 and Table 5.6). This is related to *CYP 1A1* and the *CYP 1* cluster is localized at 15q22–qter (Guengerich 1989). The delineation of the precise change responsible for the genetic variation as described by Shahidi (1968) remains to be elucidated.

Distlerath, L. M, Reilly, P. E. B., Martin, M. V., Davis, G. G., Wilkinson, G. R. & Guengerich, F. P. (1985). Purification and characterization of the human liver cytochromes P450 involved in debrisoquine 4-hydroxylation and phenacetin O-deethylation, two prototypes for genetic polymorphism in oxidative drug metabolism. *Journal of Biological Chemistry*, **260**, 9057–67.

Guengerich, F. P. (1989). Characterization of human microsomal P-450 enzymes. *Annual Review of Pharmacology and Toxicology*, **29**, 241–64.

Kahn, G. C., Boobis, A. R., Brodie, M. J., Toverud, E. L., Murray, S. & Davies, D. S. (1985). Phenacetin O-deethylase: an activity of a cytochrome P-450 showing genetic linkage with that catalysing the 4-hydroxylation of debrisoquine? *British Journal of Clinical Pharmacology*, **20**, 67–76.

Loft, S., Otton, S. V., Lennard, M. S., Tucker, G. T. & Pulsen, H. E. (1991). Characterisation of metronidazole metabolism by human liver microsomes. *Biochemical Pharmacology*, **41**, 1127–34.

Park, B. K. & Kitteringham, N. R. (1990). Assessment of enzyme induction and enzyme inhibition in humans: toxicological implications. *Xenobiotica*, **20**, 1171–85.

Rettie, A. E., Korzekwa, K. R., Kunze, K. L., Lawrence, R. F., Eddy, A. C., Aoyama, T., Gelboin, H. V., Gonzalez, F. J. & Trager, W. F. (1992). Hydroxylation of warfarin by human cDNA- expressed cytochrome P-450: a role for P-450 2C9 in the etiology of (S)-warfarin-drug interactions. *Chemistry Research and Toxicology*, **5**, 54–9.

Rollo, I. M. (1975). Drugs used in the chemotherapy of amebiasis. In *The Pharmacological Basis of Therapeutics*, 5th edition, ed. L. S. Goodman & A. Gilman, p. 1087. New York: Macmillan.

Shahidi, N. T. (1968). Acetophenetidin-induced methemoglobinemia. *Annals of the New York Academy of Sciences*, **151**, 822–32.

Sloan, T. P., Mahgoub, A., Lancaster, R., Idle, J. R. & Smith, R. L. (1978). Polymorphism of carbon oxidation of drugs and clinical implications. *British Medical Journal*, **2**, 655–7.

12   Cytochrome P450 reductase

AS was explained in the introductory section on cytochromes P450 these enzymes are at the end of an electron-transport chain. An important intermediary between NADPH and P450 is the enzyme cytochrome P450 reductase, one molecule of which is thought to service between 10 and 100 molecules of cytochrome P450 (Nebert & Gonzalez 1987).

Shephard *et al.* (1989) have isolated and sequenced cDNA clones that code for rat and human NADPH-dependent cytochrome P450 reductase. In 15 human livers there was less than 3-fold variation in the amount of the corresponding mRNA.

By studying human–rodent somatic cell hybrids with a radiolabelled 1.9 kb cytochrome P450 reductase cDNA insert the human gene was localized to the region 7q11.2.

Nebert, D. W. & Gonzalez, F. J. (1987). P450 genes: structure, evolution and regulation. *Annual Review of Biochemistry*, **56**, 945–93.

Shephard, E. A., Phillips, I. R., Santisteban, I., West, L. F., Palmer, C. N. A., Ashworth, A. & Povey, S. (1989). Isolation of a human cytochrome P450 reductase cDNA clone and localization of the corresponding gene to chromosome 7q11.2. *Annals of Human Genetics (London)*, **52**, 291–301.

13   General conclusions

AN OVERVIEW has been given in the preceding sections of the present status of knowledge regarding cytochrome P450 enzymes in pharmacogenetics. It appears that the clear cut genetic polymorphisms of debrisoquine/sparteine and mephenytoin may be exceptions. Nevertheless, it is a truism that exceptional cases frequently demonstrate widely applicable principles. There is a possibility that there exists substantial genetic variability in other pharmacologically important cytochromes P450. At present it is not possible to say how important from a clinical point of view such a variability might be.

The approach to genetic variability in pharmacology is now making an about-turn. Previously, the idea was to delineate phenotypic differences, then attempt to identify the genotypes and from them work towards the DNA. Now, information is being acquired more quickly about candidate genes themselves than on the phenotypic aspects. Techniques such as the polymerase chain reaction (see Belyavsky *et al.* 1989; Peake 1989; Vosberg 1989) as well as the other standard techniques of molecular genetics hold great promise. If the appropriate genes could be studied in the DNA extracted from the leucocytes of a blood specimen or from the cells present in a specimen of saliva, then even more rapid progress could be made in population and inter-ethnic surveys.

However, from a clinical point of view the doctor is dealing with the phenotype. So, to know about the structure of the DNA by itself is valueless. It is necessary to understand how variations in DNA structure influence the metabolism of drugs and the responses to drugs in the population. This will mean knowing about the structure and function of the relevant cytochromes P450. Even with knowledge of the genes it will still be necessary to perform *in vivo* experiments but it is possible that they may be structured more economically.

With regard to new drugs it may be possible to use *in vitro* observations to predict *in vivo* results. For example, an array of tissue culture cells, bacteria or yeasts each bearing a specific P450 activity could be used to assess the metabolism of a novel compound. In fact, cell lines containing individual human cytochromes P450 are now available for purchase from the Gentest Corporation, Woburn, MA (Gonzalez 1992). This idea has considerable similarity to the API system (Analytab Products, Plainview NY) used to identify bacteria where a number of binary pieces of information (+ or −) give a profile number which gives a percentage probability of recognition. Then from the biotransformation observed a specific hypothesis could be tested by experiments on whole human beings. There is a possibility that proceeding in this way might make superfluous a lot of the present expensive and time-consuming animal experimentation in new drug development.

The same *in vitro* technology is also applicable to the closely allied field of the study of mechanisms of carcinogenesis.

Belyavsky, A., Vinogradova, T. & Rajewsky, K. (1989). PCR based cDNA library construction: general cDNA libraries at the level of a few cells. *Nucleic Acids Research*, **17**, 2919–32.

Gonzalez, F. J. (1992). *In vitro* systems for prediction of rates of drug clearance and drug interactions. *Journal of Anesthesiology*, **7**, 413–15.

Peake, I. (1989). The polymerase chain reaction. *Journal of Clinical Pathology*, **42**, 673–6.

Vosberg, H. P. (1989). The polymerase chain reaction: an improved method for the analysis of nucleic acids. *Human Genetics*, **83**, 1–15.

PART III Cholinesterase

14 Cholinesterase

INTRODUCTION

THIS chapter is concerned with genetic variants of human cholinesterase. These genetic variants have importance in therapeutics because they influence the speed of hydrolysis of the muscle relaxant drug succinyldicholine (syn succinylcholine, suxamethonium). The now obsolete term pseudocholinesterase was coined by Mendel *et al.* (1943) to distinguish this plasma enzyme (EC 3.1.1.8) from the 'true' red cell cholinesterase now called acetylcholinesterase (EC 3.1.1.7) which hydrolyses acetylcholine.

MECHANISM OF ACTION OF SUCCINYLCHOLINE

In order to understand the clinical significance of the genetic variants of cholinesterase it is necessary first to describe briefly how succinylcholine works. This drug is a depolarizing neuromuscular blocking agent, and the normal dose for endotracheal intubation is 1 mg per kg body weight. When this dose is injected intravenously it is rapidly distributed throughout the total extracellular space, but up to 80% is rapidly hydrolysed by the plasma enzyme cholinesterase and so only a fraction of the dose administered actually reaches the neuromuscular end plates. Succinyldicholine is hydrolysed solely by cholinesterase to succinylmonocholine which has only 2 to 5% of the neuromuscular blocking activity of the original compound. Succinylmonocholine is

also hydrolysed by cholinesterase but possibly also by other enzymes.

At the neuromuscular end plate succinylcholine binds to a receptor which causes the nerve end plate to be depolarized with a loss of sensitivity to the natural transmitter acetylcholine.

Having reached the neuromuscular end plate the succinylcholine then diffuses back into the blood where it is hydrolysed, and it is this process which brings about the end of the neuromuscular blockade.

The duration of the neuromuscular blockade is thus determined by the (1) amount of succinyldicholine at the end plate, (2) binding of the drug to the receptor, (3) rate of diffusion back into the plasma, (4) hydrolysis in the plasma of this backdiffused succinylcholine and (5) muscle blood flow.

Genetic variants of plasma cholinesterase which have different activities to the usual enzyme obviously influence how much succinylcholine gets to the neuromuscular end plate in the first instance (i.e. (1) above) and also (4) above, and so determine the duration of paralysis.

ASSESSMENT OF THE DEGREE OF NEUROMUSCULAR BLOCK

During anaesthesia the degree of neuromuscular blockade can be assessed by clinical criteria such as muscular tone and movement. These signs are however influenced by other factors such as the anaesthetic employed and the ventilation.

137

An objective assessment of neuromuscular blockade can be provided by using indirect nerve stimulation (Viby Mogensen 1983). Three techniques are commonly employed: single twitch, tetanic and 'train of four' stimulation. The last consists of a series of four supramaximal 2 Hz single stimuli applied to the nerve every 12 seconds (Ritter *et al.* 1988). The 'train of four' stimulation has more appeal than the other two techniques because it is less painful in the recovery phase, gives a continuous recording of the blockade and differentiates between different types of block. The necessary apparatus is commonly available in operating rooms.

Very quickly after the intravenous injection of a single dose of 1 mg succinylcholine per kg body weight a depolarizing neuromuscular block occurs. There is at first no mechanical response to 'train of four' stimulation. Then after a few minutes (5.6 $\pm$ SD 1.05 minutes according to Viby Mogensen 1983) twitches return and gradually build up to a normal pattern in which the heights of all the four twitches in each group are the same.

Prolonged or repeated administration of the drug, however, converts this depolarizing block into a non-depolarizing block. Here 'fade' is exhibited within each group of four twitches in that the fourth is only a fraction of the height of the first. There is a great deal of inter-individual variability in the appearance of this phenomenon which depends on the dose of succinylcholine and the type of anaesthetic employed, being facilitated by halothane and enflurane.

The matter has practical importance because of the following consideration. Neostigmine can be used to overcome the non-depolarizing block because its effect is on the neuromuscular end plate. On the other hand neostigmine given before succinylcholine inhibits cholinesterase and impedes recovery (Bevan & Donati 1983).

EARLY DISCOVERIES – MULTIPLE ALLELES

Soon after succinylcholine (suxamethonium) was introduced, in 1951, into clinical practice as a short-term muscle relaxant occasional patients were found who suffered from prolonged apnoea due to their failure to recover muscle contractility. Plasma cholinesterase was known to terminate the action

of this ester drug by hydrolysis (Lehmann & Liddell 1961) (Fig. 14.1). Therefore the activity of this enzyme in plasma was measured and was found to be low in persons who had suffered from prolonged apnoea. In some patients it was apparent that the low enzymic activity was due to the existence of pregnancy or a pathological process, e.g. liver disease, poisoning by organophosphorus compounds, malnutrition, severe anaemia, hyperpyrexia, infectious disorders, cardiac failure, uraemia, catatonia and malignancy (Lehmann & Liddell 1961).

However, in many individuals there appeared to be no such pathological process and so the possibility was considered that the low plasma cholinesterase activity was an inherited characteristic. Family studies of individuals who had suffered from prolonged apnoea and who had no concurrent pathology disclosed healthy relatives who also had low plasma cholinesterase activities (Lehmann & Ryan, 1956).

The most important single step in putting the pharmacogenetics of plasma cholinesterase on a firm scientific basis was taken by Professor Werner Kalow who has published a historical account of his early work (Kalow 1990). The essential step was to augment the measurement of enzyme activity (Kalow *et al.* 1956) with the study of the effect of an enzyme inhibitor. The effect of dibucaine (Fig. 14.1) on the hydrolysis of benzoylcholine as measured spectrophotometrically provided a quick simple accurate and standard test. The percentage inhibition of enzymic activity was termed the 'dibucaine number' (DN) (Kalow & Genest 1957) (see Fig. 14.2). The 'usual' serum enzyme gave a DN of about 80 and the 'atypical' serum enzyme gave a DN of about 20 under the influence of 10^{-5} M dibucaine (i.e. the 'atypical' variant was dibucaine resistant).

Using this DN assay Kalow & Staron (1957) surveyed a population of 1556 labourers, students and patients. They found two very low values (12 and 19), 59 intermediate values (between 43 and 70) and the remainder above 70, thus constituting three distinct and separate modes. The esterase activity levels in these same sera gave a unimodal distribution, the persons with DN values below 70 lay nearer to the bottom end of the activity distribution but did not form a separate mode. The same workers made the same observations on sera from 135 members of seven unrelated families ascertained by

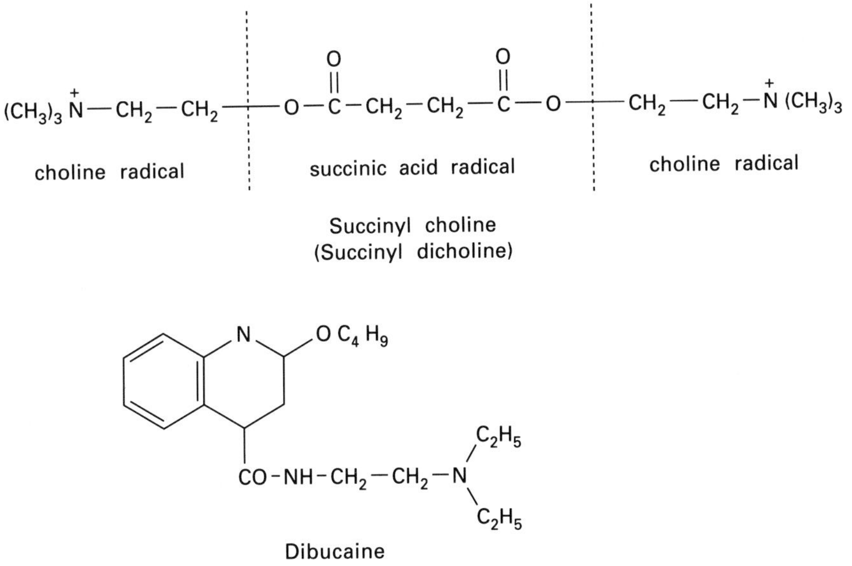

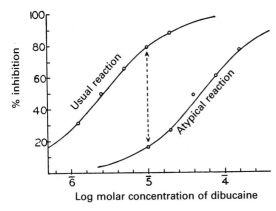

The structural formula showing:

$(CH_3)_3 \overset{+}{N}-CH_2-CH_2$ — choline radical

$O-\overset{O}{\overset{||}{C}}-CH_2-CH_2-\overset{O}{\overset{||}{C}}-O$ — succinic acid radical

$CH_2-CH_2-\overset{+}{N}(CH_3)_3$ — choline radical

Succinyl choline
(Succinyl dicholine)

Dibucaine

Fig. 14.1. The structural formulae of succinylcholine and dibucaine.

Fig. 14.2. Inhibition of cholinesterase activity in two different human sera. Cholinesterase activity was measured by ultraviolet spectrophotometry with 5×10^{-5} M benzoylcholine as substrate. The standard error of each experimental point shown in this graph is about ±2%. The dashed line indicates the region in which the results may fall if the inhibition by a standard concentration of 10^{-5} M of dibucaine is routinely tested on numerous sera. Percentage inhibition observed under these circumstances has been termed 'dibucaine number'. Inhibitions as grossly different from the usual as seen in the right-hand curve are very rare. (From Kalow & Genest 1957.)

means of probands with intermediate or low DN values (Fig. 14.3). The conclusion was that most observations in the inheritance of DN could be explained by the existence of two autosomal allelic genes, without dominance, each gene causing the formation of one of the two types of enzyme. In this classic paper some observations were made which required additional concepts for explanation, the principal one being the variation from person to person within the group with high DN values. Two possibilities were considered: (1) the existence of different types of normal alleles and (2) the existence of alleles modifying the expression of one type of normal allele. It was noted that these hypotheses were not mutually exclusive. The atypical phenotype was estimated to have a population frequency of about 1 in 2000 to 4000 persons. Another inhibitor, RO2-0683 [dimethylcarbamate of (2-hydroxy-5-phenylbenzyl) trimethyl ammonium bromide], was introduced by Liddell *et al.* (1963) and is able to recognize the same phenotypes.

The presence of two different enzyme molecules (and not a single hybrid type of molecule) in the serum of atypical heterozygotes was demonstrated by Liddell *et al.* (1962b), who used diethyl aminoethyl cellulose (DEAE) column chromatography. The same result was obtained when a mixture of sera from the two different homozygotes was applied to the column, whereas serum from one homozygote produced only one enzyme fraction.

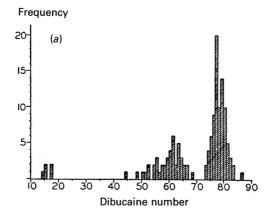

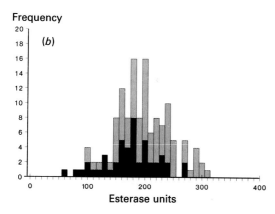

Fig. 14.3.(*a*), Frequency distribution of DNs among 135 members of seven unrelated families. (*b*), Frequency distribution of esterase levels among members of seven unrelated families. Determinations from essentially the same sera as the data shown in (*a*). The black columns show the esterase levels of sera with DN below 70. (From Kalow & Staron 1957.)

The next thrust forward in genetic analysis was made by Harris & Whittaker (1962a), who screened randomly selected adults known to have children available for study. The populations studied were from the United Kingdom, Sardinia and Northern Italy. Twenty-two individuals with the intermediate phenotype were available for study together with plasma from 19 spouses and 78 children. The samples were studied with two inhibitors, dibucaine, and fluoride at 5×10^{-5} M which these authors had earlier found to inhibit cholinesterase; the substrate was benzoylcholine at 5×10^{-5} M.

When the fluoride numbers (FN) were plotted against the dibucaine numbers a new finding emerged. Amongst individuals classified by the dibucaine method as belonging to the usual phenotype (DN 73 to 83) there appeared to be a subgroup of five individuals with dibucaine and fluoride numbers (DN 73 to 78; FN 50 to 55) lower than the remainder of the usual phenotype. Furthermore two individuals with values DN 54 and FN 33 and 34 seemed to form a subgroup of the 'intermediate' phenotype with numbers lower than the remainder of that phenotype (Fig. 14.4). Pedigree analysis showed that the 10 offspring of the latter two individuals (each of which was married to a spouse with the 'usual' phenotype: DN 78 to 82; FN 57 to 68) consisted of an equal number of children in the main group of intermediates, and in the new subgroup of intermediates. Though the suspicion was strong that these data indicated the presence of a third allele the numbers were too small to prove this hypothesis.

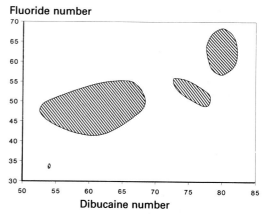

Fig. 14.4. Distributions of dibucaine and fluoride numbers in the 119 individuals studied. (From Harris & Whittaker 1962a.)

Lehmann *et al.* (1963) described a proband (detected because he had succinylcholine apnoea) and his sibling who had results DN 67 FN 34 and DN 64 FN 35 respectively which strongly suggested they were homozygous for the 'fluoride' allele. A similar family with another 'fluoride' homozygote was described by Whittaker (1964). Liddell *et al.* (1963) presented further family data indicating that the fluoride gene was allelic with the 'usual' and 'atypical' genes.

The following nomenclature was established:- E_1 for the first genetic locus identified which controlled the cholinesterase, with different superscripts, i.e. E_1^u for usual, E_1^a for atypical and E_1^f for fluoride alleles.

Meantime, Liddell et al. (1962a) had investigated some families that presented anomalous features. The anomalies arose from the fact that individuals were typed by DN as atypical homozygotes when they should, from their pedigrees, have been heterozygotes. The suggestion was therefore made that there existed a 'silent' allele. This idea was shown to be justified when a Greek woman aged 42 years had prolonged apnoea following succinylcholine administration. There was no pathological explanation, and her plasma turned out to be totally devoid of any cholinesterase activity. Two children and two siblings of this proposita had subnormal plasma cholinesterase activities and were presumably heterozygous for the silent allele, but had normal DN and FN values. The serum of the proposita had no inhibitory effect on the DN values of the sera of normal and atypical homozygotes when it was mixed with them *in vitro*. After reviewing the pedigree data available Simpson & Kalow (1964) concluded that the 'silent' gene was allelic with the 'usual' and 'atypical' genes, discounting the alternative suggestion that the 'silent' gene was a suppressor.

NEW ALLELES

New alleles controlling quantitative (rather than qualitative) properties were discovered by the study of the activities of plasma cholinesterase in families possessing E_1^a in addition to E_1^u.

The allele termed E_1^j (so designated after the name of the family) was discovered by Garry et al. (1976). This family was exceptional in the first place because it contained the three alleles E_1^u, E_1^a and E_1^f. Individuals with unexpectedly low activities were discovered in addition to the expected heterozygotes $E_1^u E_1^a$, $E_1^u E_1^f$ and $E_1^a E_1^f$. On examination of the pedigree their near relatives had lower activities than would be expected from $E_1^u E_1^u$ or $E_1^u E_1^f$. So the deduction was made that a fourth allele was present in this pedigree, which caused a reduction in the number of E_1^u controlled molecules by about 66%. The $E_1^u E_1^j$ genotype cannot be recognized with certainty.

Reduced numbers of immunologically active cholinesterase molecules were demonstrated in the

plasma of persons of the $E_1^a E_1^j$ genotype by immunodiffusion and rocket immunoelectrophoresis (Rubinstein et al., 1976). It was unclear whether the low number of molecules was due to a lower rate of synthesis than normal, or to an increased rate of degradation.

The same group (Rubinstein et al., 1978) described another two families segregating for E_1^a where again some individuals gave activities lower than would be expected from $E_1^u E_1^a$. These were considered to represent a new genotype $E_1^a E_1^k$ (naming the new allele after Professor Werner Kalow). The E_1^k allele was shown immunologically to reduce the number of E_1^u controlled molecules by about 33% and also gave lower dibucaine numbers (Figs. 14.5 and 14.6).

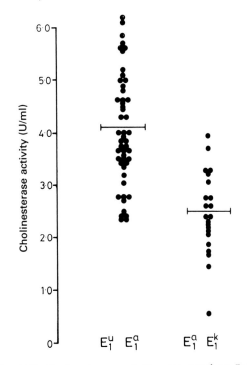

Fig. 14.5. Cholinesterase activities measured on $E_1^u E_1^a$ and $E_1^a E_1^k$ heterozygotes. (From Evans & Wardell 1984.)

Later Evans et al. (1980) described a family in which both E_1^j and E_1^k alleles could be recognized in the presence of E_1^u and E_1^a.

A further allele was identified by Whittaker & Britten (1987). Two young adults who had experienced suxamethonium sensitivity were found to

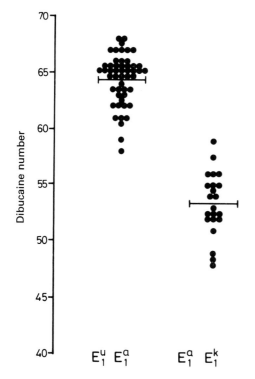

Fig. 14.6. Dibucaine numbers measured on $E_1^u E_1^a$ and $E_1^a E_1^k$ heterozygotes. (From Evans & Wardell 1984.)

have unusual RO2 numbers although the dibucaine and fluoride numbers were suggestive of an $E_1^a E_1^a$ phenotype. There was no suggestion that this finding was due to an environmental factor such as a drug, and family screening of both individuals suggested that a newly identified allele E_1^h (h for Hammersmith) was segregating with the E_1^a gene.

HETEROGENEITY OF THE 'SILENT' PHENOTYPE

Examination of two sera of the 'silent' type by Goedde et al. (1965a) revealed that there was present a protein which was bound by anti-cholinesterase antibody and also had a low level of enzymic activity (about 2 to 3% of normal). It was previously known that electrophoresis on starch gel of human serum produced four bands, termed C_1 to C_4, this being the order in which they migrated towards the anode of pH 8.6. This variety of the enzyme could be stained after starch gel electro-

phoresis in the C_4 zone only, and was inhibited by the same compounds as the 'usual' enzyme, i.e. physostigmine, acetylcholine iodide, decamethonium bromide and the neostigmine derivative RO2-0683. These observations indicated the likelihood that there was a qualitative change in the enzyme molecule (Goedde et al. 1965b).

A different result was obtained by Hodgkin et al. (1965). They found no detectable cholinesterase activity in their two index cases (who were also of Northern European extraction), and could find no immunoprecipitation with anti-cholinesterase antibody by the Ouchterlony and immunoelectrophoresis techniques. Mixing 'silent' and 'usual' sera indicated the absence of blocking activity. They could find no stainable enzyme after starch gel electrophoresis.

The issue was pursued as more individuals of the 'silent' type were discovered and Altland & Goedde (1970) were able to examine sera from 14 such persons. Heterogeneity was displayed on disc electrophoresis where nine different patterns were shown amongst 11 unrelated individuals after esterase staining. Some showed 2 to 3% of normal activity. Two sera gave a precipitate identical to the normal enzyme in the Ouchterlony test. However, all the 'silent' sera absorbed antibodies against purified human cholinesterase in a range similar to that found with normal sera. Presumably these two immunological techniques tested different antigenic activities since the latter could be separated by gel filtration of sera on Sephadex G-200.

These results indicated that a whole series of different molecular variations were capable of producing the same phenotypic character, namely a lack of enzyme activity.

A similar experience was documented by Rubinstein et al. (1970), who described patients of the silent phenotype with trace enzymic activity in Eskimos. This experience was amplified by Scott (1973) who found 11 Eskimo families in each of which there was more than one child with deficiency of cholinesterase. Some individuals were completely deficient and others had trace activity. Combining both types gave a prevalence of deficiency of about 1.2% in about 4000 Eskimo people.

Two patients with deficiency who on multiple criteria did not fit into either of these two classes were described by Lubin et al. (1973).

The subject was recently re-examined by Whittaker *et al.* (1990). They performed rocket electrophoresis, incorporating a rabbit polyclonal anti-human cholinesterase into the agarose gel, and also ELISA estimates using four different monoclonal anti-human cholinesterase antibodies. The activity of each of the 29 apparently silent gene homozygotes was assayed using butyrylthiocholine and benzoylcholine. Very considerable heterogeneity was revealed by the results. One group had no binding and very low activity; it was suggested that this was $E_1^s E_1^s$. Another group had very considerable binding properties and a low level of activity; it was suggested that this group might represent a new genotype $E_1^x E_1^x$.

The matter was carried a step further by Whittaker *et al.* (1991a) using similar techniques but in addition estimating the dibucaine number (DN) and fluoride number (FN) in family studies. The apparently silent individuals in the seven families varied. An individual with no activity and no binding was identified as $E_1^s E_1^s$. Five individuals with trace activity (or no activity) with a low level of binding were $E_1^s E_1^x$. Seven individuals with no activity (or trace activity) with high binding activity were identified as $E_1^x E_1^x$. The E_1^k allele was also present in five of these pedigrees, and heterozygotes such as $E_1^k E_1^s$, $E_1^k E_1^s$, $E_1^k E_1^x$ were also identified.

Following the discovery of so many alleles, there were, as might be expected, other reports of the identification of less common heterozygotes and homozygotes. Examples of these were as follows:

$E_1^f E_1^s$	Simpson 1967
$E_1^k E_1^f$	Burgess 1988; Whittaker *et al.* 1987
$E_1^k E_1^k$	Whittaker & Britten 1990; Whittaker & Britten 1988
$E_1^k E_1^s$	Whittaker & Britten 1988; Whittaker *et al.* 1988

THE SUCCINYLCHOLINE APNOEA-PRONE PERSON OF 'NORMAL' PHENOTYPE

About a third of persons who developed prolonged apnoea after succinylcholine administration in various series were found to have a normal phenotype on testing activity, dibucaine inhibition and fluoride inhibition (Whittaker & Vickers 1970). This suggested at that time that there were unknown factors unrevealed by the tests then extant.

Various approaches have been tried to investigate

Table 14.1. *Additional substrates and inhibitors employed to delineate cholinesterase phenotypes*

Substrates	
Succinyldicholine	Agarwal *et al.*. 1976; Goedde & Agarwal 1978

Inhibitors	
n-Butyl alcohol	Whittaker 1968a
Alkyl alcohols	Whittaker 1968b
Chloride	Whittaker 1968c
Urea	Hanel & Viby Mogensen 1971
Propanolol	Whittaker *et al.* 1982
RO2-0683[a]	Whittaker & Britten 1985
Mytelase[b]	Lubin *et al.* 1973
Quinidine	Lubin *et al.* 1973
Bambuterol[c]	Tunek *et al.* 1991

[a]RO2-0683 is [dimethylcarbamate of (2-hydroxy-5-phenyl-benzyl)-trimethyl-ammonium bromide].
[b]Mytelase is ambenonium chloride or *N,N'*-[oxalylbis (iminoethylene)]bis[(2-chlorobenzyl) diethylammonium] dichloride.
[c]1-[3,5-bis(*N,N*-dimethylcarbamoyloxy)phenyl]-2-t-butylaminoethanol hydrochloride, the pro-drug of the bronchodilator terbutaline.

this puzzle and, as has been explained earlier, the discovery of E_1^k, E_1^j and E_1^h alleles has shed some light on the problem.

Other approaches which have been tried have involved the use of different substrates and inhibitors (Table 14.1).

Using succinylcholine as a substrate and dibucaine as inhibitor, Goedde & Agarwal (1978) found that of 36 prolonged apnoea persons of the 'usual' phenotype, as determined using benzoylcholine as substrate, 30 exhibited a new variant. Probably the reason that this technique has not gained popularity is the fact that it is technically more demanding than, for example, the estimation of dibucaine numbers.

When the results of using *N*-butyl alcohol as an inhibitor were plotted against conventional dibucaine numbers, new phenotypes were revealed. Similar findings emerged when chloride was used as an inhibitor. Urea, on the other hand, separated out usual and atypical phenotypes in a manner very similar to dibucaine inhibition, as did propranolol (particularly the D-isomer). Cimetidine was found to inhibit cholinesterase competitively by Hansen & Bertl (1983) but the possibility of using this property to differentiate phenotypes was not investigated.

Table 14.2. *High activity cholinesterase*

Reference	Ethnic group	Found as a result of	Manner of inheritance	Succinylcholine resistance	DN	FN
Neitlich 1966	?	Population survey (1 in 1029)	Probably autosomal dominant but X-linked dominant not ruled out	Yes, as tested with 0.1 and 0.2 mg per kg i.v.	'Normal'	'Normal'
Yoshida & Motulsky 1969	?	Same individual as described above	Probably autosomal dominant but X-linked dominant not ruled out	–	72 to 75	–
Delbruck & Henkel 1979	German (2 probands)	Succinylcholine resistance detected clinically?	Autosomal dominant	–	Normal	Normal
Warran et al. 1987	Saudi	Succinylcholine resistance detected clinically?	Autosomal dominant	Yes with therapeutic doses of 60 and 100 mg i.v.	83	62
Krause et al. 1988	South African Afrikaner	Population screening	Probably an autosomal dominant but not possible to rule out X-linked	–	83	70.2
Yamamoto et al. 1986, 1987	Japanese	Medical check-up including measurement of cholinesterase activity	Autosomal dominant	–	85	93
Ohkawa et al. (1989)	Japanese	Population survey	Autosomal dominant	–	54% (no different to normal controls)	22% (no different to normal controls)

PAGE, polyacrylamide gel electrophoresis; DFP, di-isopropyl fluorophosphate.

ELECTROPHORETICALLY DETERMINED POLYMORPHISMS

As a result of studying cholinesterase by starch gel electrophoresis, Harris et al. (1963) showed that the enzyme produced several bands, termed C_1 to C_4 because they migrated towards the anode in that order at pH 8.6. Out of 248 unrelated individuals 13 were found to have an additional component termed C_5. The mean level of total serum cholinesterase activity in C_5+ individuals was significantly higher than that found in C_5- individuals.

Family studies revealed that the C_5+ phenotype could be due to the heterozygous or homozygous state. The C_5+/C_5- system constituted a genetic polymorphism with 10% of the British population being C_5+. The electrophoretic phenotypes neither segregated with the 'usual', 'atypical' , 'fluoride' or 'silent' alleles, nor were they statistically associated with them. Hence this polymorphism appeared to be controlled at an independent genetic locus (Robson & Harris 1966). This is the reason why the nomenclature E_1^u, E_1^a, E_1^f and E_1^s was established for the 'usual', 'atypical', 'fluoride' and 'silent' alleles

Electrophoretic pattern	DFP binding	pH optimum	Heat inactivation	K_m	Electrofocussing	Rocket immunoelectrophoresis
Densely staining additional band adjacent to C_4 but slightly closer to the origin of PAGE	Three or four times more sensitive to DFP than controls					
Extra band evident on starch gel at pH 5.3 distinguishable from C_5	No significant difference between the variant and normal enzymes in their inactivation profile					
An additional band detected closer to the origin than C_1 C_2 C_3 and C_4 on PAGE	130 to 140 nmol/U cholinesterase (same as normal)	Same as normal enzyme	Inactivated 90% at 55 °C same as normal enzyme	1.4 mM for acetyl-thiocholine iodide	Homogenous fraction at pH 3.9 to 4.0 plus six bands in region pH 4.4 to 4.9 (normal pK 3.8 to 4.0)	Normal
Slow moving extra band on PAGE						
No abnormal mobility detected on starch	The activities of the usual and variant enzymes were decreased by the same percentage at each DFP concentration		Normal half-life 101 $\pm$ 3.9 minutes at 52 °C variant 147 minutes	In range of normal for benzoyl-choline		Similar amount of immunoprecipitable cholinesterase in variant and normal plasmas
Isozyme analysis using 5% PAGE showed slow migrating band in the cathodic region between C_5 and the origin. In PAGE with different properties additional band seen between C_3 and C_4		8.0 as compared to 7.5 for normal	90% at 56 °C in 30 minutes same as control	for benzoyl-choline 0.048 M same as control	Variant pK 4.2 to 4.5 whereas normal enzyme pK 3.9 to 4.2	Relative amount of cholinesterase enzyme paralleled the activities of the enzyme in the variant and control series
C_5+ present in the proband and segregating independently of the high enzymic activity phenotype in the family						

respectively, while E_2^+ was the designation for the allele governing the appearance of the extra electrophoretic band C_5.

The existence or absence of C_5 has no bearing on the clinical phenomenon of succinylcholine apnoea.

It was found by Chautard-Freire-Maia *et al.* (1991) that persons with intensely staining C_5 bands had a significantly lower mean adult weight and variance as compared with other subjects. The significance of this observation is at present unknown.

The molecular basis of the C_5 polymorphism is unknown.

Two further electrophoretic patterns of serum cholinesterase seen using paper and starch gel electrophoresis were found in African subjects by Van Ros & Druet (1966).

The first type of unusual pattern consisted of the normal C_1 to C_4 zones plus an extra zone called C_6 which migrated faster than C_5 and stained less intensively than C_4. Furthermore, in agar gel at pH 8.4, C_6 moved towards the cathode whereas the common cholinesterase components migrated towards the anode, and C_5 was not differentiated.

The second type of unusual pattern showed the

four normal zones and two unusual slow components C_{7a} and C_{7b} in addition.

The hereditary origin of these extra bands was unproven. C_6 occurred in two out of 356 Congolese and in two out of 378 Burundis. The C_{7a} plus C_{7b} pattern was found in two out of 378 Burundis and not in the Congolese. Neither pattern was found in 312 white subjects.

There do not appear to have been any further studies on these presumably genetic African variants.

HIGH ACTIVITY CHOLINESTERASE VARIANTS

A number of healthy individuals have been found whose plasma cholinesterase activity has been much greater than normal, to the extent that they form a separate mode on a frequency distribution histogram. Some have been found as a result of resistance to the muscle-relaxing action of succinylcholine during anaesthesia, whilst others have come to light as a result of screening large numbers of sera for cholinesterase activity. The latter type of exercise has revealed that the phenotype is fairly rare. These variants are quite separate from those designated E_2^+, which posses a C_5 band and which have about 30% more activity than normal and which are described in the preceding section.

The first example was in the survey of about 1700 sera investigated by Kalow & Genest (1957). This individual like the others discussed in this section was free of disease.

The characteristics of the different variants are summarized in Table 14.2. An individual found and described by Neitlich (1966), who was also studied with his family by Yoshida & Motulsky (1969), aroused a lot of interest. The latter authors proposed that this variant should be named (like haemoglobin and G6PD variants) after its place of origin namely Cynthiana (Kentucky), but this practice did not become established for the other variants.

There are two key questions to which answers have been sought: (1) are the high activity variants detected in different parts of the world the same? (2) are these variants different in their structure to the normal enzyme, or are larger numbers of normal enzyme molecules being produced per unit time? There is some difficulty about answering the first question because different groups have used differ-

ent techniques. Nevertheless it seems the variant of Krause *et al.* (1988) was different from the others because it possessed normal electrophoretic activity, and the di-isopropyl fluorophosphate (DFP) and immunoprecipitation results did not suggest the presence of increased concentrations of cholinesterase protein but rather increased activity per active site, unlike E Cynthiana and the variant of Delbruck & Henkel (1979). The consensus view is that the high activity variants are likely to have structures different from normal.

High activity can also occur in disease states and the following list was given by Lehmann & Liddell (1961): obesity, nodular goitre, nephrosis, psoriasis and alcoholism.

GENETIC LINKAGE AND CHROMOSOMAL LOCALIZATION

Linkage between CHE1 (the locus controlling the dibucaine-resistant variant, fluoride-resistant variant, etc.) and transferrin (TF) had been suspected since the 1960s and was confirmed by Sparkes *et al.* (1984). The suspicion that this synteny might be on chromosome 1 was, however, not substantiated. Later, Kidd & Gusella (1985) showed that these loci were on chromosome 3q, a finding confirmed by Zelinksi *et al.* (1987), who also suggested that the alpha-2HS glycoprotein (AHSG) locus was separated from the CHE1 locus by the transferrin locus.

In situ hybridization experiments were carried out by Soreq *et al.* (1987), using a radioactively labelled cloned human cDNA for cholinesterase as a probe. The clone was localized at 3q21 → 26 and 16p11–16q23. The finding of two sites for hybridization suggests that there are two loci coding for human cholinesterase. More refined experiments of the same type by Zakut *et al.* (1989) revealed that there were three loci (termed CHEL 'cholinesterase-like') controlling cholinesterase, at 3q21 (CHEL1), 3q26 → ter (CHEL2) and 16q24 (CHEL3) in chromosomal preparations prepared from chorionic villi. In view of the preceding linkage studies it was felt that CHEL2 was the site most likely to carry the functional gene coding for cholinesterase.

An assimilation of all available linkage data by Marazita *et al.* (1989) indicated that 16q22 was the most likely location for CHEL2 (i.e. the genes controlling the C_5+/C_5- polymorphism (note that some confusion is created by the nomenclature of Zakut *et al.* (1989) referred to above). This conclusion matches well the information obtained from the hybridization experiments using cDNA probes.

A different result was however obtained by Eiberg *et al.* (1989) as a result of a very extensive linkage study involving 832 normal families from the Copenhagen area tested for the C_5+ polymorphism and 100 other polymorphic systems. Linkage was found between the C_5+/C_5- system and the γ-crystallin gene cluster (CRYG) at 2q33–Q35. The two loci on chromosome 16 which were examined, namely phosphoglycolate phosphatase (PGP) at 16p13–p12 and haptoglobin (HP) at 16q22, were excluded from linkage.

A further difficulty arises from the molecular genetic studies on cholinesterase which will be discussed below. The essential points are that the complete amino acid sequence of the catalytic subunit of human plasma cholinesterase was determined chemically; then using oligonucleotide probes and overlapping cDNA clones from various sources allowed complete amino acid sequence to be deduced. The two sequences thus obtained matched perfectly, indicating that most probably a single gene controls the structure of cholinesterase (Arpagaus *et al.* 1990).

Obviously more work will be required to clarify these disparities.

TECHNIQUES FOR ASSESSING CHOLINESTERASE ACTIVITY AND PHENOTYPES INCLUDING THE USE OF AUTOMATED METHODS

After the introduction of the classical dibucaine and fluoride methods for inhibiting benzoylcholine hydrolysis, considerable ingenuity was deployed in formulating tests which were less technically demanding, less time consuming and which could be performed easily on large numbers of specimens for screening purposes. Some results are shown in Table 14.3.

Of the automated methods, that of Brock (1988) seems to be the most attractive because it uses exactly the same chemistry as the classical methods with which such a large amount of information has now been assembled, and does so on a widely available apparatus.

A useful adjunct is the computer programme described by Loughlin *et al.* (1984), which can identify the genotype of the patient from the reaction rates obtained from total and inhibited assays of activity.

A mathematical approach was applied by Turner *et al.* (1985) to results obtained using benzoylcholine and butyrylthiocholine as substrates. Inhibitors employed included dibucaine, RO2-0683, urea, succinyldicholine, sodium chloride, sodium bromide, sodium fluoride and butan-1-ol. Discriminant function analysis was then applied to the results. Using benzoylcholine as substrate the combination of tests which afforded the best discrimination was RO2-0683, urea, dibucaine, chloride and fluoride number in that order of importance. Using butyrylthiocholine as substrate the best discrimination was obtained using a function which combined a series of five tests, namely RO2-0683, fluoride (100 μM), butan-1-ol, succinylcholine and fluoride (50 μM), in that order of importance. Using both substrates was superior to using only one. The authors concluded that a single inhibitor which will differentiate all genotypes may not exist.

In the last few years there have been startling new developments in the molecular biology of cholinesterase (*loc. cit*). The use of the polymerase chain reaction and specific biotinylated probes may render some of the above considerations of historical interest only.

MOLECULAR BIOLOGY OF CHOLINESTERASE

Early investigators were able to purify cholinesterase and determine its molecular weight. For example, Das & Liddell (1970), following 13 000-fold purification, could find only one protein and one cholinesterase activity band on polyacrylamide gel electrophoresis. They found the molecular weight to be about 366 000 and the isoelectric point was estimated to be pH 3.99. Similarly Boutin & Brodeur (1971) assessed the molecular weight as 348 000, made up of four identical subunits whose molecular weight was estimated as 86 000. A lower figure of 260 000 for the molecular weight was given by LaMotta & Woronick (1971). Muensch *et al.* (1976) obtained a figure by ultracentrifugation of 345 000 with the subunit weight of 85 000.

It had been deduced by Kalow (Kalow *et al.* 1956;

Table 14.3. *Some methodologies for detection of cholinesterase variants*

Reference	Purpose for which the method was developed	Substrate(s)	Inhibitor(s)	Apparatus	Additional information
Lehman & Davies 1962 Crowley & Lehmann 1962	Forensic Assessment of 'a chol test' papers for screening	Benzoylcholine	Dibucaine	UV spectrophotometer	DN genotyping on old blood spots Unreliable in detecting patients with succinylcholine induced apnoea
Harris & Robson 1963	Mass screening	α-Naphthylacetate	RO2-0683	Agar plates	Differentiated between 'usual' on the one hand, and 'atypical' and 'intermediate' on the other. Also detected low activity due to any cause.
Morrow & Motulsky 1968	Mass screening	α-Naphthylacetate	RO2-0683	Test tube method	Differentiated between the three genotypes noted above. Difficulty with fluoride and silent alleles.
Swift & LaDu 1966	Mass screening	Benzoylcholine	No inhibitor. Sodium chloride added as enhancer.	Test tube method	Sodium chloride enhances the activity of the usual enzyme only. Phenol red used as indicator.
Rostron & Higgins 1988	Detection of atypical cholinesterase variants	Butyrylthiocholine	Dibucaine	Technicon RA-1000 analyser pH stat	Separates usual, heterozygous and atypical genotypes.
Ashby et al. 1970	Detection of individuals susceptible to succinylcholine apnoea	Butyrylcholine	Dibucaine		Separated 'usual', 'intermediate' and 'atypical'.
Garry 1971a	Exploration of different substrates, inhibitors and buffer constituents	Acetylcholine, propionylcholine and butyrylcholine	Dibucaine, succinylcholine, fluoride and various other inorganic ions	Spectrophotometric	Many different techniques can differentiate the 'usual' and 'atypical' enzymes
Garry 1971b	Detection of individuals susceptible to succinylcholine apnoea (mass screening)	Butyrylthiocholine	Phosphate and TRIS buffers	Spectrophotometric using Technicon auto-analyser modules	does not use dibucaine RO2-0683 fluoride or succinylcholine. Atypical enzyme strongly inhibited. Method detects $E_1^a E_1^a$ and $E_1^s E_1^s$
Arnold 1981	Dibucaine numbers for clinical purposes	Butyrylthiocholine	Dibucaine	Du Pont Automatic Clinical Analyser (ACA) Recording UV spectrophotometer	Does not work to give fluoride numbers.
Whittaker et al. 1983	Comparison of different substrates for detection of genetic variants	Benzoylcholine Propionylthiocholine Butyrylthiocholine	Dibucaine, fluoride		Benzoylcholine best for differentiating variants. Butyrylthiocholine superior to propionylthiocholine.
Wakid et al. 1985	Detection of succinylcholine apnoea-prone patients	Succinylcholine Propionylthiocholine	Dibucaine, fluoride	UV spectrophotometer	Succinylcholine gave less overlap between $(E_1^a E_1^a + E_1^u E_1^f)$ and $(E_1^u E_1^u + E_1^u E_1^a)$
Panteghini et al. 1988	Pre-operative detection of succinylcholine apnoea-susceptible individuals	Succinylthiodicholine	Nil	Cobas Bio analyser (Hoffman La Roche)	Detects $E_1^s E_1^s$. Fluoride observed to inhibit the enzyme but the automated technique not adapted to determine DN and FN.
Brock 1988	Detection of atypical cholinesterase variants	Benzoylcholine	Dibucaine, fluoride	Cobas-Fara centrifugal analyser	Distinct separation of eight phenotypes previously authenticated by manual techniques
Lainé-Cessac et al. 1989	Identification of individuals sensitive to succinylcholine	Succinylcholine Butyrylcholine Acetylcholine	Physostigmine	Robotic unit with flow injection linked to an Apple II computer Spectrophotometer	Allowed detection of very sensitive subjects $E_1^a E_1^a$ but did not separate E_1^s from E_1^f
Alcantara et al. 1991a, b	Detection of U, UF, UA, AK, AF and A phenotypes	α-naphthyl acetate	RO2-0683 DL-propanolol	Spectrophotometer	Achieves its objective
Hangaard et al. 1991	Immunoassay for phenotyping of cholinesterase variants	Rabbit polyclonal and mouse monoclonal antibodies	Dibucaine Succinylcholine Sodium fluoride Urea	Titertek multiscan MC (Flow Laboratories) set at 450 nm	Separates most genotypes. Some difficulty distinguishing between $E_1^u E_1^a$ and $E_1^u E_1^f$. Also difficulty in detecting E_1^s in heterozygotes.

Kalow 1964) that the enzyme contained two active sites per molecule and that these sites differed in their pH dependence. A different approach measuring the DFP (di-isopropyl fluorophosphate) bound to protein used by Muensch *et al.* (1976) gave a figure approaching two active sites. It was a mystery why the whole tetrameric molecule should have two sites if each of the four constituent monomers possessed an active site, which must be the case since the monomer exhibits enzymic activity. Later research dispelled this mystery.

An approach to finding the difference between the usual and atypical enzymes was made by Yamato *et al.* (1983) who purified the relevant enzyme, then when it was bound with [³H]di-isopropylphosphate (DFP) subjected it to tryptic digestion. The DFP had bound to the active site. The peptides containing DFP were isolated by column chromatography and electrophoresis. Then their amino acid sequences were determined. The 'atypical' peptide was found to differ from the usual by the substitution of a histidine for a glutamic acid residue. This finding later turned out to be incorrect. The sequence in a 'silent' mutant did not differ from the usual. On the other hand Lockridge & La Du (1986) carried out a similar experiment on usual (UU), atypical (AA) and atypical-silent (AS) enzymes obtaining a 29-residue, a 22-residue and an 8-residue labelled peptide respectively. No amino acid substitutions were observed in these labelled peptides.

Using the information obtained about the amino acid sequence in the active site of cholinesterase and other cholinesterases, Prody *et al.* (1986) synthesized oligodeoxynucleotide probes for the six amino acid sequence Phe-Gly-Glu-Ser-Ala-Gly. These probes were then used for the isolation of a 770 nucleotide human cholinesterase cDNA clone from human fetal brain tissue. By using this technique further clones were isolated by Prody *et al.* (1987) so that the complete cDNA for the fetal human cholinesterase could be assembled, and from this the amino acid sequence was deduced.

A different approach was utilized by La Du & Lockridge (1986). They purified human cholinesterase which was then digested with several proteolytic enzymes. The resulting peptides were purified and sequenced. The complete amino acid sequence was published by Lockridge *et al.* (1987a); it contained 574 amino acids per subunit and nine carbo-

hydrate chains attached to nine asparagines. The four subunits appeared to be identical (Fig. 14.7) and each contains an active site. The active site serine was the 198th residue from the amino-terminus and only one type of active site was found. By studying the cysteine residues in the tryptic digests it was found that there were 8 cysteines in each subunit of which 6 formed 3 disulphide bridges (Lockridge *et al.* 1987b). A comprehensive account of the structure of the whole enzyme molecule was given by Lockridge (1988). The subunits form dimers by means of disulphide bridges and two of these dimers are held together by strong non-covalent bonds. The tetramer cannot be dissociated into active subunits, but the subunits can be separated by using proteolytic agents such as trypsin.

Oligonucleotide probes were constructed from the knowledge of the amino acid sequences and used

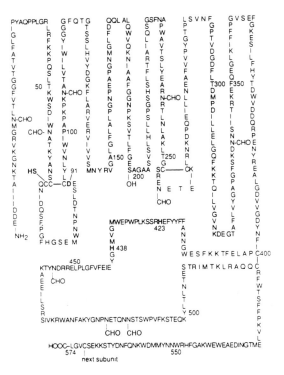

Fig. 14.7. Amino acid sequence of human cholinesterase. Carbohydrate chains are indicated by CHO; the active site serine 198 by OH; the potential free sulphydryl C$_{ys}$66 by SH. Asp 91, His 423, or His 438 may be part of the catalytic triad Asp-His-Ser though this is speculative. (From Lockridge 1988.)

to screen a human liver cDNA library and a human genomic library (La Du & Lockridge 1986). The nucleotide sequences published from the laboratories of Prody *et al.* (1987) and Lockridge were nearly identical. Developmental age and tissue of origin did not affect the nucleotide sequence. The amino acid sequence deduced from brain cDNA and liver cDNA exactly matched the amino acid sequence of the cholinesterase in serum. This led to the conclusions that (1) the cholinesterase in liver serum and brain is identical, (2) there is only one gene for cholinesterase.

The gene itself is approximately 80 kb in length and is divided into four exons by three introns at nucleotides −93, +1433 and +1600. The first of these introns is upstream from the leader peptide sequence and the other two are near the 3′-terminus of the coding region (Lockridge 1990). Each exon has been sequenced and found to agree with the cDNA sequence. If there was more than one gene then some disparity would have been expected.

Knowledge of the 'usual' cDNA was used by McGuire *et al.* (1989) in the following way. Genomic libraries were constructed from individuals homozygous for either the usual or the atypical cholinesterase genes. The libraries were screened using a previously isolated cDNA as a probe. The new clones so obtained were sequenced and DNA amplifications were effected by the polymerase chain reaction. The 2.37 kb clone from the genomic DNA of an individual homozygous for atypical cholinesterase contained 78% of the coding sequence for mature cholinesterase and was identical with the cDNA sequence from an individual of the usual phenotype except for one base change: guanine replaced adenine at nucleotide 209, producing glycine instead of aspartate at position 70 (Table 14.4). The validity of this observation was proven by repeating the whole procedure on genomic DNA from 26 individuals including 15 members of one family in which the atypical and fluoride alleles were segregating.

Similarly, a frameshift mutation was found by Nogueira *et al.* (1990) to be responsible for a silent mutant (Table 14.4) and this was again confirmed by the study of 12 individuals in two pedigrees. The same approach has shown a single base change responsible for the K variant, and two different mutations giving rise to two different 'fluoride' vari-

ants (Table 14.4). A linkage was found between the K variant mutation and the atypical mutation (Bartels *et al.* 1992a).

The Ann Arbor group have produced an important technical breakthrough in the form of biotin-labelled allele-specific probes. Briefly, the methodology is as follows. Genomic DNA from white blood cells is digested with a restriction endonuclease which produces fragments about 200 nucleotides long. These are amplified by the polymerase chain reaction. Duplicate aliquots of the amplification mixture are dot-blotted on to nitrocellulose sheets. The DNA dots are cut out as 1 cm squares. Each square is put into its own well and after washing is incubated with a specific biotin-labelled probe (biotin is the carbon dioxide carrier involved in the synthesis of oxaloacetate from pyruvate). There is an allele-specific oligonucleotide probe which will hybridize with the 'usual' allele only, another which will hybridize with the 'atypical' allele only etc. After washing away all the unattached probe an avidin-alkaline phosphatase (AP) reagent is added with an AP substrate (eg nitroblue tetrazolium). Avidin is a 70 kDa protein from egg white with a high affinity for biotin. Where the biotin-labelled probe has hybridized the avidin-(AP) will bind and the AP catalysed reaction produces a dark blue colour in 20 minutes (see Fig. 14.8). When the result is negative no colour is produced (La Du 1989; La Du *et al.* 1990).

These techniques are now being deployed to sort out a number of difficult areas concerned with cholinesterase variants such as to:-

1 detect the differences between different types of 'silent' variant, (13 have now been identified: Professor La Du 1992, personal communication);
2 identify the $E_1^k E_1^k$ homozygote;
3 differentiate between $E_1^a E_1^a$ and $E_1^a E_1^s$;
4 investigate possible heterogeneity within the apparent $E_1^u E_1^u$ phenotype;
5 find out the nature of the high activity variants.

It is also obvious that the use of non-radioactive biotinylated oligonucleotide probes following polymerase chain amplification will be an immensely powerful technique for the investigation of other pharmacogenetic conditions and inherited metabolic abnormalities (Hajra *et al.* 1992).

Table 14.4. *Molecular variants of cholinesterase*

Name of variant	Reference	Nucleotide mutation	Codon change	Amino acid change	Enzymic effect
Atypical	McGuire et al. 1989	209 A → G	70 GAT → GGT	Aspartic acid 70 → Glycine	Gives dibucaine-resistance with reduced affinity for choline esters. The aspartic acid at position 70 must be an important component of the anionic site.
Fluoride-resistant 1	La Du et al. 1990	728 C → T	243 ACG → ATG	Threonine 243 → Methionine	Fluoride-resistance
Fluoride-resistant 2	La Du et al. 1990	1169 G → T	390 GGT → GTT	Glycine 390 → Valine	Fluoride-resistance
Silent 1	Nogueria et al. 1990	351 T → AG	117 GGT → GGAG	Glycine 117 → frameshift	The protein is only 22% of the proper length. It lacks the active site and is not detected by antibodies. No enzymic activity.
Silent 2	Bartels et al. 1992a	16 A deletion	6 ATT → TT	Isoleucine 6 → frameshift	No enzymic activity
Silent 3	Bartels et al. 1992a	1500 T → A	500 TAT → TAA	Tyrosine 500 → STOP	No cholinesterase activity
K	La Du et al. 1990	1615 G → A	539 GCA → ACA	Alanine 539 → Threonine	Activity 66% of the usual enzyme
J	Bartels et al. 1992b	1615 G → A and 1470 A → T	539 GCA → ACA 497 GAA → GTA	Alanine 539 → Threonine and Glutamic acid 497 → Valine	Activity 30% of the usual enzyme
H	Bartels et al. 1992a	424 G → A	142 GTG → ATG	Valine 142 → Methionine	Activity 10% of the usual enzyme
Nucleotide 116	Arpagaus et al. 1990	116 G → A	−39 TAC → TGC Occurs in 3′-untranslated region	Cysteine 39 → Tyrosine	No known effect
Nucleotide 1914	Arpagaus et al. 1990	1914 A → G		None	No known effect

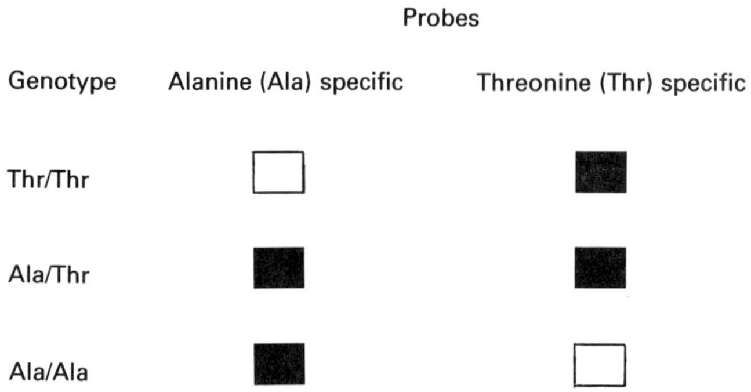

Probes

Genotype	Alanine (Ala) specific	Threonine (Thr) specific
Thr/Thr	☐	■
Ala/Thr	■	■
Ala/Ala	■	☐

Fig. 14.8. Analysis of the alanine/threonine polymorphism with allele-specific, biotinylated 19-mer oligonucleotide probes. (Adapted from LaDu *et al.* 1990.)

MISCELLANEOUS CLINICAL TOPICS

1 One of the curious aspects of cholinesterase is that persons who are homozygous for the 'silent' allele which expresses zero enzymic activity seem to be perfectly healthy and live to an advanced age. Nevertheless the enzyme is normally present in many tissues, and the gene has been conserved during the course of evolution implying that it may not be neutral, i.e. that it has some survival value.

This conundrum has been discussed by Lockridge (1990) who suggested that there may exist a back-up system of enzymes.

2 An interesting relationship of the dibucaine-detected variants to a natural phenomenon was described by Harris & Whittaker (1962b). They found that potato extracts were able to differentiate three genotypes the same as dibucaine. The alkaloids solanine and solanidine are known to occur in potatoes, particularly in the skin (solanine is the glyco-alkaloid which on hydrolysis liberates one molecule each of glucose, galactose and rhamnose leaving the alkaloid solanidine: Fig. 14.9). It was shown that solutions of solanine and solanidine also had differential effects like dibucaine and potato extracts.

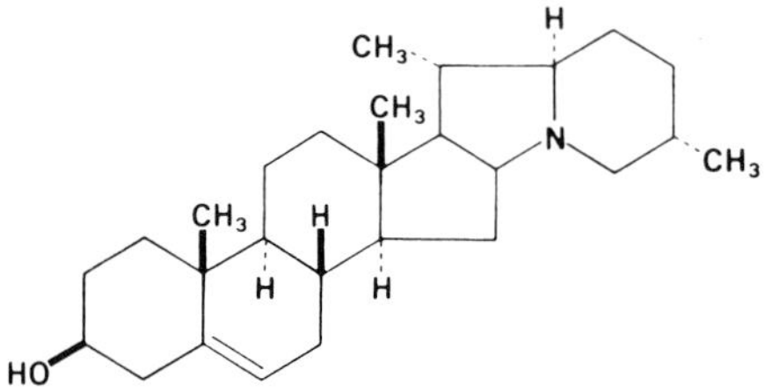

Many episodes of potato poisoning have been recorded in the past. A particularly detailed outbreak was recorded by McMillan & Thompson (1979) involving 78 schoolboys who became ill after eating potatoes. Seventeen boys required admission to hospital and three of those were dangerously ill. The main symptoms and signs were diarrhoea, vomiting, anorexia, abdominal pain, confusion, hallucinations, restlessness and septic spots. Excessive solanine was demonstrated in the relevant potatoes. Plasma cholinesterase was demonstrated to be low in 10 boys, and in nine rose during the month after recovery, but one subnormal value did not rise to the normal range. Plasma specimens showed normal dibucaine and fluoride numbers. It is not known whether the subnormal cholinesterase, which did not rise to the normal range, represented a genetic variant because family studies were not performed (Dr M. Whittaker 1991, personal communication).

3 The influence of sex and age on cholinesterase activity has been the subject of dispute. Shanor *et al.* (1961) reviewed the literature and in a survey of 100 healthy subjects found that (1) in young adults, women had only about 70% of the activity of men, (2) in old age there was no sex difference, (3) young men had levels about 24% higher than old men. The subject does not seem to have been re-examined with a knowledge of genetic variants.

4 Pregnancy is known to lower the cholinesterase

Fig. 14.9. Solanidine. (From *Clarke's Isolation and Identification of Drugs*, 1986.)

activity of the plasma by about 20%. This occurs throughout pregnancy and is independent of the age of the woman or how many pregnancies she has had previously. The chloride, fluoride and dibucaine numbers were not significantly different throughout pregnancy (Hazel & Monier 1971; Whittaker *et al.* 1991b).

5 Exposure to organophosphorus compounds which occurs particularly in agricultural workers spraying insecticides is well known to lower the plasma cholinesterase activity (e.g. Peedicayil *et al.* 1991). A striking new finding, however, is that recorded by Prody *et al.* (1989). These researchers called attention to the fact that intact cholinergic functioning appears to be important in germ-line cell development and early embryogenesis. Cholinesterase mRNA is present in developing oocytes and the enzyme is expressed early in embryogenesis. It was considered, therefore, that the cholinesterase gene was a good candidate for amplification *in vivo* where the germ-line cells are exposed to organophosphates, particularly in 'silent' homozygotes.

Examination of the peripheral blood DNA of a man who had been heavily exposed to parathion, revealed amplification of the central part of the cholinesterase gene. This man possessed the 'silent' phenotype. His son also possessed the gene amplification phenomenon. The proband's parents had both been exposed to parathion at the time he was conceived but their DNA did not show the gene amplification. The authors make the suggestion that the abnormal gene may have arisen during spermatogenesis making it inheritable. The effect of the amplified genetic material is unclear but it resembles gene disturbances found in some tumours. The paraoxonase phenotype of the proband was apparently not determined. It was suggested that the possession of a silent cholinesterase gene may have somehow created conditions under which only the amplification and overproduction of silent cholinesterase would permit survival.

6 A patient with the genotype $E_1^u E_1^a$ was subjected to orthotopic liver transplantation. Thereafter his apparent phenotype as assessed by serum studies was $E_1^u E_1^u$ (Khoury 1987, 1988; Viby-Mogensen 1988). This observation suggests that the determination of the plasma enzyme character resides entirely within the liver.

7 The use of succinylcholine as a short term muscular relaxant is not contra-indicated in persons with decreased plasma cholinesterase activity (of whatever origin), and Hickey (1987) describe experience in a patient with documented atypical cholinesterase who was given 0.04 to 0.06 mg succinylcholine per kg body weight (i.e. one twentieth of the customary dose) with satisfactory results. It may be commented that this is an important outcome of knowledge of pharmacogenetics, namely, to tailor the dose of the drug to be appropriate to the individual patient. Too often a useful drug is discarded because the average conventional dose cannot be given to every patient.

8 Hitherto no really convincing association has been described between a cholinesterase phenotype and a spontaneous disorder (see Lockridge 1990). Nevertheless, there have been one or two interesting results and leprosy deserves a mention. In India, Thomas *et al.* (1976) studied 701 normal individuals, 420 patients with lepromatous leprosy and 191 patients with tuberculoid leprosy. These workers found a higher frequency of E_1^a in the lepromatous lepers than in the other two groups. In Mexicans, Rea & Ng (1978) found no such association but Navarette *et al.* (1979) in a larger study corroborated the Indian findings. In Africans two studies can be cited; Agarwal *et al.* (1973) found no significant difference in the dibucaine numbers between 150 normal Ethiopians and 206 lepers. In a study in Zimbabwe Whittaker *et al.* (1976) found no individual with an E_1^a gene, but the frequency of E_1^f was lower in 312 patients with tuberculoid leprosy compared with 1034 healthy controls and 217 patients with lepromatous leprosy. On the other hand, the percentage of the C_5+ phenotype was lower in the tuberculoid leprosy patients than in the other groups. Although it is known that dapsone exerts no influence on the phenotyping it was not determined whether other anti-leprotic drugs might have affected the results.

9 Significant amounts of fluoride ions are known to be produced in the blood following the administration of enflurane, halothane, methoxyflurane and sevoflurane anaesthesia. The influence of fluoride concentrations *in vitro* was studied on sera with normal DN values, by Kambam *et al.* (1990). Inorganic fluoride at concentrations of 20 to 75 μM was

found to inhibit cholinesterase activity by 28 to 65% This could be of clinical importance in obese patients (in whom fluoride levels are higher) or where a second halogen-containing anaesthetic is administered within a few hours of the first one. The fluoride numbers of the plasmas were not studied. It is to be noted that the total number of plasma samples investigated was only 14.

10 Bambuterol (a bis-dimethylcarbamate of terbutaline) is a long-acting bronchodilator. The influence of this drug given pre-operatively was studied by Bang *et al.* (1990) on seven $E_1^u E_1^a$ and two $E_1^u E_1^s$ individuals. Cholinesterase activity was lowered and their recovery of neuromuscular function after succinylcholine administration was delayed. Several developed a Phase II block ('fade' of response during train of four stimulations) during recovery (which was probably a result of the bambuterol-induced depression of the normal enzyme activity permitting a larger than normal amount of succinylcholine to reach the neuromuscular end plates).

11 An interesting geographic clustering of individuals prone to develop succinylcholine apnoea was described by Milligan *et al.* (1986). The proband was a 76 year old man who had a 5 hour apnoea following 75 mg succinylcholine given for a prostatectomy. Apart from his benign prostatic hypertrophy he was healthy. Later another proband was admitted from the same small town (population 3140). Screening family members disclosed 17 $E_1^a E_1^f$ and one $E_1^f E_1^f$ amongst the relatives. Although the area was not traditionally regarded as one in which significant inbreeding occurred it seemed likely that the findings indicated genetic drift.

THE USE OF SUCCINYLDICHOLINE AS AN *IN VITRO* TEST SUBSTANCE FOR CHOLINESTERASE ASSESSMENT

A technique was designed by Goedde *et al.* (1968) whereby the capacity of cholinesterase to hydrolyse succinylcholine *in vitro* could be measured. The method involved the use of ^{14}C-labelled succinyldicholine and high voltage electrophoresis. Competitive inhibition was demonstrated between benzoylcholine and succinyldicholine. Schmidinger *et al.* (1966) of the same research group had earlier shown that succinyldicholine at a concentration below 5×10^{-5} M (which would be approximately

the expected concentration of a 50 mg dose dissolved in the plasma volume of a 70 kg man) was hydrolysed by $E_1^u E_1^u$ but not by $E_1^a E_1^a$ serum.

The hydrolysis of succinyldicholine by plasma was also investigated by Hobbiger & Peck (1969) using an isolated frog rectus abdominis preparation. It is to be noted that these workers used 0.025 mM succinyldicholine which is about the plasma concentration to be expected after giving an adult man 45 mg of the drug intravenously. They concluded that inhibition by dibucaine or sodium fluoride was not a general guide to rates of hydrolysis of succinyldicholine by different plasmas ($E_1^u E_1^u$, $E_1^a E_1^a$ and $E_1^f E_1^f$).

The idea was thus generated that it might be meaningful to use succinyldicholine in *in vitro* tests because it might predict *in vivo* events better than other compounds. McComb *et al.* (1965) found that they could clearly distinguish sera which were homozygous or heterozygous for atypical cholinesterase (as determined by DN) using *O*-nitrophenyl-butyrate as the substrate and succinyldicholine as a competitive inhibitor. By this means a 'succinyl-choline number' (the percentage of inhibition) was produced, and the values mirrored those produced by the dibucaine method.

On the other hand Agarwal *et al.* (1975) used succinyldicholine (Su) as the substrate and dibucaine as the inhibitor. Three distinct groups could be established by this method and they resembled those found using benzoylcholine as a substrate. However, applying this new method to patients who had sustained prolonged apnoea revealed differences from the phenotypes as determined using benzoylcholine (B) as the substrate. Thus of 36 usual phenotype (B), 16 were atypical (Su), 7 silent (Su) and 7 heterozygous UA (Su); 15 typed UA (B), 5 were atypical (Su) and 1 usual (Su).

In order further to investigate these 'new' phenotypes Goedde *et al.* (1979) labelled UU, UA and AA (as detected by dibucaine) with radioactively labelled di-isopropyl-fluorophosphate. Then the fragments obtained with trypsin were subjected to high-voltage electrophoresis. All the fragments from UU moved anodally indicating a strongly acidic character, all the fragments from AA moved cathodally, and fragments from UA moved in both directions. When the new variants were treated similarly all fragments moved towards the anode, which suggests that the mutational changes producing them were different to those in the dibucaine variants.

Pedigree data indicated that the new variant

seemed to be inherited as an autosomal recessive (Goedde & Agarwal 1978).

The same topic was investigated by Wakid *et al.* (1985) who compared the results obtained using propionylthiocholine and succinyldicholine as *in vitro* substrates. They found more overlap between the activities of succinylcholine-sensitive and succinylcholine-insensitive individuals using the former substrate and advocated using the latter as a predictor of predisposition to succinylcholine apnoea.

A significant negative correlation between log duration of action/activity (ordinate) and activity using propionylthiocholine as a substrate (abscissa) was demonstrated by Yücel *et al.* (1988) and this correlation could be used to compute a suitable dose for a patient with low plasma activity from whatever cause.

Perhaps the reason that the methods employing succinylcholine as a substrate have not achieved widespread popularity is because the benzoyl-choline/dibucaine method (and its variants) was already well known and simple to carry out.

CHOLINESTERASE ENZYME TREATMENT TO PREVENT APNOEA CAUSED BY SUCCINYLCHOLINE

Therapeutic possibilities of shortening the period of apnoea in persons prone to it after administration of succinyldicholine have included the administration of a cholinesterase preparation. Patients likely to benefit would include those with a normal phenotype but with low levels due to illness as well as persons with genetically defective forms of the enzyme. The idea was tested by Goedde *et al.* (1968) who infused a 1300-fold purified preparation of the enzyme from human plasma. Persons with $E_1^a E_1^a$ or $E_1^a E_1^s$ were given 1 mg succinylcholine per kg body weight with a short acting barbiturate and nitrous oxide (a) without any enzyme administration, (b) 16 minutes before the administration of the whole plasma activity of cholinesterase, calculated from individual plasma volume and normal plasma level, (c) 24 hours later. The average period of apnoea which was 120 minutes with (a), was normalized in (b), and a little prolonged in (c). The cholinesterase activity which was very low in (a) was normal in (b).

A concentrate of highly purified cholinesterase derived from human plasma is available as 'serum cholinesterase P' (Behringwerke AG, D-3550 Marburg, Germany). Its use in clinical practice is illustrated by an account of treatment of prolonged apnoea in a neonate by Benzer *et al.* (1992).

An alternative approach has been proposed by others (e.g. Liddell, 1968) who have advocated the use of plasma as a possible specific treatment for succinylcholine apnoea.

In fact neither of the two treatments has become popular. This is for three reasons: (1) fear of the transmission of viral hepatitis and more recently HIV, (2) the possibility of giving a suitably small dose of succinylcholine where the subject is known to be apnoea-prone before the operation, (3) although it is inconvenient it is safe and easy to continue the artificial ventilation until muscle tone and natural breathing return.

THE RELATIONSHIP BETWEEN CHOLINESTERASE AND PLASMA LIPOPROTEINS

The physiological function of cholinesterase is obscure but there is some evidence that it may be involved in lipoprotein metabolism. Hence if genetic variants discovered by means of aberrant drug hydrolysis have any metabolic significance, lipoprotein metabolism is possibly a relevant area.

Various authors have found correlations between plasma cholinesterase activity and different plasma lipoprotein measurements (Table 14.5). The positive correlation seems mainly to be with low density lipoprotein, and conversely a negative correlation with high density lipoprotein. Other authors have used a more complicated way of expressing their results. For example Kutty *et al.* (1981) found an increase in cholinesterase activity/high density lipoprotein cholesterol (referred to as the 'complementary risk factor' = CRF) with increasing risk of cardiovascular disease. There was a positive correlation between CRF and (1) total cholesterol/high density lipoprotein cholesterol, (2) low density lipoprotein cholesterol, and (3) triglycerides.

Although plasma cholinesterase activity was found to be slightly higher in patients with coronary artery disease than in controls by Lehtonen *et al.* (1986), its discriminating power was weak. However, the fractions lipoprotein A-1/cholinesterase activity and high density lipoprotein cholesterol/cholinesterase activity had a higher

Table 14.5. *Correlations of cholinesterase with plasma lipoproteins*

Reference	Location	TC	TG	HDLC	$\dfrac{\text{HDLC}}{\text{TC}}$	LDLC	VLDL
Cucuiano *et al.* 1968	Romania	+	+				
Nakamura *et al.* 1985	Japan				−		
Schouten *et al.* 1987	Netherlands			−		+	
Magarian & Dietz 1987	USA	+	+	−		+	+
Schouten *et al.* 1988	Netherlands		+			+	
Cucuiano 1988	Romania						+

TC, total cholesterol; TG, triglycerides; HDLC, high density lipoprotein cholesterol; LDLC, low density lipoprotein cholesterol; VLDL, very low density lipoprotein.

discriminating power, both being lower in coronary artery patients than in controls.

In the study of Nakamura *et al.* (1985) the correlation between high density lipoprotein cholesterol(HDLC)/total cholesterol(TC) (see Table 14.5) and cholinesterase was impressive at −0.86. Nevertheless, a lack of a direct relationship between lipoproteins and the enzyme has been suggested by the following observations. Schouten *et al.* (1987) found that in heterozygous familial hypercholesterolaemia a hydroxymethylglutarate-CoA reductase inhibitor MK-733 lowered low density lipoprotein cholesterol (LDLC) and increased HDLC but did not alter cholinesterase activity. Similarly, Cucuianu (1988) found that clofibrate lowered very low density lipoprotein (VLDL) by enhancing removal but cholinesterase was not reduced in parallel.

In an experimental study in rats made diabetic with streptozotocin Annapurna *et al.* (1991) found a close correlation between cholinesterase activity and low density lipoproteins but the effect of heparin was to lower the level of the latter in the serum without lowering the former.

Hence it may be concluded, as Schouten *et al.* (1988) point out, that the relationship between cholinesterase activity and serum lipoproteins, if there is any at all, is certainly not a simple one.

An interesting study of coronary disease patients, their relatives and controls was carried out by Tripathi *et al.* (1987) who found that serum cholinesterase activity (PChEA) levels increased with age and were significantly higher in myocardial infarction patients than in controls with a suggestion that they might also be higher in the relatives of patients than in controls. They propose that PChEA might be used

as an index of liability to develop coronary artery disease.

The influence of genetic variants on lipoprotein metabolism is as yet unknown. Because of the overwhelming importance of coronary artery disease on the medical scene it might be of interest to survey this unexplored territory.

INTER-ETHNIC VARIABILITY IN THE FREQUENCIES OF THE ALLELES CONTROLLING CHOLINESTERASE VARIANTS

The allele whose frequency has received most attention in different population and ethnic groups is E_1^a. Already in the early monograph of Goedde *et al.* (1967) there was a table indicating that this allele had a frequency of about 0.012 to 0.019 in various European populations. There was however an exception in that a frequency of 0.033 was found in Czechoslovakia and there was no evidence of it in 100 Japanese which had been tested.

Since then a huge number of studies have been performed and a comprehensive survey of the relevant literature was published by Whittaker (1986) in her book.

In Europeans the average frequency of E_1^a is about 0.017 (Table 14.6) so the number of persons in the population which includes one homozygote $E_1^a E_1^a$ is $1/0.017^2 = 3460$. However, as Arnaud *et al.* (1991) point out there is considerable variability in the frequency of heterozygotes in the French population. Also, in Mediterranean regions populations have been described with much higher frequencies, e.g. Valencia with an allele frequency of 0.0732 which

Table 14.6. *Frequency of E_1^a in various populations*

Reference	Population	Number tested	Number of $E_1^u E_1^a$	Frequency of E_1^a
Europe				
Goedde & Altland 1963;				
Goedde *et al.* 1963	Germans	8314	264	0.0162
Prokop 1966	Germans (Berlin)	1000	23	0.0115
Walter *et al.* 1965	Germans (Rheinland-Pfalz)	285	8	0.0141
Neumann & Walter 1968	Germans (Hessen)	137	2	0.0073
Goedde *et al.* 1972a	Germans (Marburg)	146	2	0.0069
Steegmüller 1975	Germans	280	7	0.0125
Boman 1981	Norwegians	3143	97	0.0150
Hanel *et al.* 1978	Danes	1278	32	0.0125
Neumann & Walter 1968	Icelanders[a]	128	0	0.0000
Singh *et al.* 1974	Ålanders (Finno-Swedes)	199	1	0.0025
Singh *et al.* 1971a;				
Altland *et al.* 1969	Finns	317	8	0.0158
Mkheidze *et al.* 1978	Russians (St Petersburg)	200	[b]	0.0025
Singh *et al.* 1974	Maris (USSR)	295	0	0.0000
Singh *et al.* 1971a	Finnish Lapps:			
	Sevettijarvi Skolts	349	9	0.0129
	Nellim Skolts	189	9	0.0238
	Fisher Lapps	143	2	0.0069
	Mountain Lapps	124	5	0.0125
Fraser *et al.* 1974	Dutch	800	34	0.0225
Pronk 1976	Dutch	322	14	0.0220
Van Ros & Vervoort 1973	Belgians	354	12	0.0169
Cardan & Schopp 1986	Romanians	452	19	0.0210
Schaap *et al.* 1967	French	1522	57	0.0187
Vergnes *et al.* 1967	French:			
	Haut Languedoc	39	1	0.0128
	Pays Basque	200	2	0.0050
Masson *et al.* 1979	French (Lyons)	1594	52	0.0188
Vergnes *et al.* 1981	French (South West)	2453	104	0.0253
Arnaud *et al.* 1991	French	2421	[b]	0.0213
Kattamis *et al.* 1962	British	703	27	0.0192
Whittaker 1968	British students (presumably white)	780	23	0.0160
Walter *et al.* 1965	Hungarians:			
	Ivad	276	5	0.0091
	Ungarn	196	1	0.0026
Goedde & Altland 1963;				
Goedde *et al.* 1963	Czechoslovakians	262	19	0.0362
Whittaker 1968d	Italians	382	8	0.0109
Morrow & Motulsky 1965	Greeks	561	16	0.0143
Kattamis *et al.* 1962	Greeks	360	13	0.0181
Neumann & Walter 1968	Greeks	218	10	0.0252
Fraser *et al.* 1969	Greeks	860	14	0.0081
Das *et al.* 1975	Greeks	429	38	0.0664
Steegmüller 1975	Bulgarians	108	2	0.0093
Fraser *et al.* 1969	Yugoslavians:			
	Skopje Gypsies	33	0	0.0000
	Macedonians	74	0	0.0000
	South West	94	5	0.0270
	Middle West	95	3	0.0160
	North West	67	1	0.0070

Table 14.6. (*cont*).

Reference	Population	Number tested	Number of $E_1^u E_1^a$	Frequency of E_1^a
Goedde *et al.* 1972b	Spanish:			
	Central meseta	159	3	0.0094
	Andalusia	124	1	0.0040
	Galicia	143	7	0.0279
	Basque	224	14	0.0312
Gomar *et al.* 1986	Spanish (ENT patients)	464	22	0.0237
Kattamis *et al.* 1962	Portuguese	179	6	0.0168
Cruz *et al.* 1973	Portuguese (Vilarinho da Furna)	77	2	0.0129
Middle East				
Loiselet & Srouji 1968	Lebanese	1315	42	0.0167
Szeinberg 1966	Jews (Ashkenazi)	923	29	0.0168
Szeinberg *et al.* 1972	Jews (Ashkenazi)	4196	149	0.0178
	Jews (Iraq)	1057	96	0.0482
	Jews (Iran)	159	18	0.0755
	Jews (Yemen)	459	19	0.0207
	Jews (North Africa)	1106	34	0.0163
	Jews (Balkan & Turkey)	674	36	0.0267
	Jews (Lebanon & Syria)	203	7	0.0172
	Jews (unspecified)	1652	69	0.0209
Sayek *et al.* 1967	Turks (surgical paediatric patients)	725	45	0.0344
Vergnes & Gherardi 1971	Kurds in Syria & Lebanon	162	1	0.0031
Kattamis *et al.* 1962	Jews (Morocco)	51	1	0.0098
	Berbers	55	2	0.0182
Szeinberg *et al.* 1966	Arabs (Israel)	110	2	0.0091
Bowman & Habib 1983	Egyptians	505	36	0.038
Whittaker 1968d	Arabs (Iran)	36	1	0.0143
Asia				
Rahimi *et al.* 1977	Afghans:			
	Tajiks	310	2	0.0032
	Pushtoons	210	0	0.0000
	Hazaras	172	2	0.0058
	Usbeks	124	0	0.0000
Neumann & Walter 1968	Pakistanis	121	3	0.0124
Singh *et al.* 1974	Punjabis:			
	Brahmin	106	5	0.0236
	Arora	103	6	0.0291
	Khattri	132	7	0.0265
	Jat	159	8	0.0252
Goedde *et al.* 1972c	Assamese	75	1	0.0066
Goedde *et al.* 1972c	Khasis	60	0	0.0000
Gopalam & Rao 1979	Vysyas of Andhra Pradesh (South India)	731	4	0.0027
Thomas *et al.* 1976	Vellore Indians	720	18	0.0125
Steegmüller 1975	Bengalis & Biharis	139	0	0.0000
Omoto & Goedde 1965; Altland *et al.* 1967	Japanese	371	0	0.0000
Morrow & Motulsky 1965	Japanese	140	0	0.0000
Omoto & Harada 1968	Ainu	360	0	0.0000
Bajatzadeh *et al.* 1969	Koreans	155	0	0.0000
Altland *et al.* 1967	Thais	723	0	0.0000
Simpson 1968	Thais	500	0	0.0000
Motulsky & Morrow 1968	Philippinos	427	2	0.0023

Table 14.6. (*cont*).

Reference	Population	Number tested	Number of $E_1^u E_1^a$	Frequency of E_1^a
Morrow & Motulsky 1965	Philippinos	411	2	0.0024
Morrow & Motulsky 1965	Taiwanese	340	1	0.0015
Lee & Chang 1987	Taiwanese	265	9	0.0170
Ganendran & Ogle 1975	Singaporean:			
	Malays	79 ⎫		
	Chinese	325 ⎬	0	0.0000
	Indians	175 ⎭		
Australia				
Horsfall *et al.* 1963	Aborigines	98	1	0.0050
Whittaker 1968d	Aborigines	100	0	0.0000
Africa				
Agarwal *et al.* 1973	Ethiopia	150	7	0.0233
Whittaker 1968d	Gambians	103	1	0.0049
Whittaker 1968d;				
Bouloux *et al.* 1972	Senegalese	700	0	0.0000
Whittaker 1968d	Nigerian Ibos	69	0	0.0000
Steegmüller 1975	Nigerians	33	0	0.0000
Hiernaux 1976	Southern Chad – Sara Majingay	187	1	0.0027
Ukoha *et al.* 1987	Northern Nigerians (Zaria)	345	6	0.0087
Motulsky & Morrow 1968	Zaïrians	460	1	0.0011
Kattamis *et al.* 1962	Zaïrians	585	[b]	0.0009
Demeester 1965	Zaïrians	515	0	0.0000
Van Ros & Vervoort 1973	Zaïrians	200	0	0.0000
Demeester *et al.* 1965	Congolese Bantu	515	0	0.0000
Whittaker & Lowe 1976	Rhodesians	1227	0	0.0000
Whittaker & Lowe 1976	Zambians	34	0	0.0000
Whittaker & Lowe 1976	Malawis	191	0	0.0000
Whittaker & Lowe 1976	Mozambicans	162	0	0.0000
Whittaker & Reys 1975	Mozambicans:			
	Portuguese	153	4	0.0130
	Shangana	109	0	0.0000
	Chopi	79	0	0.0000
	Ronga	96	0	0.0000
	Bitonga	52	0	0.0000
Motulsky & Morrow 1968	Ituri Pygmies	125	0	0.0000
	Babinga Pygmies	300	0	0.0000
Vergnes *et al.* 1979	Aka Pygmies	780	0	0.0000
Krause *et al.* 1987	South Africans:			
	Ashkenazi	461	16	0.0173
	Afrikaner	255	8	0.0157
	Coloured	61	0	0.0000
	Ngwato	110	0	0.0000
	Taung	213	0	0.0000
	Zulu	68	0	0.0000
	San (!Kung)	86	0	0.0000
Arctic				
Morrow & Motulsky 1965	Eskimos (American)	145	0	0.0000
Gutsche *et al.* 1967	Eskimos (Northern)	122	0	0.0000
Gutsche *et al.* 1967	Eskimos (Southern)	379	0	0.0000
Simpson 1972	Eskimos (Canadian)	100	0	0.0000
Singh *et al.* 1974	Eskimos (Greenland)	146	0	0.0000
Gutsche *et al.* 1967	Aleuts	58	1	0.0086

Table 14.6. (*cont*).

Reference	Population	Number tested	Number of $E_1^u E_1^a$	Frequency of E_1^a
North America				
McAlpine *et al.* 1974	Eskimos of Eastern Canadian Arctic (Igloolik)	298	0	0.0000
Gutsche *et al.* 1967	Athabascan Indians	141	0	0.0000
Lubin *et al.* 1971	White Mountain Apaches	111	0	0.0000
Garry 1977	Navajo	357	0	0.0000
Becker 1972	Detroit dental students (559 white, 4 negro)	463	12	0.0107
Tashian *et al.* 1967	Xavanthe Indians	285	0	0.0000
Kalow & Gunn 1959	Canadians	2017	74	0.0188
Morrow & Motulsky 1965	European Americans	246	8	0.0163
Garry 1971	Caucasians	1495	49	0.0164
	Negroes	347	1	0.0014
Lubin *et al.* 1971	Caucasians	1497	49	0.0177
Lubin *et al.* 1971	Mississippi Caucasians	142	8	0.0281
Lisker *et al.* 1964	Mexicans (Spaniards)	469	8	0.0107
Lubin *et al.* 1971	Mexican American	118	0	0.0000
Lubin *et al.* 1971	Negro Americans	347	1	0.0014
Morrow & Motulsky 1965	Negro Americans (Seattle, WA)	666	7	0.0053
Morrow & Motulsky 1965	Mixed Orientals mainly Japanese (Seattle, WA)	426	4	0.0047
Lisker *et al.* 1964	Four Mexican Indian tribes	377	7	0.0093
Lisker *et al.* 1967	13 Mexican Indian tribes	1352	13	0.0048
Lisker *et al.* 1969	Populations on East coast of Mexico:			
	Tamiahua	109	0	0.0000
	Paraiso	160	0	0.0000
	Saladero	119	6	0.0250
	El Carmen	109	0	0.0000
	Vera Cruz	147	5	0.0170
Lisker *et al.* 1966	Mexicans of Italian origin	150	2	0.0067
Rea & Ng 1978	Mexicans	30	7	0.0263
Naverette *et al.* 1979	Mexicans	133	0	0.0000
Garcia & Diaz 1972	Puerto Ricans	1739	35	0.0101
South America				
Arends *et al.* 1967	Indians	291	0	0.0000
Ashton & Simpson 1966	Mixed ethnic population of Brazil[*]	2102	60	0.0147
Chautard-Freire-Maia *et al.* 1984a	Brazilians (Negroid):			
	Curitiba	1015	15	0.0074
Chautard-Freire-Maia *et al.* 1984b	Salvador	772	13	0.0084
Chautard-Freire-Maia *et al.* 1984a	Brazilians (whites):			
	Curitiba	999	30	0.0150
Magna *et al.* 1980	South-east	406	21	0.0259
Chautard-Freire-Maia *et al.* 1984b	Salvador	84	1	0.0059
Guerreiro *et al.* 1987	Brazilian Amazonian Indians:			
	Urubu-Kaapor	210	0	0.0000
	Assurini	160	0	0.0000

Table 14.6. (*cont*).

Reference	Population	Number tested	Number of $E_1^u E_1^a$	Frequency of E_1^a
Pacific				
Propert & Brackenridge 1976	Caucasian Australian residents	1224	57	0.0233
Curtain *et al.* 1965	Papua & New Guinea populations:			
	New Britain	835	17	0.0102
	Sepik River District	636	20	0.0157
	Markham River Valley	257	2	0.0039
	Eastern Highlands	717	17	0.0118
	Southern Highlands	227	8	0.0176
	Western Highlands	59	1	0.0085

[a] Arnason *et al.* (1975) report one $E_1^a E_1^a$ amongst 1600 randomly selected Icelanders.
[b] Number not supplied.

Table 14.7. *Frequency of E_1^f in various populations*

Reference	Population	Number tested	Frequency of E_1^f
Europe			
Masson *et al.* 1979	French (Lyons)	1594	0.0103
Vergnes *et al.* 1981	French (Vallée de P'Ouzum)	292	0.0034
Steegmüller 1975	Germans	280	0.0071
Steegmüller 1975	Bulgarians	108	0.0046
Neumann & Walter 1968	Germans	137	0.0000
Neumann & Walter 1968	Icelanders	128	0.0117
Neumann & Walter 1968	Greeks	218	0.0161
Das *et al.* 1975	Greeks	429	0.0221
Whittaker 1968e	British students	780	0.0032
Whittaker & Berry 1977	British (NE England)	736	0.0109
Goedde *et al.* 1964	Germans	801	0.0075
Hanel *et al.* 1978	Danes	1278	0.0012
Arnaud *et al.* 1991	French	2421	0.0039
Whittaker & Lowe 1976	Portuguese (in Mozambique)	153	0.0030
Middle East			
Szeinberg *et al.* 1972	Jews Ashkenazi	4196	0.0004
Szeinberg *et al.* 1972	Jews Iraqi	1057	0.0009
Szeinberg *et al.* 1972	Jews Yemen	459	0.0011
Szeinberg *et al.* 1972	Jews N. Africa	1106	0.0009
Bowman & Habib 1983	Egyptians	505	0.0109
Asia			
Sayek *et al.* 1967	Turks	7725	0.0041
Singh *et al.* 1971b	Punjabis	202	0.1287
Steegmüller 1975	Bengalis & Biharis	139	0.0036
Neumann & Walter 1968	Pakistanis	121	0.0000
Lee & Chang 1987	Taiwanese	265	0.0132
Omoto & Goedde 1965	Japanese	100	0.0100
Bajatzadeh *et al.* 1969	Koreans	115	0.0000
Whittaker & Lowe 1976	Chinese (in Australia)	120	0.0000
Gopalam & Rao 1981	Vysyas (Hyderabad)	71	0.0027
Gopalam & Rao 1981	Vysyas (Andhra Pradesh)	731	0.0027

Table 14.7. (*cont*).

Reference	Population	Number tested	Frequency of E_1^f
Africa			
Whittaker & Reys 1975	SE Mozambique Bantu:		
	Portuguese	153	0.0030
	Ronga	96	0.0469
	Shangaan	109	0.0596
	Chopi	79	0.0886
	Bitonga	52	0.0481
Whittaker & Lowe 1976	Rhodesians	1227	0.0346
	Mozambiqueans	162	0.0309
	Malawis	191	0.0366
	Zambians	34	0.0441
Steegmüller 1975	Nigerians	3	0.0000
Vergnes *et al.* 1979	Aka Pygmies of Central Africa	780	0.0045
North America			
Simpson 1968	Caucasians	41	0.0118
Becker 1972	American students	563	0.0035
Garry *et al.* 1972	US Caucasians	836	0.0066
	US Negroes	168	0.0000
Garry 1977	Navajo	358	0.0000
South America			
Simpson 1968	Brazilians	216	0.0046
Australia			
Whittaker & Lowe 1976	Aborigines	100	0.0000
Propert & Brockenridge 1976	Caucasian Australian residents	1224	0.0053

Table 14.8. Frequency of E_1^s in various populations

Reference	Population	Number tested	Frequency of E_1^s
Europe			
Vergnes *et al.* 1981	French (South West France)	2325	0.0086
Arnaud *et al.* 1991	French	2421	0.0064
North America			
Simpson & Kalow 1964	Caucasians	[a]	0.0017 to 0.0028
Gutsche *et al.* 1967	Eskimos	379	0.1210
India			
Gopalam & Rao 1981	Vysyas of Andhra Pradesh	731	0.1040
Africa			
Vergnes *et al.* 1979	Aka Pygmies of Central Africa	780	0.0013
Szeinberg *et al.* 1972	North African Jews	1106	about 0.0018

[a]Computation involving frequency E_1^a.

Table 14.9. *Frequency of the C₅+ character in various populations*

Reference	Population	Number tested	% C_5+
Europe			
Robson & Harris 1966	British	1941	9.70
Robson & Harris 1966	Icelanders	25	16.00
Eiberg *et al.* 1989	Danes	1656	8.30
Altland *et al.* 1969	Germans	952	11.90
Goedde *et al.* 1972a	Germans	150	8.00
Steegmüller 1975	Germans	586	10.10
Klein *et al.* 1967	Germans	770	3.90
Trela 1967	Poles	1400	8.71
Fraser *et al.* 1978	Dutch	798	7.40
Van Ros & Vervoort 1973	Belgians	354	11.30
Altland *et al.* 1969	Czechoslovak	312	11.00
Steegmüller 1975	Bulgarians	109	8.20
Singh *et al.* 1971a	Finns	317	3.50
Altland *et al.* 1969	Skolt Lapps	330	12.00
Singh *et al.* 1971a	Lapps:		
	Svettijärvi Skolts	189	15.30
	Nellim Skolts	349	11.50
	Fisher Lapps	143	4.90
	Mountain Lapps	124	6.50
Singh *et al.* 1974	Ålanders	200	7.50
Singh *et al.* 1974	Maris (USSR)	295	9.40
Nazarova 1981	Russian (Moscow)	399	9.20
Vergnes *et al.* 1981	Pyrenean French	2766	6.98
Goedde *et al.* 1972b	Spanish:		
	Central Meseta	159	8.80
	Andalusia	124	6.50
	Galacia	143	9.90
	Basque	224	11.10
Robson & Harris 1966	Greeks:		
	Village A (Arta region)	138	9.00
	Village B (Arta region)	100	29.00
Asia			
Robson & Harris 1966	Iraqi Jews	64	0.00
Singh *et al.* 1974	Punjabis:		
	Brahmin	106	9.40
	Aroro	103	6.80
	Khattri	132	6.80
	Jat	159	10.10
Goedde *et al.* 1972c	Assamese	75	11.00
Goedde *et al.* 1972c	Khasis	59	13.30
Steegmüller 1975	Bengalis & Biharis	550	3.60
Ananthakrishnan & Kirk 1967	Madras Indians	267	0.00
Gopalam & Rao 1981	Vysyas of Andhra Pradesh	731	0.14
Rao *et al.* 1985	Hyderabad, India:		
	1 Brahmins		
	(a) Niyogi	237	5.06
	(b) Madwa	255	5.10
	(c) Dravida	172	4.65
	(d) Vadahalai	200	2.00
	(e) Tengalai	205	2.44
	(f) Vaidiki		
	(i) Eluru	90	3.33
	(ii) Amalapuram	136	1.47
	(iii) Manthini	141	2.84

Table 14.9. (*cont.*)

Reference	Population	Number tested	% C₅+
Rao *et al.* 1985	(iv) Hyderabad	200	6.50
	2 Vysyas	1498	0.20
	3 Reddy	248	1.21
	4 Kamma	103	0.97
	5 Padmasali	217	0.00
	6 Mudiraj	184	1.08
	7 Kurma	116	1.72
	8 Gowda	201	1.50
	9 Munnuru Kapu	203	0.98
	10 Besta	95	0.00
	11 Madiga	138	1.45
	12 Mala	173	0.00
	II Muslims		
	(a) Sunnis		
	(i) Hyderabad	343	1.17
	(ii) Mahboobnagar	178	11.80
	(b) Shias	40	5.00
	(c) Bohras	58	8.62
	(d) Khojas	216	1.85
	(e) Mehdwi Patans	60	0.00
Simpson 1968	Thais	81	14.00
Steegmüller 1975	Koreans	47	2.10
Omoto & Harada 1968	Japanese	237	8.43
	Ainu	195	5.64
Oimomi *et al.* 1988	Japanese	563	1.24
Australia			
Horsfall *et al.* 1963	Aborigines	104	0.00
Africa			
El Hassan *et al.* 1968	Beja of Eastern Sudan	100	1.00
Van Ros & Vervoort 1973	Zaïrians	200	3.50
Steegmüller 1975	Nigerians	68	2.90
Steegmüller 1975	Senegalese	224	2.20
Steegmüller 1975	Mozambiqueans	331	1.30
Steegmüller 1975	Angolese	303	1.30
Krause *et al.* 1987	South Africans:		
	Ashkenazim	461	8.03
	Afrikaner	255	10.59
	San (!Kung)	86	10.46
	Zulus	67	1.49
	Taung	213	3.29
	Ngwato	110	4.50
	Coloured	61	3.28
Whittaker & Lowe 1976	Rhodesian Africans	881	1.70
	Mozambique Africans	41	4.88
	Malawi Africans	102	0.98
	Zambian Africans	10	0.00
Vergnes *et al.* 1979	Aka Pygmies of Central Africa	858	12.90
Nurse & Jenkins 1977	South African desert dwellers:		
	Kuiseb Topnaar	57	0.00
	Sesfontain Topnaar	40	2.50
	Dama	91	6.60
	Dobe !Kung	98	5.10

Table 14.9. (*cont.*)

Reference	Population	Number tested	% C_5+
Eskimos			
Scott *et al.* 1970	Marshall	74	0.00
Scott *et al.* 1970	Pilot Station	99	2.00
Scott *et al.* 1970	St Marys	151	1.30
Scott *et al.* 1970	Mountain Village	151	6.00
Scott *et al.* 1970	Chevak	225	4.90
Scott *et al.* 1970	Hooper Bay	357	1.10
Scott *et al.* 1970	Emmonak	242	12.80
Scott *et al.* 1970	Kotlik	150	8.70
Scott *et al.* 1970	Unalakleet	151	2.00
Singh *et al.* 1974	Greenland Eskimos	146	11.00
Simpson 1972	Canadian Eskimos (Igloolik)	298	13.10
North America			
Lavrien *et al.* 1978	Americans		9.10
Ashton & Simpson 1966	Canadians	726	7.00
Ashton & Simpson 1966	Seattle Negroes	317	5.00
Robson & Harris 1966	Seattle Negroes	100	2.00
Tashian *et al.* 1967	Xavanthe Indians	285	0.00
Simpson 1968	Cree Indians	589	14.00
South America			
Arends *et al.* 1970	Venezuelans Makiritare	418	11.50
Arends *et al.* 1967	Venezuelans Motilon	70	1.40
Arends *et al.* 1967	Venezuelans Warrau	131	0.00
Vergnes *et al.* 1976	Bolivians Sirionó	65	0.00
Guerreiro *et al.* 1985	Brazilians Wayana-Apalai	127	7.90
Primo-Parmo *et al.* 1986	Brazilians Mura	112	1.80
Primo-Parmo *et al.* 1986	Brazilians Tenharim	23	8.70
Primo-Parmo *et al.* 1986	Brazilians Sateré-Mawé	188	0.00
Primo-Parmo *et al.* 1986	Brazilians Pacaás-Novos	219	15.10
Primo-Parmo *et al.* 1986	Brazilians Krahó	94	8.50
Primo-Parmo *et al.* 1986	Brazilians Kaingang and Guarani	27	0.00
Primo-Parmo *et al.* 1986	Brazilians Kaingang	57	24.60
Guerreiro & Santos 1987	Brazilians Munduruku	194	11.30
Guerreiro & Santos 1987	Brazilians Parakanã	123	0.00
Guerreiro *et al.* 1987	Brazilians Urubu-Kaapor	210	26.20
Guerreiro *et al.* 1987	Brazilians Assurini	162	0.00
Ashton & Simpson 1966	Brazilians (mixed population)	2102	8.10
Chautard-Freire-Maia *et al.* 1990	Blumenau Santa Catarina Brazil (mixed ethnic group)	689	6.82
Chautard-Freire-Maia *et al.* 1984c	Curitiba	320	4.69
Pacific Islands			
Simpson 1968	Easter Islanders	497	0.00
Tristan da Cunha			
Robson & Harris 1966	Islanders	214	17.00

means one person in 187 is a homozygote. A similar estimate was found for Iranian Jews. In African Negro and Oriental populations the average allele frequency is 0.0002 indicating one homozygote in 25×10^6 persons.

The E_1^j allele is rare in most populations (Table 14.7). The frequency of about 0.0021 in Europeans indicates one homozygote in 227×10^3 persons. One sample comprised of Punjabis shows an unexpectedly high frequency (Singh *et al.* 1971b). In Zimbabweans the frequency of the homozygote should be $1/0.0358^2 = 1$ in 783 (Dr M. Whittaker, personal communication).

The frequency of the homozygote $E_1^s E_1^s$ has been estimated to be 1 to 8 in 100 000 of Caucasian populations (Simpson & Kalow 1964). Very few population surveys of this gene have been conducted, and their results are shown in Table 14.8. Most surveys have been of families acertained by means of a proband who displayed the phenomenon of prolonged apnoea after succinylcholine. Examples of silent homozygotes have been recorded in American Caucasians (Lubin *et al.* 1973), Japanese (Miyamoto *et al.* 1987), Bantu (Jenkins *et al.* 1967), white South Africans (Pannall *et al.* 1976) and Icelanders (Arnason *et al.* 1975). It is likely that high gene frequencies for E_1^s in small populations of Alaskan Eskimos and inbred Vysyas of Andhra Pradesh are due to genetic drift or founder effect.

The $C_5 +$ character determined electrophoretically has a frequency of about 10% in Europeans (this figure represents the homozygous dominants plus the heterozygotes). In other ethnic groups the frequencies are lower but as with all alleles described in this chapter odd anomalies occur, for example, the high figure of 14% obtained for Thais by Simpson (1968); such instances are probably the result of a quirk of sampling (Table 14.9).

The rare C_6, C_{7a} and C_{7b} electrophoretic variants have hitherto been described in only Africans.

Gene frequency estimates for the quantitative alleles E_1^j and E_1^k are mainly available for Caucasian samples as discussed earlier. However, Alcantara *et al.* (1990), studying a sample of 49 from a mixed race population in Southern Brazil using α-naphthyl acetate as substrate and RO2-0683 and DL-propanolol as inhibitors found only one heterozygous CHE1 AK individual. They suggest that the British estimates for the E_1^k allele may be too high because of ascertainment being biased by patients who had sustained prolonged apnoea.

It seems likely that the use of allele-specific gene probes combined with the polymerase chain reaction will lead to more extensive population surveys in different ethnic groups.

The author would like to express his gratitude to Dr Mary Whittaker, Department of Environmental Sciences, Polytechnic South West, Plymouth, Devon, UK and Dr Richard F. Seed, Department of Anaesthesia, Riyadh Armed Forces Hospital, Saudi Arabia who made many helpful suggestions about the contents of this chapter.

Appendix 14.1. Reference centres for phenotyping cholinesterase variants

Anaesthetic Dept
(Dr J. J. Britten)
Royal Postgraduate Medical School
Hammersmith Hospital
Du Cane Road
Hammersmith London W12 0HS
United Kingdom

Tel. 081-743-2030 Ext. 2295
Fax. 081 743 3987

Clinical Biochemistry Dept
(Dr R. T. Coans)
St. James University Hospital
Beckett Street
Leeds LS9 7TF
United Kingdom

Tel. 0532 433144
Fax. 0532 426496

Institute of Biochemistry
(Dr R. Campbell)
Royal Infirmary
Castle Street
Glasgow G4 0SF
United Kingdom

Tel. 041-552-3535
Fax. 041-304-4889

Danish Cholinesterase Research Unit (DCRU)
Dept of Anaesthesia
(Dr F. Jensen)
Rigshospitalet
University of Copenhagen
Blegdamsvej 9
DK-2100 Copenhagen
Denmark

Tel. 45-35-45-34-74
Fax. 45-35-45-29-50

Dept. of Biological Chemistry
(Prof. H. Soreq)
Institute of Life Sciences
The Hebrew University of Jerusalem
Jerusalem 91904
Israel

Tel. 2-585-450, 585-109
Fax. 2-520-258, 666-804

(Note this is a research laboratory only, not a clinical reference centre.)

Dept of Laboratory Medicine
(Dr M. J. McQueen)
Hamilton General Division
Hamilton Civic Hospitals
237 Barton Street East
Hamilton Ontario L8L 2X2
Canada

Tel. 416-527-0271 Ext. 6101
Fax. 416-577-8027

Dept. of Anesthesiology
(Prof. B. N. La Du, Jr)
The University of Michigan Medical School R4038
Kresge II Building
Ann Arbor, MI 48109-0572.
USA

Tel. 313-763-6429
Fax. 313-936-9091, 313-763-4450

Genetics Department
(Prof. E. A. Chautard Freire Maia)
Federal University of Paraná
PO Box 19071
81531-970 Curitiba, PR
Brazil

Tel. 0055-041-2663633 Ext. 259
Fax. 0055-041 2662042

Agarwal, D. P., Goedde, H. W., Schloot, W, Flatz, G. & Rohde, R. (1973). A note on atypical serum cholinesterase and genetic factors in leprosy. *Human Heredity*, **23**, 370–3.

Agarwal, D. P., Schwenkenbecker, S., Srivastava, L. M. & Goedde, H. W. (1975). Spektrophotometrische Bestimmungsmethode für Serumcholinesterase (EC 3.1.1.8) – Varienten mit Succinylbischolin als Substrat. *Zeitschrift für Klinische Chemie und Klinische Biochemie*, **13**, 133–5.

Agarwal, D. P, Srivastava, L. M. & Goedde, H. W. (1976). A note on suxamethonium sensitivity and serum cholinesterase variants. *Human Genetics*, **32**, 85–8.

Alcantara, V. M., Chautard-Freire-Maia, E. A. & Culpi, L. (1991b). CHE1 UF serum cholinesterase phenotype in white and non-whites from southern Brazil as determined by a new method. *Human Heredity*, **41**, 103–6.

Alcantara, V. M., Chautard-Freire-Maia, E. A., Picheth, G. & Vieira, M. M. (1990). Frequency of the CHE1*K allele of serum cholinesterase in a sample from Southern Brazil. *Human Heredity*, **40**, 386–90.

Alcantara, V. M., Chautard-Freire-Maia, E. A., Picheth, G. & Vieira, M. M. (1991a). A method for serum cholinesterase phenotyping. *Revista Brasileira de Genetica*, **14**, 841–6.

Altland, K., Bucher, R., Kim, T. W., Busch, H., Brockelmann, C. & Goedde, H. W. (1969). Population genetic studies on cholinesterase polymorphism in Germany, Czechoslovakia, Finland and among Lapps. *Humangenetik*, **8**, 158–61.

Altland, K., Epple, F. & Goedde, H. W. (1967). Cholinesterase variants in Thailand and Japan. *Humangenetik*, **4**, 127–9.

Altland, K. & Goedde, H. W. (1970). Heterogeneity in the silent gene phenotype of cholinesterase of human serum. *Biochemical Genetics*, **4**, 321–38.

Ananthakrishnan, R. & Kirk, L. R. (1967). The distribution of some serum protein and enzyme group systems in two endogamous groups in South India. *Indian Journal of Medical Research*, **57**, 1011–7.

Annapurna. V., Senciall, I., Davis, A. J. & Kutty, K. M. (1991). Relationship between serum pseudocholinesterase and triglycerides in experimentally induced diabetes mellitus in rats. *Diabetologia*, **34**, 320–4.

Arends, T., Davies, D. A, & Lehmann, H. (1967). Absence of variants of usual serum cholinesterase (acylcholine acylhydrolase) in South American Indians. *Acta Genetica (Basel)*, **17**, 13–6.

Arends, T., Westkamp, L. R., Gallango, M. L., Neel, J. W. & Schultz, J. (1970). Gene frequencies and microdifferentiation among the Makiritare Indians. II. Seven serum protein systems. *American Journal of Human Genetics*, **22**, 526–32.

Arnason, A., Jensson, O. & Gudmundsson, S. (1975). Serum esterases of Icelanders I A 'silent' pseudocholinesterase gene in an Icelandic family. *Clinical Genetics*, **7**, 405–12.

Arnaud, J. Brun, H., Llobera, R. & Constans, J. (1991). Serum cholinesterase polymorphism in France: an epidemiological survey of the deficient alleles detected by an automated micro-method. *Annals of Human Biology*, **18**, 1–8.

Arnold, W. P. (1981). A rapid semi-automated method for determining dibucaine numbers. *Anesthesiology*, **55**, 676–679.

Arpagaus, M., Kott, M., Vatsis, K. P., Bartels, C. F., LaDu, B. N. & Lockridge, O. (1990). Structure of the gene for human butyrylcholinesterase. Evidence for a single copy. *Biochemistry*, **29**, 124–31.

Ashby, T. M., Suggs, J. E. & Jue, D. L. (1970). Detection of atypical cholinesterase by an automated pH stat method. *Clinical Chemistry*, **16**, 503–6.

Ashton, G. C. & Simpson, N. E. (1966). C_5-types of serum cholinesterase in a Brazilian population. *American Journal of Human Genetics*, **18**, 438–47.

Bajatzadeh, M., Neumann, S. & Walter, H. (1969). Cholinesterases and human red cell acid phosphatases in Koreans. *Humangenetik*, **7**, 91–2.

Bang, U., Viby-Mogensen, J. & Wiren, J. E. (1990). The effect of bambuterol on plasma cholinesterase activity and suxamethonium- induced neuromuscular blockade in subjects heterozygous for abnormal plasma cholinesterase. *Acta Anaesthesiologica Scandinavica*, **34**, 600–4.

Bartels, C. F., James, K. & La Du, B. N. (1992b). DNA mutations associated with the human butyrylcholinesterase J- variant. *American Journal of Human Genetics*, **50**, 1104–14.

Bartels, C. F., Jensen, F. S., Lockridge. O, van der Spek, A. F. L., Rubinstein, H. M., Lubrano, T. & La Du, B. N. (1992a). DNA mutation associated with the human butyrylcholinesterase K-variant and its linkage to the atypical variant mutation and other polymorphic sites. *American Journal of Human Genetics*, **50**, 1086–103.

Becker, C. E. (1972). Screening of 563 students for cholinesterase variants. *Clinical Chemistry*, **18**, 75–6.

Benzer, A., Luz, G., Oswald, E., Schmoigl, C. & Menardi, G. (1992). Succinylcholine-induced prolonged apnoea in a 3-week old newborn: treatment and human plasma cholinesterase. *Anesthesia and Analgesia*, **74**, 137–8.

Bevan, D.R. & Donati, F. (1983). Anticholinesterase antagonism of succinylcholine phase II block. *Canadian Anaesthetists Society Journal*, **30**, 569–72.

Boman, H. (1981). Distribution of the E_1^a gene among Norwegian blood donors studied by an automated screening method. *Human Heredity*, **31**, 308–11.

Bouloux. C,, Gomilo, J. & Langaney, A. (1972). Hemotypology of the Bedik. *Human Biology*, **44**, 289–302. (Cited by Whittaker & Reys 1975.)

Boutin, D. & Brodeur, J. (1971). Human serum cholinesterases: molecular weight estimation of a subunit structure. *Canadian Journal of Physiology and Pharmacology*, **49**, 777–9.

Bowman, H. & Habib, Z. (1983). Serum cholinesterase loci E_1 and E_2 polymorphisms among Egyptians. *Hereditas*, **99**, 1–6.

Brock, A. (1988). Plasma cholinesterase genetic variants phenotyped using a Cobas–Fara centrifugal analyser. *Journal of Clinical Chemistry and Clinical Biochemistry*, **26**, 873–5.

Burgess, A. M. (1988). Identification of the $E_1^t E_1^k$ cholinesterase genotype. *Journal of Medical Genetics*, **25**, 554–6.

Cardan, E. & Schopp, K. (1986). Plasma cholinesterase variants in a Romanian population. *European Journal of Anaesthesiology*, **3**, 481.

Chautard-Freire-Maia, E. A, Carvalho, R. D. S, daSilva, M. C. B. O., Souza, Md. G. F. & Azevedo, E. S. (1984b). Frequencies of atypical serum cholinesterase in a mixed population of North Eastern Brazil. *Human Heredity*, **34**, 364–70.

Chautard-Freire-Maia, E. A., Lourenço, M. A. C. & Jugend, R.M. (1984c). Phenotype frequencies of the CHE2 locus of serum cholinesterase in a sample collected in Curitiba. *Revista Brasileira de Genetica*, **7**, 709–15.

Chautard-Freire-Maia, E. A., Primo-Parmo, S. L., Lourenço, M. A. C. & Culpi, L. (1984a). Frequencies of atypical serum cholinesterase among Caucasians and Negroes from Southern Brazil. *Human Heredity*, **34**, 388–92.

Chautard-Freire-Maia, E. A., Primo-Parmo, S. L., Picheth, G., Lourenço, M. A. C. & Vieira, M. M. (1991). The C_5 isozyme of serum cholinesterase and adult weight. *Human Heredity*, **41**, 330–9.

Chautard-Freire-Maia, E. A., Stueber-Odebrecht, N., Junge, C., Lourenço, M. A. C., Primo-Parmo, S. L. & Carrenho, J. M. X. (1990). Phenotypes of the CHE2 locus of serum cholinesterase and adult weight in a sample from Blumenau, Santa Catarina, Brazil. *Revista Brasileira de Genetica*, **13**, 371–6.

Crowley, M. F. & Lehmann, H. (1962). Test papers for determining plasma cholinesterase. *British Medical Journal*, **3**, 609–10.

Cruz, J. M., Bender, K., Burckhardt, K., Küppers. F., Benkmann, H. G. & Goedde, H. W. (1973). Genetic studies of some red cell and serum protein polymorphisms in the population of Vilarinho da Furna (Portugal). *Anais da Faculdadi Ciencias do Porto- Extracto do fax do*, **54**, 3–15.

Cucuianu, M. (1988). Cholinesterase and lipoproteins. *Atherosclerosis*, **72**, 83–4.

Cucuianu, M., Popescu, T. A. & Haragus, St. (1968). Cholinesterase in obese and hyperlipemic subjects. *Clinica Chimica Acta*, **22**, 151–5.

Curtain, C. C., Gadjusek, D. C., Kidson, C., Gorman, J., Champness, L. & Rodrique, R. (1965). *American Journal of Tropical Medicine and Hygiene*, **14**, 671–7.

Das, P. K., Kattamis, C., Haidas, S. & Liddell, J. (1975). Validity of a screening test for typing serum cholinesterase variants among Greek populations. *Human Heredity*, **25**, 429–41.

Das, P. K. & Liddell, J. (1970). Purification and properties of human serum cholinesterase. *Biochemical Journal*, **116**, 875–81.

Delbrück, A. & Henkel, E. (1979). A rare genetically determined variant of cholinesterase in two German families with high plasma enzyme activity. *European Journal of Biochemistry*, **99**, 65–9.

Demeester, P. (1965) Fréquence de la pseudocholinestérase atypique dans le population bantoue du Congo. *Acta Anaesthesiologica Belgica*, **16**, 42–4.

Eiberg, H., Nielson, L. S., Klausen, J., Dahlen, M., Kristensen, M., Bisgaard, M. L., Møller, N. & Mohr, J. (1989). Linkage between serum cholinesterase 2 (CHE2) and γ-crystallin gene cluster (CRYG): assignment to chromosome 2. *Clinical Genetics*, **35**, 313–21.

El Hassan, A. M., Godber, M. G., Kopec, A. C., Mourant, A. E., Tills, D. & Lehmann, H. (1968). The hereditary blood factors of the Beja of the Sudan. *Man*, **3**, 272–83.

Evans, R. T., Iqbal, J., Dietz, A. A., Lubrano, T. & Rubinstein, H. M. (1980). A family segregating for E$_1^j$ and E$_1^k$ at cholinesterase locus 1. *Journal of Medical Genetics*, **17**, 464–7.

Evans, R. T. & Wardell, J. (1984). On the identification and frequency of the J and K cholinesterase phenotypes in a Caucasian population. *Journal of Medical Genetics*, **21**, 99–102.

Fraser, G. R., Grünwald, P., Kitchin, F. D. & Steinberg, A.G. (1969). Serum polymorphisms in Yugoslavia. *Human Heredity*, **19**, 57–64.

Fraser, G. R., Steinberg, A. G., Defaranas, B., Mayo, O., Stamatoyannopoulos, G. & Motulsky, A. G. (1969). Gene frequencies at loci determining blood-group and serum-protein polymorphisms in two villages in North-Western Greece. *American Journal of Human Genetics*, **21**, 46–60.

Fraser, G. R., Volkers, W. S., Bernini, L. F., Loghem, E., Meera Khan, P. & Nijenhuis, L .E. (1974). Gene frequencies in a Dutch population. *Human Heredity*, **24**, 435–40.

Ganendran, A., Ogle, C. W. (1975). Absence of abnormal variants of cholinesterase (E.C. 3.1.1.1.8.) in a Malaysian population with three major racial groups. *Singapore Medical Journal*, **16**, 256–8.

Garcia, C. H. & Diaz, P. M. (1972). Atypical cholinesterase. Frequency in a Puerto Rican population. *Anesthesiology*, **36**, 81–2.

Garry, P. J. (1971a). Serum cholinesterase variants: examination of several differential inhibitors, salts and buffers used to measure enzyme activity. *Clinical Chemistry*, **17**, 183–91.

Garry, P. J. (1971b) A manual and automated procedure for measuring serum cholinesterase activity and identifying enzyme variants. *Clinical Chemistry*, **17**, 192–8.

Garry, P. J. (1977). Atypical (E$_1^a$) and fluoride-resistant (E$_1^f$) cholinesterase genes: Absent in a native American Indian population. *Human Heredity*, **27**, 433–6.

Garry, P. J., Dietz, A. A., Lubrano, T., Ford, P. C., James, K. & Rubinstein, H. M.·(1976). New allele at cholinesterase locus 1. *Journal of Medical Genetics*, **13**, 38–42.

Garry, P. J, Own, G. M. & Lubin. A. H. (1972). Identification of serum cholinesterase fluoride variants by differential inhibition in Tris and phosphate buffers. *Clinical Chemistry*, **18**, 105–9.

Goedde, H. W, & Agarwal, D. P. (1978). Cholinesterase variation. Human genetic variation in response to medical and environmental agents: pharmacogenetics and ecogenetics. *Human Genetics*, Suppl. 1, 45–55.

Goedde, H. W., Agarwal, D. P. & Benkmann, H.-G. (1979). Pharmaco-genetics of cholinesterase: New variants and suxamethonium sensitivity. *Ärztliche Laboratorium*, **25**, 219–24.

Goedde, H. W. & Altland, K. (1963). Cholinesterase variants in Germany and Czechoslovakia. *Nature*, **189**, 1203–4.

Goedde, H. W., Altland, K. & Bross, K. (1963). Genetik und Biochemie der Cholinesterasen. *Deutsche Medizinische Wochenschrift*, **52**, 2510–22.

Goedde, H. W., Altland, K. & Schloot, W. (1968). Therapy of prolonged apnoea after suxamethonium with purified cholinesterase: new data on kinetics of the hydrolysis of succinyldicholine and succinylmonocholine and further data on *N*-acetyltransferase polymorphism. *Annals of the New York Academy of Sciences*, **151**, (Art 2), 742–52.

Goedde, H. W., Benkmann, H. G., Singh, S., Das, B, Chakravatti, M., Flatz, G. & Delbrück H. (1972c). Polymorphism of some serum proteins and blood enzymes in the population of Assam. *Human Heredity*, **22**, 331–7.

Goedde, H. W., Deoenicke, A. & Altland K. (1967). *Cholinesterasen – Pharmakogenetik, Biochemie, Klinik*, Berlin, Springer, p. 46.

Goedde, H. W., Gehring, D. & Hofmann, R. A. (1965a). On the problem of a 'silent' gene in cholinesterase polymorphism. *Biochimica et Biophysica Acta*, **107**, 391–3.

Goedde, H. W., Gehring, D. & Hofmann, R. A. (1965b). Biochemische Untersuchungen zur Frage der Existenz eines, 'Silent Gene' im Polymorphismus der Cholinesterasen. *Humangenetik*, **1**, 607–20.

Goedde, H. W., Held, K. R. & Altland, K. (1968). Hydrolysis of succinyldicholine and succinylmonocholine in human serum. *Molecular Pharmacology*, **4**, 274–87.

Goedde, H. W., Hirth, L., Benkmann, H. G., Singh, S., Stahn, M., Pellicer, A. & Pellicer, T. (1972b). Serum protein and enzyme polymorphism in four Spanish populations. *Human Heredity*, **22**, 552–60.

Goedde, H. W., Hirth, L., Benkmann, H.-G., Singh, S. & Wendt, G. (1972a). Family studies on the third component of complement (C'3) α$_1$-antitrypsin and cholinesterase polymorphism (locus E$_1$ and E$_2$) in the area of Marburg (Germany). *Humangenetik*, **17**, 85–7.

Goedde, H. W., Omoto, K., Ritter, H. & Baitsch, H. (1964). Zur formalen Genetik der Cholinesterasen.

Untersuchungen von 408 Familien. *Humangenetik*, **1**, 1–13.

Gomar, C., Doria, A., Carrasco, M. S., Cobo, I., Fernandez, M. C., Pons, M., Andreu, L., Gil, C. & Nalda y, M. A. (1986). Estudio genético de las colinesterasas plasmáticas en la poblacion adulta de Barcelona. *Revista Española de Anesthesiologia y Reanimacion*, **33**, 323–4.

Gopalam, K. B. & Rao, P. R. Genetic studies on Vysyas of Andhra Pradesh, S. (1981). India, A_1 A_2 BO, Rh(O)D, Transferrin, group specific component, haptoglobin and pseudocholinesterase types. *Acta Anthropogenetica*, **5**, 175–80.

Grobler S. M. & Potgieter, G. M. (1986). Cholinesterase variants in a South African population. *South African Medical Journal*, **70**, 319–21.

Guerreiro, J. F., dos Santos, S. E. B., Canever de Lourenço, M.A., Primo-Parmo, S.L. & Chautard-Freire-Maia, E.A. (1987). Serum cholinesterase polymorphism (CHE1 and CHE2 loci) in Indians from the Amazon region of Brazil: Urubu-Kaapor and Assurini tribes. *Revista Brasileira de Genetica*, **10**, 781–5.

Guerreiro, J. F. & Santos, S. E. B. (1987). Studies on serum cholinesterase (CHE1 and CHE2 loci) among Indians from the Amazon region of Brazil: Munduruku and Parakaña tribes. *Revista Brasileira Genetica*, **10**, 559–64.

Guerreiro, J. F., Santos, S. E. B. & Black, F. L. (1985). Frequencies of the atypical and C_5 variants of serum cholinesterase in Wayana-Apalai Indians. *Revista Brasileira Genetica*, **8**, 123–9.

Gutsche, B. B., Scott, E. M. & Wright, R. C. (1967). Hereditary deficiency of cholinesterase in Eskimos. *Nature*, **215**, 322–3.

Hajra, A., Sorenson, R. C. & La Du, B. N. (1992). Detection of human DNA mutations with non-radioactive, allele-specific oligonucleotide probes. *Pharmacogenetics*, **2**, 78–88.

Hanel, H. K. & Viby-Mogensen, J. (1971). Urea inhibition of human cholinesterase. *British Journal of Anaesthesia*, **43**, 51–3.

Hanel, H. K., Viby-Mogensen, J. & Schaffalitzky de Muckadell, O. B. (1978). Serum cholinesterase variants in the Danish populations. *Acta Anaesthesiologica Scandinavica*, **22**, 505–7.

Hangaard, J., Whittaker, M., Loft, A. G. R. & Nørgaard-Pedersen, B. (1991). Quantification and phenotyping of serum cholinesterase by enzyme antigen immunoassay: methodological aspects and clinical applicability. *Scandinavian Journal of Clinical and Laboratory Investigation*, **51**, 349–58.

Hansen, W. E. & Bertl, S. (1983). The inhibition of acetylcholinesterase and cholinesterase by cimetidine. *Arzneimittel-Forschung/Drug Research*, **33**, 161–3.

Harris, H., Hopkinson, D. A. Robson, E. B. & Whittaker, M. (1963). Genetical studies on a new variant of serum cholinesterase detected by electrophoresis. *Annals of Human Genetics (London)*, **26**, 359–82.

Harris, H. & Robson, E. B. (1963). Screening tests for the 'atypical' and 'intermediate' serum-cholinesterase types. *Lancet*, **2**, 218–21.

Harris, H. & Whittaker, M. (1962a). The serum cholinesterase variants. A study of twenty-two families selected via the 'intermediate' phenotype. *Annals of Human Genetics (London)*, **26**, 59–72.

Harris, H. & Whittaker, M. (1962b). Differential inhibition of

the serum cholinesterase phenotypes by solanine and solanidine. *Annals of Human Genetics (London)*, **26**, 73–6.

Hazel, B. & Monier, D. (1971). Human serum cholinesterase: variations during pregnancy and post-partum. *Canadian Anaesthetists Society Journal*, **18**, 272–7.

Hickey, D. R. (1987). Use of succinylcholine in patients with decreased plasma cholinesterase activity. *Anesthesia and Analgesia*, **66**, 1049-1060.

Hiernaux, J. (1976). Blood polymorphism frequencies in the Sara Majingay of Chad. *Annals of Human Biology*, **3**, 127–40.

Hobbiger, F. & Peck, A. W. (1969). Hydrolysis of suxamethonium by different types of plasma. *British Journal of Pharmacology*, **37**, 258–71.

Hodgkin, W. E., Giblett, E. R., Levine. H., Bauer. W. & Motulsky, A. G. (1965). Complete cholinesterase deficiency; genetic and immunologic characterization. *Journal of Clinical Investigation*, **44**, 486–93.

Horsfall. W. R., Lehmann, H. & Davies, D. (1963). Incidence of cholinesterase variants in Australian Aborigines. *Nature*, **199**, 1115.

Jenkins, T., Balinsky, D. & Patient, D. W. (1967). Cholinesterase in plasma. First report of absence in the Bantu. *Science*, **156**, 1748–50.

Kalow, W. (1964). The influence of pH on the hydrolysis of benzoylcholine by cholinesterase by human plasma. *Canadian Journal of Physiology and Pharmacology*, **42**, 161–8.

Kalow, W. (1990). Pharmacogenetics, Past and Future. *Life Sciences*, **47**, 1385–97.

Kalow, W. & Genest, K. (1957). A method for the detection of atypical forms of human serum cholinesterase. Determination of dibucaine numbers. *Canadian Journal of Biochemistry and Physiology*, **35**, 339–46.

Kalow, W., Genest, K. & Staron, N. (1956). Kinetic studies on the hydrolysis of benzoylcholine by human serum cholinesterase. *Canadian Journal of Biochemistry and Physiology*, **34**, 637–53.

Kalow, W. & Gunn, D. R. (1959). Some statistical data on atypical cholinesterase of human serum. *Annals of Human Genetics (London)*, **23**, 239–50.

Kalow, W. & Staron, N. (1957). On distribution and inheritance of atypical forms of human serum cholinesterase, as indicated by dibucaine numbers. *Canadian Journal of Biochemistry and Physiology*, **35**, 1305–20.

Kambam, J. R., Parris, W. C. V., Naukam, R. J., Franks, J. J. & Rama Sastry, B. V. (1990). *In vitro* effects of fluoride and bromide on cholinesterase and acetylcholinesterase activities. *Canadian Journal of Anaesthesia*, **37**, 916–9.

Kattamis, Ch., Zannus-Mariolea, L., Franco, A. P., Liddell, J., Lehmann, H. & Davies, D. (1962). Frequency of atypical cholinesterase in British and Mediterranean populations. *Nature*, **196**, 599–600.

Khoury, G. F. (1988). Atypical serum cholinesterase eliminated by orthotopic liver transplantation. *Anesthesiology*, **68**, 474.

Khoury, G. F., Brill, J., Walts, I. & Busuttil, R.W. (1987). Atypical serum cholinesterase eliminated by orthotopic liver transplantation. *Anesthesiology*, **67**, 273–4.

Kidd, K. K. & Gusella, J. (1985). Report of the committee on the genetic constitution of chromosome 3 and 4 HGM 8. *Cytogenetics and Cell Genetics (Basel)*, **40**, 107–27.

Klein, H., Ğartner, K. & Günther, R. (1967). Die Variente C₅ der cholinesterase des Serums. *Deutsche Zeitschrift für gerichtlichen Medizinsche*, **61**, 137–47. (Cited by Steegmüller 1975.)

Krause, A., Lane, A. B. & Jenkins, T. (1987). Cholinesterase variation in southern African populations. *South African Medical Journal*, **71**, 298–301.

Krause, A., Lane, A. B. & Jenkins, T. (1988). A new high activity plasma cholinesterase variant. *Journal of Medical Genetics*, **25**, 677–81.

Kutty, K. M., Jain. R., Huang, S.-N. & Kean, K. (1981). Serum cholinesterase: high density lipoprotein cholesterol ratio as an index or risk for cardiovascular disease. *Clinica Chimica Acta*, **115**, 55–61.

La Du, B. N. (1989). Identification of human serum cholinesterase variants using the polymerase chain reaction amplification technique. *Trends in Pharmacological Sciences*, **10**, 309–13.

La Du, B. N., Bartels, C. F., Nogueira, C. P., Hajra, A., Lightstone, H., Van der Spek, A. & Lockridge, O. (1990). Phenotypic and molecular biological analysis of human butyryl cholinesterase variants. *Clinical Biochemistry*, **23**, 423–31.

La Du, B. N. & Lockridge, O. (1986). Molecular biology of human serum cholinesterase. *Federation Proceedings*, **45**, 2965–69.

Lainé-Cessac, P., Turcant, A. & Allain, P. (1989). Automated determination of cholinesterase activity in plasma and erythrocytes by flow-injection analysis and application to identify subjects sensitive to succinylcholine. *Clinical Chemistry*, **35**, 77–80.

LaMotta, R. V. & Woronick, C. L. (1971). Molecular heterogeneity of human serum cholinesterase. *Clinical Chemistry*, **17**, 135–44.

Lee. J.-H. & Chang, J.-B. (1987). Determination of genetic variants of serum cholinesterase in healthy adults and patients with liver diseases. *Journal of the Formosan Medical Association*, **86**, 255–8.

Lehman, H. & Davies, D. (1962). Identification of the cholinesterase type in human blood spots. *Medicine Science and the Law*, **2**, 180–3.

Lehmann, H. & Liddell, J. (1961). The cholinesterases. In *Modern Trends in Anaesthesia 2*, ed. F.T. Evans & T. C. Gray, Chapter 8, pp 164–205. London: Butterworths.

Lehmann, H, Liddell, J, Blackwell, B., O'Connor, D. C. & Daws, A. V. (1963). Two further serum cholinesterase phenotypes as causes of suxamethonium apnoea. *British Medical Journal*, **1**, 1116–8.

Lehmann, H. & Ryan, E. (1956). The familial incidence of low cholinesterase level. *Lancet*, **2**, 124.

Lehtonen, A., Marniemi, J., Inberg, M., Maatela, J., Alanen, E. & Niittymäki, K. (1986). Levels of serum lipids, Apoli β proteins A- 1 and B and cholinesterase activity and their discriminative values in patients with coronary by-pass operation. *Atherosclerosis*, **59**, 215–21.

Liddell, J. (1968). Cholinesterase variants and suxamethonium apnoea. *Proceedings of the Royal Society of Medicine*, **61**, 168–70.

Liddell, J., Lehmann, H. & Davies, D. (1963). Harris and Whittaker's cholinesterase variant with increased resistance to fluoride – a study of four families and the identification of the homozygote. *Acta Genetica (Basel)*, **13**, 95–108.

Liddell. J., Lehmann, H., Davies, D. & Sharih, A. (1962b).

Physical separation of cholinesterase variants in human sera. *Lancet*, **1**, 463–4.

Liddell, J., Lehmann, H. & Silk, E. (1962a). A 'silent' cholinesterase gene. *Nature*, **193**, 561–2.

Lisker. B., Cordova, M. S. & Graciela Zarate, Q. B. P. (1969). Studies on several genetic hematological traits of the Mexican population. *American Journal of Physical Anthropology*, **30**, 349–54.

Lisker, R., DelMoral, C. & Loria, A. (1964). Frequency of the atypical cholinesterase in four Indian (Mexican) tribes. *Nature*, **202**, 815.

Lisker, R., Loria, A. & Zarate, G. (1967). Studies on several genetic haematological traits of the Mexican population. *Acta Genetica (Basel)*, **17**, 524–9.

Lisker, R., Reyes, G. R., Lopez, G., Peral, A. M. & Zarate, G. (1966). Caracteristicas hematologicas hereditarias de la poblacion Mexicana. *Revista de Investigacion Clinica (Mexico City)*, **18**, 11–21.

Lisker, R., Zarate, G. & Rodriguez, E. (1967). Studies on several genetic hematological traits of the Mexican population. *American Journal of Physical Anthropology*, **27**, 27–32.

Lockridge, O. (1988). Structure of human serum cholinesterase. *Bioessays*, **9**, 125–8.

Lockridge, O. (1990). Genetic variants of human serum cholinesterase influence metabolism of the muscle relaxant succinylcholine. *Pharmacology and Therapeutics*, **47**, 35–60.

Lockridge, O., Adkins, S. & La Du, B. N. (1987b). Location of disulfide bonds with the sequence of human serum cholinesterase. *Journal of Biological Chemistry*, **262**, 12945–52.

Lockridge, O., Bartels, C. F., Vaughan, T. A., Wong, C. K., Norton, S. E. & Johnson, L. L. (1987a). Complete amino acid sequence of human serum cholinesterase. *Journal of Biological Chemistry*, **262**, 549–57.

Lockridge. O, & La Du, B. N. (1986). Amino acid sequence of the active site of human serum cholinesterase from usual atypical and atypical-silent genotypes. *Biochemical Genetics*, **24**, 485–98.

Loiselet, J. & Srouji, G. (1968). Répartition de la cholin-estérase mutante parmi les communautés Libanaises. Comparison avec la répartition d'autres gènes. *Annales de Génétique (Paris)*, **11**, 152–6.

Loughlin, J. F., Tuckerman, J. F. & Henderson, A.R. (1984). A BASIC program for serum cholinesterase phenotyping using a microcomputer. *Annals of Clinical Biochemistry*, **21**, 43–4.

Lovrien, E. W., Magenis, W. E., Rivas, M., Lamvik, N., Rowe, S., Wood. J. & Hemmerlnig, J. (1978). Serum cholinesterase (E₂) linkage analysis: possible evidence for location to chromosome 16. *Cytogenetics and Cell Genetics*, **22**, 324–6.

Lubin, A. H., Garry, P. J. & Owen, G. M. (1971). Sex and population differences in the incidence of a plasma cholin-esterase variant. *Science*, **173**, 161–4.

Lubin, A. H., Garry, P. J., Owen, G. M., Prince, L. C. & Dietz, A. A. (1973). Further variation of the 'silent' cholinesterase gene. *Biochemical Medicine*, **8**, 160–9.

McAlpine. P. J., Chen, S.-H., Cox, D. W., Dossetor, J. B., Giblett, E., Steinberg, A. G. & Simpson, N. E. (1974). Genetic markers in blood in a Canadian Eskimo population with a comparison of allele frequencies in circumpolar populations. *Human Heredity*, **24**, 114–42.

McComb, R. B., LaMotta, R. V. & Wetstone, H. J. (1965).

Procedure for detecting atypical serum cholinesterase using O- nitrophenylbutyrate as substrate. *Clinical Chemistry*, **11**, 645–52.

McGuire, M. C., Nogueira, C. P., Bartels, C. F., Lightstone, H., Hajra, A., Van der Spek, A. F. L., Lockridge, O. & La Du, B. N. (1989). Identification of the structural mutation responsible for the dibucaine-resistant (atypical) variant form of human serum cholinesterase. *Proceedings of the National Academy of Sciences (USA)*, **86**, 953–7.

McMillan, M. & Thompson, J. C. (1979). An outbreak of suspected solanine poisoning in schoolboys. *Quarterly Journal of Medicine, NS*, **48**, 227–43.

Magarian, E. O. &, Dietz, A. J. (1987). Correlation of cholinesterase with serum lipids and lipoproteins. *Journal of Clinical Pharmacology*, **27**, 819–20.

Magna, L. A., Morandin, R. C., Pinto, W. Jr. & Beiguelman, B. (1980). Frequency of the atypical serum cholinesterase in South Eastern Brazilian Caucasoids. *Revista Brasileira de Genetica*, **3**, 329–37. (Cited by Chautard-Freire-Maia *et al.*, 1984a.)

Marazita, M. L., Keats, B. J. B., Spence, M. A., Sparkes, R. S., Field. L. L., Sparkes, M. C. & Crist, M. (1989). Mapping studies of the serum cholinesterase-2 locus (CHE2). *Human Genetics*, **83**, 139–44.

Masson, P., Germani, F. & Plasse, M. (1979). Fréquence de variants du locus E₁ de la butyrylcholinestérase plasmatique dans une population francaise. *Computes Rendus Academie des Sciences (Paris)*, **289**, 537–9.

Mendel, B., Mundell, D. B. & Rudney, H. (1943). Studies on cholinesterase. 3. Specific tests for true cholinesterase and pseudocholinesterase. *Biochemical Journal*, **37**, 473–6.

Milligan, K. R., Hayes, T. C., Huss, B. K. D. & Beattie, B. (1986). Atypical plasma cholinesterase – case clustering. *Anaesthesia*, **41**, 841–3.

Miyamoto, M., Maukawa, A., Ochiai, A., Ito, K., Ando, Y., Niwa, M., Kondo, H., & Harasawa, S. (1987). A case with silent type of pseuo-acholinesterasemia. *Tokai Journal of Experimental and Clinical Medicine*, **12**, 365–72.

Mkheidze, M. O., Pekarskaya, N. A. & Shaposhnikov, A. M. (1978). An express method for evaluation of the mutant forms of cholinesterase in human blood serum. *Macmynura*, **5/IV**, 359–63.

Morrow, A. & Motulsky, A. G. (1965). Population genetics of cholinesterase variants. Studies with a rapid screening test. *Clinical Research*, **13**, 266 (Abstract).

Morrow, A. C. & Motulsky, A. G. (1968). Rapid screening method for the common atypical cholinesterase variant. *Journal of Laboratory and Clinical Medicine*, **71**, 350–6.

Motulsky, A. G. & Morrow, A. (1968). Atypical cholinesterase gene E₁ᵃ: rarity in negroes and most orientals. *Science*, **159**, 202–3.

Muensch, H., Goedde, H.-W. & Yoshida, A. (1976). Human serum cholinesterase subunits and number of active sites of the major component. *European Journal of Biochemistry*, **70**, 217–23.

Nakamura, S. (1985). Total cholesterol, high density lipoprotein cholesterol and choline esterase in overseas and Japanese university students. *Tohoku Journal of Experimental Medicine*, **145**, 369–71.

Naverette, J. I., Lisker, R. & Pérez-Briceño, R. (1979). Serum atypical pseudocholinesterase and leprosy. *International Journal of Dermatology*, **18**, 822–3.

Nazarova, A. F. (1981). Human serum cholinesterase polymorphism in Moscow population. *Genetika (Moskva)*, **17**, 357–61.

Neitlich, H. W. (1966). Increased plasma cholinesterase activity and succinylcholine resistant: a genetic variant. *Journal of Clinical Investigation*, **45**, 380–7.

Neumann, S. & Walter, H. (1968). Frequencies of cholinesterase variants in Icelanders, Greeks and Pakistanis. *Nature*, **219**, 950.

Nogueira, C. P, McGuire, M. C., Graeser, C., Bartels, C. F., Arpagaus, M., Van der Spek, A. F. L., Lightstone, H., Lockridge, O. & La Du, B. N. (1990). Identification of a frameshift mutation responsible for the silent phenotype of human serum cholinesterase, Gly 117 (GGT→GGAG). *American Journal of Human Genetics*, **46**, 934–42.

Nurse, G. T. & Jenkins, T. (1977). Health and the hunter-gatherer. In *Monographs in Human Genetics*, ed. L. Beckman & M. Hague, Vol. 8, p.71. Basel: Karger.

Ohkawa, J., Oimomi, M. & Baba, S. (1989). Familial hypercholinesterasemia. *Kobe Journal of Medical Science*, **35**, 39–45.

Oimomi, M., Ohkawa, J., Saeki, S. & Baba, S. (1988). The frequency of C₅ cholinesterase in the normal Japanese population. *Clinica Chimica Acta*, **175**, 349–50.

Omoto, K. & Goedde, H. W. (1965). Cholinesterase variants in Japan. *Nature*, **205**, 726.

Omoto, K. & Harada, S. (1968). Red cell and serum protein types in the Ainu population of Shizunai Hokkaido. *8th International Congress of Anthropology and Ethnological Science, Tokyo and Kyoto*, **1**, 206–9.

Pannall, P. R., Potgieter, G. M. & Raubenheimer, M. M. (1976). Plasma cholinesterase variants – an unexpectedly high incidence of the silent allele. *South African Medical Journal*, **50**, 304–6.

Panteghini, M., Bonora, R. & Pagani, F. (1988). An alternative approach to the prevention of succinyldicholine-induced apnoea. *Journal of Clinical Chemistry and Clinical Biochemistry*, **26**, 85–90.

Peedicayil, J., Ernest, K., Thomas, M., Kanagasabapathy, A. S. & Stephen, P. M. {1991). The effect of organophosphorus compounds on serum pseudocholinesterase levels in a group of industrial workers. *Human and Experimental Toxicology*, **10**, 275–8.

Primo-Parma, S.L., Chautard-Freire-Maia, E. A., de Lourenço, M. A. C., Salzano, F. M. & Melo e Freitas, M. J. (1986). Studies on serum cholinesterase (CHE1 and CHE2) in Brazilian, Indian and admixed populations. *Revista Brasileira de Genetica*, **9**, 467–78.

Prody, C. A., Dreyfus, P., Zamir, R., Zakut, H. & Soreq, H. (1989). *De novo* amplification within a 'silent' human cholinesterase gene in a family subjected to prolonged exposure to organophosphorus insecticides. *Proceedings of the National Academy of Sciences (USA)*, **86**, 690–4.

Prody, C. A., Zevin-Sonkin, D., Gnatt, A., Goldberg, O. & Soreq, H. (1987). Isolation and characterization of full-length cDNA clones coding for cholinesterase from fetal human tissues. *Proceedings of the National Academy of Sciences (USA)*, **84**, 3555–9.

Prody, C. A., Zevin-Sonkin, D., Gnatt, A., Koch, R., Zisling, R., Goldberg, O. & Soreq, H. (1986). Use of synthetic oligonucleotide probes for the isolation of a human cholinesterase cDNA clone. *Journal of Neuroscience Research*, **16**, 25–35.

Prokop, O. (1971). *Die Menschlichen Blut- und Serumgruppen*. Stuttgart, Fischer. (Cited by Steegmüller, 1975.)

Pronk, J.C. (1976). Atypical serum cholinesterase in the Netherlands. *Human Heredity*, **26**, 128–30.

Propert, D.N. & Brackenridge, C.J. (1976). The relation of sex age smoking status birth rank and parental ages to pseudocholinesterase activity and phenotypes in a sample of Australian Caucasian adults. *Human Genetics*, **32**, 181–8.

Rahimi, A. G., Goedde, H. W., Flatz, G., Kaifie, S., Benkmann, H. G. & Delbrück, H. (1977). Serum protein polymorphisms in four populations of Afghanistan. *American Journal of Human Genetics*, **29**, 356–60.

Rao, P. R., Char, K. S. N., Theophilus, J., Parasa, L. & Hussain, S. (1985). Incidence of C_5 isozyme of serum cholinesterase (E_2 locus) in populations of Andhra Pradesh, South India. *Human Heredity*, **35**, 126–8.

Rao, P. R. & Gopalam, K. B. (1979). High incidence of the silent allele at cholinesterase locus I in Vysyas of Andhra Pradesh (S India). *Human Genetics*, **52**, 139–41.

Rea, T. H. & Ng, W. G. (1978). Serum pseudocholinesterase variants in Mexican-born patients with lepromatous leprosy. *International Journal of Leprosy*, **46**, 333–6.

Ritter, D. M., Retke, S. R., Ilstrup, D. M. & Burritt, M. F. (1988). Effect of plasma cholinesterase activity on the duration of action of succinylcholine in patients with genotypically normal enzyme. *Anesthesia and Analgesia*, **67**, 1123–6.

Robson, E. B. & Harris, H. (1966). Further data on the incidence and genetics of the serum cholinesterase phenotype C_5+. *Annals of Human Genetics (London)*, **29**, 403–8.

Rostron, P. & Higgins, T. (1988). Serum cholinesterase and dibucaine numbers as measured with the Technicon RA-1000 analyser. *Clinical Chemistry*, **34**, 1924–5.

Rubinstein, H. M., Dietz, A. A., Hodges, L. K., Lubrano, T. & Czebotar, V. (1970). Silent cholinesterase gene: variations in the property of serum enzyme in apparent homozygotes. *Journal of Clinical Investigation*, **49**, 479–86.

Rubinstein, H. M., Dietz, A. A. & Lubrano, T. (1978). E_1^k another quantitative variant at cholinesterase locus 1. *Journal of Medical Genetics*, **15**, 27–9.

Rubinstein, H. M., Dietz, A. A., Lubrano, T. & Garry, P. J. (1976). E_1^j a quantitative variant at cholinesterase locus 1: immunological evidence. *Journal of Medical Genetics*, **13**, 43–5.

Sayek, I., Karahasanoghu, A. M. & Ozand, P. (1967). Pseudocholinesterases III: The presence of pseudocholinesterase variants in a Turkish population. *Turkish Journal of Paediatrics*, **9**, 8–12.

Schaap, T., Frezal, J., Briard-Guillemot, M. L. & Lamm, M. (1967). Fréquence du gène E_1^a (cholinesterase atypique) dans une population française. *Bulletin de l'Institut National de la Santé et de la Recherche Médicale (Paris)*, **22**, 1119–27.

Schmidinger St, Held, K. R. & Goedde, H. W. (1966). Hydrolysis of succinyldicholine by cholinesterase at low concentrations. *Humangenetik*, **2**, 221–4.

Schouten, J. A., Beynen, A. C. & Mulder, C. (1988). Cholinesterase and VLDL: a reply to the letter by Cucuianu 1988;*(Atherosclerosis*, 72: 83-84). *Atherosclerosis*, **72**, 85–6.

Schouten, J. A., Mulder, C. & Beynen, A. C. (1987). Cholinesterase and serum lipoproteins. *Atherosclerosis*, **67**, 269–70.

Scott, E. M. (1973). Inheritance of two types of deficiency of human serum cholinesterase. *Annals of Human Genetics (London)*, **37**, 139–43.

Scott, E. M., Weaver, D. D. Wright, R. (1970). Discrimination of phenotypes in human serum cholinesterase deficiency. *American Journal of Human Genetics*, **22**, 363–9.

Shanor, S. P., Van Hees, G. R., Baart, N., Erdös, E. G. & Foldes, F. F. (1961). The influence of age and sex on human plasma and red cell cholinesterase. *American Journal of the Medical Sciences*, **242**, 357–61.

Simpson, N. E. (1967). A second heterozygote for 'silent' and 'fluoride resistant' genes for serum cholinesterase. *Journal of Medical Genetics*, **4**, 264–7.

Simpson, N. E. (1968). Genetics of esterases in man. *Annals of the New York Academy of Sciences*, **151**, 699–709.

Simpson, N. E. (1972). Polyacrylamide electrophoresis used for the detection of C_5+ cholinesterase in Canadian Caucasians, Indians and Eskimos. *American Journal of Human Genetics*, **24**, 317–20.

Simpson, N. E. & Kalow W. (1964). The 'silent' gene for serum cholinesterase. *American Journal of Human Genetics*, **16**, 180–8.

Singh, S., Amma, M. K. P., Sareen, K. N. & Goedde, H. W. (1971b). A study of the cholinesterase polymorphism among a Panjabi population. *Human Heredity*, **21**, 388–93.

Singh, S., Jensen, M., Goedde, H. W., Lehmann, H. W., Pyörälä, I. & Eriksson, A. W. (1971a). Cholinesterase polymorphism among Lapp populations in Finland. *Humangenetik*, **12**, 131–5.

Singh, S., Sareen, K. N. & Goedde, H. W. (1974). Investigation of some biochemical genetic markers in four endogamous groups from Panjab (NW India). *Humangenetik*, **21**, 341–6.

Singh, S., Saternus, K., Münsch, H., Altland, K., Goedde, H. W. & Eriksson, A.W. (1974). Cholinesterase polymorphism among Ålanders (Finno-Swedes), Maris (Cheremisses, USSR) and Greenland Eskimos, and the segregation of some E_1 and E_2 locus types in Finnish Lapp families. *Human Heredity*, **24**, 352–62.

Soreq, H., Zamir, R., Zevin-Sonkin, D. & Zakut, H. (1987). Human cholinesterase genes localized by hybridization to chromosomes 3 and 16. *Human Genetics*, **77**, 325–8.

Sparkes, R. S., Field, L. L., Sparkes, M. C., Crist, M., Spence, M. A., James, K. & Garry, P. L. (1984). Genetic linkage studies of transferrin, cholinesterase and chromosome 1 loci. *Human Heredity*, **34**, 96–100.

Steegmüller, H. (1975). On the geographical distribution of cholinesterase variants. *Humangenetik*, **26**, 167–85.

Swift, M. R. & La Du, B. N. (1966). A rapid screening test for atypical serum-cholinesterase. *Lancet*, **1**, 513–4.

Szeinberg, A., Pipano, S., Assa, M., Medalie, J. H. & Neufeld, H. N. (1972). High frequency of atypical cholinesterase gene among Iraqi and Iranian Jews. *Clinical Genetics*, **3**, 123–7.

Szeinberg, A., Pipano, S. & Ostfeld, E. (1966). Frequency of atypical cholinesterase in different population groups in Israel. *Acta Anaesthesiologica Scandinavica*, Suppl. **24**, 199–205.

Tashian, R. R., Brewer, G. C., Lehmann, H., Davis, D. A. & Rucknagel, D. L. (1967). Further studies on Xavanthe Indians V. Variability in some serum and erythrocyte enzymes, hemoglobin and the urinary excretion of β-aminoisobutyric acid. *American Journal of Human Genetics*, **19**, 524–31.

Thomas, M. & Job, C. K. (1972). Serum atypical pseudocholinesterase and genetic factors in leprosy. *British Medical Journal*, **3**, 390–1.

Thomas, M., Job, C. K. & Kurian, P. V. (1976). Susceptibility to leprosy and serum atypical pseudocholinesterase. *International Journal of Leprosy*, **44**, 315–8.

Trela, F. (1967). Über die neuen pseudocholinesterase-varianten C_5^+ C_5^-, identifiziert mittles stärkegelelektrophorese. *Zeitschrift Arztliche Fortbildung (Jena)*, **61**, 786–7.

Tripathi, A. K., Sikka, K. K. & Srivastava, D. K. (1987). Serum cholinesterase levels in the patients of coronary artery disease and their 'normal' first degree relatives. *Indian Heart Journal*, **39**, 9–11.

Tunek, A., Hjertberg, E. & Vigy-Mogensen, J. (1991). Interactions of bambuterol with human serum cholinesterase of the genotypes $E_u E_u$ (normal) $E_a E_a$ (atypical) and $E_u E_a$. *Biochemical Pharmacology*, **41**, 345–8.

Turner J. M., Hall, R. A., Whittaker, M., Holder, R. L. & Kricka, L. J. (1985). Application of stepwise discriminant analysis in the phenotyping of plasma cholinesterase variants. *Annals of Clinical Biochemistry*, **22**, 175–8.

Ukoha, A. I., Nwoke, U. N., Rahman, M. M. & Alam, M. S. (1987). The prevalence of atypical serum cholinesterase in a Nigerian population. *Tropical and Geographical Medicine*, **39**, 169–72.

Van Ros, G. & Druet, R. (1966). Uncommon electrophoretic patterns of serum cholinesterase (cholinesterase). *Nature*, **212**, 543–4.

Van Ros, G. & Vervoort, T. (1973). Frequencies of the 'atypical' and C_5 variants of serum cholinesterase in Zarians and Belgians. Detection of the C_5 variant by agar gel electrophoresis with an acid buffer. *Annales de la Société Belge de Médécine Tropicale (Antwerpen)*, **53**, 633–44.

Vergnes, H., Colombies, P. & Hobbe, Th. (1967) Les pseudocholienstérases sériques:, résultats dans les populations du haut-languedoc et du pays Basque. *Bulletins et Mémoires de la Societé d'Anthropologie de Paris*, **1(12)**, 249–55.

Vergnes, H. & Gherardhi, M. (1971). Les enzymotypes erythrocytaires et seriques dans un groupe de Kurdes. *Annales de Génétique (Paris)*, **14**, 199–205.

Vergnes, H. & Quilici, J. C. (1970). Le gène E_1^a de la pseudo-cholinesterase serique (ACAH) chez les Amérindiens. *Annales de Génétique (Paris)*, **13**, 96–9.

Vergnes, H., Quilici, J. C., Gherardi, M. & Bejarano, G. (1976). Serum and red cell enzyme variants in an Amerindian tribe the Sirionós (Eastern Bolivia). *Human Heredity*, **26**, 252–62.

Vergnes, H., Sevin, J. & Peralta, M. (1981). Plasma cholinesterase variants in population samples from south-west France. *Annals of Human Biology*, **8**, 59–63.

Vergnes, H., Sevin, A., Sevin, J. & Jaeger, G. (1979). Population genetic studies of the Aka pygmies (Central Africa). *Human Genetics*, **48**, 343–55.

Viby-Mogensen, J. (1983). Cholinesterase and succinyl-choline. *Danish Medical Bulletin*, **30**, 129–50.

Viby-Mogensen, J. (1988). Atypical serum cholinesterase eliminated by orthotopic liver transplantation. *Anesthesiology*, **68**, 474.

Wakid, N. W., Tubbeh, R. & Baraka, A. (1985). Assay of serum cholinesterase with succinylcholine and propionyl-thiocholine as substrates. *Anesthesiology*, **62**, 509–12.

Walter, H., Neumann, S., Backhausz, R. & Nemeskeri, J. (1965). Populations genetische Untersuchingen uber die Cholinesterase-Varienten bei Ungarn und Deutschen. *Humangenetik*, **1**, 551–6.

Warran, P., Theeman, M., Bold, A. M. & Jones, S. (1987). Hypercholinesterasemia and suxamethonium resistance. *Anaesthesia*, **42**, 855–7.

Whittaker, M. (1964). The cholinesterase variants: esterase levels and increased resistance to fluoride. *Acta Genetica (Basel)*, **14**, 281–5.

Whittaker, M. (1968e). The frequency of the fluoride resistant gene in a population of British students. *Acta Genetica (Basel)*, 18; 563–6.

Whittaker, M. (1968a). Differential inhibition of human serum cholinesterase with *n*-butyl alcohol: recognition of new phenotypes. *Acta Genetica (Basel)*, **18**, 335–40.

Whittaker, M. The cholinesterase variants. (1968b). Differentiation by means of alkyl alcohols. *Acta Genetica (Basel)*, **18**, 325–34.

Whittaker, M. (1968c) An additional cholinesterase phenotype occurring in suxamethonium apnoea. *British Journal of Anaesthesia*, **40**, 579–82.

Whittaker, M. (1968d). Frequency of atypical cholinesterase in groups of individuals of different ethnographical origin. *Acta Genetica (Basel)*, **18**, 567–72.

Whittaker, M. (1980). Plasma cholinesterase variants and the anaesthetist. *Anaesthesia*, **35**, 174–97.

Whittaker, M. (1986). Cholinesterase. In *Monographs in Human Genetics*, Vol. 11, ed. L. Beckman. Basel: Karger.

Whittaker, M. & Berry, M. (1977). The plasma cholinesterase variants in mentally ill patients. *British Journal of Psychiatry*, **130**, 397–404.

Whittaker, M. & Britten, J. J. (1985). Plasma cholinesterase variants. Family studies of the E_1^k gene. *Human Heredity*, **35**, 364–8.

Whittaker, M. & Britten, J. J. (1987). E_1^h a new allele at cholinesterase locus 1. *Human Heredity*, **37**, 54–8.

Whittaker, M., Britten, J. J., Vyas, A. B. & Hayes, T. C. (1988). Family studies of the E_1^k E_1^k genotype for plasma cholinesterase. *Human Heredity*, **38**, 228–32.

Whittaker, M. & Britten, J. J. (1988). Recognition of two new phenotypes segregating the E_1^k allele for plasma cholinesterase. *Human Heredity*, **38**, 233–9.

Whittaker, M. & Britten, J. J. (1990). Recognition of the E_1^k E_1^k homozygote for plasma cholinesterase. *Human Heredity*, **40**, 247–9.

Whittaker, M., Britten, J. J. & Dawson, P. J. G. (1983). Comparison of a commercially available assay system with two reference methods for the determination of plasma cholinesterase variants. *Clinical Chemistry*, **29**, 1746–51.

Whittaker, M., Jones, J. & Braven, J. (1990). Heterogeneity of the silent gene for plasma cholinesterase. *Human Heredity*, **40**, 153–8.

Whittaker, M., Jones, J. W. & Braven, J. (1991a). Immunological studies of families segregating the silent gene for plasma cholinesterase. *Human Heredity*, **41**, 77–83.

Whittaker, M., Jones, J. W. & Braven, J. (1991b). Immunological studies of plasma cholinesterase during pregnancy and the puerperium. *Clinica Chimica Acta*, **199**, 223–30.

Whittaker, M. & Lowe, R. F. (1976). The cholinesterase variants found in some African tribes living in Rhodesia. *Human Heredity*, **26**, 380–93.

Whittaker, M., Lowe, R. F. & Ellis, B. P. B. (1976). Serum cholinesterase variants in African leprosy patients resident in Rhodesia. *Human Heredity*, **26**, 372–9.

Whittaker, M. & Reys, L. (1975). Plasma cholinesterase studies on South-Eastern Bantu of Mozambique. *Human Heredity*, **25**, 296–301.

Whittaker, M., Taylor, F. & Battersby, E. F. (1987). Recognition of the $E_1^k E_1^j$ cholinesterase genotype in a family segregating thee rare genes E_1^k, E_1^j and E_1^a. *Human Heredity*, **37**, 82–5.

Whittaker, M. & Vickers, M. D. (1970). Initial experiences with the cholinesterase research unit. *British Journal of Anaesthesia*, **42**, 1016–20.

Whittaker, M., Wicks, R. J. & Britten, J. J. (1982). Studies on the inhibition by propanolol of some human erythrocyte membrane enzymes and plasma cholinesterase. *Clinica Chimica Acta*, **119**, 107–14.

Yamato, K., Huang, I.-Y., Muensch, H., Yoshida, A., Goedde H.W. & Agarwal D. P. (1983). Amino acid sequence of the active site of human cholinesterase. *Biochemical Genetics*, **21**, 135–45.

Yamamoto, K., Morito, F., Motomura, M., Kaneoka, H. & Sakai, T. (1986). A case of familial hyper-cholinesterasemia associated with isozyme variant band. *Gastroenterologica Japonica*, **21**, 379–84.

Yamamoto, K., Morito, F., Nobutaka, I., Setoguchi, Y., Fuji, S., Kariya, T. & Sakai, T. (1987). Characterization of serum cholinesterase in familial hypercholinesterasemia associated with an isozyme variant band. *Gastroenterologica Japonica*, **22**, 187–93.

Yoshida, A. & Motulsky, A. G. (1969). A cholinesterase variant (E Cynthiana) associated with elevated plasma enzyme activity. *American Journal of Human Genetics*, **21**, 486–98.

Yücel, D., Top, S., Erdemli, Ö. & Öğüs, H. (1988). Relationship between serum cholinesterase activity and duration of succinylcholine action in subjects with the 'usual' phenotype for the enzyme. *Clinical Chemistry*, **34**, 2579–80.

Zakut, H., Zamir, R., Sindel, L. & Soreq, H. (1989). Gene mapping on chorionic villi chromosomes by hybridization *in situ*: localization of cholinesterase cDNA binding sites to chromosome 3q21, 3q26-ter and 16q21. *Human Reproduction*, **4**, 941–6.

Zelinski, T., Kaita, H., Lewis, M., Coghlan, G. & Craig, D. (1987). The sequence of chromosome 3 loci AHSG:TF:CHE1. *Human Heredity*, **37**, 1–6.

PART IV   Alcohol and alcoholism

15   Alcohol and alcoholism

THE OBJECTIVES OF THIS CHAPTER

TO SHOW that genetic factors:

1 influence the occurrence of alcoholism;
2 determine the physiological responses to alcohol (ethanol) ingestion;
3 control alcohol dehydrogenase;
4 control acetaldehyde dehydrogenase (ALDH);
5 determine specific variants of ALDH which control the amount of alcohol consumed and so determine who becomes alcoholic in Japanese populations;
6 determine the deleterious sequelae of excessive alcohol consumption.

HISTORICAL BACKGROUND

The familial aggregation of alcoholics is a phenomenon known since antiquity (Legrain 1889, cited by Cruz-Coke 1983). Goodwin (1980) cites Aristotle who declared that drunken women 'bring forth children like themselves' and Plutarch, who said 'one drunkard begets another'.

In the nineteenth century, when drunkenness had become a serious social problem, emphatic views were expressed by the Society for the Study of Inebriety (founded in 1884). On the basis of a Lamarckian view of heredity and with a eugenic perspective it was suggested that one way to curb the problem was to discourage the 'congenital inebriate' from procreating (anonymous editorial: *British Journal of Addiction*, 1984).

In the present century ideas derived from Darwin and Galton displaced Lamarckian notions of genetics. Crothers (1909) stated

There is one conclusion which the clinician is profoundly impressed with namely: alcoholic ancestors transmit to the next generation not only states of exhaustion, low vitality, and feeble resisting power but also marked impulses to use alcohol for its pleasing narcotic effects.

The great and sharp rise in the incidence of alcohol-related disorders following the Second World War caused opinions to swing away from heredity and to favour environmental causation.

Now more recently has come the realization that alcoholism, like other chronic disorders, results from an interplay between a genetically determined constitution and environmental influences.

A PHARMACOGENETIC APPROACH

Even though the idea of pharmacogenetics has been in existence since the late 1950s its application to alcohol-related problems is a quite recent development.

Von Wartburg (1980) stated

Pharmacogenetic phenomena are the expression of pre-existing inborn differences among individuals which become apparent upon exposure of the body to drugs. If alcohol is considered to be a drug and the differences in biological sensitivity have a genetic origin they may be called pharmacogenetic.

Propping (1983a) utilized the electroencephalogram (EEG) as a tool which detects variants in the population. After observing different effects of alcohol on genetically determined EEG patterns he concluded that alcoholism is under genetic influence not only at the metabolic but also at the pharmacodynamic level.

Murray *et al.* (1983) utilized pharmacogenetic concepts as related to tetraisoquinolines in alcoholism whilst Crabbe (1984), in discussing pharmacogenetic strategies, proposed the study of animal models of alcoholism. Radouco-Thomas *et al.* (1984) with a similar philosophy and considerable foresight proposed the investigation of alcohol-related problems by applying recombinant DNA technology. Associations might be found between specific alcohol-related clinical phenomena and particular phenotypes within genetic polymorphisms of DNA. This theme was further expounded by Worton (1991).

In a general review Agarwal & Goedde (1986) state

The study of pharmacogenetics and ecogenetics among different individuals and populations offers an unique opportunity to understand multiple, simultaneously-occurring interactions between genes and environment and the subsequent expression of heritable characters.

Their success in applying this concept to the study of alcoholism will be described below.

DEFINITIONS

It is a common observation that there are different types of alcohol-related problems and there has been no uniformity of views on how to define and classify them (Cooper 1983). It is often unclear what a particular author has studied, and the comparison of the results of different authors becomes uncertain. Goodwin (1981) has graphically referred to 'definitional chaos'. Examples of different definitions each of which has some merit are those given by: WHO Expert Committee on Mental Health (1951), Jellinek (1952), Kennedy & Fish (1958), Edwards & Gross (1976), Gurling *et al.* (1981), Goedde *et al.* (1983a), Freund (1984) and Schuckit (1986).

The American Psychiatric Association DSM III (DSM = Diagnostic and Statistical Manual) is now widely used as an operational tool by psychiatrists. It contains descriptions and criteria for various alcohol-related syndromes amongst which are abuse and dependence. Brief descriptions are as follows:

The essential feature of alcohol abuse is a pattern of pathological use for at least a month that causes impairment in social or occupational functioning. The essential features of Alcohol Dependence are either a pattern of pathological alcohol use or impairment in social or occupational functioning due to alcohol and either tolerance or withdrawal. Alcohol dependence has also been Alcoholism.

It would be helpful in the future if researchers were all to use one set of definitions and probably the best choice would be those given by DSM III (the 1987 revision DSM III-R is somewhat more discursive). An alternative would be the very recently formulated definition given by Morse *et al.* (1992) on behalf of the National Council on Alcoholism and Drug Dependence, and the American Society of Addiction Medicine.

ALCOHOL-RELATED PROBLEMS ARE INFLUENCED BY HEREDITY AND ENVIRONMENT

The main purpose of this book is to explore the genetic reasons why persons vary in their responses to drugs. However, in the case of alcohol-related problems it is relevant to point out that environment is very important. Upbringing in the home, friends, type of work, general availability of alcohol, money to purchase it, encouragement to drink it (or otherwise) are all powerful influences in determining the outcome. The interplay of these environmental factors with heredity has been the subject of a debate between Heather (1992) and Jurd (1992).

It is generally agreed that, given the same level of environmental influences, the propensity of individuals to develop alcohol-related problems varies greatly. An important reason for this variation is genetic endowment. However, there are many inter- related facets which were recognized by Omenn & Motulsky (1972) when they defined different levels of genetic influence:

1 susceptibility to intoxication effects;
2 metabolism of alcohol;
3 adaptation to chronic intake;
4 predisposing personality factors;
5 susceptibility to medical complications.

Some of these facets have been the subject of extensive scientific research which will now be summarized.

Table 15.1. *Characteristics of Type I versus Type II alcoholism*

Distinguishing characteristic	Type I	Type II
Alcohol-related problems:		
Age of onset (years)	After 25	Before 25
Spontaneous alcohol seeking (inability to abstain)	Infrequent	Frequent
Alcohol-related legal problems (fighting, arrests)	Infrequent	Frequent
Psychological dependence (loss of control)	Frequent	Infrequent
Guilt and fear (about dependence)	Frequent	Infrequent
Personality traits:		
Novelty seeking	Low	High
Harm avoidance	High	Low
Reward dependence	High	Low

From: Devor & Cloninger 1989.

Familial studies

The category of 'familial alcoholism' was proposed by Jellinek (1940) and characterized by an early age of onset and a particularly severe course. In the ensuing sections the terms 'alcoholism' and 'alcoholic' will be used as synonyms for the DSM II-R term 'alcohol dependence'. There have been two types of studies to test whether this idea is true; these are (1) analysis of the families of alcoholics and (2) adoption studies.

The former type of survey was carried out by Goodwin (1985), Cook & Winokur (1985), Cloninger (1985) and Penick *et al.* (1987). Persons with family histories were found to have an earlier onset of alcoholism, greater severity and more complications. It is, however, possible that assortative mating between alcoholics (see Hall *et al.* 1983a, b) may account for some of the differences between familial and non-familial alcoholics. Opinion has swung against the idea that there is a strong association between alcoholism and other psychiatric disorders. Three types of alcoholics have been defined (Cloninger 1985) as milieu-limited (Type I), male-limited (Type II) and antisocial behaviour disorder. The most important features of the two major subtypes are shown in Table 15.1.

The most impressive evidence supporting the importance of genetic factors in alcoholism comes from adoption studies. The practice of placing the offspring of alcoholics with unrelated families for raising gave an opportunity to separate the effects of 'nature' from 'nurture'. Controls were children of non-alcoholics matched for age and circumstances of adoption. Studies of the type have been carried out in Missouri (Schuckit *et al.* 1972), Sweden (Bohman 1978), Iowa (Cadoret & Gath 1978) and Denmark (Goodwin 1983).

Type II alcoholism shown in Table 15.1 – which is predominantly a male phenomenon – was shown to be strongly influenced by genetic factors. One study gave a nine-fold risk (compared with the risk in controls) regardless of environment for the sons of fathers of this type to develop the same syndrome. The females in these families have recurrent headache, backache, abdominal pain and other somatic complaints from a young age.

Twin studies

Another method, originally proposed by Galton, of disentangling the effects of heredity from those of environment is by the study of twins. The basic idea is that differences between monozygous twins are purely environmental, whereas differences between dizygous twins are due to an amalgam of environmental and genetical influences. The simplest way of expressing the results is by the 'concordance rate'. $C/(C + D)$, where C = total number of concordant pairs, D = number of discordant pairs (see Emery 1976).

There have been a number of large twin studies of alcohol-related problems which are summarized in Table 15.2. So it can be stated that twin research on (a) amount of alcohol consumed and (b) alcohol-related problems has yielded some conflicting

Table 15.2. *Some surveys in twins of amount of alcohol consumed and alcohol-related problems*

Reference	Location	Number of twin pairs	Variable examined	Result
Murray *et al.* 1983	London	494	Total weekly alcohol consumption	Additive genetic factors accounted for 40% of the variance
Hayakawa 1987	Osaka	407 MZ 136 DZ	Alcohol consumption	MZ: 131 concordant 89 discordant DZ: 42 concordant 43 disordant
Kaprio *et al.* 1987	Helsinki	879 MZ 1940 DZ males	Frequency of beer consumption Frequency of spirits consumption Density of drinking (number of bouts of heavy drinking per month) Quantity drunk	0.387 0.302 0.396 ⎬ Heritabilities 0.362
Kaij 1960	Sweden	174 male	Alcohol abuse	One third of variance under direct genetic control
Partanen *et al.* 1966	Finland	729 male	Lack of control of consumption Amount Density (number of bouts of heavy drinking per month)	0.14 0.36 ⎬ Heritabilities 0.39
Hrubec & Omenn 1981	USA	15 924 male twin probands	Alcohol related disorders (alcoholism)	MZ twins had significantly greater number than DZ ($p < 0.001$)
Gurling *et al.* 1981; Murray *et al.* 1983	London	56 incl. female	Severe and moderate types of alcohol dependence	No genetic predisposition suggested

MZ, Monozygous; DZ, Dizygous.
Heritability: The component of total variance which is due to the additive effects of genes (Falconer 1960).

results but the balance of evidence favours an important measure of genetic susceptibility. It is not entirely clear why the London study of Murray *et al.* (1983) disagreed with the others; possibly this may have been due to sampling selection (for example the London sample included females) and the inclusion of different types of alcoholism. It must be remembered that twin studies are much more complicated than at first appreciated (e.g. MZ twins share a more common environment than DZ twins).

THE ATTRIBUTES OF PERSONS GENETICALLY SUSCEPTIBLE TO ALCOHOLISM: 'AT RISK' INDIVIDUALS

In view of the foregoing it appears highly probable that genetic factors are of considerable importance in making some persons much more prone than

others to alcohol abuse and alcohol dependence. So the questions are: (1) What phenotypic properties do the relevant genes control? (2) What differences might there be in the response to alcohol in 'at risk' individuals as compared with controls?

The psychological attributes of 'at risk' individuals

Extensive researches have been made into the psychological attributes of persons (especially males) who later become alcoholics, and also of the sons of alcoholics.

Some workers claim to have delineated certain psychological attributes which characterize at risk individuals (e.g. Sehr & Levinson 1982; Tarter *et al.* 1985) and they are summarized in Table 15.3. However, other workers (as reviewed by Nagoshi & Wilson 1987) failed to find significant differences

Table 15.3. *Some psychological attributes which are more prominent in persons with positive family histories for alcoholism than in persons who have negative family histories*

High activity level
Less able to sustain attention or concentration
Susceptibility to become easily and intensely distressed
Excitability and aggressiveness
Antisocial behaviour
Emotional immaturity, low frustration tolerance and
    moodiness
Lower verbal and abstracting/problem solving abilities

between family history positive and family history negative non-alcoholics in a range of personality dimensions.

Much remains to be discovered about the psychological factors which lead to alcoholism. The paucity of long-term follow-up studies was emphasized by Hammond (1981) who pointed out that a wide range of behaviour is associated in one group or another with heavy drinking at the age of 20 years. It was pointed out by Cooper (1983) that socio-cultural factors may be more accurate predictors of alcohol abuse than psychological variables. The interactions between psychological phenotypes and environmental factors to produce individuals with alcohol-related problems were reviewed by Braucht (1983).

Physiological markers

The approach to these aspects has been to study the offspring of alcoholics who had not established the alcohol habit, and compare them with matched offspring of non-alcoholics. The numbers of subjects varied from nine to 34 in both groups. The principal results are shown in Table 15.4. It should be explained that brain stem auditory event-related potentials are obtained by subjecting an individual to regular stimuli. Then an unusual stimulus, e.g. an auditory stimulus of different frequency, is applied. This unusual stimulus produces a positive brain-wave termed P300 (often abbreviated to P3) on the EEG. There is a conflict of evidence with regard to the evoked P3. O'Connor *et al.* (1986) and Begleiter & Porjesz (1988) found reduced P3 voltages in response to auditory and visual stimuli in high risk subjects without the administration of

alcohol. *Per contra* Polich *et al.* (1988a, b) found that P3 amplitude and latency in response to a visual stimulus was not different in family history positive and family history negative undergraduate matched pairs who had not been exposed to alcohol.

Although the physiological and biochemical observations noted in Table 15.4 were interesting because they show organic differences between high risk individuals versus controls, they are of little predictive or clinical value.

Alcohol and the electroencephalogram

It has been pointed out by Propping (1983a) that the electroencephalogram (EEG) is a tool which offers several advantages for the geneticist. In a given individual it has a constant and typical pattern. It reflects the degree of vigilance or central activity, and it can be used as a sensitive indicator of the central effects of drugs. Many drugs can be investigated pharmacogenetically using the same apparatus. A great deal of the pharmacogenetic researches carried out hitherto has been concerned with inherited variations in the biotransformation of drugs, whereas much less attention has been paid to the genetic bases of variability in tissue responses to drug medications. The EEG offers a technique whereby this imbalance can be addressed.

In an early investigation 26 monozygous (MZ) twin pairs and 26 dizygous (DZ) twin pairs received an acute dose of alcohol under standardized experimental conditions. In the EEG, alcohol improved activity in the alpha and theta band and decreased beta activity, an effect described as synchronization. MZ twins reacted identically to alcohol, but the EEGs of DZ twins became more dissimilar after alcohol (Kopun & Propping 1977). This experiment provided proof that the differential reaction of the EEG to alcohol is under genetic control.

It has been reported in the past that alcoholics, on the average, when compared with healthy controls have less alpha activity in their EEGs. A survey of 115 alcoholics (see Propping 1983b) compared with controls revealed no difference in the males. The female alcoholics, however, exhibited poor EEG synchronization compared with matched controls. In order to decide whether this was an effect of alcohol or the expression of a genetic trait, the first degree relatives of the alcoholics were examined. The relatives exhibited the same tendency in their

Table 15.4. *Studies of physiological and biochemical responses to alcohol in 'at risk' individual (A) and control (B)*

Reference	Variable investigated	Result
Begleiter *et al.* 1984	P3 component of event-related potential without alcohol	P3 voltage reduced in A
Schuckit 1984	Self-rating of intoxication recorded for 24 minutes after: (1) placebo (2) 0.75 alcohol ml/kg } schedule Θ (3) 1.1 alcohol ml/kg	Less intense feelings of intoxication in A
Schuckit 1985b	Levels of body sway estimated after: (1) placebo (2) 0.75 ml 95% alcohol/kg (3) 1.1 ml 95% alcohol/kg	Body sway after alcohol less intense in A
Schuckit 1987a	Plasma cortisol levels following alcohol (schedule Θ)	Lower cortisol levels in A especially after 1.1 ml alcohol/kg
Schuckit *et al.* 1987b	Serum prolactin levels following alcohol (schedule Θ)	Lower serum prolactin levels in A after 0.75 and 1.1 ml alcohol/kg
Schuckit *et al.* 1988a	Plasma ACTH levels following alcohol (schedule Θ)	Lower plasma ACTH levels in A after 1.1 ml alcohol/kg
Schuckit *et al.* 1988b	Event-related brain potential recorded after alcohol (schedule Θ)	The P3 potential was evaluated at baseline and 70 minutes after alcohol. The only significant difference was a quicker return towards baseline of P3 latency in A than in B
Neulin & Thomson 1991	Various physiological measurements after 0.5 g alcohol /kg on 3 occasions (heart rate, finger temperature, finger pulse, attitude, skin conductance and motor activity)	Sensitization (i.e. increased effects) common in A. Tolerance (i.e. diminished effects) common in B
Schuckit *et al.* (1991)	Levels of body sway estimated after: (1) 5 ml alcohol p.o. and placebo i.v. (2) 5 ml alcohol p.o. and 0.12 mg/kg diazepam i.v. (3) oral placebo and 0.20 mg/kg diazepam i.v. (4) oral 0.75 ml/kg of 95% alcohol and placebo i.v.	No differences in responses between A and B after both dosage levels of diazepam.

EEGs as did the index cases, which was interpreted as favouring a genetic basis for the EEG abnormality (however, it is not clear whether the relatives investigated were non-alcoholics).

It is possible that persons possessing a certain type of 'abnormal' EEG with lack of alpha activity and a preponderance of small, fast beta waves may be more vulnerable than persons with 'normal' EEGs, not only to alcoholism but also to schizophrenia and other behavioural disorders (Propping 1983b).

Biochemical markers

Two biochemical measurements which have received a lot of attention have been platelet monoamine oxidase (MAO) and platelet adenylate cyclase; both have been reviewed by Tabakoff & Hoffmann (1988) and Devor & Cloninger (1989).

The brain contains both A and B types of MAO;

the latter type is found in platelets and is thought to mirror the activity of the B type in the brain. Low values of platelet MAO activities have been found in alcoholics, even those who have been abstinent for a long time, so that even though the enzyme is inhibited by alcohol, the low level may indicate an inherent characteristic of alcoholics, (particularly Type II: von Knorring *et al.* 1985; Whelan 1992).

Similarly, adenylate cyclase (AC) activity which can be stimulated by fluoride and other agents has been found to be lower in the platelets and lympho-cytes of alcoholics than in controls, even after the former had been abstinent for long periods.

Discriminant analysis using the values for alcohol-inhibited MAO activity and fluoride-stimulated AC activity was able to provide correct classification of 75% of alcoholics and 73% of con-trols (Tabakoff & Hoffman 1988).

Nevertheless, the drawback to all the studies mentioned in this section is that they deal with continuous variables and thus the differences between alcoholics and controls have to be defined in terms of means and variances. This is a similar problem to the definition of hypertension. There is an obvious superiority in being able to study the discontinuous variables in a polymorphism so that phenomena can be analysed in terms of frequencies, and that is the new thrust provided by the pharmacogenetic approach which will be explored in the sections which follow.

Genetic control of a brain mechanism which responds to alcohol – a first attempt

An interesting development was marked by the paper of Blum *et al.* (1990). They set out to see if there was a statistical association between any of the genotypes detected in a TaqI restriction fragment length polymorphism of the human dopamine D$_2$ receptor gene (recently mapped to 11q22–q23: Grandy *et al.* 1989) with alcoholism. A significant association of one genotype (termed A$_1$) with alcoholism was claimed. However, this claim has been refuted by the more carefully conducted studies of Bolos *et al.* (1990) and Gelernter *et al.* (1991).

It was pointed out by Gordis *et al.* (1990) that there were some difficulties with the experiment of Blum *et al.* (1990). The numbers of subjects were small, the criteria for diagnosis of alcoholism unclear, the status of the controls vague and DNA could have been obtained more easily from blood leucocytes than from brain. Nevertheless the work of Blum *et al.* (1990) is of some interest because it was an attempt to apply the 'new genetics' to the elucidation of the basis of alcoholism as forecast by Radouco-Thomas *et al.* (1984).

GENETIC CONTROL OF THE METABOLISM AND EFFECTS OF ALCOHOL

Twin studies of the metabolism of alcohol

An early and carefully performed study was that of Luth (1939), who investigated various pharmacokinetic parameters previously established by Widmark on 10 monozygous and 10 dizygous male twinships. The fall in blood alcohol concentration

per ml per minute was measured over 200 minutes following an oral dose. The author concluded that the metabolism of alcohol was largely (but not entirely) governed by hereditary factors.

The plasma elimination half-life was used as an index of alcohol metabolism by Vesell *et al.* (1971), who studied 14 pairs of twins. Their conclusion was that the heritability value for the alcohol elimination rate was 0.98, indicating that the rate was almost totally controlled by genetic factors.

Likewise, Kopun & Propping (1977) carried out a study on 40 pairs of twins (19 MZ and 21 DZ) and found a much lower heritability (h^2) for elimination of 0.46. Both these studies were criticized by Gurling *et al.* (1981) because of the small numbers of twins used and the biometric analysis employed.

It has been pointed out by Gibson & Oakeshott (1981) that for the above two studies the 95% confidence limits of the heritability estimates did not lie within the range 0.0 to 1.0.

A similar twin study comparing six monozygous and eight dizygous twin pairs was reported by Forsander & Eriksson (1974) (cited by Goodwin 1980). A heritability value of 0.8 was found by them for alcohol elimination rate.

A much larger and superbly analysed experiment was conducted by Martin *et al.* (1985) who studied blood alcohol concentrations (BAC) in 206 pairs of 18 to 34 year old twins; heritabilities of 0.62 ± 0.06 were found for peak BAC and 0.50 ± 0.07 for rate of elimination (Table 15.5). These estimates did not differ significantly from the repeatabilities of the BAC parameters, indicating that all repeatable variation among people in the way they metabolize alcohol is genetically determined.

So this large experiment indicates that the rates of alcohol metabolism are controlled to a substantial degree by both genetic and environmental factors.

Inter-ethnic variability in the effects of alcohol

The susceptibility of Oriental subjects, particularly Japanese, to develop objective phenomena such as flushing, and subjective phenomena such as headache and nausea after consuming what is, by European standards, a small amount of alcohol, has been known for a long time (Kalow, 1962).

The matter has been scientifically assessed by a number of workers in various ways. Wolff (1972,

Table 15.5. *Observed mean squares for parameters of blood alcohol metabolism*

	D.F.	Time to peak	Peak BAC	Rate of elimination ($\times 10^6$)
MZ females				
Between	42	1038	371	27.12
Within	43	353	89	8.56
MZ males				
Between	41	1471	361	27.08
Within	42	496	92	9.10
DZ females				
Between	43	1316	294	31.72
Within	44	440	226	18.44
DZ males				
Between	37	959	336	15.28
Within	38	448	131	12.17
DZ opposite sex				
Between	38	735	373	20.76
Within[a]	38	948	170	16.17

[a]Corrected for mean sex difference.
Time to peak (minutes) computed from $t_{max} = \frac{1}{k_1} \ln(k_1 Ao/k_2)$ computed for each individual where k_1 = rate constant for absorption; k_2 = rate constant for elimination; Ao = notional blood alcohol concentration if the dose were instantly ingested and spread throughout the body at zero time.
Peak BAC = blood alcohol concentration (B) at t_{max}.
Rate of elimination = $[\hat{B} (3 \text{ h}) - \hat{B}(t_{max})]/(3 \text{ h} - t_{max})$.
From: Martin *et al.* 1985

1973) tested the cutaneous vasomotor changes by means of optical densitometry of the earlobe, skin temperature of the cheek, finger plethysmography and visual inspection of the face (Table 15.6). Pronounced flushing was found in only 5% of Caucasians, but was present in 83% of Japanese, Taiwanese and Koreans, and in 80% of Algonquin Indians. Americans of Orientals extraction who were born and reared in the United States entirely on Western diets responded the same way as persons of the same ethnic group raised in the Far East. Offspring of marriages between Orientals and Europeans gave responses the same as pure Orientals.

Similar investigations were carried out by Ewing *et al.* (1974) but they scored individual symptoms on Oriental and Occidental subjects after they had ingested a standard dose of alcohol. Objective assessments of flushing, earlobe densitometry, blood-pressure and heart rate were made as well. Some symptoms occurred with the same frequency in the two groups (e.g. dizziness, sleepiness). Other symptoms occurred with significantly different frequencies. Pounding in the head was commoner in Orientals, whilst euphoric symptoms such as relaxa-

tion, confidence and happiness were commoner in Occidentals. Eleven of 24 Oriental, and three of 24 Occidental subjects had five or more symptoms indicating dysphoria (especially dizziness, pounding in the head, muscle weakness and tingling sensations). Blood acetaldehyde levels were measured and tended to be higher in Orientals than in Occidentals. Ewing *et al.* (1974) suggest that 'the general level of discomfort experienced by many Oriental people on drinking small amounts of alcohol would seem to offer them protection from overusing alcoholic beverages as a psychological escape mechanism'.

The subject of alcoholism among the Chinese is discussed by Lin & Lin (1982). They offer two counter-arguments to the 'physiological protection' hypothesis advanced above. First, not all Chinese have heightened sensitivity to alcohol, and even some of those who do have it still drink heavily despite having it. Secondly, Amerindians and Japanese who also have a high prevalence of alcohol sensitivity nevertheless have a significant problem with alcoholism in their societies. Lin & Lin (1982) opt in favour of socio-cultural rather than

Table 15.6. *Flushing responses, and increases of optical density and pulse pressure in the earlobe, after ingestion of alcohol. In each case, the Caucasoid population is compared with a corresponding Mongoloid group. Since only records free of artifacts were tabulated, whereas mean changes of optical density were calculated for the entire subgroup, the magnitude of flushing responses among Korean subjects appears to be less than that among other Mongoloid subgroups. This conclusion is not warranted by the results.*

Group	Sample size (No.)	Visible flushing (No.)	Optical density		Pulse pressure	
			Increase >5 mm (No.)	Mean increase for total (mm)	Measurable increase (No.)	Mean increase for total (%)
Caucasoid						
Adults	34	1	2	1.1	1(?)	5(?)
Infants	20	1	1	1.7	0	
Japanese						
Adults	38	32[a]	34[a]	36.8[b]	33[a]	257[b]
Infants	25	17[a]	17[a]	16.8[b]	9	
Taiwanese						
Adults	24	19[a]	20[a]	37.7[b]	19[a]	246[b]
Infants	10	9[a]	9[a]	14.6[b]	4	
Korean						
Adults	20	14[a]	10[a,c]	17.4[b,c]	9[a,c]	161[b]

[a]Ethnic group differences are significant at $p < 0.001$, χ^2 test.
[b]$p < 0.001$, t-test.
[c]The records of six Korean subjects could not be analysed reliably because of line-voltage disturbances.
From: Wolff 1972.

physiological factors being responsible for the low incidence of alcoholism among Chinese societies (even those who have been 'Westernized' to some extent).

In this connection an interesting study was carried out in Hawaii by Wilson *et al.* (1978). They ascertained the usage of alcoholic beverages in adults of Chinese, Japanese, Filipino, Caucasian, Hawaiian or part Hawaiian or mixed Oriental and Caucasian (Hapa Haole) ancestry. The term Hapa Haole refers to persons who reported one Caucasian parent and one Oriental (Chinese, Korean or Japanese) parent.

Flushing was much more common in Chinese, Japanese or Hapa Haole than in Caucasians. Compared with Caucasians a smaller proportion of Orientals reported ever using alcohol and the overall amount they consumed was somewhat smaller. Current or former use of alcohol was reported by 83% of the Hapa Haoles, similar to that found in Caucasians but different from either Oriental group. With respect to the estimated amount consumed Hapa Haoles were intermediate between the Orientals and the Caucasians, though few reported very heavy drinking. There was a close similarity between the Hapa Haoles and the Orientals in the frequency of flushing after the ingestion of alcohol. So it would seem that the social and/or physiological differences which underlined the lesser use of alcohol by Orientals are largely overcome in the Hapa Haole by the admixture of Caucasian genes, or social mores or both.

Inter-ethnic comparisons of the rates of alcohol metabolism

The rate of metabolism of alcohol is most frequently assessed by estimating the rate of elimination of alcohol from the plasma following a single oral dose. Reed (1978) points out that not much attention had been given by researchers to the inter-ethnic variability in this parameter until recently. At the same time, he points out that the inter-ethnic variability must be assessed against the background of the variability within a single ethnic group — which is considerable.

The variability within, and the variability between ethnic groups will be made up of genetic and environmental components. Consequently, particular value attaches to studies of different ethnic groups which are living in a common environment, but opportunities to perform such studies are obviously uncommon.

Environmental factors identified as influencing the rate of metabolism of alcohol were:

> chronic intake of alcohol (regular drinkers have higher rates) nutrition; drugs such as barbiturate and nicotine which increase rates; obesity which decreases rates.

Even bearing in mind the difficulties encountered in the studies due to recognizable environmental factors it did seem that Amerindians metabolized alcohol slightly, but significantly, faster than whites. In the study of Reed *et al.* (1976) Chinese subjects appeared to be intermediate between the other two ethnic groups. The calculated rates of alcohol metabolism were: Caucasians 103.6 mg/kg per hour, Chinese 136.6 mg/kg per hour, Ojibwa Amerindians 182.7 mg/kg per hour. Mean acetaldehyde values paralleled the rates of alcohol metabolism. Hanna (1978) obtained similar figures, namely, Japanese 133.6, Chinese 127.0 and Europeans 108 mg/kg per hour. The relationship between the ethnic groups remained very much the same after the figures were adjusted for body mass.

Reed (1978) discusses four other similar studies which reach much the same conclusions as regards comparing Amerindians with white subjects.

Segal & Lawrence (1992) found that the rate of elimination of alcohol from the blood was significantly higher in Alaskan natives than in whites or American Indians.

ALCOHOL DEHYDROGENASE

The metabolism of alcohol in man

Ethyl alcohol is metabolized by means of a number of enzymic pathways particularly in the liver, which include cytosolic alcohol dehydrogenase (ADH) the microsomal oxidizing system and catalase.

The microsomal alcohol oxidizing system (MEOS) is of importance because it is inducible by alcohol; this induction is responsible for the enhanced rate of metabolism of alcohol found in regular heavy drinkers. This oxidation is now known to be catalysed by the enzyme cytochrome P450 2E1 which is also induced by alcohol (see p.

15). A *Dra*I fragment length polymorphism in an intron of the governing *CYP 2E1* gene was described by Uematsu *et al.* (1991). There have been as yet no published studies of the molecular genetics of this enzyme in the field of alcoholism.

However, alcohol dehydrogenase is considered to be the major agent responsible for the metabolism of alcohol and has received most attention in genetic studies.

Alcohol dehydrogenase (EC 1.1.1.1) oxidizes alcohol to acetaldehyde, and the essential co-factor is NAD which becomes reduced to NADH in the process. This enzyme has zero-order kinetics, i.e. the speed of the reaction is not greater with an increased concentration of substrate. For this reason the manner of disappearance of a dose of alcohol from the plasma is unusual in that the fall in concentration is linear with time, unlike the customary exponential curve.

A variant form of alcohol dehydrogenase

An important advance was made when Von Wartburg *et al.* (1965) described a variant form of the enzyme in man. This enzyme had a considerably higher specific activity, a lower pH optimum and a greater sensitivity to inhibition by thiourea than the normal isozyme. It was found that about 5 to 20% of Caucasians possessed this atypical isozyme. It was thought possible that the atypical enzyme in an individual might lead to a greater capacity to metabolize alcohol *in vivo*. This should give a faster rate of disappearance of alcohol from the plasma after taking a single dose. The idea was tested out in Caucasians and the results are shown in Table 15.7. The expected enhanced metabolism was not observed. A possible explanation for this finding will be discussed below.

It was later found that the frequency of the atypical alcohol dehydrogenase was much greater in Oriental than in Caucasian populations (see Table 15.8). Frequencies of 85 to 98% have been found in surveys of Japanese, Chinese and Vietnamese.

A complex genetic polymorphism

Further investigations revealed that the liver alcohol dehydrogenases of man represent a very complex situation. There are three classes of ADH enzymes

Table 15.7. *Investigations of ethanol metabolism* in vivo *in individuals possessing typical and atypical liver alcohol dehydrogenase*

Reference	Alcohol degradation rate (mg/kg body weight/h)			
	Typical ADH		Atypical ADH	
	M	F	M	F
Edwards & Evans 1967	99.0 108.0	95.3	113.6	125.0
	118.7 107.6	90.1		
	121.9 101.5	89.7		
	108.1 118.0	107.0		
	115.6 113.0			
	108.9 107.0			
	101.3 126.0			
	119.8 118.0			
	101.2			
Von Wartburg & Schurch 1968	Sex not stated		Sex not stated	
	90		141	
Schulz *et al.* 1976	No data		Sex not stated	
			117	
			93	
			86	
			118	
			140	

ADH, Alcohol dehydrogenase; M, Male; F; Female.

Table 15.8. *Frequency of atypical ADH in different populations*

Subject group	% atypical individuals
Swiss	20
English	5–10
Americans, white	<5
Germans	9–14
Japanese	85–98
Americans, black	<10
Chinese	89
Bahia (Brazil)	2.8
Asian Indians	0
American Indians (Sioux, Navajo, Pueblo)	0

Adapted from: Agarwal & Goedde 1990. See also Chen *et al.* 1992.

differentiated from each other because they can be separated by various techniques such as ion-exchange resin and affinity chromatography. Class I enzymes (which are inhibited by pyrazole) are thought to be the most important in dealing with alcohol. Class II (π; pyrazole-insensitive) enzymes

are synthesized in the liver and stomach; even though they have a higher K_m for alcohol they are thought to be of importance in its metabolism. Class III (χ) enzymes have a very low affinity for alcohol and are thought to be involved more in the metabolism of long chain alcohols and ω-hydroxy fatty acids. They are the only ADH isozymes present in the brain (Bosron & Li 1986).

We are here concerned with Class I enzymes. They are constructed by random association to form dimers of three types of polypeptide subunits α, β and γ. These three peptide subunits are controlled by three separate gene loci *ADH1*, *ADH2* and *ADH3*. On this basis there were thought to exist six combinations: three homodimers and three heterodimers. However the situation was found to be much more complicated because there are three forms of β (β_1, β_2 and β_3) and two forms of γ (γ_1 and γ_2) in the population. This means there are 21 possible combinations, six of which are homodimers (see Fig. 15.1).

The 'atypical' *ADH* described by von Wartburg *et al.* (1965) contains the subunit β_2 whereas the 'typical' *ADH* is $\beta_1 \beta_1$. Since the variant allele *ADH2²* has a low frequency in Caucasian populations most of

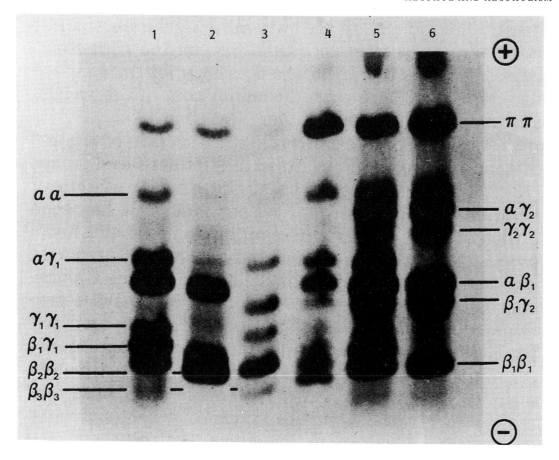

Fig. 15.1. Starch gel electrophoresis of ADH in human liver homogenate supernatants. Electrophoresis of six livers with different ADH phenotypes was performed according to Bosron et al. (1986). The ADH phenotype of the liver in *Lane 1* is ADH$_2$ 1–1, ADH$_3$ 1–1; *Lane 2* is ADH$_2$ 2–2, ADH$_3$ 1–1; *Lane 3* is ADH$_2$ 3–3, ADH$_3$ 1–1; *Lane 4* is ADH$_2$ 3–1, ADH$_3$ 1–1; *Lane 5* is ADH$_2$ 1–1, ADH$_3$ 2–1, and *Lane 6* is ADH$_2$ 1–1; ADH$_3$ 2–2. (From Bosron & Li 1986.)

the people who exhibit 'atypical' dehydrogenase on testing the liver enzymatically are heterozygotes (Smith *et al.* 1972).

Variants of the different subgroups of Class I ADH enzymes as studied by classical amino acid sequencing methods have been found to differ considerably. For example the β_1 subunit differs from the γ_1 subunit at 21 positions, 16 in the substrate binding domain and five in the coenzyme-binding domain (Buhler *et al.* 1984). On the other hand, within a given subclass a single amino acid substitution has been found to be responsible for the altered kinetic characteristics.

The variant dimer called β_2 Berne and β_2 Honolulu was shown to differ from β_1 by possessing a histidine residue at position 47 instead of arginine.

A variant β_3 β_3 (formerly called β Indianapolis) has been described, controlled by an allele which has a frequency of 0.16 in American blacks. This variant differed markedly from β_1 β_1 in its catalytic properties. For example, K_m for alcohol was 0.048 for β_1 β_1 and 64 for β_3 β_3 (Smith 1986). Also the K_m for NAD of β_3 β_3 was 70 times and the K_i value for NADH 35 times greater than for β_1 β_1. Sequencing of the β_3 subunit showed that there was substitution of cysteine for arginine at position 369. This amino acid change probably reduces the affinity of the enzyme for the nicotinamide phosphate moiety of NADH, thus accounting for the changed kinetic properties (Burnell *et al.* 1987).

Variation has also been described in the *ADH3* isozyme patterns due to the different dimers γ_1 and γ_2. In Europeans the respective frequencies of the structural alleles responsible, namely, *ADH3[1]* and *ADH3[2]* were found to be 0.6 and 0.4 respectively. In Japanese, however, the corresponding figures were 0.91 and 0.09. The allele *ADH3[2]* appears to be relatively infrequent in populations of African origin.

It is essential to know the three-dimensional structure of the enzyme in order to understand how amino acid substitutions at different positions exert their effects. The structure of human β_1 β_1 alcohol dehydrogenase has been determined by X-ray crystallography (Hurley *et al.* 1991). Previously only the horse enzyme had been crystallographically analysed and in order to overcome this deficiency conformational models were constructed using computer graphics (Eklund *et al.* 1990). It has been shown that within human Class I ADH only 1 to 3 residues vary out of eleven constituting the substrate-binding site. Between the three classes the substrate binding site varies greatly with 8 to 11 replacements, but one amino acid residue Val 295 is conserved throughout.

All the ADH isozymes have had their amino acid sequences determined. Now progress is being made very rapidly in the elucidation of the structure of the controlling genes.

Molecular genetics of ADH

The relevance of the many different types of alcohol dehydrogenase to clinical alcohol-related problems has not as yet been determined. As Bosron & Li (1986) pointed out, this has been because of lack of non-invasive and reliable methods of determining the phenotypes and genotypes since hitherto liver or other inaccessible tissue has been required to obtain the information. Now, however, as will be demonstrated below, the situation is undergoing a fundamental change.

A concise account of the molecular genetics is given by Smith (1986). Essential tools are restriction endonucleases and DNA probes. Probes have been developed by two techniques. First working from a segment of the known amino acid sequence of β_1

ADH a corresponding radiolabelled nucleotide was obtained and used to screen a human liver cDNA library. A clone was identified containing 1110 base pairs to which the probe hybridized. This clone was called pADH 12. Further work on the clone revealed that its DNA sequence predicted exactly the previously known sequence of the 3'-terminal 91 amino acids in β ADH. Secondly, an independent method using antibodies against ADH led to the recognition of a 1.7 kilobase (kb) insert in one human clone which represented a full length cDNA for ADH.

Chromosomal localization

Hybrid cells can be produced by fusing cells derived from rodents with those derived from humans. These cells tend progressively to lose human chromosomes as they are grown in tissue culture. The remaining human chromosomes are recognizable by their banding morphology. The radiolabelled probe pADH 12 will not bind to rodent chromosomes. When hybrid cells were examined only those containing human chromosome 4 hybridized to the probe. When a hybrid cell which contained only human chromosome 4 was hybridized to pADH 12 and then split up with *Eco*RI the same size fragments as from human genomic DNA were obtained. Eventually by these techniques it was shown that α, β and γ ADH are mapped on the long arm of chromosome 4 at q21 to q24. It seems likely that these three genes are not immediately adjacent to each other (Smith 1988).

Using similar techniques Rathna Giri *et al.* (1989) have produced evidence which suggests that the allele *ADH5* encoding Class III (χ) alcohol dehydrogenase is on human chromosome 4.

Gene organization

The three genes *ADH1*, *ADH2* and *ADH3* have a similar construction, each consisting of nine exons and they are about 10 to 15 kb long. There is a high degree of resemblance (about 95%) in the primary protein structures, coding cDNA sequences and even in their untranslated regions (Yoshida *et al.* 1988).

Some examples of sequencing information will now be described.

The complete sequence of *ADH2[1]* and *ADH2[2]* exons are now known and they differ only by one

Table 15.9. *Frequencies of* Xba*I,* Rsa*I and* Msp*I polymorphisms of alcohol dehydrogenase in random Caucasian and Oriental individuals*

Probe	Restriction enzyme	Location of polymorphic segment	Fragment sizes (kb)	Frequency	Population	Number of chromosomes
pADH74	*Xba*I	5′-end of ADH3	4.4 and 3.3	0.52 and 0.48	C	112
				0.91 and 0.09	O	22
pADH73	*Msp*I	3′-end of ADH3	12 and 10	0.65 and 0.35	C	46
				0.91 and 0.09	O	24
pADH36	*Rsa*I	5′-end of ADH2 (β)	1.0 and 0.5	0.78 and 0.22	C	78
				0.18 and 1.82	O	44

C, Caucasian; O, Oriental. *From:* Smith, 1986 (Ch. 5), 1988.

exonic nucleotide. The triplet responsible for amino acid 47 is CGC which codes for arginine in *ADH2*[1]. This is changed to CAC in *ADH2*[2] which codes for histidine (Matsuo *et al.* 1989). By means of site-directed mutagenesis and expression in *E. coli*, Hurley *et al.* (1990) showed that the substitution of arginine at position 47 by histidine gave a V_{max} which was 100 times higher even though K_m values were also increased.

The work of Carr *et al.* (1989) also illustrates very clearly how single nucleotide substitutions may or may not alter the gene product. The gene *ADH2*[3] has four nucleotide substitutions as compared with *ADH2*[1].

1 In exon 9 thymine is substituted for cytosine at the base position 159 which is the start of the triplet which codes for amino acid 369. Hence CGT (which is one of the six triplets which code for arginine) is altered to TGT which codes for cysteine.

2 In intron 5, twelve base pairs before the start of exon 6, cytosine is substituted for thymine. Since the bases in the intron do not code for an amino acid there is no change in the gene product.

3 In exon 6 at base position 67 a substitution of thymine for cytosine changes the triplet GTC which codes for valine into GTT, which is one of the other three triplets which code for valine which is amino acid 203 in the enzyme.

4 In exon 6 at base position 208 thymine is substituted for cytosine giving ATT which codes for isoleucine, instead of ATC which (with ATA) also codes for isoleucine which is amino acid 250 in the enzyme.

The single amino acid substitution at position 369 is responsible for the kinetic differences between β_1 and β_3 isozymes.

There are other factors apart from gene structure (and hence enzyme structure) which control the activity of ADH in the liver. Examples which are listed by Hittle & Crabb (1988) are:

1 rate of gene transcription;
2 selection of alternative promoters or transcription start sites;
3 variations in RNA processing;
4 mRNA stability;
5 efficiency of translation;
6 protein stability.

Some of these processes have been shown to be variable in other species but as yet there is no evidence of such phenomena in humans.

Restriction fragment length polymorphisms

By using various restriction endonucleases and ADH probes human leucocyte DNA can be explored. It has been possible to identify RFLPs which have very different allele frequencies in Oriental and Caucasian populations (Table 15.9).

ADH genotyping using DNA from leucocytes

Oligonucleotide probes were synthesized by Ikuta *et al.* (1988). These were constructed specifically to detect the DNA structures of *ADH2*[1] and *ADH2*[2] (Fig. 15.2). The DNA was obtained from peripheral blood leucocytes. The DNA was digested using the restriction endonucleases *Eco*RI and *Pvu*II and the restriction fragments were separated by agarose gel electrophoresis. The gel was then successively exposed to the two probes which had been labelled at the 5′-

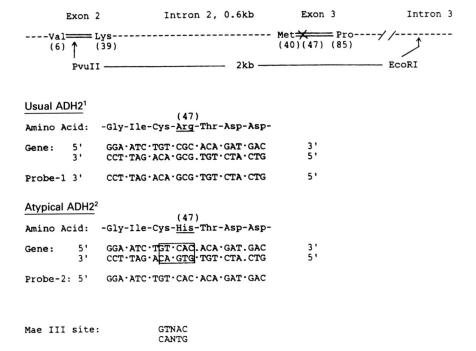

Fig. 15.2. Restriction map of the mutation region of the *ADH2* gene and amino acid sequences, nucleotide sequences, and the specific synthetic probes for the usual *ADH¹* and the atypical *ADH²* genes. Exons are shown by double lines, and introns are shown by dashed lines. Positions of amino acid residues from the N-terminal are given in parentheses. The position of the mutation is marked 'X'. (From Ikuta *et al.* 1988.)

end with ³²P. Finally, radioautographs were prepared. As Fig. 15.3 reveals genotyping information is readily obtainable on individuals by this means. In a survey of 49 unrelated Japanese individuals using this method, Ikuta *et al.* (1988) found that the frequencies of the two alleles were *ADH2¹* 0.29 and *ADH2²* 0.71.

It has been pointed out by Groppi *et al.* (1990) that using the polymerase chain reaction (PCR) and RFLPs, the genotypes at *ADH2* and *ADH3* can be determined from blood samples unambiguously and quickly.

Application and speculation

There are a number of applications of this new knowledge. For example Smith (1988) details the use of ADH genotyping information in the analysis of hepatomas. Of more immediate interest however, would be the possibility of re-examining the question of whether the possession of the enzyme β₂ confers upon an individual the ability more rapidly to oxidize alcohol to acetaldehyde. It is no longer necessary to establish the phenotype using liver biopsy specimens, as the genotype can be established directly using blood. The evidence which has already been discussed above shows that Orientals have more rapid blood alcohol disappearance rates than Caucasians. As shown by the results of Ikuta *et al.* (1988) about half of Japanese individuals are homozygous *ADH2²/ADH2²*. In a phenotyping survey of 90 livers in Hong Kong Chinese, 83 were found to possess 'atypical' ADH by Fong *et al.* (1989) which gives almost exactly the same genotype frequencies. So maybe the β₂ β₂ Oriental is capable of producing acetaldehyde more quickly than the β₁ β₁ Caucasian and it would be valuable to know this for reasons which will come apparent later.

The relationships of the *ADH* genotypes to various alcohol-induced disorders wait to be explored; similarly the part played by different *ADH* genotypes in the metabolism of substrates other than alcohol (Table 15.10).

ALDEHYDE DEHYDROGENASE

Different types of acetaldehyde dehydrogenase

When alcohol is metabolized by means of the enzyme alcohol dehydrogenase, acetaldehyde is produced. The acetaldehyde is in turn metabolized by acetaldehyde dehydrogenase (aldehyde:NAD^+ oxidoreductase, EC 1.2.1.3) to acetate.

Attention became focused on aldehyde dehydrogenase (ALDH) relatively later than alcohol dehydrogenase and a keynote paper was that of Greenfield & Pietruszko (1977), who purified two forms of the enzyme from human liver to apparent homogeneity using classical chromatographic methods. Then on starch gel electrophoresis they found that the enzyme migrating more slowly towards the anode (enzyme 1), had at pH 9.5 a K_m of 0.1 mM for acetaldehyde and was very strongly inhibited by disulfiram (K_i of 0.2 µM at pH 7.0). In contrast, the faster migrating enzyme 2 had a K_m of 2 to 3 µM for acetaldehyde at pH 9.5 and was not inhibited by disulfiram at pH 7.0. Polyacrylamide gel electrophoresis gave molecular weight estimates of 245 000 for enzyme 1 and 225 000 for enzyme 2.

Table 15.10. *Compounds other than ethanol which are metabolized by liver alcohol dehydrogenase*

Methanol	
Ethylene glycol	
1,2-propandiol	
Digoxin	
Digitoxin	Converted to 3-keto derivatives[a]
Gitoxin	
Steroids	
Bile acids	
Short chain alcohols responsible for food flavours	Proposed

[a]Simultaneous ethanol consumption has the possibility via competitive inhibition to cause toxicity due to cardiac glycosides.
Compiled using information from: Agarwal & Goedde 1990.

At this point it should be explained that there have been two ways of classifying human ALDH. This may create some confusion on reading the literature. Some workers, e.g. Greenfield & Pietruszko (1977) labelled the cytosolic liver enzyme as 1 and the mitochondrial enzyme as 2. Others, e.g. Goedde & Agarwal (1987) labelled the enzymes

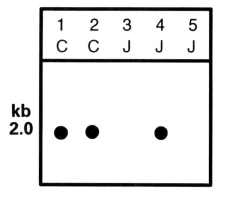

Probe 1

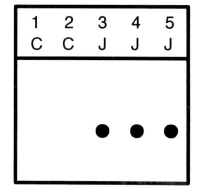

Probe 2

Fig. 15.3. Hybridization of human genomic DNA prepared from blood, with oligonucleotide probes. Probe 1 detects *ADH2¹* whereas Probe 2 detects *ADH2²*. C, Caucasian; J, Japanese. Individuals 1 and 2 are homozygous *ADH2¹/ADH2¹*; individuals 3 and 5 are homozygous *ADH2²/ADH2²* and individual 4 is a heterozygote. (From Ikuta *et al.* 1988.)

according to their electrophoretic mobility and since the mitochondrial enzyme moves fastest it was called ALDH1. Now following the publication 'Nomenclature of mammalian aldehyde dehydrogenases' (1989) the former nomenclature has become standard. In this book this standardized nomenclature is used throughout.

A little after the publication of Greenfield & Pietruszko (1977) it was shown by Harada *et al.* (1978) that ALDH exhibited complex electrophoretic patterns in human tissues. The same group (Goedde *et al.* 1979) found in studies of liver ALDH in Japanese that 21 of 40 liver specimens showed only the slower migrating isozyme band, whereas under the same circumstances 68 postmortem livers from German individuals showed two isozyme bands (Fig. 15.4).

It will be recalled that the 'atypical' alcohol dehydrogenase was found in 85% of Japanese liver specimens, and it was found that the frequency of the unusual pattern of ALDH was independent of the alcohol dehydrogenase polymorphism.

As has been mentioned earlier, it was already known that flushing and associated phenomena were observable in about half of Japanese subjects following alcohol ingestion. Goedde *et al.* (1979) made the suggestion that the polymorphic nature of ALDH in Japanese livers might be of particular importance in connection with the ethnic variation in alcohol sensitivity. The initial vasomotor flushing after alcohol ingestion in Japanese might be due to their inability to metabolize acetaldehyde quickly and effectively in the absence of the faster migrating isozyme of ALDH. Consequently subjects possessing the unusual ALDH phenotype would be exposed to elevated blood acetaldehyde concentration until it was oxidized by the slower migrating enzyme which had a low affinity for acetaldehyde.

A huge amount of detailed information on the pharmacogenetics of ALDH was provided by Goedde & Agarwal (1990). The discussion in this book is limited to the exploration of the main point, which is that genetically determined interindividual variability determines the outcome of exposure to alcohol.

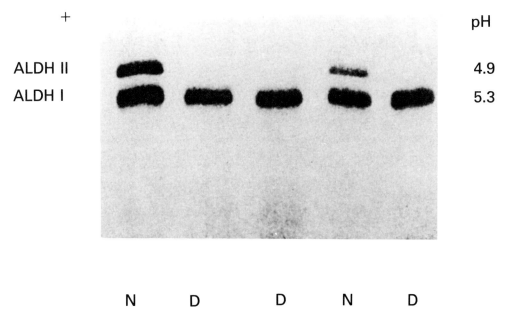

Fig. 15.4. Isoelectric focusing pattern of human liver ALDH isozymes. N, normal type; D, deficient type. The Roman numerals have been reversed from the original so that they appear according to the current standard nomenclature. (From Agarwal & Goedde 1987a.)

Table 15.11. *The properties of two human liver aldehyde dehydrogenases*

	Cytosolic ALDH1	Mitochondrial ALDH2
Composition	Homotetramer	Homotetramer
M_r	245 000	225 000
K_m for acetaldehyde	0.1 mM at pH 9.5	2 to 3 µM at pH 9.5
Preferred coenzyme NAD$^+$	K_m 8 µM at pH 9.5	K_m 70 µM at pH 9.5
Inhibition by disulphiram	K_i 0.2 µM at pH 7.0	No inhibition at pH 7.0 considered partially sensitive to disulfiram, but sensitive to its metabolites
Precipitation by antibodies	Specific antibodies, i.e. not cross-reacting, can be produced	Specific antibodies, i.e. not cross-reacting, can be produced
Chromosomal localization	9q21	12q24
Genomic structure	Partial cDNA sequencing reveals about 66% homology in coding regions	

Cytosolic and mitochondrial liver aldehyde dehydrogenase

The two ALDH enzymes differ with regard to many structural and functional properties (Table 15.11). It is possible that the segregation of the two enzymes inside the liver cell is not absolute (Meier-Tackmann *et al.* 1988) but it is difficult to be sure that the presence of the two enzymes in one subcellular compartment is not due to artefact; for example, following freezing and thawing. Both enzymes have a K_m in the micromolar range but the value for the mitochondrial enzyme is lower. At a 1 mM concentration the cytosolic enzyme is inhibited *in vitro* by disulfiram isoniazid and benzyl isothiocyanate, whilst the mitochondrial enzyme is inhibited by isoniazid. No inhibition was demonstrated (Agarwal *et al.* 1987) to metronidazole, moxalactam, tolbutamide, cimetidine, ranitidine, lithium, haloperidol or diazepam. It is, however, possible that metabolites of drugs may be inhibitory – for example diethylamine formed from disulfiram is inhibitory to the mitochondrial enzyme.

A technical advance in studying the acetaldehyde dehydrogenase phenotype

A technical step forward was made by Goedde *et al.* (1980). The studies on liver samples obtained by biopsies at surgical operations, and at autopsies, had advanced knowledge of both alcohol dehydrogenase and ALDH. Nevertheless, it was obviously impossible to make large population surveys on living persons. This difficulty was overcome by the finding that by using sensitive micro-methods these enzymes and their variant forms could be detected in human hair-root cells. It was shown that in an individual a similar pattern was obtained from liver and hair-roots (Fig. 15.5). Family studies suggested that the Japanese ALDH2 electrophoretic banding pattern was a genetic polymorphism controlled by two autosomal alleles. Much later the ALDH bands were also shown to be present in human lymphocytes and their patterns parallel those of hair roots (Dyck 1990).

Ethnic distribution

Using the hair-root technique, surveys of the ALDH polymorphism have been carried out in numerous ethnic groups (Table 15.12). The highest incidence of ALDH2 deficiency occurs in Japanese, Han Chinese, Vietnamese and South American Indians. Oddly enough, North American Indians, although they are believed to have an Oriental ancestry have a low incidence of ALDH2 deficiency (Goedde *et al.* 1986a). Using more sophisticated genotyping methods, O'Dowd *et al.* (1990) cast doubt on the accuracy of the phenotyping data obtained by hair root enzymic analysis in Mapuche Indians. Taiwanese Malayo–Polynesian 'aborigines' had deficiency frequencies of 4/63 (6.4%), 2/52 (3.9%) and 0/42 in Atayal, Paiwan and Yami tribes respectively, significantly less than their Chinese (Han) neighbours who were 51% deficient (Chen *et al.* 1991).

In view of the reports of Wilkin (1988) and Mura-

Table 15.12. *Frequency of mitochondrial ALDH isozyme deficiency in Asian Mongoloids, American Indians and other populations.*

Population	Sample size	% deficient
Orientals		
Japanese	184	44
Chinese		
Mongolian	198	30
Zhuang	106	25
Han	120	45
Korean (Mandschu)	209	25
Koreans (South)	75	27
Vietnamese	138	53
Indonesians	30	39
Thais (North)	110	8
Phillipinos	110	13
Ainu	80	20
South American Indians		
Shuara (Ecuador)	99	42
Atacamenos (Chile)	133	43
Mapuche (Chile)	64	41
North American Indians		
Sioux (North Dakota)	90	5
Navajo (New Mexico)	56	2
Mexican Indians		
Mestizo (Mexico City)	43	4
Other populations		
Germans	300	0
Egyptians	260	0
Sudanese	40	0
Kenyans	23	0
Liberians	184	0
Fangs	37	0
Turks	65	0
Israeli	77	0
Hungarians	177	0
Matyo	106	0
Roman	84	0
Asian Indians	50	0

From: Goedde & Agarwal 1986. See also Chen *et al.* 1992.

matsu *et al.* (1989) an alcohol skin patch test may enable population surveys to be performed with much greater ease. Muramatsu *et al.* (1989) showed a correlation between the ALDH2-deficient electrophoretic pattern from hair-roots with the erythema produced after applying a small alcohol-soaked patch to the upper arm for 7 minutes. Wilkin (1988) showed that the cutaneous vascular response to alcohol could be blocked by 4-methylpyrazole, an inhibitor of alcohol dehydrogenase Class I.

Molecular genetics

Oriental livers of the ALDH2-deficient type were studied with antibodies to the enzyme and were found to contain cross-reactive material. This gene product which is an inactive enzyme differed from the active enzyme in that at the 14th position from the C-terminal end (and 487th position from the amino terminal end) glutamic acid was substituted with lysine (Yoshida *et al.* 1984; Hsu *et al.* 1985). This is due to a change from guanine to adenine as the first base of the coding triplet in the DNA in this position (Hempel *et al.* 1985).

Genomic clone analysis has led to the structure of the ALDH2 gene being elucidated. It is about 44 kb in length and contains at least 13 exons which encode 517 amino acids. The amino acid sequence deduced from the exons coincided with the reported primary structure of ALDH plus an N-terminal signal peptide of 17 amino acids which is absent from the mature enzyme (Yoshida *et al.* 1988).

A full-length ALDH2 cDNA has been cloned and introduced into a rabbit reticulocyte lysate in the presence of ^{35}S-methionine. The synthesized polypeptide migrated similarly to the authentic ALDH2 on SDS-PAGE. This indicated the absence of major post-translational modifications (Braun *et al.* 1987).

Synthetic oligonucleotides have been prepared which are specific for the two forms of ALDH2, so that under adequate hybridization conditions the genotype of an individual can be determined using DNA prepared from circulating blood leucocytes (Yoshida *et al.* 1988).

This technique was deployed by Goedde *et al.* (1989) who proceeded as follows. The ALDH phenotypes were determined in hair-root samples. One microgram of DNA from white cells was taken for polymerase chain reaction (PCR) amplification. Forty cycles of amplification were performed using the 21-mer primers 5'-CAAATTACAGGGTCA-ACTGCT and 5'-CCACACTCACAGTTTTCACTT which encompass exon 12 of the mitochondrial *ALDH* gene. The product was rendered single stranded then dot-blotted and hybridized with the γ-^{32}P-ATP 5'-end-labelled oligonucleotide probes 3'-CCGTATGTGACTTCACTTTTG-5' and 5'-GGCATACACTAAAGTGAAAAC-3' corresponding to the normal and mutant DNA sequences in exon 12. The pattern obtained is shown in Fig. 15.6. A population of 218 South Koreans contained 62

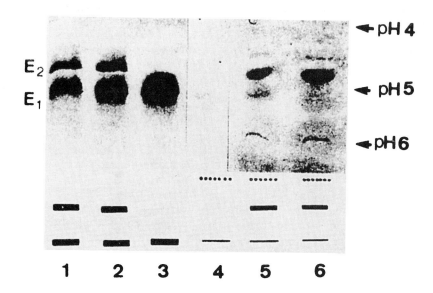

Fig. 15.5. Isoelectric focusing pattern of ALDH in liver (1–3) and hair-root extracts (4–6) from Japanese. Lanes 1, 2, 5 and 6 show the usual phenotype and lanes 3 and 4 the unusual phenotype. (From Agarwal *et al.* 1981.)

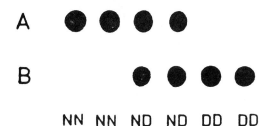

Fig. 15.6. Genotyping of mitochondrial ALDH. Dot blot patterns of six individuals. Amplified DNA was hybridized with allele-specific oligonucleotide probes corresponding to normal sequence (A) and mutant sequence (B). *NN* Normal homozygote, *ND* heterozygote, *DD* deficient homozygote. (From Goedde *et al.* 1989.)

apparently deficient phenotypes (as determined by hair-root analysis) shown by genomic analysis to be 58 heterozygotes and 4 homozygotes. So the deficient phenotype, strangely enough, is the dominant one. Similar techniques were deployed by Crabb *et al.* (1989) and Singh *et al.* (1989), yielding the same results.

The way in which the possession of one defective allele confers dominance invites some sort of explanation, and one is offered by Crabb *et al.* (1989) as follows. The enzyme ALDH2 is a homotetrameric enzyme. Random association of active and inactive subunits, present in equal numbers, would produce one normal tetramer in every 16 tetramers. It is possible that the other heterotetramers are inactive and/or unstable.

Chromosomal localization

Southern blot hybridization of DNA samples obtained from a panel of rodent–human hybrid cells with cDNA probes (Fig. 15.7) and also hybridization *in situ*, showed that the cytosolic *ALDH1* gene is located at 9q21 and the mitochondrial *ALDH2* gene is located at 12q24 (Hsu *et al.* 1986). A third class of cytoplasmic isozyme aldehyde dehydrogenase called ALDH3, which is found in human stomach, lung and hepatocellular carcinoma, has been mapped to chromosome 17 (see Agarwal & Goedde 1987b).

The pharmacological effects of alcohol in relation to aldehyde dehydrogenase type

The suggestion made by Goedde *et al.* (1979) that ALDH2-deficient individuals might be more prone to flushing after alcohol ingestion than non-

Table 15.13. *Genotypes of aldehyde dehydrogenase-2 locus (ALDH2) in alcohol flushers and non-flushers. The difference in gene frequency between flushers and non-flushers is statistically significant (p < 0.01)*

	Genotypes			Gene frequency	
	1-1	1-2	2-2	1	2
Flushers (*n* = 9)	0	7	2	0.39	0.61
Non-flushers (*n* = 6)	5	1	0	0.92	0.08
Total (*n* = 16)	5	8	2	0.60	0.40

From: Shibuya *et al.* 1989.

Table 15.14. *Peak blood acetaldehyde and ethanol levels in normal and deficient Japanese after an acute dose of ethanol*

	Peak values (mean ± SD) of	
Aldehyde dehydrogenase isozyme pattern	Acetaldehyde (µM)	Alcohol (mM)
Normal (*n* = 25)	2.1 ± 1.7	10.30 ± 1.85
Deficient (*n* = 19)	35.4 ± 12.8	10.93 ± 2.31

Dose = 0.5 g alcohol/kg body weight orally.
From: Harada *et al.* 1981.

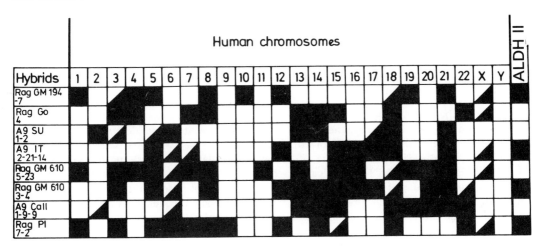

Fig. 15.7. Segregation of human ALDH 2 in a panel of human–mouse somatic cell hybrids. Filled spaces indicate the presence of the chromosome; half-filled spaces indicate that part of the chromosome is present; empty spaces indicate that the chromosome was not detected by biochemical and cytogenetic analysis. ALDH 2 segregates concordantly with chromosome 12.

When chromosome 12 was present the ALDH 2 probe hybridized solely with it. This was not so for any other chromosome. (From Braun *et al.* 1986.)

deficients, was tested by Shibuya *et al.* (1989). They determined the ALDH2 genotypes of 15 healthy Japanese individuals using leucocyte DNA. Their response to alcohol as flushers or non-flushers as described by themselves or according to a physician's observation were recorded and this information was not known to the genotype analyst. The results are shown in Table 15.13 and indicate that alcohol flushing is strongly associated with the

ALDH2² allele.

The way in which ALDH2 deficiency produces flushing after alcohol ingestion has been shown by Harada *et al.* (1981, 1985), who demonstrated in healthy individuals that whilst the mean blood alcohol level was the same in Japanese ALDH2 normal and ALDH2-deficient individuals (as shown by hair-root cell analysis) the mean blood acetaldehyde level was 15 times higher in the ALDH2-deficient individuals than the normals following a single oral dose of alcohol (see Table 15.14).

A further refinement of this information has been supplied by Enomoto *et al.* (1991a). They genotyped and phenotyped persons for ALDH status. After moderate amounts of alcohol the acetaldehyde levels were the same in ALDH2 heterozygotes and homozygotes, but after small amounts of alcohol the peak acetaldehyde levels were nearly four times higher in the latter.

Table 15.15. *Drinking habits in ALDH2 normal and deficient subjects*

		ALDH2 normal (59)	ALDH2 deficient (42)
Both sexes	Drinking +	29	8
	−	30	34[a]
Males	+	19	7
	−	6	12[b]
Females	+	10	1
	−	24	22[b]

[a]$p < 0.01$.
[b]$p < 0.05$.
From: Ohmori *et al.* 1986.

Table 15.16. *Frequency of ALDH2 deficiency in alcoholics, normal controls and other diagnostic categories in Japan*

Subjects	Number	Percentage with ALDH2 deficiency
Normal controls	105	41.0
Alcoholics (total)	175	2.3
Alcoholics with liver disorder	72	2.8
Alcoholics with mental disorder	103	1.9
Schizophrenics	86	41.9
Drug dependents	47	48.9

Adapted from: Harada *et al.* 1982.

Alcohol consumption in relation to the Japanese ALDH2 polymorphism

The relationship of the ALDH2 polymorphism to the quantity of alcohol consumed by Japanese was investigated by Ohmori *et al.* (1986). Out of 101 persons tested 42% were ALDH2-deficient. The subjects were classified as 'drinking habits +' indicating subjects who drink every day or almost every day, and 'drinking habits −' which included subjects who drink sometimes, only occasionally or not at all. The results are shown in Table 15.15. About half of the ALDH2-positive subjects have drinking habits whereas only 19% of ALDH2-deficient subjects have such habits. The same type of conclusion was reached for both sexes but the association may be stronger in women.

A survey of 282 Japanese by Higuchi *et al.* (1992) correlated alcohol consumption with ALDH phenotype as determined by the hair-root method. They showed in both men and women that ALDH2-deficient persons drank significantly less alcohol than those who possessed an active ALDH2.

An association of an acetaldehyde dehydrogenase phenotype with alcoholism

When 175 Japanese alcoholics (diagnostic criteria not specified) were compared with 133 Japanese non-alcoholics and 105 Japanese healthy controls Harada *et al.* (1982) found that only about 2% of the alcoholics had the hair-root ALDH2-deficiency

pattern compared with 41 to 49% in the other two groups (Table 15.16). Similar results were also obtained in a further series of 261 abstinent alcoholics.

Possession of ALDH2 (as determined by hair-root examination) was associated with alcohol abuse and alcohol dependence in Han Chinese in Taiwan, but not in their Formosan aborigine neighbours who have a significant incidence of alcohol problems but a low frequency of ALDH2 deficiency (Chen *et al.* 1991).

Using genomic analysis of leucocyte DNA with oligonucleotide probes Shibuya & Yoshida (1988) studied 49 healthy unrelated Japanese and 23 unrelated patients with alcoholic liver diseases (based on histological criteria). In the control group 21 of 49 individuals were homozygous 1-1 (i.e. Caucasian type), 22 heterozygous 1-2 and six were 2-2. Amongst the alcoholics 20 out of 23 were of genotype 1-1 and three were 1-2. There were no 2-2 atypical homozygotes.

So the evidence is very strongly in favour of the following view. In the Japanese ALDH2 polymorphism the deficient phenotype is relatively unable to metabolize acetaldehyde to acetate. This leads to higher blood acetaldehyde concentrations following a dose of alcohol. This acetaldehyde causes symptoms and signs such as nausea and flushing, which have been shown to be associated with the ALDH2-deficient phenotype. Presumably because of this chain of events the individual with the ALDH2 deficient phenotype has been shown to drink less alcohol and presumably because of their lower alcohol consumption ALDH2-deficient individuals are less prone to alcoholism and its sequelae than ALDH2 non-deficient persons.

There was a possibility that Oriental persons who are ADH β_2 β_2 and also ALDH2-deficient, who constitute over 40% of Japanese and Chinese (Fong *et al.* 1989) populations, may have higher acetaldehyde levels than other ALDH2-deficients and so have more flushing and possibly more protection against alcohol dependence.

This idea has now been tested by a survey of 49 Chinese alcoholics (alcohol-dependent by DSM III criteria) and 47 normal Chinese in Taipei. The genotypes at *ADH2*, *ADH3*, and *ALDH2* loci were determined by PCR amplification and allele specific probe techniques. The allelic frequencies in the controls were similar to those previously described in Chinese and Japanese populations. The *ADH2²* and *ADH3¹* alleles were less frequent among the alcoholics than among the non-alcoholics (93% of non-alcoholics had one or more *ADH2²* alleles as compared with 64% of alcoholics) and this pattern remained true if *ALDH2¹* homozygotes were examined in isolation (Thomasson *et al.* 1991). Perhaps the data presented in Table 15.7, which were obtained in Caucasians where *ADH2²* homozygotes are rare do not represent the situation in Orientals where such homozygotes are frequent.

Some further considerations concerning ALDH deficiency

Quite separate from the ALDH2-deficiency polymorphism there is also an ALDH1-deficiency polymorphism in Japanese. A few per cent of the Japanese population has an ALDH1-deficiency phenotype (Yoshida *et al.* 1983a, b) and examples have also been found in a Chinese and a Thai (Eckey *et al.* 1986).

The relationship of this ALDH1-deficiency polymorphism to clinical phenomena such as alcohol-flushing, alcohol addiction, alcohol dependence and alcohol abuse is quite unknown. Similarly it is not known if the ALDH1-deficiency and the ALDH2-deficiency phenotypes, when they coexist, have additive effects.

In fact it is rather uncertain what are the relative importances of ALDH1 and ALDH2 in the metabolism of alcohol. The striking phenomena, described above, which occur in ALDH2 deficiency have given

rise to the idea that it is this mitochondrial enzyme which is by far the more important. That this view may not be entirely correct is suggested by the following observation.

The problem of alcohol-induced flushing in Caucasians (which affects some 5 to 10% of the population) is clearly unsolved by the work on ALDH2-deficiency in Japanese because this phenotype does not occur in Caucasians.

In an attempt to shed light on this mystery, Yoshida *et al.* (1989) investigated nine Caucasian alcohol-flushers for their ALDH1 characteristics. It had been demonstrated by Agarwal *et al.* (1989) that the amino acid sequences of erythrocytic and liver cytosolic ALDH1 are identical. So studying the red cells reveals the properties of the liver enzyme. Two of the nine Caucasian alcohol-flushers were found to have variant forms of the enzyme. One had very low activity (10 to 20% of control) and the other moderately low activity (60% of control). They also had abnormal electrophoretic mobilities and in the first example the same abnormal enzyme was found in the proband's daughter.

So it appears that the explanation for at least some Caucasian alcohol-flushers may be defective ALDH1 activity.

It is interesting to note that the symptoms produced when a Caucasian ingests alcohol while he is receiving disulfiram are very similar to the symptoms produced in a Japanese ALDH2-deficient individual when he drinks alcohol. The explanation for this is that diethylamine (a degradation product of disulfiram) inhibits the low K_m ALDH2 which is present in the Caucasian thus making him metabolically similar to the ALDH2-deficient Japanese (Goedde *et al.* 1983b).

The very impressive work on the relationship between the ALDH2-deficiency polymorphism and alcoholism in Japanese sheds no light on the enormous social problem of alcohol-related disease in Caucasians. However it is a stimulus to further studies of acetaldehyde-metabolizing and other enzymes to see if a disease-prone diathesis can be delineated.

A final problem concerns the relationship between the ALDH enzymes and the phenomenon of chlorpropamide–alcohol flushing (CPAF), which is discussed in Chapter 28. Very little work has been carried out in this area, which is a pity because the alleged protection of CPAF positives from diabetic complications makes the topic one of considerable clinical importance.

TWO NEW ASSOCIATIONS OF PHENOTYPES WITHIN POLYMORPHISMS WITH ALCOHOLISM

Harada *et al.* (1987) have reported preliminary findings on two new associations in Japanese.

The first concerns salivary ALDH electrophoresed on polyacrylamide gel. Four different isozyme sets were detected in different individuals, and the phenotypes were tentatively designated 0, 1, 2-1 and 2. The first, phenotype 0, has no detectable activity in the saliva. It was found to be very common (67.8%) among healthy subjects but less frequent among alcoholics (32.9%). The 2-1 and 2 phenotypes together accounted for 4.7% of the healthy subjects and 30.3% of alcoholics.

Glutathione-S-transferase (GST) was found to give four isozyme patterns in random autopsy liver extracts. The patterns were designated 0, 1, 2-1 and 2, where pattern 0 exhibited no detectable enzyme activity. The same four enzymic patterns were also detectable using lysates of peripheral blood lymphocytes. In both tissues the frequency of the 0 phenotype was significantly higher in alcoholics than in healthy controls, whereas 1 and 2-1 combined occurred in 43.9% of controls and only in 17.2% of alcoholics.

These results will have to be confirmed on larger numbers, and the genetics of the phenotypes will have to be studied in families. Families of alcoholic probands will also need to be studied to see if the putative association holds up within them. However it is possible that these new discoveries may help build up an enzymic 'profile' of individuals who are particularly at risk of becoming alcoholics in Japanese society.

GENETIC PREDISPOSITION TO THE SEQUELAE OF ALCOHOLISM

It was previously mentioned that Omenn & Motulsky (1972) in their comprehensive genetic model of alcoholism included amongst other considerations the possibility that genetic factors might determine the susceptibility to medical complications.

This idea was explored by Hrubec & Omenn

(1981) who examined the medical histories of 15 924 male twin pairs in the USA National Academy of Sciences–National Research Council Twin Registry. The prevalences of alcoholism, alcoholic psychosis and liver cirrhosis were similar in monozygous (MZ) and dizygous (DZ) proband twins. The prevalences in percentage among co-twins of diagnosed subjects, i.e. case-wise twin concordance rates, were for alcoholism 26.3 MZ, 11.9 DZ; for alcoholic psychosis 21.1 MZ, 6.0 DZ; and for liver cirrhosis 14.6 MZ, 5.4 DZ. The greater concordance for alcoholic psychosis and liver cirrhosis among MZ than among DZ twins could not be explained by the difference in the concordance for alcoholism between them. As the authors state the results provide evidence in favour of genetic predisposition to organ-specific complications of alcoholism and should serve to stimulate searches for the underlying biochemical mechanisms.

In Japanese startling figures were produced by Enomoto *et al.* (1991b), who genotyped 47 patients with alcoholic liver disease for *ALDH*. Forty were *ALDH2*[1] homozygotes and seven *ALDH2*[1]/*ALDH2*[2] heterozygotes with no *ALDH2*[2] homozygotes, which was significantly different from the population distribution. So in Japanese it seems clear that the possession of even one mutant *ALDH* allele protects against cirrhosis, and possibly two mutant alleles are even more protective.

A biochemical basis has emerged to explain the susceptibility of certain individuals to the well-known Wernicke–Korsakoff syndrome (WKS) which is characterized by a profound and chronic memory disorder, particularly affecting short-term memory, usually with nystagmus and ataxia.

Two clinical facts suggested that this disorder might be a result of the interplay of genetic susceptibility and environmental influence. While it was known to be due to thiamine deficiency it only occurred in a few (about 5%) alcoholics and other severely malnourished persons. Also it occurred more frequently in Europeans than in non-Europeans on similar thiamine-deficient diets. With these thoughts in mind Blass & Gibson (1977) studied transketolase in cultured fibroblasts from four patients with WKS and six controls. The enzyme from the cells of WKS patients bound thiamine pyrophosphate less avidly than that from the controls (Table 15.17). The apparent K_m was 195 ± 31 and 16 ± 2 respectively for the two groups,

Table 15.17. K_m values for thiamine pyrophosphate for transketolase from WKS patients and controls[a]

K_m for TPP (μM)			
Patients		Controls	
Case 1	$281 \pm 79(5)$	No. 1	$20 \pm 9(4)$
Case 2	$196 \pm 45(4)$	No. 2	$20 \pm 4(8)$
Case 3	$156 \pm 40(4)$	No. 3	$15 \pm 5(5)$
Case 4	$146 \pm 45(5)$	No. 4	$15 \pm 5(5)$
		No. 5	$12 \pm 3(5)$
Mean	195 ± 31	No. 6	$11 \pm 3(4)$
		Mean	16 ± 2

[a]The apparent K_m for thiamine pyrophosphate (TPP) was determined in ammonium sulphate extracts of cultured skin fibroblasts from the 4 patients with the Wernicke–Korsakoff syndrome and six control lines. Values are means ± SEM. The number of cultures studied for each subject is given in parentheses. Differences between the group of patients and the group of controls were highly significant ($p < 0.001$). Values for each patient also differed from values for the group of controls ($0.01 > p > 0.001$). Values similar to those in control fibroblasts were found in lysed red cells from 6 other clinically normal controls.
From: Blass & Gibson 1977.

strongly suggesting the presence of a structural variant. So it would appear that the low-affinity enzyme would cause metabolic disruption in the nervous system only when dietary thiamine was in short supply, whereas the high-affinity enzyme would continue to function under the same circumstances.

Further work on the thiamine-dependent transketolase of cultured fibroblasts has been published by Mukherjee *et al.* (1987). They investigated 41 subjects including three alcoholism-associated WKS, seven familial chronic alcoholic males and seven of their sons, and ten individuals in three generations of an Amish family without any history of alcoholism (Fig. 15.8).

The variant of transketolase with high K_m for thiamine pyrophosphate (TPP) occurred more frequently among familial chronic alcoholic males and their offspring (who had no prior history of alcohol abuse) than among non-alcoholic families. The abnormal enzyme was present in both male and female members of the family. It is possible that the inheritance may be as an autosomal recessive character in a polymorphic system.

The phenotype of 'high K_m transketolase' would appear to confer greater risk of developing WKS

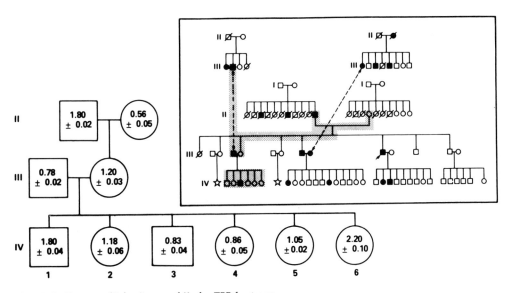

Fig. 15.8. Pattern of inheritance of K_m for TPP for transketolase in three generations of a family. The shaded portion of the pedigree has been studied. Note that the abnormal K_m occurs in both male and female members of this pedigree. (From Mukherjee *et al.* 1987.)

when thiamine becomes scarce than 'low K_m transketolase'. Usually this thiamine scarcity occurs in malnutrition accompanying alcoholism, but one WKS diabetic with high K_m transketolase was also recorded by Mukherjee *et al.* (1987).

A different approach was employed by Nixon *et al.* (1984), who studied erythrocyte transketolase from WKS patients and controls. Preparations of erythrocyte haemolysates were subjected to isoelectric focusing and stained for transketolase activity. It was claimed that a certain isoenzyme pattern was statistically associated with WKS but these results could not be confirmed by Kaufmann *et al.* (1987) who suggested that there were difficulties with the chromatographic preparation of the erythrocytic haemolysates prior to isoelectric focusing.

The observation was made by Hulyalkar *et al.* (1984) that electrophoretic variants of arylsulphatase A in blood leucocytes occurred in 12 of 56 hospitalized alcoholics, but only in one out of 100 normal controls, and in one of 95 patients with schizophrenia. It is not yet proved if these abnormalities are genetic, but if they are, then similar variant enzymes in the brain may render the subjects more liable to become alcoholic, or to be hospitalized if alcoholic.

The exact mechanism responsible for damaging the liver in alcoholics is not known (Thompson 1986). For example it is not clear whether the damage is caused by alcohol itself or by acetaldehyde. Consequently, the nature of the genetic factors conferring susceptibility or resistance is unknown. There is no good evidence to date of an association between HLA antigen status and susceptibility to alcohol-induced cirrhosis (Faizallah *et al.* 1982).

THE EFFECTS OF ALCOHOL ON CHROMOSOMES AND CHROMATIDS

Populations of 'still-drinking' and 'dry' alcoholics were studied by Obe *et al.* (1980) for chromosome and chromatid abnormalities in peripheral blood lymphocytes. Since most alcoholics are smokers, and since smoking is known to damage the chromosomes and chromatids, it was not possible statistically to dissociate the effects of these two environmental agents. Nevertheless it was shown that 'still-drinking' alcoholics exhibited both chromosomal

abnormalities (e.g. dicentric chromosomes; ring chromosomes) and chromatid type exchanges at a greater frequency than controls. In contradistinction the 'dry' alcoholics exhibited only the increased frequency of the chromosomal abnormalities and not of chromatid type changes.

A similar set of findings was reported as a result of a detailed analysis by Badr & Hussain (1982). They, too, comment on the difficulty of dissociating the influences of smoking from those of alcohol.

Bohlke *et al.* (1983) were able to show that acetaldehyde *in vitro* causes a dose-dependent linear increase in the induction of sister chromatid exchanges in lymphocytes. It was previously known that alcohol itself does not cause this effect.

At present it is unknown what is the significance of these observations in the production, for example, of organ damage in chronic alcoholism or gametic effects transmitted to offspring.

THE FETAL ALCOHOL SYNDROME

Physical and behavioural abnormalities are observable in children born to severe, chronically alcoholic mothers who consume large amounts of alcohol whilst they are pregnant. The main features are:

stunted growth; delayed development, impaired fine motor functioning and low intelligence quotient; irritability, decreased sucking performance in infancy and poor performance in school later on; malformations typically microcephaly, short palpebral fissures, epicanthal folds and various other deformities, including some affecting the hand, the heart and other organs.

Some of these abnormalities exist before birth and are recognizable at birth – termed the 'fetal alcohol syndrome'.

The existence of this disorder would seem likely to be due to the effects of alcohol or its metabolites crossing the placenta from the mother's circulation. There may also be other factors such as malnutrition and genetic endowment from the mother and possibly (on the basis of assortative mating) from the father also. Up to the present there have been no investigations on the possible effects of the genetic factors discussed earlier on the occurrence and severity of the 'fetal alcohol syndrome'. (Schenker *et al.* 1990).

A RESUMÉ AND A PERSPECTIVE

Alcoholism (or alcohol dependence) is to be regarded as a disease.

There is clear evidence that the familial form of the disease is the resultant of both genetic and environmental factors, as shown particularly by adoption studies.

'At risk' individuals, namely, the sons of known alcoholics, exhibit different psychomotor responses to alcohol as compared with controls, as well as different EEG responses.

Twin studies reveal that there is a substantial genetic contribution to the control of alcohol metabolism as shown by the rate of elimination of alcohol from the blood.

Amongst Orientals there is a much greater frequency than amongst Europeans of individuals who exhibit marked flushing and other vasomotor responses after consuming alcohol.

Different ethnic groups also metabolize alcohol at different rates, Orientals having higher rates than Europeans.

A great deal of work has been done on the biochemistry and molecular genetics of human alcohol dehydrogenase.

An 'atypical' variant which has the ability to metabolize alcohol more rapidly *in vitro*, does not seem to confer a correspondingly enhanced *in vivo* metabolic capacity on Europeans who possess it. However, this phenotype is much more frequent in Orientals and the metabolic consequences in them has not, as yet, been fully determined.

Aldehyde dehydrogenase has also been extensively investigated with particularly fruitful results. A genetically determined deficiency variant which is common in Japanese has been found to be rare amongst Japanese alcoholics. Possession of this variant renders the subject liable to develop higher blood acetaldehyde concentrations after ingesting alcohol. It is thought possible that the symptoms generated by the acetaldehyde (flushing, nausea, etc.) may be the reason why the individual seems protected from becoming alcoholic. This is particularly significant in view of the fact that with the increasing affluence of Japanese society in the last 30 years alcoholism has become an important social problem.

Recently two new enzymic polymorphisms have been described in Japanese: first, of salivary aldehyde dehydrogenase and secondly, of glutathione-S-transferase. Preliminary observations indicate that particular phenotypes within these two polymorphisms may be associated with alcoholism. These observations will need to be confirmed, and if they are confirmed they may help build up a biochemical–genetical profile of 'at risk' subjects. This would be valuable for counselling purposes.

These developments in knowledge in Japanese do not shed light on the enormous problem of alcoholism in populations of European extraction (the financial burden of alcohol ·dependence in the USA alone was estimated in 1988 to be $116 billion per annum: Larson 1991). Nevertheless, they may form models on which future pharmacogenetic approaches to this problem may be based.

It seems likely that amongst heavy drinkers, genetic factors dictate which persons will suffer from specific deleterious effects, such as liver cirrhosis, cerebral disorders, haematological effects, cardiomyopathy, etc. A specific enzymic defect, probably genetically determined, namely, transketolase with a high K_m for thiamine, has been found to be associated with the Wernicke–Korsakoff syndrome.

As has been emphasized previously (Evans, 1987), since alcoholism is a pharmacogenetic phenomenon, the environmental and genetic components are both of great importance. The statistics of alcohol consumption are striking. According to von Wartburg (1980), in Switzerland as in many other countries about 10% of the population drink approximately half of the total alcohol consumed in the whole country. In contradistinction 80% of the population drink only a few grams of alcohol on a daily average.

It is well known that the total alcohol consumption is rising. In parallel with this is the proportion of people becoming alcoholic. Jewish communities were previously regarded as having a low incidence of alcohol-related problems, but now these problems have become a significant social phenomenon in young Israeli Jews (Rawat 1983). Even Islam, possibly the most powerful anti-alcohol influence that the world has ever seen, does not wholly prevent the occurrence of alcoholism in populations of its adherents.

As pointed out in an editorial by Hamburg & Nightingale (1987), alcohol constitutes a huge public health problem in both the developed and the developing world. It probably needs a research approach by a combination of the biomedical and behavioural sciences to reach a better understanding of the condition. Since alcoholism is such a common and widespread disorder methodologies developed to study it may prove useful to look at other multifactorial disorders.

The author would like to express his gratitude to Dr Richard B. McConnell, Department of Medicine, University of Liverpool, UK and Dr Anthony I. Morris, Gastroenterology Department, Royal Liverpool Hospital, UK who made many helpful suggestions about the contents in this chapter.

Agarwal, D. P., Cohn, P., Goedde, H. W. & Hempel, J. (1989). Aldehyde dehydrogenase from human erythrocytes' structural relationship to the liver cytosolic isozyme. *Enzyme*, **42**, 47–52.

Agarwal, D. P. & Goedde, H. W. (1986). Pharmacogenetics and ecogenetics. *Experientia*, **42**, 1148–54.

Agarwal, D. P. & Goedde, H. W. (1987a). Genetic variation in alcohol metabolizing enzymes: implications in alcohol use and abuse. In *Genetics and Alcoholism*, ed. H. W. Goedde & D. P. Agarwal. *Progress in Clinical and Biological Research*, **241**, 121–39. New York: Alan R Liss.

Agarwal, D. P. & Goedde, H. W. (1987b). Human aldehyde dehydrogenase isozymes and alcohol sensitivity. In *Isozymes: Agriculture, Physiology and Medicine*, ed. M. C. Rattazzi, J. G. Scandalio & G. S. Whitt. *Current Topics in Biological and Medical Research*, **16**, pp. 21–48. New York: Alan R. Liss.

Agarwal, D. P. & Goedde, H. W. (1990). Pharmacogenetics of alcohol dehydrogenase (ADH). *Pharmacology and Therapeutics*, **45**, 69–83.

Agarwal, D. P., Harada, S. & Goedde, H. W. (1981). Racial differences in biological sensitivities to ethanol: the role of alcohol dehydrogenase and aldehyde dehydrogenase isozymes. *Alcoholism: Clinical and Experimental Research*, **5**, 12–16.

American Psychiatric Association (1980): *Diagnostic and Statistical Manual of Mental Disorders*, 3rd edition, pp. 169–170. Washington, DC: American Psychiatric Association.

American Psychiatric Association (1987): *Diagnostic and Statistical Manual of Mental Disorders*, 3rd edition (revised), p. 173. Washington, DC: American Psychiatric Association.

Anonymous. (1984). Editorial: alcoholism, genetics and society. *British Journal of Addiction*, **79**, 353.

Badr, F. M. & Hussain, F. H. (1982). Chromosomal aberrations in chronic male alcoholics. *Alcoholism: Clinical and Experimental Research*, **6**, 122–9.

Begleiter, H. & Porjesz, B. (1988). Potential biological markers in individuals at high risk for developing alcoholism. *Alcoholism: Clinical and Experimental Research*, **12**, 488–93.

Begleiter, H., Porjesz, B., Bihari, B. & Kissin, B. (1984). Event-related brain potentials in boys at risk for alcoholism. *Science*, **225**, 1493–6.

Blass, J. P. & Gibson, G. E. (1977). Abnormality of a thiamine-requiring enzyme in patients with Wernicke–Korsakoff syndrome. *New England Journal of Medicine*, **297**, 1367–70.

Blum, K., Noble, E. P., Sheridan, P. J., Montgomery, A., Ritchie, T., Jagadeeswaran, P., Nogami, H., Briggs, H. & Cohn, J. B. (1990). Allelic association of human dopamine D_2 receptor gene in alcoholism. *Journal of the American Medical Association*, **263**, 2055–60.

Bohlke, J. U., Singh, S. & Goedde, H. W. (1983). Cytogenetic effects of acetaldehyde in lymphocytes of Germans and Japanese: SCE clastogenic activity and cell cycle delay. *Human Genetics*, **63**, 285–9.

Bohman, M. (1978). Some genetic aspects of alcoholism and criminality. *Archives of General Psychiatry*, **35**, 269–76.

Bolos, A. M., Dean, M., Lucas-Derse, S., Ramsburg, M., Brown, G. L. & Goldman, D. (1990). Population and pedigree studies reveal a lack of association between the dopamine D_2 receptor gene and alcoholism. *Journal of the American Medical Association*, **264**, 3156–60.

Bosron, W. F. & Li, T.-K. (1986). Genetic polymorphism of human liver alcohol and aldehyde dehydrogenases and their relationship to alcohol metabolism and alcoholism. *Hepatology*, **6**, 502–10.

Braucht, G. N. (1983). How environments and persons combine to influence problem drinking. *Recent Developments in Alcoholism*, **1**, 79–103.

Braun, T., Bober, E., Singh, S., Agarwal, D. P. & Goedde, H. W. (1987). Evidence for a signal peptide at the amino-terminal end of human mitochondrial aldehyde dehydrogenase. *Federation of European Biochemical Societies Letters*, **215**, 233–6.

Braun, T., Grzeschik, K. H., Bober, E., Singh, S., Agarwal, D. P. & Goedde, H. W. (1986). The structural gene for the mitochondrial aldehyde dehydrogenase maps to chromosome 12. *Human Genetics*, **73**, 365–7.

Bühler, R., Hempel, J., Kaiser, R., von Wartburg, J. P. & Nallee, B. L. (1984). Human alcohol dehydrogenase: Structural differences between beta and gamma sub-units suggest parallel duplications in isoenzyme evolution and predominant expression of separate gene descendants in livers of different mammals. *Proceedings of the National Academy of Sciences (USA)*, **81**, 6320–4.

Burnell, K. J. C., Carr, L. G., Divulet, F. E., Edenberg, H. J., Li, T.-K. & Bosron, W. F. (1987). The human β_3 alcohol dehydrogenase subunit differs from β_1 by a cys for ARG - 369 substitution which decreases NAD(H) binding. *Biochemical and Biophysical Research Communications*, **146**, 1227–33.

Cadoret, R. J. & Gath, A. (1978). Inheritance of alcoholism in adoptees. *British Journal of Psychiatry*, **132**, 252–8.

Carr, L. C., Xu, Y., Ho, W.-H. & Edenberg, H. J. (1989). Nucleotide sequence of the $AHD2^3$ gene encoding the human alcohol dehydrogenase β_3 subunit. *Alcoholism: Clinical and Experimental Research*, **13**, 594–6.

Chen, C.-C., Hwu, H.-G., Yeh, E.-K., Morimoto, K. & Otsuki, S. (1991). Aldehyde dehydrogenase deficiency, flush patterns and prevalence of alcoholism: an interethnic comparison. *Acta Medica Okayama*, **45**, 409–15.

Chen, S.-H., Zhang, M. & Scott, C. R. (1992). Gene frequencies of alcohol dehydrogenase$_2$ and aldehyde dehydrogenase in Northwest Coast Amerindians. *Human Genetics*, **89**, 351–2.

Cloninger, C. R. (1985). Genetics of alcoholism. *Alcoholism: Clinical and Experimental Research*, **9**, 479–482 (In Schuckit et al., 1985a).

Cook, B. L. & Winokur, G. (1985). A study of familial positive versus familial negative alcoholics. *Journal of Nervous and Mental Disease*, **173**, 175–8.

Cooper, S. E. (1983). Survey of studies on alcoholism. *International Journal of the Addictions*, **18**, 971–85.

Crabb, D. W., Edenberg, H. J., Bosron, W. F. & Li, T.-K. (1989). Genotypes for aldehyde dehydrogenase deficiency and alcohol sensitivity. *Journal of Clinical Investigation*, **83**, 314–6.

Crabbe, J. C. (1984). Pharmacogenetic strategies for studying alcohol dependence. *Alcohol*, **1**, 185–91.

Crothers, T. D. (1909). Heredity in the causation of inebriety. *British Medical Journal*, **2**, 659–61.

Cruz-Coke, R. (1983). Genetics and alcoholism. *Neurobehavioural Toxicology and Teratology*, **5**, 179–80.

Devor, E. J. & Cloninger, C. R. (1989). Genetics of alcoholism. *Annual Review of Genetics*, **23**, 19–36.

Dyck, L. E. (1990). Isoenzymes of aldehyde dehydrogenase in human lymphocytes. *Alcoholism: Clinical and Experimental Research*, **14**, 534–8.

Eckey, R., Agarwal, D. P., Saha, N. & Goedde, H. W. (1986). Detection and partial characterization of a variant form of cytosolic aldehyde dehydrogenase isozyme. *Human Genetics*, **72**, 95–7.

Edwards, J. A. & Evans, D. A. P. (1967). Ethanol metabolism in subjects possessing typical and atypical liver alcohol dehydrogenase. *Clinical Pharmacology and Therapeutics*, **8**, 824–9.

Edwards, G. & Gross, M. M. (1976). Alcohol dependence: provisional description of a clinical syndrome. *British Medical Journal*, **1**, 1058–61.

Eklund, H., Müller-Wille, P., Horjales, E., Futer, O., Holmquist, B., Vallee, B. L., Höög, J.-O., Kaiser, R. & Jörnvall, H. (1990). Comparison of three classes of human liver alcohol dehydrogenase. Emphasis on different substrate binding pockets. *European Journal of Biochemistry*, **193**, 303–10.

Emery, A. E. H. (1976). *Methodology in Medical Genetics – an Introduction to Statistical Methods*, p. 84. Edinburgh: Churchill-Livingstone.

Enomoto, N., Takase, S., Yasuhara, M. & Takada, A. (1991a). Acetaldehyde metabolism in different aldehyde dehydrogenase-2 genotypes. *Alcoholism: Clinical and Experimental Research*, **15**, 141–4.

Enomoto, N., Takase, S., Takada, N. & Takada, A. (1991b). Alcoholic liver disease in heterozygotes of mutant and normal aldehyde dehydrogenase-2 genes. *Hepatology*, **13**, 1071–5.

Evans, D. A. P. (1987). A pharmacogenetic approach to alcoholism. In *Genetics and alcoholism*, ed. H. W. Goedde & D. P. Agarwal. *Progress in Clinical and Biological Research*. **241**, 319–22. New York: Alan R Liss.

Ewing, J. A., Bose, B. A. & Pellizzari, E. D. (1974). Alcohol sensitivity and ethnic background. *American Journal of Psychiatry*, **131**, 206–10.

Faizalla, R., Woodrow, J. C., Krasner, N. K., Walker, R. J. & Morris, A. I. (1982). Are HLA antigens important in the development of alcohol-induced liver disease? *British Medical Journal*, **285**, 533–4.

Falconer, D. S. (1960). *Introduction to Quantitative Genetics*. (reprinted with amendments, 1967), pp. 135, 163. Edinburgh: Oliver & Boyd.

Fong, W. P., Ho, Y. W., Lee, C. Y. & Keung, W. M. (1989). Liver alcohol and aldehyde dehydrogenase isozymes in a Chinese population in Hong Kong. *Human Heredity*, **39**, 185–91.

Forsander, O. & Eriksson, K. (1974). Forekommer det etnologiska skillnader i alkoholens amnesomsattningen. *Alkoholpolitik*, **37**, 315. (Cited by Goodwin 1980.)

Freund, G. (1984). Biomedical causes of alcohol abuse. *Alcohol*, **1**, 129–31.

Gelernter, J., O'Malley, S., Risch, N., Kranzler, H. R., Krystal, J., Merikangas, K., Kennedy, J. L. & Kidd, K. K. (1991). No association between an allele at the D_2 dopamine receptor gene (DRD2) and alcoholism. *Journal of the American Medical Association*, **266**, 1801–07.

Gibson, J. B. & Oakeshott, J. G. (1981). Genetics of biochemical and behavioural aspects of alcohol metabolism. *Australian and New Zealand Journal of Medicine*, **11**, 128–31.

Goedde, H. W. & Agarwal, D. P. (1986). Aldehyde oxidation: ethnic variations in metabolism and response. In *Ethnic Differences in Reactions to Drugs and Xenobiotics*, ed. W. Kalow, H. W. Geodde & D. P. Agarwal. *Progress in Clinical and Biological Research*, **214**, 113–38. New York: Alan R. Liss.

Goedde, H. W. & Agarwal, D. P. (1987). Aldehyde dehydrogenase polymorphism: molecular basis and phenotypic relationship to alcohol sensitivity. *Alcohol and Alcoholism*, Suppl. **1**, 47–54.

Goedde, H. W. & Agarwal, D. P. (1990). Pharmacogenetics of aldehyde dehydrogenase (ALDH). *Pharmacology and Therapeutics*, **45**, 345–71.

Goedde, H. W., Agarwal, D. P. & Harada, S. (1980). Genetic studies on alcohol-metabolizing enzymes: detection of isozymes in human hair roots. *Enzyme*, **25**, 281–6.

Goedde, H. W., Agarwal, D. P. & Harada, S. (1983b). The role of alcohol dehydrogenase and aldehyde dehydrogenase isozymes in alcohol metabolism, alcohol sensitivity and alcoholism. In *Isozymes. Cellular Localization Metabolism and Physiology*, ed. M. C. Rattazzi, J. G. Scandalios & G. S Witt. *Current Topics in Biological and Medical Research*, **8**, 175–93. New York: Alan R. Liss.

Goedde, H. W., Agarwal, D. P., Harada, S., Rothhammer, F., Whittaker, J. O. & Lisker, R. (1986). Aldehyde dehydrogenase polymorphism in North American, South American and Mexican Indian populations. *American Journal of Human Genetics*, **38**, 395–9.

Goedde, H. W., Harada, S. & Agarwal, D. P. (1979). Racial differences in alcohol sensitivity: a new hypothesis. *Human Genetics*, **51**, 331–4.

Goedde, H. W., Hoo, J. J. & Agarwal, D. P. (1983a). Addictive disorders. In *Principles and Practice of Medical Genetics*, Vol. 1, ed. A. E. Emery & D. L. Rimoin, pp. 342–51. London: Churchill-Livingstone.

Goedde, H. W., Singh, S., Agarwal, D. P., Fritze, G., Stapel, K & Paik, Y. K. (1989). Genotyping of mitochondrial aldehyde dehydrogenase using allele specific oligonucleotides in blood samples: comparison with phenotyping in hair roots. *Human Genetics*, **81**, 305–7.

Goodwin, D. W. (1980). The genetics of alcoholism. *Substance and Alcohol Actions/Misuse*, **1**, 101–17.

Goodwin, D. W. (1981). Family studies of alcoholism. *Journal of Studies on Alcohol*, **42**, 156–62.

Goodwin, D. W. (1983). Familial alcoholism: a separate entity? *Substance and Alcohol Actions/Misuse*, **4**, 129–36.

Goodwin, D. W. (1985). Alcoholism and genetics: the sins of the fathers. *Archives of General Psychiatry*, **42**, 171–4.

Gordis, E., Tabakoff, B., Goldman, D. & Berg, K. (1990). Finding the gene(s) for alcoholism. *Journal of the American Medical Association*, **263**, 2094–6.

Grandy, D. K., Litt, M., Allen, L., Bunzow, J. R., Marchionni, M., Makam, H., Reed, L., Magenis, R. E. & Civelli, O. (1989). The human dopamine D₂ receptor gene is located on chromosome 11 at q22-q23 and identifies a Taq1 RFLP. *American Journal of Human Genetics*, **45**, 778–85.

Greenfield, N. J. & Pietruszko, R. (1977). Two aldehyde dehydrogenases from human liver. Isolation via affinity chromatography and characterization of the isozymes. *Biochimica et Biophysica Acta*, **483**, 35–45.

Groppi, A., Begueret, J. & Iron, A. (1990). Improved methods for genotype determination of human alcohol dehydrogenase (ADH) at ADH2 and ADH23 loci by using polymerase chain reaction-directed mutagenesis. *Clinical Chemistry*, **36**, 1765–8.

Gurling, H. M. D., Murray, R. M. & Clifford, C. A. (1981). Investigations into the genetics of alcohol dependence and into its effects on brain function. In *Progress in Clinical and Biological Research*, Vol. 69, Part C. *Twin Research 3. Epidemiological and Clinical Studies*, pp. 77–87. New York: Alan R. Liss.

Hall, R. L., Hesselbrock, V. M. & Stabenau, J. R. (1983a). Familial distribution of alcohol use I. Assortative mating in the parents of alcoholics. *Behaviour Genetics*, **13**, 361–72.

Hall, R. L., Hesselbrock, V. M. & Stabenau, J. R. (1983b). Familial distribution of alcohol use II. Assortative mating of alcoholic probands. *Behaviour Genetics*, **13**, 373–82.

Hamburg, D. A. & Nightingale, E. O. (1987). Conjunction of biomedical and behavioural sciences: Can research on alcoholism show the way? *Alcoholism: Clinical and Experimental Research*, **11**, 229–33.

Hammond, S. B. (1981). Alcohol-related behaviour patterns. *Australian and New Zealand Journal of Medicine*, **11**, 115–7.

Hanna, J. M. (1978). Metabolic responses of Chinese, Japanese and Europeans to alcohol. *Alcoholism: Clinical and Experimental Research*, **2**, 89–92.

Harada, S., Agarwal, D. P. & Goedde, H. W. (1978). Isozyme variations in acetaldehyde dehydrogenase (EC 1,2,1,3) in human tissue. *Human Genetics*, **44**, 181–5.

Harada, S., Agarwal, D. P. & Goedde, H. W. (1981). Aldehyde dehydrogenase deficiency as cause of facial flushing reaction to alcohol in Japanese. *Lancet*, **2**, 982.

Harada, S., Agarwal, D. P. & Goedde, H. W. (1985). Aldehyde dehydrogenase polymorphism and alcohol metabolism in alcoholics. *Alcohol*, **2**, 391–2.

Harada, S., Agarwal, D. P. & Goedde, H. W. (1987). Aldehyde dehydrogenase and glutathione-S-transferase polymorphism: association between phenotype frequencies and alcoholism. In *Genetics and Alcoholism*, ed. H. W. Goedde & D. P. Agarwal. *Progress in Clinical and Biological Research*, **241**, 241–50. New York: Alan R. Liss.

Harada, S., Agarwal, D. P., Goedde, H. W., Tagaki, S. & Ishikawa, B. (1982). Possible protective role against alcoholism for aldehyde dehydrogenase isozyme deficiency in Japan. *Lancet*, **2**, 827.

Hayakawa, K. (1987). Smoking and drinking discordance and health condition: Japanese identical twins reared apart and together. *Acta Geneticae Medicae et Gemellologiae*, **36**, 493–501.

Heather, J. (1992). Why alcoholism is not a disease. *Medical Journal of Australia*, **156**, 212–15.

Hempel, J., Kaiser, R. & Jornvall, H. (1985). Mitochondrial aldehyde dehydrogenase from human liver. Primary structure, differences in relation to the cytosolic enzyme and functional correlations. *European Journal of Biochemistry*, **153**, 13–28.

Higuchi, S., Muramatsu, T., Shigemore, K., Saito, M., Kono, H., Dufour, M. C. & Harford, T. C. (1992). The relationship between low Kₘ aldehyde dehydrogenase phenotype and drinking behaviour in Japanese. *Journal of Studies on Alcohol*, **53**, 170–5.

Hrubec, Z. & Omenn, G. S. (1981). Evidence of genetic predisposition to alcoholic cirrhosis and psychosis: Twin concordances for alcoholism and its biological end points by zygosity among male veterans. *Alcoholism: Clinical and Experimental Research*, **5**, 207–15.

Hsu, L. C., Tani, K., Fujiyoshi, T., Kurachi, K. & Yoshida, A. (1985). Cloning of cDNAs for human aldehyde dehydrogenases 1 and 2. *Proceedings of the National Academy of Sciences (USA)*, **82**, 3771–5.

Hsu, L. C., Yoshida, A. & Mohandas, T. (1986). Chromosomal assignment of the genes for human aldehyde dehydrogenase-1 and aldehyde dehydrogenase-2. *American Journal of Human Genetics*, **38**, 641–8.

Hulyalkar, A. R., Nora, R. & Manowitz, P. (1984). Arylsulfatase A variants in patients with alcoholism. *Alcoholism: Clinical and Experimental Research*, **8**, 337–41.

Hurley, T. D., Bosron, W. F., Hamilton, J. A. & Amzel, L. M. (1991). Structure of human β₁ β₁ alcohol dehydrogenase: catalytic effects of non-active-site substitutions. *Proceedings of the National Academy of Sciences (USA)*, **88**, 8149–53.

Hurley, T. D., Edenberg, H. J. & Bosron, W. F. (1990). Expression and kinetic characterization of variants of human β₁β₁ alcohol dehydrogenase containing substitutions at amino acid 47. *Journal of Biological Chemistry*, **265**, 16366–72.

Ikuta, T., Shibuya, A. & Yoshida, A. (1988). Direct determination of usual (Caucasian-type) and atypical (Oriental-type) alleles of the class I human alcohol dehydrogenase-2 locus. *Biochemical Genetics*, **26**, 519–25.

Jellinek, E. M. & Jolliffe, N. (1940). Effect of alcohol on the individual. *Quarterly Journal of Studies on Alcohol*, **1**, 110–81. (Cited by Goodwin 1983.)

Jellinek, E. M. (1952). Phase of alcohol addiction. *Quarterly Journal of Studies on Alcohol*, **13**, 673–784. (Cited by Cooper 1983.)

Jurd, S. M. (1992). Why alcoholism is a disease. *Medical Journal of Australia*, **156**, 215–17.

Kaij, L. (1960). *Alcoholism in Twins. Studies on the Aetiology and Sequels of Abuse of Alcohol*. Stockholm: Almqvist & Wiksell. (Cited by Cloninger & Reich 1983.)

Kalow, W. (1962). *Pharmacogenetics*, p. 209. Philadelphia: Saunders.

Kaprio, J, Koskenvuo, M., Langinvaino, H., Romanov, K., Sarna, S. & Rose, R. J. (1987). Genetic influences on use and abuse of alcohol: a study of 5638 adult Finnish twin brothers. *Alcoholism: Clinical and Experimental Research*, **11**, 349–56.

Kaufmann, A,. Uhlhaas, S., Friedl, W. & Propping, P. (1987). Human erythrocyte transketolase: no evidence for variants. *Clinica Chimica Acta*, **162**, 215–19.

Kennedy, A. & Fish, F. J. (1958). Alcoholism, alcoholic addiction and drug addiction. *Recent Progress in Psychiatry*, **3**, 277–302.

Kopun, M. & Propping, P. (1977). The kinetics of ethanol

absorption and elimination in twins and supplementary repetitive experiments in singleton subjects. *European Journal of Clinical Pharmacology*, **11**, 337–44.

Larson, E. W. (1991). Alcoholism: The disease and the diagnosis. *American Journal of Medicine*, **91**, 107–9.

Legrain, F. *Heredité el Alcoolisme*. Paris: Masson. (Cited by Cruz-Coke 1983.)

Lin, T.-Y. & Lin, D. T. C. (1982). Alcoholism among the Chinese. Further observations of a low-risk population. *Culture, Medicine and Psychiatry*, **6**, 109–16.

Lüth, K. F. (1939). Untersuchungen über die alkohol-blutkonzentration nach Alkoholgaben bei 10 eineiigen und 10 zweieiigen zwillingspaaren. *Deutsche Zeitschrift für gerichtlichen Medizinische*, **32**, 145–64.

Martin, N. G., Perl, J., Oakeshott, J. G., Gibson, J. P., Starmer, G. A. & Wilks, A. V. (1985). A twin study of ethanol metabolism. *Behaviour Genetics*, **15**, 93–109.

Matsuo, Y., Yokohama, R. & Yokohama, S. (1989). The genes for human alcohol dehydrogenases β_1 and β_2 differ by only one nucleotide. *European Journal of Biochemistry*, **183**, 317–20.

Meier-Tackmann, D., Korenke, G. C., Agarwal, D. P. & Goedde, H. W. (1988). Human liver aldehyde dehydrogenase: subcellular distribution in alcoholics and nonalcoholics. *Alcohol*, **5**, 73–80.

Morse, R. M. & Flavia, D. K. (1992). The definition of alcoholism. *Journal of the American Medical Association*, **268**, 1012–14.

Mukherjee, A. B., Svoronos, S., Ghazanfari, A., Martin, P. R., Fisher, A., Roecidein, B., Rodbard, D., Staton, R., Behar, D., Berg, C. J. & Manjunath, R. (1987). Transketolase abnormality in cultured fibroblasts from familial chronic alcoholic men and their male offspring. *Journal of Clinical Investigation*, **79**, 1039–43.

Muramatsu, T., Higuchi, S., Shigemori, K., Saito, M., Sasao, M., Harada, S., Shigeta, Y., Yamado, K., Muraoka, H., Takagi, S., Maruyama, K. & Kono, H. (1989). Ethanol patch test – a simple and sensitive method for identifying ALDH phenotype. *Alcoholism: Clinical and Experimental Research*, **13**, 229–31.

Murray, R. M., Clifford, C., Gurling, H. M. D., Topham, A., Clow, A. & Bernadt, M. (1983). Current genetic and biological approaches to alcoholism. *Psychiatric Developments*, **2**, 179–92.

Nagoshi, C. T. & Wilson, J. R. (1987). Influence of family alcoholism history on alcohol metabolism, sensitivity and tolerance. *Alcoholism: Clinical and Experimental Research*, **11**, 392–8.

Newlin, D. B. & Thomson, J. B. (1991). Chronic tolerance and sensitization in sons of alcoholics. *Alcoholism: Clinical and Experimental Research*, **15**, 399–405.

Nixon, P. F., Kaczmarek, M. J., Tate, J., Kerr, R. A & Price, J. (1984). An erythrocyte transketolase isoenzyme pattern associated with the Wernicke–Korsakoff syndrome. *European Journal of Clinical Investigation*, **14**, 278–81.

Nomenclature of Mammalian Aldehyde Dehydrogenases (1989). In *Enzymology and Molecular Biology of Carbonyl Metabolism 2. Aldehyde dehydrogenase, alcohol dehydrogenase and aldo-keto reductase*, XIX–XXI. New York: Alan R. Liss.

Obe, G., Gobel, D., Engeln, H., Herha, J. & Natarajan, A. T. (1980). Chromosomal aberrations in peripheral lymphocytes of alcoholics. *Mutation Research*, **73**, 377–86.

O'Connor, S., Hesselbrock, V. & Tasman, A. (1986). Correlates of increased risk for alcoholism in young men.

Progress in Neuro-psychopharmacology and Biological Psychiatry, **10**, 211–18.

O'Dowd, B. F., Rothhammer, F. & Israel, Y. (1990). Genotyping of mitochondrial aldehyde dehydrogenase locus of native American Indians. *Alcoholism: Clinical and Experimental Research*, **14**, 531–3.

Ohmori, T., Koyama, T., Chen, C.-C., Yeh, E. K. Reyes, B. V. & Yamashita, I. (1986). The role of aldehyde dehydrogenase isozyme variance in alcohol sensitivity, drinking habits formation, and the development of alcoholism in Japan, Taiwan and the Philippines. *Progress in Neuro-Psychopharmacology and Biological Psychiatry*, **10**, 229–35.

Omenn, G. S. & Motulsky, A. G. (1972). A biochemical and genetic approach to alcoholism. In *Nature and Nurture in Alcoholism*, ed. F. A. Sexias, G. S. Omenn, E. D. Burke & S. A. Eggleston. *Annals of the New York Academy of Sciences*, **197**, 16–23.

Partanen, J., Bruun, K. & Markkanen, T. (1966). Inheritance of drinking behaviour – a study of intelligence, personality and use of alcohol in adult twins. *Helsinki Finnish Foundation for Alcohol Studies*, **4**, 159. (Cited by Gurling *et al.* 1981.)

Penick, E. C., Powell, B. J., Bingham, S. F., Liskow, B. I., Miller, N. S. & Read, M. R. (1987). A comparative study of familial alcoholism. *Journal of Studies on Alcohol*, **48**, 136–46.

Polich, J., Burns, T. & Bloom, F. E. (1988a). P300 and the risk for alcoholism: family history, task difficulty and gender. *Alcoholism: Clinical and Experimental Research*, **12**, 248–54.

Polich, J., Haier, R. J., Buchsbaum, M. & Bloom, F. E. (1988b). Assessment of young men at risk for alcoholism with P300 from a visual discrimination task. *Journal of Studies on Alcohol*, **49**, 186–90.

Propping, P. (1983a). Pharmacogenetics of alcohol's CNS effect: Implications for the etiology of alcoholism. *Pharmacology, Biochemistry and Behaviour*, **18** (Suppl.1), 549–53.

Propping, P. (1983b). Pharmacogenetics of alcohol and its CNS effects – a digest. *Neuropharmacology*, **22**, 559–60.

Radouco-Thomas, S., Garcin, F., Murthy, M. R. V., Faure, N., Lemay, A., Forest, J. C. & Radouco-Thomas, C. (1984). Biological markers in major psychosis and alcoholism: Phenotype and genotype markers. *Journal of Psychiatric Research*, **18**, 513–39.

Rathna, Giri P., Krug, J. F., Kozak, C., Moretti, T., O'Brien, S. J., Seuanez, H. N. & Goldman, D. (1989). Cloning and comparative mapping of a human class III (χ) alcohol dehydrogenase cDNA. *Biochemical and Biophysical Research Communications*, **164**, 453–60.

Rawat, A. K. (1983). Genetic aspects of ethanol disposition and dependence. *Neurobehavioural Toxicology and Teratology*, **5**, 193–99.

Reed, T. E. (1978). Racial comparisons of alcohol metabolism: Background problems and results. *Alcoholism: Clinical and Experimental Research*, **2**, 83–7.

Reed, T. E., Kalant, H.,. Gibbins, R. J., Kapur, B. M. & Rankin, J. G. (1976). Alcohol and acetaldehyde metabolism in Caucasians, Chinese and Amerinds. *Canadian Medical Association Journal*, **115**, 851–2.

Schenker, S., Becker, H. C., Randall, C. L., Phillips, D. K., Baskin, G. S. & Henderson, G. I. (1990). Fetal alcohol syndrome: current status of pathogenesis. *Alcoholism: Clinical and Experimental Research*, **14**, 635–47.

Schuckit, M. A. (1984). Subjective responses to alcohol in sons of alcoholics and controls. *Archives of General Psychiatry*, **41**, 879–84.

Schuckit, M. A. (1985b). Ethanol-induced changes in body sway in men at high alcoholism risk. *Archives of General Psychiatry*, **42**, 375–9.

Schuckit, M. A. (1986). Genetic and clinical implications of alcoholism and affective disorder. *American Journal of Psychiatry*, **143**, 140–7.

Schuckit, M. A, Duthie, L. A., Mahler, H. I. M., Irwin, M. & Monteiro, M. G. (1991). Subjective feelings and changes in body sway following diazepam in sons of alcoholics and control subjects. *Journal of Studies on Alcohol*, **52**, 601–8.

Schuckit, M. A., Gold, E. O., Croot, K., Finn, P. & Polich, J. (1988b). P300 latency after ethanol ingestion in sons of alcoholics and in controls. *Biological Psychiatry*, **24**, 310–15.

Schuckit, M. A., Gold, E. & Risch, C. (1987a). Plasma cortisol levels following ethanol in sons of alcoholics and controls. *Archives of General Psychiatry*, **44**, 942–5.

Schuckit, M. A., Gold, E. & Risch, C. (1987b). Serum prolactin levels in sons of alcoholics and control subjects. *American Journal of Psychiatry*, **144**, 854–9.

Schuckit, M. A., Goodwin, D. A. & Winokur, G. (1972). A study of alcoholism in half siblings. *American Journal of Psychiatry*, **128**, 1132–6.

Schuckit, M. A., Li, T.-K., Cloninger, C. R. & Deitrich, R.A. (1985a). Genetics of alcoholism. *Alcoholism: Clinical and Experimental Research*, **9**, 475–92.

Schuckit, M. A., Risch, S. C. & Gold, E. O. (1988a). Alcohol consumption ACTH level and family history of alcoholism. *American Journal of Psychiatry*, **145**, 1391–5.

Schulz, Von W., Kreuzberg, S., Neymeyer, H. G., Schwarz, U. & Pachaly, A. (1976). Über die haufigkeit der atypischen ADH in leberbiopsiematerial und den einfluss auf den athanolumsatz *in vivo*. *Kriminalistik und forensische Wissenschaften*, **26**, 109–11.

Segal, B. & Duffy, L. K. (1992). Ethanol elimination among different racial groups. *Alcohol*, **9**, 213–17.

Sher, K. J.& Levenson, R. W. (1982). Risk of alcoholism and individual differences in the stress-response-dampening effect of alcohol. *Journal of Abnormal Psychology*, **91**, 350–67.

Shibuya, A., Yasunami, M. & Yoshida, A. (1989). Genotypes of alcohol dehydrogenase and aldehyde dehydrogenase loci in Japanese alcohol flushers and non-flushers. *Human Genetics*, **82**, 14–16.

Shibuya, A. & Yoshida, A. (1988). Genotypes of alcohol-metabolizing enzymes in Japanese with alcohol liver diseases: A strong association of the usual Caucasian-type aldehyde dehydrogenase gene (ALDH$_2^1$) with the disease. *American Journal of Human Genetics*, **43**, 744–8.

Singh, S., Fritze, G., Fang, B., Harada, S., Paik, Y. K., Echey, R., Agarwal, D. P. & Goedde, H. W. (1989). Inheritance of mitochondrial aldehyde dehydrogenase: genotyping in Chinese, Japanese and South Korean families reveals dominance of the mutant allele. *Human Genetics*, **83**, 119–21.

Smith, M. (1986). Genetics of human alcohol and aldehyde dehydrogenases. In *Advances in Human Genetics*, Vol. 15, ed. H. Harris & K. Hirschorn, pp. 249–90.

Smith, M. (1988). Molecular genetic studies on alcohol and aldehyde dehydrogenase individual variation, gene

mapping and analysis of regulation. *Biochemical Society Transactions*, **16**, 227–30.

Smith, M, Hopkinson, D. A. & Harris, H. (1972). Alcohol dehydrogenase isozymes in stomach and liver. Evidence for activity of the ADH3 locus. *Annals of Human Genetics (London)*, **35**, 243–53.

Tabakoff, B. & Hoffman, P. L. (1988). Genetics and biological markers of risk for alcoholism. *Public Health Reports*, **103**, 690–8.

Tarter, R. E., Alterman, A. I. & Edwards, K. L. (1985). Vulnerability to alcoholism in men: A behaviour-genetic perspective. *Journal of Studies on Alcohol*, **46**, 329–56.

Thomasson, H. R., Edenberg, H. J., Crabb, D. W., Mai, X. L., Jerome, R. E., Li, T.-K., Wang, S.-P., Lin, Y.-T., Lu, R.-B. & Yin, S.-J. (1991). Alcohol and aldehyde dehydrogenase genotypes and alcoholism in Chinese men. *American Journal of Human Genetics*, **48**, 677–81.

Thompson, R. P. H. (1986). Measuring the damage – ethanol and the liver. *GUT*, **27**, 751–5.

Uematsu, F., Kikuchi, H., Motomiya, M., Abe, T., Sagami, I., Ohmachi, T., Wakui, A., Kanamaru, R. & Watanabe, M. (1991). Association between restriction fragment length polymorphism of the human cytochrome P450 II E1 gene and susceptibility to lung cancer. *Japanese Journal of Cancer Research*, **82**, 254–6.

Vesell, E. S., Page, J. G. & Passananti, G. T. (1971). Genetic and environmental factors affecting ethanol metabolism in man. *Clinical Pharmacology and Therapeutics*, **12**, 192–201.

von Knorring, A.-L., Bohman, M., von Knorring, L. & Oreland L. (1985). Platelet MAO activity as a biological marker in subgroups of alcoholism. *Acta Psychiatrica Scandinavica*, **72**, 51–8.

von Wartburg, J. P. (1980). Alcohol metabolism and alcoholism – pharmacogenetic considerations. *Acta Psychiatrica Scandinavica*, (Suppl.) **286**, 179–88.

von Wartburg, J. P., Papenburg, J. & Aebi, H. (1965). An atypical human alcohol dehydrogenase. *Canadian Journal of Biochemistry*, **43**, 889–98.

von Wartburg, J. P. & Schurch, P. M. (1968). Atypical human liver alcohol dehydrogenase. *Annals of the New York Academy of Sciences*, **151**, 936–46.

Whelan, G. (1992). Biological markers of alcoholism. *Australian and New Zealand Journal of Medicine*, **22**, 209–13.

WHO Technical Report Series No. 48 (1951). (Cited by Kennedy & Fish 1958.)

Wilkin, J. K. (1988). 4-methylpyrazole and the cutaneous vascular sensitivity to alcohol in Orientals. *Journal of Investigative Dermatology*, **91**, 117–19.

Wilson, J. R., McClearn, G. E. & Johnson, R. C. (1978). Ethnic variation in use and effects of alcohol. *Drug and Alcohol Dependence*, **3**, 147–51.

Wolff, P. H. (1972). Ethnic differences in alcohol sensitivity. *Science*, **175**, 449–50.

Wolff, P. H. (1973). Vasomotor sensitivity to alcohol in diverse Mongoloid populations. *American Journal of Human Genetics*, **25**, 193–9.

Worton, R. G. (1992). Molecular genetic approaches to the study of individual risk in alcoholism. *Alcohol and Alcoholism* (Suppl. 1), 19–25.

Yoshida, A., Hsu, L. C., Ikuta, T., Kikuchi, I., Shibuya, A. & Mohandas, T. K. (1988). Molecular genetics of alcohol-metabolizing enzymes. *Biochemical Society Transactions*, **16**, 230–2.

Yoshida, A., Dave, V., Ward, R. J. & Peters, T. J. (1989). Cytosolic aldehyde dehydrogenase (ALDH1) variants found in alcohol flushers. *Annals of Human Genetics (London)*, **53**, 1–7.

Yoshida, A., Huang, I. Y. & Ikawa, M. (1984). Molecular abnormality of an inactive aldehyde dehydrogenase variant commonly found in Orientals. *Proceedings of the National Academy of Sciences (USA)*, **81**, 258–61.

Yoshida, A., Wang, G. & Dave, V. (1983a). Determination of genotypes of human aldehyde dehydrogenase $ALDH_2$ locus. *American Journal of Human Genetics*, **35**, 1107–16.

Yoshida, A., Wang, G. & Dave, V. (1983b). A possible structural variant of human cytosolic aldehyde dehydrogenase with diminished enzyme activity. *American Journal of Human Genetics*, **35**, 1115–16 (Appendix).

PART V *N*-Acetyltransferase

16 *N*-Acetyltransferase

SUMMARY

THE *N*-acetyltransferase polymorphism in man was discovered as a result of studying the fate of isoniazid in tuberculous patients and later was shown to be genetically controlled by observations on healthy families. Acetylation was demonstrated to be the basis, by (1) *in vitro* experiments using liver samples from persons typed *in vivo*, (2) the concordant acetylation of sulphamethazine and isoniazid in the different phenotypes. Subsequently, other drugs including hydralazine, sulphapyridine, aminoglutethimide, dapsone and metabolites of caffeine and nitrazepam were also shown to be polymorphically acetylated.

In general, slow acetylators of these therapeutic drugs are more susceptible to adverse effects than are rapid acetylators because the drugs are cleared from the body less well and so are present in higher concentrations. On the other hand, in some instances it is the rapid acetylator which is at a therapeutic disadvantage.

The exact molecular genetic basis and enzymic basis of this human polymorphism have now been determined.

Considerable differences exist in allele frequencies between ethnic groups, with the allele controlling slow acetylation present at a high level in the Middle East whilst the allele controlling rapid acetylation is present at a high level in Eskimos and Japanese.

Knowledge of this polymorphism leads to some practical implications, e.g. (1) under some circumstances there may be an advantage in phenotyping patients at the beginning of prolonged courses of treatment, (2) the questionable validity of transferring treatment regimens from one ethnic group to another and (3) in the construction of therapeutic trials when the numbers of patients involved are small.

Associations have been sought between acetylator phenotypes and spontaneous disorders. Slow acetylators are 30% more prone to develop bladder cancer and much more so with heavy industrial exposure to known carcinogens. There are strong suggestions of associations between the slow acetylator phenotype and silicosis and periodic disease. The rapid acetylator phenotype is associated with both types of diabetes in Caucasians. These associations may shed light on aetiologic mechanisms.

INTRODUCTION AND INITIAL DISCOVERY OF THE POLYMORPHISM

Isoniazid (1-isonicotinyl hydrazide) was first synthesized by Meyer and Mally in 1912 but its antituberculosis properties were not found until 40 years later. Robitzek *et al.* (1952) gave isoniazid to 92 'hopeless' patients with extensive bilateral far-advanced progressive caseous-pneumonic pulmonary tuberculosis who had failed to show improvement after any therapy. The authors report, 'The mortally ill patients we have studied have obtained therapeutic benefit beyond anything we have ever seen with any of the chemotherapeutic or antibiotic agents previously utilized by us.' These reports were confirmed and extended by Selikoff & Robitzek (1952).

Following this dramatic debut, isoniazid quickly attained widespread popularity, and various research groups investigated its metabolic fate in the human body.

When isoniazid metabolism was first evaluated in large groups of patients it became apparent that there were inter-individual differences in its metabolism which were suggestive of a polymorphism. The first such account was that of Bonicke & Reif (1953), who found that 86 persons could be divided into two types, i.e. (1) those in whom 68% of the administered dose appeared in the urine in a conjugated microbiologically inactive form and (2) those in whom a smaller proportion was excreted conjugated. These types delineated via the urine also showed, respectively, low and high plasma tuberculostatic activity. However, these authors did not produce evidence of a clearly bimodal distribution of unconjugated isoniazid in blood or urine.

A great contribution was made by Hughes et al. (1955), who found in 11 normal subjects that (1) essentially all of the isoniazid ingested could be accounted for in the urine in some form, (2) the amount of unchanged isoniazid varied from 1 to 17% of the dose, (3) the major excretory products were acetylisoniazid and nicotinic acid and (4) in persons who excreted small amounts of unchanged isoniazid there were more metabolites and vice versa. The same research group showed that the pattern of metabolism of isoniazid remained constant in the same individual when examined sequentially over several weeks.

The first clear bimodal frequency distribution histogram was published by Biehl (1957), who studied the percentage of the dose excreted in the urine by a chemical method in 122 patients. His frequency distribution histogram for this parameter following a 20 mg per kg body weight daily dose shows an antimode at 12–16%.

Similarly, Mitchell & Bell (1957) had formed the view that patients could be classified as 'slow' (about 60% of the population), 'rapid' (25%) and 'intermediate' inactivators of isoniazid, on the results of their serum concentrations of the microbiologically active drug, 6 hours following the ingestion of 4 mg isoniazid per kg body weight. So

the idea that there was a polymorphism in the metabolism of the compound came into being.

Genetic investigations

The percentage of the oral dose of isoniazid which was excreted in the urine in 24 hours was estimated by both microbiological and chemical assays by Bonicke and Lisboa (1957) in five pairs of monozygous and five pairs of dizygous twins. A much greater variability was found in the latter group. The microbiological and chemical assays correlated well. These results suggested the presence of genetic influences, but the authors did not observe a bimodality and did not consider control of the metabolism by alleles at one locus.

The first published suggestion of a genetic basis for the polymorphism of isoniazid metabolism in man was in the paper of Mitchell et al. (1958), who stated:

That human variations in isoniazid inactivation may have a genetic background is suggested by certain ... observations: 15 Sioux Indians have proven predominantly to be 'rapid' isoniazid inactivators as compared with the rest of the population treated at Colorado General and Denver General Hospitals; in addition Japanese patients so tested have shown the same phenomenon.

Harris et al. (1958) investigated 25 Nisei (American citizens of Japanese descent, born in the USA) and compared them with 25 US citizens from North European stock. Only three of the Japanese group gave free serum isoniazid concentrations indicating slow inactivation, compared with 13 of the European group who fell in the same category. The authors comment:

This distribution does not suggest the bell-shaped curve of biologic variation but rather suggests a discontinuous system such as is frequently seen in the segregation of Mendelian genes.

Knight et al. (1959) carried out family studies to find out if the polymorphism was genetically determined. Their results, in 20 families tested by a microbiological method to estimate serum isoniazid, suggested that slow inactivation of the drug was recessive to rapid inactivation and, moreover, that the genes concerned were autosomal. However, there was a very considerable overlap between the two

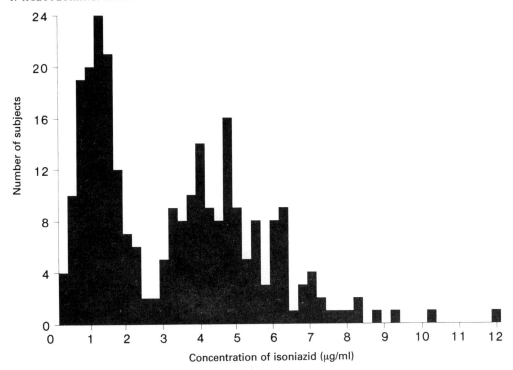

Fig. 16.1. Plasma isoniazid concentrations 6 hours after drug ingestion. Results obtained in 267 members of the 53 complete family units investigated are shown. All these subjects received approximately 9.8 mg of isoniazid per kg body weight. (From Evans *et al.* 1960.)

classes and the scoring of some individuals was doubtful. Evans *et al.* (1960) studied 267 members of 53 complete two-generation Caucasian family units with a chemical assay of plasma isoniazid concentration 6 hours following the ingestion of 10 mg/kg body weight. The results (Fig. 16.1, Table 16.1 and Table 16.2) confirmed that slow inactivation was an autosomal recessive character and there was a 'dosage' effect in that the mean concentration values for known heterozygotes differed from those of other dominants (which would contain all the homozygotes). A similar family study in Nigerians has recently been published by Odeigah & Okunowo (1989).

Meanwhile, in Japan, Sunahara (1961) and Sunahara *et al.* (1961) investigated 78 Japanese families with 162 children. With his microbiological assay, three genotypes (slow homozygotes, intermediate heterozygotes and rapid homozygotes) could be recognized with no dominance. The disparity between these results and those obtained in Europeans was not explained until the very recent work on molecular biology (*vide infra*).

The family data of Evans *et al.* (1960) have been re-examined twice with different aspects in mind.

Evans (1968) pointed out that in families consisting entirely of slow inactivators, a positive regression is present for mean offspring plasma isoniazid concentration upon mean parent concentration. No correlation exists between the concentrations in mothers and fathers. When families in which the mother is a slow inactivator and the father is a rapid inactivator are examined, a similar result is obtained. Insufficient numbers are present to examine the converse mating. In the mating of a slow inactivator with a rapid inactivator which has produced slow inactivator offspring, all the rapid inactivators are heterozygous. Here again, although the result fails to attain significance, there is a positive regression of mean rapid inactivator offspring plasma isoniazid concentration upon rapid inactivator parent concentration.

Table 16.1. *Numbers of observed matings compared with those expected by application of the Hardy–Weinberg law*

Phenotypic matings	Genotypic matings	Expected frequency of matings		Expected occurrence in 53 matings	Observed occurrence
S × S	$I_r I_r \times I_r I_r$	p^4 0.2728		14.46	17
R × S	$\begin{cases} I_R I_R \times I_r I_r \\ I_R I_r \times I_r I_r \end{cases}$	$\begin{array}{ll} 2p^2q^2 & 0.0803 \\ 4p^3q & 0.4187 \end{array}$ 0.4990		26.45	23
R × R	$\begin{cases} I_R I_R \times I_R I_R \\ I_R I_R \times I_R I_r \\ I_R I_r \times I_R I_r \end{cases}$	$\begin{array}{ll} q^4 & 0.0059 \\ 4q^3p & 0.0616 \\ 4q^2p^2 & 0.1606 \end{array}$ 0.2281		12.09	13
		0.9999		53.00	53

I_R = The allele controlling the dominant character; $\chi^2 = 0.964$; D.F. = 2; $p > 0.5$.
From: Evans *et al.* 1960.

Table 16.2. *Expected numbers of children of each phenotype compared with those observed*

Phenotypic matings	Number of matings	Number of children	Number of children of each phenotype				χ^2	D.F.
			Rapid		Slow			
			Exp.	Obs.	Exp.	Obs.		
S × S	17	54	Nil	4	54	50	–	–
R × S	23	67	38.88	40	28.10	27	0.075	1
R × R	13	38	31.30	31	6.68	7	0.018	1
	53	159		75		84	0.093	2

The hypothesis is made that slow-inactivator persons are genetically homozygous recessives.
From: Evans *et al.* 1960.

Taken as a whole, these results suggest that secondary genetic influences are present which modify the expression of the major genetic polymorphism.

Iselius & Evans (1983) published the results of complex segregation analysis of the family data which shows the existence of a gene controlling the recessive character and a multifactorial background. The phenotype is also influenced by age, sex and weight.

An approximate mean value for the homozygous dominants can be obtained by a method published by Evans *et al.* (1980) (Appendix 1).

A study of 16 families (Kilbane *et al.* 1990) indicates that the individual genotypes can be detected using a caffeine test.

DRUGS OTHER THAN ISONIAZID WHICH ARE POLYMORPHICALLY ACETYLATED

After the genetic nature of the isoniazid 'inactivation' polymorphism had been determined, a number of new problems required to be solved. One of the foremost of these was to ascertain what biochemical processes the responsible alleles controlled.

The early, careful work of Hughes *et al.* (1954) had indicated that the amount of acetylisoniazid excreted in the urine varied widely between people, and that those who produced a lot of the metabolite were the ones with the low plasma concentrations.

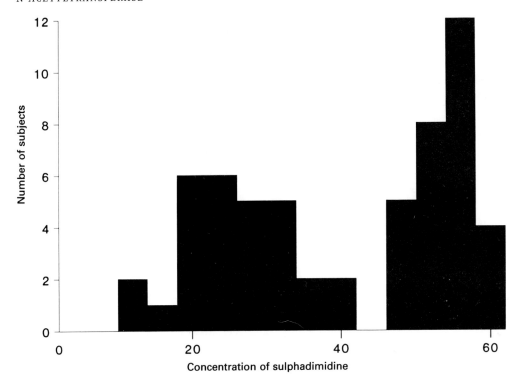

Fig. 16.2. Concentration of free sulphadimidine as a percentage of the total sulphadimidine in the urine excreted 8 hours after drug ingestion. (From Evans 1962.)

Since the principal group of drugs which were known to be metabolized by acetylation were the sulphonamides, attention was directed to these compounds: this decision was also strengthened by the advice of Dr E. K. Marshall, Jr, of the Johns Hopkins Hospital and Dr Spinks of ICI, UK who had both observed wide variability between individuals in the acetylation of sulphonamides. Sulphamethazine (SMZ-*syn* sulphadimidine) was chosen because its acetylation was rapid and extensive and it was then not known to be subject to any other biotransformation (Fig. 16.2).

After persons who had previously been typed using isoniazid were shown to be similarly polymorphic for their acetylation of SMZ, two things followed: (1) the genes responsible for the polymorphism were known to control acetylation, (2) the 'typed panel' approach was established as an investigative procedure whereby other drugs could

be examined. The results are shown in Table 16.3.

The N-acetyltransferase polymorphism has been demonstrated to be independent of the debrisoquine/sparteine P450-dependent oxidation polymorphism, by Harmer *et al.* (1986) and Sardas *et al.* (1988).

TECHNIQUES FOR DETERMINING THE ACETYLATOR PHENOTYPE

Over the last 30 years a number of techniques have been used to determine the acetylator phenotype. A lot of the early work was carried out by means of microbiological assays of isoniazid using tubercle bacilli, a method which was obviously inappropriate for widespread use and so was fairly quickly supplanted by chemical assays.

Even though genotyping tests have now become available, there is still a requirement to study phenotypic features.

There are certain desiderata for phenotyping procedures. They should ideally be quick, easy, not painful or hazardous, and give an unequivocal classification. There is no test which is quick and easy.

Table 25.2. *Mutations in the human G6PD gene*

	Name	Exon	Nucleotide number	Nucleotide substitution	Codon change	Amino acid number	Amino acid substitution	WHO class	Reference
1	Gaohe[a]	2	95	A → G	CAC → CGC	32	His → Arg	III	Chao et al. 1991
2	Sunderland	2	105–107	Deletion	–CTC	35	–Ile	I	MacDonald et al. 1991
3	Aures	3	143	T → C	ATC → ACC	48	Ile → Thr	II	Nafa et al. 1993
4	Metaponto	4	172	G → A	GAT → AAT	58	Asp → Asn	III	Vulliamy et al. 1988
5	A–[b]	4,5	202	G → A	GTG → ATG	68	Val → Met	III	Hirono & Beutler 1988
			376	A → G	AAT → GAT	126	Asn → Asp		
6	Swansea	4	224	T → C	CTC → CCC	75	Leu → Pro	I	MacDonald et al. unpublished
7	Konan[c]	4	241	C → T	CGC → TGC	81	Arg → Cys	III	Hirono et al. 1992
8	Lagosanto	4	242	G → A	CGC → CAC	81	Arg → His	III	Ninfali et al. unpublished
9	Vancouver	4,6,6	317	C → G	TCC → TGC	106	Ser → Lys	I	Maeda et al. 1992
			544	T → C	CGG → TGG	182	Arg → Trp		
			592	C → T	CGC → TGC	198	Arg → Cys		
10	A	5	376	A → G	AAT → GAT	126	Asn → Asp	IV	Takizawa et al. 1987
11	Chinese-4	5	392	G → T	GGG → GTG	131	Gly → Val		Chiu et al. 1991a
12	Ilesha	5	466	G → A	GAG → AAG	156	Glu → Lys	III	Vulliamy et al. 1988
13	Mahidol	6	487	G → A	GGC → AGC	163	Gly → Ser	III	Vulliamy et al. 1989
14	Plymouth	6	488	G → A	GGC → GAC	163	Gly → Asp	I	Town et al. unpublished
15	Chinese-3	6	493	A → G	AAC → GAC	165	Asn → Asp	II	Tang et al. 1992
16	Santamaria	6,5	542	A → T	GAC → GTC	181	Asp → Val	II	Beutler et al. 1991a
			376	A → G	AAT → GAT	126	Asn → Asp		
17	Mediterranean[d]	6	563	C → T	TCC → TTC	188	Ser → Phe	II	Vulliamy et al. 1988
18	Coimbra	6	592	C → T	CGC → TGC	198	Arg → Cys	II	Cocoran et al. 1992
19	Santiago	6	593	G → C	CGC → CCC	198	Arg → Pro	I	Beutler et al. 1992a
20	Sibari	6	634	A → G	ATG → GTG	212	Met → Val	III	Calabro et al. 1992
21	Minnesota[e]	6	637	G → T	GTG → TTG	213	Val → Leu	III	Beutler et al. 1991b
22	Harilaou	7	648	T → G	TTT → TTG	216	Phe → Leu	I	Poggi et al. 1990
23	Mexico City	7	680	G → A	CGG → CAG	227	Arg → Gln	III	Beutler et al. 1992a
24	A–	7,5	680	G → T	CGG → CTG	227	Arg → Leu	III	Beutler et al. 1989
			376	A → G	AAT → GAT	126	Asn → Asp		
25	Stonybrook	7	724–729	Deletion	–GGCACT	242–243	–Gly, Thr	I	Beutler et al. unpublished
26	Wayne	7	769	C → G	CGG → GGG	257	Arg → Gly	I	Beutler et al. 1991c
27	Chinese-1	8	835	A → T	ACC → TCC	279	Thr → Ser	II	Beutler et al. 1992b
28	Seattle[f]	8	844	G → C	GAT → CAT	282	Asp → His	III	DeVita et al. 1989
29	Montalbano	8	854	G → A	CGT → CAT	285	Arg → His	III	Viglietto et al. 1990
30	Viangchan[g]	9	871	G → A	GTG → ATG	291	Val → Met	II	Beutler et al. 1991c
31	Kalyan[h]	9	949	G → A	GAG → AAG	317	Glu → Lys	III	Ahluwalia et al. 1991
32	A–[i]	9,5	968	T → C	CTG → CCG	323	Leu → Pro	III	Beutler et al. 1989
			376	A → G	AAT → GAT	126	Asn → Asp		
33	Chatham	9	1003	G → A	GCC → ACC	335	Ala → Thr	III	Vulliamy et al. 1988
34	Chinese-5	9	1024	C → T	CTC → TTC	342	Leu → Phe	I	Chiu et al. 1991a
35	Ierapetra	10	1057	C → T	CCC → TCC	353	Pro → Ser	II	Beutler et al. 1992a
36	Loma linda	10	1089	C → A	AAc → AAA	363	Asn → Lys		Beutler et al. 1991b
37	Tomah	10	1153	T → C	TGC → CGC	385	Cys → Arg	I	Hirono et al. 1989
38	Iowa[j]	10	1156	A → G	AAG → GAG	386	Lys → Glu	I	Hirono et al. 1989

Hydralazine	Antihypertensive	Plasma concentration of hydralazine lower in R than in S	SM	Shepherd *et al.* 1981
Hydralazine	Antihypertensive	Mean areas under the curve of MTP higher in R, and bioavailability of hydralazine after oral doses higher in S. HPPAH major plasma metabolite in S and MTP in R following oral doses	SM	Reece *et al.* 1980
DDS	Antileprotic	Plasma ratio of MADDS/DDS	SM and isoniazid	Peters & Levy 1971
DDS	Antileprotic	Plasma ratio of MADDS/DDS	SM and isoniazid	Gelber *et al.* 1971
DDS	Antileprotic	Plasma ratio of MADDS/DDS	SM	Peters *et al.* 1975
Nitrazepam metabolite	Hypnotic	Percentage acetylation of 7-amino nitrazepam in urine	SM	Karim & Evans 1976
Prizidilol	Precapillary vasodilator and β-adrenergic blocker	Plasma levels of prizidilol higher in S	SM	Larsson *et al.* 1981
Amrinone	Positive inotropic with vasodilator properties	Plasma concentrations of amrinone higher in S and urinary acetyl amrinone/amrinone higher in R	Isoniazid	Hamilton *et al.* 1986
Endralazine	Antihypertensive	Plasma concentrations of endralazine slightly higher in S and area under the curve of plasma acetyl endralazine higher in R	SM	Reece *et al.* 1982
Dipyrone	Analgesic Antipyretic Anti-inflammatory	Mean plasma concentration, peak time and half-live greater for parent drug in S. Mean plasma concentration for acetyl metabolite greater in R	DDS	Levy *et al.* 1984
Clonazepam metabolite	Anti-epileptic	7-acetylamino clonazepam in urine greater in R	SM	Miller *et al.* 1981
Clonazepam metabolite	Anti-epileptic	N-acetylation by human liver homogenates polymorphic	None	Peng *et al.* 1984
Aminoglutethimide	Inhibitor of adrenal steroid synthesis and peripheral aromatization of androgens	Urinary excretion of unchanged aminoglutethimide less and of acetylaminoglutethimide more in R than in S	SM	Coombes *et al.* 1982
Aminoglutethimide	Inhibitor of adrenal steroid synthesis and peripheral aromatization of adrenal androgens	Greater plasma ratio, area under curve acetylaminoglutethimide/area under curve glutethimide in R. More unchanged drug in urine in S	DDS	Adam *et al.* 1984
Aminoglutethimide	Inhibitor of adrenal steroid synthesis and peripheral aromatization of adrenal androgens	More unchanged drug in the serum of S and more acetyl metabolite in the serum of R	None	Demers *et al.* 1987
Caffeine metabolite	Stimulant	Urinary ratio of, 5-acetylamino-6-formyl amino-3-methyluracil/L-methylxanthine	SM	Grant *et al.* 1984
Amonafide	Antineoplastic agent	Plasma concentration of N-acetylamonafide 24 hours after a dose	Caffeine	Ratain *et al.* 1991

HPPAH, hydralazine pyruvic acid hydrazone; NAc HPZ, 4-N-acetyl hydrazinophthalazin-1-one; TP, S-triazolo[3,4-a]phthalazine; PZ, phthalazinone; HH, hydralazine acid-labile hydrazones; OH MTP, 3-hydroxy-methyl-triazolo[3,4-a]phthalazine; Ac SM, acetyl-sulphamethazine; SM, sulphamethazine; SP, sulphapyridine; MADDS, 4-amino-4'-acetamidodiphenyl-sulphone (mono-acetyldapsone); DDS, 4,4'-diaminodiphenyl-sulphone (dapsone); R, rapid acetylator; S, slow acetylator.

All involve the subject concerned ingesting, or having administered intravenously, a foreign compound (even caffeine). Most do not give an unequivocal characterization of the phenotype.

It is self-evident that a very accurate test which is elaborate (say, involving a number of timed blood specimens) can be carried out only on a limited number of people. So it may be necessary to settle for a simpler though less accurate test when a large number of subjects is to be investigated.

Some comments will now be made concerning the more popular of the tests which have been employed.

Isoniazid tests

These tests have generally relied on the oral ingestion of a dose of isoniazid following which specimens of blood and/or urine have been collected. In some instances the drug has been given intravenously or intramuscularly; this does not seem to be a wise idea because isoniazid is absorbed from the gut completely and quickly, and meets the polymorphic *N*-acetyltransferase, which the test is supposed to evaluate, immediately. After intramuscular injections particularly, absorption into the systemic circulation may be erratic (Scott *et al.* 1969).

Isoniazid half-lives using a chemical technique of measurement were used by Jenne (1960) who used an i.v. injection of 5 mg per kg body weight and sampled the blood at 30, 90 and 150 minutes thereafter. Excellent discrimination between the phenotypes was given by this method. In order to phenotype large numbers of people, Evans *et al.* (1960) used the plasma concentration of isoniazid 6 hours following the ingestion of 10 mg/kg. Slight overlapping at the antimode occurred which implied a small degree of misclassification. It was shown by Evans *et al.* (1961) that giving the drug according to metabolically active mass (weight$^{0.7}$) minimized the overlap and using this oral dosage schedule and a half-life compiled with 2 and 6 hour plasma concentrations gave satisfactory discrimination of phenotypes (Gow & Evans 1964).

Many other workers since have produced new isoniazid tests and modifications of those mentioned above (Table 16.4).

Sulphamethazine tests

Sulphamethazine was introduced by Evans (1962) as an alternative to isoniazid as a test substance because the Bratton–Marshall analytical method used to measure it was much simpler than the methods then available for the analysis of isoniazid.

When both blood and urine are analysed and the percentage acetylation of SMZ is plotted in a two-dimensional scattergram, a very clear separation of phenotypes results (Evans 1969). This test has been used in very large populations with success (e.g. Viznerova *et al.* 1973; Fig. 16.3). Modifications have been described using (1) filter paper to collect the blood sample (which can then be mailed: Weber & Brennan 1974; Hoo *et al.* 1977), (2) no instrumentation (Schroder 1972) and (3) an autoanalyser technique for analysis (Eze & Evans 1972).

Since the original experiments of Evans (1962) and Evans & White (1964), many groups have confirmed the correspondence between isoniazid and SMZ test results, the latest being Seth *et al.* (1988).

The argument is sometimes raised as to whether blood or urine is the better liquid to sample. If only one can be obtained, plasma (or serum) is superior to urine. However, even though the phenotypic separation using urine is not as satisfactory as with serum (it can be influenced by renal factors), it still gives some extra gap between the two phenotypes in two dimensions. When a clear separation is not obtained by this two-liquids technique it means that there has not been sufficient attention to detail in performing the test. For example, subjects must be fasting and be observed to swallow the SMZ, the timing of the specimens should be exact, analytical techniques must be carefully controlled and specimens analysed in duplicate.

There are disadvantages to the SMZ test, for example, it cannot be performed on persons who have a history of sulphonamide hypersensitivity, and even in the absence of such a history, a transient rash very rarely occurs; also, the drug is not freely available in the USA.

More recently, attention has turned in two directions: (1) the replacement of the Bratton–Marshall analytical technique with high-pressure liquid chromatography and (2) more sophisticated pharmacokinetics.

The objections to the Bratton–Marshall technique are that (1) it is labour-intensive, (2) some of the

Table 16.4. *Isoniazid phenotyping procedures*

References	Dose	Sample(s)	Expression of results	Comments
Scott et al. 1969	4 mg/kg bw p.o.	Serum 2 and 6 h	Rate constant of inactivation and $t_{1/2}$	Seem to give similar phenotypic separation
	2 mg/kg bw i.m.	Serum 0.5, 1.5 and 2.5 h	Rate constant of inactivation and $t_{1/2}$	
Tiitinen 1969a	5 mg/kg i.v.	Serum 0.5, 1.0 and 3 h	$t_{1/2}$	Similar result to single 6 h value
Russell 1970	3 spaced doses of 100 mg p.o.	Urine next morning	AcINH/INH	Simple. Assessed on 19 subjects only
Eidus et al. 1971	8 mg/kg i.m.	Urine at 2, 4, 6, 8 and 10 h	AcINH/INH at 6–8 h	Satisfactory separation of phenotypes in 35 persons
Eidus & Hodgkin 1973	10 mg/kg p.o.	Urine 6–8 h	AcINH/INH	Satisfactory separation of 25 selected S from 25 selected R
Varughese et al. 1974	10 mg/kg p.o.	Urine 6–8 h	AcINH/total hydrazides by autoanalyser	Excellent separation
Ellard et al. 1973b	5 mg INH/kg i.m.	Urine 0–3 h	AcINH/acid labile INH	Ditto and may be able to detect homozygous R
Raghupati Sarma et al. 1976	3 mg/kg i.m.	Urine 3–4 h	Acetyl INH/INH	Fairly good separation of phenotypes
Hutchings & Routledge 1986	200 mg p.o.	Blood at 2, 3, 4, 5 and 6 h	$t_{1/2}$INH AcINH/INH at 3 h	The ratio at 3 h appears to give an equal separation of phenotypes. The ratio may be detecting 2 homozygous R out of 32 subjects
Inaba & Arias 1987	10 mg/kg p.o.	Urine 6–8 h	INH/AcINH probit	A new way of defining a unique antimode for each population
Miscoria et al. 1988	Unclear	Plasma 3 h	AcINH/INH	Satisfactory separation
Hutchings et al. 1988	200 mg INH	Saliva at 2, 3, 4, 5 and 6 h	Salivary INH $t_{1/2}$	Correlates with simultaneously determined plasma INH $t_{1/2}$

bw, Body weight; p.o., by mouth; $t_{1/2}$, half-life; i.m., intramuscular; i.v., intravenous; AcINH, acetylisoniazid; INH, isoniazid; S, slow acetylator; R, rapid acetylator.

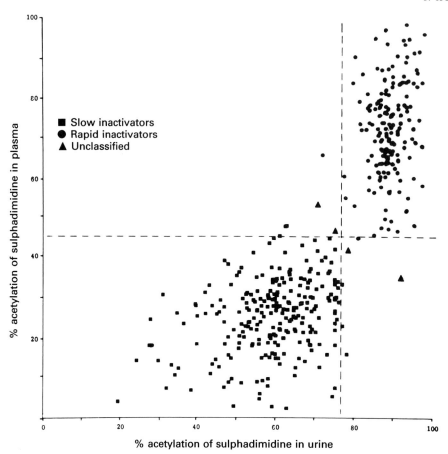

Fig. 16.3. Distribution of 421 patients according to the percentage of sulphadimidine acetylated in the plasma and urine (using method II of Evans 1969). (From Viznerova *et al.* 1973.)

compounds are destroyed when boiled with acid, which can in some instances give apparently 'negative' concentrations of acetyl SMZ (or percentage SMZ acetylated). The high-pressure liquid chromatography (HPLC) method requires sophisticated and expensive apparatus but is not labour-intensive and, since it does not require the specimens to be boiled with acid, should give accurate values for the concentrations of SMZ and acetyl SMZ. Whelpton *et al.* (1981) and Olsen (1982a) have investigated this problem and indicate that HPLC is superior, but no rigorous mathematical proof has yet been provided from surveys under field conditions.

It can be seen in Table 16.5 that the methods of du Souich *et al.* (1979a,b), Chapron *et al.* (1980), Vree *et al.* (1980) and Lee & Lee (1982) all require many blood samples and urine samples. The method of Vree *et al.* (1980) is the most economical, but still requires five blood samples. The result of this is that these methods are not applicable for the investigation of large numbers of subjects, though they are valuable as special procedures on selected small numbers of people.

Sulphapyridine

The acetylation of sulphapyridine exactly parallels that of SMZ (Schröder & Evans 1972a). The principal value of this observation is that the sulphapyridine (SP) released from salicylazosulphapyridine (SASP) can be used to phenotype patients whilst they are receiving the drug for therapeutic purposes (see section on SASP, p. 244).

Table 16.5. *Isoniazid phenotyping procedures*

References	Dose	Sample(s)	Expression of results	Comments
Evans 1962	160 mg/kg MAM (i.e. per kg$^{0.7}$)	Urine passed during the 8 h following drug ingestion	% Free SMZ/Total SMZ	Clear bimodality
Evans & White 1964	60 mg/kg MAM (i.e. per kg$^{0.7}$)	Urine passed during the 8 h following drug ingestion	% SMZ acetylated	Clear bimodality
Evans 1969	Method II approx 11 mg/kg bw or 40 mg/kg MAM	Blood at 6 h and urine passed 5–6 h after drug ingestion	Two dimensional plot of % SMZ acetylated	Wide separation of the two phenotypes
Rao et al. 1970	44 mg/kg bw	Blood and urine at 6 h	% SMZ acetylated	Separation of phenotypes not as clear as in above
Sen et al. 1982	44 mg/kg bw	Blood at 6 h, urine at 5–6 h	% SMZ acetylated	Very poor discrimination between phenotypes.
du Souich et al. 1979a, b	10 mg/kg bw	Blood at 0, 0.5, 1, 2, 3, 4, 6, 8, 12, 18 and 24 h Urine hourly for 8 h then paralleling the blood collections	Plasma SMZ $t_{1/2}$ and % N-acetyl SMZ in plasma at 6 h. % Acetylation of SMZ in 5–6 h urine or 6 h urine	6 h plasma % N-acetyl SMZ most reliable
Chapron et al. 1980	20 mg/kg	Plasma samples at 1 h intervals for 8 h. Urine for 72 h	Acetylation clearance. Metabolic rate constant. Overall elimination rate constant	All 3 define 3 phenotypes in 19 subjects (9 Oriental). Segregates rapid acetylators into 2 non-overlapping groups
Vree et al. 1980	500 mg	Finger tip blood hourly for first 10 h then at more widely spaced intervals up to 35 h	Plasma conc. SMZ $t_{1/2}$ and % SMZ acetylated	Reckon SMZ most useful compound for phenotyping but at least 2 plasma samples at different times and % SMZ acetylated required
Lee & Lee 1982	1 g	Venous blood at 6, 7, 8, 9 and 10 h. Urine at 7–8 h	SMZ conc. in all samples. AcSMZ/SMZ in 6 h blood sample. Compute metabolic clearance	Elimination rate constant, total body clearance and metabolic clearance appeared to give three modes in 10 Chinese subjects
Hombhanje 1991	Various doses 250 mg to 1 g	Urine 5–6 h after drug ingestion	% SMZ acetylated	Clear bimodality most pronounced with 750 mg dose

MAM, metabolically active mass (bw to the power of 0.7); SMZ, sulphamethazine; bw, body weight; $t_{1/2}$, half-life.

There are some disadvantages to sulphapyridine, namely: (1) it is deacetylated in the body (Schroder 1973), which seems to be a less important phenomenon for sulphamethazine; (2) it is polymorphically hydroxylated to a considerable degree (Schroder & Evans 1972a), whereas sulphamethazine is hydroxylated to a lesser extent (Vree *et al.* 1986); (3) it is probably a more toxic compound.

Other phenotyping methods

Other phenotyping methods using SASP hydralazine, caffeine and dapsone are discussed in sections dealing with these individual drugs.

Attempts have been made to use human cells *in vitro* for phenotyping. It was shown by Evans & White (1964) that it can be done with small liver biopsies but this is useless for large-scale surveys. The same authors investigated white cell preparations but obtained no acetylation of SMZ.

Motulsky & Steinmann (1962) found that human erythrocytes will acetylate *p*-aminosalicylic acid and *p*-aminobenzoic acid (PABA), but not isoniazid or sulphanilamide. Likewise, McQueen & Weber (1980) tested lymphocyte *N*-acetyltransferase for ability to acetylate SMZ, benzocaine, procainamide and PABA. Only for the last was activity detected. The lymphocyte *N*-acetyltransferase metabolizing PABA was less stable in rapid than in slow acetylators, possibly indicating a structural difference.

Jejunal mucosa has the ability to acetylate isoniazid (Jenne 1963) and could probably be used for phenotyping *in vitro*, but this is a method which could be of use only under the most special circumstances.

The search for a genotyping test

Ever since the genetics of the acetylator polymorphism were worked out, there has been one unsatisfactory feature. The early microbiological methods seemed capable of detecting the three genotypes. However, prior to the advent of caffeine tests (see below) no worker had convincingly demonstrated the identification of the three genotypes using chemical methods. Claims that a particular method might be able to achieve this objective have been made by Ellard *et al.* (1973b) with a urinary

AcINH/acid labile INH test, and by both Chapron *et al.* (1980) and Lee & Lee (1982) with multi-sample tests. No specific claim was made by the authors but it seems possible that Hutchings & Routledge (1986) with a plasma AcINH/INH ratio were able to separate the rapid acetylators into two groups. Sunahara *et al.* (1963a) were able to show a trimodal distribution curve in the Japanese population and to prove that they represented the three genotypes with family studies. A similar trimodal curve was obtained by testing a Thai population (which has a much lower percentage of homozygous rapid individuals) with the same technique, i.e. 4 mg INH per kg dosage and microbiological assessment of blood INH level at 6 hours (Sunahara *et al.* 1963b). The method of Hutchings & Routledge (1986) is the most similar to that of Sunahara *et al.* (1963a).

Recently Horai & Ishizaki (1988) found an apparently trimodal frequency distribution of 3 hour plasma MADDS/DDS ratios in Japanese, but unfortunately the numbers of subjects in the three modes were not in accordance with the Hardy–Weinberg distribution. Grant *et al.* (1984) considered the possibility that their caffeine test may be able to separate the three genotypes, but found that the Hardy–Weinberg equilibrium was not obeyed in their population and that some family data did not support the hypothesis.

Using a new technique of assaying caffeine metabolites in the urine, Tang *et al.* (1987, 1991) suggested the possibility that they might be able to detect the individual genotypes. Likewise, Gascon *et al.* (1987), who plotted the frequency distribution of urinary AFMU/IX following the ingestion of a cup of coffee by each of 63 medical personnel, demonstrated three clear modes (Fig. 16.4), the numbers of subjects in which were in keeping with the Hardy–Weinberg equilibrium. A 16 family study employing the caffeine test and expressing the results as AAMU/1X has been published by Kilbane *et al.* (1990) and gives convincing evidence that this procedure can detect genotypes.

FACTORS INFLUENCING ACETYLATOR PHENOTYPING TESTS

The evidence is condensed in Table 16.6. Only when liver function and renal function are severely

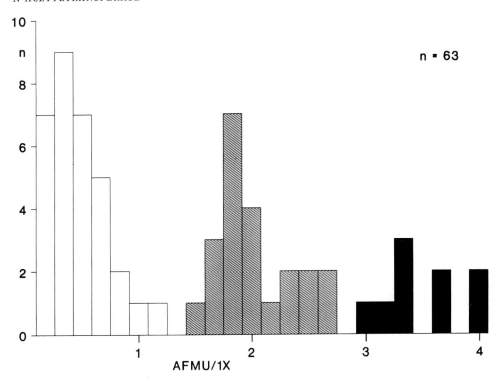

Fig. 16.4. Frequency distribution of the metabolic ratio AFMU/1X in the urine of 63 healthy subjects, 4 hours after the consumption of a cup of coffee. Those individuals with a ratio of less than 1.2 (32/63) are the slow acetylators. The others are the heterozygous and homozygous rapid acetylators. (From Gascon *et al.* 1987.)

impaired do they affect the outcome of conventional phenotyping tests. The data of Pacifici *et al.* (1990) suggest that the enzymic activity of liver N-acetyltransferase is greatly depressed by severe cirrhosis in rapid acetylators so that they come to resemble slow acetylators.

Glucose speeds the metabolism of acetylated compounds such as isoniazid and SMZ, but the effect is not sufficient to interfere with the usual phenotyping tests when carried out in diabetics. The effect is thought to be mediated by enhancing the supply of 'active acetate' (i.e. acetyl CoA). Similarly, ethanol has a marked influence on the acetylation of test drugs.

It was shown by Lindsay & Baty (1988) that the addition of acetyl CoA to human blood samples increased their acetylation capacity significantly; and the addition of glucose *in vitro* to rat blood had the same effect (Lindsay & Baty 1990). On the other hand, the induction of diabetes with streptozotocin significantly reduced the *in vivo* acetylation capacity of the rat (Lindsay & Baty 1990); the explanation for this apparent paradox is unclear.

Conversely, other drugs which are known to be acetylated, particularly *p*-aminosalicylic acid, slow the acetylation rate of a test compound such as isoniazid. This influence could be mediated by a reduced supply of acetyl CoA.

Some of these phenomena in humans can be reproduced in experimental animals (see Table 16.6). Another intriguing observation in animals is the increase in the acetylation of SMZ *in vivo* and *in vitro* in rabbits and rats, which is produced by Freund's adjuvant. The mechanism is unknown but it is possible that the phenomenon may have some relationship to the enhanced acetylation reported by Chekharina *et al.* (1978) in patients with lymphoma.

Table 16.6. *Factors assessed for their influence on acetylator phenotyping tests and acetylation processes in humans and animals*

References	Phenotyping tests	Influencing factor instigated	Effect
Levi et al. 1968	INH $t_{1/2}$	Liver disease	Bimodal frequency distribution curve blurred when serum bilirubin >2 mg/100 ml
Lester 1965	INH $t_{1/2}$	Pretreatment with drugs	No effect
		Alcoholism	Bimodal frequency distribution curve unimpaired 30% decrease in INH $t_{1/2}$
Lilyin et al. 1984	SMZ acetylation	Alcohol (0.02–0.04% in the blood)	Bimodal frequency distribution curve unimpaired by
		Alcoholism	some increase in % acetylation
Olsen & Morland 1978	SMZ acetylation	Alcohol (1 g/l in blood)	20% decrease in $t_{1/2}$ SMZ
Olsen & Morland 1982	Procainamide $t_{1/2}$	Alcohol (about 16 mM in blood)	12.6% decrease in $t_{1/2}$
Hutchings et al. 1984	MADDS/DDS	Alcohol (650–1180 mg/ml in blood)	No significant change
Fine & Sumner 1975	SMZ acetylation	Uraemia	Acetylation induced but acetyl SMZ not excreted as well as normal. Hence simple test such as Evans (1969) may give erroneous phenotyping
Hall 1981	SMZ acetylation (Evans 1969)	Uraemia	Acetyl SMZ not excreted as well as normal when creatinine clearance low but phenotyping unimpaired with serum values
Talseth & Landmark 1977	SMZ acetylation (Evans 1969)	Uraemia	Acetyl SMZ not excreted as well as normal when creatinine clearance low but phenotyping unimpaired with serum values
Shastri 1982	SMZ acetylation (Evans 1969)	Undernourishment	No effect
Buchanan 1979	INH $t_{1/2}$	Kwashiorkor	Impaired elimination
Suhardjono et al. 1986	SMZ acetylation in blood and urine	Glucose	Minor changes in SMZ clearance but unlikely to alter phenotypic acetylation status
Zysset & Peretti 1986	SMZ acetylation (Evans 1969)	Isoniazid	Acetylation diminished in rapid acetylators. Could lead to errors in phenotyping
Ylitalo et al. 1984	SMZ acetylation in urine	Isoniazid	No effect
Thom et al. 1981	INH $t_{1/2}$	Glucose	Reduction of 24% which might under some circumstances affect the determination of acetylator phenotype
Ahmad et al. 1981	MADDS/DDS in plasma	INH or SMZ	Ratio changed, could change phenotype
	MADDS/DDS in plasma	Hydralazine	Insignificant changes
	% Acetylation of SMZ in plasma and urine	Hydralazine	Insignificant changes
Jenne et al. 1961	INH $t_{1/2}$	PAS	Prolongation
Hanngren et al. 1970	INH $t_{1/2}$	PAS	Prolongation
Vas et al. 1990	K_{el} SMZ	Pantothenic acid 1100 mg (200 TID PO + 500 mg i.v.)	In general no significant change (except one rapid acetylator became a slow)
		Ethanol during the SMZ test	No significant change
Tiitinen 1969b	INH $t_{1/2}$	PAS	INH $t_{1/2}$ prolonged and serum INH concentration increased in both phenotypes
		SMZ	INH $t_{1/2}$ prolonged in S only

Reference		Agent	Effect
Mattila & Takki 1969	INH $t_{1/2}$	Chlorpromazine	INH $t_{1/2}$ prolonged
		Phenyramidol	INH $t_{1/2}$ prolonged
		Sodium salicylate	INH $t_{1/2}$ shortened
Wright et al. 1984	MADDS/MADDS+DDS in plasma	Cimetidine	No effect
Timbrell et al. 1985	Isoniazid and metabolites in urine	Rifampicin	7 days therapy no affect
Animal Studies			
Zidek et al. 1977	Percentage SMZ in urine (rat)	Freund's adjuvant 21 days before test	Increase in males
	Liver N-acetyltransferase activity (rat)	Freund's adjuvant 21 days before test	No change
du Souich & Courteau 1981	SMZ acetylation in blood and urine (rabbits)	Complete Freund's adjuvant Hydrocortisone	Increased 60% in R and 135% in S Increased 30%
Ryazanov et al. 1985	SMZ acetylation (rats)	Oestrogen Tetracycline Reopyrine Phenobarbital	All increased rate of acetylation
Olsen & Morland 1978	SMZ acetylation by rat liver cells in vitro	Ethanol	30% increase
Olsen 1982b	Procainamide acetylation by rat liver cells in vitro	Ethanol	Unchanged
Peters et al. 1966	INH acetylation (rat)	Glucose	Increased
	PAS acetylation (rat)	Glucose	Decreased
Reeves et al. 1988, 1989	SMZ acetylation (rabbits)	Hydrocortisone	Acetylation induced because of hypertrophy of hepatic tissue and increased liver blood flow
Littley et al. 1988	INH acetylation	Thyrotoxicosis	No change in phenotype
Svensson & Knowlton 1989	Procainamide acetylation (rats)	Tilorone	Acetylation increased
Kang et al. 1989	Procaine acetylation in rat liver	Clofibrate	Acetylation increased at low concentrations
Pieters et al. 1988	Dapsone	Rifamicin	Reduction in $t_{1/2}$ and plasma concentration
	Dapsone	Clofazimine	No effect on pharmacokinetics
Philip et al. 1989	Plasma MADDS/DDS	Cancer chemotherapy	Mainly increase in MADDS/DDS including some individuals with apparent change of phenotype. Ratio decreased in some patients

INH, isoniazid; $t_{1/2}$ half-life of concentration in plasma; SMZ, sulphamethazine; MADDS, monoacetyldiaminodiphenylsulphone; DDS, diaminodiphenylsulphone; PAS, p-aminosalicylic acid; R, rapid acetylator; S, slow acetylator.

The effect of age on the N-acetylation process and its polymorphism

The white American family data of Evans *et al.* (1960) was originally analysed only in terms of acetylator phenotype frequency and no age effect was observed. Re-examination of the same data by more refined statistical techniques (Iselius & Evans 1983) revealed that an age effect was present. Subsequently, other groups have contributed information on the subject throughout the span of life.

Using PABA as a substrate, Pacifici *et al.* (1986) showed that the acetylation activity (expressed as nmol of product formed per min per mg protein: mean ± SE) was 1.10 ± 0.59 in the fetal liver of Swedish subjects and 3.87 ± 0.053 in the adult liver cytosol. Similar values (0.71 ± 0.11 and 3.80 ± 0.34) were obtained for fetal and adult intestinal mucosa, respectively. Unfortunately PABA is not subject to polymorphic acetylation in man, so this information, which is interesting in that it does show that some acetylating activity is present in fetal life, does not give information about the polymorphism.

Meisel *et al.* (1986) studied the acetylation capacities of fetal livers using procainamide. Unfortunately they could not study single individuals because it was necessary to pool hepatic tissues from different individuals. The activities found in fetal livers were higher than the lowest single values of adult slow and rapid acetylator livers. So it is possible that the polymorphism is expressed during intra-uterine life.

A hundred Hungarian babies aged 2–3 days old were investigated by Szorady *et al.* (1987). They used a sulphadimidine phenotyping test and the differentiation between phenotypes was poor. The percentage of slow acetylators was said to be 83% in the babies as compared with 48% in children and young adults, 50% in the age range 19–59 years and 66.4 in the elderly. A possibility is that a relative pantothenic acid deficiency may exist in the newborn and that this is a limiting factor on coenzyme A formation, so leading to an apparent deficiency in expressing the rapid acetylation phenotype.

A caffeine metabolism test was performed by Carrier *et al.* (1988) on four premature newborn and 10 older infants. The AFMI/1X ratio was very low in 10 of the babies and below 0.4 (the interphenotypic dividing antimode in adult studies) in 13. One baby

was tested at both 54 and 196 days after birth and she was phenotyped as slow and rapid on the first and second occasions respectively. The suggestion is made by the authors that some rapid acetylators only establish their phenotypic status well on in the first year of life.

Patients in Buffalo of unspecified racial origin, with ulcerative colitis and Crohn's disease, were studied by Clarke *et al.* (1982). Twenty-one children aged 12 ± 3 years required daily SASP therapy for treatment and they were phenotyped by determining the percentage of acetylated sulphapyridine metabolites in plasma. Another group of 24 patients aged 9 to 62 years, who had quiescent inflammatory bowel disease not requiring therapy, were given sulphasalazine daily for at least one week to bring them into steady state for the purpose of this survey. Then they were phenotyped as described above. Age had no effect on apparent SP clearance (which is lower in slow than in rapid acetylators, and lower in disease remission than with active disease).

A hundred and fifty-six children aged from 8 months to 15 years, comprising of 73 white Europeans, 79 white Moroccans, two blacks and two Asiatics were studied by Paire *et al.* (1984) with an isoniazid elimination test (using an inactivation index where slow metabolism gives high values and rapid metabolism low values). The frequency distribution histogram shows a rather poor bimodal curve; but when compared with a histogram derived form 204 adults using the same methodology, the children's histogram indicated lower values. Within the children's data those aged below 6 years had lower values than those aged above 6 years, who resembled adults. The phenotype frequency seemed similar, in children above 6 years of age, to that seen in the adults studied under similar circumstances. On the basis of the unsatisfactorily bimodal frequency distribution histogram, it is claimed that children below 6 years of age had a significantly higher percentage of rapid acetylation.

Indian children were studied in Bombay by Desai *et al.* (1973) and Bajaj *et al.* (1988). In the first paper 97 individuals were studied but the definition of the antimode was suspect. In the second study 276 children were studied with an isoniazid test and 17% were rapid acetylators.

Swedish patients were studied by means of an isoniazid plasma half-life test by Paulsen & Nilsson (1985). They definitely showed an increase in the half-life values in older men. However, when it came to computing the phenotype frequency they continued to use the dividing antimodal value obtained from the histogram of individuals under 53 years of age. As a result they found a smaller percentage frequency of rapid acetylators in the older age groups. This finding might not have been obtained if they used a different dividing value for the age groups <53 years and >53 years, as is clearly suggested by their Fig. 16.1a.

Using the sulphadimidine phenotyping test II of Evans (1969), 253 Caucasian Hungarian patients aged 19 to 91 years were phenotyped by Gachalyi et al. (1984). Unfortunately they do not display their phenotyping data in their article. They arbitrarily divided their subjects into those below 60 years of age and those above 60 years of age. It seems that they applied the same phenotype separation criteria to both groups. They claim there were 50% slow acetylators in 128 subjects aged less than 60 years and 66.4% slow in 125 subjects aged over 60 years ($\chi_1^2 = 6.99$, $p < 0.01$).

The conclusion of Gachalyi et al. (1984) was challenged by Pontiroli et al. (1985), who used a very similar test to investigate 55 normal subjects aged 15 to 77 years and 92 patients with type II diabetes aged 31 to 80 years. No significant regression of acetylation rate upon age was found in either group, but it must be pointed out that it would have been better to have computed the regressions separately for the two phenotypes (similar to the method used in another context in the paper of Evans et al. 1961). Gachalyi et al. (1985), in their criticism of Pontiroli et al. (1985) fail to take up this point.

In the large study of French patients by Kergueris et al. (1986), this difficulty was avoided. They computed the regression of various pharmacokinetic parameters on age independently in the two phenotypes. Total body clearance, half-life and volume of distribution of isoniazid all decreased with age in slow acetylators but not in rapid acetylators.

The authors comment that the variation conferred by age is slight in comparison with that of genetic origin. It would not appear that the effect of age changes the phenotypic pattern. Similar conclusions were reached by Walubo et al. (1991), who also used isoniazid.

The acetylation of dapsone, as determined by the ratio of mono-acetyldapsone (MADDS) to dapsone (DDS) in plasma following a single dose of DDS in

337 white British subjects (193 female, 144 male), was studied by Philip et al. (1987a). In the elderly group (65 years and over) 51.3% of 191 individuals were found to be slow acetylators. This was not significantly different from the 60.3% of the 146 individuals aged below 30 years of age who were slow acetylators. It is fair to comment that the antimodal separation of phenotypes is very blurred, and also that the percentage of individuals with MADDS/DDS> 0.60 was 9.6% in the young group and 17.8% in the elderly group. This would be in keeping with some diminution of acetylating capacity with advanced age.

So the conclusion is that there is some diminution of acetylating capacity with age but that this is insufficient to interfere with the phenotyping procedure. The situation in unborn and young children is at present unclear.

Height and weight

The heights and weights of both healthy controls, and of diabetics were shown not to differ significantly between acetylator phenotypes by Evans et al. (1985).

THE METABOLIC BASIS OF THE POLYMORPHISM

It was suspected from the pioneering work of Hughes et al. (1954) that the metabolic activity controlled by the isoniazid inactivator alleles might be acetylation. This suspicion was strengthened by the fact that when other compounds such as p-amino-salicylate (PAS) and sulphonamides (which were also known to be acetylated), were administered together with isoniazid, higher plasma levels resulted than were obtained with isoniazid alone.

The approach of the present author and his colleagues was a dual one:

1 to investigate the metabolism of sulphamethazine, a drug known to be extensively acetylated and not then known to have any other fate;

2 to investigate the capacity of healthy liver biopsies from individuals of known phenotype to metabolize isoniazid and other drugs in vitro.

The results showed:

1 that sulphamethazine acetylation (as shown by the percentage acetylated in plasma and urine) was

bimodal and the phenotypes so found were identical with the phenotypes detected using isoniazid.

2 that the ability of liver homogenates to acetylate isoniazid and sulphamethazine *in vitro* was also polymorphic mirroring the previously determined phenotypes of the donors (Evans & White 1964) (see Fig. 16.5).

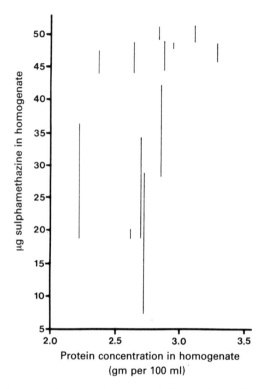

Fig. 16.5. Sulphamethazine metabolism by human liver homogenates. Fresh liver was supplied with acetyl CoA in addition to sulphamethazine. The top and bottom of each line represent the estimated weight of substrate shortly after the start of incubation at 37 °C and 2 hours afterwards. (From Evans & White 1964.)

Jenne (1963, 1965) also studied human liver and jejunal mucosal enzyme preparations from persons of known phenotype, which had been purified by ammonium sulphate precipitation followed by Sephadex G-100 and DEAE columns. The enzyme obtained from both inactivator phenotypes, which was competitively inhibited by PAS and hydralazine (the latter being 100 times as strong as the former), showed no difference in apparent Michaelis constant, and in other respects behaved identically in the two phenotypes. The specific activities for isoni-

azid acetylation of both liver and jejunal mucosal enzyme preparations correlated with the phenotypes of the donors as determined *in vivo*. The author concluded that it was probably different numbers of enzyme molecules of the same type that accounted for the difference between the phenotypes.

Peters *et al.* (1965) demonstrated a parallelism between the ratio of acetylated to parent drug excreted in the urine for isoniazid and SMZ in both phenotypes. They also noted that the acetylation of sulphanilamide was the same in both phenotypes *in vivo*, matching the results obtained using homogenates *in vitro* by Evans & White (1964).

After the above events, many drugs have been shown to have their acetylation controlled by the genetic polymorphism using the 'typed panel' approach. For many of these drugs different pharmacokinetic parameters (depending on acetylation) have been shown to be polymorphic.

Enzymic studies of the polymorphism took a new direction after the progress that has been described above, and will be discussed in the next section.

Further studies on the molecular nature of the enzyme polymorphism

One of the key dilemmas concerning human *N*-acetyl-transferase is based on the following facts. Isoniazid, sulphamethazine, hydralazine and other substrates are acetylated polymorphically by humans *in vivo*. On the other hand PAS (Fig. 16.6), PABA and sulphanilamide are monomorphically acetylated *in vivo* (Evans 1963; Peters *et al.* 1965) and so also are sulphamethoxazole (Bozkurt *et al.* 1990a) and sulpha-2-monomethoxine (Vree *et al.* 1992). Human red cells exhibit monomorphic acetylation of PAS and PABA *in vitro*, whereas they do not acetylate isoniazid or SMZ. Furthermore, these compounds do not inhibit the acetylation of PAS or PABA by red cells (Motulsky & Steinmann 1962). Human lymphocytes from both phenotypes can acetylate PABA. One difference was found between the phenotypes, namely that the lymphocyte enzyme from rapid acetylators was less stable than that from slow acetylators, suggesting that there might be a structural difference (McQueen & Weber 1980). *In vitro* PAS has the ability to inhibit isoniazid acetylation by liver enzyme preparations (but hydralazine is 100 times more powerful: Jenne 1965). Homogenates from frozen livers which polymorphically metabolized isoniazid sulphamethazine

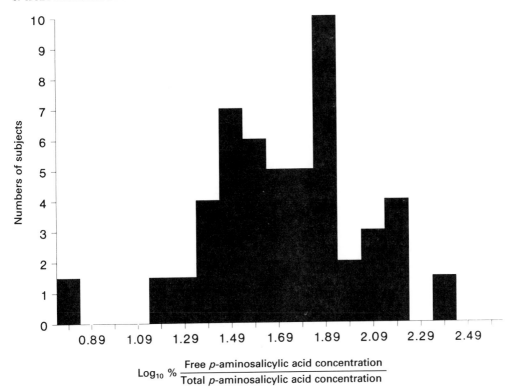

Fig. 16.6. The unimodal frequency distribution of a parameter of *p*-aminosalicylic acid metabolism in man. (From Evans 1963.)

and hydralazine failed to metabolize PABA and sulphanilamide (Evans & White 1964; Gunawardhana *et al.* 1991). So two sets of questions were posed as a result of these data.

(a) With regard to drugs which were monomorphically acetylated:

1 was there a separate system of enzymes which dealt with them (possibly in addition to some contribution from the polymorphic system); or
2 did these substrates have the same affinities to the polymorphic enzymes in the two phenotypes?

(b) With regard to the drugs that were polymorphically acetylated:

1 were there enzymes of different structures controlled by the two alleles responsible for the polymorphism;

   or

2 were there different numbers of enzyme molecules of the same structure in the two phenotypes?

Even these questions could not be as clear cut as posed above because, for example, for sulphamethoxypyridazine there was only a slight influence of the acetylator polymorphism on its metabolism, as shown by an increased percentage acetylation in the urine in rapid, as compared with slow, acetylators (White & Evans, 1968).

Curiously, very little further work was published for a long time on human liver acetylating enzymes. Most investigative efforts were devoted to studying polymorphic acetylating systems in animals. However, Weber *et al.* (1978) studied SMZ and PAB acetylation by human liver preparations and confirmed for the former a ×3.7 difference between the phenotypes but no difference for the latter. For various carcinogenic amines the ratio varied from 5.2 for α-naphthylamine to 13 for 2-aminofluorene.

The system which closely resembles the human is the rabbit polymorphic acetylation system first described by Frymoyer & Jacox (1963a,b). Most of the subsequent work on the rabbit acetylation polymorphism has been carried out by Dr Wendell W. Weber and his group and their experience is condensed in his monograph (Weber 1987).

MOLECULAR BIOLOGY

Very swift progress has taken place recently in our understanding of the basic mechanisms of the human acetylation polymorphism. Grant *et al.* (1990) investigated liver biopsy material from 26 surgical patients who had been phenotyped using a caffeine test. Liver specimens were also available from 24 organ donors who were typed with an *in vitro* sulphamethazine test. Slow acetylation was found to be associated with a decrease in the quantity of immunodetectable N-acetyltransferase protein in liver cytosol using a polyclonal rabbit antiserum raised against a highly active enzyme preparation derived from human liver.

A cDNA for the polymorphic N-acetyltransferase was obtained from rabbits. This DNA, after radiolabelling, was used by Blum *et al.* (1990) as a probe to identify complementary sequences in fragments obtained from a human genomic library prepared from an obligate heterozygote as identified by pedigree status. Restriction mapping with a series of restriction endonucleases revealed that the 18 positive clones fell into three non-overlapping clusters. These were termed *NAT1, NAT2* and *NATP* and were intronless sequences. The clones *NAT1* and *NAT2* each contained a single open reading frame of 870 base pairs. There was 87% homology between *NAT1* and *NAT2* and this homology extended upstream from the initiation codon and downstream from the stop codon.

NAT1 and *NAT2* were chromosomally mapped by Southern blot analysis of a panel of human rodent somatic cell hybrid DNAs. The characteristic DNA fragments for both *NAT1* and *NAT2* segregated concordantly indicating that they were on the same chromosome and were unambiguously associated with the presence of chromosome 8. More detailed examinations resulted in both genes being assigned to 8pter–qll.

The fragments of DNA containing the individual genes were transferred into COS-1 cells. After 50 to 70 hours the cytosol of these cells exhibited N-acetyltransferase activity as tested with sulphamethazine. The NAT so manufactured had electrophoretic and immunoreactive features identical to those obtained from liver cytosol. The apparent molecular masses were 33 and 31 kDa for *NAT1* and *NAT2*, respectively.

The recombinant enzyme *NAT1* had marked kinetic selectivity (both high affinity and high maximal velocity) for the monomorphic substrates PAS and PABA, while recombinant *NAT2* was equally specific for the polymorphic substrates SMZ and procaine amide (Grant *et al.* 1991). This exactly parallels findings on human liver cytosol.

The third gene, *NATP*, has accumulated a large number of mutations presumably leading to loss of function and can therefore be considered a pseudogene.

Mutant alleles at the *NAT2* gene locus were identified by restriction fragment length polymorphism (RFLP) analysis on genomic DNA of 26 *in vivo* phenotyped healthy individuals and additional 22 DNAs from organ donors of known *NAT2* activity. The most informative restriction endonuclease was *Kpn*I. The 'wild type' (wt) allele responsible for rapid acetylation gave bands of 15 and 5 kilobases (kb). The mutant allele Ml had lost the *Kpn*I site giving a single 20 kb fragment whereas mutant M2 gave bands of 15 and 4.4 kb. Two additional mutants did not reveal *Kpn*I RFLPs; M3 revealed a *Bam*HI RFLP and M4 had not been analysed (Blum *et al.* 1990b; and see Table 16.7).

Very similar researches were carried out by Ohsako & Deguchi (1990). They found that a cDNA fragment termed D24 conferred in Chinese hamster ovary cells the ability to acetylate PABA but not SMZ. This corresponded to *NAT1* of the Swiss workers. Fragments 07 and D14 conferred the ability to acetylate SMZ but not PABA. Deguchi *et al.* (1990) carried this work forward and, using restriction fragment length polymorphisms, delineated three alleles of the polymorphic acetyltransferase, and correlated them with the INH-determined acetylator phenotypes.

Hickman & Sim (1991) phenotyped 22 Caucasians with sulphamethazine. Then the genomic DNA from their white cells was amplified with the polymerase chain reaction using specific oligonucleotide primers. The DNA was then subjected to the action of restriction endonucleases. Three enzymes sufficed to differentiate between the four alleles at the polymorphic N-acetyltransferase locus as shown in Table 16.7.

The monomorphic N-acetyltransferase was characterized by the absence of both the *Kpn*I and the *Bam*HI restriction sites.

The data from all three groups of researchers are condensed in Table 16.8.

Table 16.7. *Restriction fragment length polymorphism at the NAT2 N-acetyltransferase locus*

Allele designation	Presence of restriction site and fragment sizes (bp)			
Hickman & Sim 1991	Blum *et al.* 1991	*Kpn*I	*Taq*I	*Bam*HI
F1	*wt*	Present	Present	Present
		520 and 480	230 and 170	850 and 150
S1	*M1*	Absent	Present	Present
		1000	230 and 170	850 and 150
S2	*M2*	Present	Absent	Present
		520 and 480	400	850 and 150
S3	*M3*	Present	Present	Absent
		520 and 480	230 and 170	1000

wt, Wild type.
Constructed from: data in Fig. 3 of Hickman & Sim 1991. The fragments were obtained by digestion of a 1000 bp portion of the gene amplified by the polymerase chain reaction.

Table 16.8. *Alleles for polymorphic N-acetyltransferase*

Allele (nomenclature of Blum *et al.* 1991)		Nucleotide change[a]	Amino acid change	Frequency (%)		
				Caucasian		Japanese
				Hickman & Sim (1991) based on 62 alleles	Blum *et al.* (1991) based on 88 alleles	Deguchi *et al.* (1990)[b] based on 172 alleles
wt	(1)	–	–	25.8	26.1	68.6
M1	(2)	341 T → C	114 Ile → Thr	45.2	34.1	NIL
		481 C → T	NIL			
M2	(3)	282 C → T	NIL	27.4	36.4	24.4
		590 G → A	197Arg → Gln			
M3	(4)	857 G → A	286 Gly → Glu	1.6	3.4	7.0

[a]Nucleotide numbering refers to the coding exon.
[b]Computed from Fig. 2(b) of Deguchi *et al.* (1990).
(1) F1 of Hickman & Sim (1991), allele 1 of Deguchi *et al.* (1990) and 07 of Ohsako & Deguchi (1990).
(2) S1 of Hickman & Sim (1991), absent in Japanese.
(3) S2 of Hickman & Sim (1991), allele 3 of Deguchi *et al.* (1990).
(4) S3 of Hickman & Sim (1991), allele 2 of Deguchi *et al.* (1990) and D14 of Ohsako & Deguchi (1990).

Similar researches were carried out by Vatsis *et al.* (1991). Genomic DNA was isolated from four liver samples whose phenotypes had been determined *in vitro* and from three blood leucocyte samples whose phenotypes had been determined *in vivo*. The *NAT2* gene was amplified by the polymerase chain reaction and subjected to direct sequencing.

Four of the nucleotide changes shown in Table 16.8 were discovered, but the 857 G → A change was not observed. A nucleotide change 803 A → G, causing an amino acid change 268 Lys → Arg was observed, which was not reported in the studies shown in Table 16.8.

Allele r_2 of Vatsis *et al.* (1991) was the same as *M2* of Blum *et al.* (1991), *S2* of Hickman & Sim (1991) and allele 3 of Deguchi *et al.* (1990). Allele r_3 of Vatsis *et al.* (1991) was similar to *M1* of Blum *et al.* (1992) and *S1* of Hickman & Sim (1991) and eliminated a *Kpn*I site, but had in addition the nucleotide change at position 803.

Various combinations of alleles were observed, e.g. $r_2 r_3$. Disparities were found between genotyping and phenotyping results, which were ascribed to inaccuracies in the latter procedure.

By studying a population of 26 Caucasian rheumatoid arthritis patients and 22 healthy Caucasian subjects, Hickman *et al.* (1992) showed that the r_3 gene of Vatsis *et al.* (1991), containing the 341 T → C, 481 C → T and 803 A → G mutations, accounted for the majority of the S1 category in Table 16.8. Alleles containing only the first two or the last two of these mutations were much less frequent.

The most striking fact is the absence of the S1(M1) mutant in Japanese. This accounts for the differences which have been observed over the years, namely (1) the high proportion of rapid acetylators in the Japanese population as compared with Caucasians, (2) the fact that Sunahara *et al.* (1963a, b) and others subsequently (e.g. Deguchi *et al.* 1990) were able clearly to discern heterozygotes, which has only been proved possible only in Caucasians using caffeine.

Probably there are other rare mutants in addition to those shown in Table 16.8 which need to be defined. Clues to the existence of further mutants are:

1 Allele *M4* with a calculated frequency of 1% referred to by Blum *et al.* (1990b).
2 Deguchi *et al.* (1990) found two individuals with intermediate phenotype who appeared to be homozygous for their 'gene 1' (*syn F1, wt*: see Table 16.7).
3 One individual in the series of Hickman & Sim (1991) had the slow acetylator phenotype but appeared to have the *S1 F1* genotype (see Table 16.7).

The way in which the structural changes in the mutant alleles are related to the performance of the eventual gene product has been investigated. The amount of mRNA formed appeared to be much the same for all alleles (Ohsako & Deguchi 1990; Blum *et al.* 1991). The genes were expressed in monkey kidney COS-1 cells. With *M1* little protein seemed to be made, indicating a translation defect, whereas with *M2* the enzyme formed had a greatly diminished half-life (6 hours as compared with 22), indicating impaired stability. The K_m values for both sulphadimidine and acetyl CoA were very similar for *wt, M1* and *M2* (Blum *et al.* 1991).

The construction of chimeric alleles by Blum *et al.* (1991) showed that both nucleotide substitutions of *M1* were required to cause the diminished production of protein presumably by defective translation. However, in the *M2* allele the amino acid change Arg 197 → Gln alone was responsible for the production of a less stable protein than the 'wild type'. These mechanisms will require further study.

The allele-specific amplification by means of PCR as described by Blum *et al.* (1991) and the restriction endonuclease fragment patterns following PCR described by Hickman & Sim (1991) both offer the possibility of genotyping large numbers of people. Similarly, a non-radioactive biotinylated allele-specific probe has been developed by Hajra *et al.* (1992), which detects the 857 G → A point mutation in PCR-amplified DNA by means of a directly read colour change. In the future for individuals to be tested it will be necessary neither to swallow chemical substances nor to provide timed samples of blood and urine. The new techniques will be particularly useful for pharmaco-epidemiological surveys, for example (1) to detect individuals prone to adverse reactions, (2) to re-examine the associations between acetylator status and various cancers and (3) to ascertain the acetylator status of individuals in whom illness may interfere with the results of *in vivo* phenotyping tests.

ASSOCIATIONS OF CLINICAL RESPONSES TO DRUGS WITH ACETYLATOR PHENOTYPES

The clinical phenomena of greatest interest which have been associated with acetylator phenotypes are (1) adverse reactions and (2) therapeutic responses.

The principal items of information are summarized in Table 16.9. For some drugs there are special considerations which will be discussed in separate sections below.

Isoniazid

Soon after the discovery of the human polymorphism for the 'inactivation' of isoniazid (INH), a great deal of effort was expended in trying to determine whether the rapid acetylator fared less well than the slow as regards the response of the tuberculosis to treatment with INH.

The idea was very thoroughly tested by Harris (1961), who studied 744 patients with pulmonary

Table 16.9. *Clinical responses and adverse reactions to drugs related to the acetylation polymorphism*

Drug	Acetylator phenotype	Clinical phenomenon observed in the phenotype noted	Reference
Isoniazid	Slow	More prone to develop peripheral neuropathy on conventional doses	Hughes et al. 1954 Devadatta et al. 1960
	Slow	More prone to phenytoin adverse effects when the patient is being simultaneously treated with isoniazid	Kutt 1971
	Slow	More prone to elevation of plasma bilirubin concentration and transaminases when the patient is being treated with isoniazid and rifampicin in non-Oriental individuals	see appropriate section in text (page 235)
	Rapid	In Japanese and Chinese subjects hepatotoxic effects are more common	Menon et al. 1968
	Rapid	Less favourable results of treating open pulmonary tuberculosis with a once-weekly isoniazid dosage regimen	Mitchison 1971
Hydralazine	Slow	Develop antinuclear antibodies and systemic lupus erythematosus-like syndrome	Perry et al. 1970 Strandberg et al. 1976 Batchelor et al. 1980 Zacest & Koch-Weser 1972 Pasanen et al. 1973 Shepherd et al. 1981 Ramsay et al. 1984
	Rapid	Require higher doses to control hypertension	
SASP	Slow	Slightly better response of rheumatoid arthritis	Amos et al. 1986 – disputed by Pullar & Capell 1986
	Slow	Increased incidence of various adverse reactions principally hematological and gastrointestinal	Schröder & Evans 1972b Das et al. 1973 Sharp et al. 1981 Pullar et al. 1985 Pullar & Capell 1986 Rahav et al. 1990
DDS	Rapid	Methaemoglobin concentrations higher	Azad Khan et al. 1983
	Slow	More haematological adverse effects	Ellard et al. 1974a
	Rapid	Higher doses needed to control dermatitis herpetiformis	Forstrom et al. 1974 – disputed by Ellard et al. 1974a
Procainamide	Slow	More prone to the development (or earlier appearance) of systemic lupus erythematosus-like syndrome	Henningsen et al. 1975 Bernstein 1979 Woosley et al. 1978 – disputed by Davies et al. (1975), Sonnhag et al. 1979 and Ylitalo et al. 1983
	Rapid	More ventricular premature beats in cardiac patients treated with standard doses	Schroder et al. 1979
Sulphonamides	Slow	Hypersensitivity reactions	Shear et al. 1986
Amonafide	Rapid	Leucopenia	Rieder et al. 1991 Ratain et al. 1991

tuberculosis on standardized treatment schedules. There was a tendency for cavity closure and sputum conversion (i.e. disappearance of tubercle bacilli) to occur earlier in slow acetylators, but the eventual outcome after 6 months of treatment was the same in both phenotypes.

Similarly, Gow & Evans (1964) found that neither acetylator phenotype was associated with reversion (i.e. reappearance of tubercle bacilli in the urine) following a course of therapy for genito-urinary tuberculosis.

Thus, as anticipated by McDermott (1960), the acetylator polymorphism does not seem to influence the outcome of tuberculosis treated by standard schedules which include isoniazid.

This finding has been confirmed by many workers in underdeveloped countries. The various trials in which the British Medical Research Council has collaborated in India, Africa, Singapore and Hong Kong may be cited as outstanding examples.

The acetylator polymorphism, however, turned out to be of great importance when intermittent dosage regimens were employed (*British Medical Journal* 1967). Previously untreated patients with INH-sensitive organisms on admission were studied at the Tuberculosis Chemotherapy Centre, Madras. Treatment was given for one year. Patients with bacteriologically quiescent disease at the end of the year were said to have a favourable response if they had negative cultures at 10, 11 and 12 months, or only one positive culture out of about nine set up during these months. Patients with an unfavourable response may have remained positive during treatment or had a relapse, or may have deteriorated and had their treatment changed; a few died from their tuberculosis.

When the medications (including isoniazid) were given twice weekly the acetylator phenotype did not influence the treatment. In all the once-weekly regimens the rapid acetylators responded much less well than the slow acetylators (Tuberculosis Chemotherapy Centre 1970).

The acetylator phenotype was shown by Donald *et al.* (1992) to influence isoniazid concentrations in the cerebrospinal fluids of 96 children with tuberculous meningitis. Rapid acetylators had lower levels than slow acetylators, but this did not prevent therapeutically effective concentrations being achieved with conventional treatment schedules.

There is no association between the development of isoniazid-resistant tubercle bacilli and either acetylator phenotype (Biehl 1957; Harris 1961).

A clinically apparent systemic lupus erythematosus-like syndrome uncommonly occurs in the large numbers of people treated with isoniazid for tuberculosis (Alarcon-Segovia 1969). It has been observed that tuberculous patients treated with isoniazid exhibited positive anti-nuclear factor (ANF) tests more commonly than controls (Cannat & Seligman 1966). ANF can be considered a forerunner of the drug-induced SLE syndrome (Alarcon-Segovia 1969).

Both the development of ANF during treatment, and acetylator phenotypes were determined by Evans *et al.* (1972) in 95 tuberculous patients. The incidence of ANF was approximately 17% which was considerably higher than the incidence commonly found in random population surveys. For example, Wren *et al.* (1967) found only one man with a positive ANF serum amongst 67 fathers of Down's syndrome children and none amongst 66 fathers of normal children. These men had a similar mean age to the tuberculosis patients, lived in the same area and were tested in the same laboratory by the same technique. This result was in keeping with those of Cannat & Seligman (1966) and Alarcon-Segovia (1969).

There was no association of either acetylator phenotype with ANF development. It was noted, however, that the patients who developed ANF were significantly older than those who did not do so.

Patients with intracerebral tuberculomata are prone to epilepsy, and therefore require treatment both for the tuberculosis and to prevent fits. Sometimes the coincidence of other types of tuberculosis (e.g. pulmonary) with fits also requires combined treatment. Slow acetylators of INH were shown by Kutt (1971) to be more prone to diphenylhydantoin (DPH) toxicity than rapid acetylators when they were receiving combined treatment (see Chapter 10, p. 120).

An apparently similar interaction has been reported between carbamazepine and isoniazid, leading to carbamazepine intoxication (Valsalan & Cooper 1982), but this has not been associated with the slow acetylator phenotype. Theophylline clearance is also reduced by isoniazid pretreatment but not significantly more so in six slow acetylators as compared with seven rapid acetylators in the survey of Samigun *et al.* (1990).

The combination of rifampicin and isoniazid was

shown to reduce vitamin D metabolite 1,25-$(OH)_2D$ serum concentrations more in fast than slow acetylators after 4 weeks of treatment (Brodie *et al.* 1982).

The acetylator phenotype and hepatotoxicity due to isoniazid

This subject, which is of clinical importance, has become complicated because the information is available in several categories which have generated confounding factors.

Isoniazid has been given alone as a chemo-prophylactic measure to persons at risk of contracting tuberculosis who have been found to have a positive Mantoux test. This chemo-prophylaxis has been given to various ethnic groups.

Isoniazid is given as one constituent of a number of drugs (commonly three) for active tuberculosis. In the first years of the usage of isoniazid the drug PAS was a frequent component of combined chemotherapy and PAS was already known to be hepatotoxic. Later, chemotherapeutic regimens commonly had both isoniazid and rifampicin present in them.

Of course, these various chemotherapeutic regimens have been deployed in different ethnic groups and in environmental circumstances which varied with regard to many factors but especially with regard to nutrition.

Then again, it depends what one means by 'hepatotoxicity'. In some studies it has been taken to mean merely elevation of transaminases on routine biochemical screening, whilst in others it is taken to mean a clinical illness (which has occasionally even proved to be fatal).

Isoniazid given alone

The six patients on whom isoniazid was originally studied (at a dosage level of 3 mg/kg per day, given for a period of 4–16 weeks) had their hepatic function estimated every 2 weeks by bromsulphophthalein retention, bilirubin concentration, thymol turbidity and alkaline phosphatase activity. No abnormality was found (Elmendorf *et al.* 1952).

A report of the American Trudeau Society's Committee on Therapy (1953) analysed the experience of the toxicity of isoniazid then available (from about 2 years of usage). The statement with regard to the liver is brief: 'Results of liver function tests were fairly frequently abnormal but became normal when the drug was discontinued. A few cases of clinical jaundice were reported.'

The subject received only scant attention for the next few years and then interest was reawakened in the late 1960s. The review of Snider & Caras (1992) reveals that hepatotoxicity due to isoniazid alone is still occurring, but they do not comment on the role of acetylator phenotypes.

Maddrey & Boitnott (1973) described the clinical features of hepatitis occurring in people given isoniazid alone as a prophylactic because of a positive tuberculin skin test. The picture resembled viral hepatitis, but recurred in a much more florid (and sometimes fatal) form on rechallenge with isoniazid following recovery from the initial episode. They considered that the evidence strongly indicated that the lesion was a hypersensitivity reaction. Curiously, they did not consider what part the acetylator phenotype might play in the predisposition to this illness.

A large patient population (i.e. 13 838 patients who were admitted to the USPHS surveillance programme during the period July 1971–November 1972, and who received 300 mg of isoniazid daily) was examined in detail by Black *et al.* (1975). The records of 224 patients suspected of having 'isoniazid hepatitis' were analysed and categorized into five groups:

1 Probable isoniazid-related hepatic injury: 87 cases
2 Possible isoniazid-related hepatic injury: 76 cases
3 Hepatobiliary disease unrelated to isoniazid administration: 18 cases
4 No apparent hepatic disease: 20 cases
5 Patients with insufficient data: 23 cases

A patient was deemed to fall into the 'probable' group when there was a substantial elevation of transaminases and bilirubin without any other identifiable cause of hepatocellular injury and when recovery followed the withdrawal of the drug.

Unfortunately 27 patients with isoniazid hepatitis from other sources were added to the 87 probable patients mentioned above, and because the structure of the populations from which they were derived was not known it is not possible to compute the incidence in each ethnic group. The analysis of Brown (1976) disregards this fact and is consequently erroneous.

It was, however, known that the drop-out rate was substantially lower amongst the Oriental than amongst the other ethnic groups in the USPHS programme. Furthermore, there were no deaths in the Oriental group whereas nine of the 13 deaths that did occur were in black females. In Mitchell et al. (1976, p. 186), there is a statement ascribed to Dr Phyllis Edwards that Orientals were more susceptible than other racial groups to liver injury from isoniazid in this large survey.

Black et al. (1975) considered that the liver injury was very similar to that seen in viral hepatitis, and also point out that the accepted hallmarks of allergy, such as skin rash and peripheral eosinophilia, were uncommon and that a febrile onset of the disease was absent in most patients. In addition, (1) the variable and prolonged exposure before liver injury occurred was unlike the fairly brief period associated with an allergic mechanism, and (2) the mild liver injury which occurs in 12 to 20% of consumers of isoniazid shows that the phenomenon is not restricted to rare idiosyncratic or allergic subjects. An alternative suggestion was put forward, namely that the liver injury was due to the toxic metabolite acetylhydrazine. The implication was made that this toxic metabolite might be more abundant in rapid acetylators.

Mitchell et al. (1975a) were able to investigate, by means of an SMZ test, the acetylator phenotypes of 21 non-Oriental persons who had recovered from 'probable' hepatitis occurring during a large trial using isoniazid (alone) as preventative therapy. Eighteen of these individuals were rapid acetylators and three were slow acetylators. The authors emphasized that this was consistent with the finding that in large isoniazid-alone prophylactic trials 'isoniazid hepatitis occurred more commonly in Oriental populations which are known to have a much higher frequency of rapid acetylators than American white and black populations.'

Inmates at a psychiatric institution who were found to be tuberculin positive after being in contact with tuberculosis patients were investigated by Mitchell et al. (1975b) during a supervised prophylactic isoniazid regimen. The concentration of isoniazid in the serum 6 hours after the ingestion of 300 mg isoniazid in 147 patients indicated, according to the authors, no direct relationship between the rapid acetylator phenotype and susceptibility to subclinical liver injury (as shown by SGOT levels). It must be pointed out, however, that the authors' phenotyping procedure was not satisfactory, Nevertheless, the observation led to the suggestion that

the moderate increase in exposure to acetylhydrazine experienced by rapid acetylators is a significant risk factor only for those susceptible persons who will progress to severe hepatitis. In other words, the authors were suggesting that there may be some important factor other than acetylator phenotype which determines whether an individual is prone to isoniazid hepatitis.

A prospective survey of 113 patients, who took isoniazid (INH) alone for at least 2 months and whose acetylator phenotypes were known at the outset, was conducted by Dickinson et al. (1981). Twelve started with abnormal liver function tests and 12 were alcoholic. Of the remaining 89, 15 met the criteria for significant liver test abnormality developing during treatment. The commonest major liver test abnormality was a raised SGOT.

Of the 101 subjects starting INH with normal liver function tests, 53 were slow, 47 were rapid acetylators and one was not phenotyped. Fifty-four were under 35 years of age. Sixty-eight were black, 31 white and two Oriental. Excluding 12 alcoholics, it was clear that age and slow acetylator phenotype were two factors influencing the result, as shown in Table 16.10.

Direct proof in healthy volunteers that there was more hydrazine present in the plasma of four slow acetylators than in four rapid acetylators after 2 weeks' ingestion of 300 mg isoniazid daily was provided by Blair et al. (1985). The plasma hydrazine concentrations of the rapid acetylators were not significantly higher after 2 weeks' therapy than they were following the first dose, in contradistinction to the situation in the slow phenotype.

Similarly, Peretti et al. (1987a) showed that following a single 300 mg dose of isoniazid in healthy volunteers there was a significantly higher urinary excretion of hydrazine and acetylhydrazine in slow acetylators compared with rapid acetylators.

Hydrazine is known to be a carcinogen, a mutagen and toxic to the central nervous system and the liver. Whether the plasma concentrations of hydrazine achieved after isoniazid ingestion are sufficient to produce toxicological sequelae is at present unclear (Blair et al. 1985).

The present evidence therefore indicates that acetylhydrazine and hydrazine are likely candidates as the agents causing hepatotoxicity following isoniazid treatment. As indicated above, disease states, concomitantly administered drugs and ethnic factors as well as acetylator phenotype need to be taken

Table 16.10. *Predicted probability of developing liver test abnormalities based on logistic regression equation*[a]

Age (years)	Acetylation phenotype	Number of patients with normal baseline laboratory studies[b]	Number developed significant liver dysfunction (%)[c]	Probability of developing significant liver dysfunction
<35	Rapid	24	1 (4.2%)	3.7%
<35	Slow	24	3 (12.5%)	13.0%
≥35	Rapid	16	2 (12.5%)	13.2%
≥35	Slow	24	9 (37.5%)	37.0%

[a]$\text{Log}_e\ (\theta)/(1 - \theta) = -1.90434 + 1.37376X_1 - 1.35344X_2$, where θ is the probability of developing significant liver damage, $X_1 = 1$ if age >35, and 0 if age <35; $\chi_2 = 1$ if rapid acetylation phenotype and 0 if slow acetylation phenotype.
[b]Excluding 12 subjects who drank an excess of alcohol.
[c]$\chi^2 = 10.5$; D.F. = 3; $p = 0.015$.   *From:* Dickinson *et al.* (1981).

into account to explain the final clinical consequences of treatment regimens.

Regimens containing isoniazid plus other drugs but no rifampicin

A comprehensive review of the hepatic toxicity of various antituberculous regimens was published by Girling (1978).

With regard to prophylactic treatment with isoniazid alone, it was concluded that there was a definite risk of hepatitis, particularly in individuals over 35 years old.

The risk of hepatitis during standard chemotherapy of active tuberculosis could be assessed with a fair degree of accuracy from the controlled clinical trials conducted in collaboration with local treatment services by the British Medical Research Council. Eleven cases of hepatitis occurred amongst 1666 patients treated in Britain with various combinations of isoniazid with other drugs in five trials. (It is of interest that five cases occurred in 112 patients treated with rifampicin as one of the components of one regime.)

The results of the other trials are summarized in Table 16.11. There is a suggestion in this table that Oriental populations may be more susceptible than European and African populations to developing hepatitis on isoniazid, which is confirmed when the data are condensed (Table 16.12).

A retrospective analysis of the results of treating 1757 slow acetylators and 1238 rapid acetylators with eight different regimens (one of which contained rifampicin) in Madras was published by Gurumurthy *et al.* (1984). Clinically evident jaundice occurred in 34 slow acetylators (11.9%) and

15 rapid acetylators (1.2%) – a non-significant difference. The elevation of transaminases also showed a similar incidence in the two phenotypes.

Regimens containing both isoniazid and rifampicin

Smith *et al.* (1972) reported a planned survey of 181 patients admitted to hospital in Glasgow with tuberculosis. One hundred and twenty-three (67.9%) were slow (S) and 58 (32.1%) rapid acetylators (R). Of these patients 126 (90S and 36R) were treated with rifampicin and isoniazid. Twenty-nine (20S 9R) showed a rise of transaminases only, whereas 14 (13S 1R) showed a rise of both transaminases plus bilirubin. The sole rapid acetylator who had elevated serum bilirubin levels was the only patient whose liver function disturbance occurred during a drug hypersensitivity reaction which gave rise to rigors, pyrexia, circulatory collapse and oliguria.

This study indicated clearly that there was no difference in the frequency of raised transaminases alone between the phenotypes, but that the occurrence of raised bilirubin levels in addition was overwhelmingly associated with the slow acetylator phenotype.

A very similar survey to that of Smith *et al.* (1972) was carried out in a North Indian population by Husain *et al.* (1973). These workers state 'There was no toxicity attributable to isoniazid' and 'the present study failed to provide any evidence of the influence of rate of inactivation of isoniazid on therapeutic efficacy and toxicity of treatment given in the form of triple therapy including isoniazid.' It must be pointed out that these authors did not perform routine serial liver function tests on their patients.

Table 16.11. *Trials of various antituberculosis regimens, including isoniazid, conducted in collaboration with the British Medical Research Council*

Location	Number of trials	Number of patients treated	Number of patients with hepatitis	%
Britain	5	1666	11	0.66
(including	1	112	5	4.46) Rifampicin
Madras	5	1090	16	1.47
East Africa	5	2054	12	0.58
Hong Kong	1	250	9	3.60
Singapore	1	359	10	2.79

Based on data from: Girling 1978.

Table 16.12. *Condensed data from Table 16.11*

	Did not develop hepatitis	Did develop hepatitis	Total
European and African	4664	34 (0.44%)	4698
Oriental	590	19 (3.12%)	609
Total	5254	53	5307

(Omitting the 112 patients who received rifampicin with isoniazid and of whom 5 developed hepatitis in one trial in Britain.)
$\chi_1^2 = 59.7$ (with Yates correction); $p < 0.001$.

Girling (1978) reviewed the occurrence of hepatitis on regimens including both rifampicin and isoniazid. He pointed out that apparent differences in incidence occurred amongst some relatively small studies, but when pooling four surveys from the literature the incidence of hepatitis was 21 out of 596 patients (3.52%). As a result of an extensive literature review Steele *et al.* (1991) conclude that regimes containing isoniazid plus rifampicin are significantly more hepatotoxic than with isoniazid alone or with regimes combining rifampicin with drugs other than isoniazid.

Consecutive tuberculous patients receiving isoniazid and rifampicin were studied in Finland by Gronhagen-Riska *et al.* (1978). These authors were particularly interested in comparing small, usually spontaneously receding increases in transaminases and large increases which were often combined with serious symptoms and demands for change in therapy. The aim was to determine which factors if any differentiated a seemingly harmless hepatic reaction from a potentially dangerous one. The acetylator phenotypes are shown in Table 16.13, where it is clear that slow acetylators are more prone to the more severe reactions whereas neither phenotype is more prone to mild reactions.

A prospective study of 95 German patients with active tuberculosis was carried out by Musch *et al.* (1982). The patients were treated with isoniazid, rifampicin and ethambutol. The transaminases were elevated in 26 out of 56 slow acetylators, but only in four of 30 rapid acetylators. The 12 patients with more severe hepatotoxicity, as shown by elevated serum transaminase activities, were all slow acetylators.

It has been proposed by Mitchell *et al.* (1975b) that rapid acetylators were more at risk of developing isoniazid hepatitis because they form more acetylisoniazid, which in turn gives rise to acetylhydrazine which is metabolized in a P450 dependent reaction to form the toxic metabolite.

Eichelbaum *et al.* (1982), studying patients on triple therapy for tuberculosis, point out that although rapid acetylators form more acetylhydrazine (40% of the dose) than slow acetylators (25% of the dose) they also convert more of it (70%) to diacetylhydrazine compared with 27% in slow acetylators. Renal excretion of acetylhydrazine and its hydrazones accounted for 2.3% of the isoniazid dose in rapid acetylators and 3.5% in slow acetylators among their patients.

In slow acetylators, 68% of acetylhydrazines (corresponding to 17.5% of the isoniazid dose) was oxidatively metabolized, whereas in rapid acetylators the corresponding percentages were 30 and 12%, respectively. Hence these authors propose

Table 16.13. *Isoniazid acetylator phenotype distribution among patients developing increases in transaminase during therapy with isoniazid (INH) and rifampicin*

Liver function	Slow INH acetylators		Rapid INH acetylators		Slow and rapid acetylators	
	Number	%	Number	%	Number	%
A. SGOT and/or SGPT 45–149 μ/l	38	51	37	49	75	100
B. SGOT and/or SGPT >150 μ/l	33	73	12	27	45	100
C. Normal	148	57	113	43	261	100

For comparison of B with C, $p < 0.05$; for A compared with C, difference not significant.
From: Gronhagen-Riska *et al.* (1978).

that the higher incidence of hepatotoxicity in slow acetylators under the conditions of their study was due to the formation of larger amounts of toxic metabolite (see Fig. 16.7). An already complex situation was further complicated by the report of Peretti *et al.* (1987b) that the excretion of $^{15}N_2$-acetylhydrazine in humans was inhibited by the presence of isoniazid

in the plasma and this occurred in both acetylator phenotypes.

Beever *et al.* (1982) investigated four slow and four rapid healthy acetylators who took isoniazid and rifampicin for 15 days on an experimental basis. Both total and free plasma hydrazide levels were higher in slow than in rapid acetylators.

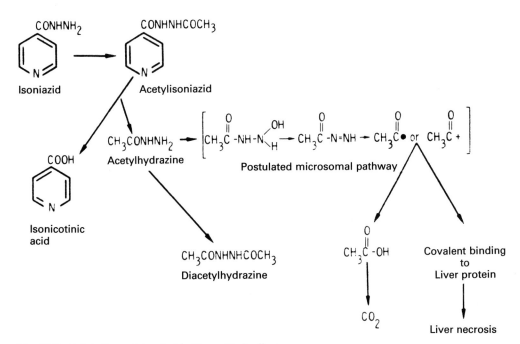

Fig. 16.7. Metabolism of isoniazid. (From Timbrell *et al.* 1985.)

Seventy-three tuberculous Spanish children treated with isoniazid and rifampicin were studied by Martinez-Roig *et al.* (1986). The distribution of the acetylator phenotype in the 27 patients with biochemical (22) or clinical (5) signs of hepatoxicity showed the same percentage (11% of rapid acetylators) as that found in the total population studied. Furthermore, there were no differences between the two acetylator phenotypes in the time at which hepatotoxicity occurred. However, it does need to be pointed out that the five patients with both clinical and biochemical signs of liver damage were all slow acetylators.

A review of the results of treating 1686 tuberculous South Indian patients in various trials was presented by Parthasarathy *et al.* (1986). Hepatitis, nearly always with jaundice, was higher in incidence in patients treated with daily regimens of isoniazid and rifampicin, and occurred more often in slow (11% of 317) than in rapid (1% of 244) acetylators.

However, the liver enzymes AST and ALT plus total bilirubin levels were closely similar over 7 months' therapy in 177 slow and 135 rapid acetylator children treated by Swamy *et al.* (1987) with regimes containing both rifampicin and isoniazid. Likewise, in 178 slow and 126 rapid acetylator children treated with regimes which contained isoniazid but no rifampicin, there were no differences in the liver function test results between the phenotypes. The liver enzymes SGOT and SGPT were closely similar over 12 months of therapy with isoniazid and rifampicin in 46 slow and 20 rapid acetylator children observed by Seth & Beotra (1989). Maybe the toxicity of these regimens is different in children from that in adults.

An investigation of the metabolites of isoniazid with and without concomitant rifampicin was conducted in normal volunteers by Raghupati Sarma *et al.* (1986). They investigated the ratio (isonicotinic acid + isonicotinoyl glycine)/acetylisoniazid in the urine. The idea behind this was that the compounds in the numerator are formed from isoniazid by isoniazid hydrolase and from acetylisoniazid by acetylisoniazid hydrolase. The action of the hydrolase was considered to be the release of hydrazide. The basal value after isoniazid alone was greater in slow acetylators. An increase in the ratio was seen in both phenotypes after rifampicin had been given to the subjects, but the rise in the ratio was much greater for slow acetylators taking isoniazid than in the other groups. On this basis the authors suggest that hydrazide fulfils the requirements of a toxic compound made from isoniazid which is present more in slow than in rapid acetylators, and which is increased in amount much more by rifampicin in slow acetylators than in rapid acetylators. Nevertheless, the hypothesis is based on indirect proof because they did not actually demonstrate the hydrazide.

Hepatitis as indicated by raised serum transaminase levels was studied in Japanese tuberculosis patients by Yamamoto *et al.* (1986). Elevated serum aminotransferase levels were found in 35 out of 74 isoniazid + rifampicin + streptomycin patients, and in 17 out of 69 isoniazid + *p*-aminosalicylate + streptomycin patients; this difference was significant ($\chi_1^2 = 7.9$). The elevation in transaminase levels was mild and the patients did not have clinical symptoms. When the liver function tests were normal, the serum acetylisoniazid to isoniazid ratio was estimated in 18 patients from the rifampicin treatment group who had previously raised transaminases, and in 18 patients from the same group whose transaminases had not been elevated. The serum acetylisoniazid/isoniazid ratio distribution indicated the phenotypes 11 slow (S) and seven rapid (R) acetylators in the non-hepatitic, and 4S and 14R acetylators in the hepatitic groups ($\chi_1^2 = 5.6$). The authors interpret these data to indicate that the rapid acetylator is more at risk to developing hepatitis on isoniazid + rifampicin in Japanese people, and suggest that the toxic agent may be formed from acetylisoniazid, which is present in significantly greater amounts in the sera of the R acetylator as compared with the S acetylator patients. There is suspicion about the phenotyping data because if the hepatitis group contained such a preponderance of rapid acetylators, the serum isoniazid level 3 hours after dosing should have been lower in this group than in the controls, and it was not. So perhaps the patients in the hepatitis group were unable to metabolize the acetylisoniazid as an effect of their disorder.

Conclusions

Despite the finding of Mitchell *et al.* (1975b) which remains unexplained, it seems probable that when isoniazid is given alone, slow acetylators are more prone to hepatotoxicity than rapid acetylators in whites and blacks.

Using regimens which contain isoniazid with other drugs but no rifampicin, Orientals are more susceptible to hepatotoxicity than European and African populations. In Indians the two acetylator phenotypes seem equally prone to liver toxicity.

When regimens which contain both isoniazid and rifampicin are used, it is clear that in Caucasian populations (1) the incidence of hepatotoxicity is higher than it is with either isoniazid alone or with isoniazid plus drugs other than rifampicin and (2) slow acetylators are more prone to liver toxicity, particularly of severe grades, than are rapid acetylators. It seems likely that a derivative of acetyl-hydrazine or hydrazide may be the toxic agent responsible for the liver toxicity in Caucasian and Indian subjects. (See Steele *et al.* 1991 for a recent meta-analysis of the hepatotoxicity of isoniazid plus rifampicin.)

On the basis of the study of Yamamoto *et al.* (1986) it would appear that (1) liver toxicity is significantly more common (nearly ×2) in regimens which combine isoniazid and rifampicin and (2) among Oriental patients receiving isoniazid and rifampicin, rapid acetylators may be significantly associated with biochemical (but not clinical) hepatotoxicity.

Hydralazine

Hydralazine, though it has been in use for nearly 40 years, is still quite a popular drug for the treatment of hypertension.

After the polymorphism for the metabolism of isoniazid had been discovered, it appeared that hydralazine might be another candidate drug for the same genetically controlled acetylation. This idea was attractive, not only because hydralazine is a mono-substituted hydrazide, but also because it had been shown by Douglass *et al.* (1957) to inhibit the in vitro acetylation of sulphanilamide in pigeon liver extracts.

As indicated in Table 16.3 the first direct indication that its metabolism was governed by the polymorphism was its differential metabolism in liver homogenates obtained from persons with the two phenotypes. Thereafter, as more sophisticated chemical methodologies became available, direct proof of its polymorphic acetylation *in vivo* was obtained.

The control of hypertension by hydralazine is directly related to the concentration in the plasma, and it was clear that for a given dose this concentration (and hence the hypotensive effect) was more marked in the slow than in the rapid phenotype (Shepherd *et al.* 1980). However, Rowell & Clarke (1990) tested eight slow acetylators and 12 rapid acetylators, all with bronchial carcinomas, with oral hydralazine. Falls in peripheral resistance were greater in slow than in rapid acetylators but the difference did not reach statistical significance.

A clinical phenomenon, which gained attention fairly soon after the introduction of the drug into practice, was the development in patients treated with it of a complete mimic of systemic lupus erythematosus.

A survey of Cameron & Ramsay (1984) revealed the incidence of this complication amongst 281 patients treated over 51 months. There were no cases in patients taking 50 mg daily, and incidences of 5.4% with 100 mg daily, and 10.4% with 200 mg daily. The incidence was higher in women than in men. In the whole population the incidence was 6.7% (confidence limits 3.2 to 10.2%). There is ample evidence to show that the development of this syndrome is overwhelmingly a disorder of slow acetylators (Table 16.14), and it is also commoner in women than in men.

Since the disease is so unusual in rapid acetylators it is worth focusing on these exceptional patients. The two patients of Strandberg *et al.* (1976) who were not clearly slow acetylators are interesting. One was a woman who continued to have the disorder for 4 years after the drug was discontinued. So she suffered coincidentally from spontaneous SLE. The second was a woman who had a high titre of antibodies to *Yersinia enterocolitica* on complement-fixation testing. About $2\frac{1}{2}$ months after the onset of symptoms (and discontinuation of hydralazine) the symptoms and the laboratory abnormalities disappeared. So this was a complicated clinical situation, added to which the acetylator phenotyping data were equivocal.

Another possible explanation is provided by a recent careful study of hydralazine metabolism conducted in four groups of patients. Slow and rapid

Table 16.14. *Acetylator phenotyping of hydralazine-induced systemic lupus erythematosus patients*

Reference	Location where study conducted	Ethnic group	Technique of phenotyping	Total number of patients phenotyped	Number of slow acetylators
Perry *et al.* 1970	St Louis and La Jolla	Caucasian	Percentage acetylation of SMZ in urine	12	12
Strandberg *et al.* 1976	Stockholm and Lulea	Presumably Caucasian	Isoniazid half-life	31[a]	29
Batchelor *et al.* 1980	London, Stoke-on-Trent and Leicester	Presumably Caucasian	Percentage acetylation of SMZ in plasma and in urine (Evans 1969–Method 2)	26	25
Mansilla-Tinoco *et al.* 1982 and S.J. Harland, personal communication	London	Caucasian Black	Percentage acetylation of SMZ in plasma and in urine (Evans 1969–Method 2)	12 1	11 1

[a]See text for discussion of two of these patients.

acetylators who had been treated for a long period with hydralazine and who had, or had not, developed an SLE-like syndrome were investigated (Timbrell *et al.* 1984). The one rapid acetylator hydralazine–SLE patient showed a different metabolic pattern from the control rapid acetylators (Harland *et al.* 1980). The excretion of phthalazinone was higher, and hydralazine hydrazones and methyltriazolophthalazine were also excreted in slightly larger amounts; conversely, triazophthalazine excretion was lower. As regards phthalazine, the percentage of the dose excreted thus by this rapid acetylator hydralazine–SLE patient resembled the excretion of the slow acetylator hydralazine–SLE patients. It would be interesting to see if other rapid acetylator hydralazine–SLE patients also have a toxic metabolic pathway causing phthalazinone production, as occurs in slow acetylators. By this means the actual chemical compound responsible for the production of the syndrome might be identified (see Fig. 16.8).

It would seem that the acetylator phenotype is not a factor of importance in determining the outcome of therapy where hydralazine is used as one element of a 'triple therapy' regime with a β-blocker and a diuretic (Vandenburg *et al.* 1982).

Another question of practical importance is whether it would be worth determining the acetylator phenotype as a guide to treatment of hypertension with hydralazine. Slow acetylators would want smaller doses than rapid acetylators to control their disease. The measurement of plasma levels of hydralazine itself is a much more expensive laboratory procedure than determining the acetylator phenotype by one of the methods described elsewhere in this chapter. Opinion is divided; Shepherd *et al.* (1981) are in favour on the grounds that the knowledge might enable the correct dose to be given more frequently and more speedily to control the hypertension, especially in rapid acetylators. Cameron & Ramsay (1984) and Ramsay *et al.* (1984) are in favour under certain

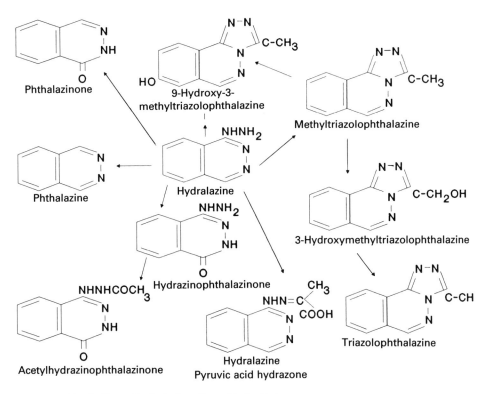

Fig. 16.8. Metabolism of hydralazine. (From Timbrell *et al.* 1984.)

circumstances. They point out that if all Caucasian hypertensives were phenotyped the effort would be wasted in 65%. Hence they suggest phenotyping individuals whose blood pressure is uncontrolled by 200 mg daily. It must be realized that since they wrote this the situation has changed, in that nifedipine and captopril have now shown themselves to be very effective antihypertensives for many years and so there is no need for high dose hydralazine or for the use of the phenotyping test in routine practice.

Dihydralazine and endralazine

These two hypertensive drugs are derivatives of hydralazine and so it was an attractive idea to see what influence the acetylator polymorphism had on their metabolism and clinical effect.

Dihydralazine was studied by Iisalo *et al.* (1979) in 19 hypertensive acetylator-phenotyped hypertensives. It was found that there were no significant differences between the two phenotypes in (1) the daily dose of dihydralazine needed to control the blood pressure, (2) the concentrations of dihydralazine achieved in plasma, (3) the dose–concentration relationship of dihydralazine or (4) in the appearance of side effects. The authors did not study the metabolites of the drug but suggest that pathways other than acetylation should be considered in its metabolism.

Endralazine was found to be acetylated and the influence of the polymorphism on its metabolism was investigated by Reece *et al.* (1982). They used a SMZ phenotyping test and assumed that this detects genotypes, which has not been proven. They found no significant difference between the plasma concentration half-lives of rapid and slow acetylators, but they did find that the mean area under the plasma concentration/time curve (AUC) was 18.2% lower after a 5 mg dose and 11% lower after a 10 mg dose in rapid than in slow acetylators.

Also the AUC of acetylendralazine, although small, was significantly higher in rapid acetylators than in slow. The authors suggest that the terminal half-life in the plasma which is the same for the two acetylator phenotypes (and much longer than for hydralazine) depends on hydrazone formation by a chemical reaction with endogenous ketone bodies, mainly pyruvic acid, in the plasma.

No influence of the acetylator polymorphism on the response of hypertension to endralazine was

found by Holmes *et al.* (1983) in 34 slow and 16 fast acetylators, treated with the drug in combination with pindolol (to which they had previously not responded adequately). Neither the lowering of the blood pressure nor the average dosage of endralazine required differed significantly between the two phenotypes. This was ascribed to the fact that 10% or less of the drug is metabolized by acetylation.

Nineteen phenotyped hypertensives treated with endralazine for 3 years showed no serious adverse effects and a low incidence of development of antinuclear antibody. There were no differences between the phenotypes in the dosage of endralazine required or in the incidence of adverse effects (Bogers & Meems 1983).

Sulphapyridine – a metabolite of salicylazosulphapyridine

Sulphapyridine is not now used by itself as an antimicrobial, but nevertheless has clinical importance because it is a metabolite of salicylazosulphapyridine (sulphasalazine, SASP) which is used to treat ulcerative colitis, Crohn's disease, rheumatoid arthritis and occasionally other rheumatic disorders such as ankylosing spondylitis (Feltelius & Hallgren 1986).

This drug, which was introduced by Dr Svartz in Stockholm in the early 1940s, was used for nearly 30 years before its fate in the body was properly understood. It was known early on that the drug was split in the human body leading to the release of sulphapyridine (SP) and 5-aminosalicylic acid. Much later, Schroder & Campbell (1972) showed that a considerable proportion of the SP as well as some of the unsplit sulphasalazine was absorbed, whilst most of the 5-aminosalicylic acid was excreted largely unchanged in the faeces. The absorbed SP was shown to undergo acetylation (and hydroxylation) in man so that SP, acetylated SP and hydroxylated SP (as the glucuronide) appeared in the urine. Only a small proportion of the unsplit SASP was absorbed from the jejunum and excreted in the urine. A little absorbed 5-aminosalicylate appeared in the urine, also in the acetylated form (see Fig. 16.9).

It was shown by Schroder *et al.* (1973), Das *et al.* (1974) and Azad Khan *et al.* (1982) that if the colon was removed the urinary excretion of SASP remained unchanged whilst the urinary excretion of

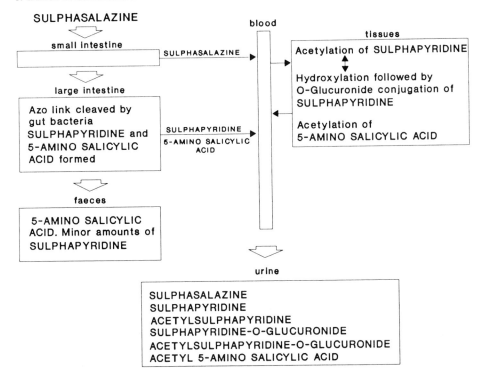

Fig. 16.9. The pharmacokinetics of sulphasalazine in man. (From Schröder & Evans 1972b.)

SP and its metabolites (which had been 42% of the dose) fell to a very low level.

The relevance of the acetylator polymorphism in the clinical use of SASP arises form the fact that sulphapyridine is polymorphically acetylated (Schroder & Evans 1972a; Das & Eastwood 1975). In healthy subjects, on repeated SASP administration, the effect of the polymorphism is shown within 4 days of starting. The serum SP concentration becomes higher in slow than in rapid acetylators (Schroder & Evans 1972b). In patients with ulcerative colitis on chronic treatment with SASP a similar phenomenon is shown. For example, Das & Dubin (1976) give the free serum sulphapyridine concentration as $42.2 \pm$ SD 24.4 µg/ml in slow and 8.5 ± 2.8µg/ml in rapid acetylators – a highly significant difference. Similarly Azad Khan *et al.* (1983) showed the free SP serum level to be $18.5 \pm$ SD 8.2 µg/ml in slow, and 7.5 ± 4.3 µg/ml in rapid acetylators – again a highly significant difference.

The occurrence of adverse reactions after the administration of SASP has been studied in relation to the acetylator phenotype in healthy volunteers and in patients, principally those with ulcerative colitis, Crohn's disease and rheumatoid arthritis. These studies have been facilitated by the finding that the phenotype can be determined by measuring the free and acetylated SP in the plasma and urine of patients on their standard SASP therapeutic regimens (see, for example, Lee & Ang 1986).

Schroder & Evans (1972b) found that slow acetylator healthy subjects given SASP reported adverse effects earlier, and of a more pronounced nature than the rapid acetylators. These symptoms (nausea, headache, abdominal discomfort, etc.) correlated with the serum free SP concentration.

Similarly, Das *et al.* (1973) reported 28 patients with side effects. The majority of them were taking 4 g SASP per day or more. The authors state that 'about ⅔ of the patients studied ($n = 133$) and 86% of those with side effects had slow acetylator phenotypes.' This is a significant association. The patients with side effects had serum free SP concentrations of $46.5 \pm$ SD 15.6 µg/ml whilst those without had a value of 28.6 ± 20.3 µg/ml.

The range of adverse effects found in the patients was much larger than in the healthy volunteers. This would be expected because they were on the treatment for very much longer. The list included vomiting, rashes, 'cyanosis', haemolysis, transient reticulocytosis, agranulocytosis, headache and dizziness.

Other workers have found results along the same lines as those reported above. Cowan *et al.* (1977) studied ulcerative colitics receiving SASP, and found that out of 43 in remission, 32 had serum SP levels greater than 20 μg/ml. In comparison, out of 21 with active disease, 10 were taking inadequate doses of SASP as shown by lower serum SP levels. These authors comment that high serum SP levels produce adverse effects, and therefore slow acetylators need lower doses of SASP. They advocate both identifying the patient's phenotype and thereafter monitoring serum SP levels for the two purposes of tailoring the dose and assessing compliance.

Goldstein *et al.* (1979) also studied 15 paediatric outpatients with chronic inflammatory disease receiving 1 to 4 g of SASP daily. They claim to have identified acetylator phenotypes by the percentage of SP acetylated in serum. Their conclusions are not to advocate phenotyping prior to commencing therapy; but they do suggest acetylator phenotyping and monitoring serum SP concentrations in 'non-responders'.

Sharp *et al.* (1981) also found that 19 slow acetylators receiving SASP treatment for inflammatory bowel disease had higher serum concentrations of SP than nine rapid acetylators. The incidence of adverse effects in the slow acetylators was higher but not significantly so, but the serum concentrations of SP were significantly higher in patients with symptoms of toxicity (23.2 ± 15.9 μg/ml) than in those without (13.9 ± 9.5 μg/ml). A significant correlation between clinical status of disease and serum drug concentrations was apparent only for rapid acetylators. It was considered that this was probably a secondary effect in that less rapid transit allows greater SP absorption. These workers advocate initial acetylator phenotyping and subsequent monitoring of SP levels to avoid toxic effects and to get the best response.

Clarke *et al.* (1982) studied 17 children and four adolescents with chronic inflammatory bowel disease; there were 15 slow and six rapid acetylators.

Higher SP serum levels and lower acetyl SP levels were found in slow acetylators than in rapid acetylators. Five out of six rapid acetylators and seven out of 15 slow acetylators developed side effects, and the mean SP levels in patients with and without side effects were almost the same. Why these workers' findings differ from those of others is unclear.

Bondesen *et al.* (1986) found that the metabolism and disposition of SASP and its metabolites were very similar in paediatric and adult patients, except that the amount of SASP and its metabolites excreted via the faeces was lower.

The haemolysis which occurred on treating 36 adults with chronic inflammatory bowel disease with 4.5–6.0 g SASP daily was studied by Van Hees *et al.* (1979). They determined the acetylator phenotype by means of a sulphamethazine test. Nineteen patients had haemolysis (serum haptoglobin > 0.8 g/l); their serum level of free SP was 53.8 ± SD 24.5 as compared with 15.9 ± 12.3 in those without haemolysis. Only 1 of 12 rapid acetylators had adverse effects ($p < 0.001$). These authors favour acetylator typing and monitoring the serum free SP levels (since haemolysis is frequent with serum free SP levels of more than 55 μg/ml).

Turning to rheumatoid arthritis therapy, Pullar *et al.* (1985) as the result of three very extensive surveys found the following. Side effects, especially nausea and vomiting, were more common amongst 66 slow acetylators than amongst 83 rapid acetylators in one series, and there were more 'drop-outs' amongst the slow acetylators also. In another planned trial they gave 40 rapid acetylators 3 g SASP daily and found that after 24 weeks they showed marked improvement, whereas 20 slow acetylators showed no improvement on 1.5 g daily over the same period. They conclude that routine acetylator phenotyping is not of value.

In the matter of adverse reactions a dissenting experience was that of Chalmers *et al.* (1990) who found no correlation with acetylator phenotype.

The general problem of serious sulphonamide toxicity was examined by Shear *et al.* (1986). They examined six patients who had suffered toxicity to the skin, five of whom had sustained damage to internal organs also after exposure to a triple sulphonamide preparation (sulphadiazine, sulphamethazine and sulphamerazine). All six were slow acetylators. *In vitro* lymphocyte cytotoxicity tests to sulphonamide were positive in all six, and were also positive in many family members. Likewise, Rieder *et al.* (1991) found 19 slow acetylators amongst 21 patients who had suffered various hypersensitivity reactions to sulphonamides. These authors put forward the view that more than one genetic factor may interact to produce a clinical adverse effect (in the context of chronic inflammatory bowel disease it must be pointed out that the milder 'toxic' reactions are much commoner than the more severe 'idiosyncratic' reactions). Their findings are comparable with the observations of Palatis *et al.* (1973), who tested 18 persons who had skin reactions to sulphamethoxypyridazine (SMP) by ascertaining their isoniazid half-lives. There was no increase in frequency of either acetylator phenotype, a finding which is consistent with the known fact that the acetylator polymorphism exerts very little influence on the metabolism of SMP (White & Evans 1968).

Nitrazepam

After the polymorphic acetylation of the amino metabolite of nitrazepam had been demonstrated by Karim & Evans (1976) there was speculation as to whether either phenotype was more prone to the drowsiness, hangover and confusion which sometimes arise after this drug is taken in 5 mg or 10 mg doses in the elderly (Viukari *et al.* 1983).

The problem was investigated by Swift *et al.* (1980), who phenotyped 24 healthy young Caucasian subjects with SMZ. They then investigated plasma levels of nitrazepam and residual effects at 12 hours following both 5 and 10 mg doses. The residual effects were determined first by means of an 'alert/drowsy' visual analogue rating and secondly by a tapping test.

There were no significant differences between the two phenotypes as regards (1) plasma nitrazepam concentrations, (2) plasma nitrazepam half-lives, or (3) residual effects.

The authors suggest that the acetylation of the amino metabolite is not a rate-limiting step in the elimination of the drug. Their observations are at variance with those of Eze (1987), who found that 95% of his 57 slow acetylators complained of drowsiness, a hangover feeling and lightheadedness on the day following a dose of 10 mg nitrazepam as compared with 14% of 22 rapid acetylator subjects. This may have something to do with differences between the two ethnic groups studied in the two experiments.

Aminoglutethimide

Aminoglutethimide, the amino derivative of the hypnotic glutethimide, was first introduced as a potential anticonvulsant over 20 years ago. In 1966, adrenal insufficiency was noted in two children being treated in this way. The next year the drug was introduced with the express therapeutic purpose of causing adrenal suppression in postmenopausal advanced breast cancer (Plowman, 1987). Its use, with dexamethasone to prevent the secondary rise in ACTH, is now established as an effective second line breast cancer treatment.

The most important action is to inhibit aromatase which converts adrenal androgens to oestrogens in many tissues including adipose tissue, muscle, skin and breast cancer.

The most common adverse effects encountered are in three groups: (1) dose-dependent, e.g. dizziness, somnolence, lethargy, nausea, vomiting and diarrhoea; (2) non-dose-dependent drug rash which may disappear on continued treatment; (3) non-dose-dependent thrombocytopenia leucopenia and agranulocytosis.

The drug is a primary aromatic amine and the urinary excretion of the *N*-acetyl derivative accounts for 4 to 25% of the ingested dose. For this reason, Coombes *et al.* (1982) investigated the metabolism of aminoglutethimide in five rapid and five slow acetylators of sulphamethazine. They found that the rapid acetylators excreted a greater percentage of the dose as *N*-acetylaminoglutethimide (NAG) in the urine than the slow acetylators, and (with one exception) less of the parent compound. In addition, they discovered that the percentage of the dose excreted as nitroglutethimide was higher in the slow than in the rapid acetylators, but that the mean excretion of *N*-formylaminoglutethimide was the same in the two phenotypes.

The same group (Jarman *et al.* 1983) found that 4-hydroxyaminoglutethimide was also present in the urine of patients being treated with the drug.

An extensive analysis of the effect of the acetylator phenotype on the disposition of aminoglutethimide was published by Adam *et al.* (1984). They were able to investigate the parent drug and its acetyl metabolite in plasma. It was found that the drug was rapidly absorbed and then very quickly the acetyl metabolite appeared in the plasma. After a few hours an equilibrium had been established between the two compounds; after this in a given subject their elimination rates from the plasma were the same. Hence at any subsequent time point (whilst the compounds were measurable) the ratio of their concentrations would be the same.

After a week's continuous therapy the plasma half-lives were shortened to the same extent in a given individual and this occurred in both acetylator phenotypes. These effects were ascribed to an induction effect of aminoglutethimide (AG) on oxidation enzymes involved in its metabolism.

The acetylation polymorphism was found to influence the plasma NAG/AG ratio (which was higher in rapid acetylation); and the rapid acetylators excreted a lower percentage of the dose of AG

ingested and more NAG in the urine than did the slow acetylators.

A paradoxical and hitherto unexplained finding was that the plasma elimination half-lives of both AG and NAG were shorter in slow acetylators than in rapid.

The maximum plasma AG concentrations attained were not significantly different in the two phenotypes.

Although it is clear that the acetylator polymorphism influences AG metabolism significantly, there are no published results of the NAG/AG ratio in a large population to show the presence or absence of bimodality. Perhaps it should not be expected that the distribution would be bimodal in view of the complex pathways (Fig. 16.10) of metabolism involved (Dalrymple & Nicholls 1988).

An investigation of side effects in relation to the acetylator polymorphism was carried out by Demers *et al.* (1987) in 38 breast cancer patients. They found the symptoms to be correlated with higher plasma

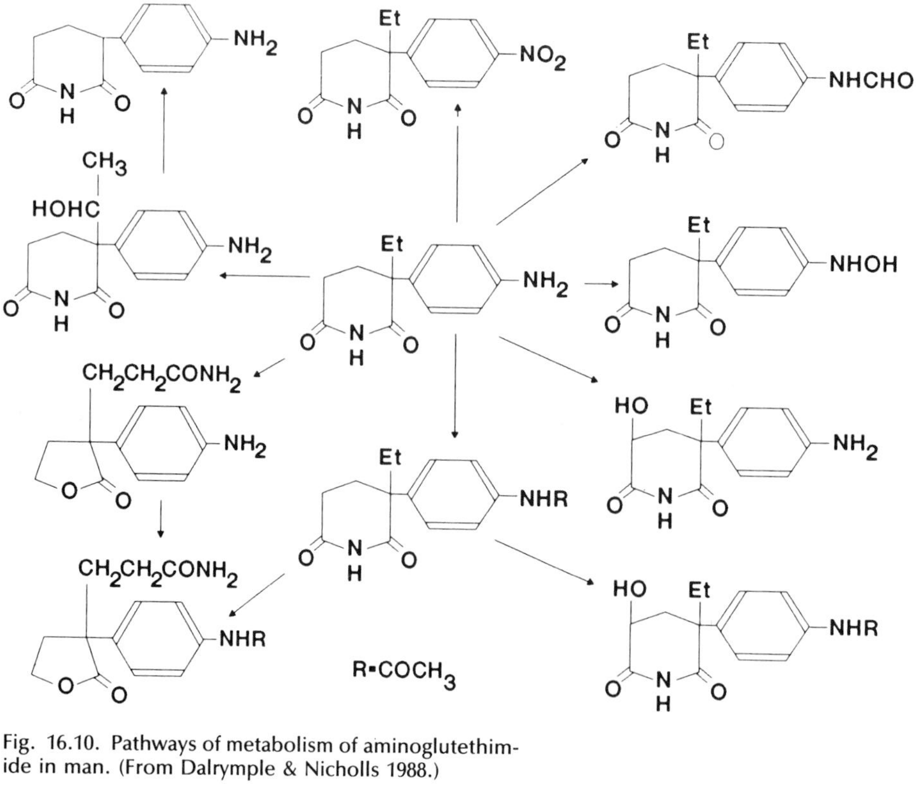

Fig. 16.10. Pathways of metabolism of aminoglutethimide in man. (From Dalrymple & Nicholls 1988.)

AG levels but not to be related to the acetylator phenotype.

Bone marrow damage is a well recognized hazard of aminoglutethimide therapy producing leucopenia, agranulocytosis and thrombocytopenia (Buzdar *et al.* 1984; Harris *et al.* 1986). It is thought to be a direct toxic effect on the marrow (Harris *et al.* 1986). No attempt has been made to look at these phenomena in relation to the acetylation polymorphism.

Procainamide

The polymorphic acetylation of procainamide (PA) in man has been amply demonstrated (Karlsson & Molin 1975; Gibson *et al.* 1975; Ylitalo *et al.* 1983). These studies were carried out in healthy subjects and in patients with cardiac disorders, principally myocardial infarction and ventricular premature beats. The reference phenotyping techniques included sulphapyridine acetylation, isoniazid half-life, MADDS/DDS in plasma and sulphamethazine acetylation. The indices of PA metabolism were percentage acetylation of the drug in both plasma and urine.

It should be noted in the study of Karlsson *et al.* (1975) that the separation between the phenotypes for percentage urinary PA acetylated was blurred. This might have been because the 41 patients studied had suspected or proven myocardial infarction with ventricular arrhythmias and some of them had renal functional impairment. When 29 patients with normal renal function were examined separately, the phenotype separation was more distinct (Karlsson *et al.* 1974). Likewise in 25 patients who had recent myocardial infarcts with dysrhythmias, SMZ phenotyping was impaired by concomitant PA therapy (Campbell *et al.* 1976).

A more detailed investigation of the pharmacokinetics of PA was carried out by Lima *et al.* (1979) and they emphasize that the two variables which most affect the plasma concentrations of both PA and acetyl PA are renal function and acetylator phenotype. In the opinion of these authors 'phenotyping patients before dosing is impractical and unnecessary'.

The question of efficacy of PA as a medication for ventricular arrhythmias became complicated by the discoveries that the metabolite *N*-acetyl PA had effects on the heart similar to the parent drug

(Drayer *et al.* 1974; Elson *et al.* 1975) and that the two compounds were approximately equipotent. It was also suggested that there might be some antagonism between the two substances, possibly due to competitive inhibition at the same receptor sites (Schroder *et al.* 1979). As a result of these findings it was considered that monitoring the plasma levels of PA was not useful to control therapy.

A study of *N*-acetyl procainamide (acecainide) by Coyle *et al.* (1991) in three rapid and three slow acetylators showed that the non-renal clearance was greater in the latter (i.e. inversely related to the sulphapyridine acetylation used as the phenotyping procedure). The explanation for this finding is unclear but it could be artefactual from the method of computation.

Another aspect of great clinical interest arising from the continued use of procainamide as a prophylactic against arrhythmias is the development of a mimic of SLE. Woosley *et al.* (1978) investigated patients who had developed the syndrome and found that the duration of therapy required for induction in four slow and three rapid acetylators was 12 ± SD 6 and 54 ± 18 months respectively. When combined with other data from the literature, corresponding figures were for 14 slow and seven rapid acetylators, 12 ± SD 5 and 48 ± 22 months respectively ($p < 0.002$).

The same authors also studied 11 slow and nine rapid acetylators to find out the speed with which they develop anti-nuclear antibodies (ANA). The times needed for development of antinuclear antibodies in 50% of the slow and rapid acetylators were 2.9 and 7.3 months respectively ($p < 0.002$). The median cumulative dosages consumed at the time ANA were detected in the slow and rapid acetylators were 1.5 and 6.1 g/kg, respectively ($p < 0.02$).

It can be noted that the phenotype distribution in the population of patients who developed the procainamide-SLE syndrome appeared not to be significantly different to that in the general population. Small sample sizes may lead to erroneous conclusions. Compare, for example, the findings of Davies *et al.* (1975), who amongst seven patients with the SLE syndrome found five rapid and two slow acetylators, with those of Sonnhag *et al.* (1979), who amongst nine patients with the syndrome found two rapid and seven slow acetylators.

It therefore seems that both phenotypes will develop the syndrome on long term procainamide, but slow acetylators will develop it sooner than rapid acetylators. It is presumed that the procainamide itself is the agent responsible for producing the immunologic disorder, but it is possible that non-acetyl metabolites may also play a part (Woosley *et al.* 1978; Ylitalo *et al.* 1983).

Dapsone

Dapsone has been used in the treatment of leprosy since 1942, but for many years relatively little was known about its metabolism in man. The discovery that it was acetylated on a primary aromatic amine group led Gelber *et al.* (1971) to see whether this acetylation was polymorphic. They investigated 19 subjects by means of an isoniazid half-life determination, an SMZ test in which the percentage of the drug acetylated in urine was determined, and the ratio of the concentration of the metabolite MADDS to that of the parent compound (MADDS/DDS) in the plasma. They found complete agreement between the phenotyping results achieved by the three methods.

Ancillary experiments revealed the following.

The DDS acetylation results were reproducible from one occasion to another.
Very little of an ingested dose of dapsone emerged in the urine. Some emerged unchanged and this was the same in both phenotypes. More MADDS was excreted by rapid than by slow acetylators but the data did not provide a clear separation of the phenotypes.
MADDS was deacetylated, since after its oral administration the plasma DDS level rose rapidly. The two compounds were cleared from the plasma at about the same rate and so once equilibrium had been achieved the MADDS/DDS ratio remained constant.
This equilibrium was achieved after about 4 hours in a rapid and after about 6 hours in a slow acetylator after MADDS ingestion. The same equilibrium was achieved within half an hour after DDS ingestion. This means that the acetylation of DDS and the deacetylation of MADDS are both going on simultaneously all the time with the former occurring at a much faster rate.
The half-lives of the disappearance of MADDS and DDS from the serum (which were approximately the same) were independent of the speed of acetylation.

The same group (Peters *et al.* 1972) conducted further extensive investigations on subjects in the Philippines. Again SMZ and dapsone acetylation (as shown by plasma MADDS/DDS) were compared. On this occasion the acetylation of SMZ was studied in plasma as well as in urine. The percentage of sulphamethazine acetylated in plasma appeared to be the best of the three measurements for separating the phenotypes. The plasma DDS concentration was independent of its percentage acetylation. The plasma MADDS concentration was positively correlated with the percentage of DDS acetylated in plasma.

The assessment of plasma MADDS/DDS was utilized by Reidenberg *et al.* (1973, 1975) as the calibratory acetylator phenotyping procedure in their investigations of the polymorphic metabolism of hydralazine and procainamide.

The use of the plasma MADDS/DDS ratio to assess acetylator phenotype was investigated by Carr *et al.* (1978). By this time high performance liquid chromatography (HPLC) was available to measure DDS and MADDS (after a preliminary extraction step), replacing the previous calorimetric and fluorimetric assays. In 50 healthy Caucasian volunteers they achieved a satisfactory separation of the two acetylator phenotypes. The MADDS/DDS ratio obtained in phenotyping tests was shown not to be affected by concurrent cimetidine administration by Wright *et al.* (1984) indicating that the acetylation biotransformation is independent of hepatic mixed function enzymes (P450). However, 94% of the inter-individual variability in dapsone clearance is accounted for by differences in *N*-hydroxylation indicating that acetylation is a relatively minor pathway (May *et al.* 1990). Strangely, Wiggan *et al.* (1991), also like Carr *et al.* (1978) using a 100 mg DDS dose and estimating MADDS/DDS in plasma 3 hours later by an HPLC method, were unable to find a bimodal distribution in the population and question the validity of this phenotyping procedure.

Peters *et al.* (1975) investigated 50 South Indians with SMZ and DDS acetylation tests. They again concluded that the percentage acetylation of SMZ in plasma was a better phenotype discriminator than either plasma MADDS/DDS or percentage acetylation of SMZ in urine.

Philip *et al.* (1984) devised a simple protein precipitation step to replace the extraction techniques used previously and employed high pressure liquid chromatography to measure the plasma concentrations of DDS and MADDS. This new rapid assay for acetylator phenotype has been used by this group in various population surveys and investigations of patients.

The DDS test of acetylator phenotyping has quite naturally been applied in clinical areas in which the drug is used, the most important being leprosy.

Gelber & Rees (1975) found no significant association between acetylator phenotype and DDS-resistant leprosy. They also reported that rifampicin (a stimulator of mixed function oxidases) does not affect dapsone acetylation but does halve its half-life. This was one more piece of evidence to show that acetylation kinetics and plasma dapsone clearance are unrelated. Peters *et al.* (1974) studied DDS-resistant leprosy patients in different racial groups. They were phenotyped using both SMZ and DDS. The DDS plasma half-lives were shorter in resistant patients. Adequate numbers of controls of the appropriate racial groups were not available to decide whether either phenotype was more prone to develop DDS-resistant leprosy. Similar observations were made by Ellard *et al.* (1972) on Chinese patients. Fifteen out of 21 DDS-resistant patients were rapid acetylators, a proportion similar to that found in healthy Chinese populations (see a later section for a fuller discussion of this aspect).

According to Venkatesa (1989) the acetylation polymorphism has no effect on dapsone handling by leprosy patients and Garg *et al.* (1988) concluded that 100 mg dapsone daily maintained plasma therapeutic concentrations in Indian lepers.

The amount of DDS required to control dermatitis herpetiformis was studied by Forstrom *et al.* (1974). They found that out of 24 rapid acetylators, 13 needed more than 100 mg DDS daily, whereas this was the case in only three out of 22 slow acetylators ($p < 0.001$). They found that haemolysis (as shown by haptoglobin levels) was not correlated with acetylator phenotype. Ellard *et al.* (1974a) found that methaemoglobin total denatured protein and Heinz bodies correlated better with peak DDS plasma concentrations than with the daily dose of dapsone being taken. In contradistinction to Forstrom *et al.* (1974), it was found by Swain *et al.* (1983) in similar patients that the dose of DDS required to control the dermatitis herpetiformis was not significantly different in eight rapid acetylators as compared with 16 slow acetylators.

Dapsone has also been used to treat rheumatoid arthritis. An attempt was made to correlate clinical efficacy with acetylator phenotype by Crook *et al.*

(1983) and no such correlation was found. The same group found that there was no association between either phenotype and adverse effects. Likewise, Kelly & Griffiths (1981) failed to find any association between severity of haemolysis during dapsone treatment for rheumatoid arthritis and either acetylator phenotype.

Caffeine

Caffeine is thought to be the most widely consumed drug. It has been found that it undergoes a complicated series of biotransformations in the human being, mainly by oxidative demethylation and hydroxylation. Ring opening converts the xanthine of the parent structure into uracil. In the urine of a subject who has ingested caffeine there appears a whole series of methylated derivatives of xanthine and uracil (Fig. 16.11).

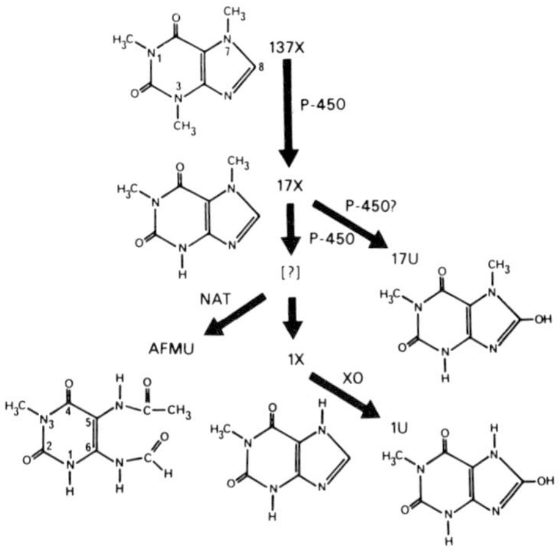

Fig. 16.11. Proposed pathways of formation of the five major metabolites of caffeine in man. Enzymes responsible for the metabolic steps are shown beside the arrows; P-450, cytochrome(s) P450; NAT, N-acetyltransferase; XO, xanthine oxidase. Question mark denotes a postulated ring-opened intermediate. Abbreviations: 137X, caffeine; 17X, 1,7-dimethylxanthine; 17U, 1,7-dimethyluric acid; 1X, 1-methylxanthine; 1U, 1-methyluric acid; AFMU, 5-acetylamino-6-formylamino-3-methyluracil. (From Grant *et al.* 1984.)

The compound 5-acetylamino-6-amino-3-methyluracil (AAMU) had been identified in urine by Fink *et al.* (1964) who noted that, although it was present in small amounts in the urine of caffeine-free individuals, a lot more appeared after caffeine consumption.

Not much attention was devoted to the subject until 1983, by which time many new useful chemical techniques were available. The same compound was detected in the urine as a metabolite of caffeine by Branfman *et al.* (1983). Radiolabelled caffeine was given by mouth to 12 non-smoking adults by Callahan *et al.* (1983) and the same subjects were phenotyped by means of an isoniazid test. It was found that the AAMU excreted accounted for about 19% of the administered dose of caffeine, and that this compound and another unidentified diaminouracil caffeine derivative were excreted in larger amounts by the two rapid acetylators than by the other subjects.

Similarly, Tang *et al.* (1983) identified 5-acetylamino-6-formylamino-3-methyluracil (AFMU) in the urine of persons who had ingested caffeine. This compound was shown to be unstable, giving rise to the deformylated AAMU. Grant *et al.* (1983a), in a major study of 68 unrelated healthy non-smoking subjects in whom urinary caffeine metabolites and acetylator phenotype were determined, were able to present convincing evidence that the acetylation step which produces AFMU is polymorphic. This evidence was based on the distribution of AFMU/(1U + 1X + 17U + 17X + AFMU) as a molar fraction in the urine excreted in 24 hours after ingesting 300 mg caffeine (1U, 1-methyluric acid; 1X, 1-methylxanthine; 17U, 1,7-dimethyluric acid; 17X, 1,7-dimethylxanthine). This ratio was clearly bimodal and persons with values in the upper mode were rapid acetylators on a sulphamethazine test, and persons with values in the lower mode were slow acetylators (Fig. 16.12). Later the same research group (Grant *et al.* 1983b) simplified the situation by showing that the distribution of log AFMU/1X in the urine was bimodal with separate low and high value modes representing slow and rapid acetylators, respectively in both Caucasians and Orientals (see Fig. 16.12).

The stability of the phenotype thus determined by the urinary AFMU/1X ratio was demonstrated by Grant *et al.* (1984), who examined urines produced by eight individuals who had ingested coffee on five random occasions over a 3 week period. The authors suggest that the rapid acetylators identified by the AFMU/1X ratio may form two modes representing the two constituent genotypes. The suggested

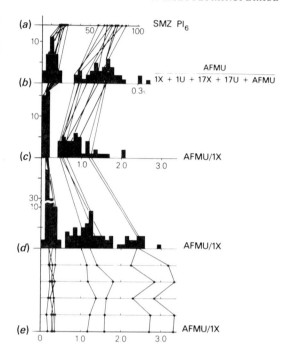

Fig. 16.12. Relationship between methods used for determining acetylator phenotype. Solid lines connect data points from subjects taking part in more than one study. (a) Sulphamethazine plasma acetylation index, PI_6, denoting the percentage of SMZ in plasma in the acetylated form for 20 subjects. (b) Frequency histogram of data (n = 72) from caffeine population study. Abscissa denotes the fraction of the five major recoverable urinary caffeine metabolites present as AFMU in 24 h pooled urine samples after ingestion of 300 mg caffeine. (Data in a and b adapted from Grant *et al.* 1983a). (c) Frequency histogram of data from study in b above; abscissa is the molar ratio of AFMU to 1X. (d) Frequency histogram of data from simplified acetylator phenotyping method (n = 146); abscissa is the molar ratio of AFMU to 1X. (e) Consistency of the simplified method in d for eight selected subjects. Five replicates of the method were performed for each subject over a period of 3 weeks; abscissae as in c and d. (From Grant *et al.* 1984.)

reason for this was that there was no upper limit to the value of the ratio. This is in contradistinction to, for example, percentage sulphamethazine acetylated in plasma, where there is a maximum value of 100% and so differences between the two rapid acetylator genotypes might be obscured.

As mentioned previously AFMU is unstable, particularly in alkaline urines, and there is therefore the possibility that some of it may change to AAMU before the analysis is performed, thereby giving erroneously low values for the ratio AFMU/1X. For this reason Tang et al. (1986) published a new analytical method, based on high performance exclusion chromatography, in which all the AFMU was initially changed by exposure to pH 10 to AAMU and then the AAMU/1X measured in the urine as an index of acetylation capacity.

The results of using this new technique and ratio in a population of 49 Caucasians were published by Tang et al. (1987). Again, complete correspondence with the results of a sulphamethazine test was shown for 10 rapid and 10 slow acetylators. In the population there was a suggestion that the three genotypes were detectable with the caffeine technique. This suggestion was based on the following: (1) two natural 'breaks' in the probit plot and (2) agreement of the numbers in the three hypothesized modes with the Hardy–Weinberg equilibrium. Of course (as the authors themselves pointed out), in order to prove whether genotypes are detectable required family studies. A similar, much larger study (178 unrelated healthy subjects) was published by Tang et al. (1991) and this paper includes several useful practical hints.

Gascon et al. (1987) using the AFMU/1X analytical method in 63 persons produced a convincingly trimodal frequency distribution histogram (Fig. 16.4). The numbers of subjects in the three modes were in keeping with the Hardy–Weinberg equilibrium. Fairly good phenotypic separation was achieved by Roots et al. (1988) using the AFMU/1X test, apparently better separation by Morris et al. (1989) using the AAMU/1X test, and definitely better separation by Hildebrand & Seifert (1989) using the AFMU/1X test.

Unfortunately a number of groups have had difficulty in reproducing these results. For example, the phenotypic separation by two assessments was unconvincing in the survey of El-Yazigi et al. (1989a, b). Hardy et al. (1988), using a 300 mg caffeine dose and HPLC analytic method showed a clear phenotypic separation in 46 individuals of undefined ethnic origin. However, over a 5 week period four persons changed their apparent phenotype and intra-individual variability was computed as 19%. There are two main sources of difficulty. First, as pointed out by Lorenzo & Reidenberg (1989) AFMU will be lost in basic urines prior to voiding and whilst 1X is stable under all conditions it is precipitated by storage of the urine at −80°C and may subsequently be difficult to re-dissolve. Another source of difficulties lies in the chromatography itself, for two main reasons: (1) the very small differences in physico-chemical properties between the various caffeine metabolites and (2) the presence of interfering background substances in the urines. This method is worthy of a lot more effort to get it to succeed because caffeine is not popularly regarded as a serious drug, and so there are no ethical objections to asking people to ingest it (as coffee, for example), such as may be raised against giving other test compounds (e.g. SMZ, isoniazid and DDS) to persons who do not need them for their own good.

As mentioned earlier, Kilbane et al. (1990) have published a study of 16 informative families showing that genotypes can be detected using urinary AAMU/1X; however, their Fig. 4 – a population frequency distribution histogram – is not as convincing as regards phenotype definition as the scattergram of Viznerova (1973) using sulphamethazine (see Fig. 16.3 above) or the histogram of Gascon et al. (1987) using caffeine (see Fig. 16.4 above).

Phenelzine

The original idea that phenelzine might be a substrate for the human acetylation polymorphism arose because it is a mono-substituted hydrazide, like isoniazid. At that time no suitable chemical analytical techniques were available with which to investigate the possibility directly. However, a clinical study was mounted in which patients with both endogenous and neurotic depression had their phenotype determined, and were then treated with phenelzine, and the outcome observed (Evans et al. 1965). The expectation was that there might be differences between the phenotypes in clinical response or adverse effects. It was found that side effects were more common in slow acetylators but there was no difference in clinical outcome between the two phenotypes. Rose (1982) points out that the dose of phenelzine used was inadequate by modern standards.

Six further studies of a somewhat similar type have been carried out subsequently and are critically discussed by Rose (1982). In four of these studies no significant difference in response of the depression to treatment with phenelzine was observed between the acetylator phenotypes. In the other two surveys, the slow acetylators showed a significantly better psychiatric response than did the rapid acetylators. Meanwhile biochemical studies were proceeding.

Patients who were under treatment with phenelzine were acetylator phenotyped with sulphamethazine by Caddy et al. (1976). Phenelzine was assayed in plasma and urine by gas chromatography of the acetonide derivative. By this technique phenelzine could not be detected in the plasma of patients (but could be found in the plasma of a person who had taken an overdose as attempted suicide). In the urine, slow acetylators excreted more than rapid acetylators.

The complete absence of evidence that phenelzine is acetylated in humans was emphasized by Marshall (1976).

An interesting drug interaction was described by Harris & McIntyre (1981) in a man who had been taking phenelzine. He was then prescribed nitrazepam, and thereafter developed severe postural hypotension. After recovery a phenotyping test showed that he was a slow acetylator. It was suggested that the clinical effect occurred because the second drug given led to an increased concentration of the first. This might have been due to direct competition for acetylation or to inhibition of other metabolic pathways.

Phenelzine is a substrate for human N-acetyltransferase in vitro (Tilstone et al. 1979) whilst Naraismhachari et al. (1980) claim to have detected N-acetylphenelzine in human urine using combined gas chromatography/mass spectrometry in the selected ion mode. After the intraperitoneal administration of high doses of phenelzine to rats, N-acetylphenelzine was found in the blood and brain by Mozayani et al. (1988) and Coutts et al. (1991).

Hein & Weber (1982) performed in vitro work using highly purified preparations of rabbit liver N-acetyltransferase (which is polymorphic, resembling the human situation). Acetylation of phenelzine was shown to be polymorphic, and the responsible enzymic activity co-purified with that responsible for the acetylation of isoniazid. The heat inactivation patterns of phenelzine and sulphamethazine acetylating enzymes were indistinguishable.

Despite all this, Robinson et al. (1985) produced a much more definitive experiment using site-specific, stable, isotope-labelled phenelzine analogues in metabolic and pharmacokinetic studies in humans with gas chromatography/mass spectrometry detection. The authors were able to detect the labelled phenelzine and labelled phenylacetic acid and p-hydroxyphenylacetic acid in plasma but were unable to detect N-acetylphenelzine in any plasma or urine samples from the six patients studied. The major metabolites, phenylacetic acid and p-hydroxyphenylacetic acid, constituted 79% of the administered dose excreted via the urine in the first 96 hours. It must be pointed out that, as their patients were not acetylator-phenotyped, they may not have studied any rapid acetylator who might have the ability to acetylate the compound, when the slow acetylator could not do so.

Another antidepressive compound which has been investigated with the most modern methods is maprotiline. No correlation of the metabolite pattern with the acetylator phenotype was found in 44 individuals (26 of whom were slow acetylators) by Baumann et al. (1988). This finding is not surprising because the compound is a secondary aliphatic amine.

Miscellaneous observations

The observations of Young (1980) are difficult to interpret. He investigated the effects of thymoxamine on 30 patients with labyrinthine vertigo and also ascertained their acetylator phenotypes. He found that slow acetylators responded better than rapid acetylators. The reason why this finding is difficult to understand arises from a consideration of the structural formula. The only nitrogen atom is in a dimethylamino-ethoxy group and so it is unlike any of the compounds known to be acetylated even by a secondary metabolic step. The scheme of metabolism proposed by Duchene et al. (1988) does not include an acetylation step.

After a dose of 6 mg per kg body weight of prizidilol, slow acetylators had greater antihypertensive effects than rapid acetylators, a finding which was accompanied by higher plasma levels. Since the molecule has a hydrazide moiety it is highly likely that it is polymorphically acetylated (Larsson et al. 1981).

The use of cotrimazine (a combination of sulphadiazine and trimethoprim) to treat paracoccidioidomycosis was investigated in 22 patients who were phenotyped with isoniazid (Barraviera et al.

1989). The highest free sulphadiazine levels were obtained in slow acetylator patients, a result which would be expected from the careful pharmaco-kinetic studies of Vree *et al.* (1980).

The clinical significance of the polymorphic acetylation of dipyrone amrinone and the amino metabolite of clonazepam remain unexplored.

WHEN SHOULD ONE DO AN ACETYLATOR PHENOTYPING TEST IN CLINICAL PRACTICE?

This question has been addressed in detail by Clark (1985). There is one situation where this author regards phenotyping as definitely advantageous, namely for SASP therapy. Three situations are designated 'possibly advantageous', namely:

1 simultaneous therapy with phenytoin and isoniazid;
2 before treating tuberculosis with a once-weekly regimen;
3 before treating hypertension with high doses of hydralazine.

Regarding procainamide therapy, Clark (1985) is of the opinion that phenotyping is not necessary because the therapeutic effect (on arrhythmia) and serum concentrations of procainamide and *N*-acetyl procainamide can be monitored.

Since hydralazine is usually given in small doses combined with other drugs for hypertension the determination of acetylator phenotype is not required in all hypertensives to be treated. Knowledge of the phenotype may, however, be useful (as suggested by Ramsay *et al.* 1984), where it is desired to increase the dose of hydralazine above 200 mg/day.

The advocates of phenotyping patients receiving high doses of sulphasalazine were van Hees *et al.* (1979), who found that the majority of slow acetylators taking 4.5 to 6.0 g sulphasalazine daily will reach haemolytic plasma concentrations of sulphapyridine. They observed that 18 of 19 patients with haemolysis were slow acetylators, and of 17 patients without haemolysis there were only six slow acetylators.

The cost–benefit analysis of doing a phenotyping test before instituting therapy with both phenytoin and an antituberculous regimen containing isoniazid has not been ascertained. It could be argued that in most hospitals the phenytoin level will be monitored sequentially whatever the phenotyping test would have revealed, which makes the rationale for its deployment tenuous.

The case may be stronger for phenotyping before giving once-weekly treatment for tuberculosis. This is because the desire to institute such a treatment occurs in communities where financial resource are meagre. It might well be advantageous to phenotype – using, for example, the colorimetric test of Schröder (1972) and give twice-weekly treatment to rapid acetylators only.

Amonafide (5-amino-2-(2-(dimethylamino-ethyl)-1H-benz(de)-isoquinoline-1,3(2H)-dione; NSC 308847) is a new site-specific deoxyribonucleic acid (DNA) intercalating agent with apparent anti-tumour activity in carcinomas of breast and pro-state. The *N*-acetyl metabolite is active. Ratain *et al.* (1991) demonstrated that the production of this metabolite was correlated with the acetylator phenotype (as determined with a caffeine test). They also showed that rapid acetylators were particularly prone to the toxic effect of leucopenia from which the slow acetylators were protected. This situation is analogous to the treatment of childhood acute lymphatic leukaemia with azathioprine, which is referred to in the chapter on methylation reactions. It is not clear whether the anti-tumour effect with a fixed dosage regimen was greater in rapid acetylators, but now there is a proposal to give amonafide doses based on acetylator phenotype (Ratain *et al.* 1991).

THE GLOBAL DISTRIBUTION OF ALLELE FREQUENCY

In the early days of the study of the acetylation poly-morphism it was observed with regard to phenotype distribution that:

1 American Negroes did not differ much from American Caucasians (Evans *et al.* 1960);
2 Japanese were very different from Caucasians, in that about 90% of Japanese were rapid acetylators (Harris *et al.* 1958).

Soon after this, Sunahara (1961) observed that there was a 'cline' in the frequency of q (the allele controlling slow acetylation) along the Pacific Asian littoral in that the value rose steadily from a very low level in the far north to a fairly high level in Thailand.

Table 16.15. *Geographic distribution of the frequency of the allele controlling slow acetylation in the Pacific*

Reference	Ethnic group	Location collected	Latitude	q	SE (q)
North Pacific					
Sunahara & Urano 1963	Japanese	Hokkaido	43	0.31	0.05
Sunahara & Urano 1963	Korean	Korea	37	0.33	0.06
Kang & Lee 1973	Korean	Korea	37	0.34	0.02
Paik *et al.* 1988	Korean	Seoul	37	0.49	0.02
Shin *et al.* 1992	Korean	Seoul	37	0.43	0.07
Sunahara & Urano 1963	Japanese	Japan	35	0.34	0.01
Mitchell *et al.* 1960	Japanese (T)	Denver Colorado	35[a]	0.45	0.04
Knight *et al.* 1959	Japanese (T)	Salt Lake City	35[a]	0.35	0.09
Dufour *et al.* 1964	Japanese (T)	Tokyo	35	0.31	0.03
Horai *et al.* 1982	Japanese	Tokyo	35	0.32	0.11
Horai *et al.* 1989	Japanese	Tokyo	35	0.25	0.03
Xu & Jiang 1990	Chinese	Shanghai	31	0.44	0.04
Horai *et al.* 1988	Chinese	Changsa	28	0.36	0.04
Sunahara & Urano 1963	Ryukyuans	Ryukyuan Islands	27	0.40	0.04
Ellard & Gammon 1977	Chinese (T)	Singapore	23[a]	0.46	0.02
Sunahara *et al.* 1963b	Chinese	Taiwan	23	0.41	0.04
Evans 1963	Chinese	Liverpool	23[a]	0.47	0.06
Kukonaviriyapan *et al.* 1984	Thais	Kohn Kaen	16	0.67	0.03
Sunahara & Urano 1963	Thais	Thailand	14	0.54	0.04
Peters *et al.* 1972	Philippinos	Cebu	10	0.82	0.04
Ellard &Gammon 1977	Malays (T)	Singapore	1	0.65	0.04
South Pacific					
Cook *et al.* 1986	Papua, New Guineans	Lae	6	0.11	0.04
Hombhanje 1991	Papua, New Guineans	Boroko	6	0.32	0.15
Penketh *et al.* 1983	Papua, New Guineans	Highland and coastal provinces	6	0.16	0.05
	Indigenous population	New Britain	6	0.33	0.16
	Indigenous population	North Solomon Islands	8	0.80	0.09
Hayward 1975	Polynesians	Auckland	37	0.33	0.04

[a]Population ascribed to latitude other than that at which it was collected.
T, tuberculosis patients.
Modified from: Karim *et al.* (1981)

Now many more estimates of q are available and so it is possible to investigate the relationship between geographical location and q more fully.

However, as has been pointed out previously (Karim *et al.* 1981), the results of some surveys cannot be used for this purpose for a variety of reasons, as follows.

1 The division between the slow and rapid acetylators is not sufficiently sharp so that the estimates of allele frequency are not acceptable.
2 In otherwise excellent studies the ethnic structure of the population is not clearly defined.
3 The populations studied moved to their present locations only a few generations ago. This category included, for example, all North American and Australian Caucasian samples.
4 The population sample contains patients with a vari-

ety of disorders. Only samples of patients with tuberculosis have been included as representative of the population since there is evidence that allele frequencies do not differ in them from samples of healthy subjects.
5 The population is known to be an amalgam of different ethnic groups in unknown proportions. This objection applies to all North American Negro samples, and there is also a problem with Eskimos and Amerindians.

Some ethnic groups remain isolated in their new environment and for this reason Japanese in North America have been ascribed to Tokyo and Chinese in Singapore to Canton.

The Pacific Asian littoral data are displayed in Table 16.15 and Fig. 16.13. The frequency of q is low near the Arctic and increases towards the

Pacific

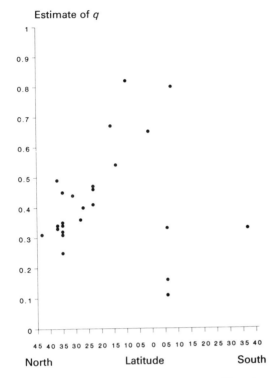

Fig. 16.13. Frequency of q (the allele controlling slow acetylation) as related to latitude in the Pacific.

Equator. The regression is $q = 0.74 - 0.0109x$ (where x = latitude North). The points south of the equator were not included in this computation. The correlation coefficient $r = 0.83$ ($p < 0.001$).

South of the Equator the pattern in the Pacific is incomplete because there are few data. Nevertheless, it is clear that the properties of the populations of Papua New Guinea do not fit the pattern of the Asian Pacific littoral because even though they are near the Equator, their frequency of q is very low. This finding might be explained by genetic drift.

With regard to the African continent (Table 16.16, Fig. 16.14) the value of q falls from North to South across the Equator; $r = 0.56$ ($p < 0.01$) and $q = 0.54 - 0.0047x$ (where x = latitude + 25° N), but a lot of the weight in this relationship is provided by the low value of q from !Kung Bushmen.

There is insufficient information available to assess the relationship between q and latitude in the subcontinent of India, in Europe, and in the Americas. No clear pattern emerges and there is no evidence of any cline with latitude. It would appear that the highest values for q are found in Arab/Middle Eastern populations (Tables 16.17, 16.18 and 16.19).

Africa

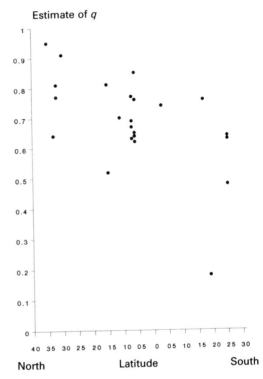

Fig. 16.14. Frequency of q (the allele controlling slow acetylation) as related to latitude in Africa.

The information available from South America is very meagre and shows no consistent pattern. In Bolivia, Lopez & de Claure (1987) observed the population frequency histogram for the plasma isoniazid concentration 6 hours after ingestion of a dose of 8–10 mg/kg. In Santa Cruz, at an elevation of 470 m above sea level, the antimodal value was very similar to that in other published series. In La Paz at an altitude of 3600 m the antimodal value was very much lower. They suggest that this might

Table 16.16. *Geographic distribution of the frequency of the allele controlling slow acetylation in Africa*

Reference	Ethnic group	Location collected	Latitude (°)	q	SE (q)
Hir *et al.* 1964	Moroccans (T)	Tangier	35 N	0.95	0.05
Bouayad *et al.* 1982	Moroccans	Casablanca	33 N	0.64	0.04
Karim *et al.* 1981	Libyans	Benghazi	32 N	0.81	0.05
Ali & Bashir 1991	N. Sudanese	Benghazi	32 N	0.77	0.04
Hashem *et al.* 1969	Egyptians	Cairo	30 N	0.91	0.03
Evans 1963	Non-Arab Sudanese	Khartoum	15 N	0.81	0.03
Homeida *et al.* 1986	Arab Sudanese	Khartoum	15 N	0.52	0.05
Fawcett & Gammon 1975	Northern Nigerians (T*)	Zaria	11 N	0.70	0.03
Salako & Aderounmu 1977	Nigerians	Ibadan	7 N	0.77	0.03
Jeyakumar & French 1981	Yoruba Nigerians	Ibadan	7 N	0.67	0.03
Jeyakumar & French 1986	Nigerians	Ibadan	7 N	0.63	0.03
Jeyakumar *et al.* 1990	Nigerians	Ibadan	7 N	0.69	0.07
Eze & Obidoa 1978	Nigerians	Nsukka	6 N	0.64	0.04
Eze 1987	Nigerians	Nsukka	6 N	0.85	0.03
Odeigah & Okunowo 1989	Nigerians	Lagos	6 N	0.62	0.02
Afonja *et al.* 1979	Yoruba Nigerians	Lagos	6 N	0.65	0.03
	Nigerians (Ibos)	Lagos	6 N	0.76	0.05
Ellard *et al.* 1975	Kenyan (T)	East Africa	3 S	0.74[a]	0.05
	Ugandan				
	Tanzanian			0.74[b]	0.02
	Zambian				
Nhachi 1988	Zimbabweans	Harare	17 S	0.76	0.03
Jenkins *et al.* 1974	Kung	Tsumkwe	19 S	0.18	0.09
Hodgkin *et al.* 1979	S African Blacks (T)	Pretoria	25 S	0.64	0.03
Glatthar 1977	S African Blacks (T)	Pretoria	25 S	0.48	0.06
Eidus *et al.* 1979	S African Blacks	Pretoria	25 S	0.64	0.04

T, tuberculosis patients; T*, mixture of healthy subjects and tuberculosis patients.
[a] 57 patients; [b] 204 patients, both being random selection (treatment group 4 of East African/British Medical Research Council Short Course Study, 1974) from 953 patients studied in 35 centres in East Africa. The latitude stated has been calculated as a weighted mean obtained by taking the number of patients of each nationality and the latitude of the four capitals. The individual details of the patients concerned are not now available. The 57 subjects were phenotyped with both sulphadimidine and matrix isoniazid, while the 204 subjects were phenotyped with matrix isoniazid only.
Modified from: Karim *et al.* (1981).

have been due to hypoxia, but also that it might have some relationship to the different estimates of q obtained from the two populations of tuberculous subjects (0.67 and 0.35, respectively).

A logical interpretation for geographic variability would have to be based on a knowledge of the natural substrates of the polymorphic N-acetyltransferase but hitherto no information is available on this point.

It may be speculated that along the Asian Pacific littoral, latitude might influence q by means of the chemical environment (e.g. food), or by means of the physical environment (e.g. temperature, radiation or magnetosphere).

Completion of the global pattern requires technically satisfactory surveys of indigenous populations in South America, the South Pacific and hitherto neglected areas of Africa.

ASSOCIATIONS BETWEEN ACETYLATOR PHENOTYPES AND SPONTANEOUS DISORDERS

It has been shown in the preceding section that there are significant associations between drug-induced effects and acetylator phenotypes. In this section the evidence will be reviewed for associations between acetylator phenotypes and 'spontaneous' (i.e. non-drug-induced) disorders. This subject has previously been reviewed (Evans 1984) but now quite a lot of new data have emerged.

There are a number of points which have to be considered when evaluating studies of associations between the acetylator polymorphism phenotypes and spontaneous disorders; the most important are discussed below.

Table 16.17. *Geographic distribution of the frequency of the allele controlling slow acetylation in Asia excluding Pacific Littoral*

Reference	Ethnic group	Location collected	Latitude (°N)	q	SE (q)
Sardas *et al.* 1986a	Turkish	Ankara	40	0.78	0.03
Bozkurt *et al.* 1990b	Turkish	Ankara	40	0.78	0.02
Goedde *et al.* 1977a	Puchtoons	Afghanistan	34	0.82	0.03
	Tajiks	Afghanistan	34	0.78	0.03
	Hazaras	Afghanistan	34	0.65	0.03
	Usbeks	Afghanistan	34	0.51	0.04
Sardas *et al.* 1993	Iranians	Ankara (but ascribed to latitude of Estfahan)	32	0.88	0.03
Irshaid *et al.* 1991	Jordanians	Irbid	32	0.82	0.02
Nair *et al.* 1984	Indians	Chandigarh	30	0.78	0.03
Gupta *et al.* 1984	Indians	Chandigarh	30	0.78	0.03
Husain *et al.* 1973	Indians (T)	Bikaner	28	0.85	0.02
Evans *et al.* 1985	Saudi Arabians	Riyadh	24	0.82	0.03
Sinha *et al.* 1978	Indians (T)	Ranchi	23	0.76	0.02
Sen *et al.* 1982	Indians (T)	Calcutta	22	0.74	0.02
Islam 1982	Saudi Arabians	Jeddah	21	0.82	0.03
Desai *et al.* 1973	Indians	Bombay	19	0.44	0.07
Smith & Kyi 1968	Burmese	Rangoon	16	0.61	0.04
Devadatta *et al.* 1960	Indians (T)	Madras	13	0.76	0.03
Gangadharam *et al.* 1961	Indians (T)	Madras	13	0.78	0.02
Rao *et al.* 1970	Indians (T)	Madras	13	0.71	0.03
Peters *et al.* 1975	Indians (T)	Madras	13	0.80	0.04
Raghupati Sarma *et al.* 1976	Indians (T)	Madras	13	0.77	0.02
Gurumurthy *et al.* 1984	Indians (T)	Madras	13	0.77	0.006
Parthasarathy *et al.* 1986	Indians (T)	Madras	13	0.75	0.02
Ellard & Gammon 1977	Indians (T)	Singapore	1	0.87	0.03

T, tuberculosis patients.
The low estimate of q given by Desai *et al.* (1973) may result from a methodological difficulty.
The many reports from Madras Tuberculosis Chemotherapy Centre may not represent completely independent series.
Modified from: Karim *et al.* (1981).

Table 16.18. *Geographic distribution of the frequency of the allele controlling slow acetylation in North and South America*

Reference	Ethnic group	Location collected	Latitude (°)	q	SE (q)
Eidus *et al.* 1974	Eskimos	Coppermine	67 N	0.77	0.03
Scott *et al.* 1969	Eskimos (T)	Anchorage	61 N	0.46	0.04
	Athabascan Indians	Anchorage	61 N	0.62	0.06
Armstrong & Peart 1960	Eskimos (T)	Hudson and James Bay	57 N	0.22	0.03
Jeanes *et al.* 1972	Eskimos	Edmonton	53 N	Nil	–
	Canadian Indians	Edmonton	53 N	0.29	0.14
Mitchell *et al.* 1960	American Indians (T)	Denver	39 N	0.47	0.05
Inaba & Arias 1987	Panamanian Indians:				
	Teribe	Bocas del Toro	9 N	0.53	0.05
	Cuna	Bocas del Toro	9 N	0.49	0.06
Goedde *et al.* 1977b	Shuara Indians	Ecuador	2 S	0.47	0.05
Lopez & de Claure 1987	Bolivians	La Paz	16 S	0.67	0.04
	Bolivians	Santa Cruz	17 S	0.35	0.06
Goedde *et al.* 1984	Atacameno Indians	Toconao	22 S	0.45	0.05
Ligueros *et al.* 1989	Chilians (T)	Santiago	33 S	0.62	0.06

T, tuberculosis patients.
Modified from: Karim *et al.* (1981).

Table 16.19. *Geographic distribution of the frequency of the allele controlling slow acetylation in Europe*

Reference	Ethnic group	Location collected	Latitude (°N)	(q)	SE (q)
Tiitinen et al. 1967	Lapps	Inari	69	0.62	0.06
Ellard et al. 1973a	Lapps	Inari	69	0.55	0.09
Mattila & Tiitinen 1967	Finns (T)	Helsinki	60	0.86	0.03
Tiitinen 1969c	Finns (T)	Helsinki	60	0.77	0.03
Tiitinen 1969a	Finns (T*)	Helsinki	60	0.76	0.02
Tiitinen et al. 1967	Finns	Helsinki	60	0.78	0.05
Frislid et al. 1976	Norwegians	Oslo	60	0.74	0.08
Talseth & Landmark 1977	Norwegians	Oslo	60	0.72	0.08
Chekharina et al. 1978	Russians	Leningrad	60	0.82	0.03
Hanngren et al. 1970	Swedish (T)	Stockholm	59	0.82	0.02
Molin et al. 1977	Swedish	Linkoping	58	0.72	0.06
Lower et al. 1979	Danish	Copenhagen	55	0.72	0.04
	Swedish	Lund	55	0.82	0.03
Paulsen & Nilsson 1985	Swedish	Lund	55	0.77	0.02
Lilyin et al. 1983	Russian	Moscow	55	0.70	0.03
Siegmund et al. 1988	Presumably Germans	Greifswald	54	0.71	0.03
Siegmund et al. 1991	Germans	Greifswald	54	0.74	0.02
Hoo et al. 1977	German	Hamburg	53	0.72	0.08
Hanssen et al. 1985	German	Hamburg	53	0.65	0.06
Evans Series 1 1969	British White (T*)	Liverpool	53	0.79	0.03
Karim & Evans 1976	British White	Liverpool	53	0.83	0.05
Evans et al. 1972	British White (T)	Liverpool	53	0.81	0.03
Eze & Evans 1972	British White	Liverpool	53	0.77	0.05
Schröder & Evans 1972a	British White	Liverpool	53	0.75	0.05
Schröder & Evans 1972b	British White	Liverpool	53	0.75	0.06
Gow & Evans 1964	British White	Liverpool	53	0.81	0.03
Bartmann & Massmann 1960	German	Berlin	52	0.71	0.08
Iwainsky 1961	German	Berlin	52	0.70	0.03
Hildebrand & Seiferi 1989	Caucasians	Berlin	52	0.78	0.01
Tomaskiewicz et al. 1979	Polish	Poznan	52	0.67	0.06
Orzechowska-Juzwenko et al. 1986	Polish	Warsaw	52	0.70	0.05
Skretkowicz et al. 1981	Polish	Lodz	51	0.68	0.06
Orzechowska-Juzwenko et al. 1990	Polish	Wroclaw	51	0.70	0.05
Schmeidel 1960	German	Leipzig	51	0.76	0.01
Ellard et al. 1975	British White	London	51	0.78	0.04
Philip et al. 1987a	British White	London and Orpington	51	0.78	0.02
Viznerova et al. 1973	Czech	Prague	50	0.77	0.02
Ellard et al. 1973b	Czech	Prague	50	0.77	0.07
Drozdz et al. 1987	Polish	Katowice	50	0.78	0.03
Hykes & Elis 1980	Czech	Kladno	50	0.72	0.05
Bernard et al. 1961	French	Paris	49	0.78	0.02
Hadasova et al. 1990	Czech	Brno	49	0.78	0.03
Stoll et al. 1989	Presumably French	Strasbourg	48	0.71	0.03
Bressollette et al. 1990	Breton	Brest	48	0.81	0.05
	Bigouden	Brest	48	0.82	0.06
Kergueris et al. 1986	French	Nantes	47	0.80	0.01
Pontiroli et al. 1985	Italian	Milan	45	0.84	0.04
Fantoli et al. 1963	Italian	Rome	42	0.74	0.03
de March & Garcia 1966	Spanish	Barcelona	41	0.75	0.05
Podymov et al. 1988	Armenians	Yerevan	40	0.82	0.03
Ladero et al. 1979	Spanish	Madrid	40	0.75	0.03
Jimenez-Nieto et al. 1989	Spanish	Madrid	40	0.76	0.03
Ladero et al. 1989	Spanish	Madrid, Badajez	40, 39	0.76	0.03

T, tuberculosis patients; T*, mixture of tuberculous patients and healthy subjects.
Modified from. Karim et al. 1981).

1 Was the disease entity being investigated adequately defined? It is preferable to define the disease entity using some internationally accepted criterion. For example, systemic lupus erythematosus (SLE) can be defined according to the American Rheumatological Association criteria (Tan *et al.* 1982). There was very little value in, for example, publishing the phenotypes of 100 patients with various lung disorders without providing details of the diagnoses (Walsted 1975).

2 Was the ethnic composition of both patient and control groups defined? It is essential to know the ethnic composition of the patient and control groups. For example, in the otherwise excellent paper of Zacest & Koch-Weser (1972) the ethnic composition of the group of 20 hypertensives studied in Boston, Massachusetts is not stated. Sometimes an arbitrary assumption with regard to ethnic group seems warranted, for example presumably Lawson *et al.* (1979) were studying SLE and rheumatoid arthritis in white Glasgow citizens.

3 Was the patient sample a stratum (that is, derived from a selected group within the population)? It is preferable that the sample of the disorder being investigated is as unselected as possible. Sometimes, however, a selection is inevitable. For example, it is possible that a particularly severely afflicted group is studied simply because the patients attend a special hospital clinic for their disorder.

4 Was the phenotyping test performed in a technically satisfactory manner: that is, was the phenotype definition satisfactory? It is clear that ambiguous results (subjects with 'intermediate' status) are best avoided by rigorous attention to detail. For example when using the sulphamethazine test of Evans (1969) some investigators omit the collection of the blood sample and rely solely on the urine specimen. Obviously the same confidence cannot be placed in the results as if both specimens were collected and their results demonstrated to be in agreement with each other, in the form of a scattergram. The separation between the two phenotypes must be clear. When a diagram is constructed from the data in Godeau *et al.* (1973), for example, it is not possible to assess the phenotype frequencies in their lupus erythematosus patients, so this study is not considered further.

5 Did the disorder being investigated interfere with the phenotyping test? This aspect has been discussed in an earlier section. The group of patients and the group of controls should both be tested under circumstances which are as similar as possible. The position and activity of the persons phenotyped may be of importance. For example, Levi *et al.* (1968) found that isoniazid half-lives in patients with liver disease are increased by about 20% by the change from lying to walking. On the other hand, pretreatment with other drugs (mainly barbiturates) had no effect on the distribution curve of plasma isoniazid half-lives in normal subjects.

6 Satisfactory control series for comparison. Satisfactory control series are required (as mentioned above) before any association between phenotype and disorder can be assessed. This is probably the most difficult point of all. It is generally considered that unaffected siblings constitute the most satisfactory control group for studies of associations between disorders and genetic phenotypes (Clarke *et al.* 1956; Mayo & Street 1986). Other possible controls which may be used are unrelated domiciliary controls (Evans *et al.* 1982) or general population controls. Using other patients who do not suffer from the disease being investigated is generally not considered a good idea because their illness may have some relationship to the polymorphism in question. A considerable body of data is required to rule out such a possibility.

7 Reproducibility of the statistical association. Because of the difficulties outlined above, confidence in the validity of an association increases when similar results have been obtained by different investigators in widely different locations and in different ethnic groups.

Studies of associations between various disorders and acetylator phenotypes are reviewed in the sections which follow.

Bladder cancer

The expectation of an association in this disorder (which is, perhaps, not really correctly described as 'spontaneous') arose principally from the basic observation of Glowinski *et al.* (1978) that various carcinogenic amines, particularly benzidine and β-naphthylamine, were polymorphically acetylated

Table 16.20. Association of the slow acetylator phenotype with bladder cancer

Reference	Location of study	Number of Subjects — Bladder cancer Slow (h)	Bladder cancer Rapid (k)	Controls Slow (H)	Controls Rapid (K)	Approximate relative risk (x)	$\log_e x$ (y)	Sampling variance (V)	Weight $\left(\frac{1}{V} = w\right)$	Significance of difference from zero (wy^2)	wy
Lower et al. 1979	Copenhagen	46	25	38	36	1.7288	0.5474	0.1124	8.8962	2.6660	4.8700
Lower et al. 1979	Lund	80	35	79	39	1.1267	0.1193	0.0776	12.8826	0.1832	1.5365
Cartwright et al. 1982	Huddersfield	74	37	118	89	1.5005	0.4058	0.0592	16.9025	2.7832	6.8587
Woodhouse et al. 1982	Newcastle	21	9	16	11	1.5774	0.4557	0.2876	3.4769	0.7222	1.5846
Evans et al. 1983	Liverpool	66	34	510	342	1.2932	0.2571	0.0484	20.6748	1.3669	5.3160
Lower 1983	Deepwater NJ	13	5	11	8	1.8142	0.5957	0.4325	2.3119	0.8203	1.3771
Miller & Cosgriff 1983	Rochester NY	12	14	18	8	0.3961	-0.9394	0.3073	3.2538	2.7908	-3.0134
Cartwright 1984	Portugal	14	33	10	25	1.0512	0.0499	0.2254	4.4356	0.0110	0.2214
Ladero et al. 1985	Madrid	83	47	90	67	1.3111	0.2709	0.0584	17.1136	1.2559	4.6360
Hanssen et al. 1985	Hamburg	65	40	18	24	2.1418	0.7617	0.1322	7.5658	4.3890	5.7625
Mommsen & Aagaard 1986	Arhus	145	83	54	46	1.4867	0.3966	0.0582	17.1783	2.7017	6.8126
Karakaya et al. 1986	Ankara	9	14	67	42	0.4125	-0.8855	0.2046	4.8869	3.8317	-4.3272
Kaisary et al. 1987	Bristol	59	39	54	56	1.5616	0.4457	0.0774	12.9211	2.5669	5.7591
Bicho et al. 1988	Lisbon	21	28	35	49	1.0519	0.0506	0.1277	7.8299	0.0200	0.3961
Roots et al. 1989	Berlin	67	35	149	143	1.8251	0.6016	0.3339	2.9952	1.0841	1.8020
Horai et al. 1989	Tokyo	3	48	13	190	1.0183	0.1816	0.3471	2.8812	0.0009	0.0523
								Totals	146.2064	27.1939	39.6443

Weighted mean value of $y = Y = \frac{\Sigma wy}{\Sigma w} = 0.2711$; antilog $= X = 1.3115$; SE $(Y) = \sqrt{\frac{1}{\Sigma w}} = 0.0827$.

95% fiducial limits of $Y = 0.4474$ and 0.0949.

Equivalent X values to the 95% fiducial limits of $Y = 1.5642$ and 1.0996.

Significance of difference of X from unity $= \chi_1^2 = \frac{(\Sigma wy)^2}{\Sigma w} = 10.7497$ ($p < 0.001$).

Heterogeneity estimate $= \chi_{15}^2 = \Sigma wy^2 - \frac{(\Sigma wy)^2}{\Sigma w} = 16.4443$ ($p > 0.30$).

The calculations were made to 6 decimal places. The numbers shown here have been rounded off to 4 decimal places.

Source: Modification by Haldane (1955) of the method of Woolf (1954).

in human and rabbit livers. These compounds are well known to be carcinogenic in humans.

It has also been shown by Flammang *et al.* (1987) that the carcinogen 2-aminofluorene is polymorphically *N*-acetylated by human liver cytosolic preparations.

The first surveys of acetylator phenotypes in bladder cancer were carried out by Lower *et al.* (1979) in Denmark and Southern Sweden. After this group had revealed a significant association between the slow acetylator phenotype and bladder cancer, other groups made similar surveys. The results are shown in Table 16.20 and indicate that in 16 series the slow acetylator phenotype is about 30% more associated with bladder cancer than would be expected at random. Furthermore, there is no significant heterogeneity between the series.

The question of controls is of paramount importance. The nature of the control group has varied between different samples. In some series (e.g. Cartwright *et al.* 1982; Kaisary *et al.* 1987) urological patients who did not have cancer were used as controls. In other series, geriatric patients (Woodhouse *et al.* 1982), patients with non-malignant disorders (Lower *et al.* 1979) and the spouse or an unrelated friend of each proband (Miller & Cosgriff 1983) were studied. In the study of Cartwright *et al.* (1982) both a population control group and a non-cancer patient control group were shown to be closely similar with regards to acetylator gene frequency. It was pointed out many years ago by Penrose (see Clarke *et al.* 1956) that the best form of control in association studies of this type is a non-affected sibling of each proband. A control group of this nature would obviously be very difficult to assemble for bladder cancer patients who have an average age of over 60 years. In the absence of this ideal, it gives some credence to the association that it is found consistently using various other types of control groups.

The overall finding needs closer scrutiny. First, it is known that bladder cancer occurs more commonly in urban and industrial environments than in rural settings. Sub-populations from Table 16.20, known to be derived from industrial environments, can be examined separately. This has been done in Table 16.21, and the result for the association does not differ much.

To take a highly selected group may be revealing. Amongst the 23 persons who had specifically been employed in the dye industry, who had developed

bladder cancer and who were phenotyped by Cartwright *et al.* (1982), only one was a rapid acetylator. This observation suggests that a high exposure to specific aromatic amines over a number of years is required to differentiate between the two acetylator phenotypes.

Five series give the acetylator phenotype distribution within grades of bladder cancer. When these are examined (Table 16.22) there is a hint in four series that the frequency of the slow acetylators is less with the more severe grades, but the trend is otherwise in the Danish series.

The idea was put forward by Evans *et al.* (1983) that, since the studies of associations had been largely conducted on patients attending urology clinics, one explanation for the findings might be that slow acetylators survive longer than rapid acetylators after having contracted the disease. (This was an alternative hypothesis to the favoured one, i.e. that the rapid acetylators, being more efficient at detoxifying the causative amines, were protected from developing the disease.) Evidence against this alternative hypothesis was supplied by Ladero *et al.* (1985) who found that the time interval between diagnosis and determination of the acetylator phenotype did not differ between the patients of the two phenotypes.

It was in 1895 that Rehn first described bladder cancer in three men engaged in the manufacture of magenta and he subsequently described other similar cases. He considered aniline to be the cause. However, it is now known that it is not. The aniline employed in Rehn's time was impure and contained numerous other compounds (Gorrod & Manson 1986).

In the 1920s and 1930s attention was focused on aromatic amines, especially naphythylamine and benzidine. These chemicals were used especially in the rubber industry. In 1949, practices were changed in the manufacture of new rubber so as to reduce exposure to these injurious chemicals (Whitty 1987), but the recycling of rubber made by the previously used processes may have to some extent defeated the object of the exercise.

In 1954, Case & Pearson showed that the age of death from bladder cancer in workers who handled aromatic amines and especially those working in the rubber industry was almost 15 years lower than in the general population. The mean induction period was about 16 years for benzidine and β-naphthyl-

Table 16.21. *Association of the slow acetylator phenotype with bladder cancer. Subpopulations exposed to urban and industrial environments*

Reference	Location of study	Number of Subjects Bladder cancer Slow (h)	Bladder cancer Rapid (k)	Controls Slow (H)	Controls Rapid (K)	Approximate relative risk (x)	$\text{Log}_e\ x$ (y)	Sampling variance (V)	Weight $\left(\frac{1}{V}=w\right)$	Significance of difference from zero (wy^2)	wy
Cartwright et al. 1982	Huddersfield	74	37	118	89	1.5005	0.4058	0.0592	16.9025	2.7832	6.8587
Evans et al. 1983	Liverpool	11	8	510	342	0.9077	−0.0968	0.1993	5.0171	0.0470	−0.4895
Lower 1983	Deepwater, NJ	13	5	11	8	1.8142	0.5956	0.4225	2.3119	0.8202	1.3771
Miller & Cosgriff 1983	Rochester, NY	6	9	18	8	0.3144	−1.1572	0.4066	2.4594	3.2934	−2.8460
Ladero et al. 1985	Madrid	41	14	90	67	2.1347	0.7583	0.1168	8.5652	4.9255	6.4952
Hanssen 1985	Hamburg	19	8	18	24	3.0382	1.1113	0.2537	3.7410	4.8668	4.3795
								Totals	39.1971	16.7361	15.7786

Weighted mean value of $Y = y = \dfrac{\Sigma wy}{\Sigma w} = 0.4025$; antilog $= X = 1.4596$; SE of $Y = \sqrt{\dfrac{1}{\Sigma w}} = 0.1597$.

95% fiducial limits of $Y = 0.8131$ and -0.0079.

The equivalent X values to the 95% fiducial limits of $Y = 2.2549$ and 0.9921.

Significance of difference of X from unity $= \chi_1^2 = \dfrac{(\Sigma wy)^2}{\Sigma w} = 6.3516$ $(p = 0.02)$.

Heterogeneity estimate $= \chi_5^2 = \Sigma wy^2 - \dfrac{(\Sigma wy)^2}{\Sigma w} = 10.3845$ $(p > 0.05)$.

The calculations were made to 6 decimal places. The numbers shown here have been rounded off to 4 decimal places.
Source: Modification by Haldane (1955) of the method of Woolf (1954).

Table 16.22. *Category of bladder cancer and acetylator phenotype*

Reference	Description of tumour category	Tumour category	Number of patients		% Slow acetylators
			Slow acetylators	Rapid acetylators	
Cartwright *et al.* 1982	Stage	T *in situ*	9	1	90
		T$_1$	47	20	70
		T$_2$	19	6	76
		T$_3$/T$_4$	5	2	71
Evans *et al.* 1983	Grades	1	40	20	67
		2, 3 and 4	20	12	63
Hanssen *et al.* 1985	Grading	I	14	4	78
		II	30	18	63
		III	21	18	54
Mommsen & Aagaard 1986	'T Category'	T$_a$	58	39	60
		T$_1$	30	22	58
		T$_2$	14	8	63
		T$_3$	30	10	75
		T$_4$	13	4	76
Kaisary *et al.* 1987	Stage	Non-aggressive I and II	42	23	65
		Aggressive III	17	16	52
Bicho *et al.* 1988	TMN classification	T$_1$	9	7	56
		T$_2$ and T$_3$	2	2	50

amine and about 22 years for α-naphthylamine (Gorrod & Manson 1986).

The situation with regard to tobacco smoking and bladder cancer has some elements of similarity to occupational exposure but at a much lower level of risk. Cartwright *et al.* (1983) reviewed the previous evidence, and in a large and carefully conducted survey concluded that smoking accounted for under one-third of the attributable risk to developing bladder cancer. The previous studies had indicated that the risk from smoking was somewhat higher (Koroltchouk *et al.* 1987).

It is known that many carcinogenic substances, including many aromatic amines (such as β-naphthylamine) and nitrosamines, are present in tobacco smoke, and the urine of smokers has been found to be mutagenic (Cartwright *et al.* 1983). Also 4-aminobiphenyl, known to be a powerful bladder carcinogen, forms haemoglobin adducts in persons who smoke certain types of tobacco (Ronco *et al.* 1990). The suggestion has been made, therefore, that aromatic amines like β-naphthylamine from tobacco smoke may, over a long period, be responsible for the increased risk of developing bladder cancer in smokers.

Other types of amines are also known to be carcinogenic. For example, 2-amino-3-methylimidazo

(4,5-f) quinoline (IQ) and 2-amino-3,8-dimethylimidazo (4,5-f) quinoxaline (MeIQx). These and similar heterocyclic amines are produced in cooked food as well as in cigarette smoke and are known to be carcinogenic. They accumulate in the plasmas of uraemic patients who are known to be more liable to develop cancers (Yanagisawa & Wada 1989). Thus IQ and MeIQx may represent natural carcinogenic substrates for polymorphic acetylation.

The acetylation of IQ, MeIQx and similar molecules has been investigated using COS-1 cells in which various human genes were expressed singly and in combination. It was found that N-hydroxylation was carried out by both *CYP 1A1* and *CYP 1A2*. Acetylation was of three types, namely, N-acetylation, O-acetylation and N–O-transacetylation, and these reactions were preferentially catalysed by polymorphic NAT2. The result of these reactions was the production of N-acetyoxy-N-arylamine which is presumed to be spontaneously degraded via unstable arylnitrenium ions to the production of carcinogenic DNA adducts. The highest activity was obtained with the combination of *CYP 1A2* and *NAT2* (Minchin *et al.* 1992; Probst *et al.* 1992).

On the other hand, the monomorphic NAT1 was able to N-acetylate the aromatic amines 2-aminofluorene and 4-aminobiphenyl and also to O-acetyl-ate the N-hydroxy derivatives (Minchin et al. 1992).

The relationship of these metabolic capacities to the acetylation polymorphism in vivo needs to be further explored. It would be interesting to see the metabolism of compounds as discussed above in tissues derived from humans of different genotypic constitutions (see Hein 1988 for a further discussion).

Two views may be taken regarding the relationship between the acetylation phenotype and bladder cancer. First, it may be considered that in rapid acetylators aromatic amines will be acetylated in the liver and intestinal mucosa to such a degree that very few, if any, free compounds will reach the bladder; whereas, in slow acetylators, free amines are more likely to reach the bladder. Secondly, it may be considered that the bladder mucosa itself may exhibit polymorphic N-acetyltransferase activity, so that in rapid acetylators free aromatic amines would be locally acetylated and eliminated more efficiently than in slow acetylators.

Carcinogenic arylamine acetylation activities have been examined in bladder mucosal cytosols from human organ donors by Kirlin et al. (1989) and have been found to be polymorphic. This finding was not, however, fully supported by the observations of Land et al. (1989) or Pacifici et al. (1988). In an analogous N-acetyltransferase polymorphism in Syrian hamsters, Hein et al. (1987) have shown that bladder mucosal enzyme activity was completely concordant with liver enzyme activity. So it seems likely that the polymorphic enzyme activity in both liver and bladder mucosa contribute to the differential phenotypic risk of developing bladder cancer.

As pointed out by Schulte (1988), the carcinoma of the bladder incidence in Japan is low (6.3 per 100 000), paralleling a low frequency of the slow acetylator phenotype in the population (11%); this is to be compared with the situation in the USA where the figures are 25.8 per 100 000 and 58%, respectively. In this context the study of Horai et al. (1989), who phenotyped 51 patients with non-occupational bladder cancer, is of interest. Only three slow acetylators were found, compared with 13 out of 203 healthy control individuals – a non-significant difference. The grade of cancer was not associated with acetylator phenotype. This finding

strengthens the idea that it is slow acetylators who are heavily exposed to carcinogens, particularly at work, who are more liable to develop bladder cancer.

Occupational exposure to polymorphically acetylated compounds

Interesting data, which are related to the studies described above on cancer of the bladder, come from studies from the occupational medicine field.

Dewan et al. (1986) studied workers in a chemical plant in India who were engaged in the manufacture of benzidine hydrochloride. The acetylator status of workers was established with a sulpha-dimidine test. The urinary benzidine concentration was determined both before and after a work shift. The results before the work shift show a clear separation of the two phenotypes (6S,5R) and the urinary benzidine concentrations were significantly higher in the slow acetylators. The results at the end of the shift did not reveal a clear separation between phenotypes, but all the workers showed a raised level of urinary benzidine concentration as compared with the pre-shift values – particularly those with a higher percentage value of acetylsulpha-methazine in blood on the phenotyping test.

This publication provides strong support for benzidine being polymorphically acetylated in humans. The slow acetylator's bladder mucosa would seem to be more consistently exposed to higher concentrations of benzidine. The authors make the following provocative statement at the end of their discussion:

Perhaps it may also be worthwhile to carry out acetylator phenotyping as a preplacement investigation for the prevention of occupational bladder cancer in countries where exposure to benzidine remains a serious health hazard.

Support for the general idea is also provided by Peters et al. (1990) who found there was a correlation between percentage acetylation of benzidine and sulphamethazine in 10 human liver samples (though their differentiation between rapid and slow acetylator livers was not as good as that of Evans & White 1964).

The mutagenicity of urine from dye workers was found to be higher in slow acetylators than in rapid acetylators by Sinues *et al.* (1992).

Lewalter & Korallus (1985) were interested in investigating the chemical stresses to which the contents of erythrocytes are subjected in industrial workers handling aniline. From the acetanilide excretion observed in the urine during 'normal' industrial exposure, they were able to segregate the workers they studied into slow and rapid acetylators. The intra-erythrocytic aniline concentration was much higher in the former and the methaemoglobin (Met Hb) level marginally so. The urinary free aniline excretion was very small in the rapid acetylators, but appreciable (270–560 µg/g creatinine) in the slow acetylators. A rapid and a slow acetylator were studied after accidental high industrial exposure to aniline. The former had a Met Hb level of 7% and a urinary acetanilide excretion of 11 mg/g creatinine, whereas the latter had figures of 45% and 100 µg/g, respectively. All workers observed by the authors with Met Hb levels of >30% were slow acetylators. Erythrocyte conjugates were at a high level and urinary acetanilide excretion at a lower level in slow acetylators as compared with rapid acetylators, when workers with a Met Hb level of 5% were examined. These changes within erythrocytes could not be reproduced *in vitro*. From these observations it could be deduced that the chemical stress caused within the body (as exemplified by the red cell) was much greater in slow than in rapid acetylators.

A recent paper (Kawakubo *et al.* 1988) demonstrated polymorphic acetylation of 2-aminofluorene in the skin of hamsters and considerable arylamine *N*-acetylation activity in human skin. These findings suggest the possibility that the acetylator polymorphism might be of importance in some occupationally determined skin cancers.

An interaction between occupational exposure and the personal habit of smoking is suggested by the finding of Vineis *et al.* (1990) that 4-aminobiphenyl-haemoglobin adduct concentrations were higher in slow acetylators when the users of two different types of tobacco were surveyed.

Colorectal carcinoma

Four studies are available in which patients with colorectal carcinoma and controls have had their acetylator phenotypes determined (Table 16.23).

They do not substantiate the hypothesis that rapid acetylation is statistically associated with this disorder. Kirlin *et al.* (1991) studied colonic surgical specimens from 12 non-cancer patients and 23 cancer patients. They claimed to be able to establish the acetylator genotypes from the specimens using a variety of substrates. The distributions of genotypes were not significantly different in the two groups.

These are disappointing results in view of the enzymological and biochemical background. The enzymic characteristics of the human colonic mucosa are different from those of the bladder mucosa. In the bladder there are high levels of *N*-acetyltransferase (NAT) activity with low levels of *N*-hydroxyarylamine *O*-acetyltransferase (OAT) activity. In the colon both enzymic activities are high (Hein 1988; Kirlin *et al.* 1991). This distinction could be important in as much as whilst the bladder NAT inactivates carcinogenic amines, the colonic mucosa activates hydroxyarylamines.

It has been suggested that *O*-acetylation of *N*-hydroxyarylamine metabolites converts them into DNA-reactive derivatives which could initiate large bowel cancer (Lang *et al.* 1986). In this context it is interesting that Wohlleb *et al.* (1990) found that eating bacon and barbecued, smoked and cured meats seemed to enhance the risk of developing colorectal cancer. Some of these foods contain heterocyclic arylamines which are known to be carcinogenic. Possibly such compounds may be activated to a greater degree by rapid, compared with slow, acetylators.

It is of great interest in this context that Flammang *et al.* (1987), using 35 human liver cytosol preparations were able to show a correlation between sulphamethazine *N*-acetylation activity (which indicated the phenotype) and the acetyl CoA-dependent *N*-hydroxy-2-aminofluorene *O*-acetyltransferase activity. The latter activity was determined by a DNA binding assay.

In theory there is a possibility, therefore, that the rapid acetylator has a greater capacity than the slow to activate a carcinogenic *N*-hydroxyarylamine to form arylamine-DNA adducts.

Nevertheless, the observed facts (i.e. no significant association of colonic cancer with the rapid acetylation phenotype) are in keeping with an epidemiologic observation. Japanese populations which have a very high frequency of rapid

Table 16.23. *Test of the association of the rapid acetylator phenotype with colorectal cancer*

Reference	Location of study	Number of Subjects				Approximate relative risk (x)	$\text{Log}_e x$ (y)	Sampling variance (V)	Weight $\left(\frac{1}{V} = w\right)$	Significance of difference from zero (wy^2)	wy
		Colorectal cancer		Controls							
		Slow (h)	Rapid (k)	Slow (H)	Rapid (K)						
Lang et al. 1986	Little Rock, AR	20	20	28[a]	11	2.4783	0.9076	0.2130	4.6936	3.8660	4.2597
Ilett et al. 1987	Western Australia	22	27	26[a]	19[a]	1.6610	0.5074	0.1662	6.0158	1.5488	3.0524
Roots et al. 1989	Berlin	67	53	149	143	0.7981	−0.2255	0.0468	21.3515	1.0857	−4.8148
Ladero et al. 1991	Madrid & Badajoz	60	49	56	40	1.1414	0.1323	0.0783	12.7670	0.2234	1.6887
								Totals	44.8280	6.7239	4.1860

[a]Young controls.

Weighted mean value of $y = \bar{y} = Y = \dfrac{\Sigma wy}{\Sigma w} = \dfrac{4.1860}{44.8280} = 0.0934$; antilog of $Y = X = 1.0979$.

$\text{SE}\,(Y) = \sqrt{\dfrac{1}{\Sigma w}} = 0.1494.$

95% fiducial limits of $Y = 0.5686$ and -0.3819.
Equivalent X values to the 95% fiducial limits of $Y = 1.7658$ and 0.6826.

Significance of difference of X from unity $= \chi_1^2 = \dfrac{(\Sigma wy)^2}{\Sigma w} = 0.3909$ $(p > 0.50)$.

Heterogeneity estimate $= \chi_3^2 = \Sigma wy^2 - \dfrac{(\Sigma wy)^2}{\Sigma w} = 6.3330$ $(p > 0.10)$.

The calculations were made to 6 decimal places. The numbers shown here have been rounded off to 4 decimal places.
Source: Modification by Haldane (1955) of the method of Woolf (1954).

acetylators exhibit a very low incidence of colorectal cancer (Connor *et al.* 1986).

Carcinoma of the larynx

The acetylator phenotype distribution of patients with epidermoid cancer of the larynx was compared with that of normal individuals in the Polish population by Drozdz *et al.* (1987). Slow acetylators were much more frequent amongst the patients than among the controls.

Furthermore, when cigarette smokers were compared with non-smokers it was found that (1) both phenotypes had a higher relative risk of being associated with the disease than non-smokers and (2) slow acetylator smokers had a much higher (× 10.9) relative risk than rapid acetylator smokers of being associated with the disease.

The former finding is in keeping with the previously known facts (Brownson & Chang 1987).

However, the results of Drozdz *et al.* (1987) were not confirmed by Roots *et al.* (1989): see Table 16.24.

Bronchial carcinoma

The same ideas underlie the examination of populations of patients with bronchial carcinoma for the frequency of the acetylator phenotypes, as for carcinoma of the bladder and larynx. All three diseases are known to be statistically associated with smoking. Cigarette smoke contains carcinogenic aromatic amines − and these aromatic amines are polymorphically acetylated in man.

As far as the author is aware, however, it has not been determined whether the bronchial mucosa itself actually exhibits polymorphic *N*-acetyltransferase activity. Four surveys of acetylator phenotype in bronchial carcinoma patients and controls yield no hint of the association of either phenotype with the disorder (Table 16.25).

Cancer of the breast

Seven studies are available of the acetylator phenotypes of women with breast cancer. The first study to be published was that of Bulovskaya *et al.* (1978), who found a much greater frequency of rapid acetylators amongst patients than in a control group of 'healthy females some of them with age-associated cardiovascular disturbances who matched the cancer patients by age'. These workers also found an increase in the acetylating capacity of the carcinoma patients. Rather disconcertingly, six patients apparently changed their phenotypes after chemotherapy. In three the slow phenotype became rapid and in three the opposite change occurred. The authors suggest that this change occurred after therapy because of the lessening of some hormonal or metabolic influence of the tumour. Bulovskaya *et al.* (1978) also describe a general increase in the acetylating capacity of breast carcinoma patients.

The results of six other series are incorporated in Table 16.26. The overall analysis shows a significant association between rapid acetylation and carcinoma of the breast. However, when the rather strange results of Bulovskaya *et al.* (1978) are removed from the computation the association is no longer significant.

Lymphoma

Two reports give the acetylation phenotypes of lymphoma patients and appropriate controls. Chekharina *et al.* (1978) in Leningrad found 40% rapid acetylators in 57 lymphoma patients compared with 32% in 84 healthy controls. Philip *et al.* (1987c) in London found 53% of 94 lymphoma patients compared with 45% of 337 controls. The results hint that there might be an association between the disease and the rapid acetylator phenotype but do not attain statistical significance.

An interesting side-product of the investigations of Chekharina *et al.* (1978) was the finding that patients with advanced lymphomas (grades III and IV) had higher acetylation rates than those with less extensive disease (grades I and II). Furthermore, whilst repeat observations of the acetylation rates in 10 controls differed only from −7 to +8% of the original values, repeat measurements in 16 patients showed substantial diminution of acetylation with improvement and increase in the rates with deterioration. It is a pity that the authors do not make it clear exactly how these rates were computed.

These findings have some similarity to the effect of carcinoma of the breast in enhancing acetylating activity, which was described by the same group (Bulovskaya *et al.* 1978) but not found by Ladero *et al.* (1987).

Table 16.24. *Test of the association of the slow acetylator phenotype with carcinoma of the larynx*

Reference	Location of study	Cancer of larynx Slow (h)	Cancer of larynx Rapid (k)	Controls Slow (H)	Controls Rapid (K)	Approximate relative risk (x)	$\log_e x$ (y)	Sampling variance (V)	Weight ($\frac{1}{V} = w$)	Significance of difference from zero (wy^2)	wy
Drozdz et al. 1987	Katowice	107	21	64	42	3.2946	1.1923	0.0933	10.7119	15.2272	12.7716
Roots et al. 1989	Berlin	33	37	149	143	0.8575	−0.1538	0.0701	14.2743	0.3375	−2.1948
								Totals	24.9862	15.5647	10.5768

Weighted mean value of $y = Y = \dfrac{\Sigma wy}{\Sigma w} = 0.4233$; antilog of $Y = \dot{X} = 1.5270$.

$\mathrm{SE}\,(Y) = \sqrt{\dfrac{1}{\Sigma w}} = 0.2000$.

95% fiducial limits of $Y = 2.9652$ and -2.1186.
Equivalent X values to the 95% fiducial limits of $Y = 19.3987$ and 0.1208.

Significance of difference of X from unity $= \chi_1^2 = \dfrac{(\Sigma wy)^2}{\Sigma w} = 4.4772$ ($p < 0.05$).

Heterogeneity estimate $= \chi_1^2 = \Sigma wy^2 - \dfrac{(\Sigma wy)^2}{\Sigma w} = 11.0875$ ($p < 0.001$).

The calculations were made to 6 decimal places. The numbers shown here have been rounded off to 4 decimal places.
Source: Modification by Haldane (1955) of the method of Woolf (1954).

Table 16.25. *Test of the association of the rapid acetylator phenotype with carcinoma of the bronchus*

Reference	Location of study	Number of Subjects				Approximate relative risk (x)	$\log_e x$ (y)	Sampling variance (V)	Weight $\left(\frac{1}{V} = w\right)$	Significance of difference from zero (wy^2)	wy
		Carcinoma of bronchus		Controls							
		Slow (h)	Rapid (k)	Slow (H)	Rapid (K)						
Burgess & Trafford 1985	Brighton, UK	32	21	18	13	0.9065	−0.0981	0.1998	5.0045	0.0482	−0.4910
Philip et al. 1988	London, Leeds & Pontefract	58	68	138	135	1.1969	0.1797	0.0460	21.7443	0.7022	3.9076
Roots et al. 1989	Berlin	136	141	149	143	1.0800	0.0769	0.0279	35.7756	0.2118	2.7524
Ladero et al. 1991	Madrid	48	39	54	39	1.1237	0.1166	0.2522	3.9647	0.0539	0.4624
									Totals 95.6505	1.4383	10.5334

Weighted mean value of $y = Y = \frac{\Sigma wy}{\Sigma w}$ = 0.1101; antilog of $Y = X = 1.1164$.

$SE\ (Y) = \sqrt{\frac{1}{\Sigma w}}$ = 0.1022.

95% fiducial limits of Y = 0.4355 and −0.2152.
Equivalent X values to the 95% fiducial limits of Y = 1.5457 and 0.8063.

Significance of difference of X from unity = $\chi_1^2 = \frac{(\Sigma wy)^2}{\Sigma w}$ = 1.1600 $(p > 0.20)$.

Heterogeneity estimate = $\chi_3^2 = \Sigma wy^2 - \frac{(\Sigma wy)^2}{\Sigma w}$ = 0.278357 $(p > 0.95)$.

The calculations were made to 6 decimal places. The numbers shown here have been rounded off to 4 decimal places.
Source: Modification by Haldane (1955) of the method of Woolf (1954).

Table 16.26. *Test of the association of the rapid acetylator phenotype with carcinoma of the breast*

Reference	Location of study	Carcinoma of breast Slow (h)	Rapid (k)	Controls Slow (H)	Rapid (K)	Approximate relative risk (x)	Log_e x (y)	Sampling variance (V)	Weight ($\frac{1}{V} = w$)	Significance of difference from zero (wy^2)	wy
Bulovskaya et al. 1978	Leningrad	13	28	24	14	3.5670	1.2717	0.2126	4.7041	7.6081	5.9824
Cartwright 1984	Leeds	42	51	65	47	1.6710	0.5134	0.0785	12.7436	3.3589	6.5425
Ladero et al. 1987	Madrid	49	32	45	30	0.9795	−0.0207	0.1043	9.5877	0.0041	−0.1989
Philip et al. 1987b	London	99	82	189	148	1.0581	0.0564	0.0340	29.3927	0.0936	1.6591
Webster et al. 1989	Wales	57	43	59	41	1.0846	0.0813	0.0804	12.4310	0.0821	1.0101
Ilett et al. 1990	Western Australia	25	20	31	17	1.4471	0.3695	0.1729	5.7842	0.7899	2.1374
Sardas et al. 1990	Ankara	11	17	33	18	2.7556	1.0136	0.2209	4.5263	4.6505	4.5880
								Totals	79.1696	16.5872	21.7206

Weighted mean value of $y = Y = \frac{\Sigma wy}{\Sigma w} = 0.2744$; antilog of $Y = X = -1.2933$.

$\text{SE}(Y) = \sqrt{\frac{1}{\Sigma w}} = 0.1124$.

95% fiducial limits of $Y = 0.5633$ and -0.0146.
Equivalent X values to the 95% fiducial limits of $Y = 1.7565$ and 0.9855.

Significance of difference of X from unity $= \chi_1^2 = \frac{(\Sigma wy)^2}{\Sigma w} = 5.9592$ ($p < 0.02$).

Heterogeneity estimate $= \chi_6^2 = \Sigma wy^2 - \frac{(\Sigma wy)^2}{\Sigma w} = 10.6280$ ($p > 0.05$).

The calculations were made to 6 decimal places. The numbers shown here have been rounded off to 4 decimal places.
Source: Modification by Haldane (1955) of the method of Woolf (1954).

Complete Freund's adjuvant and hydrocortisone administration result in 'induction' of the acetylation of sulphadimidine in the rabbit (du Souich & Courteau, 1981). It seems probable that this effect is mediated via the hepatocytes rather than the reticulo-endothelial system. Also, Rya-zonov et al. (1985) have described an increase in the rate of acetylation of sulphadimidine in rats by oestrone, tetracycline, reopyrine and phenobarbital. The effects of such compounds on phenotyping human patients are at present unknown.

Lavigne *et al.* (1977) report on increased acetylation of *p*-aminosalicylate (PAS) in patients with lymphosarcoma and acute and chronic leukaemia. It is known that PAS is monomorphically and not polymorphically acetylated in man. Nevertheless the possibility exists that there may be a general enhancement of acetylating capability in some neoplastic disorders.

Rheumatoid arthritis

A number of groups have investigated three aspects: (1) statistical associations between the occurrence of the disorder and the acetylator phenotypes, (2) whether the disease exhibits any different clinical manifestations in the two phenotypes and (3) responses to therapy in the two phenotypes.

The information on the first point is condensed in Table 16.27. No significant association with either phenotype is demonstrated. It is to be regretted that four groups failed to produce adequate control phenotypic frequencies. There is a hint that if more substantial numbers were studied with proper controls, rapid acetylation might be associated with rheumatoid arthritis.

Five groups have contributed on the second aspect. Ehrenfeld *et al.* (1983) described an earlier age of onset in rapid acetylation, but other clinical features were the same in both phenotypes. The latter evaluation is mirrored by Oka & Seppala (1978) and Crook *et al.* (1983).

Leden *et al.* (1981) studied the acetylator phenotype status in patients who had rheumatoid arthritis with and without Sjögren's syndrome. In the former group there were 21 slow (S) and six rapid (R) whereas in the latter group there 15S and 19R, the two distributions being significantly different. As the authors point out this finding might explain disparities in acetylator phenotype distribution between various series, since generally the patients were not subdivided into those with and those without Sjögren's syndrome.

With regard to the response to therapy, Pullar *et al.* (1985) in an exhaustive analysis, found no differences in the improvement of clinical parameters in the two phenotypes when treated with SASP. In one of their surveys the rapid acetylators were given a higher dose of the drug. In keeping with other series, upper gastrointestinal side effect symptoms (nausea, vomiting) were commoner in the slow acetylators.

Systemic lupus erythematosus

The idea that slow acetylators might be more prone than rapid acetylators to developing spontaneous SLE arose from the following train of thought. It is quite clear that for many of the drugs which are polymorphically acetylated, slow acetylators are more prone to develop adverse effects at conventional doses. For hydralazine (and to a lesser extent for procainamide), systemic lupus as a drug-induced adverse reaction is largely a disorder of slow acetylators. It is possible that naturally occurring primary amine and hydrazide compounds may be the environmental agents responsible for causing SLE. If that is so then slow acetylators may be more prone to develop the disorder. This hypothesis was put forward by Godeau *et al.* (1973) and Reidenberg & Martin (1974).

Now a considerable body of evidence has accumulated whereby this hypothesis can be tested.

Unfortunately the results of some surveys cannot be analysed. For example, Godeau *et al.* (1973) have unconvincing phenotyping data, while Fishbein & Alarcon-Segovia (1979), Foad *et al.* (1977), Larsson *et al.* (1977), Morris *et al.* (1979) and Orlowska-Westwood *et al.* (1980) have no controls accompanying their series of SLE patients.

The results of the analysable series obtained by a variety of phenotyping methods are shown in Table 16.28. In some instances a few individuals were classified as 'intermediate', i.e. assignable to neither slow nor rapid phenotype, and these have been excluded from the analysis.

The results of Kumana *et al.* (1990) have not been included in Table 16.27 because of the very poor definitions of the phenotypes. However, the overall shapes of the distributions were very similar in 36

Table 16.27. *Acetylator phenotypes in rheumatoid arthritis*

Reference	Location of study	Number of Subjects Rheumatoid arthritis Slow (h)	Rapid (k)	Controls Slow (H)	Rapid (K)	Approximate relative risk (x)	$\text{Log}_e x$ (y)	Sampling variance (V)	Weight $\left(\frac{1}{V}=w\right)$	Significance of difference from zero (wy^2)	wy
Oka & Sappala 1978	Finland	16	23	9	11	0.849944	−0.162585	0.283824	3.523306	0.093135	−0.572937
Lawson et al. 1979	Glasgow	18	−7	16[a]	9[a]	1.420202	0.350799	0.336455	2.972157	0.365754	1.042630
Ehrlich et al. 1979	Philadelphia	19	6								
Leden et al. 1981	Lund	15	19	None given	None given						
Kelly & Griffiths 1981	Newcastle upon Tyne	5	8	None given	None given						
Ehrenfield et al. 1983	Israel	28	15	21	21	1.838710	0.609064	0.187892	5.322178	1.974310	3.241548
Crook et al. 1978	Stoke on Trent	34	20	None given	None given						
Pullar et al. 1985	Glasgow	66	83	None given	None given						
								Totals	11.817641	2.433199	3.711341

Analysed according to the hypothesis that there is an association between the slow acetylator phenotype and rheumatoid arthritis.

[a] 5 controls said to be divide 50/50 between the acetylator phenotypes!

Weighted mean value of $y = Y = \frac{\Sigma wy}{\Sigma w} = 0.3141$, antilog $X = 1.3690$.

$\text{SE}(Y) = \sqrt{\frac{1}{\Sigma w}} = 0.2909$.

95% fiducial limits of $Y = +1.5649$ and -0.9368.
Equivalent X values to the 95% fiducial limits of $Y = 4.7822$ and 0.3919.

Significance of difference of X from unity $= \chi_1^2 = \frac{(\Sigma wy)^2}{\Sigma w} = 1.1656$ $(p > 0.10)$.

Heterogeneity estimate $= \chi_6^2 = \Sigma wy^2 - \frac{(\Sigma wy)^2}{\Sigma w} = 1.2676$ $(p > 0.50)$.

Source: Modification by Haldane (1955) of the method of Woolf (1954).

Table 16.28. *The acetylator polymorphism and systemic lupus erythematosus*

Reference	Location of study	Ethnic group	Systemic lupus erythematosus — Slow (h)	Rapid (k)	Controls — Slow (H)	Rapid (K)	Approximate relative risk (x)	$\mathrm{Log}_e\,x$ (y)	Sampling variance (V)	Weight $\left(\frac{1}{V}=w\right)$	Significance of difference from zero (wy^2)	wy
Reidenberg & Martin 1974	Philadelphia	Not stated	11	2	10	11	5.0381	1.6170	0.5909	1.6924	4.4252	2.7366
Johansson et al. 1976	Helsinki	Finnish	29	13	16	3	0.4635	−0.7689	0.4136	2.4179	1.4295	−1.8591
Lawson et al. 1979	Glasgow	Presumably Scottish	16	6	16	9	1.4615	0.3795	0.3605	2.7740	0.3995	1.0527
Reidenberg et al. 1980	Israel	Various as explained in the chapter	16	10	14	13	1.4631	0.3805	0.2877	3.4743	0.5031	1.3221
Horai et al. 1982	Tokyo	Japanese	3	16	2	17	1.4848	0.3953	0.6977	1.4333	0.2240	0.5666
Marsden et al. 1985	Newcastle upon Tyne	Presumably English	14	13	29	22	0.8192	−0.1992	0.2149	4.6532	0.1847	−0.9270
Lee et al. 1985	Singapore	Chinese	13	29	109	351 [a]	1.4690	0.3846	0.1167	8.5694	1.2675	3.2957
Baer et al. 1986	Nashville	44 white / 2 Oriental / 18 black	19 / 5	24 / 13	30 / 18 / 5	27 HV / 21 CP / 6 CP	0.8298	−0.1866	0.1308	7.6443	0.2661	−1.4263
Sardas et al. 1986b	Ankara	Turkish	12	9	67	42	0.8285	−0.1882	0.2149	4.6537	0.1648	−0.8758
									Totals	39.1384	9.8397	2.5508

[a] Pooling figures from Ellard & Gammon (1977) and Lee & Lim (1981).
HV, healthy volunteers; CP, control patients.

Weighted mean value of $y = Y = \dfrac{\Sigma wy}{\Sigma w} = 0.6517$, antilog $= X = 1.9189$.

$\mathrm{SE}\,(Y) = \sqrt{\dfrac{1}{\Sigma w}} = 0.1598$.

95% fiducial limits of $Y = 1.0130$ and 0.2905.
The equivalent X values to the 95% fiducial limits of $Y = 2.7538$ and 1.3371.

Significance of difference of X from unity $= \chi_1^2 = \dfrac{(\Sigma wy)^2}{\Sigma w} = 0.1662$ ($p > 0.50$).

Heterogeneity estimate $= \chi_8^2 = \Sigma wy^2 - \dfrac{(\Sigma wy)^2}{\Sigma w} = 9.6735$ ($p > 0.10$).

The calculations were made to 6 decimal places. The numbers shown here have been rounded off to 4 decimal places.
Source: Modification by Haldane (1955) of the method of Woolf (1954).

Hong Kong Chinese with systemic lupus and 36 Hong Kong Chinese controls.

It will be seen that a variety of Caucasian, black and Oriental series are represented in Table 16.27. The analysis has been conducted on the hypothesis that there is an association between systemic lupus erythematosus and the slow acetylator phenotype. The result shows that no such association has been demonstrated. This conclusion, reached on the basis of phenotyping tests, has now been corroborated in Japanese by Shiokawa et al. (1992) using a polymerase chain reaction genotyping method. Fourteen out of 48 patients and 18 out of 53 healthy controls were slow acetylators; thus there was no significant difference between the frequencies in the two groups.

The clinical manifestations of the disease were noted in both acetylator phenotypes by Foad et al. (1977). No statistical difference was noted between the acetylator phenotypes with regard to the clinical manifestations of SLE or the activity of the disease. A speckled anti-nuclear pattern was more frequent in rapid than in slow acetylators. Slow acetylators had lower lymphocytic responses to PHA-M, ConA and PWM compared with rapid acetylators. It is known that persons with spontaneous SLE differ from those with drug-induced SLE in that HLA-DR4 is uncommon in the former and seems to predispose to the latter (Batchelor et al. 1980; Reinertsen et al. 1984).

Marsden et al. (1985) found that the median number of skin lesions was higher amongst slow acetylators with discoid plus SLE than amongst rapid acetylators with the same combined disorder. This phenotypic difference was not present in patients with SLE alone.

As far as discoid lupus erythematosus itself is concerned Ladero et al. (1988) on examining a series of 37 patients, found them not to be significantly different in phenotype distribution to the control Spanish population.

Clinical and laboratory manifestations of SLE were compared between the two phenotypes by Baer et al. (1986) and no significant differences were found.

Diabetes

The first study of acetylator phenotype in diabetics was that of Mattila & Tiitinen (1967) who called

attention to the fact that 'Relatively more rapid acetylators were found among the diabetics especially among diabetic children.'

Subsequently other groups have investigated the problem with different motivations. Shenfield et al. (1982), for example, were looking to see if there was an association between diabetic peripheral neuropathy and acetylator status; none was found. Burrows et al. (1978) had the same idea and produced a similar result. McLaren et al. (1977), on the other hand, investigating the same problem, found a higher proportion of rapid acetylators in the diabetic neuropathics than in either diabetics without neuropathy or in the control population. Bodansky et al. (1981) sought to clarify the relationship of the acetylator phenotype with Type I diabetes and its microvascular complications; no such association was found. Ladero et al. (1982) were looking only for an association between the genetic marker and the disorder (both juvenile and maturity onset types) but in their analysis of the results were unable to show any association between acetylator phenotype and diabetic complications. Bonisolli et al. (1985) had as one aim the defining of the prevalence of chlorpropamide–alcohol flushing (CPAF) and acetylator phenotype in a large series of Type I and Type II diabetics. They found an association between the rapid acetylator phenotype and CPAF in Type II but not in Type I diabetics; rapid acetylators were more frequently CPAF-positive while slow acetylators were more frequently CPAF-negative. In addition, a linear relationship was found between the rate of acetylation and the speed of ascent of facial skin temperature after chlorpropamide and alcohol in Type II diabetics, but not Type I diabetics. The meaning of this association was unclear. The series of Bonisolli et al. (1985) seems to be an expansion of the series of Pontiroli et al. (1984) since the controls are the same in both. The same group (Pontiroli et al. 1987) has shown that neither acetylator phenotype is more prone to the micro- or macro-angiopathic complications of diabetes.

The three UK diabetic series were not accompanied by their own control series, so a large control series was assembled from data in 15 published papers as explained by Evans (1984).

Many of the papers indicated whether their patients were Type I or Type II diabetics. Some authors use the terms 'juvenile' and 'maturity-onset', and for the present purpose these are taken to be the same as Type I and Type II.

Using the data from all these series, Table 16.29 and Table 16.30 have been compiled. It should be noted that in both Type I and Type II diabetes there is an association with the rapid acetylator phenotype. This phenotype is twice as likely as it would be, by chance, to be associated with Type I diabetes. In the case of Type II diabetes the association is not as strong. In neither type do the 95% fiducial limits of the association include zero, nor is there significant heterogeneity between the series.

The possibility was raised by Shenfield *et al.* (1982) that a high plasma glucose concentration might cause greater acetylation in diabetics. It is true (as is discussed elsewhere in this review) that a high glucose level can enhance acetylation capacity. However the effect of such a factor, which would vary considerably between patients, would be to increase the variance of the acetylation parameter in both phenotypes. Shenfield *et al.* (1982) published neither histogram nor scattergram. The scattergram of Bodansky *et al.* (1981) shows no increased spread of the data points in the two phenotypes. Mattila & Tiitinen (1967) present a histogram of isoniazid half-lives which shows a clear bimodality; the mean isoniazid half-life in both phenotypes in diabetics closely resembled those found in non-diabetics. Likewise Bonisolli *et al.* (1985) show histograms of percentage acetylation in serum which indicate clear bimodal curves in the patients as in the controls (though the antimode is shifted to a slightly lower level in the diabetics).

All the above studies were carried out in Europeans. Diabetes is a common disorder among Saudi Arabians. One notable clinical feature differentiating them from Europeans is the ability of many Saudi diabetics to tolerate grossly raised plasma glucose concentrations without symptoms (Kingston & Skoog 1986).

Two series of Saudi Arabian diabetics have been acetylator phenotyped, each with its own control group (Evans *et al.* 1985; El-Yazigi *et al.* 1992). The two series yielded different associations for Type I diabetics probably because of the small numbers involved. The pooled Type I diabetics did not differ significantly in phenotype frequencies from the pooled controls (which were not significantly different from each other). Similarly, the pooled Type II diabetics did not differ in phenotype frequencies from the pooled controls. More data are required from non-European populations.

Miscellaneous disorders

Two series (Platzer *et al.* 1978; Siegmund *et al.* 1991) show a highly significant association between the slow acetylator phenotype and Gilbert's disease (Table 16.31).

In a study of Graves' disease (Ladero & Cano 1983) it was found that the phenotype frequencies did not differ from those of the general population. Slow acetylators, however, developed the disease at a significantly younger mean age than rapid acetylators (29.5 as compared with 39.5 years). Siegmund *et al.* (1988) found slow acetylators to be significantly more common in hyperthyroid patients aged over 50 years.

Roots *et al.* (1989) surveyed a series of cancers for associations with acetylator status. The data for colon, bronchial, laryngeal and bladder cancers have already been cited. A series of 203 gastric cancers showed 64.1% slow acetylators (odds ratio 1.76, 95% confidence limits 1.20–2.58, $p = 0.002$). Also a series of 109 pharyngeal cancers showed 62.4% slow acetylators (odds ratio 1.59, 95% confidence limits 0.99–2.75, $p = 0.027$). It would be interesting to see if other series, studied in other locations, confirm these two associations of the slow acetylator phenotype with cancers.

For many miscellaneous conditions the data available do not suggest any significant association with either acetylator phenotype, but in many instances the ethnic group is not defined and adequate controls were not studied (Table 16.32). A remarkable association between the slow acetylator phenotype and periodic disease was demonstrated by Podymov *et al.* (1988).

With regard to leprosy there is no reliable comparison group for the Malawi patients (Karim *et al.* 1981; Hodgkin *et al.* 1979; Glatthaar *et al.* 1977; Eidus *et al.* 1979). So the association with acetylator phenotype cannot be assessed in them. For the Chinese patients the pooled estimate is $q = 0.6383 \pm$ SE 0.0370 (Table 16.32). The three available Chinese control groups (Table 16.33) give very consistent estimates, and when they are pooled, $q = 0.4662 +$ SE 0.0162. This suggests that in Chinese the slow acetylators may be more prone than rapid acetylators to develop leprosy (Table 16.34).

Table 16.29. *Test of the association between Type I or juvenile diabetes and the rapid acetylator phenotype*

Reference	Location of study	Number of Subjects				Approximate relative risk (x)	$\log_e x$ (y)	Sampling variance (V)	Weight $\left(\frac{1}{V} = w\right)$	Significance of difference from zero (wy^2)	wy
		Diabetes		Controls							
		Slow (h)	Rapid (k)	Slow (H)	Rapid (K)						
Mattila & Tiitinen 1967	Helsinki	2	7	43	20	6.3658	1.8509	0.5287	1.8915	6.4803	3.5011
McLaren et al. 1977	Sheffield, Leicester	22	27								
Burrows et al. 1978	Oxford			556	375	1.6617	0.5078	0.0423	23.6340	6.0947	12.0018
Bodansky et al. 1981	Liverpool	27	28								
Shenfield et al. 1982	Perth, W. Australia	12	35	58	54	3.0484	1.1146	0.1398	7.1514	8.8849	7.9712
Ladero et al. 1982	Madrid	15	17	90	67	1.5137	0.4146	0.1437	6.9565	1.1957	2.8841
Bonisolli et al. 1985	Milan	57	53	39	16	2.2274	0.8008	0.1196	8.3625	5.3632	6.6970
Stryjek-Kaminska et al. 1988	Warsaw	29	51	56	44	2.2165	0.7959	0.0923	10.8307	6.8615	8.6206
Hadasova et al. 1990	Brno	29	19	50	32	1.0271	0.02686	0.1332	7.5050	0.0054	0.2008
								Totals	66.3316	34.8858	41.8765

Weighted mean value of $y = Y = \frac{\Sigma wy}{\Sigma w} = 0.6313$, antilog $= X = 1.8801$.

SE $(Y) = \sqrt{\dfrac{1}{\Sigma w}} = 0.1228$.

95% fiducial limits of $Y = 0.9321$ and 0.3305.
The equivalent X values to the 95% fiducial limits of $Y = 2.5399$ and 1.3917.

Significance of difference of X from unity $= \chi_1^2 = \dfrac{(\Sigma wy)^2}{\Sigma w} = 26.4375$ ($p < 0.001$).

Heterogeneity estimate $= \chi_6^2 = \Sigma wy^2 - \dfrac{(\Sigma wy)^2}{\Sigma w} = 8.4482$ ($p > 0.10$).

The calculations were made to 6 decimal places. The numbers shown here have been rounded off to 4 decimal places.
Source: Modification by Haldane (1955) of the method of Woolf (1954).

Table 16.30. *Test of the association between Type II or adult onset diabetes and the rapid acetylator phenotype*

Reference	Location of study	Number of Subjects Diabetes Slow (h)	Diabetes Rapid (k)	Controls Slow (H)	Controls Rapid (K)	Approximate relative risk (x)	$\text{Log}_e x$ (y)	Sampling variance (V)	Weight $\left(\frac{1}{V} = w\right)$	Significance of difference from zero (wy^2)	wy
Mattila & Tiitinen 1967	Helsinki	13	6	43	20	1.0217	0.0214	0.0284	63.5133	0.0016	0.0754
McLaren et al. 1977	Sheffield, Leicester	39	42	556	375	1.8429	0.6113	0.0356	28.1021	10.5021	17.1794
Burrows et al. 1978	Oxford	18	29								
Bodansky et al. 1981	Liverpool										
Shenfield et al. 1982	Perth, W. Australia	27	42	58	54	1.6589	0.5061	0.0941	10.6269	2.7224	5.3787
Ladero et al. 1982	Madrid	37	50	90	67	1.8055	0.5909	0.0716	13.9628	4.8745	8.2500
Bonisolli et al. 1985	Milan	91	55	39	16	1.4521	0.3730	0.1126	8.8849	1.2360	3.3139
Stryjek-Kaminska et al. 1988	Warsaw	34	46	56	44	1.7113	0.5372	0.0896	11.1590	3.2208	5.9951
					Totals				76.2489	22.5576	40.1925

Weighted mean value of $y = Y = \frac{\Sigma wy}{\Sigma w} = 0.5271$, antilog $= X = 1.6940$.

$\text{SE}\ (Y) = \sqrt{\frac{1}{\Sigma w}} = 0.1145.$

95% fiducial limits of $Y = 0.8214$ and 0.2328.
The equivalent X values to the 95% fiducial limits of $Y = 2.2738$ and 1.2621.

Significance of difference of X from unity $= \chi_1^2 = \frac{(\Sigma wy)^2}{\Sigma w} = 21.1863\ (p < 0.001).$

Heterogeneity estimate $= \chi_5^2 = \Sigma wy^2 - \frac{(\Sigma wy)^2}{\Sigma w} = 1.3712\ (p > 0.90).$

The calculations were made to 6 decimal places. The numbers shown here have been rounded off to 4 decimal places.
Source: Modification by Haldane (1955) of the method of Woolf (1954).

Table 16.31. *Test of the association between Gilbert's disease and the slow acetylator phenotype*

| | | | Number of Subjects | | | | | | | | |
| | | | Gilbert's disease | | Controls | | | | | | |
Reference	Location of study	Ethnic group	Slow (h)	Rapid (k)	Slow (H)	Rapid (K)	Approximate relative risk (x)	$\text{Log}_e\,x$ (y)	Sampling variance (V)	Weight $\left(\frac{1}{V}=w\right)$	Significance of difference from zero (wy^2)	wy
Platzer *et al.* 1978	Berne	Swiss	21	6	39	37	3.1402	1.1443	0.2396	4.1731	5.4643	4.7753
Siegmund *et al.* 1991	Greifswald	German	40	14	135	112	2.3190	0.8411	0.1073	9.3231	6.5962	7.8420
									Totals	13.4963	12.0605	12.6173

Weighted mean value of $y = Y = \overline{Y} = \dfrac{\Sigma wy}{\Sigma w} = 0.9349$, antilog $= X = 2.5469$.

$\text{SE}\;(Y) = \sqrt{\dfrac{1}{\Sigma W}} = 0.2722$.

95% fiducial limits of $Y = 4.3946$ and -2.5248.
The equivalent X values to the 95% fiducial limits of $Y = 81.0100$ and 0.0800.

Significance of difference of X from unity $= \chi_1^2 = \dfrac{(\Sigma wy)^2}{\Sigma w} = 11.7956$ $(p < 0.05)$.

Heterogeneity estimate $= \chi_1^2 = \Sigma wy^2 - \dfrac{(\Sigma wy)^2}{\Sigma w} = 0.2649$ $(p > 0.80)$.

The calculations were made to 6 decimal places. The numbers shown here have been rounded off to 4 decimal places.
Source: Modification by Haldane (1955) of the method of Woolf (1954).

Table 16.32. Studies of association between acetylator phenotypes and spontaneous disorders – miscellaneous disorders

Reference	Disease category	Location survey conducted	Ethnic group	Number of patients	Number of slow acetylators	q	SE (q)
Mental disorders							
Mattila & Takki 1969	Chronic schizophrenics on neuroleptics	Helsinki	Finns	29	21	0.851	0.049
Price 1971	Schizophrenics	Liverpool	British whites	78	51	0.809	0.033
Evans et al. 1965	Neurotic depression	Newcastle	British whites	25	16	0.800	0.060
	Endogenous depression	Newcastle	British whites	25	17	0.825	0.057
Marshall et al. 1978	Neurotic depression	Newcastle	British whites	29	19	0.809	0.055
	Neurotic anxiety states	Newcastle	British whites	28	17	0.779	0.059
	Phobic anxiety states	Newcastle	British whites	23	15	0.808	0.061
Caddy et al. 1976	Neurotic depression	Glasgow	Presumably British whites	27	12	0.667	0.072
Johnstone & Marsh 1973	Neurotic depression	Glasgow	British whites	97	51	0.725	0.034
Airaksinen et al. 1969	Down's syndrome	Helsinki	Finns	61	41	0.820	0.037
Morris et al. 1989	[a] Down's syndrome	Buffalo, NY	White	22	7	0.564	0.088
Gastrointestinal disorders							
Evans 1967	Duodenal ulcer	Liverpool	British whites	50	28	0.748	0.046
Mattila et al. 1969b	Postgastrectomy syndrome	Oulu and Helsinki	Finns	13	8	0.784	0.086
Schröder et al. 1973	Ulcerative colitis (17) and Crohn's disease of ileum and colon (2)	Liverpool	British whites	19	11	0.761	0.074
Das & Eastwood 1975	Ulcerative colitis (84) and Crohn's disease (38)	Edinburgh	British whites	122	87	0.844	0.024
Sharp et al. 1981	Crohn's disease (14), ulcerative colitis (10) and undifferentiated CIBD (4)	Saskatoon	Canadian	28	19	0.824	0.054
Clarke et al. 1982	Ulcerative colitis (20) and Crohn's disease (25)	Buffalo	Not stated	45	28	0.789	0.046
Azad Khan et al. 1983	Ulcerative colitis	Oxford	British whites	181	112	0.787	0.023
Reidenberg et al. 1980	Colitis on sulphasalazine	Israel	Israeli (derivation not stated)	63	30	0.690	0.046
Fisher & Klotz 1979	Ulcerative colitis and Crohn's disease	Stuttgart	Not stated	65	40	0.785	0.038
Leprosy							
Ellard et al. 1974b	Leprosy	Malawi	Malawis	17	8	0.686	0.088
Ellard et al. 1972	Leprosy	Malaysia	Chinese	24	16	0.817	0.059
Gelber et al. 1975	DDS-resistant leprosy	Sungei Buloh Selangor, Malaysia	Chinese	40	16	0.632	0.061
	Non-DDS-resistant leprosy	Sungei Buloh Selangor, Malaysia	Chinese	44	12	0.522	0.064

Table 16.32. (*cont.*)

Reference	Disease category	Location survey conducted	Ethnic group	Number of patients	Number of slow acetylators	q	SE (q)
Raj *et al.* 1988	DDS-sensitive leprosy	Tamil Nadu	Indian	11	4	0.603	0.120
	DDS-resistant leprosy	Tamil Nadu	Indian	16	7	0.661	0.094
Dermatitis herpetiformis							
Ellard *et al.* 1974a	Dermatitis herpetiformis	London	British whites	10	7	0.837	0.087
Forstrom *et al.* 1974	Dermatitis herpetiformis	Helsinki	Finns	50	28	0.748	0.046
Swain *et al.* 1983	Dermatitis herpetiformis	London	British whites	28	19	0.809	0.054
Hypertension[b]							
Perry *et al.* 1970	Hypertension (24 accelerated)	St Louis	Caucasian	27	18	0.816	0.056
			Negro	30	15	0.707	0.065
Zacest & Koch-Weser 1972	Hypertension	Boston	Not stated	20	13	0.806	0.066
Jounela *et al.* 1975	Hypertension	Helsinki	Finns	23	12	0.722	0.072
Iisalo *et al.* 1979	Hypertension	Turku	Finns	21	9	0.655	0.083
Hall 1981	Hypertension	Vasteras	Swedes	57	30	0.725	0.046
Mansilla Tinoco *et al.* 1982	Hypertension	London	Caucasian	123	62	0.710	0.037
			Black	30	16	0.730	0.062
			Indian	10	8	0.894	0.070
Facchini and Timbrell 1981	Hypertension	London	Not stated	13	6	0.679	0.102
Pasanen *et al.* 1973	Hypertension	Helsinki	Not stated	8	4	0.707	0.125
Vandenburg *et al.* 1982	Hypertension	London	Not stated	25	12	0.693	0.072
Ramsay *et al.* 1984	Hypertension	Sheffield	Not stated	57	31	0.737	0.049
Shepherd *et al.* 1984	Hypertension	Austin and San Antonio, Texas	Not stated	9	5	0.745	0.111
Holmes *et al.* 1983	Hypertension	European multi-center	Not stated	50	34	0.825	0.040
Larsson *et al.* 1981	Hypertension	Linkoping	Not stated	12	5	0.645	0.110
Huynor 1975	Hypertension	Sydney	Not stated	26	20	0.877	0.047
Cardiac							
Schröder *et al.* 1979	Ventricular premature beats	Odense	Danes	18	12	0.816	0.068
Molin *et al.* 1977	Cardiac and/or renal disease	Linkoping	Swedes	21	17	0.900	0.048
Campbell *et al.* 1976	Myocardial infarction	Glasgow	Presumably British whites	19	12	0.795	0.070
Campbell *et al.* 1976	Ventricular dysrhythmia	Glasgow	Presumably British whites	25	12	0.693	0.072
Ylitalo *et al.* 1983	Ventricular dysrhythmia following myocardial infarction	Tampere	Presumably Finns	35	19	0.737	0.057

Reference	Disease	Location	Ethnic group				
Woosley et al. 1978	Various cardiac arrhythmias	Nashville	Not stated	20	11	0.742	0.075
Lima et al. 1979	Ventricular arrhythmias	Buffalo	Whites	20	13	0.806	0.066
Sonnhag et al. 1979	Ventricular arrhythmias	Linkoping	Presumably Swedish	40	33	0.908	0.033
Skretkowicz et al. 1981	Hypertension and arrhythmias	Lodz	Polish	60	26	0.658	0.049
Evans et al. 1991	[a]Coronary artery atheroma	Riyadh	Saudi Arabs	101	65	0.802	0.030
Renal							
Williams et al. 1968	Uremia before dialysis	Cardiff	Presumably British whites	10	6	0.775	0.100
Fine & Sumner 1975	Uremia on dialysis	Glasgow	British whites	10	6	0.775	0.100
Hepatic							
Ladero et al. 1981	Porphyria cutanea tarda	Madrid	Presumably Spanish	51	33	0.804	0.042
Alcoholics							
Lester 1965	Alcoholics	Metuchen, NJ	Not stated	28	14	0.707	0.067
Lilyin et al. 1984	[a]Alcoholics	Moscow	Russians	75	42	0.748	0.038
Guthrie et al. 1989	Alcoholics	Bethesda, MD	Caucasians	37	17	0.678	0.060
Miscellaneous							
Olszewska et al. 1980	Psoriasis	Lodz	Polish	105	65	0.787	0.030
Jimenez-Nieto et al. 1989	[a]Familial psoriasis	Madrid	Spanish	27	22	0.903	0.041
	Sporadic psoriasis	Madrid	Spanish	37	18	0.697	0.059
Hykes & Elis 1980	[a]Silicosis	Kladno	Czeck	27	24	0.942	0.032
Tomaskiewicz et al. 1979	[a]Carcinoma cervix	Poznan	Polish	37	12	0.569	0.068
	Endometrial cancer	Poznan	Polish	13	6	0.679	0.120
	Malignant ovarian neoplasms	Poznan	Polish	29	18	0.788	0.057
Ladero et al. 1989	[a]Parkinson's disease	Madrid and Badajoz	Spanish	100	69	0.830	0.028
Orzechowska-Juzwenko et al. 1986	[a]Allergic disorders	Warsaw	Polish	31	20	0.803	0.053
Stoll et al. 1989	Mothers of OWCM	Strasbourg	Presumably French	81	44	0.737	0.037
	Fathers of OWCM			77	41	0.730	0.039
Siegmund et al. 1988	[a]Graves' hyperthyroidism	Greifswald, GDR	Presumably Germans	87	50	0.758	0.035
	Toxic multinodular goitre	Greifswald, GDR	Presumably Germans	38	20	0.725	0.056
Podymov et al. 1988	[a]Periodic disease	[d]Yerevan	Armenians	29	28	0.983	0.017

[a]Corresponding control series are shown in Table 16.19.
[b]Details of early studies of small numbers of patients given by Talseth (1977).
[c]Recurrent polyserositis, familial Mediterranean fever.
[d]Assumed location in view of the ethnic group.
CIBD, Chronic inflammatory bowel disease; OWCM, Offspring with congenital malformations.

Table 16.33. *Chinese control subjects*

Reference	Disease category	Location survey conducted	Technique of phenotyping	Number of subjects	Number of slow acetylators	q	SE (q)	Upper confidence limit	Lower confidence limit
Sanhara *et al.* 1963a	Healthy	Taiwan	Plasma INH concentration	121	27	0.4724	0.0401	0.5525	0.3923
Ellard & Gammon 1977	Tuberculosis	Singapore, Hong Kong	Sulphadimidine and INH	386	83	0.4637	0.0225	0.5088	0.4186
				184	40	0.4663	0.0326	0.6315	0.4010
Evans 1963	Healthy	Liverpool	Plasma INH concentration	59	13	0.4694	0.0575	0.5844	0.3544

INH, isoniazid.
Reprinted from: Evans (1984) with permission of the copyright holder, British Medical Association, London.

Table 16.34 *Acetylator phenotypes in Chinese leprosy patients and controls*

| | Acetylator phenotype | | |
	Slow	Rapid	Total
Leprosy patients	44	64	108
Control subjects	163	587	750
Total	207	651	858

$\chi_1^2 = 17.6$.
Reprinted from: Evans (1984) with permission of the copyright holder, British Medical Association, London.

However, in 27 lepers in Tamil Nadu q was 0.638 (Raj *et al.* 1988), which is lower than the range of values for Madras samples shown in Table 16.17.

An innovative study by Saiz-Ruiz & Aguilera (1985) describes how 75 healthy individuals were acetylator phenotyped and assessed on the Eysenck Personality Inventory (EPI) and the Minnesota Multiphasic Personality Inventory (MMPI). It was found that rapid acetylator females obtained higher scores on the EPI neuroticism scale than slow acetylator females. Also, for the whole group, higher scores were obtained by the rapid acetylators on the MMPI hypochondriasis scale.

Discussion

The interpretation of the association between bladder cancer and the slow acetylator phenotype rests upon the knowledge that carcinogenic amines are polymorphically acetylated (Glowinski *et al.* 1978).

With regard to the other associations described with Gilbert's disease, diabetes mellitus, age of onset of Graves' disease and leprosy, there is no logical interpretation possible at present. The natural substrates for the polymorphic *N*-acetyltransferase enzyme are unknown. It may be speculated that acetyl-accepting molecules such as hydrazines, aromatic amines or aminomethyluracils may be involved in the production of the disorders mentioned above. The results of association studies presented here may stimulate researchers to investigate such possibilities.

CONCLUSIONS

The pharmacogenetic polymorphisms illustrate in clinical settings that what happens to an individual is a result of interaction between his genetically determined constitution and the environmental influence to which he is subjected. This theme is common throughout biology. In modern medicine it has taken a central place in the concepts of aetiology. Pharmacogenetics indicates that the same holds true in therapeutics, in this case the environmental influences under consideration being medicinal drugs.

The genetic polymorphism in the metabolism of isoniazid was discovered by observing the interindividual variability in the metabolism of the drug, and by subsequent family studies.

Until recently individuals could be phenotyped only by ingesting a test compound (e.g. isoniazid, SMZ, DDS or caffeine) and subsequently having the drug and its metabolite in blood and/or urine analysed. Now direct genotyping is possible using mutation-specific primers for allele-specific amplification of small amounts of DNA from leucocytes by the polymerase chain reaction.

The enzymic basis of the polymorphism lies in different activities of cytosolic *N*-acetyltransferase in the jejunal mucosa and liver. The molecular basis has now been shown to be due to three mutant alleles in addition to the 'wild type' allele.

The polymorphism must have a profound ecological significance because the frequencies of the two phenotypes vary greatly. The Eskimos and Japanese populations have over 90% rapid acetylators whereas some Arab, Indian and European populations have 70% slow acetylators. However, the details of interplay of the polymorphism with the natural environment remain unknown because there is no knowledge about the nature of the natural substrate(s).

From a clinical point of view there are two groups of phenomena of great interest. The first concerns the relationship of the polymorphism to adverse reactions and therapeutic effects. The second concerns statistical associations between phenotypes within the polymorphism and spontaneous disorders.

Interest in the first aspect is heightened by the fact that using the 'typed panel' approach a number of different drugs have been found to be metabolized polymorphically by the relevant *N*-acetyltransferase. As well as the original isoniazid, the list includes SMZ, hydralazine, SP (from SASP), procainamide, DDS, aminorone, aminoglutethimide, dipyrone and the metabolites formed by the reduction of the nitro-groups of nitrazepam and clonazepam.

Generally speaking, at a given dose, the occurrence of adverse reactions is greater in slow acetylators. This is because some adverse reactions are correlated with the concentration of the drug in the plasma (a fact which is not true of adverse reactions which have hypersensitivity as their basis).

Therapeutic effects may be suboptimal in rapid acetylators when they are taking dosages appropriate to slow acetylators. Examples are (1) the response of tuberculosis to once-weekly isoniazid-containing regimes, which are satisfactory in slow acetylators but quite unacceptable in rapid acetylators and (2) the treatment of hypertension with hydralazine.

Since neither phenotype is rare in the population this polymorphism emphasizes the fact that in clinical trials adequate numbers of people (chosen preferably at random) should be studied to make sure that both the phenotypes are adequately represented.

In some instances, e.g. treatment of tuberculosis in developing countries, treatment of ulcerative colitis with SASP and treatment of hypertension with hydralazine, it might be of value to acetylator-phenotype patients before commencing treatment.

An association has been shown between slow acetylation and bladder cancer. This is understandable because the aromatic amines which are the cause of the cancer are polymorphically acetylated in the liver Other associations have been found as follows: slow acetylation is associated with Gilbert's disease, younger mean age of onset in Graves' disease and leprosy in Chinese, silicosis and periodic disease; rapid acetylation is associated with diabetes mellitus of both types in Europeans. In order to understand these purely statistical facts properly it will be necessary to determine what are the natural substrate(s) for the polymorphic enzyme.

The author would like to express his gratitude to the Pergamon Press, which gave permission to reproduce this chapter which first appeared in *Pharmacogenetics of Drug Metabolism*, ed. W. Kalow, New York, Pergamon, 1992 [ISBN 0-08-041175-4].

Adam, A. M., Rogers, H. J., Amiel, S. A. & Rubens, R. D. (1984). The effect of acetylator phenotype on the disposition of amnoglutethimide. *British Journal of Clinical Pharmacology*, **18**, 495–505.

Afonja, A. O., Arharwarien, E. D., Okotore, R. O. & Femi-Pearse, D. (1979). Isoniazid acetylator phenotypes of Nigerians. *Nigerian Medical Journal*, **9**, 86–8.

Ahmad, R. A., Rogers, H. J., Vandenberg, M. & Wright, P. (1981). Effects of concurrent administration of other substrates of N-acetyltransferase on dapsone acetylation. *British Journal of Clinical Pharmacology*, **12**, 664–681.

Airaksinen, E., Mattila, M. J. & Olilla, O. (1969). Inactivation of isoniazid and sulphadimidine in Mongoloid subjects. *Annales Medicinae Experimentalis et Biologiae Fennicae*, **47**, 303–7.

Alarcon-Segovia, D. (1969). Drug-induced lupus syndromes. *Mayo Clinic Proceedings*, **44**, 664–81.

Ali, B. H. & Bashir, A. A. (1991). Polymorphic acetylation of sulphadimidine in healthy Northern Sudanese. *Annals of Saudi Medicine*, **11**, 483–4.

American Trudeau Society. (1953). The toxicity of isoniazid. A report of the Committee on therapy. *American Review of Tuberculosis*, **68**, 302–5.

Amos, R. S., Pullar, T., Bax, D. E., Situnayake, D., Capell, H. A. & McConkey, B. (1986). Sulphasalazine for rheumatoid arthritis: toxicity in 774 patients monitored for one to 11 years. *British Medical Journal*, **293**, 420–2.

Armstrong, A. R. & Peart, H. E. (1960). A comparison between the behaviour of Eskimos and non-Eskimos to the administration of isoniazid. *American Review of Respiratory Diseases*, **81**, 588–94.

Azad Khan, A. K., Nurazzaman, M. & Truelove, S. C. (1983). The effect of the acetylator phenotype on the metabolism of sulphasalazine in man. *Journal of Medical Genetics*, **20**, 30–6.

Azad Khan, A. K., Truelove, S. C. & Aronson, J. K. (1982). The disposition and metabolism of sulphasalazine (salicylazosulpha-sulphapyridine) in man. *British Journal of Clinical Pharmacology*, **13**, 523–8.

Baer, A. N., Woolsey, R. L. & Pincus, T. (1986). Further evidence for the lack of association between acetylator phenotype and systemic lupus erythematosus. *Arthritis and Rheumatism*, **29**, 508–14.

Bajaj, R. T., Desai, M. P., Desai, N. K. & Sheth, U. K. (1988). Isoniazid acetylator status in children. *Indian Paediatrics*, **25**, 775–9.

Barraviera, B., Pereira, P. C. M., Mendes, R. P., Machado, J. M., Lima, C. R. G. & Meira, D. A. (1989). Evaluation of acetylator phenotype, renal function and serum sulfadiazine levels in patients with paracoccidioidomycosis treated with cotrimazine (a combination of sulfadiazine and trimethoprim). *Mycopathologia*, **108**, 107–12.

Bartmann, K. & Massmann, W. (1960). Der Blutspiegel des INH bei Erwachsenen und Kindern. *Beitrage zur klinischen Neurologie und Psychiatrie*, **122**, 239–50.

Batchelor, J. R., Welsh, K. I., Mansilla-Tinoco, R., Dollery, C. T., Hughes, G. R. V., Bernstein, R., Ryan, P., Naish, P. F., Aber, G. M., Bing, R. F. & Russel, G. I. (1980). Hydralazine-induced systemic lupus erythematosus: influence of HLA-DR and sex on susceptibility. *Lancet*, **1**, 1107–9.

Baumann, P., Bosshart, P., Gabris, G., Gastpar, M. & Koeb, L. (1988). Acetylation of maprotiline and desmethylmaprotiline in depressive patients phenotyped with sulfadimidine, debrisoquine and mephenytoin. *Arzneimittel-Forschung*, **38**, 292–6.

Beever, I. W., Blair, I. A. & Brodie, M. J. (1982). Circulating hydrazine during treatment with isoniazid rifampicin in man. *British Journal of Clinical Pharmacology*, **13**, 599P.

Bernard, E., Israel, L., Pariente, D., Sausy, J. & Taux, D'I. N. H. (1961). Libre residuel et resultants therapeutiques chez 104 tuberculeux pulmonaires 'neufs'. *Revue de tuberculose et de pneumologie*, **25**, 319–38.

Bernstein, R. E. (1979). Procainamide, acetyl procainamide and drug-induced lupus erythematosus. *Lancet*, **2**, 1076.

Bicho, M. P., Breitenfeld, L., Carvalho, A. A. & Manso, C. F. (1988). Acetylation phenotypes in patients with bladder carcinoma. *Annales de Génétique (Paris)*, **31**, 167–71.

Biehl, J. P. (1957). Emergence of drug resistance as related to the dosage and metabolism of isoniazid. *Transactions, 16th Conference Chemother Tuberc.* pp. 108–13. Washington, DC: US Veterans Adm Army Navy.

Black, M., Mitchell, J. R., Zimmerman, H. J., Ishak, K. G. & Epler, G. R. (1975). Isoniazid-associated hepatitis in 114 patients. *Gastroenterology*, **69**, 289–302.

Blair, I. A., Mansilla Tinoco, R., Brodie, M. J., Clare, R. A., Dollery, C. T., Timbrell, J. A. & Beever, I. A. (1985). Plasma hydrazine concentrations in man after isoniazid and hydralazine administration. *Human Toxicology*, **4**, 195–202.

Blum, M., Demierre, A., Grant, D. M., Heim, M. & Meyer, U. A. (1991). Molecular mechanism of slow acetylation of drugs and carcinogens in humans. *Proceedings of the National Academy of Sciences (USA)*, **88**, 5237–41.

Blum, M., Grant, D. M., McBride, W., Heim, M. & Meyer, U. A. (1990). Human arylamine N-acetyltransferase genes: isolation chromosomal location and functional expression. *DNA and Cell Biology*, **9**, 193–203.

Bodansky, H. J., Drury, P. L., Cudworth, A. G. & Evans, D. A. P. (1981). Acetylator phenotypes and Type I (insulin-dependent) diabetics with microvascular disease. *Diabetes*, **30**, 907–10.

Bogers, W. A. J. L. & Meems, L. (1983). Endralazine, a new peripheral vasodilator. Evaluation of safety and efficacy over a 3 year period. *European Journal of Clinical Pharmacology*, **24**, 301–5.

Bondesen, S., Nielsen, O. H., Schou, J. B., Jensen, P. H., Lassen, L. B., Binder, V., Krasilnikoff, P. A., Dano, P., Honore, S., Hansen, S., Norby-Rasmussen, S. & Hvidberg, E. F. (1986). Steady state kinetics of 5-aminosalicylic acid and sulfapyridine during sulfasalazine prophylaxis in ulcerative colitis. *Scandinavian Journal of Gastroenterology*, **21**, 693–700.

Bonicke, R. & Lisboa, B. P. (1957). Über die Erbbedingtheit der intraindividuellen Konstanz der Isoniazidaus-scheidung beim Menschen (Untersuchungen an eineiigen und zweieiigen Zwillingen). *Naturwissenshaften*, **44**, 314.

Bonicke, R. & Reif, W. (1953). Enzymatische Inaktivierung von Isonicotinsäurehydrazid im menschlichen und tierischen Organismus. *Archiv für experimentelle Pathologie und Pharmakologie (Naunyn-Schmiedeberg)*, **220**, 321–33.

Bonisolli, L., Pontiroli, A. E., de Pasqua, A., Calderara, A., Maffi, P., Gallus, G., Radaelli, G. & Pozza, G. (1985). Association between chlorpropamide-alcohol flushing and fast acetylator phenotype in Type I and Type II diabetes. *Acta Diabetologica Latina*, **22**, 305–15.

Bouayad, Z., Chevalier, B., Maurin, R. & Bartal, M. (1982). Phénotype d'acetylation de l'isoniazide au Moroc. Etude preliminaire sur 100 cas. *Revue Marocaine de médécine et santé*, **4**, 13–18.

Bozkurt, A., Basci, N. E., Isimer, A., Tuner, M., Erdal, R. & Kayaalp, S. O. (1990a). Sulphamethoxazole acetylation in fast and slow acetylators. *International Journal of Clinical Pharmacology, Therapy and Toxicology*, **28**, 164–6.

Bozkurt, A., Basci, N. E., Kalan, S., Tuncer, M. & Kayaalp, S. O. (1990b). N-acetylation phenotyping with sulphadimidine in a Turkish population. *European Journal of Clinical Pharmacology*, **38**, 53–6.

Branfman, A. R., McComish, M. F., Bruni, R. J., Callahan, M. M., Robertson, R. & Yesair, D. W. (1983). Characterization of diaminouracil metabolites of caffeine in human urine. *Drug Metabolism and Disposition*, **11**, 206–10.

Bressollette, L., Berthou, F., Riche, C., Mottier, D. & Floch, H. H. (1990). Polymorphisme génétique d'acetylation et d'hydroxylation dans la population bretonne. *Therapie*, **45**, 99–103.

British Medical Journal (1967). Middle articles: Conferences and Meetings: Chemotherapy of tuberculosis in developing countries. *British Medical Journal*, **4**, 230–1.

Brodie, M. J., Boobis, A. R., Hillyard, C. J., Abeyasekara, C., Stevenson, J. C., MacIntyre, I. & Park, B. K. (1982). Effect of rifampicin and isoniazid on vitamin D metabolism. *Clinical Pharmacology and Therapeutics*, **32**, 525–30.

Brown, A. (1976). Risks of isoniazid therapy [letter]. *Annals of Internal Medicine*, **85**, 828.

Brownson, R. & Chang, J. C. (1987). Exposure to alcohol and tobacco and the risk of laryngeal cancer. *Archives of Environmental Health*, **42**, 192–6.

Buchanan, H. (1979). Isoniazid pharmacokinetics in kwashiorkor *South African Medical Journal*, **56**, 299–300.

Bulovskaya, L. N., Krupkin, R. G., Bochina, T. A., Shipova, A. A. & Pavlova, M. V. (1978). Acetylator phenotype in patients with breast cancer. *Oncology*, **35**, 185–8.

Burgess, E. J. & Trafford, J. A. P. (1985). Acetylator phenotype in patients with lung carcinoma – a negative report. *European Journal of Respiratory Diseases*, **67**, 17–19.

Burrows, A. W., Hockaday, T. D. R., Mann, J. I. & Taylor, J. G. (1978). Diabetic dimorphism according to acetylator status. *British Medical Journal*, **1**, 208–10.

Buzdar, A. V., Fraschini, G. & Blumenschein, G. R. (1984). Hematologic adverse effects of aminoglutethimide. *Annals of Internal Medicine*, **100**, 159.

Caddy, B., Tilstone, W. J. & Johnston, E. C. (1976). Phenelzine in urine: assay and reaction to acetylator status. *British Journal of Clinical Pharmacology*, **3**, 633–7.

Callahan, M. M., Robertson, R. S., Branfman, A. R., McComish, M. F. & Yesair, D. W. (1983). Comparison of caffeine metabolism in three nonsmoking populations after oral administration of radiolabeled caffeine. *Drug Metabolism and Disposition*, **11**, 211–17.

Cameron, H. A. & Ramsay, L. E. (1984). The lupus syndrome induced by hydralazine: a common complication with low dose treatment. *British Medical Journal*, **289**, 410–12.

Campbell, W., Tilstone, W. J., Lawson, D. H., Hutton, I. & Lawrie, T. D. V. (1976). Acetylator phenotype and the clinical pharmacology of low-release procainamide. *British Journal of Clinical Pharmacology*, **3**, 1023–6.

Cannat, A. & Seligman, M. (1966). Possible induction of antinuclear antibodies by isoniazid. *Lancet*, **1**, 185–7.

Carr, K., Oates, J. A., Nies, A. S. & Woolsey, R. L. (1978). Simultaneous analysis of dapsone and monoacetyldapsone employing high performance liquid chromatography: a rapid method for determination of acetylator phenotype. *British Journal of Clinical Pharmacology*, **6**, 421–7.

Carrier, O., Pons, G., Rey, E., Richard, M. O., Moran, C.,

Badoual, J. & Olive, G. (1988). Maturation of caffeine metabolic pathways in infancy. *Clinical Pharmacology and Therapeutics*, **44**, 145–51.

Cartwright, R. A. (1984). Epidemiological studies on N-acetylation and C-center ring oxidation in neoplasia. In *Genetic Variability in Responses to Chemical Exposure*, ed. G. S. Omenn & H. V. Gelboin. Banbury Report 16, pp. 359–65. Cold Spring Harbor Laboratory.

Cartwright, R. A., Adib, R., Appleyard, I., Glashan, R. W., Gray, B., Hamilton-Stewart, P. A., Robinson, M. & Barham-Hall, D. (1983). Cigarette smoking and bladder cancer: an epidemiological inquiry in West Yorkshire. *Journal of Epidemiology and Community Health*, **37**, 256–63.

Cartwright, R. A., Glasham, R. W., Rogers, H. J., Ahmad, R. A., Barham-Hall, D., Higgins, E. & Khan, M. A. (1982). Role of N-acetyltransferase phenotypes in bladder carcinogenesis: a pharmacogenetic epidemiological approach to bladder cancer. *Lancet*, **2**, 842–6.

Chalmers, I. M., Sitar, D. S. & Hunter, T. (1990). A one-year, open, prospective study of sulfasalazine in the treatment of rheumatoid arthritis: adverse reactions and clinical response in relation to laboratory variables, drug and metabolite serum levels, and acetylator status. *Journal of Rheumatology*, **17**, 764–70.

Chapron, D. J., Kramer, P. A. & Mercik, S. A. (1980). Kinetic discrimination of three sulfamethazine acetylation phenotypes. *Clinical Pharmacology and Therapeutics*, **27**, 104–13.

Chekharina, Y. A., Bulovskaya, L. N., Pavlova, M. V. & Krupkin, R. G. (1978). Activity of N-acetyltransferase in patients with malignant lymphomas. *Neoplasma*, **25**, 471–5.

Clark, D. W. J. (1985). Genetically determined variability in acetylation and oxidation. *Drugs*, **29**, 342–75.

Clarke, C. A., Edwards, J. W., Haddock, D. R. W., Howel-Evans, A. W., McConnell, R. B. & Sheppard, P. M. (1956). ABO blood groups and secretor character in duodenal ulcer. Population and sibship studies. *British Medical Journal*, **2**, 725–31.

Clarke, D. F., George, D., Milsap, R. L., Pogonowska-Wala, E., Owerbach, J., Lebenghal, E. & Jusko, W. J. (1982). Sulfasalazine metabolite pharmacokinetics in pediatric patients with inflammatory bowel disease. *Pediatric Pharmacology*, **2**, 323–33.

Connor, A., Altorki, N. & Moossa, A. R. (1986). Tumours of the colon, rectum and anus: Clinical features and surgical treatment. In *Comprehensive Textbook of Oncology*, ed. A. R. Moosa, M. C. Robson & S. C. Schimpff. **97a**, 1063–79. Baltimore: Williams and Wilkins.

Cook, J. F., Cochrane, J. P. & Edstein, M. D. (1986). Race-linked differences in serum concentrations of dapsone monoacetyldapsone and pyrimethamine during malaria prophylaxis. *Transactions of the Royal Society of Tropical Medicine and Hygiene*, **80**, 897–901.

Coombes, R. C., Foster, A. B., Harland, S. J., Jarman, M. & Nice, E. C. (1982). Polymorphically acetylated aminoglutethimide in humans. *British Journal of Cancer*, **46**, 340–5.

Coutts, R. T., Mozayani, A., Danielson, T. J. & Baker, G. B. (1991). Tissue levels and some pharmacological properties of an acetylated metabolite of phenelzine in the rat. *Journal of Pharmaceutical Science*, **80**, 765–7.

Cowan, G. O., Das, K. M. & Eastwood, M. A. (1977). Further studies of sulphasalazine metabolism in the

treatment of ulcerative colitis. *British Medical Journal*, **2**, 1057–9.

Coyle, J., Boudoulas, H. & Lima, J. J. (1991). Acecainide pharmacokinetics in normal subjects of known acetylator phenotype. *Biopharmaceutics and Drug Disposition*, **12**, 599–612.

Crook, P. R., Hortas, C., Roberts, J. M., Swinson, D. R., Mucklow, J. C. & Shadforth, M. F. (1983). Acetylator phenotype and the effect of dapsone in rheumatoid arthritis. *Journal of Rheumatology*, **10**, 805–8.

Dalrymple, P. D. & Nicholls, P. J. (1988). Metabolism profiles and excretion of C-aminoglutethimide in several animal species and man. *Xenobiotica*, **18**, 75–81.

Das, K. M. & Dubin, R. (1976). Clinical pharmacokinetics of sulphasalazine. *Clinical Pharmacokinetics*, **1**, 406–25.

Das, K. M. & Eastwood, M. A. (1975). Acetylation polymorphism of sulfapyridine in patients with ulcerative colitis and Crohn's disease. *Clinical Pharmacology and Therapeutics*, **18**, 514–20.

Das, K. M., Eastwood, M. A., McManus, J. P. A. & Sircus, W. (1973). Adverse reactions during salicylazosulfapyridine therapy and the relation with drug metabolism and acetylator phenotype. *New England Journal of Medicine*, **289**, 491–5.

Das, K. M., Eastwood, M. A., McManus, J. P. A. & Sircus, W. (1974). The role of the colon in the metabolism of salicylazosulphapyridine. *Scandinavian Journal of Gastroenterology*, **9**, 137–41.

Davies, D. M., Beedie, M. A. & Rawlins, M. D. (1975). Antinuclear antibodies during procainamide treatment and drug acetylation. *British Medical Journal*, **3**, 682–3.

De March, A. P. & Garcia, J. N. (1966). Metabolismo de la isoniazida. I Aspecto antropologico. *Revista Clinica Española*, **102**, 32–41.

Deguchi, T., Mashimo, M. & Suzuki, T. (1990). Correlation between acetylator phenotypes and genotypes of polymorphic arylamine N-acetyltransferase in human liver. *Journal of Biological Chemistry*, **265**, 12757–60.

Demers, L. M., Boucher, A. E. & Santen, R. J. (1987). Aminoglutethimide therapy in breast cancer: relationship of blood levels to drug-related side effects. *Clinical Physiology and Biochemistry*, **5**, 287–91.

Desai, M., Jariwala, G., Khokhani, B., Desai, N. K. & Sheth, U. K. (1973). Isoniazid inactivation in Indian children. *Indian Pediatrics*, **10**, 373–6.

Devadatta, S., Gangadharam, P. R. J., Andres, R. H., Fox, W., Ramakrishnan, C. V., Selkon, J. B. & Vela, S. (1960). Peripheral neuritis due to isoniazid. *Bulletin of the World Health Organisation*, **23**, 587–98.

Dewan, A., Jani, J. P., Shah, K. S. & Kashyab, S. K. (1986). Urinary excretion of benzidine in relation to the acetylator status of occupationally exposed subjects. *Human Toxicology*, **5**, 95–7.

Dickinson, D. S., Bailey, W. C., Hirschowitz, B. I., Soong, S.-J., Eidus, L. & Hodgkin, M. M. (1981). Risk factors of isoniazid (INH)-induced liver dysfunction. *Journal of Clinical Gastroenterology*, **3**, 271–9.

Donald, P. R., Gent, W. L., Seifart, H. I., Lamprecht, J. H. & Parkin, D. P. (1992). Cerebrospinal fluid isoniazid concentrations in children with tuberculous meningitis: the influence of dosage and acetylation status. *Pediatrics*, **89**, 247–50.

Douglass, C. D., Dillaha, C. J., Dillaha, J. & Kountz, S. L. (1957). Inhibition of biologic acetylation by l-hydrazinophthalazine. *Journal of Laboratory and Clinical Medicine*, **49**, 561–5.

Drozdz, M., Gierek, T., Jendryczko, A., Pilch, J. & Pierkarska, J. (1987). N-acetyltransferase of patients with cancer of the larynx. *Neoplasma*, **34**, 481–4.

Duchene, P., LeDily, J., Bromet-Petit, M., Mosser, J. & Feniou, C. (1988). High-performance liquid chromatographic assay of the metabolites of thymoxamine. *Journal of Chromatography*, **424**, 205–10.

Dufour, A. P., Knight, R. A. & Harris, H. W. (1964). Genetics of isoniazid metabolism in Caucasian, Negro and Japanese populations. *Science*, **145**, 391.

Du Souich, P. & Courteau, H. (1981). Induction of acetylating capacity with complete Freund's adjuvant and hydrocortisone in the rabbit. *Drug Metabolism and Disposition*, **9**, 279–83.

Du Souich, P., Lalka, D., Slaughter, R., Elvin, A. T. & McLean, A. J. (1979b). Mechanisms of non-linear disposition kinetics of sulfamethazine. *Clinical Pharmacology and Therapeutics*, **26**, 172–88.

Du Souich, P., McLean, A. J., Stoeckel, K., Ohlendorf, D. & Gibaldi, M. (1979a). Screening methods using sulfamethazine for determining acetulator phenotype. *Clinical Pharmacology and Therapeutics*, **26**, 757–65.

East African/British Medical Research Council (1974). Controlled clinical trial of four short-course (6 month) regimens of chemotherapy for treatment of pulmonary tuberculosis. *Lancet*, **2**, 1100–6.

Ehrenfeld, M., Zylber-Katz, E, & Levy, M. (1983). Acetylator phenotype in rheumatoid arthritis. *Israel Journal of Medical Sciences*, **19**, 368–70.

Ehrlich, G. E., Freeman-Narrod, M. & Winebrugh, G. S. (1979). Predominance of slow acetylators among patients with rheumatoid arthritis. *European Journal of Rheumatology and Inflammation*, **2**, 196–8.

Eichelbaum, M., Musch, E., Castro-Parra, M. & von Sassen, W. (1982). Isoniazid hepatotoxicity in relation to acetylator phenotype and isoniazid metabolism. *British Journal of Clinical Pharmacology*, **14**, 575P–6P.

Eidus, L., Glatthaar, E., Hodgkin, M. M., Nel, E. E. & Kleeberg, H. H. (1979). Comparison of isoniazid phenotyping of black and white patients with emphasis on South African blacks. *International Journal of Clinical Pharmacology and Biopharmacy*, **17**, 311–16.

Eidus, L., Harenanansingh, A. M. T. & Jessamine, A. G. (1971). Urine test for phenotyping isoniazid inactivators. *American Review of Respiratory Disease*, **104**, 587–91.

Eidus, L. & Hodgkin, M. M. (1973). Simplified screening test for phenotyping of isoniazid inactivators. *International Journal of Clinical Pharmacology, Therapy and Toxicology*, **7**, 82–6.

Eidus, L., Hodgkin, M. M., Schaefer, O. & Jessamine, A. G. (1974). Distribution of isoniazid inactivators determined in Eskimos and Canadian college students by a urine test. *Revue Canadienne de Biologie (Montreal)*, **33**, 117–23.

El Yazigi, A., Chaleby, K. & Martin, C. R. (1989a). Acetylator phenotypes of Saudi Arabians by a simplified caffeine metabolites test. *Journal of Clinical Pharmacology*, **29**, 246–50.

El Yazigi, A., Chaleby, K. & Martin, C. R. (1989b). A simplified and rapid test for acetylator phenotyping by use of the peak height ratio of two urinary caffeine metabolites. *Clinical Chemistry*, **35**, 848–51.

El-Yazigi, A., Johansen, K., Raines, D. A. & Dossing, M. (1992). N-acetylation polymorphism and diabetes mellitus among Saudi Arabians. *Journal of Clinical Pharmacology*, **32**, 905–10.

Ellard, G. A. & Gammon, P. T. (1977). Acetylator phenotyping of TB patients using matrix isoniazid or sulphadimidine and its prognostic significance for treatment with several intermittent isoniazid containing regimes. *British Journal of Clinical Pharmacology*, **4**, 5–14.

Ellard, G. A., Gammon, P. T. & Harris, J. M. (1974b). The appliction of urine tests to monitor the regularity of dapsone self-administration. *Leprosy Review*, **45**, 224–34.

Ellard, G. A., Gammon, P. T., Helmy, H. S. & Rees, R. J. W. (1972). Dapsone acetylation and the treatment of leprosy. *Nature*, **239**, 159–60.

Ellard, G. A., Gammon, P. T., Polansky, F., Viznerova, A., Havlik, I. & Fox, W. (1973b). Further studies on the pharmacology of a slow-release matrix preparation of isoniazid (Smith and Nephew Hs 82) of potential use in the intermittent treatment of tuberculosis. *Tubercle*, **54**, 57–66.

Ellard, G. A., Gammon, P. T., Savin, J. A. & Tan, R. S. H. (1974a). Dapsone acetylation in dermatitis herpetiformis. *British Journal of Dermatology*, **90**, 441–4.

Ellard, G. A., Gammon, P. T. & Tiitinen, H. (1973a). Determination of the acetylator phenotype from the ratio of urinary excretion of acetyl-isoniazid to acid-labile isoniazid: a study in Finnish Lapland. *Tubercle*, **54**, 201–10.

Ellard, G. A., Gammon, P. T. & Tiitinen, H. (1975). Determination of the acetylator phenotype using matrix isoniazid. *Tubercle*, **56**, 203–9.

Elmendorf, D. F. Jr., Cawthon, W. U., Muschenheim, C. & McDermott, W. (1952). The absorption distribution excretion and short-term toxicity of isonicotinic acid hydrazide (Nydrazid) in man. *Annual Review of Tuberculosis*, **65**, 429–42.

Evans, D. A. & White, T. A. (1964). Human acetylation polymorphism. *Journal of Laboratory and Clinical Medicine*, **63**, 394–403.

Evans, D. A. P. (1962). Pharmacogénétique. *Médecine et Hygiène (Genève)*, **20**, 905–8.

Evans, D. A. P. (1963). Pharmacogenetics. *American Journal of Medicine*, **34**, 639–62.

Evans, D. A. P. (1967). The acetylator phenotypes of duodenal ulcer patients. *Scandinavian Journal of Gastroenterology*, **2**, 289–92.

Evans, D. A. P. (1968). Genetic variations in the acetylation of isoniazid and other drugs. *Annals of the New York Academy of Sciences*, **151**, 723–33.

Evans, D. A. P. (1969). An improved and simplified method of detecting the acetylator phenotype. *Journal of Medical Genetics*, **6**, 405–7.

Evans, D. A. P. (1984). Survey of the human acetylator polymorphism in spontaneous disorders. *Journal of Medical Genetics*, **21**, 243–53.

Evans, D. A. P., Bullen, M. F., Houston, J., Hopkins, C. A. & Vetters, J. M. (1972). Antinuclear factor in rapid and slow acetylator patients treated with isoniazid. *Journal of Medical Genetics*, **9**, 53–6.

Evans, D. A. P., Davison, K. & Pratt, R. T. C. (1965). The influence of acetylator phenotype on the effects of treating depression with phenelzine. *Clinical Pharmacology and Therapeutics*, **6**, 430–5.

Evans, D. A. P., Donohoe, W. T. A., Hewitt, S. & Linaker, B. D. (1982). Le^a blood group substance degeneration in the human alimentary tract and urine Le^a in coeliac disease. *Vox Sanguinis*, **43**, 177–87.

Evans, D. A. P., Eze, L. C. & Whibley, E. J. (1983). The association of the slow acetylator phenotype with bladder cancer. *Journal of Medical Genetics*, **20**, 330–3.

Evans, D. A. P., Mahgoub, A., Sloan, T. B., Idle, J. R. & Smith, R. L. (1980). A family and population study of the genetic polymorphism of debrisoquine oxidation in a white British population. *Journal of Medical Genetics*, **17**, 102–5.

Evans, D. A. P., Manley, K. A. & McKusick, V. A. (1960). Genetic control of isoniazid metabolism in man. *British Medical Journal*, **2**, 485–91.

Evans, D. A. P., Paterson, S., Francisco, P. & Alvarez, G. (1985). The acetylator phenotypes of Saudi Arabian diabetics. *Journal of Medical Genetics*, **22**, 479–83.

Evans, D. A. P., Storey, P. B. & McKusick, V. A. (1961). Further observations on the determination of isoniazid inactivator phenotype. *Bulletin of the Johns Hopkins Hospital*, **108**, 60–6.

Evans, D. A. P., Wicks, J., Higgins, J. & Assisto, M. (1991). The acetylator phenotypes of Saudi Arabians with coronary arterial atheroma. *Journal of Medical Genetics*, **3**, 192–3.

Eze, L. C. (1987). High incidence of the slow nitrazepam acetylator phenotype in a Nigerian population. *Biochemical Genetics*, **25**, 225–9.

Eze, L. C. & Evans, D. A. P. (1972). The use of the 'autoanalyser' to determine the acetylator phenotype. *Journal of Medical Genetics*, **9**, 57–9.

Eze, L. C. & Obidoa, O. (1978). The acetylation of sulphamethazine in a Nigerian population. *Biochemical Genetics*, **16**, 1073–7.

Facchini, V. & Timbrell, J. A. (1981). Further evidence for an acetylator phenotype difference in the metabolism of hydralazine in man. *British Journal of Clinical Pharmacology*, **11**, 345–51.

Fantoli, U., Cattaneo, C., Ritis, G. C. D. & Belasio, L. (1963). Metabolismo dell'idrazide dell'acido isonicotinoco. *Annali dell Istituto Carlo Forlanini*, **23**, 115–42.

Fawcett, I. W. & Gammon, P. T. (1975). Determination of the acetylator phenotype in a Northern Nigerian population. *Tubercle*, **56**, 119–201.

Feltelius, N. & Hallgren, R. (1986). Sulphasalazine in ankylosing spondylitis. *Annals of the Rheumatic Diseases*, **45**, 396–9.

Fine, A. & Sumner, D. J. (1975). Determination of acetylator status in uraemia. *British Journal of Clinical Pharmacology*, **2**, 475–6.

Fink, K., Adams, W. S. & Pfleiderer, W. (1964). A new urinary pyrimidine, 5-acetylamino-6-amino-3-methyluracil. *Journal of Biological Chemistry*, **239**, 4250–6.

Fishbein, E. & Alarcon-Segovia, D. (1979). Slow acetylation phenotype in systemic lupus erythematosus. *Arthritis and Rheumatism*, **22**, 95–6.

Fisher, C. & Klotz, U. (1979). High performance liquid chromatographic determination of aminosalicylate, sulfapyridine and their metabolites. Its application for pharmacokinetic studies with salicylazosulfapyridine in man. *Journal of Chromatography*, **162**, 237–43.

Flammang, T. J., Yamazoe, Y., Guengerich, F. P. & Kadlubar, F. F. (1987). The S-acetyl coenzyme A-dependent metabolic activation of the carcinogen *N*-hydroxy-2-aminofluorene by human liver cytosol and its relationship to the aromatic amine N-acetyltransferase phenotype. *Carcinogenesis*, **8**, 1967–70.

Foad, B., Litwin, A., Zimmer, H. & Hess, E. V. (1977). Acetylator phenotype in systemic lupus erythematosus. *Arthritis and Rheumatism*, **20**, 815–18.

Forstrom, L., Mattila, M. J. & Mustakallio, K. K. (1974). Acetylator phenotype minimal maintenance dose and haemolytic effect of dapsone in dermatitis herpetiformis. *Annals of Clinical Research*, **6**, 308–10.

Frislid, K., Berg, M., Hansteen, V. & Lunde, P. K. M. (1976). Comparison of the acetylation of procainamide and sulfadimidine in man. *European Journal of Clinical Pharmacology*, **9**, 433–8.

Frymoyer, J. W. & Jacox, R. F. (1963a). Investigation of the genetic control of sulfadiazine and isoniazid metabolism in the rabbit. *Journal of Laboratory and Clinical Medicine*, **62**, 891–904.

Frymoyer, J. W. & Jacox, R. F. (1963b). Studies of genetically controlled sulfadiazine acetylation in rabbit livers. *Journal of Laboratory and Clinical Medicine*, **62**, 905–9.

Gachalyi, B., Vas, A., Hajos, P. & Kaldor, A. (1984). Acetylator phenotypes: Effect of age. *European Journal of Clinical Pharmacology*, **26**, 43–5.

Gachalyi, B., Vas, A. & Kaldor, A. (1985). Ageing and the acetylator phenotype. *European Journal of Clinical Pharmacology*, **29**, 377–8.

Gangadharam, P. R. J., Bhatia, A. L., Radhakrishna, S. & Selkon, J. B. (1961). Rate of inactivation of isoniazid in South Indian patients with pulmonary tuberculosis. *Bulletin of the World Health Organisation*, **25**, 765–77.

Garg, S. K., Kumar, B., Bakaya, V., Lal, R., Shukla, V. K. & Kaur, S. (1988). Plasma dapsone and its metabolite monoacetyl dapsone in leprotic patients. *International Journal of Clinical Pharmacology, Therapy and Toxicology*, **26**, 552–4.

Gascon, M. P., Leeman, T. & Dayer, P. (1987). Evaluation d'un test á la caféine pour déterminer le phénotype de la N-acétyltransférase (NAT). *Schweizerische Medizinische Wochenschrift*, **117**, 1974–6.

Gelber, R., Peters, J. H., Gordon, G. R., Glazko, A. J. & Levy, L. (1971). The polymorphic acetylation of dapsone in man. *Clinical Pharmacology and Therapeutics*, **12**, 225–38.

Gelber, R. H. & Rees, R. J. W. (1975). Dapsone metabolism in patients with dapsone-resistant leprosy. *American Journal of Tropical Medicine and Hygiene*, **24**, 963–7.

Gibson, T. P., Matusik, E., Nelson, H. A., Wilkinson, J. & Briggs, W. A. (1975). Acetylation of procainamide in man and its relationship to isonicotinic acid hydrazide acetylation phenotype. *Clinical Pharmacology and Therapeutics*, **17**, 395–9.

Girling, D. J. (1978). The hepatic toxicity of antituberculosis regimens containing isoniazid, rifampicin and pyrazinamide. *Tubercle*, **59**, 13–32.

Glatthaar, E., Gartig, D., Staner, M. F. & Kleeberg, H. H. (1977). Isoniazid levels in black patients dosed with a matrix preparation (Tebesium). *Praxis der Pneumologie Vereinigt mit der Tuberkuloseartz (Stuttgart)*, **31**, 885–9.

Glowinski, I. B., Radtke, H. E. & Weber, W. W. (1978). Genetic variation in N-acetylation of carcinogenic arylamines by human and rabbit liver. *Molecular Pharmacology*, **14**, 940–9.

Godeau, P., Aubert, M., Imbert, J.-C. & Herreman, G. (1973). Lupus erythemateux dissemine et taux d'isoniazide actif. *Annales de Médecine Internal*, **124**, 181–6.

Goedde, H. W., Benkmann, H. G., Agarwal, D. P. &,
Kroeger, A. (1977b). Genetic studies in Ecuador,
acetylator phenotypes, red cell enzyme and serum protein
polymorphisms of Shuara Indians. *American Journal of
Physical Anthropology*, **47**, 419–25.

Goedde, H. W., Flatz, G., Rahimi, A. G., Kaifie, S.,
Benkmann, H. G., Kriese, G. & Delbruck, H. (1977a). The
acetylator polymorphism in four populations of
Afghanistan. *Human Heredity*, **27**, 383–8.

Goedde, H. W., Rothhammer, F., Benkmann, H. G. &
Bogdanski, P. (1984). Ecogenetic studies in Atacameno
Indians. *Human Genetics*, **67**, 343–6.

Goldstein, P. D., Alpers, D. H. & Keating, J. P. (1979).
Sulfapyridine metabolites in children with inflammatory
bowel disease receiving sulfasalazine. *Journal of Pediatrics*,
95, 639–40.

Gorrod, J. W. & Manson, D. (1986). The metabolism of
aromatic amines. *Xenobiotica*, **16**, 933–55.

Gow, J. G. & Evans, D. A. P. (1964). A study of the
influence of the isoniazid inactivator phenotype on
reversion in genitourinary tuberculosis. *Tubercle*, **45**, 136–
43.

Grant, D. M., Blum, M., Beer, M. & Meyer, U. A. (1991).
Monomorphic and polymorphic human arylamine *N*-
acetyltransferases: a comparison of liver isozymes and
expressed products of two cloned genes. *Molecular
Pharmacology*, **39**, 184–91.

Grant, D. M., Morike, K., Eichelbaum, M. & Meyer, U. A.
(1990). Acetylation pharmacogenetics. The slow acetylator
phenotype is caused by decreased or absent arylamine
N-acetyltransferase in human liver. *Journal of Clinical
Investigation*, **85**, 968–72.

Grant, D. M., Tang, B. K. & Kalow, W. (1983a).
Polymorphic *N*-acetylation of a caffeine metabolite. *Clinical
Pharmacology and Therapeutics*, **33**, 355–9.

Grant, D. M., Tang, B. K. & Kalow, W. (1983b). Variability
in caffeine metabolism. *Clinical Pharmacology and
Therapeutics*, **33**, 591–602.

Grant, D. M., Tang, B. K. & Kalow, W. (1984). A simple test
for acetylator phenotype using caffeine. *British Journal of
Clinical Pharmacology*, **17**, 459–64.

Gronhagen-Riska, C., Hellstrom, P. E. & Frosetti, B. (1978).
Predisposing factors in hepatitis induced by
Isoniazid-Rifampicin treatment of tuberculosis. *American
Review of Respiratory Disease*, **118**, 461–6.

Gunawardhana, L., Barr, J., Weir, A. J., Brendel, K. & Sipes,
I. G. (1991). The *N*-acetylation of sulfamethazine and
p-aminobenzoic acid by human liver slices in dynamic
organ culture. *Drug Metabolism and Disposition*, **19**, 648–
54.

Gupta, R. C., Nair, C. R., Jindal, S. K. & Malik, S. K. (1984).
Incidence of isoniazid acetylation phenotypes in North
Indians. *International Journal of Clinical Pharmacology,
Therapy and Toxicology*, **22**, 259–64.

Gurumurthy, P., Krishnamurthy, M. S., Nazareth, O.,
Parthasarathy, R., Raghupati Sarma, G., Somasundaram,
P. R., Tripathy, S. P. & Ellard, G. A. (1984). Lack of
relationship between hepatic toxicity and acetylator
phenotype in three thousand South Indian patients during
treatment with isoniazid for tuberculosis. *American Review
of Respiratory Disease*, **129**, 58–61.

Guthrie, S. K., Lane, E. A. & Linnoila, M. (1989).
Acetylation phenotype in abstinent alcoholics. *Alcoholism:
Clinical and Experimental Research*, **13**, 66–8.

Hadasova, E., Brysova, V. & Kadlcakova, E. (1990). *N*-

acetylation in healthy and diseased children. *European
Journal of Clinical Pharmacology*, **39**, 43–7.

Hajra, A., Sorenson, R. C. & LaDu, B. N. (1992). Detection
of human DNA mutations with non-radioactive
allele-specific oligonucleotide probes. *Pharmacogenetics*, **2**,
78–88.

Haldane, J. B. S. (1955). The estimation and significance of
the logarithm of a ratio of frequence. *Annals of Human
Genetics (London)*, **20**, 309–11.

Hall, S. (1981). Evaluation of the sulphadimidine acetylator
phenotyping test in patients with reduced renal function.
Acta Medica Scandinavica, **209**, 505–7.

Hamilton, R. A., Kowalskuy, S. F., Wright, E. M., Cernak,
P., Benziger, D. P., Stroshane, R. M. & Edelson, J. (1986).
Effect of the acetylator phenotype on amrinone
pharmacokinetics. *Clinical Pharmacology and Therapeutics*,
40, 615–19.

Hanngren, A., Borga, O. & Sjoqvist, F. (1970). Inactivation
of isoniazid (INH) in Swedish tuberculous patients before
and during treatment with para-amino-salicylic acid
(PAS). *Scandinavian Journal of Respiratory Disease*, **51**,
61–9.

Hanssen, H. P., Agarwal, D. P., Goedde, H. W., Bucher, H.,
Huland, H., Brachmann, W. & Ovenbeck, R. (1985).
Association of *N*-acetyltransferase polymorphism and
environmental factors with bladder carcinogenesis.
European Urology, **11**, 263–6.

Hardy, B. G., Lemieux, C., Walker, S. E. & Bartle, W. R.
(1988). Interindividual and intraindividual variability in
acetylation: characterization with caffeine. *Clinical
Pharmacology and Therapeutics*, **44**, 152–7.

Harland, S.J., Facchini, V. & Timbrell, J. A. (1980).
Hydralazine-induced lupus erythematosus-like syndrome
in a patient of the rapid acetylator phenotype. *British
Medical Journal*, **281**, 273–4.

Harmer, D., Evans, D. A. P., Eze, L. C., Jolly, M. & Whibley,
E. J. (1986). The relationship between the acetylator and
the sparteine hydroxylation polymorphisms. *Journal of
Medical Genetics*, **23**, 155–6.

Harris, A. L., Hughes, G., Barrett, A. J., Abusrawil, S.,
Dowsett, M. & Smith, I. E. (1986). Agranulocytosis
associated with aminoglutethimide; pharmacological and
marrow studies. *British Journal of Cancer*, **54**, 119–12.

Harris, A. L. & McIntyre, N. (1981). Interaction of
phenelzine and nitrazepam in a slow acetylator. *British
Journal of Clinical Pharmacology*, **12**, 254–55.

Harris, H. W. (1961). High dose isoniazid compared with
standard-dose isoniazid with PAS in the treatment of
previously untreated cavitary pulmonary tuberculosis. In
Trans 20th Conf Chemother Tuberc, pp. 39–68. Washington
DC: US Veterans Adm Army Navy.

Harris, H. W., Knight, R. A. & Selin, K. J. (1958).
Comparison of isoniazid concentrations in the blood of
people of Japanese and European descent. *American
Review of Tuberculosis*, **78**, 944–8.

Hashem, H., Khalifa, S. & Nour, A. (1969). The frequency of
isoniazid acetylase enzyme deficiency among Egyptians.
American Journal of Physical Anthropology, **31**, 97–101.

Hayward, G. A. (1975). Human acetylation polymorphism in
Polynesians. *Proceedings of the University of Otago Medical
School*, **53**, 67–8.

Hein, D. W. (1988). Acetylator genotype and
arylamine-induced carcinogenesis. *Biochimica et Biophysica
Acta*, **948**, 37–66.

Hein, D. W., Kirlin, W. G., Yerokun, T., Trinidad, A. &

Ogolla, F. (1987). Inheritance of acetylator genotype-dependent arylamine N-acetyltransferase in hamster bladder cytosol. *Carcinogenesis*, **8**, 647–52.

Hein, D. W. & Weber, W. W. (1982). Polymorphic N-acetylation of phenelzine and monoacetylhydrazine by highly purified rabbit liver isoniazid N-acetyltransferase. *Drug Metabolism and Disposition*, **10**, 225–9.

Henningsen, N. C., Cederberg, A,. Hanson, A. & Johansson, B. W. (1975). Effects of long-term treatment with procainamide. *Acta Medica Scandinavica*, **198**, 475–82.

Hickman, D., Risch, A., Camilleri, J. P. & Sim, E. (1992). Genotyping human polymorphic arylamine N-acetyltransferase: identification of new slow allotypic variants. *Pharmacogenetics*, **2**, 217–26.

Hickman, D. & Sim, E. (1991). N-acetyl transferase polymorphism. *Biochemical Pharmacology*, **42**, 1007–14.

Hildebrand, M. & Seifert, W. (1989). Determination of acetylator phenotype in Caucasians with caffeine. *European Journal of Clinical Pharmacology*, **37**, 525–6.

Hir, M. R., Chicou, J., Hetrick, G., Mercier, A., Neel, R. & Rise, N. (1964). Essai clinique controle de trois types de traitement oral de la tuberculose pulmonaire. *Bulletin of the World Health Organisation*, **30**, 701–32.

Hodgkin, M. M., Eidus, L. & Bailey, W. C. (1979). Isoniazid phenotyping of black as well as white patients. *Canadian Journal of Physiology and Pharmacology*, **57**, 760–3.

Holmes, D. G., Bogers, W. A. J. L., Wideros, T.-E., Huuman-Seppala, A. & Wideroe, B. (1983). Endralazine, a new peripheral vasodilator: absence of effect of acetylator status on antihypertensive effect. *Lancet*, **1**, 670–1.

Hombhanje, F. (1991). Possible optimization of sulphadimidine dosage for acetylator phenotyping. *Japanese Journal of Pharmacology*, **56**, 531–4.

Homeida, M., Abboud, O. I., Dawi, O., Rahama, A. M., Awad, E. H. & Ahmed, O. M. (1986). The acetylator phenotype of Sudanese subjects. *Arab Journal of Medicine*, **5**, 30–1.

Hoo, J. J., Hussein, L. & Goedde, H. W. (1977). A simplified micro-method for the determination of the acetylator phenotype. *Journal of Clinical Chemistry and Clinical Biochemistry*, **15**, 329–31.

Horai, Y., Fujita, K. & Ishizaki, T. (1989). Genetically determined N-acetylation and oxidation capacities in Japanese patients with non-occupational urinary bladder cancer. *European Journal of Clinical Pharmacology*, **37**, 581–7.

Horai, Y. & Ishizaki, T. (1988). N-acetylation polymorphism of dapsone in a Japanese population. *British Journal of Clinical Pharmacology*, **25**, 487–94.

Horai, Y., Ishizaki, T., Sasaki, T., Koya, G., Matsuyama, K. & Iguelin, S. (1982). Isoniazid disposition, comparison of isoniazid phenotyping methods in an acetylator distribution of Japanese patients with idiopathic lupus erythematosus and control subjects. *British Journal of Clinical Pharmacology*, **13**, 361–74.

Horai, Y., Zhou, H. H., Ahang, L. M. & Ishizaki, T. (1988). N-acetylation phenotyping with dapsone in a mainland Chinese population. *British Journal of Clinical Pharmacology*, **25**, 81–7.

Hughes, H. B., Biehl, J. P., Jones, A. P. & Schmidt, L. H. (1954). Metabolism of isoniazid in man as related to the occurrence of peripheral neuritis. *American Review of Tuberculosis*, **70**, 266-273.

Hughes, H. B., Schmidt, L. H. & Biehl, J. P. (1955). The metabolism of isoniazid, its implications in therapeutic use. In *Trans 14th Conf Chemother Tuberc*. pp. 217–22. Washington, DC: US Veterans Adm Army Navy.

Hunyor, S. N. (1975). Hydralazine and beta-blockade in refractory hypertension with characterization of acetylator phenotype. *Australian and New Zealand Journal of Medicine*, **5**, 530–6.

Husain, S. A., Mathur, K. C. & Jhamaria, J. P. (1973). Incidence of rapid and slow isoniazid inactivators with special reference to clinical response and toxicity of the drug amongst sputum positive pulmonary tuberculosis cases. *Indian Journal of Tuberculosis*, **20**, 20-25.

Hutchings, A., Monie, R. D., Spragg, B. & Routledge, P. A. (1984). Acetylator phenotyping. The effect of ethanol on the dapsone test. *British Journal of Clinical Pharmacology*, **18**, 98–100.

Hutchings, A. D., Monie, R. D., Spragg, B. P. & Routledge, P. A. (1988). Saliva and plasma concentrations of isoniazid and acetyl-isoniazid in man. *British Journal of Clinical Pharmacology*, **25**, 585–9.

Hutchings, A. & Routledge, P. A. (1986). A simple method for determining acetylator phenotype using isoniazid. *British Journal of Clinical Pharmacology*, **22**, 343–5.

Hykes, P. & Elis, J. (1980). Vyskyt uhlokopske pneumokoniozy u rychlych a pomalych acetylatoru sulfadimidinu. *Casopis Lekaru Ceskych*, **119**, 313–14.

Iisalo, E., Laine, T., Lehtonen, A. & Sellman, R. (1979). Dihydralazine therapy and acetylator phenotype. *International Journal of Clinical Pharmacology and Biopharmacy*, **17**, 119–24.

Ilett, K. F., David, B. M., Detchon, P., Catleden, W. M. & Kwa, R. (1987). Acetylation phenotype in colorectal carcinoma. *Cancer Research*, **47**, 1466–9.

Ilett, K. F., Detchon, P., Ingram, D. M. & Castleden, W. M. (1990). Acetylation phenotype is not associated with breast cancer. *Cancer Research*, **50**, 6649–51.

Inaba, T. & Arias, T. D. (1987). On phenotyping with isoniazid. The use of urinary acetylation/ratios and the uniqueness of antimodes found in two Amerindian populations. *Clinical Pharmacology and Therapeutics*, **42**, 493–7.

Irshaid, Y. M., Al-Hadidi, H. F., Abuirjeie, M. A. & Rawashdeh, N. M. (1991). N-acetylation phenotyping using dapsone in a Jordanian population. *British Journal of Clinical Pharmacology*, **32**, 289–93.

Iselius, L. & Evans, D. A. P. (1983). Formal genetics of isoniazid metabolism in man. *Clinical Pharmacokinetics*, **8**, 541–4.

Islam, S. I. (1982). Polymorphic acetylation of sulphamethazine in rural Bedouin and urban-dwellers in Saudi Arabia. *Xenobiotica*, **12**, 323–8.

Iwainsky, H., Gerloff, W. & Schmeidel, A. (1961). Die differenzierung zwischen INH-Inaktivierern under normal abbauenden patienten mit hilfe eines einfachen testes. *Bieträge zur Klinik der Tuberkulose und Spezifischen Tuberkulose forschung*, **124**, 384–9.

Jarman, M., Foster, A. B., Goss, P. E., Griggs, L. J., Howe, I. & Coombes, R. C. (1983). Metabolism of aminoglutethimide in humans; identification of hydroxyaminoglutethimide as an induced metabolite. *Biomedical Mass Spectrometry*, **10**, 620–5.

Jeanes, C. W. L., Schaefer, O. & Eidus, L. (1972). Inactivation of isoniazid by Canadian Eskimos and Indians. *Canadian Medical Association Journal*, **106**, 331–5.

Jenkins, T., Lehmann, H. & Nurse, G. P. (1974). Public health and genetic constitution of the San ('Bushmen'): carbohydrate metabolism and acetylator status of the Kung of Tsumkwe in the North-Western Kalahari. *British Medical Journal*, **2**, 23–6.

Jenne, J. W. (1960). Studies of human patterns of isoniazid metabolism using an intravenous fall-off technique with a chemical method. *American Review of Respiratory Disease*, **81**, 1-8.

Jenne, J.W. (1963). Isoniazid acetylation by human liver and intestinal mucosa. *Federation Proceedings (Abstract)*, **22**, 540.

Jenne, J. W. (1965). Partial purification and properties of the isoniazid transacetylase in human liver. Its relationship to the acetylation of *p*-aminosalicylic acid. *Journal of Clinical Investigation*, **44**, 1992–2002.

Jenne, J. W., McDonald, F. M. & Mendoza, E. (1961). A study of the renal clearances, metabolic inactivation rates and serum fall-off interaction of isoniazid and para-aminosalicylic acid in man. *American Review of Respiratory Disease*, **84**, 371–8.

Jeyakumar, L. H., Arowoshegbe, U. A., Akinuinka, O. O., Akinbami, F. O. & Bababunmi, E. A. (1990). Acetylator status of Kwashiorkor children in Ibadan (South-West Nigeria). *European Journal of Drug Metabolism and Pharmacokinetics*, **15**, 57–62.

Jeyakumar, L. H. & French, M. R. (1981). Polymorphic acetylation of sulphamethazine in a Nigerian (Yoruba) population. *Xenobiotica*, **11**, 319–21.

Jeyakumar, L. H. & French, M. R. (1986). Acetylator phenotype among individuals with glucose-6-phosphate dehydrogenase variants. *Xenobiotica*, **16**, 1129–32.

Jimenez-Nieto, L. C., Ladero, J. M., Fernandez-Gondin, M. J. & Robledo, A. (1989). Acetylator phenotype in psoriasis. *Dermatologica*, **178**, 136–7.

Johansson, E. A., Mustakallio, K. K., Mattila, M. M. & Tiilikairen, A. (1976). Cutaneous reactions to drugs, acetylation phenotype and HLA antigens in patients with and without systemic lupus erythematosus (SLE). *Annals of Clinical Research*, **8**, 126–8.

Johnstone, E. D. & Marsh, W. (1973). Acetylator status and response to phenelzine in depressed patients. *Lancet*, **1**, 567–70.

Jounela, A. J., Pasanen, M. & Mattila, M. J. (1975). Acetylator phenotype and the anti-hypertensive response to hydralazine. *Acta Medica Scandinavica*, **197**, 303–6.

Kaisary, A., Smith, P., Jaczq, E., McAllister, C. B., Wilkinson, G. R., Ray, W. A. & Branch, R. A. (1987). Genetic predisposition to bladder cancer: Ability to hydroxylate debrisoquine and mephenytoin as risk factors. *Cancer Research*, **47**, 5488–93.

Kang, E. S., Deaton, P. R., Epstein, D., Ingram, L. A. & Mirvis, D. M. (1989). Procainamide *N*-acetyltransferase: modulation by clofibrate and microsomal form. *General Pharmacology*, **20**, 223–7.

Kang, Y. S. & Lee, C. C. (1973). The researches of the Korean population genetics – studies on the frequencies and distributions of some human enzyme deficient traits. *Journal of the National Academy of Sciences, Republic of Korea, Natural Sciences Series*, **12**, 115–37.

Karakaya, A. E., Cok, I., Sardas, S., Gogus, O. & Sardas, O. S. (1986). N-acetylation phenotype of patients with bladder cancer. *Human Toxicology*, **5**, 333–5.

Karim, A. K. M. B., Elfellah, M. S. & Evans, D. A. P. (1981). Human acetylator polymorphism: estimate of allele frequency in Libya and details of global distribution. *Journal of Medical Genetics*, **18**, 325–30.

Karim, A. K. M. B & Evans, D. A. P. (1976). Polymorphic acetylation of nitrazepam. *Journal of Medical Genetics*, **13**, 17–19.

Karlsson, E., Aberg, G., Collste, P., Molin, L., Norlander, B. & Sjöqvist, F. (1975). Acetylation of procaine amide in man. A preliminary communication. *European Journal of Clinical Pharmacology*, **8**, 79–81.

Karlsson, E. & Molin, L. (1975). Polymorphic acetylation of procaine amide in healthy subjects. *Acta Medica Scandinavica*, **197**, 299–302.

Karlsson, E., Molin, L., Norlander, B. & Sjoqvist, F. (1974). Acetylation of procainamide in man studied with a new gas chromatographic method. *British Journal of Clinical Pharmacology*, **1**, 467–75.

Kawakubo, Y., Manabe, S., Yamazoe, Y., Nishikawa, T. & Kato, R. (1988). Properties of cutaneous acetyltransferase catalyzing *N*-and *O*-acetylation of carcinogenic arylamines and *N*-hydroxyarylamine. *Biochemical Pharmacology*, **37**, 265–70.

Kelly, C. & Griffiths, I. D. (1981). Dapsone in rheumatoid arthritis. *Annals of the Rheumatic Diseases*, **40**, 630–2.

Kergueris, M. F., Bourin, M. & Larousse, C. (1986). Pharmacokinetics of Isoniazid: influence of age. *European Journal of Clinical Pharmacology*, **30**, 335–40.

Kilbane, A. J., Silbart, L. K., Manis, M., Beitins, I. Z. & Weber, W. W. (1990). Human *N*-acetylation genotype determination with urinary caffeine metabolites. *Clinical Pharmacology and Therapeutics*, **47**, 470–7.

Kingston, M. & Skoog, W. C. (1986). Diabetes in Saudi Arabia. *Saudi Medical Journal*, **7**, 130–42.

Kirlin, W. G., Ogolla, F., Andrews, A. F., Trinidad, A., Ferguson, R. J., Yerokun, T., Mpezo, M. & Hein, D. W. (1991). Acetylator genotype-dependent expression of arylamine *N*- acetyltransferase in human colon cytosol from non-cancer and colorectal cancer patients. *Cancer Research*, **51**, 549–55.

Kirlin, W. G., Trinidad, A., Yerokun, T., Ogolla, F., Ferguson, R. J., Andrews, A. F., Brady, P. K. & Hein, D. W. (1989). Polymorphic expression of acetyl coenzyme A dependent arylamine *N*-acetyltransferase and acetyl coenzyme A dependent *O{O}*-acetyltransferase mediated activation of *N*-hydroxyarylamines by human bladder cytosol. *Cancer Research*, **49**, 2448–54.

Knight, R. A., Selin, M. J. & Harris, H. W. (1959). Genetic factors influencing isoniazid blood levels in humans. In *Trans 18th Conf Chemother Tuberc.*, pp. 52–8. Washington, DC: US Veterans Adm Army Navy.

Koroltchouk, V., Stanley, K., Stjernsward, J. & Mott, K. (1987). Bladder cancer: approaches to prevention and control. *Bulletin of the World Health Organization*, **65**, 513–20.

Kukongviriyapan, V., Lulitamoud, V., Arrejitanusorn, C., Kongyingyose, B. & Laupattarakasem, P. (1984). *N*-acetyl transferase polymorphism in Thailand. *Human Heredity*, **34**, 246–9.

Kumana, C. R., Chan, M. M. Y., Wong, K.-L., Wong, R. W. S., Kon, M. & Lander, I.J. (1990). Lack of association between slow acetylator status and spontaneous lupus erythematosus. *Clinical Pharmacology and Therapeutics*, **48**, 208–13.

Kutt, H. (1971). Biochemical and genetic factors regulating

dilantin metabolism in man. *Annals of the New York Academy of Sciences*, **179**, 702–22.

Ladero, J. M., Arrojo, A., De Salamanca, R. E., Gomez, M., Cano, F. & Alfonso, M. (1982). Hepatic acetylator phenotype in diabetes mellitus. *Annals of Clinical Research*, **14**, 187–9.

Ladero, J. M. & Cano, F. (1983). Fenotipo acetilador en la enfermedad de Basedow. *Nuevos archivos de la Facultad de Medicina*, **41**, 79–81.

Ladero, J. M., De Salamanca, R. E. & Chinarro, S. (1981). Hepatic acetylator phenotype in porphyria cutanea tarda. *Archives of Dermatological Research*, **270**, 171–3.

Ladero, J. M., Fernandez, M. J., Palmeiro, R., Munoz, J. J., Jara, C., Lazaro, C. & Perez-Manga, G. (1987). Hepatic acetylator polymorphism in breast cancer patients. *Oncology*, **44**, 341–4.

Ladero, J. M., Gonzalez, J. F., Benitez, J., Vargas, E., Fernandez, M. J., Baki, W. & Diaz-Rubio, M. (1991). Acetylator polymorphism in human colorectal carcinoma. *Cancer Research*, **51**, 2098–100.

Ladero, J. M., Jimenez, F. J., Benitez, J., Fernandez-Gundin, M. R., Martinez, C., Llerena, A., Cobaleda, J. & Munoz, J. J. (1989). Acetylator polymorphism in Parkinson's disease. *European Journal of Clinical Pharmacology*, **37**, 391–3.

Ladero, J. M., Jiminez, L. C., Fernandez, M. J. & Robledo, A. (1988). Acetylator polymorphism in discoid lupus erythematosus. *European Journal of Clinical Pharmacology*, **34**, 307–8.

Ladero, J. M., Kwok, C. K., Jara, C., Fernandez, L., Silmi, A. M., Tapia, D. & Uson, A. C. (1985). Hepatic acetylator phenotype in bladder cancer patients. *Annals of Clinical Research*, **17**, 96–9.

Ladero Quesada, J. M., Romero, A. A. & Garcia, G. (1979). Acetilaction hepatica en la poblacíon Española. *Gastroenteriologia y Hepatologia (Barcelona)*, **2**, 236–40.

Ladero Quesada, J. M., Sanchez, C. J., Rodriquez, J. B., Gondin, M. J. F., Castrillon, E. V., Gonzalez, J. J. M., Ruiz, A., Le Polo, J. C. & Perez-Manga, G. (1991). Polimorfismo acetilador en el cáncer de pulmón. *Annales de Medicina Interna (Madrid)*, **8**, 66–8.

Land, S. J., Zukowski, K., Lee, M.-S., Debiec-Rychter, M., King, C. M. & Wang, C. Y. (1989). Metabolism of aromatic amines: relationship of N-acetylation O-acetylation N, O-acetyltransfer and deacetylation in human liver and urinary bladder. *Carcinogenesis*, **10**, 727–31.

Lang, N. P., Chu, D. Z. J., Hunter, C. F., Kendall, D. C., Flammang, T. J. & Kadlubar, F. F. (1986). Role of aromatic amine acetyltransferase in human colorectal cancer. *Archives of Surgery*, **121**, 1259–61.

Larsson, R., Karlberg, B. E., Norlander, B. & Wirsen, A. (1981). Prizidilol, an antihypertensive with precapillary vasodilator and β-adrenoceptor blocking actions in primary hypertension. *Clinical Pharmacology and Therapeutics*, **29**, 588–93.

Larsson, R., Karlsson, E. & Molin, L. (1977). Spontaneous systemic lupus erythematosus and acetylator phenotype. *Acta Medica Scandinavica*, **201**, 223–6.

Lavigne, J.-G., Barry, A., D'Auteuil, C. & Delage, J.-M. (1977). *p*-Aminosalicylate metabolism in cancer patients sensitive and resistant to chemotherapy. *British Journal of Cancer*, **35**, 580–6.

Lawson, D. H., Hanry, D. A., Lowe, J., Reavey, P., Rennie,

J. A. N. & Solomon, A. (1979). Acetylator phenotype in spontaneous SLE and rheumatoid arthritis. *Annals of the Rheumatic Diseases*, **38**, 171–3.

Leden, I., Hanson, A., Melander, A., Sturfelt, G., Svensson, B. & Wahlin-Boll, E. (1981). Varying distribution of acetylation phenotypes in RA patients with and without Sjogren's syndrome. *Scandinavian Journal of Rheumatology*, **10**, 253–5.

Lee, E. J. C. & Ang, S. B. (1986). A simple and sensitive HPLC assay for sulfapyridine and acetylsulfapyridine in serum and urine. *Asia-Pacific Journal of Pharmacology*, **1**, 59–62.

Lee, E. J. C. & Lee, L. K. H. (1982). A simple pharmacokinetic method for separating the three acetylation phenotypes. A preliminary report. *British Journal of Clinical Pharmacology*, **13**, 375–8.

Lee, E. J. D. & Lim, J. M. E. (1981). A study of the acetylator phenotype in normal subjects. *Singapore Medical Journal*, **22**, 117–20.

Lee, E. J. D., Lim, J. M. E. & Feng, P. H. (1985). Acetylator phenotype in Chinese patients with spontaneous systemic lupus erythematosus. *Singapore Medical Journal*, **26**, 295–9.

Lester, D. (1965). The acetylation of isoniazid in alcoholics. *Quarterly Journal of Studies on Alcohol*, **25**, 541–3.

Levi, A. J., Sherlock, S. & Walker, D. (1968). Phenylbutazone and isoniazid metabolism in patients with liver disease in relation to previous drug therapy. *Lancet*, **1**, 1275–9.

Levy, M., Flusser, D., Zylber-Katz, E. & Granit, L. (1984). Plasma kinetics of dipyrone metabolites in rapid and slow acetylators. *European Journal of Clinical Pharmacology*, **27**, 453–8.

Lewalter, J. & Korallus, U. (1985). Blood protein conjugates and acetylation of aromatic amines. *International Archives of Occupational and Environmental Health*, **56**, 179–96.

Ligueros, M. S., Cruz-Coke, R. M., Neira, S. U., Saavedra, H. C., Kramer, V. A. Prieto, J. C. D., Gelman, M. B., Saavedra, A. G., Nunez, A. & Pescio, S. S. (1989). Polimorfismo genetico de acetilacion de isoniazida en pacientes tuberculosos Chileños. *Revista Medica de Chile*, **117**, 1339–43.

Lilyin, E. T., Korunskaya, M. P., Meksin, V. A., Drozdov, E. S., Nasarov, V. V. & Monastyrskaya, A. R. (1984). The distribution of acetylator phenotypes of normal individuals and the patients suffering from alcoholism among Moscow urban population. *Genetika (Moskva)*, **20**, 1557–9.

Lilyin, E. G., Korsunskaya, M. P., Meksin, V. A., Taelicheva, L. V. & Shapiro, E. F. (1983). The distribution of acetylator phenotypes in Moscow population. *Genetika (Moskva)*, **19**, 1378–80.

Lima, J. J., Conti, D. R., Goldfarb, A. L., Tilstone, W. J., Golden, L. H. & Jusko, W. J. (1979). Clinical pharmacokinetics of procainamide infusions in relation to acetylator phenotype. *Journal of Pharmacokinetics and Biopharmaceutics*, **7**, 69–85.

Lindsay, R. M. & Baty, J. D. (1988). Inter-individual variation of human blood N-acetyl transferase activity *in vitro*. *Biochemical Pharmacology*, **37**, 3915–21.

Lindsay, R. M. & Baty, J. D. (1990). The effect of streptozotocin-induced diabetes on the *in vivo* acetylation capacity and the *in vitro* blood N-acetyl transferase activity of the adult male Sprague-Dawley rat. *Biochemical Pharmacology*, **39**, 1193–97.

Littley, M. D., Hutchings, A., Spragg, B. P., Routledge, P. A. & Lazarus, J. H. (1988). The effect of thyrotoxicosis on isoniazid acetylation. *British Journal of Clinical Pharmacology*, **26**, 103–6.

Lopez, G. T. & De Claure, M. L. N. (1987). Acetilacion de isoniacida su relacion con factores geneticos y ambientales de altura. *Archivos de Biologia y Medicina Experimentales*, **20**, 13–19.

Lorenzo, B. & Reidenberg, M. M. (1989). Potential artefacts in the use of caffeine to determine acetylation phenotype. *British Journal of Clinical Pharmacology*, **28**, 207–8.

Lower, G. Jr. (1983). Molecular epidemiology of arylamine-induced urinary bladder cancer: some theoretical considerations. In *Relationship of acetylator status to isoniazid toxicity, lupus erythematosus and bladder cancer*, ed. W. W. Weber, D. W. Hein, A. Litwin & G. M. Lower Jr. *Federation Proceedings*, **42**, 3086–97.

Lower, G. M. Jr., Nilsson, T., Nelson, C. E., Wolf, H., Gamsky, T. E. & Bryan, G. T. (1979). *N*-acetyltransferase phenotype and risk in urinary-bladder cancer: approaches in molecular epidemiology. Preliminary results in Sweden and Denmark. *Environmental Health Perspectives*, **29**, 71–9.

Maddrey, W. C. & Boitnott, J. K. (1973). Isoniazid hepatitis. *Annals of Internal Medicine*, **79**, 1–12.

Mansilla-Tinoco, R., Harland, S. J., Ryan, P. J., Bernstein, R. M., Dollery, C. T., Hughes, G. R. V., Bulpitt, C. J., Morgan, A. & Jones, J. M. (1982). Hydralazine antinuclear antibodies and the lupus syndrome. *British Medical Journal*, **284**, 936–9.

Marsden, J. R., Mason, G. G. F., Coburn, P. R., Rawlins, M. D. & Schuster, S. (1985). Drug acetylation and expression of lupus erythematosus. *European Journal of Clinical Pharmacology*, **28**, 387–90.

Marshall, E. F. (1976). The myth of phenelzine acetylation. *British Medical Journal*, **2**, 817.

Marshall, E. F., Mountjoy, C. Q., Campbell, I. C., Garside, R. F., Leitch, I. M. & Roth, M. (1978). The influence of acetylator phenotype on the outcome of treatment with phenelzine in a clinical trial. *British Journal of Clinical Pharmacology*, **6**, 247–54.

Martinez-Roig, A., Cami, J., Llorens-Terol, J., de la Torre, R. & Perich, F. (1986). Acetylation phenotype and hepatoxicity in the treatment of tuberculosis in children. *Pediatrics*, **77**, 912–15.

Mattila, M. J., Frimen, A., Larmi, T. K. I. & Koskinen, R. (1969b). Absorption of ethionamide, isoniazid and aminosalicylic acid from the post-resection gastrointestinal tract. *Annales Medicinae Experimentalis et Biologiae Fennicae*, **47**, 209–12.

Mattila, M. J. & Takki, S. (1969). Half-lives of isoniazid and salicylic acid in serum and their modification by different drugs in psychiatric patients. *Annales Medicinae Experimentalis et Biologiae Fennicae*, **47**, 124–8.

Mattila, M. J. & Tiitinen, H. (1967). The rate of isoniazid inactivation in Finnish diabetic and non-diabetic patients. *Annales Academiae Scientiarum Fennicae*, **45**, 423–7.

Mattila, M. J., Tiitnen, H. & Alhava, E. (1969a). Acetylation pattern of different sulphonamides in rapid and slow isoniazid inactivators. *Annales Medicinae Experimentalis et Biologiae Fennicae*, **47**, 308–15.

May, D. G., Porter, J. A., Uetrecht, J. P., Wilkinson, G. R. & Branch, R. A. (1990). The contribution of *N*-hydroxylation and acetylation to dapsone pharmacokinetics in normal subjects. *Clinical Pharmacology and Therapeutics*, **48**, 619–27.

Mayo, O. & Street. D. J. (1986). Heterogeneity in disease associations. *Human Heredity*, **36**, 89–92.

McDermott, W. (1960). Antimicrobial therapy of pulmonary tuberculosis. *Bulletin of the World Health Organisation*, **23**, 427–61.

McLaren, E. H., Burden, A. C. & Moorhead, P. J. (1977). Acetylator phenotype in diabetic neuropathy. *British Medical Journal*, **2**, 291–93.

McQueen, C. A. & Weber, W. W. (1980). Characterization of human lymphocyte *N*-acetyltransferase and its relationship to the isoniazid acetylator polymorphism. *Biochemical Genetics*, **18**, 889–904.

Meisel, M., Schneider, T., Siegmund, W., Nikschick, S., Kebingat, K.-J. & Scherber, A. (1986). Development of human polymorphic *N*-acetyltransferase. *Biological Research in Pregnancy and Perinatology (Munchen-Diesenhofen)*, **7**, 74–6.

Menon, N. K. (1968). Madras study of supervised once-weekly chemotherapy. *Bulletin of the International Union against Tuberculosis and Lung Disease*, **41**, 316–21.

Meyer, H. & Mally, J. (1912). Über hydrazinderivate der pyridincarbonsussen. *Monatshefte fuer Chemie and Verwandte Teile Anderer Wissenschaften*, **33**, 393–414.

Miller, M. E. & Cosgriff, J. M. (1983). Acetylator phenotype in human bladder cancer. *Journal of Urology*, **130**, 65–6.

Miller, M. E., Garland, W. A., Min, B. H., Ludwick, B. T., Ballard, R. H. & Levy, R. H. (1981). Clonazepam acetylation in fast and slow acetylators. *Clinical Pharmacology and Therapeutics*, **30**, 343–7.

Minchin, R. F., Reeves, P. T., Teitel, C. H. McManus, M. E., Mojarrabi, B., Ilett, K. F. & Kadlubar F. F. (1992). *N*- and *O*-acetylation of aromatic and heterocyclic amine carcinogens by human monomorphic and polymorphic acetyltransferases expressed in COS-1 cells. *Biochemical and Biophysical Research Communications*, **185**, 839–44.

Miscoria, G., Leneveu, A., Walle, C. & Roux, A. (1988). Application d'une methode de dosage de l'isoniazide et de l'acetylisoniazide par chromatographie liquide haute performance a la determination due phenotype d'acetylation. *Annales de Biologie Clinique*, **46**, 734–40.

Mitchell, J. R., Long, M. W., Thorgeirsson, U. P. & Jollow, D. J. (1975b). Acetylation rates and monthly liver function tests during one year of isoniazid preventive therapy. *Chest*, **68**, 181–90.

Mitchell, J. R., Thorgeirsson, U. P., Black, M., Timbrell, J. A., Snodgrass, W. R., Potter, W. Z., Jollow, D. J. & Kelser, H. R. (1975a). Increased incidence of isoniazid hepatitis in rapid acetylators, possible relation to hydrazine metabolites. *Clinical Pharmacology and Therapeutics*, **18**, 70–9.

Mitchell, J. R., Zimmerman, H. J., Ishak, K. G., Thorgeirsson, U. P., Timbrell, J. A., Snodgrass, W. R. & Nelson, S. D. (1976). Isoniazid liver injury: clinical spectrum, pathology and possible pathogenesis. *Annals of Internal Medicine*, **84**, 181–92.

Mitchell, R. S. & Bell, J. C. (1957). Clinical implications of isoniazid PAS and streptomycin blood levels in pulmonary tuberculosis. *Transactions of the American Clinical and Climatological Association*, **69**, 98–105.

Mitchell, R. S., Bell, J. C. & Reimensnider, D. K. (1960). Further observations with isoniazid inactivation tests. In *Trans 19th Conf Chemother Tuberc*, pp. 62–6. Washington, DC: US Veterans Adm Army Navy.

Mitchell, R. S., Riemensnider, D. K., Harsch, J. R. & Bell, J. C. (1958). New information on the clinical implications of individual variations in the metabolic handling of antituberculous drugs particularly isoniazid. In *Trans 17th Conf Chemother Tuberc*, pp. 77–85. Washington, DC: US Veterans Adm Army Navy.

Mitchison, D. A. (1971). Clinical applications of antibiotic and chemotherapeutic agents. *Proceedings of the Royal Society of Medicine*, **64**, 537–40.

Molin, L., Larsson, R. & Karlsson, E. (1977). Evaluation of the sulphapyridine acetylator phenotyping test in healthy subjects and in patients with cardiac and renal disease. *Acta Medica Scandinavica*, **201**, 217–22.

Mommsen, S. & Aagaard, J. (1986). Susceptibility in urinary bladder cancer. Acetyltransferase phenotypes and related risk factors. *Cancer Letters*, **32**, 199–205.

Morris, M. E., Griener, J. C. & Msall, M. E. (1989). N-acetylator variability in Down's syndrome: characterization with caffeine. *Clinical Pharmacology and Therapeutics*, **46**, 359–66.

Morris, R. J., Freed, C. R. & Kohler, P. F. (1979). Drug acetylation phenotype unrelated to development of spontaneous systemic lupus erythematosus. *Arthritis and Rheumatism*, **22**, 777–80.

Motulsky, A. G. & Steinmann, L. (1962). Arylamine acetylation in human red cells. *Journal of Clinical Investigation*, **41**, 1387.

Mozayani, A., Coutts, R. T., Danielson, T. J. & Baker, G. B. (1988). Metabolic acetylation of phenelzine in rats. *Research Communications in Chemical Pathology and Pharmacology*, **62**, 397–406.

Musch, E., Eichelbaum, M., Wang, J. K., von Sassen, W., Castro-Parra, M. & Dengler, J. H. (1982). Die Häufigkeit hepatotoxischer Nebenwirkungen der tuberculostatischen kombinations therapie (INH RMP EMB) in Abhangigkeit vom acetyliererp̂hanotype. *Klinische Wochenschrift*, **60**, 513–19.

Nair, C. R., Gupta, R. C., Varshneya, A. K. & Malik, S. K. (1984). Correlation of sulphadimidine acetylation test in urine and blood for isoniazid phenotyping. *International Journal of Clinical Pharmacology, Therapy and Toxicology*, **22**, 646–7.

Narasimhachari, N., Chang, S. & Davis, J. M. (1980). A test for 'acetylator status' hypothesis for antidepressant response to phenelzine. *Research Communications in Psychology, Psychiatry and Behaviour*, **5**, 199–204.

Nhachi, C. F. B. (1988). Polymorphic acetylation of sulphamethazine in a Zimbabwe population. *Journal of Medical Genetics*, **25**, 29–31.

Odeigah, P. G. C. & Okunowo, M. A. (1989). High frequency of the rapid isoniazid acetylator phenotype in Lagos (Nigeria). *Human Heredity*, **39**, 26–31.

Ohsako, S. & Deguchi, T. (1990). Cloning and expression of cDNA's for polymorphic and monomorphic arylamine N-acetyltransferases from human liver. *Journal of Biological Chemistry*, **265**, 4630–4.

Oka, M. & Seppala, O. (1978). Acetylation phenotype in rheumatoid arthritis. *Scandinavian Journal of Rheumatology*, **7**, 29–30.

Olsen, H. (1982a). Colorimetric or HPLC method for acetylator phenotyping with sulfadimidine? *Acta Pharmacologica Toxicologia*, **50**, 75–7.

Olsen, H. (1982b). Interaction between drug acetylation and ethanol, acetate, pyruvate, citrate and L(-)carnitine in isolated rat liver parenchymal cells. *Acta Pharmacologica et Toxicologica*, **50**, 67–74.

Olsen, H. & Morland, J. (1978). Ethanol-induced increase in drug acetylation in man and isolated rat cells. *British Medical Journal*, **2**, 1260-1262.

Olsen, H. & Morland, J. (1982). Ethanol-induced increase in procainamide acetylation in man. *British Journal of Clinical Pharmacology*, **13**, 203–8.

Olsewska, Z., Orlowsak-Westwood, B., Orszulak, D., Jablkowska-Gajdzinska, J. & Skretkowiccz, J. (1980). Fenotyp acetylacji w luszczycy, *Przeglad Dermatologiczny (Warszawa)*, **67**, 19–22.

Orlowska-Westwood, B., Skretkowicz, J., Orszulak, D., Krykowski, E. & Mazurowa, A. (1980). Fenotyp acetylacji u chorych na toczen rumieniowaty ukladowy. *Polskie Archiwum Medycyny Wewnetrznej*, **64**, 431–4.

Orzechowska-Juzwenko, K., Milejski, P., Patowski, J. & Malolepszy, J. (1986). Fenotyp acetylacji i jego znaczenie w chorobach alergicznych. *Polski Tygodnik Lekarski*, **41**, 25–8.

Orzechowska-Juzwenko, K., Milejski, P., Patkowski, J., Nittner-Marszalska, M. & Malolepszy, J. (1990). Acetylator phenotype in patients with allergic diseases and its clinical significance. *International Journal of Clinical Pharmacology, Therapy and Toxicology*, **28**, 420–5.

Pacifici, G. H., Bencini, C. & Rane, A. (1986). Acetyltransferase in humans: development and tissue distribution. *Pharmacology*, **32**, 283–91.

Pacifici, G. M., Franchi, M., Bencini, C., Repetti, F., diLascio, N. & Muraro, G. B. (1988). Tissue distribution of drug metabolizing enzymes in humans. *Xenobiotica*, **18**, 849–56.

Pacifici, G. M., Viani, A., Franchi, M., Santerini, S., Temellini, A., Giuliani, L. & Carrai, M. (1990). Conjugation pathways in liver disease. *British Journal of Clinical Pharmacology*, **30**, 427–35.

Paik, Y. K., Cho, Y. H., Kim, I. K., Benkmann, H. G. & Goedde, H. W. (1988). Pharmacogenetic studies in South Korea: serum cholinesterase and N-acetyltransferase polymorphism. *Korean Journal of Genetics*, **10**, 272–8.

Paire, M., Lavarenne, J. & Rodet, M. F. (1984). Inactivation de l'isoniazide chez l'enfant. *Therapie*, **39**, 625–31.

Palatsi, R., Jansen, C. T. & Hopsu-Havu, V. K. (1973). Inactivator status of cutaneous reactors to sulphonamide. *Scandinavian Journal of Clinical and Laboratory Investigation*, **31** (Suppl. 130), 13.

Parthasarathy, R., Raghupati Sarma, G., Janardhanam, B., Ramachandran, P., Santha, T., Sivasubramaian, S., Somasundaram, P. R. & Tripathy, S. P. (1986). Hepatic toxicity in South Indian patients during treatment of tuberculosis with short-course regimens containing isoniazid, rifampicin and pyrazinamide. *Tubercle*, **67**, 99–108.

Pasanen, M., Pasanen, A. & Jounela, A. (1973). Effect of acetylation phenotype on the antihypertensive response to hydralazine. *Scandinavian Journal of Clinical and Laboratory Investigation*, **31** (Suppl. 130), 12.

Paulsen, O. & Nilsson, L. G. (1985). Distribution of acetylator phenotype in relation to age and sex in Swedish patients. *European Journal of Clinical Pharmacology*, **28**, 311–15.

Peng, D. R., Birgersson, C., von Bahr, C. & Rane, A. (1984). Polymorphic acetylation of 7-amino-clonazepam in human liver cytosol. *Pediatric Pharmacology*, **4**, 155–9.

Penketh, R. J. A., Gibreig, S. F. A., Nurse, G. T. & Hopkinson, D. A. (1983). Acetylator phenotypes in Papua New Guinea. *Journal of Medical Genetics*, **20**, 39–40.

Peretti, E., Karlaganis, G. & Lauterburg, B. H. (1987a). Increased urinary excretion of toxic hydrazine metabolites of isoniazid by slow acetylators: effect of a slow-release preparation of isoniazid. *European Journal of Clinical Pharmacology*, **33**, 283–6.

Peretti, E., Karlaganis, G. & Lauterburg, B. H. (1987b). Acetylation of acetylhydrazine the toxic metabolite of isoniazid in humans. Inhibition by concomitant administration of isoniazid. *Journal of Pharmacology and Experimental Therapeutics*, **243**, 686–9.

Perry, H. H., Tan, E. M., Carmody, S. & Sakamoto, A. (1970). Relationship of acetyl transferase activity to antinuclear antibodies and toxic symptoms in hypertensive patients treated with hydralazine. *Journal of Laboratory and Clinical Medicine*, **76**, 114–25.

Peters, J. H., Gill, M. & Hayes, V. E. (1966). The influence of D-glucose and p-aminosalicylic acid on the metabolism of isoniazid. *Archives internationales de Pharmacodynamie*, **159**, 340–52.

Peters, J. H., Gordon, G. R. & Brown, P. (1965). The relationship between the capacities of human subjects to acetylate isoniazid sulfanilamide and sulfamethazine. *Life Sciences*, **4**, 99–107.

Peters, J. H,. Gordon, G. T., Ghoul, D. C., Tolentino, J. C., Walsh, G. P. & Levy, L. (1972). The disposition of the antileprotic drug dapsone (DDS) in Philippine subjects. *American Journal of Tropical Medicine and Hygiene*, **21**, 450–7.

Peters, J. H., Gordon, G. T. & Karat, A. B. A. (1975). Polymorphic acetylation of the anti-bacterials, sulfamethazine and dapsone, in South Indian subjects. *American Journal of Tropical Medicine and Hygiene*, **24**, 641–8.

Peters, J. H., Gordon, G. R., Levy, L., Storkan, M. A., Jacobson, R. R., Euna, C. D. & Kirchheimer, W. F. (1974). Metabolic disposition of dapsone in patients with dapsone-resistant leprosy. *American Journal of Tropical Medicine and Hygiene*, **23**, 222–30.

Peters, J. H., Gordon, G. R., Lin, E., Green, C. E. & Tyson, C. A. (1990). Polymorphic N-acetylation of sulfamethazine by human liver: implication for cancer risk? *Anticancer Research*, **10**, 225–30.

Peters, J. H. & Levy, L. (1971). Dapsone acetylation in man. Another example of polymorphic acetylation. *Annals of the New York Academy of Sciences*, **179**, 660–6.

Philip, P. A., Fitzgerald, D. L., Cartwright, R. A., Peake, M. D. & Rogers, H. J. (1988). Polymorphic N-acetylation capacity in lung cancer. *Carcinogenesis*, **9**, 491–3.

Philip, P. A., Gayed, S. L., Rogers, H. J. & Crome, P. (1987a). Influence of age, sex and body weight on the dapsone acetylation phenotype. *British Journal of Clinical Pharmacology*, **23**, 709–13.

Philip, P. A., Harper, P. G. & Rogers, H. J. (1989). Effect of cancer chemotherapy on dapsone N-acetylation in man. *Cancer Chemotherapy and Pharmacology*, **23**, 395–6.

Philip, P. A., Roberts, M. S. & Rogers, H. J. (1984). A rapid method for determination of acetylator phenotype using dapsone. *British Journal of Clinical Pharmacology*, **17**, 465–9.

Philip, P. A., Rogers, H. J. & Harper, P. G. (1987c). Acetylation and oxidation phenotypes in malignant lymphoma. *Cancer Chemotherapy and Pharmacology*, **20**, 235–8.

Philip, P. A., Rogers, H. J., Millis, R. R., Rubens, R. D. & Cartwright, R. A. (1987b). Acetylator status and its relationship to breast cancer and other diseases of the breast. *European Journal of Cancer and Clinical Oncology*, **11**, 1701–6.

Pieters, F. A. J. M., Woonink, F. & Zuidema, J. (1988). Influence of once-monthly rifampicin and daily clofazimine on the pharmacokinetics of dapsone in leprosy patients in Nigeria. *European Journal of Clinical Pharmacology*, **34**, 73–6.

Platzer, R., Kupfer, A., Bircher, J. & Preisig, R. C. (1978). Polymorphic acetylation and aminopyrine demethylation in Gilbert's syndrome. *European Journal of Clinical Investigation*, **8**, 219–23.

Plowman, P. N. (1987). Aminoglutethimide: a toxic object lesson in the endocrine management of cancer. *Human Toxicology*, **6**, 187–8.

Podymov, V. K., Vinogradova, O. M., Kovaleva, V. L., Kochueei, L. N. & Galstian, S. M. (1988). Acetylation phenotype in patients with periodic disease. *Terapevticheskii Arkhiv*, **60**, 95–8.

Pontiroli, A. E., Calderara, A., Bonisolli, L., de Pasqua, A., Maffi, P., Margonato, A., Radaelli, G., Gallus, G. & Pozza, G. (1987). Risk factors for micro-and macro-angiopathic complications in Type 2 diabetes: lack of association with acetylator phenotype, chlorpropamide alcohol flush and ABO and Rh blood groups. *Diabète Metabolisme (Paris)*, **13**, 444–9.

Pontiroli, A. E., de Pasqua, A., Bonisolli, L. & Pozza, G. (1985). Ageing and acetylator phenotype as determined by administration of sulphadimidine. *European Journal of Clinical Pharmacology*, **28**, 485–6.

Pontiroli, A. E., Mosca, A., de Pasqua, A., Alcini, D. & Pozza, G. (1984). The fast acetylator phenotype in diabetes mellitus; abnormal prevalence and association with the ABO blood groups. *Diabetologia*, **27**, 235–7.

Price, J. (1971). *Demethylation, methylation and schizophrenia. A pharmacogenetic study*. MD thesis, University of London.

Probst, M. R., Blum, M, Fasshaver, I., D'Orazio, D., Meyer, U. A. & Wild, D. (1992). The role of the human acetylation polymorphism in the metabolic activation of the food carcinogen 2-amino-3-methylimidazo [4,5-f] quinolone (IQ). *Carcinogenesis*, **13**, 1713–17.

Pullar, T. & Capell, H. A. (1986). Variables affecting efficacy and toxicity of sulphasalazine in rheumatoid arthritis. *Drugs*, **32** (Suppl. 1), 54–7.

Pullar, T., Hunter, J.A. & Capell, H. A. (1985). Effect of acetylator phenotype on efficacy and toxicity of sulphasalazine in rheumatoid arthritis. *Annals of the Rheumatic Diseases*, **44**, 831–7.

Raghupati Sarma, G., Immanuel, C., Kailasam, S., Narayana, A. S. L. & Venkatesan, P. (1986). Rifampicin-induced release of hydrazine from isoniazid. *American Review of Respiratory Disease*, **133**, 1072–5.

Raghupati Sarma, G., Kailsam, S., Kannapiran, M., Krishnaswami, K. V., Thomas, L., Nair, N. G. K. & Narayana, A. S. L. (1976). Classification of subjects as slow or rapid inactivators of isoniazid based on the ratio of acetylisoniazid to isoniazid in urine determined by a simple colorimetric method. *Indian Journal of Medical Research*, **64**, 1456–61.

Rahav, G., Zylber-Katz, E., Rachmilewitz, D. & Levy, M. (1990). Relationship between acetylator phenotype, plasma sulfapyridine levels and adverse effects during treatment with salicylazosulfapyridine in patients with chronic bowel diseases. *Israel Journal of Medical Sciences*, **26**, 31–4.

Raj, P. P., Aschoff, M., Lilly, L. & Balakrishnan, S. (1988). Influence of acetylator phenotype of the leprosy patient on the emergence of dupsoner resistant leprosy. *Indian Journal of Leprosy*, **60**, 400–6.

Ramsay, L. E., Silas, J. H., Ollerenshaw, J. D., Tucker, G. T., Phillips, F. C. & Freestone, S. (1984). Should the acetylator phenotype be determined when prescribing hydralazine for hypertension? *European Journal of Clinical Pharmacology*, **26**, 39–42.

Rao, K. V. N., Mitchison, D. A., Nair, N. G. K., Prema, K. & Tripathy, S. P. (1970). Sulphadimidine acetylation test for classification of patients as slow or rapid inactivators of isoniazid. *British Medical Journal*, **3**, 495–7.

Ratain, M. J., Mick, R., Berezin, F., Janisch, L., Schilsky, R. L., Williams, S. F. & Smiddy, J. (1991). Paradoxical relationship between acetylator phenotype and amonafide toxicity. *Clinical Pharmacology and Therapeutics*, **50**, 573–9.

Reece, P. A., Cozamanis, I. & Zacest, R. (1980). Kinetics of hydralazine and its main metabolites in slow and fast acetylators. *Clinical Pharmacology and Therapeutics*, **28**, 769–78.

Reece, P. A., Cozamanis, I. & Zacest, R. (1982). Influence of acetylator phenotype on the pharmacokinetics of a new vasodilator antihypertensive, endralazine. *European Journal of Clinical Pharmacology*, **23**, 523–7.

Reeves, P. T., Minchin, R. F. & Ilett, K. F. (1988). Induction of sulfamethazine acetylation by hydrocortisone in the rabbit. *Drug Metabolism and Disposition*, **16**, 110–15.

Reeves, P. T., Minchin, R. F. & Ilett, K. F. (1989). In vivo mechanisms for the enhanced acetylation of sulfamethazine in the rabbit after hydrocortisone treatment. *Journal of Pharmacology and Experimental Therapeutics*, **248**, 348–52.

Reidenberg, M. M., Drayer, D., de Marco, A. L. & Bello, C. T. (1973). Hydralazine elimination in man. *Clinical Pharmacology and Therapeutics*, **14**, 970–7.

Reidenberg, M. M., Drayer, D. E., Leym, M. & Warner, H. (1975). Polymorphic acetylation of procainamide in man. *Clinical Pharmacology and Therapeutics*, **17**, 722–30.

Reidenberg, M. M., Levy, M., Drayer, D. E., Zylber-Katz, E. & Robbins, W. C. (1980). Acetylator phenotype in idiopathic systemic lupus erythematosus. *Arthritis and Rheumatism*, **23**, 569–73.

Reidenberg, M. M. & Martin, J. H. (1974). The acetylator phenotype of patients with systemic lupus erythematosus. *Drug Metabolism and Disposition*, **2**, 71–3.

Reinertsen, J. L., Klippel, J. N., Johnson, A. N., Steinberg, A. D., Decker, J. L. & Mann, D. L. (1984). B lymphocyte alloantigens associated with systemic lupus erythematosus. *New England Journal of Medicine*, **299**, 515–18.

Rieder, M. J., Shear, N. H., Kanee, A., Tang, B. K. & Spielberg, S. P. (1991). Prominence of slow acetylator phenotype among patients with sulfonamide hypersensitivity reactions. *Clinical Pharmacology and Therapeutics*, **49**, 13–17.

Robinson, D. S., Cooper, T. B., Jindal, S. P., Corcella, J. & Lutz, T. (1985). Metabolism and pharmacokinetics of phenelzine, lack of evidence for acetylation pathway in humans. *Journal of Clinical Psychopharmacology*, **5**, 333–7.

Robitzek, E. H., Selikoff, I. J. & Ornstein, G. G. (1952). Chemotherapy of human tuberculosis with hydrazine derivatives of isonicotinic acid. *Quarterly Bulletin Sea View Hospital New York*, **13**, 27–51.

Ronco, G., Vineis, P., Bryant, M. S., Skipper, P. L. & Tannenbaum, S. R. (1990). Haemoglobin adducts formed by aromatic amines in smokers: Sources of inter-individual variability. *British Journal of Cancer*, **61**, 534–8.

Roots, I., Drakoulis, N., Brockmoller, J., Janicke, I., Cuprunov, M. & Ritter, J. (1989). Hydroxylation and acetylation phenotypes as genetic risk factors in certain malignancies. In *Xenobiotic Metabolism and Disposition*, ed. R. Kato, R. W. Estabrook & M. N. Cayen. pp. 499–506. London: Taylor & Francis.

Roots, I., Drakoulis, N., Ploch, M., Heinemyer, G., Loddenkemper, R., Mines, T., Nitz, M., Otte, F. & Koch, M. (1988). Debrisoquine hydroxylation phenotype, acetylation phenotype and ABO blood groups as genetic host factors of lung cancer risk. *Klinische Wochenschrift*, 66(Suppl. XI): 87–97.

Rose, S. (1982). The relationship of acetylation phenotype to treatment with MAOIS: A review. *Journal of Clinical Psychopharmacology*, **2**, 161–4.

Rowell, N. P. & Clark, K. (1990). The effects of oral hydralazine on blood pressure, cardiac output and peripheral resistance with respect to dose, age and acetylator status. *Radiotherapy and Oncology*, **18**, 293–8.

Russell, D. W. (1970). Simple method for determining isoniazid acetylator phenotype. *British Medical Journal*, **3**, 324–5.

Ryazanov, E. M., Tretyakov, A. V. & Alexander, V. A. (1985). Induction of acetylation by pharmacological means. *Voprosy Meditsinskoi Khimii*, **31**, 112–14.

Saiz-Ruiz, J. & Aguilera, J. C. (1985). Personality traits and acetylator status. *Biological Psychiatry*, **20**, 1138–40.

Salako, L. A. & Aderounmu, A. F. (1977). Determination of the isoniazid acetylator phenotype in a West African population. *Tubercle*, **58**, 109–12.

Samigun M. Santoso, B. (1990). Lowering of theophylline clearance by isoniazid in slow and rapid acetylators. *British Journal of Clinical Pharmacology*, **29**, 570–3.

Sardas, S., Cok, I., Sardas, O. S., Ilhan, O. & Karakaya, A. E. (1990). Polymorphic *N*-acetylation capacity in breast cancer patients. *International Journal of Cancer*, **46**, 1138–9.

Sardas, S., Karakaya, A. E. & Cok, I. (1986a). Determination of the acetylator phenotype in a Turkish population. *Clinical Genetics*, **29**, 185–6.

Sardas, S., Karakaya, A. E. & Idle, J. R. (1988). Are the traits for drug acetylation and oxidation co-inherited. *Clinical Genetics*, **34**, 143–4.

Sardas, S., Karakaya, A. E. & Sardas, O. S. (1986b). Acetylator phenotype in patients with systemic lupus erythematosus. *Arthritis and Rheumatism*, **29**, 1412–13.

Sardas, S., Lahijany, B., Cok, I. & Karakaya, A.E. (1993). *N*-acetylation phenotyping with sulfamethazine in an Iranian population. *Pharmacogenetics*, **3**, 131–4.

Schmeidel, A. (1960). Weitere Untersuchungen über das

Wesen und die klinische Bedeutung der hochgradigen Isoniazid- inakkivierung im Korper. *Beiträge zur Klinik der Tuberkulose und Spezifischen Tuberkulose forschung*, **122**, 232–8.

Schröder, H. (1972). Simplified method for determining acetylator phenotype. *British Medical Journal*, **3**, 506–7.

Schröder, H. (1973). Deacetylation of sulphapyridine in man. *Journal of Pharmacy and Pharmacology*, **25**, 591–2.

Schröder, H. & Campbell, D. E. S. (1972). Absorption metabolism and excretion of salicylazosulfapyridine in man. *Clinical Pharmacology and Therapeutics*, **13**, 539–51.

Schröder, H. & Evans, D. A. P. (1972a). The polymorphic acetylation of sulphapyridine in man. *Journal of Medical Genetics*, **9**, 168–71.

Schröder, H. & Evans, D. A. P. (1972b). Acetylator phenotype *and* adverse effects of sulphasalazine in healthy subjects. *Gut*, **13**, 278–84.

Schröder, H., Lewkonia, R. M. & Evans, D. A. P. (1973). Metabolism of salicylazosulfapyridine in healthy subjects and in patients with ulcerative colitis. *Clinical Pharmacology and Therapeutics*, **14**, 802–9.

Schröder, P., Klitgaard, N. A. & Simonsen, E. (1979). Significance of the acetylation phenotype and the therapeutic effect of procainamide. *European Journal of Clinical Pharmacology*, **15**, 63–8.

Schulte, P. A. (1988). The role of genetic factors in bladder cancer. *Cancer Detection and Prevention*, **11**, 379–88.

Scott, E. M., Wright, R. C. & Weaver, D. D. (1969). The discrimination of phenotypes for rate of disappearance of isonicotinoyl hydrazide from serum. *Journal of Clinical Investigation*, **48**, 1173–6.

Selikoff, I. J. & Robitzek, E. H. (1952). Tuberculosis chemotherapy with hydrazine derivatives of isonicotinic acid. *Diseases of the Chest*, **21**, 385–38.

Sen, P. K., Chatterjee, R. & Saha, J. R. (1982). Use of sulphadimidine acetylation test in determining isoniazid inactivation rate in tuberculous patients. *Indian Journal of Medical Research*, **60**, 28–39.

Seth, V. & Beotra, A. (1989). Hepatic function in relation to acetylator phenotype in children treated with antitubercular drugs. *Indian Journal of Medical Research*, **89**, 306–9.

Seth, V., Seth, S. D., Beotra, A. & Singh, U. (1988). Comparison between serum isonicotinic acid hydrazide (INH) levels and urinary sulfadimidine (sulfamethazine) acetylation as predictions of INH acetylator status. *Developmental Pharmacology and Therapeutics*, **11**, 32–6.

Sharp, M. E., Wallace, S. M., Hindmarsh, K. W. & Brown, M. A. (1981). Acetylator phenotype and serum levels of sulfapyridine inpatients with inflammatory bowel disease. *European Journal of Clinical Pharmacology*, **21**, 243–50.

Shastri, R. A. (1982). Undernourished adults and acetylation phenotype. *International Journal of Clinical Pharmacology, Therapy and Toxicology*, **20**, 194–6.

Shear, N. H., Spielberg, S. P., Grant, D. M., Tang, B. K. & Kalow, W. (1986). Differences in metabolism of sulphonamides predisposing to idiosyncratic toxicity. *Annals of Internal Medicine*, **105**, 179–84.

Shenfield, G. M., McCann, V. J. & Tjokresetio, R. (1982). Acetylator status and diabetic neuropathy. *Diabetologia*, **22**, 441–4.

Shepherd, A. M. M., Irvine, N. A., Ludden, T. M., Lin, M.-S. & McNay, J. L. (1984). Effect of oral dose size on hydralazine kinetics and vasodepressor response. *Clinical Pharmacology and Therapeutics*, **36**, 595–600.

Shepherd, A.M. M., Ludden, T. M., McNay, J. L. & Lin, M. S. (1980). Hydralazine kinetics after single and repeated oral doses. *Clinical Pharmacology and Therapeutics*, **28**, 804–11.

Shepherd, A. M. M., McNay, J. L., Ludden, T. M., Min-Shung, L. & Musgrave, G.E. (1981). Plasma concentration and acetylator phenotype determine response to oral hydralazine. *Hypertension*, **3**, 580–5.

Shin, J. G., Shin, S. G., Jang, I. J. Kim, Y. S., Lee, K. H., Han, J. S., Kim, S. & Lee, J. S. (1992). Comparisons of isoniazid phenotyping methods and acetylation distribution in 43 native Korean subjects. *Asia Pacific Journal of Pharmacology*, **7**, 1–8.

Shiokawa, S., Yasuda, M. & Nobunaga, M. (1992). Genotypes of polymorphic arylamine N-acetyltransferase in systemic lupus erythematosus. *Arthritis and Rheumatism*, **35**, 1397–9.

Siegmund, W., Fengler, J. D., Franke, G., Zschiesche, M., Eike, O., Eike, E., Meisel, P. & Wulkow, R. (1991). N-acetylation and debrisoquine hydroxylation polymorphisms in patients with Gilbert's syndrome. *British Journal of Clinical Pharmacology*, **32**, 467–72.

Siegmund, W., Franke, G., Meng, S., Gothe, P. & Meng, W. (1988). N-acetylator phenotypes in hyperthyroidism. *International Journal of Clinical Pharmacology, Therapy and Toxicology*, **26**, 397–9.

Sinha, C. P., Sinha, S. & Sinha, K. P. (1978). The incidence of the acetylator phenotype of isoniazid in healthy and in pulmonary tuberculosis subjects in Bihar. *Journal of the Association of Physicians of India*, **26**, 353–60.

Sinues, B., Perez, J., Bernal, M. I., Saenz, M. A., Lanuza, J. & Bartolome, M. (1992). Urinary mutagenicity and N-acetylation phenotype in textile industry workers exposed to arylamines. *Cancer Research*, **52**, 4885–9.

Skretkowicz, J., Mazurowa, A. & Orsulak, D. (1981). Fenotyp acetylacji w grupie ludzi pochodzacych Z, regionu lodzkiego. *Polski Tygodnik Lekarski*, **36**, 89–91.

Smith, J., Tyrrell, W. F., Gow, A., Allan, G. W. & Lees, A. W. (1972). Hepatotoxicity in Rifampicin-Isoniazid treated patients related to their rate of isoniazid inactivation. *Chest*, **61**, 587–8.

Smith, S. E. & Kyi, T. (1968). Inactivation of isoniazid in Burmese subjects. *Nature*, **217**, 1273.

Snider, Jr, D. E. & Caras, G. J. (1992). Isoniazid-associated hepatitis deaths: a review of available information. *American Review of Respiratory Disease*, **145**, 494–7.

Sonnhag, C., Karlsson, E. & Hed, J. (1979). Procainamide-induced lupus erythematosus-like syndrome in relation to acetylator phentoype and plasma levels of procainamide. *Acta Medica Scandinavica*, **206**, 245–51.

Steele, M. A., Burke, R. F. & DesPrez, R. M. (1991). Toxic hepatitis with isoniazid and rifampicin. A meta-analysis. *Chest*, **99**, 465–71.

Stoll, C., Roth, M.-P., Dott, B., Doumit, N., Alembik, Y., Welsch, M. & Imbs, J.-L. (1989). Acetylator phenotype and congenital malformations. *European Journal of Clinical Pharmacology*, **36**, 151–3.

Strandberg, I., Boman, G., Hassler, L. & Sjöqvist, F. (1976). Acetylator phenotype in patients with hydralazine-induced lupoid syndrome. *Acta Medica Scandinavica*, **200**, 367–71.

Stryjek-Kaminska, D., Malczewski, B., Kopec, A. & Rowinska-Marcinska, K. (1988). Acetylator phenotypes in diabetes mellitus. *Acta Diabetologica Latina*, **25**, 41–8.

Suhardjono, D., Boutagy, J. & Shenfield, G. M. (1986). The effect of glucose in acetylation status. *British Journal of Clinical Pharmacology*, **22**, 401–8.

Sunahara, S. (1961). Genetical geographical and clinical studies on isoniazid metabolism. *Proceedings of the XVIth International Tuberculosis Conference*, Toronto, Canada, 15–20 September. Excerpta Med. Int. Congr. Ser. **44**, 513–40.

Sunahara, S. & Urano, M. (1963). Les problèmes du metabolisme de l'isoniazid. *Medicine Thoracalris (Basel)*, **20**, 289–312.

Sunahara, S., Urano, M., Lin, H. T., Cheg, T. J. & Jarumlinda, A. (1963b). Further observations on trimodality of frequency distribution curve of biologically active isoniazid blood levels and 'cline' in frequencies of alleles controlling isoniazid inactivation. *Acta Tuberculosea et Pneumologica Scandinavica*, **43**, 181–95.

Sunahara, S., Urano, M. & Ogawa, M. (1961). Genetical and geographical studies on isoniazid inactivation. *Science*, **134**, 1530–1.

Sunahara, S., Urano, M., Ogawa, M., Yoshida, S., Mukoyama, H. & Kawai, K. (1963a). Genetical aspect of isoniazid metabolism. *Japanese Journal of Human Genetics*, **8**, 93–111.

Svensson, C. K. & Knowlton, P. W. (1989). Effect of the immunomodulator tilorone on the *in vivo* acetylation of procainamide in the rat. *Pharmaceutical Research*, **6**, 477–80.

Swain, A. F., Ahmad, R. A., Rogers, H. J., Leonard, J. N. & Fry, L. (1983). Pharmacokinetic observations on dapsone in dermatitis herpetiformis. *British Journal of Dermatology*, **108**, 91–8.

Swamy, R., Acharyiulu, G. S., Duraipandian, M., Jawahar, M. S., Ramachandran, R. & Raghupati Sarma, G. (1987). Liver function tests during treatment of tuberculosis with short-course regimens containing isoniazid, rifampicin and pyrazinamide. *Indian Journal of Medical Research*, **86**, 549–57.

Swift, C. G., Hewick, D. S., Ogg, G. & Stevenson, I. H. (1980). Acetylator phenotype nitrazepam plasma concentrations and residual effects. *British Journal of Clinical Pharmacology*, **9**, 312p – 13p.

Szorady, I., Santa, A. & Veress, I. (1987). Drug acetylator phenotypes in newborn infants. *Biological Research in Pregnancy and Perinatology (Munchen-Diesenhofen)*, **8**, 23–5.

Talseth, T. Studies on hydralazine I. (1976). Serum concentrations of hydralazine in man after a single dose and at steady-state. *European Journal of Clinical Pharmacology*, **10**, 183–7.

Talseth, T. & Landmark, K. H. (1977). Polymorphic acetylation of sulphadimidine in normal and uraemic man. *European Journal of Clinical Pharmacology*, **11**, 33–6.

Tan, E. M., Cohen, A. S., Fries, J. F., Masi, A. T., McShane, D. J., Rothfield, N. F., Schaller, J. G., Talal, N. & Winchester, R. J. (1982). The 1982 revised criteria for the classification of systemic lupus erythematosus. *Arthritis and Rheumatism*, **25**, 1271–7.

Tang, B. K., Grant, D. M. & Kalow, W. (1983). Isolation and identification of 5-acetylamino-6-formylamino-3-methyluracil as a major metabolite of caffeine in man. *Drug Metabolism and Disposition*, **11**, 218–20.

Tang, B. K., Kadar, D. & Kalow, W. (1987). An alternative

test for acetylator phenotyping with caffeine. *Clinical Pharmacology and Therapeutics*, **42**, 509–13.

Tang, B. K., Zubovits, T. & Kalow, W. (1986). Determination of acetylated caffeine metabolites by high-performance exclusion chromatography. *Journal of Chromatography*, **375**, 170–3.

Tang, B.-K., Kadar, D., Qian, L., Iriah, J., Yip, J. & Kalow, W. (1991). Caffeine as a metabolic probe: validation of its use for acetylator phenotyping. *Clinical Pharmacology and Therapeutics*, **49**, 648–57.

Thom, S., Farrow, P. R., Santoso, B., Alberti, K. G. M. M. & Rawlins, M. D. (1981). Effects of oral glucose in lime juice on isoniazid kinetics. *British Journal of Clinical Pharmacology*, **1**, 423p.

Tiitinen, H. (1969a). Isoniazid and ethionamide serum levels and inactivation in Finnish subjects. *Scandinavian Journal of Respiratory Diseases*, **50**, 110–24.

Tiitinen, H. (1969b). Modification by para-aminosalicylic acid and sulfamethazine of the isoniazid inactivation in man. *Scandinavian Journal of Respiratory Diseases*, **50**, 281–90.

Tiitinen, H. (1969c). Isoniazid inactivation status and the development of chronic tuberculosis. *Scandinavian Journal of Respiratory Diseases*, **50**, 227–34.

Tiitinen, H., Mattila, M. J. & Eriksson, A. W. (1967). Isoniazid inactivation in Finns and Lapps. *Bulletin of the European Society of Human Genetics*, **1**, 77–8.

Tilstone, W. J., Margot, P. & Johnstone, E. C. (1979). Acetylation of phenelzine. *Psychopharmacology*, **60**, 261–3.

Timbrell, J. A., Facchini, V., Harland, S. J. & Mansilla-Tinoco, R. (1984). Hydralazine-induced lupus – Is there a toxic metabolic pathway? *European Journal of Clinical Pharmacology*, **27**, 555–9.

Timbrell, J. A., Harland, S. J. & Facchini, V. (1980). The polymorphic acetylation of hydralazine in man. *Clinical Pharmacology and Therapeutics*, **28**, 350–5.

Timbrell, J. A., Park, B. K. & Harland, S. J. (1985). A study of the effects of rifampicin on isoniazid metabolism in human volunteer subjects. *Human Toxicology*, **4**, 279–85.

Tomaszkiewicz, T., Markowska, J., Simm, S. & Herwichowska, K. (1979). Polimorficzna acetylacja u kobiet chorych na nowotwory narzadow plciowych. *Polski Tygodnik Lekarski*, **34**, 1521–4.

Tuberculosis Chemotherapy Centre. (1970). A controlled comparison of a twice-weekly and three once-weekly regimens in the initial treatment of pulmonary tuberculosis. *Bulletin of the World Health Organisation*, **43**, 143–206.

Valsalan, V. C. & Cooper, G. L. (1982). Carbamazepine intoxication caused by interaction with isoniazid. *British Medical Journal*, **285**, 261–2.

Van Hees, P. A., Van Elferen, L. W., Van Rossum, J. M. & Van Tongeren, J. H. (1979). Hemolysis during salicylazosulfa-pyridine therapy. *American Journal of Gastroenterology*, **70**, 501–5.

Vandenburg, M. J., Wright, P., Holmes, J., Rogers, H. J. & Ahmad, R. A. (1982). The hypotensive response to hydralazine in triple therapy is not related to acetylator phenotype. *British Journal of Clinical Pharmacology*, **13**, 747–50.

Varughese, P., Hamilton, E. J. & Eidus, L. (1974). Mass phenotyping of ioniazid inactivators by automated determination of acetylisoniazid in urine. *Clinical Chemistry*, **20**, 639–41.

Vas, A., Gachalyi, B. & Kaldor, A. (1990). Pantothenic acid, acute ethanol consumption and sulphadimidine acetylation. *International Journal of Clinical Pharmacology, Therapy and Toxicology*, **28**, 111–14.

Vatsis, K. P., Martell, K. J. & Weber, W. W. (1991). Diverse point mutations in the human gene for polymorphic N-acetyltransferase. *Proceedings of the National Academy of Sciences (USA)*, **88**, 6333–7.

Venkatesan, K. (1989). Clinical pharmacokinetic considerations in the treatment of patients with leprosy. *Clinical Pharmacokinetics*, **16**, 365–86.

Vineis, P., Caporaso, N., Tannenbaum, S. R., Skipper, P. L., Glogowski, J., Bartsch, H., Coda, M., Tulaska, G. & Kadlubar, F. (1990). Acetylation phenotype, carcinogen-hemoglobin adducts and cigarette smoking. *Cancer Research*, **50**, 3002–4.

Viukari, M., Jaatinen, P. &, Kylmamaa, T. (1983). Flunitrazepam, nitrazepam and psychomotor skills in psychogeriatric patients. *Current Therapeutic Research, Clinical and Experimental (New York)*, **33**, 828–34.

Viznerova, A., Slavikova, Z. & Ellard, G. A. (1973). The determination of the acetylator phenotype of tuberculosis patients in Czechoslovakia using sulphadimidine. *Tubercle*, **54**, 67–76.

Vree, T. B., Beneken-Kolmer, E. W. J., Hekster, Y. A., Shimoda, M., Ono, M. & Mivra, T. (1992). Pharmacokinetics and acetylation of sulfa-2-monomethoxine in humans. *Biopharmaceutics and Drug Disposition*, **13**, 55–68.

Vree, T. B., Beneken-Kolmer, E. W. J., Martea, M., Bosch, R., Hekster, Y. A. & Shimoda, M. (1990). Pharmacokinetics, N1- glucuronidation and N4-acetylation of sulfadimethoxine in man. *Pharmaceutisch Weekblad. Scientific Edition*, **12**, 51–9.

Vree, T. B., Hekster, C. H., Baakman, M., Janssen, T., Oosterbaan, M., Termond, E. & Tijhuis, M. (1983). Pharmacokinetics acetylation-deacetylation, renal clearance and protein binding of sulphamerazine N-acetylsulphamerazine and N-trideutero-acetylsulphamerazine in 'fast' and 'slow' acetylators. *Biopharmaceutics and Drug Disposition*, **4**, 271–291.

Vree, T. B., Hekster, Y. A., Nouws, J. F. M. & Baakman, M. (1986). Pharmacokinetics metabolism and renal excretion of sulfadimidine and its N-acetyl and hydroxy metabolites in humans. *Therapeutic Drug Monitoring*, **8**, 434–9.

Vree, T. B., O'Reilly, W. J., Hekster, Y. A., Damsma, J. E. & van der Kleun, E. (1980). Determination of the acetylator phenotype and pharmacokinetics of some sulphonamides in man. *Clinical Pharmacokinetics*, **5**, 274–94.

Walstad, R. A. (1975). Inaktivering av medikamenter ved acetylering. *Tidsskrift for den norske Laegeforening*, **2**, 100–3.

Walubo, A., Chan, K., Woo, J., Chan, H. S. & Wong, C. L. (1991). The disposition of antituberculous drugs in plasma of elderly patients. I Isoniazid and hydrazine metabolite. *Methods and Findings in Experimental and Clinical Pharmacology*, **13**, 545–50.

Weber, W., Tannen, R., McQueen, C. & Glowinksi, I. (1978). New methods and models for the isoniazid acetylation polymorphism. In *Advances in Pharmacology and Therapeutics (Clinical pharmacology)*, Vol. 6, ed. P. Duchene-Marsullaz. pp. 41–50. New York: Pergamon.

Weber, W. W. (1987). *The Acetylator Genes and Drug Response*. New York: Oxford University Press.

Weber, W. W. & Brennan, W. (1974). A filter paper method for determining isoniazid acetylator phenotype. *American Journal of Human Genetics*, **26**, 467–73.

Webster, D. J. T., Flook, D., Jenkins, J., Hutchings, A. & Routledge, P. A. (1989). Drug acetylation in breast cancer. *British Journal of Cancer*, **60**, 236–7.

Whelpton, R., Watkins, G. & Curry, S. H. (1981). Bratton-Marshall and liquid-chromatographic methods compared for determination of sulfamethazine acetylator status. *Clinical Chemistry*, **27**, 1911–14.

White, T. A. & Evans, D. A. P. (1968). The acetylation of sulfamethazine and sulfamethoxypyridazine by human subjects. *Clinical Pharmacology and Therapeutics*, **9**, 80–8.

Whitty, F. (1987). Bladder cancer in rubber workers. *British Journal of Industrial Medicine*, **44**, 647.

Wiggan, E. B., Dennis, S., Reele, S. B. & Luke, D. R. (1991). Reassessment of dapsone as a marker of acetylator phenotypes. *International Journal of Clinical Pharmacology, Therapy and Toxicology*, **29**, 262–8.

Williams, D. M., Wimpenny, J. & Asscher, A. W. (1968). Renal clearance of sodium sulphadimidine in normal and uraemic subjects. *Lancet*, **2**, 1058–60.

Wohlleb, J. C., Hunter, C. F., Blass, B., Kadlubar, F. F., Chu, D. Z. J. & Lang, N. P. (1990). Aromatic amine acetyltransferase as a marker for colorectal cancer, environmental and demographic associations. *International Journal of Cancer*, **46**, 22–30.

Woodhouse, K. W., Adams, P. C., Clothier, A., Mucklow, J. C. & Rawlins, M. D. (1982). N-acetylation phenotype in bladder cancer. *Human Toxicology*, **1**, 443–5.

Woolf, B. (1954). On estimating the relation between blood group and disease. *Annals of Human Genetics (London)*, **19**, 251–3.

Woosley, R. L., Drayer, D. E., Reidenberg, M. M., Nies, A. S., Carr, K. & Oates, J. A. (1978). Effect of acetylator phenotype on the rate at which procainamide induces antinuclear antibodies and the lupus syndrome. *New England Journal of Medicine*, **298**, 1157–9.

Wren, P. J. J., Evans, D. A. P., Vetters, J. M. & Chew, A. (1967). Autoimmune antibodies in mongol families. *Lancet*, **2**, 186–8.

Wright, J. T. Jr, Goodman, R. P., Bethel, A. M. M. & Lambert, C. M. (1984). Cimetidine and dapsone acetylation. *Drug Metabolism and Disposition*, **12**, 782–3.

Xu, X.-M. & Jiang, W.-D. (1990). Debrisoquine hydroxylation and sulfamethazine acetylation in a Chinese population. *Acta Pharmacologica Sinica*, **11**, 385–8.

Yamamoto, T., Suou, T. & Hirayama, C. (1986). Elevated serum aminotransferase induced by isoniazid in relation to isoniazid acetylator phenotype. *Hepatology*, **6**, 295–8.

Yanagisawa, H. & Wada, O. (1989). Significant increase of IQ-type heterocyclic amines, dietary carcinogens in the plasma of patients with uraemia just before induction of hemodialysis treatment. *Nephron*, **52**, 6–10.

Ylitalo, P., Auterinen, L., Marttinen, A. & Koivula, T. (1984). Acetylator phenotyping with sulphadimidine in patients receiving isoniazid. *International Journal of Clinical Pharmacology Research*, **4**, 141–4.

Ylitalo, P., Ruosteenoja, R., Leskinen, O. & Metsa-Ketela, T. (1983). Significance of acetylator phenotype in pharmacokinetics and adverse effects of procainamide. *European Journal of Clinical Pharmacology*, **25**, 791–5.

Young, J.R. (1980). Acetylator status and liver function profile changes in labyrinthine ischaemia patients treated with thymoxamine. *Journal of International Medical Research*, **8**, 356–7.

Zacest, R. & Koch-Weser, J. (1972). Relation of hydralazine plasma concentration to dosage and hypotensive action. *Clinical Pharmacology and Therapeutics*, **13**, 420–5.

Zidek, Z., Friebova, M., Janku, I. & Elis, J. (1977). Influence of sex and of Freund's adjuvant on liver N-acetyltransferase activity and elimination of sulphadimidine in urine of rats. *Biochemical Pharmacology*, **26**, 69–70.

Zysset, Th. & Peretti, E. (1986). Effect of concomitant isoniazid administration on determination of acetylator phenotype by sulphadimidine. *European Journal of Clinical Pharmacology*, **30**, 463–6.

PART VI   Miscellaneous Phase II reactions showing genetic variability in drug metabolism

17   The glucosidation of amobarbital

INTRODUCTION

STUDIES on the variability in amobarbital metabolism in man started with attempts to correlate the
plasma elimination half-lives of four drugs amongst
themselves and with 6β-hydroxycortisol urinary
excretion. The latter was included because it was
thought that it might be a general indicator of
hydroxylation capacity in man (Kadar *et al.* 1973).
The results showed that amobarbital half-life correlated with that of sulphinpyrazone. Neither the half-
lives of these two drugs nor those of glutethimide
and antipyrine correlated with 6β-hydroxycortisol
urinary excretion.

The metabolite 3'-hydroxyamobarbital was
already known, and a new metabolite thought to
be N-hydroxyamobarbital was found by Tang *et al.*
(1975). This metabolite was subsequently found to
be N-(1-β-D-glucopyranosyl) amobarbital (Kalow *et
al.* 1978) (see Fig. 17.1).

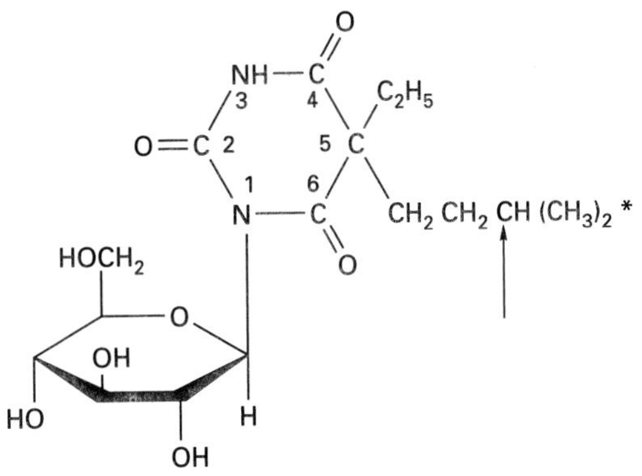

The proposition was made that amobarbital was
a very attractive drug for use as a probe for the study
of hydroxylation in man. This was because of its
pharmacokinetic properties, which included almost
complete intestinal absorption, absence of a first
pass effect, elimination by first-order kinetics, small
intra-individual variation in plasma clearance, small
inter-individual variation in binding to plasma proteins, four-fold inter-individual variability in half-
lives, three-fold variability in clearances and almost
complete conversion into two identifiable urinary
metabolites (Inaba *et al.* 1976).

In view of these properties, genetic influences on

Fig. 17.1. *N*–(1–β–D–glucopyranosyl)   amobarbital.
*This side chain is variously described as 3-methylbutyl,
or isoamyl, or isopentyl. The site of hydroxylation is
indicated by the arrow.

kinetic parameters were assessed by Endrenyi *et al.*
(1976) in the members of seven identical and seven
fraternal twinships who ingested 120 mg amobarbital. Serial blood samples were taken but the results
of analyses of urine samples were not reported. The
elimination rate constant gave a Holzinger's H factor
of 0.91 and a lower boundary of broad sense heritability h_L^2 of 0.88, indicating a very substantial genetic control of this parameter. The plasma clearance
also gave a statistically significant H factor of 0.83.

A NEW APPROACH

A radical change of approach in pharmacogenetic
studies was heralded by the study of Kalow *et al.*

(1977). Having established, as explained above that for amobarbital the overall kinetics were largely controlled by genetic factors they switched their attention to the formation of individual metabolites. They found a pair of female identical twins who produced only traces of N-glucoamobarbital in the urine following an oral dose. Their families were investigated and the results were shown in Fig 17.2. The data were consistent with control of the N-glucosidation of amobarbital by two autosomal alleles. The percentage of the dose excreted as 3-hydroxyamobarbital and the salivary half-lives of amobarbital were not unusual in the two probands. This paper gave a great impetus to the study of pharmacogenetics of single defined biotransformations by examining the metabolic product, rather than by measuring an index of the overall pharmacokinetic behaviour such as plasma half-lives or elimination rate constant.

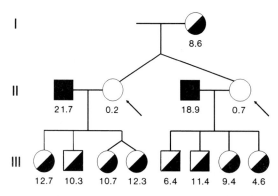

Fig. 17.2. Familial deficiency of N-glucosidation of amobarbital. The numbers represent the percentage of the oral dose recovered in the urine in 48 hours as N-glucoamobarbital. The symbols indicate genotypes based on the assumption that the capacity for N-glucosidation is determined by two autosomal alleles. The completely white fields indicate homozygous deficient individuals and the completely black fields homozygous normal individuals. (Adapted from Fig. 1 of Kalow et al. 1977.)

INTER-ETHNIC STUDIES

The glucosidation of amobarbital was assessed in a population of 129 students by examining a sample of urine voided 36 hours following a bedtime dose of 60 mg (Kalow et al. 1979). There were wide and independent inter-individual variabilities in the excretion of N-glucoamobarbital (N-Glu) and 3'-hydroxyamobarbital (C-OH). One individual was found who excreted practically nil of the former metabolite. Of the 14 who excreted more N-Glu than C-OH, four were Oriental, whereas only six of the 115 with the reverse ratio were Oriental (χ_i^2 with Yates' correction 6.26, $p < 0.02$). In a confirmatory experiment 10 out of 20 Orientals had N-Glu > C-OH compared with 1 out of 20 Caucasians ($\chi_i^2 = 10.1, p < 0.01$).

A meticulous determination of the metabolic rate constants for N-Glu and C-OH was made by Tang et al. (1982). Multiple serial blood samples and urine collections up to 120 hours after drug ingestion were analysed. The rates of decline of serum concentration of amobarbital paralleled the excretion rates of these two metabolites in urine. The rates followed simple first-order kinetics after the distributive phase. The elimination rate constants for both metabolites could be determined. The authors emphasized that though a simplified procedure was essential for large population surveys, two 12 hour night-time samples on the second and fifth day after drug intake were required for accurate determinations of the rate constants. Nevertheless, Tang et al. (1983) surveyed 52 healthy subjects by collecting urine 96 to 120 hours after the ingestion of 120 mg amobarbital. The results showed that smoking greatly elevates C-OH formation; also, they confirmed yet again that Orientals differed from Caucasians in that they formed more N-Glu and less C-OH.

THE POSSIBILITY OF *IN VITRO* STUDIES OF GLUCOSIDATION

Micromethods were developed with which to estimate amylobarbitone hydroxylation (Frazer *et al.* 1976) and glucosidation (Tang & Carro-Ciampi 1980) *in vitro* by samples of human liver. Nevertheless these methods were not applied in wide-scale surveys or in inter-ethnic comparisons or on *in vivo/in vitro* phenotyping correlations.

STEREOISOMER FORMATION

More recent work has focused on the fact that when D-glucose is coupled to either nitrogen of amobarbital, asymmetry is conferred at C_5 of the barbiturate ring (Fig. 17.1) and the N-glucose conjugates of amobarbital exist as two diastereomeric or epimeric metabolites. The S form (see p. 68) is the predominant metabolite, and the R form accounts for less than 0.2% of the dose of amobarbital. Measuring the S-form specifically in the urine with an HPLC method confirmed that the rate constant of formation (as deduced from the elimination rate constant) was 50% higher in Orientals than in Caucasians (Soine *et al.* 1990).

GLUCOSE CONJUGATION OF OTHER DRUGS

Apart from amobarbital, the following drugs are known to form glucosides in man: phenobarbital, sulphamethazine, sulphamerazine, sulphamethoxozole. The amounts of sulphonamides excreted in this form are less than 3% of the dose (Tang 1990). It would be expected, in view of the molecular similarity, that phenobarbital glucosidation would be under the same genetic control as amobarbital.

EPILOGUE

There appears to be no information about the enzymic mechanism responsible for the glucosidation of amobarbital. Inter-ethnic assessments do not seem to have been extended beyond the Caucasian/Oriental comparisons referred to above. Nothing is known about the relevance of glucosidation mechanisms in the genesis of drug-induced or spontaneous disorders.

Endrenyi, L., Inaba, T. & Kalow, W. (1976). Genetic study of amobarbital elimination based on its kinetics in twins. *Clinical Pharmacology and Therapeutics*, **20**, 701–14.

Fraser, H. S., Williams, F. M., Davies, D. L., Draffan, G. H. & Davies, D. S. (1976). Amylobarbitone hydroxylation kinetics in small samples of rat and human liver. *Xenobiotica*, **6**, 465–72.

Inaba, T., Tang, B. K., Endrenyi, L. & Kalow, W. (1976). Amobarbital – a probe of hepatic drug oxidation in man. *Clinical Pharmacology and Therapeutics*, **20**, 439–44.

Kadar, D., Inaba, T., Endrenyi, L., Johnson, G. E. & Kalow, W. (1973). Comparative drug elimination capacity in man – glutethimide amobarbital antipyrine and sulfinpyrazone. *Clinical Pharmacology and Therapeutics*, **14**, 552–60.

Kalow, W., Endrenyi, L., Inaba, T., Kadar, D. & Tang, B. (1979). Pharmacogenetic investigation of amobarbital disposition. In *Advances in Pharmacology and Therapeutics*, Vol. 6, ed. P. Duchene-Marullaz, pp. 31–40.

Kalow, W., Inaba, T. & Tang, B. K. (1977). A case of deficiency of N-hydroxylation of amobarbital. *Clinical Pharmacology and Therapeutics*, **21**, 530–5.

Kalow, W., Tang, B. K., Kadar, D. & Inaba, T. (1978). Distinctive patterns of amobarbital metabolites. *Clinical Pharmacology and Therapeutics*, **24**, 576–82.

Soine, W. H., Soine, P. J., Wireko, F. C. & Abraham, D. J. (1990). Stereochemical characterization of the diastereomers of the amobarbital N-glucosides excreted in human urine. *Pharmaceutical Research*, **7**, 794–800.

Tang, B.-K. (1990). Drug glucosidation. *Pharmacology and Therapeutics*, **46**, 53–6.

Tang, B. K. & Carro-Ciampi, G. (1980). A method for the study of N-glucosidation *in vitro* – amobarbital-N-glucoside formation in incubations with human liver. *Biochemical Pharmacology*, **29**, 2085–8.

Tang, B. K., Inaba, T. & Kalow, W. (1975). N-hydroxyamobarbital: the second major metabolite of amobarbital in man. *Drug Metabolism and Disposition*, **3**, 479–86.

Tang, B. K., Kalow, W., Endrenyi, L. & Chan, F. Y. (1982). An assessment of short-cut procedures for studying drug metabolism in vivo using amobarbital as a model drug. *European Journal of clinical Pharmacology*, **22**, 229–33.

Tang, B. K., Kalow, W., Inaba, T. & Kadar, D. (1983). Variation in amobarbital metabolism: evaluation of a simplified population study. *Clinical Pharmacology and Therapeutics*, **34**, 202–6.

18   Glucuronosyltransferases

INTRODUCTION

THE FORMATION of conjugates of foreign compounds with glucuronic acid is a chemical reaction which has been known for a century to occur in animals. There is quite an extensive discussion of the subject in Williams (1959).

One important aspect of glucuronide formation is the variety of molecular structures which can be involved. Examples from amongst common medicines are:

1 hydroxyl groups including primary, secondary and tertiary alcohols and aromatic compounds, e.g. oxazepam (Fig. 18. 1), aspirin, paracetamol, morphine, menthol, chloramphenicol (Fig. 18.2) giving 'ether' β-glucuronides;
2 carboxyl groups, e.g. aspirin, valproate, zomepirac (now withdrawn), benoxaprofen, ibufenac, alcofenac, indoprofen and clofibric acid (Fig. 18.3), giving 'ester' β-glucuronides;
3 aliphatic and aromatic amino groups, e.g. sulphadimethoxine, diaminodiphenylsulphone (dapsone), cyproheptadine ('periactin'), tripelennamine (pyribenzamine), giving N-β-glucuronides, (see Fig. 18.4).

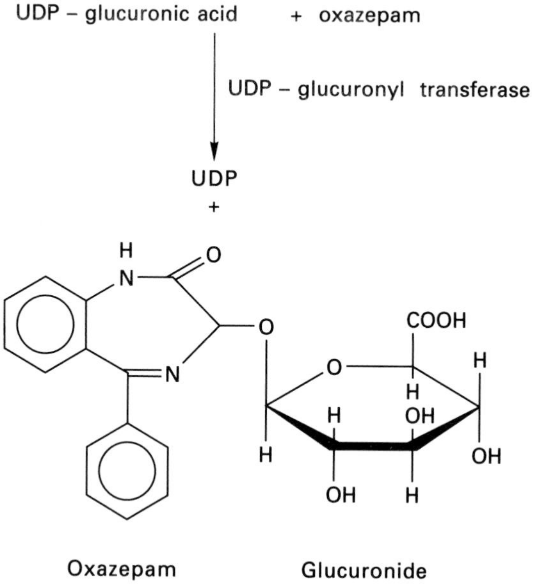

A list of drugs extensively glucuronidated in humans is given in Table 18.1.

Glucuronide conjugates are formed by a wide variety of endogenous as well as exogenous molecules, examples being bilirubin, steroids and bile acids.

Since the glucuronide conjugates are more water-soluble than the unconjugated substrates they are

Fig. 18.1. Formation of oxazepam glucuronide. UDP, uridine diphosphate.

more readily excreted from the body. For this reason glucuronide formation is usually considered to be a classical detoxication mechanism. Sometimes a compound has to be oxidized first to form a hydroxyl group (Phase 1 reaction) and subsequently conjugated with glucuronide (Phase 2 reaction) before being eliminated. However, some drugs already possess hydroxyl groups (e.g. oxazepam, menthol and morphine) and they can be glucuronidized directly.

306

Table 18.1. Drugs extensively glucuronidated in humans

Alclofenac	Mexiletine
Alprenolol	Morphine
Amitryptyline	Nalidixic acid
Benoxaprofen	Naloxone
Bornopralol	S-Naproxen
Bromperido	Nitecaponel
Carprofen	Oxaprozin
Chloramphenicol	Oxazepam
Ciclopiroxolamine	Oxprenolol
Ciramadol	Paracetamol
Clofibric acid	Phenprocoumon
Codeine	Phenylbutazone
Cyclobenzaprine	Picenadol
Cyproheptadine	Pirprofen
Desethylbemitradine	Probenecid
Diflunisal	Propofol
DP-1904	Ritodrine
Etodolac	Salicylamide
Fenofibric acid	Salicylic acid
Fenoprofen	Sulphadimethoxine
Feprazone	Sulphinpyrazone
Isoxepac	Suprofen
Ketoprofen	Temazepam
Ketorolac	Tiaprofenic acid
Ketotifen	Tocainide
L1(1.2-dimethyl-3-hydroxypyrid-4-one)	Tripelennamine
Labetalol	Valproic acid
Lamotrigine	Zidovudine
Lorazepam	Zomepirac
Meptazinol	

From: Miners & Mackenzie 1991.

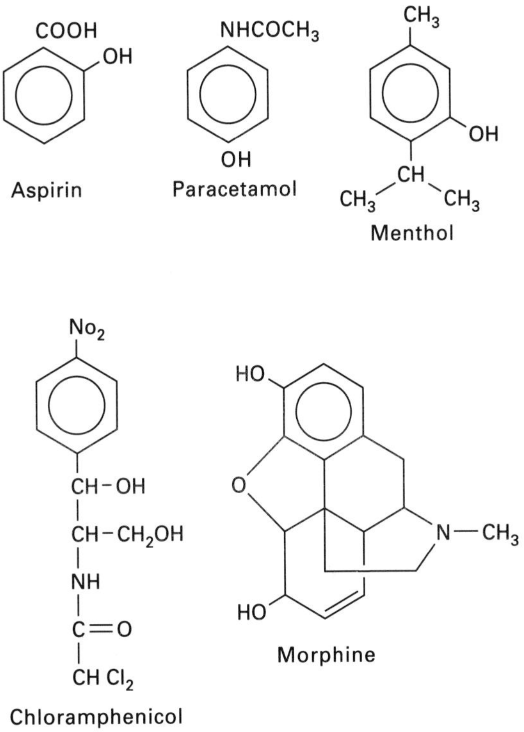

Fig. 18.2. Drugs forming 'ether' glucuronides because they possess hydroxyl groups.

Not all glucuronides are less toxic or less active than the original compound. The 6β-glucuronide of morphine has a higher affinity for the receptor in the brain than morphine itself (Osborne *et al.* 1988). The glucuronides of ethinyloestradiol and harmol are cholestatic. The acyl glucuronides of benoxaprofen and zomepirac can bind covalently to cellular proteins *in vivo* and the combination may form a hapten which sets off an immunological reaction which may be anaphylactic (Samuel 1981; Smith *et al.* 1986).

The glucuronyl moiety is transferred from a donor, uridine diphosphoglucuronic acid (UDPGA) to the acceptor molecule under the influence of UDP-glucuronyl transferase (UDPGT: Fig. 18.1). This enzyme has mainly been studied in the liver where it is located in the endoplasmic reticulum. However, UDPGT enzymes also occur in the nasal mucosa, intestine and kidney – those in the last two sites may be of importance in drug metabolism. The

fact that it is membrane-bound has been responsible for most of the difficulty in studying this transferase *in vitro*. Detergents are required to solubilize it, the experimental conditions are difficult to standardize and in many instances the resulting enzyme preparation has been unstable.

RELATIONSHIP OF DRUG GLUCURONIDATION TO SPONTANEOUSLY OCCURRING GENETIC DISORDERS

The two conditions in man in which defective bilirubin glucuronidation is the main feature are Gilbert's syndrome and Crigler–Najjar syndrome (CNS). The former is a heterogenous condition varying in severity, and the disturbances of physiology may include membrane transport defects as well as UDPGT defects. The latter has been subdivided by Arias *et al.* (1969) into two types (Table 18.2). There

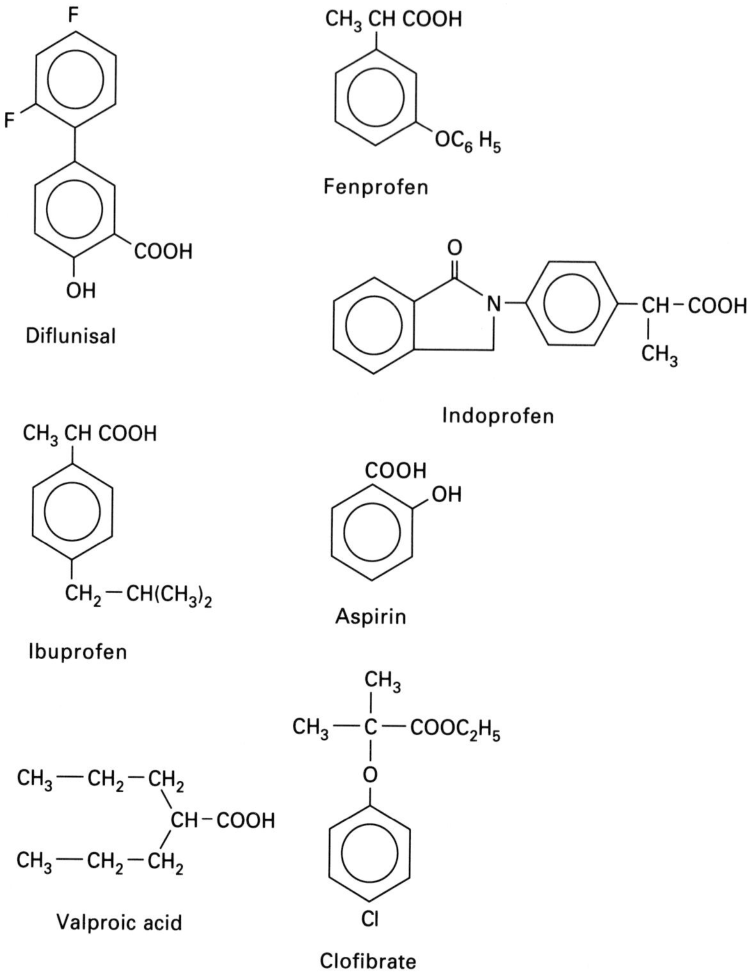

F

F

COOH

OH

Diflunisal

CH_3 CH COOH

OC_6H_5

Fenprofen

CH_3 CH COOH

$CH_2-CH(CH_3)_2$

Ibuprofen

O

N

CH-COOH

CH_3

Indoprofen

COOH

OH

Aspirin

$CH_3-CH_2-CH_2$

CH-COOH

$CH_3-CH_2-CH_2$

Valproic acid

CH_3

$CH_3-C-COOC_2H_5$

O

Cl

Clofibrate

Fig. 18.3. Drugs which form 'ester' glucuronides.

may be a relationship between Type II CNS and Gilbert's syndrome in that the clinical pictures may overlap, and both conditions may occur in the same family. It has been suggested as a possibility that CNS Type II may be the homozygous condition for which Gilbert's syndrome is the heterozygote.

Currently studies of UGT genes and their products are beginning to dispel some of the mystery surrounding these two conditions and these studies will be referred to briefly below.

Clues to the probable complexity of the genetic and biochemical systems involved in the glucuron-idation of bilirubin and various drugs shown in Table 18.2 are provided by anomalies. For example Kreek & Sleisenger (1968) described abnormal menthol metabolism in an anicteric relative of a patient who had congenital non-haemolytic unconjugated hyperbilirubinaemia, whilst a person was discovered with normal bilirubin glucuronidation but defective paracetamol glucuronidation by DeMorais et al. (1992).

The relevance of this information to the main subject matter being discussed in this book is as follows: the variability in the glucuronidation of a few drugs studied because of these genetic conditions makes it very likely that there exists genetic variability in the glucuronidation of other drug compounds.

Table 18.2. *Drug metabolism studies in unconjugated hyperbilirubinaemia*

Characteristic investigated	Gilbert's syndrome	Crigler–Najjar syndrome type I	Crigler–Najjar syndrome type II
Population frequency	2 to 5%	rare	rare
Inheritance	probably autosomal dominant	autosomal recessive **10**	unclear may be autosomal dominant or recessive **10, 17**
Severity of illness	benign	severe **10**	severe **24**
Unconjugated serum bilirubin concentration	up to about 100 μM	>340 μM **10**	<340 μM **10**
Bilirubin glucuronidation	partial reduction	nil	very low or nil
Bilirubin response to barbiturates phethbarbital & dicophane	serum bilirubin concentration reduced **1, 2, 3, 4, 5, 6**	no response **10, 11, 12, 13**	dramatic response (in some) **2, 5, 10, 19, 22, 23, 24, 25, 26, 27, 28**
Bilirubin response to glutethimide	serum unconjugated bilirubin concentration reduced **4**	no response **14**	dramatic response
Paracetamol glucuronidation *in vivo*	decreased **7**	defective **15, 16, 17**	impaired **13**
Testosterone glucuronidation *in vivo*		normal **13**	
Menthol glucuronidation *in vivo*	usually decreased **8**	defective **10, 13, 18**	defective **3, 10, 25, 26, 29**
Salicylamide glucuronidation	decreased or normal **9**	impaired **19**	defective **23, 26**
Response of salicylamide glucuronidation to phenobarbital		defective **20, 21, 22**	enhanced
Tetrahydrohydrocortisone glucuronidation *in vivo*		defective **21, 22, 23**	
Salicylate glucuronidation *in vivo*		defective **21**	
Trichloroethanol glucuronidation *in vivo*			

Sources: **1.** Black & Sherlock 1970; **2.** Hunter *et al.* 1971; **3.** Thompson *et al.* 1969; **4.** Blaschke *et al.* 1974a; **5.** Sinaasappel & Jansen 1991; **6.** Black *et al.* 1974; **7.** DeMorais *et al.* 1992; **8.** Beck & Kiani 1960; **9.** Barniville & Misk 1959; **10.** Arias 1969; **11.** Blumenschein *et al.* 1968; **12.** Burchell *et al.* 1987; **13.** Bloomer *et al.* 1971; **14.** Blaschke *et al.* 1974b; **15.** Axelrod *et al.* 1957; **16.** Schmid & Hammaker 1963; **17.** Hunter *et al.* 1973; **18.** Szabo & Ebrey 1963; **19.** Kline & Rosenkranz 1972; **20.** Peterson & Schmid 1957; **21.** Childs *et al.* 1959; **22.** Francois *et al.* 1962; **23.** Yaffe *et al.* 1966; **24.** Gollan *et al.* 1975; **25.** Kreek & Sleisenger 1968; **26.** Whelton *et al.* 1968; **27.** Gordon *et al.* 1976; **28.** Crigler & Gold 1969; **29.** Sleisinger *et al.* 1967. See also Schmid & McDonagh 1978.

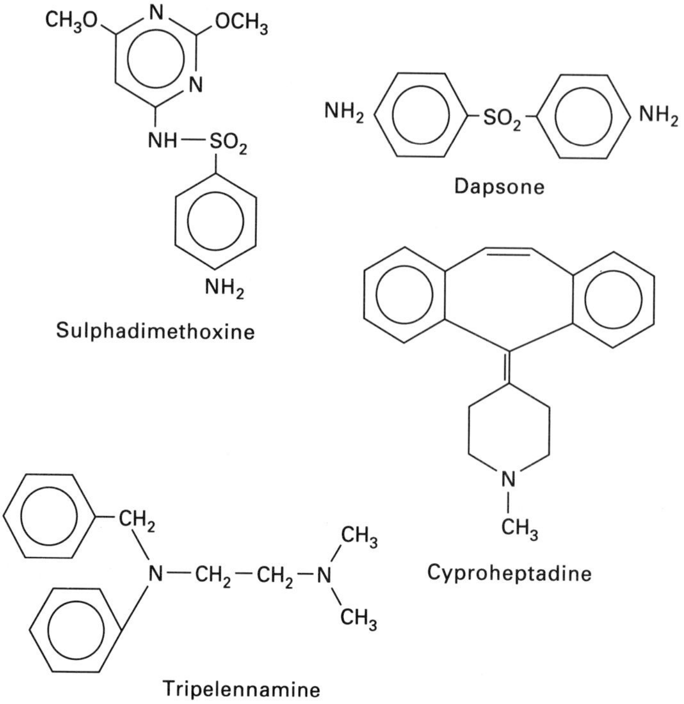

Fig. 18.4. Drugs which form *N*-glucuronides.

A very considerable difference has been found by Yue *et al.* (1989) in the proportion of a single dose of codeine which was excreted in the urine as glucuronides by Chinese, compared with Caucasians. The former excreted about one third less than the latter. This difference may be due to environmental influences (e.g. diet) but may represent a genetic difference in glucuronidizing enzymes.

SIMILARITIES TO THE CYTOCHROME P450 SYSTEM

A great deal of work has been done in the rat, and also to a lesser extent in other animals (see Burchell & Coughtrie 1989), as a result of which it has become apparent that there are considerable similarities between the UDPGT system of enzymes and the cytochrome P450 system which is described in Chapter 4. Individual rat UDPGTs have been isolated and purified, the effect of inducing agents on them studied and their cDNAs cloned. Furthermore, in some instances a rat cDNA has been transfected

in a plasmid into mammalian cells and the resulting enzyme characterised.

Consequently it can be seen that the UDPGT system and the cytochrome P450 system both consist of multiple membrane-bound enzymes. The production of various enzymes in both systems responds in different degrees to inducing agents. Both systems are characterized by overlapping specificities: one transferase can glucuronidize several different molecular structures, and one substrate can be glucuronidized by more than one transferase (see Tephly & Burchell 1990).

There is every reason to believe that the general organization of the UDPGT isoenzyme system in man is closely similar to that of the rat.

All the known cDNAs for UDPGT enzymes were analysed by Burchell *et al.* (1991) in a similar fashion to that described elsewhere for cytochromes P450. The resulting phylogenetic tree is shown in Fig. 18.5. There is a gene superfamily which is divisible into families. Within a single family the protein sequences exhibit > 50% resemblance (and within a subfamily > 60%), whereas between families the resemblance is ≤ 50%. The nomenclature for the genes has been standardized as UGT followed by an

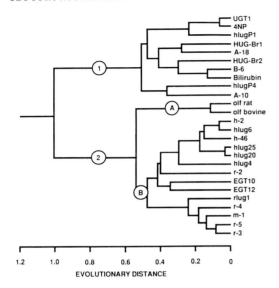

UGT1
4NP
hlugP1
HUG-Br1
A-18
HUG-Br2
B-6
Bilirubin
hlugP4
A-10
olf rat
olf bovine
h-2
hlug6
h-46
hlug25
hlug20
hlug4
r-2
EGT10
EGT12
rlug1
r-4
m-1
r-5
r-3

1.2   1.0   0.8   0.6   0.4   0.2   0
EVOLUTIONARY DISTANCE

Fig. 18.5. Unweighted-group-method of analysis (UPGMA) phylogenetic tree of the UDP-glucuronosyltransferase (*UGT*) superfamily. To date, 26 deduced protein sequences from distinct cDNAs have been characterized in human, rat, mouse, rabbit and cow. The evolutionary distance *d* on the abscissa is a measurement of time before the present, but cannot be considered linear. For a more detailed description see the section on *CYP* genes which control cytochromes P450. (From Fig. 1, Burchell *et al.* 1991.)

Arabic numeral for the family, a letter designating the subfamily and another Arabic numeral representing the individual gene within the subfamily or family (all of which parallels the CYP system for the cytochromes P450).

RECENT ADVANCES IN THE MOLECULAR BIOLOGY OF UDP GLUCURONOSYLTRANSFERASE ENZYMES

The last few years has seen a tremendous surge of knowledge concerning the UDP-GT enzymes. The increased understanding of the human enzymes has followed a great deal of basic work in the rat. The report by Jansen *et al.* (1992) of a workshop on the topic held in the Netherlands in April 1991 pulls many of the threads together.

Rat cDNAs and anti-rat UGT antibodies have been used to investigate the relevant human genes.

Human *UGT* cDNA clones have been transiently expressed in COS-7 cells and have also been expressed in a stable manner in cloned cell cultures. Chimeric genes have been expressed in V79 Chinese hamster cells. These techniques have enabled the properties of the gene products to be examined individually in isolation. By this means a start has been made to delineate their substrate specificities which show considerable degrees of overlap.

As Fig. 18.5 reveals the *UGT* genes belong to two families and the products of members of both families have now been studied in humans. Table 18.3 condenses the currently available information. *HlugP1, HlugP4, HUG-Br1* and *HUG-Br2* belong to *UGT* family 1 whereas *UDPGTh2* and *Hlug25* belong to *UGT* family 2. As is inevitable in such a rapidly advancing field of science, there may be some degree of confusion caused, for example, by different workers using different names for the same gene or enzyme. The standardization of the nomenclature according to Burchell *et al.* (1991) will help overcome this type of difficulty. The general picture that emerges is that the products of the genes in family 1 metabolize diverse compounds such as bilirubin and various phenols, whereas the products of family 2 metabolize steroids and bile acids. Comparatively few therapeutic drugs have been investigated by these means, most of the emphasis having been on 'model' organic compounds, but it seems likely that some drugs will be metabolized by enzymes coded by genes in both families.

It is to be noted that HLUGP1 gene product is not active towards morphine, bilirubin or 4-hydroxybiphenyl. Paracetamol plasma clearance is known to be correlated with the clearance of glucuronidated lorazepam, oxazepam and temazepam, so these benzodiazepines may be substrates for the 'paracetamol' UDPGT enzyme.

There is a possibility that compounds which inhibit the activity of a particular enzyme *in vitro* may also be substrates for it, but it is unlikely that compounds which do not inhibit the activity are substrates.

At the *UGT1* locus there is an arrangement which produces six isoforms of UDP-glucuronosyltransferase enzymes. Each isoform is coded by five exons. The four exons at the 3'-end are common to all forms. The exon at the 5'-end is one out of a row of six each with its own promoter. The products of *UGT1A* and *UGT1D* are bilirubin UDP-

Table 18.3. *Known human variants of UDP-glucuronosyltransferases*

Gene	Molecular weight of product	Amino acid composition of product	Substrates	Inducers	Inhibitors of activity of product	Activity of product not inhibited by
Enzymes whose drugs specificities have been characterized by purification or cloning and expression of cDNAs						
HLUGP1[a]	55 kDa	1593 base pairs code for 531 residues	1-naphthol 4-methyl umbelliferone 4-nitrophenol (planar phenols) but not testosterone, androsterone, oestrone (-)morphine, 4-hydroxybiphenyl	3 methyl cholanthrene	possibly by: R- and S- fenoprofen oxazepam salicylic acid temazepam (which may be alternative substrates)	Chloramphenicol, clofibric acid, ibuprofen, probenecid. (-) morphine, naproxen, paracetamol, ketoprofen, salicylamide, valproic acid.
HLUG4		Amino acids 45% similar to HLUGP1	Oestrol (low level activity) 4-methyl umbelliferone 4-nitrophenol naphthylamine bulky phenols			
UDPGTh2	52 kDa	75% similar to HLUG4	3-4 catechol oestrogens, oestriol propionic acid, non-steroidal anti-inflammatory drugs			
HLUG25[b]	52 kDa	83% similar to HLUG4 86% similar to UDPGTh2	hyodeoxycholic acid 4-hydroxyestrone estriol (much less active than UDPGTh2) but not lithocholic acid or androsterone			
HUG-BR1[c] HUG-BR2[d]		533 amino acids 534 amino acids	bilirubin bilirubin	phenobarbitone phenytoin clofibrate		
Enzymes postulated on the basis of human liver microsomal kinetic and inhibitor studies						
morphine UDPGT high affinity			morphine			4-methyl umbelliferone, 1-naphthol, 4-nitrophenol
morphine UDPGT low activity			morphine & also probably codeine		chloramphenicol, naloxone, oxazepam, amitriptyline, probenecid	
paracetamol UDPGT (possibly more than 1)[e]			paracetamol	moderate induction (two-fold) by phenobarbital and phenytoin[f]		planar phenols morphine chloramphenicol 4-hydroxybiphenyl

[a]Harding *et al.* 1988a.
[b]Harding *et al.* 1988b.
[c]Probably the same as HlugP2.
[d]Probably the same as HlugP3.
[e]Miners *et al.* 1990.
[f]Bock & Bock-Hennig 1987.
Information also derived from: Jansen et al. 1992; Miners & Mackenzie 1991.

glucuronosyltransferases whereas *UGT1F* encodes a phenol-specific isoform (Ritter *et al.* 1992).

It follows that lesions in one of the four exons at the 3′ end will affect all the isoforms. The following mutations have been found in Crigler–Najjar Type I patients. (1) A 13 base pair deletion in exon 2 (Ritter *et al.* 1992). (2) A C → T mutation in exon 4 consistent with a change of amino acid from serine to phenylalanine (Bosma *et al.* 1992) (3) A C → T mutation in exon 2 giving a premature stop codon (Bosma *et al.* 1992).

The *UGT1* family of genes has been mapped to chromosome 2 by Moghrabi *et al.* (1992).

THE SEARCH FOR GENETIC POLYMORPHISMS OF DRUG GLUCURONIDATION IN MAN

Comparatively little progress was made since R. T. Williams's book was published in 1959 until just recently, in detecting genetic variants of human UDPGT enzymes (Mulder, 1992). Possible reasons why they have not been recognized are: (1) the difficulties of handling the enzymes *in vitro*, (2) overlapping specificities make it difficult to examine the properties of one enzyme *in vivo*: take paracetamol as an example – it is metabolized by sulphate conjugation as well as glucuronidization, and it is possible that the latter process may be mediated by more than one transferase; (3) different individuals may have their UDPGT enzymes set at different levels of induction; (4) very small populations of healthy individuals have been studied with *in vivo* tests. The biggest such population was that described by Evans & Clarke (1961), who studied serum salicylic acid concentrations in 100 persons following an oral dose; the frequency distribution curve was normal. An oral menthol test was carried out by Szabo & Ebrey (1963) and the percentage of the dose excreted as urinary glucuronide estimated in 25 healthy individuals; there was no hint of the existence of a polymorphism.

From studies which have been performed on rats there is every reason to believe that genetic variants may occur in humans, but it is of course entirely unknown what clinical relevance might be possessed by such variants.

A 10-fold variability in drug glucuronidation is known to exist in humans (Tephly & Burchell

1990). Also different UDPGT enzymes are known to vary independently.

A study of six monozygous and six dizygous twins by Nash *et al.* (1984) gave the rate constant for the formation of the glucuronide for paracetamol. The computed heritability was low, and this is not surprising in view of the fact that many other processes were going on at the same time which would contribute to the variances within both groups.

Despite the previous lack of success in finding a genetic polymorphism of glucuronidation, what appears to be a breakthrough has occurred recently. Liu *et al.* (1991) investigated the urinary metabolic ratio fenofibric acid/fenofibryl glucuronide (Fig. 18.6*a*) in a urine sample collected over 8 hours following an oral dose of 100 mg fenofibrate. A total of 72 healthy individuals were studied, and women were found to excrete more glucuronide than men (sex hormones increase some glucuronidation reactions: see Miners & Mackenzie 1991). When the metabolic ratios were corrected for sex the frequency distribution very obviously contained two separate modes and possibly even three (Fig. 18.6*b*).

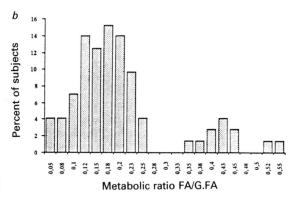

Fig. 18.6.(a) Molecular structure of fenofibryl β(D)-glucuronide. (b) Frequency distribution histogram of the urinary metabolic ratio of fenofibric acid/ fenofibryl glucuronide (FA/G.FA). (From Liu *et al.* 1991.)

Family studies are currently proceeding to assess whether this polymorphism is genetically determined (Galteau, personal communication 1992). Clofibrate did not exhibit the same phenomenon.

Perhaps a fifth reason should be added to the four listed above explaining why genetic polymorphisms have not been found: namely, that the correct drugs have not been investigated!

DIFFERENTIAL INDUCTION OF DRUG GLUCURONIDATION

Inhibition studies demonstrate the specificity and independence of individual liver UDPGTs. A clinically relevant example is the specific and competitive inhibition *in vitro* of morphine 3-glucuronidation by diazepam (de Villar *et al.* 1981; Vega *et al.* 1984; Rane *et al.* 1986). Oxazepam, lorazepam and nitrazepam had a much inferior effect, whilst the glucuronidization of *p*-nitrophenol and testosterone were not affected by diazepam.

Examples of inducibility differences are known, for example, paracetamol glucuronidation is induced with phenytoin and rifampicin, whilst morphine and chloramphenicol glucuronidation are not induced by phenytoin and phenobarbitone. Paracetamol and clofibric acid glucuronidations are induced by oral contraceptive steroids. Salicylamide and salicylate were given as test drugs by Yaffe *et al.* (1966) to an infant with unconjugated hyperbilirubinaemia. Under the influence of phenobarbitone the percentage of a salicylamide dose excreted as glucuronide doubled to a normal level but salicylate metabolism and excretion were hardly affected.

Inducibility is of importance in considering the Crigler–Najjar (CN) and Gilbert's syndromes.

It is considered likely that deficient bilirubin glucuronidization is due to a lesion in the promoter region of *HUG-Br1*, giving complete absence in CN Type II and partial absence in Gilbert's disease. The expression of *HUG-Br2* must be unaffected because the serum bilirubin level is dramatically lowered by phenobarbital induction.

In CN Type I there is a complete defect of glucuronidation of bilirubin and a decreased activity for planar phenols. There is usually no lowering of serum bilirubin levels by phenobarbital induction. It was shown by Van Es *et al.* (1990) that CN Type I was a heterogeneous condition in that at least three isoforms were missing in some patients whereas only the bilirubin isoform was missing in others.

Robertson *et al.* (1991) showed a complete absence of UDP glucuronosyltransferase activity for bilirubin in CN Type I syndrome and a very low level in CN Type II. There was preservation of the activity for 1-naphthol in both syndromes. Immunoblot studies revealed a pattern of missing transferases which varied between patients. The exact DNA defects which have been described earlier account for some of these observations on CN Type I. The DNA defects responsible for CN Type II are not known at present.

There seems little doubt, therefore, that the CN syndromes are due to defects in the UGT genes that control the glucuronidation of bilirubin. This leads to the speculation that there may be genetic polymorphisms due to variations in the UGT genes which control drug-glucuronidizing enzymes.

POSSIBLE FUTURE DEVELOPMENTS

With the advent of the techniques of modern molecular genetics the same remark can be made about the glucuronidization of drugs as about other biotransformations discussed in this volume. It may be possible by examining the DNA derived from blood leucocytes to determine genetic variants. These should then be correlated with phenotypic clinical events. However, it would seem that there may also be scope for the deployment of the less sophisticated methodology of direct phenotyping using drug ingestion, and selecting substrates from the different chemical classes that are subject to glucuronidation.

Arias, I. M., Gartner, L. M., Cohen, M., Ben Ezzer, J. & Levi, A. J. (1969). Chronic nonhemolytic unconjugated hyperbilirubinemia with glucuronyl transferase deficiency. *American Journal of Medicine*, **47**, 395–409.

Axelrod, J., Schmid, R. & Hammaker, L. (1957). A biochemical lesion in congenital non-haemolytic jaundice. *Nature*, **180**, 1426–7.

Barniville, H. T. F. & Misk, R. (1959). Urinary glucuronic acid excretion in liver disease and the effect of a salicylamide load. *British Medical Journal*, **1**, 337–40.

Beck, K. & Kiani, B. (1960). Zur frage derrglucuronbildung bei der funktionellen hyperbilirubiñamie unter berücksichtigung der renalen glucuronid-clearance. *Klinische Wochenshrift*, **38**, 428–33.

Black, M,. Fevery, J., Parker, D., Jacobson, J., Billing, B. H. & Carson, E. R. (1974). Effect of phenobarbitone on plasma [¹⁴C] bilirubin clearance in patients with unconjugated hyperbilirubinaemia. *Clinical Science and Molecular Medicine*, **46**, 1–17.

Black, M. & Sherlock, S. (1970). Treatment of Gilbert's syndrome with phenobarbitone. *Lancet*, **1**, 1359–62.

Blaschke, T. F., Berk, B. D., Rodkey, F. L., Scharschmidt, B. F., Collison, H. A. & Waggoner, J. G. (1974a). Drugs and the liver. I Effects of glutethimide and phenobarbital on hepatic bilirubin clearance, plasma bilirubin turnover and carbon monoxide production in man. *Biochemical Pharmacology*, **23**, 2795–806.

Blaschke, T. F., Berk, P. D., Scharschmidt, B. F., Guyther, J. R., Vergalla, J. M. & Waggoner, J. G. (1974b). Crigler–Najjar syndrome: an unusual course with development of neurologic damage at age eighteen. *Pediatric Research*, **8**, 573–90.

Bloomer, J. R., Berk, P. D., Howe, R. B. & Berlin, N. I. (1971). Bilirubin metabolism in congenital nonhemolytic jaundice. *Pediatric Research*, **5**, 256–64.

Blumenschein, S. D., Kallen, R. J., Storey, B., Natzschka, J. C., Odell, G. B. & Childs, B. (1968). Familial nonhemolytic jaundice with late onset of neurological damage. *Pediatrics*, **42**, 786–92.

Bock, K. W. & Bock-Hennig, B. S. (1987). Differential induction of human liver UDP-glucuronosyl transferase activities by phenobarbital-type inducers. *Biochemical Pharmacology*, **36**, 4137–43.

Bosma,, P. J., Chowdhury, J. R., Huang, T.-J., Lahiri, P., Elferink, R. P. J. O., Van Es, H. H. G., Lederstein, M., Whitington, P. F., Jansen, P. L. M. & Chowdhury, N. R. (1992). Mechanisms of inherited deficiencies of multiple UDP-glucuronosyltransferase isoforms in two patients with Crigler–Najjar syndrome, type I. *FASEB Journal*, 2851–63.

Burchell, B. & Coughtrie, M. W. H. (1989). UDP-glucuronosyl-transferases. *Pharmacology and Therapeutics*, **43**, 261–89.

Burchell, B., Coughtrie, M. W. H., Jackson, M. R., Shepherd, S. R. P., Harding, D. & Hume, R. (1987). Genetic deficiency of bilirubin glucuronidation in rats and humans. *Molecular Aspects of Medicine*, **9**, 429–55.

Burchell, B., Nevert, D. W., Nelson, D. R., Bock, K. W., Iyanagi, T., Jansen, P. L. M., Lancet, D., Mulder, G. H., Roy Chowdhury, J., Siest, G., Tephly, T. R. & Mackenzie, P. I. (1991). The UDP glucuronosyl-transferase gene superfamily: suggested nomenclature based on evolutionary divergence. *DNA and Cell Biology*, **10**, 487–94.

Childs, B., Sidbury, J. B. & Migeon, C. J. (1959). Glucuronic acid conjugation by patients with familial non-hemolytic jaundice and their relatives. *Pediatrics*, **23**, 903–13.

Crigler, J. F. & Gold, N. I. (1969). Effect of sodium phenobarbital on bilirubin metabolism in an infant with congenital non-hemolytic unconjugated hyperbilirubinemia and kernicterus. *Journal of Clinical Investigation*, **48**, 42–55.

de Morais, S. M. F., Uetrecht, J. P. & Wells, P. G. (1992). Decreased glucuronidation and increased bioactivation of acetaminophen in Gilbert's syndrome. *Gastroenterology*, **102**, 577–86.

del Villar, E., Sanchez, E., Letelier, M. E. & Vega, P. (1981). Differential inhibition by diazepam and nitrazepam of UDP-glucuronyltransferases activities in rats. *Research Communications in Chemical Pathology and Pharmacology*, **33**, 433–47.

Evans, D. A. P. & Clarke, C. A. (1961). Pharmacogenetics. *British Medical Bulletin*, **17**, 234–40.

Francois, R., Bertholon, M. A., Bertrand, J. & Quincy, C. L. (1962). La maladie de Crigler–Najjar. *Revue Internationale de Hepatologie*, **12**, 753–76.

Gollan, J. L., Huang, S. N., Billing, B. & Sherlock, S. (1975). Prolonged survival in three brothers with severe type 2 Crigler–Najjar syndrome. *Gastroenterology*, **68**, 1543–55.

Gordon, E. R., Shaffer, E. A. & Sass-Kortsak, A. (1976). Bilirubin secretion and conjugation in the Crigler–Najjar syndrome type II. *Gastroenterology*, **70**, 761–5.

Harding, D., Fournel-Gigleux, S., Jackson, M. R. & Burchell, B. (1988a). Cloning and substrate specificity of a human phenol UDP-glucuronosyltransferase expressed in COS-7 cells. *Proceedings of the National Academy of Sciences (USA)*, **85**, 8381–5.

Harding, D., Jackson, M. R., Wooster, R., Fournel-Gigleux, S. & Burchell, B. (1988b). Cloning of human UDP-glucuronosyl-transferase cDNAs. In *Cellular and Molecular Aspects of Glucuronidation*, ed. G. Siest, J. Magdalou & B. Burchell. Colloque INSERUM/John Libbey Eurotext Ltd, **173**, 13–20.

Hunter, J., Thompson, R. P. H., Rake, M. O. & Williams, R. (1971). Controlled trial of phethbarbital, a non-hypnotic barbiturate in unconjugated hyperbilirubinaemia. *British Medical Journal*, **2**, 497–9.

Hunter, J. O., Thompson, R. P. H., Dunn, P. M. & Williams, R. (1973). Inheritance of type 2 Crigler–Najjar hyperbilirubinaemia. *Gut*, **14**, 46–9.

Irshaid, Y. M. & Tephly, T. R. (1987). Isolation and purification of two human liver UDP-glucuronosyl-transferases. *Molecular Pharmacology*, **31**, 27–34.

Jansen, P. L. M., Mulder, G. J., Burchell, B. & Bock, K. W. (1992). New developments in glucuronidation research: Report of a workshop on 'Glucuronidation, its role in health and disease'. *Hepatology*, **15**, 532–44.

Kline, W. & Rosenkranz, A. (1972). Klinische und biochemische studien zum Crigler–Najjar-syndrom. *Monatsschrift Kinderheilkunde (Berlin)*, **119**, 555–8.

Kreek, M. J. & Sleisenger, M. H. (1968). Reduction of serum-unconjugated-bilirubin with phenobarbitone in adult congenital non-haemolytic unconjugated hyperbilirubinaemia. *Lancet*, **2**, 73–8.

Liu, H. F., Vincent-Viry, M., Galteau, M. M., Guéguen, R., Magdalou, J., Nicolas, A., Leroy, P. & Siest, G. (1991). Urinary glucuronide excretion of fenofibric and clofibric acid glucuronides in man. Is it polymorphic? *European Journal of Clinical Pharmacology*, **41**, 153–9.

Miners, J. O., Lillywhite, K. J., Yoovathaworn, K., Pongmarutai, M. & Birkett, D. J. (1990). Characterization of paracetamol UDP-glucuronosyltransferase activity in human liver microsomes. *Biochemical Pharmacology*, **40**, 595–600.

Miners, J. O. & Mackenzie, P. I. (1991). Drug glucuronidation in humans. *Pharmacology and Therapeutics*, **51**, 347–69.

Moghrabi, N., Sutherland, L., Wooster, R., Povey, S., Boxer, M. & Burchell, B. (1992). Chromosomal assignment of human phenol and bilirubin UDP-glucuronosyltransferase genes (UGT1A-subfamily). *Annals of Human Genetics (London)*, **56** 81–91.

Mulder, G. J. (1992) Glucuronidation and its role in regulation of biological activity of drugs. *Annual Review of Pharmacology and Toxicology*, **32**, 25–49.

Nash, R. M., Stein, L., Penno, M. B., Passananti, G. T. & Vesell, E. S. (1984). Sources of interindividual variations in acetaminophen and antipyrine metabolism. *Clinical Pharmacology and Therapeutics*, **36**, 417–30.

Osborne, R., Joel, S., Trew, D. & Slevin, M. (1988). Analgesic activity of morphine-6-glucuronide. *Lancet*, **1**, 828.

Peterson, R. E. & Schmid, R. (1957). A clinical syndrome associated with a defect in steroid glucuronide formation. *Journal of Clinical Endocrinology*, **17**, 1485–8.

Rane, A., Sawe, J., Pacifici, G. M., Svensson, J.-O. & Kager, L. (1986). Regioselective glucuronidation of morphine and interactions with benzodiazepines in human liver. In *Advances in Pain Research and Therapy*, Vol. 8, ed. K. M. Foley & C. E. Inturrisi, pp. 57–64. New York: Raven Press.

Ritter, J. K., Yeatman, M. T., Ferreira, P. & Owens, I. S. (1992). Identification of a genetic alteration in the code for bilirubin UDP-glucuronosyltransferase in the *UGT1* gene complex of a Crigler–Najjar type I patient. *Journal of Clinical Investigation*, **90**, 150–5.

Robertson, K. J., Clarke, D., Sutherland, L., Wooster, R., Coughtrie, M. W. H. & Burchell, B. (1991). Investigation of the molecular basis of the genetic deficiency of UDP-glucuronosyltransferase in Crigler–Najjar syndrome. *Journal of Inherited Metabolic Diseases*, **14**, 563–79.

Samuel, S. A. (1981). Apparent anaphylactic reaction to Zomepirac (Zomax). *New England Journal of Medicine*, **304**, 978.

Schmid, R. & McDonagh, A. F. (1978). Hyperbilirubinaemia. In *The Metabolic Basis of Inherited Disease*, 4th edition, ed. J. B. Stanbury, J. B. Wyngarden & D. S. Fredrickson, pp. 1221–57. New York: McGraw-Hill.

Schmid, R. & Hammaker, L. (1963). Metabolism and disposition of C^{14}-bilirubin in congenital non-hemolytic jaundice. *Journal of Clinical Investigation*, **42**, 1720–34.

Sinaasappel, M. & Jansen, P. L. M. (1991). The differential diagnosis of Crigler–Najjar disease, types 1 and 2 by bile pigment analysis. *Gastroenterology*, **100**, 783–9.

Sleisinger, M. H., Kahn, I., Barniville, H., Rubin, W., Ben Ezzer, J. & Arias, I. M. (1967). Nonhemolytic unconjugated hyperbilirubinemia with hepatic glucuronyl transferase deficiency: a genetic study in four generations. *Transactions of the Association of American Physicians (Philadelphia)*, **80**, 259–66.

Smith, P. C., McDonagh, A. F. & Benet, L. Z. (1986). Irreversible binding of zomepirac to plasma protein in vitro and in vivo. *Journal of Clinical Investigation*, **77**, 934–9.

Szabo, L. & Ebrey, P. (1963). Studies on the inheritance of Crigler–Najjar's syndrome by the menthol test. *Acta Paediatrica Hungarica (Budapest)*, **4**, 153–8.

Tephly, T. R. & Burchell, B. (1990). UDP-glucuronosyltransferases: a family of detoxifying enzymes. *Trends in Pharmacological Sciences*, **11**, 276–9.

Thompson, R. P. H., Pilcher, C. W. T., Robinson, J., Stathers, G. M., McLean, A. E. M. & Williams, R. (1969). Treatment of unconjugated jaundice with dicophane. *Lancet*, **2**, 4–6.

Van Es, H., Goldhoorn, B. G., Paul-Abrahamse, M., Oude Elferink, R. P. J. & Jansen, P. L. M. (1990). Immunochemical analysis of uridine diphosphate-glucuronosyltransferase in four patients with the Crigler–Najjar syndrome type I. *Journal of Clinical Investigation*, **85**, 1199–205.

Vega, P., Carrasco, M., Sanchez, E. & del Villar, E. (1984). Structure–activity relationship in the effect of 1,4-benzodiazepines on morphine aminopyrine and oestrone metabolism. *Research Communications in Chemical Pathology and Pharmacology*, **44**, 179–98.

Whelton, M. J., Krustev, L. P. & Billing, B. H. (1968). Reduction in serum bilirubin by phenobarbital in adult unconjugated hyperbilirubinaemia. *American Journal of Medicine*, **45**, 160–4.

Williams, R. T. (1959). *Detoxication Mechanisms*, p. 287. London: Chapman & Hall.

Yaffe, S. J., Levy, G., Matsuzawa, T. & Baliah, T. (1966). Enhancement of glucuronide-conjugating capacity in a hyperbilirubinaemic infant due to apparent enzyme induction by phenobarbital. *New England Journal of Medicine*, **275**, 1461–5.

Yue, Q. Y., Svensson, J.-O., Alm, C., Sjöqvist, F. & Šawe, J. (1989). Interindividual and interethnic differences in the demethylation and glucuronidation of codeine. *British Journal of Clinical Pharmacology*, **28**, 629–37.

19   Glutathione-S-transferase

INTRODUCTION

GLUTATHIONE is a tripeptide which is made up from glycine, cysteine and γ-glutamic acid (Fig. 19.1) and it can exist in the reduced and oxidized forms. Reduced glutathione is regenerated from oxidized glutathione by reaction with NADPH under the influence of glutathione reductase (Fig. 19.2).

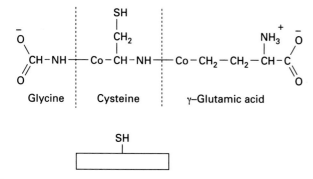

Fig. 19.1. Glutathione.

The importance of glucose-6-phosphate dehydrogenase (G6PD) in regenerating NADPH for this purpose has been emphasized in another chapter. In the red cells reduced glutathione 'protects' haemoglobin and other macromolecules from oxidation.

Glutathione has other functions including (1) acting non-catalytically as an intracellular binding molecule for a large number of lipophilic compounds that include bilirubin and steroids (Marcus *et al.* 1978; Vos & Van Bladeren 1990), (2) detoxifying endogenous and exogenous electrophilic compounds. Examples of such endogenous compounds are lipid hydroperoxides, prostaglandins and leukotriene A_4 (Tsuchida *et al.* 1990), also 4-hydroxy alkenals (Danielson *et al.* 1987). A large number of xenobiotics, including drugs, are biotransformed in the body into electrophilic intermediary compounds which are potentially harmful to cell constituents but which are rendered harmless by conjugation with glutathione under the influence of the enzyme glutathione-S-transferase (EC 2.5.1.18).

An example is paracetamol; after an oral dose of

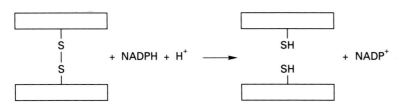

Fig. 19.2. The reduction of the oxidized form of glutathione.

317

20 mg/kg about 55% is recovered in the urine as the glucuronide, 30% as the sulphate ester, 8% as glutathione-derived adducts (mercapturic and cysteine conjugates) and only 3% as the unchanged drug (Prescott 1980). Glutathione conjugation rapidly inactivates an electrophilic metabolite formed in the liver. The compound so formed is hydrolysed by the removal of the glycine and γ-glutamyl moieties by appropriate peptidases and then acetylated on the amino group of the cysteine molecule (Habig *et al.* 1974). The resulting *N*-acetyl cysteine (i.e. mercapturic acid) derivative is excreted in the urine (Fig. 19.3).

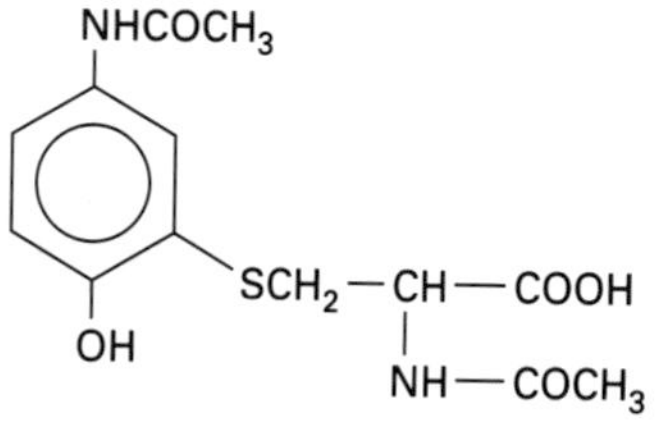

Fig. 19.3. The mercapturic (i.e. *N*-acetyl cysteine) derivative of paracetamol.

With small doses of paracetamol this mechanism works well, but if there is insufficient glutathione or excessive amounts of paracetamol the electrophilic arylating metabolites are not detoxified. In this situation they bind covalently to macromolecules such as cell proteins and DNA to cause irreversible damage.

An illustration of this damaging effect was provided by the work of Spielberg (1980) who demonstrated that paracetamol metabolites generated by mouse hepatic microsomes depleted human lymphocyte glutathione content and produced toxicity. With increasing paracetamol concentrations cell glutathione content was progressively depleted and toxicity was greater. Similarly, Spielberg *et al.* (1981) showed that lymphocytes from persons with glutathione synthetase deficiency (5-oxoprolinuria) were particularly vulnerable to paracetamol metabolites generated by an *in vitro* microsomal system.

It has become apparent, however, that conjugation with glutathione is not invariably a detoxication process. For example, the conjugate itself may be reactive (e.g. 2-bromoethylglutathione) or may be further metabolized to a toxic species (e.g. hexachloro-butadiene). These exceptions to the general rule were discussed by van Bladeren (1988), and further examples were extensively discussed by Koob & Dekant (1991). These mechanisms have not yet been identified in clinical settings.

The production of mercapturic derivatives after the administration of various foreign compounds to animals has been known for a century (see Williams 1959). However, it is only recently that glutathione-S-transferases have been closely studied, and a very complex organization has been found to exist in human and animal cells and tissues. Only a few therapeutically used drugs have been studied, since most of the work has been carried out with model organic substrates for the transferases. Nevertheless there are indications that the genetic diversity which has been found could be of importance in the metabolism of commonly used drugs. The glutathione-S-transferases also seem likely to have a role in the aetiologic mechanisms of disease.

In addition to glutathione-S-transferase activity itself, the selenium-independent glutathione-peroxidase activity (Fig. 19.4) found in the cytosol of many tissues has also been attributed to the same enzymic molecules. However, this is not true in erythrocytes (Del Boccio *et al.* 1986).

$$R - O - OH + 2GSH \longrightarrow R - OH + GSSG + H_2O$$

Fig. 19.4. Peroxidase reaction. R, organic group. The reaction is thought to proceed by two steps. First, reduced glutathione reacts with the organic peroxide to form the corresponding alcohol and the sulphenic acid of glutathione GSOH. Secondly, the sulphenic acid reacts with another molecule of reduced glutathione producing oxidized glutathione and water.

DIFFERENT CLASSES OF GLUTATHIONE-S-TRANSFERASES

The glutathione-S-transferases (GST) are a family of multifunctional proteins which are inducible and which have overlapping specificities. About 3% of the weight of protein in the human liver consists of these enzymes.

There are alternative systems of nomenclature which are confusing (see Max 1990; Morrow & Cowan 1990). The numerical system originated from laboratories working with starch gel electrophoresis, whereas the lower case Greek letter system came from biochemical laboratories working on enzyme purification. A generally accepted classification is the designation of three different classes of cytosolic enzymes as mu, alpha and pi (based on structural, evolutionary, immunological and enzymatic properties), which are encoded at three distinct genetic loci, GST1, GST2 and GST3, respectively (Board 1981; Mannervik et al. 1985). Dimeric combinations of non-identical 23 to 29 kDa subunits make up the proteins in each class (Campbell et al. 1990). The subunits which go to make enzymes of the different classes are as follows. For alpha B_1 and B_2; for mu μ and Ψ; less is known about the microsomal GST enzymes which are trimers made up of 17 kDa subunits (Morrow & Cowan 1990).

Recently a further class of soluble liver GST has been described called 'theta' (Meyer et al. 1991), which unlike the other cytosolic GST enzymes lacks activity towards the model substrate 1-chloro-2,4-dinitrobenzene (CDNB). This new class represents only a small proportion of liver-soluble GST molecules. A recent publication by 14 experts on the nomenclature of the human glutathione transferases should help standardize future articles on the topic (Mannervik et al. 1992).

GENETIC POLYMORPHISMS

A striking observation made concerning the mu class of GST was that they were present in the livers of only some people (Warholm et al. 1980, 1981).

Electrophoretic studies of human liver homogenates on starch gel (Board 1981) disclosed the following. The mu class of enzymes were those components acting powerfully on CDNB and migrating towards the anode. These enzymes are classed as GST1. Different patterns representing phenotypes termed 1, 1-2, 2 and 0-0 could be discerned. The last category lacked this enzyme activity and accounted for 26 out of 40 Caucasians.

Another polymorphism was observed in the enzyme molecules which migrated towards the cathode, which are classed as alpha or GST2. GST2 types 1 and 2 have been recognized; they are not allelic. They differ by 11 amino acids and are products of different loci which are separated by as little as 2 kb. Also, an RFLP has been found in GST by Cooke & Connor (1991) using BstEII/TaqI double digest. The allele frequencies of the polymorphic 3 kb and 2.8 kb fragments were 0.5.

Weakly staining activity migrating very fast toward the anode was termed pi or GST3 and was not polymorphic as revealed by this electrophoretic technique.

It is to be noted that Board (1981) tested his data for agreement with the Hardy–Weinberg equilibrium but did not present family data to prove the genetic nature of the polymorphism of GST1 (mu).

An interesting, more recent finding (Seidegård et al. 1985) was that the genetic differences in the hepatic expression of GST1, mu-class enzymes was reflected in mononuclear leucocytes. The population frequency distribution of monocytic GST activity towards trans-stilbene oxide (tSBO: Fig. 19.5) disclosed three separate modes (Fig. 19.6). Eight families were studied by Seidegård & Pero (1985) at a time before they were able to differentiate between the two high activity modes, so that they were dealing with only two phenotypes with low and high activities. The data were consistent with the interpretation that the activity was controlled by two allelic autosomal genes with high activity being dominant.

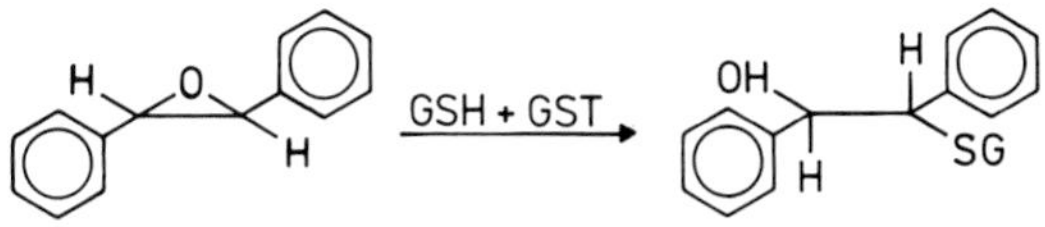

Fig. 19.5. Conjugation of trans-stilbene oxide by glutathione transferase. (Supplied through the kindness of Dr J. Seidegård.) GSH, reduced glutathione; GST, glutathione-S-transferase.

Later, Seidegård et al. (1988) were also able to show an identity of expression of GST1 in blood monocytes and liver. They used mouse and human GSTmu DNA probes to examine the RNA content of liver samples. Only persons whose monocytes had GST-tSBO activity possessed mu-class GST in their livers, whereas alpha-class GST was present in all livers. The GST-tSBO polymorphism has been demonstrated in arterial tissue, venous tissue and cultured fibroblasts (Pessah-Rasmussen et al. 1990), and in kidney and adrenal (Seidegård & Pero 1988).

Quite a lot of the confusion caused by different workers having different nomenclatures has been dispelled by the clear demonstration by Seidegård and his group that GST1, GSTmu and GST-tSBO are identical.

The same workers used a human mu-class GST cDNA probe to hybridize with restriction fragments

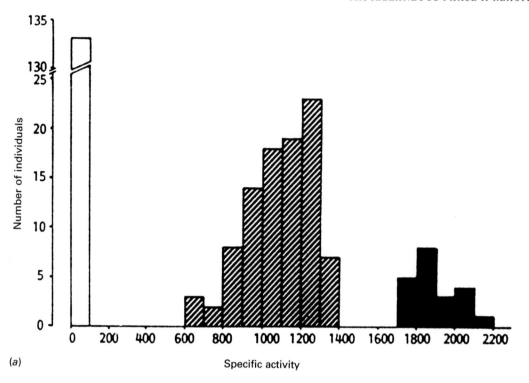

(a)

Specific activity

Fig. 19.6.(a) The distribution of glutathione transferase activity towards *trans*-stilbene oxide in a population consisting of 248 individuals. The specific activities are expressed as pmol conjugate formed/min/10^7 cells. (b) The distribution of glutathione transferase activity towards 1-chloro-2,4-dinitrobenzene in a population consisting of 214 individuals. The specific activities are expressed as nmol conjugate formed/min/10^7 cells. The individuals measured here were also assayed for their glutathione transferase activity towards *trans*-stilbene oxide. Individuals with low activity towards this latter substrate are presented in this figure as open bars, individuals with high activity are presented as striped bars and individuals with very high activity are presented as filled bars. (From Seidegård *et al.* 1985.)

of human DNA obtained from leucocytes. *Bam*HI and *Eco*RI digests either possessed or lacked 11.5 or 8.0 kb fragments, respectively, depending on the GST-tSBO status of the individual (those who possessed GST-tSBO activity possessed the fragment, others lacked both the activity and the fragment). Seidegård *et al.* (1988) therefore deduced that the basis of the polymorphism lay in a gene deletion. This was confirmed by Board *et al.* (1990).

The use of sub-fragments of the probe with vari-

ous restriction endonuclease digests of leucocyte-derived DNA suggested the presence of at least three mu-class GST enzymes in individuals expressing GST-tSBO. In addition to the products of alleles *1* and *2* mentioned above, similar mu-class GST molecules have been identified in muscle (GST4) (Board *et al.* 1988) and brain (GST5) (Campbell *et al.* 1990; Board *et al.* 1990).

The same *GST* polymorphism in monocytes was demonstrated by a different technique by Vos *et al.* (1991) who used monoclonal antibodies against GSTµ. Nine persons gave a positive and three persons gave a negative result.

Immunohistological techniques were used by Campbell *et al.* (1991), who demonstrated alpha GST in hepatocytes, proximal convoluted renal tubules, the deep reticular layer of the adrenal gland, interstitial cells of the testis and oxyntic cells of the stomach. They showed pi-class GST in ductular liver cells, pancreas, salivary gland and kidney. Mu-class GST was demonstrable in half the cases of liver, kidney, adrenal, testis, stroma and vessels of ovary, pancreas and epidermis, but was absent from placenta, fallopian tubes, endometrium, salivary

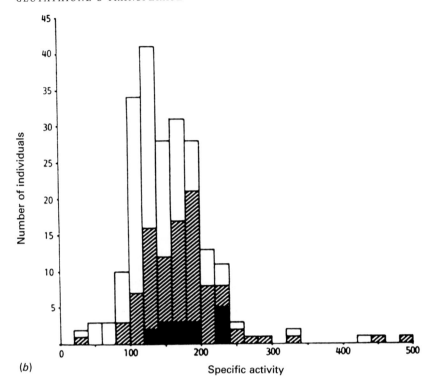

(b)

Specific activity

Fig. 19.6 (cont.).

gland and stomach. The pi class was most commonly represented in various neoplasms, whereas the mu class was the least common.

Scott & Wright (1980) investigated the genetics of erythrocytic GST. No electrophoretic variants were found amongst 294 individuals. GST activity to CDNB was examined by the techniques of quantitative genetics. There was no correlation between spouses (eliminating the effect of shared environment), but there was a positive offspring–parent correlation ($r = 0.511$, D.F.$=41$), indicating a significant genetic control of the activity.

Enzymes of the alpha class of GST are built of two subunits, termed B_1 and B_2. Thus three isozymes $B_1 B_1$, $B_1 B_2$ and $B_2 B_2$ are found (Hayes et al. 1991). The ratio of B_1 and B_2 subunits as determined by HPLC was found to vary considerably, with a suggestion of two groups with mean ratios 1.6 ± 0.3 and 3.8 ± 0.6 (Van Ommen et al. 1990), indicating a polymorphism. As Von Bladeren & Van Ommen (1991) point out, this potential polymorphism merits further attention.

GENE STRUCTURE

The cDNAs for two mu-class GST molecules have been isolated by De Jong et al. (1988) and Seidegård et al. (1988). The former cDNA was 1128 bp long, plus 10 nucleotides of A residues. The longest open reading frame spanned nucleotides 25 to 678 encoding a protein of 217 amino acids plus the N-terminal methionine. The latter was 1100 bp long and encoded a protein of 217 amino acids.

If one neglects the initiation ATG (methionine) codon of De Jong et al. (1988) codon 172 is AAG encoding lysine. In the corresponding position in the sequence of Seidegård et al. (1988) is the codon AAC encoding asparagine. There is a charge difference between these two amino acids which suggests (as pointed out by Board et al. 1990) that these two published structures are those of GST1*1 (or Ψ: Seidegård et al. 1988) and GST 1*2 (or μ: De Jong et al. 1988).

A similar (but quite separate) family of genes is likely to exist for the alpha class (basic) GST2 subunits (Rhoads et al. 1987).

GENE LOCALIZATION

The mu class *GST1* gene isolated by them was localized by hybridization studies by De Jong *et al.* (1988) to 1p31, but subsequently the genetic localizations for the various subunits were shown by De Jong *et al.* (1991) to be on chromosomes 1, 6 and 13. There is also a '*GST3*-like' locus at 12q13–14. Laisney *et al.* (1984) localized the structural gene for *GST3* (pi) to chromosome 11 and this has been subsequently refined to 11q13 (Board *et al.* 1990). The alpha-class *GST2* gene was localized at 6p12 (Board *et al.* 1990).

TISSUE DISTRIBUTION

The GST enzymes which have principally been studied in the liver have also a widespread distribution in the body, and have been studied in some human extra-hepatic locations.

In erythrocytes the GST is of the pi class and can conjugate CDNB (Marcus *et al.* 1978; Awasthi *et al.* 1983; Del Boccio *et al.* 1986), ethacrynic acid (see Fig. 19.7) (Marcus *et al.* 1978) and 4-dimethyl-aminophenol (Eckert & Eyer 1986), but is not active in the denitration of nitrite esters (Marcus *et al.* 1978). There is a transport mechanism to remove

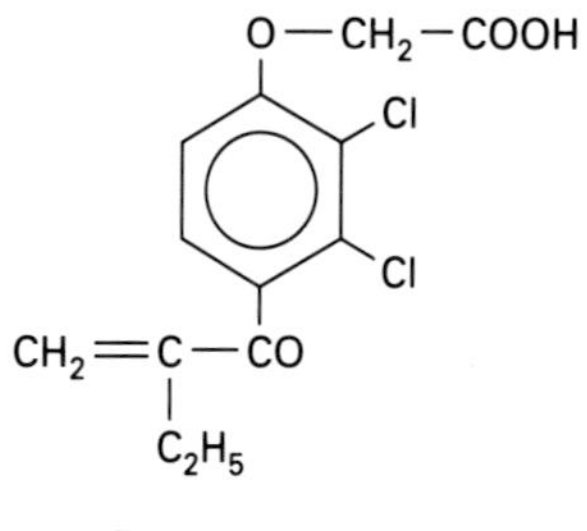

Ethacrynic acid

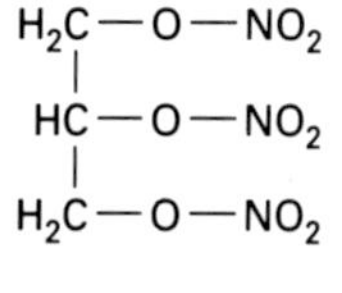

Glyceryl trinitrate
(nitroglycerine)

Fig. 19.7. Structural formulae of ethacrynic acid and glyceryl trinitrate.

the conjugates from the inside of the cell. The molecular mass and pI of the GST have been estimated as 24 000 kDa and 4.51 (Marcus *et al.* 1978) and 23 000 kDa and 4.6 (Del Boccio *et al.* 1986). The erythrocyte GST did not give precipitin bands with specific antibodies to purified liver GSTs (Marcus *et al.* 1978).

A separate type of erythrocytic GST has been described by Peter *et al.* (1989) and Hallier *et al.* (1990). The two types of GST can be separated by column chromatography (Hallier *et al.* 1992). The newly discovered GST, which does not metabolize CDNB, is active against methyl chloride, methyl bromide and methyl iodide forming S-methyl gluta-thione. The striking aspect of this discovery is that whereas 27 persons out of 45 tested possessed this enzymic activity ('conjugators') the other 18 had nil activity ('non-conjugators') (Peter *et al.* 1989). Evidence was produced by Thier *et al.* (1991) that methylene chloride metabolites were found in the plasma of 'conjugators' after the compound was incubated with blood: none was found in the plasma of 'non-conjugators'. Similarly, Föst *et al.* (1991) found that the disposition of ethylene oxide differed greatly between the two phenotypes. The genetics of this polymorphism have not yet been investigated.

The catalytic activity of blood mononuclear cells has already been mentioned. Neutrophil leucocytes were examined by Scott *et al.* (1990) and seemed to have a similar activity to erythrocytes in that they conjugated CDNB and the conjugate was expelled from the cells by an active transport mechanism.

The jejunum and ileum were found to be richly endowed with GST, the cytosolic activity assessed with CDNB being 60% of that of liver. All three classes (alpha, mu and pi) were found to be present in one jejunum by Özer *et al.* (1990) whilst de Waziers *et al.* (1990) found that the presence or absence of mu paralleled the situation in the liver. The colon had cytosolic CDNB activity 26% that of liver.

Human testis and brain were found by Campbell *et al.* (1990) to have GSTmu activity even when it was absent in liver. It was found that testis GSTmu had a blocked and extended amino-terminus and three additional amino acids at the carboxy-terminus. In the coding region the mRNA was 75% homologous with the liver form. These findings suggest that testis and liver GSTmu enzymes are the products of different genes.

Another highly complex picture was revealed by Tsuchida *et al.* (1990), who studied human heart and aorta. Pi was the predominant form of GST and this did not metabolize nitroglycerin (Fig. 19.7). There were, however, also five forms of GST which were of the mu class and these catalysed the formation of nitrous acid and glyceryl dinitrate from nitroglycerin. This activity was inhibited by bromosulphthalein, which is known to inhibit the relaxation of rabbit aorta produced by nitroglycerin. It is not yet clear if persons who lack GST mu in the liver also have an absence of the enzyme in heart and aorta.

The subcellular distribution of GST was studied in the fetal liver by Lei & Peng (1990). At 4 to 8 months of age they found cytosolic activity for CDNB and microsomal activity for ethacrynic acid.

INDUCTION AND INHIBITION

Some other enzyme systems described in this book (e.g. glucuronyltransferases, cytochromes P450, porphyrin pathway enzymes) are prone to induction and inhibition. The same is true of GST. Most of the work on this aspect has hitherto been carried out on rat enzymes.

Phenobarbital, 3-methyl cholanthrene, *trans*-stilbene oxide, hexachlorobenzene, disulfiram and constituents of diet such as cabbage and brussels sprouts have been shown to produce induction (Vos & Van Bladeren 1990; Sparnins *et al.* 1982). *Trans*-stilbene oxide, mentioned earlier, is an inducing agent for GST activity in rat liver (Seidegård *et al.* 1979).

Studies of mRNA in cultured rat hepatocytes have revealed that phenobarbital increases the transcriptional activity of *GST* genes and has a stabilizing effect *in vitro* on *GST* mRNAs (Vandenberghe *et al.* 1991).

A minor portion of liver GST activity is in the endoplasmic reticulum. It was shown by Haenen *et al.* (1991) that when α-methyldopa and NADPH were added to rat liver microsomes, the microsomal GST was activated. This effect was shown to be due to the metabolites of α-methyldopa (semi-ortho-quinone radical or ortho-quinone of α-methyldopa). The most likely mechanism of this activation was arylation of the free sulphydryl group of microsomal GST by these metabolites. This finding raises the interesting possibility that the products of Phase I metabolism mediated by cytochrome P450 in the endoplasmic reticulum induce the adjacent GST to mediate a Phase II reaction.

As yet there is no clear evidence of these induction and inhibition phenomena having clinical significance, but this is an area of knowledge which is relatively unexplored.

INTER-ETHNIC DISTRIBUTION

Comparatively little work has been published on the inter-ethnic distribution of the *GST* alleles. The available information on *GST1* and *GST2* is shown in Table 19.1.

As far as the author is aware there is no information on the *trans*-stilbene oxide polymorphism itself in non-Caucasian populations but the frequency of *GST1*0* has been estimated in various populations by other means (Table 19.1).

THE GST MU POLYMORPHISM AND SPONTANEOUS DISORDERS

There is a strong suspicion that since electrophilic compounds are conjugated by glutathione the propensity of many of them to carcinogenesis may be curtailed by that mechanism. Consequently the hypothesis was formed that persons who were deficient in *trans*-stilbene oxide–glutathione conjugation might be more prone to lung cancer. The Swedish data of Seidegård *et al.* (1990) support this idea. Amongst 191 lung cancer smokers, 121 lacked the enzymic activity in mononuclear leucocytes compared with 80 out of 192 control smokers ($\chi^2 = 18.05$; relative incidence, as computed by the method of Woolf 1954 as modified by Haldane 1955 = 2.41). However, Zhong *et al.* (1991) using both radio-immunoassay of GSTmu of leucocytes and genotyping by RFLP analysis found contrary results. Out of 225 controls, 94 (42%) were *GSTmu* null, as compared with 98 (43%) of 228 patients with lung cancers. When the cancers were subdivided by cell type 52% of 100 squamous cell carcinoma were in null individuals, as compared with 29% of 56 adeno-carcinomas.

Likewise, Heckbert *et al.* (1992), using an enzymic assay with *trans*-stilbene oxide as a substrate, found the null phenotype to be present in 69 out of 120 controls, 68 out of 113 smoking-related cancers (and 64% of lung cancers) and 29 out of 50 patients with other cancers. The distributions did not differ

Table 19.1. *Ethnic distributions of GST alleles*

Reference	Ethnic or national group	Number	GST1*1	GST1*2	GST1*0	GST1*3	GST2*1	GST2*2
Board 1981	Chinese	96	0.1709	0.0646	0.7645	Nil	0.8125	0.1875
Board 1981	Indian	43	0.1614	0.2790	0.5596	Nil	0.7791	0.2209
Board 1981	Caucasian	40	0.1061	0.0784	0.8154	Nil	0.8375	0.1625
Laisney *et al.* 1984	French	56	0.0740	0.2790	0.6470	Nil	–	–
Strange *et al.* 1984	Northern Europeans	49	0.1300	0.2300	0.6400	Nil	–	–
Seidegård & Pero 1985[a]	Swedish	248	–	–	0.7320	–	–	–
Seidegård *et al.* 1986	American	78	–	–	0.7679	–	–	–
Harada *et al.* 1987[a]	Japanese	168	0.2520	0.0570	0.6910	0.0070	–	–
Hussey *et al.* 1987[a]	Scotland	42	–	–	0.6726	–	–	–
Afanasyeva & Spitsyn 1990	Russian	100	0.0510	0.2510	0.6970	Nil	–	–
Board *et al.* 1990[a]	Micronesian	37	–	–	1.0000	–	–	–
Board *et al.* 1990[a]	Melanesian	49	–	–	0.7950	–	–	–
Board *et al.* 1990[a]	Polynesian	49	–	–	0.9040	–	–	–
Seidegård *et al.* 1990[a]	American	114	–	–	0.7609	–	–	–
Groppi *et al.* 1991[a]	French	45	–	–	0.6831	–	–	–
Zhong *et al.* 1991[a]	? Scottish	225	–	–	0.6464	–	–	–
Brockmöller *et al.* 1992	German	145[b]	–	–	0.7428	–	–	–
Seidegård & Evans 1992[a] ⎫	Saudi Arabians	333	–	–	0.7187	–	–	–
Unpublished observations ⎬	Filipinos	82	–	–	0.7962	–	–	–

[a]These studies yielded estimates of the frequency of the null allele, but did not provide information on the frequencies of the other alleles.
[b]Included 49 lung cancer patients.

between these groups of individuals.

As a result of a survey using both genotypic and enzymic assessments Brockmöller *et al.* (1992) say that their data 'revealed no trend of over-representation of *GSTPR* class mu deficient individuals among the special group of 49 lung cancer patients.'

It is not clear why there should be a difference between the Swedish result on the one hand and the USA/UK and German results on the other.

Results in Japanese matching the Swedish conclusions were found by Hayashi *et al.* (1992). Amongst 116 patients with smoking-associated lung cancers they found 62.1% *GSTmu* null individuals compared with 46.6% in the controls ($\chi_1^2 = 8.3$, $p < 0.01$). In the same patients there was also an abnormal distribution of polymorphic *CYP 1A1* alleles as described in Chapter 5.

In view of the idea that GST may detoxify mutagens, Wiencke *et al.* (1990) exposed lymphocytes *in vitro* to *trans*-stilbene oxide (TSO) and assessed the sister chromatid exchange (SCE) induction. The GST mu activity was also measured. There was a trimodal distribution of SCEs produced per cell. Relative insensitivity to TSO induction of SCEs was observed only in individuals who expressed GST mu activity for TSO. *Cis*-stilbene oxide was an equally effective inducer of SCEs but the results in this case were not correlated with the GSTmu activity for TSO. In another similar study Van Poppel *et al.* (1992) observed the number of SCEs in the lymphocytes of healthy male smokers. Significantly greater numbers were observed in 71 GSTmu-deficient individuals compared with 83 non-deficient persons. These data are persuasive that GSTmu may be protective against the carcinogenic effects of some environmental chemicals.

The binding of aflatoxin B_1 to DNA in a human liver microsomal system was investigated by Liu *et al.* (1991) using human liver cytosols *in vitro*. Cytosols from persons with high lymphocyte GSTmu activity inhibited the binding significantly more than cytosols from persons with low lymphocyte GSTmu activity. Consequently the latter phenotype may be more susceptible to develop liver cancer.

The TSO polymorphism was assessed by an immunohistochemical technique on liver sections from alcoholic patients by Harrison *et al.* (1990).

They determined the presence or absence of GST mu using a specific rabbit antiserum whose binding was visualized using biotinylated anti-rabbit IgG and an avidin–biotin detection system. Their results indicated the absence of GSTmu in six of nine cases of steatosis, six of 15 cases of alcoholic hepatitis and two of 16 cases of cirrhosis. Afanasyeva & Spitsyn (1990) found the gene frequencies for GST1*1, GST1*2 and GST1*0 to be 0.020, 0.100 and 0.879, respectively in liver biopsies from 22 alcoholic hepatitis patients. Harada *et al.* (1987) studied 41 Japanese liver patients with an electrophoretic technique on liver biopsies and found the following frequencies of the null phenotype: acute hepatitis 4 out of 6, chronic hepatitis 13 out of 17, alcoholic liver 6 out of 8 and liver carcinoma 8 out of 10 with controls 6 out of 12.

It is not possible to be sure about the meaning of these results because the enzyme distribution might be perturbed by the disease process and even if that were not so the numbers are too small to draw any definite conclusions.

A superior study was that of Groppi *et al.* (1991) who used a PCR/DNA method on blood samples. Amongst 45 healthy subjects 21 (47%) had the null genotype as compared with 22 out of 45 individuals with liver conditions.

The null phenotype at the *GST1* locus was determined by an enzymatic assay on liver tissue in 44 primary biliary cirrhosis patients and 69 control patients without liver disease (Davies *et al*, 1992). There was no significant difference between the two frequencies (39% and 46% respectively). The phenotyping was confirmed by PCR genotyping in 10 and 12 individuals from the patients and controls, respectively. The authors concluded that a chemical detoxified by GSTmu was unlikely to be an aetiological agent in the causation of primary biliary cirrhosis.

Pessah-Rasmussen *et al.* (1990) showed that a population of 73 patients with intermittent claudication contained a higher proportion of individuals lacking GST-tSBO than various control groups.

Strange *et al.* (1984) described a liver specimen totally lacking GST2 from a patient who died following a cardiac infarction. GST1 was present so postmortem changes were not responsible for the absence of GST2. A patient with Rotor's syndrome (familial conjugated hyperbilirubinaemia) was described by Adachi & Yamamoto (1987); this patient had less than 0.2% of normal liver GST activity. It seems likely that GST1 and GST2 were both absent, and so bilirubin binding may have been deficient.

With the idea in mind that absence of erythrocytic GST activity might shed light on the function of this enzyme, Beutler *et al.* (1988) assayed all blood samples coming into their laboratory using CDNB as the substrate. After 513 unrelated patients had been examined a man was found with an activity only about 15% of normal. This man was well apart from having a mild haemolytic anaemia. He was an orphan and so family studies could not be made; it could not be assumed that the haemolysis was due to the enzyme deficiency.

GLUTATHIONE-S-TRANSFERASES AND DRUG EFFECTS

Glutathione and its metabolizing enzymes are known to detoxify reactive metabolites of sulphonamides. Also peripheral blood mononuclear cells which lack glutathione synthetase are more sensitive than normal cells to toxic sulphonamide metabolites. Because of this background Riley *et al.* (1991) investigated the relationship between the GST activity of monocytes and their viability in the presence of sulphamethoxazole metabolites generated by an *in vitro* system. There was no relationship between the two variables, either in cells from normal persons or in those from patients who had suffered hypersensitivity reactions to sulphonamides.

Ethacrynic acid is both an inhibitor and a substrate for GST, and its glutathione conjugate is also an inhibitor of the enzyme. Ploemen *et al.* (1990) investigated the inhibition of the major GST isozymes by both ethacrynic acid and its glutathione conjugate, and found that both, and especially the latter, to be powerful inhibitors of human mu class GST. This inhibition was reversible.

Both chlorambucil and melphalan (Fig. 19.8) are substrates for GST mainly but not exclusively of the alpha class. It has been found that non-toxic concentrations of ethacrynic acid can potentiate the cytotoxic activity of chlorambucil in Walker 256 rat breast carcinoma cells with acquired resistance to nitrogen mustards, and in human colon carcinoma cell lines (Tew *et al.* 1988; Kuzmich *et al.* 1992). Ethacrynic acid, at concentrations similar to

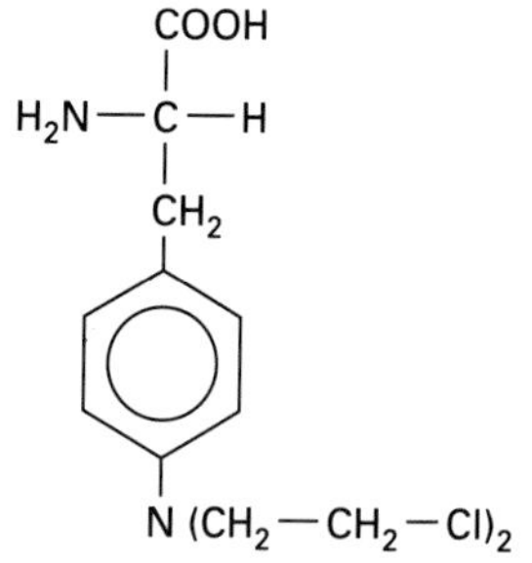

COOH
|
H₂N—C—H
|
CH₂
|
[benzene ring]
|
N (CH₂—CH₂—Cl)₂

Melphalan

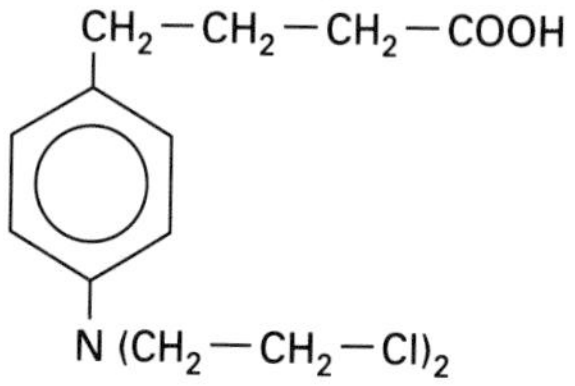

CH₂—CH₂—CH₂—COOH
|
[benzene ring]
|
N (CH₂—CH₂—Cl)₂

Chlorambucil

Fig. 19.8. The structural formulae of mephalan and chlorambucil.

clinically achievable serum values, was shown by Ciaccio *et al.* (1991) to inhibit the conjugation of chlorambucil to glutathione under the influence of alpha GST (and to a lesser extent pi GST).

Yang *et al* (1992) showed similar results in resistant N50-4 cells, a neoplastic line developed from the mouse fibroblast cell line NIH 3T3. Ethacrynic acid or indomethacin (GST inhibitors) and buthionine sulphoxamine (GSH depleting agent) both enhanced chlorambucil toxicity. The combination of both mechanisms almost completely abolished resistance. On the other hand, Rhodes & Twentyman (1992) found that the human lung cancer cell lines NCI-H69 (small cell), COR-L23 (large cell) and MOR (adenocarcinoma) were not less resistant to mephalan or cisplatin in the presence of ethacrynic acid. It is curious that this ethacrynic acid effect does not seem to have been investigated in either human GSTmu-possessing and GST mu-lacking cells or in relation to the ratio of B_1 and B_2 subunits of alpha GST to assess the influence of these genetic polymorphisms.

Similar considerations apply to the results obtained with anti-neoplastic drugs such as melphalan, BCNU (1,3-bis(2-chloroethyl)-1-nitrosourea), and mitoxanthrone, which are known to be inactivated by GST-mediated reactions (Morrow & Cowan 1990).

RELEVANCE OF GST TO OCCUPATIONAL MEDICINE

Methyl chloride is used an an industrial methylating agent, and acute overexposure produces a condition simulating drunkenness. Methyl bromide (which is odourless) is used as a fumigant and produces with acute toxicity malaise, headache, nausea and vomiting (Raffle *et al.* 1987). Methylene chloride (dichloromethane) is widely used as a solvent for stripping paint, as an industrial cleaning agent, for coating pills in the pharmaceutical industry and in the decaffeination of coffee (Their *et al.* 1991). Ethylene oxide is used in very large amounts for a variety of purposes such as:

production of ethylene glycol, and higher alcohols used as plasticizers, lubricants and synthetic materials;
ethoxylation of fatty alcohols in anionic detergent production;
dry sterilization (e.g. surgical instruments in hospitals);
a fumigant for foodstuffs and textiles;
an agricultural fungicide.

Adverse effects due to exposure to ethylene oxide are increased abortion rates and chromosomal aberrations and a suspicion of leukaemia and increased incidence of tumours (Raffle *et al.* 1987).

The incubation of blood samples with ethylene oxide was followed by the demonstration of a marked increase in sister chromatid exchanges only in 'non-conjugators' (Hallier *et al* 1992). It seems quite possible that erythrocytic 'conjugators' may be at less risk to develop other toxic effects after exposure to the compounds listed above.

The author would like to express his gratitude to Dr Jan-Eric Seidegård, Department of Molecular Ecogenetics, The Wallenberg Laboratory, Lund, Sweden who made many helpful suggestions about the contents of this chapter.

Adachi, Y. & Yamamoto, T. (1987). Partial defect in hepatic glutathione S-transferase activity in a case of Rotor's syndrome. *Gastroenterologia Japonica*, **22**, 34–8.

Afanasyeva, I. S. & Spitsyn, V. A. (1990). Glutathione S-transferase hereditary polymorphism in normal and alcoholic hepatitis liver. *Genetika (Moskva)*, **26**, 1309–15.

Awasthi, Y.C., Misra, G., Rassin, D. K. & Srivastava, S. K. (1983). Detoxification of xenobiotics by glutathione S-transferases in erythrocytes: the transport of the conjugate of glutathione and 1-chloro-2,4-dinitro-benzene. *British Journal of Haematology*, **55**, 419–25.

Beutler, E., Dunning, D., Dabe, I. B. & Forman, L. (1988). Erythrocyte glutathione S-transferase deficiency and hemolytic anemia. *Blood*, **72**, 73–7.

Board, P., Coggan, M., Johnston, P., Ross, V., Suzuki, T. & Webb, G. (1990). Genetic heterogeneity of the human glutathione transferases: a complex of gene families. *Pharmacology and Therapeutics*, **48**, 357–69.

Board, P. G. (1981). Biochemical genetics of glutathione-S-transferase in man. *American Journal of Human Genetics*, **33**, 36–43.

Board, P. G., Suzuki, T. & Shaw, D. C. (1988). Human muscle glutathione S-transferase (GST-4) shows close homology to human liver GST-1. *Biochimica et Biophysica Acta*, **953**, 214–7.

Brockmöller, J., Gross, D., Kerb, R., Drakoulis, N. & Roots, J. (1992). Correlation between *trans*-stilbene oxide-glutathione conjugation activity and the deletion mutation in the glutathione S-transferase class Mu gene detected by polymerase chain reaction. *Biochemical Pharmacology*, **43**, 647–50.

Campbell, E., Takahashi, Y., Abramovitz, M., Peretz, M. & Listowsky, I. (1990). A distinct human testis and brain μ-class glutathione S-transferase. *Journal of Biological Chemistry*, **265**, 9188–93.

Campbell, J. A. H., Corrigall, A. V., Guy, A. & Kirsch, R. E. (1991). Immunohistologic localization of alpha, Mu, and Pi class glutathione S-transferases in human tissues. *Cancer*, **67**, 1608–13.

Ciaccio, P. J., Tew, K. D. & LaCreta, F. P. (1991). Enzymatic conjugation of chlorambucil with glutathione by human glutathione S-transferases and inhibition by ethacrynic acid. *Biochemical Pharmacology*, **42**, 1504–7.

Cooke, A. & Connor, J. M. (1991). Glutathione S-transferase 2 shows an RFLP with Bst EII/Taq I double digest. *Nucleic Acids Research*, **19**, 5101.

Danielson, U. H., Esterbauer, H. J. & Mannervik, B. (1987). Structure-activity relationships of 4-hydroxyalkenals in the conjugation catalyzed by mammalian glutathione transferases. *Biochemical Journal*, **247**, 703–13.

Davies, M. H. Acharya, S. K., Elias, E., Cotton, W., Faulder, G. C. & Strange, R. C. (1992). The GTS1 0 polymorphism at the glutathione S-transferase 1 locus: phenotype and genotype studies in patients with primary biliary cirrhosis. Abstract, British Society of Gastroenterology, Autumn meeting, 1992.

De Jong, J. L., Chang, C.-M., Whang-Peng, J., Knutsen, T. & Tu, C.-P. D. (1988). The human liver glutathione S-transferase gene super-family:-expression and chromosome mapping of an Hb subunit cDNA. *Nucleic Acids Research*, **16**, 8541–54.

De Jong, J. L., Mohandas, T. & Tu, C.-P. D. (1991). The human Hb (MU) class glutathione S-transferases are encoded by a dispersed gene family. *Biochemical and Biophysical Research Communications*, **180**, 15–22.

Del Boccio, G., Casalone, E., Saccheta, P., Pennelli, A. & Di Ilio, C. (1986). Isoenzyme patterns of glutathione transferases from mammalian erythrocytes. *Biochemical Medicine and Metabolic Biology*, **36**, 306–12.

de Waziers, I., Cugnenc, P. H., Yang, C. S., Leroux, J.-P. & Beaune, P. H. (1990). Cytochrome P450 isoenzymes, epoxide hydrolase and glutathione transferases in rat and human hepatic and extrahepatic tissues. *Journal of Pharmacology and Experimental Therapeutics*, **253**, 387–94.

Eckert, K.-G. & Eyer, P. (1986). Formation and transport of xenobiotic glutathione-S-conjugates in red cells. *Biochemical Pharmacology*, **35**, 325–9.

Föst, U., Hallier, E., Ottenwalder, H., Bolt, H. M. & Peter, H. (1991). Distribution of ethylene oxide in human blood and its implications for biomonitoring. *Human Experimental Toxicology*, **10**, 25–31.

Groppi, A., Contelle, C., Fleury, B., Iron, A., Beguneret, J. & Couzigou, P. (1991). Glutathione S-transferase class μ in French alcoholic cirrhotic patients. *Human Genetics*, **87**, 628–30.

Habig, W. H., Pabst, M. J. & Jakoby, W. B. (1974). Glutathione S-transferases. The first enzymic step in mercapturic acid formation. *Journal of Biological Chemistry*, **249**, 7130–9.

Haenen, G. R. M. M., Jansen, F. P., Vermeulen, N. P. E. & Bast, A. (1991). Activation of the microsomal glutathione S-transferase by metabolites of α methyldopa. *Archives of Biochemistry and Biophysics*, **287**, 48–52.

Haldane, J. B. S. (1955). The estimation and significance of the logarithm of a ratio of frequence. *Annals of Human Genetics (London)*, **20**, 309–11.

Hallier, E., Deutschmann, S., Reichel, C., Bolt, H. M. & Peter, H. (1990). A comparative investigation of the metabolism of methyl bromide and methyl iodide in human erythrocytes. *International Archives of Occupational and Environmental Health*, **62**, 221–5.

Hallier, E., Schröder, K. R., Müller, A., Goergens, H. W. & Bolt, H. M. (1992). Modulation of methyl bromide and ethylene oxide toxicity by a new glutathione transferase. *Fourth North American International Society for the Study of Xenobiotics (ISSX) Meeting*, 2–6 November 1992, Bal Harbour, Florida. Vol. 2, Abstract 117.

Harada, S., Abei, M., Tanaka, N., Agarwal, D. P. & Goedde, H. W. (1987). Liver glutathione S-transferase polymorphism in Japanese and its pharmacogenetic importance. *Human Genetics*, **75**, 322–5.

Harrison, D. J., May, L., Hayes, P. C., Haque, M. M. & Hayes, J. D. (1990). Glutathione S-transferases in alcoholic liver disease. *Gut*, **31**, 909–12.

Hayashi, S.-I., Watanabe, J. & Kawajiri, K. (1992). High susceptibility to lung cancer analyzed in terms of combined genotypes of P450 IA1 and Mu-class glutathione S-transferase genes. *Japanese Journal of Cancer Research*, **83**, 866–70.

Hayes, P. C., Bouchier, I. A. D. & Beckett, G. J. (1991). Glutathione S-transferase in humans in health and disease. *Gut*, **32**, 813–18.

Hussey, A. J., Hayes, J. D. & Beckett, G. J. (1987). The polymorphic expression of neutral glutathione S-transferase in human mononuclear leucocytes as measured by specific radioimmunoassay. *Biochemical Pharmacology*, **36**, 4013–15.

Koob, M. & Dekant, M. (1991). Bioactivation of xenobiotics by formation of toxic glutathione conjugates. *Chemico-Biological Interactions*, **77**, 107–36.

Kuzmich, S., Vanderveer, L. A., Walsh, E. S., LaCreta, F. P. & TW, K. D. (1992). Increased levels of glutathione S-transferase π transcript as a mechanism of resistance to ethacrynic acid. *Biochemical Journal*, **281**, 219–24.

Laisney, V., Van Cong, C., Gross, M. S. & Frezal, J. (1984). Human genes for glutathione S-transferases. *Human Genetics*, **68**, 221–7.

Lei, S.-B. & Peng, R.-X. (1990). Subcellular distribution of glutathione-S-transferase in Chinese fetal liver. *Acta Pharmacologica Sinica*, **11**, 389–91.

Liu, Y. H., Taylor, J., Linko, P., Lucier, G. W. & Thompson, C. L. (1991). Glutathione S-transferase μ in human lymphocyte and liver: role in modulating formation of carcinogen-derived DNA adducts. *Carcinogenesis* **12**, 2269–75.

Mannervik, B., Ålin, P., Guthenberg, C., Jensson, H., Tahir, M. K., Warholm, M. & Jörnvall, H. (1985). Identification of three classes of cytosolic glutathione transferase common to several mammalian species; correlation between structural data and enzymatic properties. *Proceedings of the National Academy of Sciences (USA)*, **82**, 7202–6.

Mannervik, B., Awasthi, C., Board, P. G., Hayes, J. D., Di Ilio, C., Ketterer, B., Listowsky, I., Morgernstern, R., Muramatsu, M., Pearson, W. R., Pickett, C. B., Sato, K., Widersten, M. & Wolf, C. R. (1992). Nomenclature for human glutathione transferases. *Biochemical Journal*, **282**, 305–8.

Marcus, C. J., Habig, W. H. & Jakoby, W. B. (1978). Glutathione transferase from human erythrocytes. Nonidentity with the enzymes from liver. *Archives of Biochemistry and Biophysics*, **188**, 287–93.

Max, B. (1990). This and that: genetics, statistics and common sense. *Trends in Pharmacological Sciences*, **11**, 311–14.

Meyer, D. J., Coles, B., Pemble, S. E., Gilmore, K. S., Fraser, G. M. & Ketterer, B. (1991). Theta, a new class of glutathione transferases purified from rat and man. *Biochemical Journal*, **274**, 409–14.

Morrow, C. S. & Cowan, K. H. (1990). Glutathione S-transferases and drug resistance. *Cancer Cells*, **2**, 15–22.

Özer, N., Erdemli, Ö., Sayek, I. & Özer, I. (1990). Resolution and kinetic characterization of glutathione S-transferases from human jejunal mucosa. *Biochemical Medicine and Metabolic Biology*, **44**, 142–50.

Pessah-Rasmussen, H., Stavenow, L., Seidegard, J., Solem, J.-O. & Israelsson, B. (1990). Lack of glutathione transferase activity in intermittent claudication. *International Angiology*, **9**, 70–4.

Peter, H., Deutschmann, S., Reichel, C. & Hallier, E. (1989). Metabolism of methyl chloride by human erythrocytes. *Archives of Toxicology*, **63**, 351–5

Ploeman, J. H. T. M., Van Ommen, B. & Van Bladeren, P. J. (1990). Inhibition of rat and human glutathione S-transferase isoenzymes by ethacrynic acid and its glutathione conjugate. *Biochemical Pharmacology*, **40**, 1631–5.

Prescott, L. F. (1980). Kinetics and metabolism of paracetamol and phenacetin. *British Journal of Clinical Pharmacology*, **10**, 291S–8S.

Raffle, P. A. B., Lee, W. R., McCallum, R. I. & Murray, R.

(1987). *Hunter's Diseases of Occupations*, 6th edn. London: Hodder & Stoughton.

Rhoads, D. M., Zarlengo, R. P. & Tu, C.-P. D. (1987). The basic glutathione S-transferases from human livers are products of separate genes. *Biochemical and Biophysical Research Communications*, **145**, 474–81.

Rhodes, T. & Twentyman, P. R. (1992). A study of ethacrynic acid as a potential modifier of melphalen and cisplatin sensitivity in human lung cancer parental and drug-resistant cell lines. *British Journal of Cancer*, **65**, 684–90.

Riley, R. J., Cribb, A. E. & Spielberg, S. P. (1991). Glutathione transferase μ deficiency is not a marker for predisposition to sulphonamide toxicity. *Biochemical Pharmacology*, **42**, 696–8.

Scott, E. M. & Wright, R. C. (1980). Variability of glutathione S-transferase of human erythrocytes. *American Journal of Human Genetics*, **32**, 115–16.

Scott, R. B., Matin, S. & Hamilton, S. C. (1990). Glutathione, glutathione S-transferase and transmembrane transport of glutathione conjugate in human neutrophil leukocytes. *Journal of Laboratory and Clinical Medicine*, **116**, 674–81.

Seidegård, J., De Pierre, J. W. & Pero, R. W. (1985). Hereditary inter-individual differences in the glutathione transferase activity towards trans-stilbene oxide in resting human mononuclear leukocytes are due to a particular isozyme(s). *Carcinogenesis*, **6**, 1211–16.

Seidegård, J., Morgenstern, R., DePierre, J. W. & Ernster, L. (1979). Trans-stilbene oxide: a new type of inducer of drug-metabolizing enzymes. *Biochimica et Biophysica Acta*, **586**, 10–21.

Seidegård, J. & Pero, R. W. (1985). The hereditary transmission of high glutathione transferase activity towards trans-stilbene oxide in human mononuclear leukocytes. *Human Genetics*, **69**, 66–8.

Seidegård, J. & Pero, R. W. (1988). The genetic variation and the expression of human glutathione μ. *Klinische Wochenschrift*, **66**, (Suppl XI): 125–6.

Seidegård, J., Pero, R. W., Markowitz, M. M., Roush, G., Miller, D. G. & Beattie, E. J. (1990). Isoenzyme(s) of glutathione transferase (class Mu) as a marker for the susceptibility to lung cancer: a follow up study. *Carcinogenesis*, **11**, 33–6.

Seidegård, J., Pero, R. W., Miller, D. G. & Beattie, E. J. (1986). A glutathione transferase in human leucocytes as a marker for the susceptibility to lung cancer. *Carcinogenesis*, **7**, 751–3.

Seidegård, J., Vorachek, W. R., Pero, R. W. & Pearson, W. R. (1988). Hereditary differences in the expression on the human glutathione transferase active in trans-stilbene oxide are due to a gene deletion. *Proceedings of the National Academy of Sciences (USA)*, **85**, 7293–7.

Sparnins, V.L., Venegas, P. L. & Wattenberg, L. W. (1982). Glutathione S-transferase activity: enhancement by compounds inhibiting chemical carcinogenesis and by dietary constituents. *Journal of the National Cancer Institute*, **68**, 493–6.

Spielberg, S. P. (1980). Acetaminophen toxicity in human lymphocytes *in vitro*. *Journal of Pharmacology and Experimental Therapeutics*, **213**, 395–8.

Spielberg, S. P. & Gordon, G. B. (1981). Glutathione synthetase-deficient lymphocytes and acetaminophen toxicity. *Clinical Pharmacology and Therapeutics*, **29**, 51–5.

Strange, R. C., Faulder, C. G., Davis, B. A., Hume, R., Brown, J. A. H., Cotton, W. & Hopkinson, D. A. (1984). The human glutathione S-transferases: studies on the tissue distribution and genetic variation of the GST1, GST2 and GST3 isozymes. *Annals of Human Genetics (London)*, **48**, 11–20.

Tew, K. B., Bomber, A. M. & Hoffman, S. J. (1988). Ethacrynic acid and piripost as enhancers of cytotoxicity in drug resistant and sensitive cell lines. *Cancer Research*, **48**, 3622–5.

Thier, R., Foest, U., Feutschmann, S., Schroeder, K. R., Westphal, G., Hallier, E. & Peter, H. (1991). Distribution of methylene chloride in human blood. Recent developments in toxicology, trends, methods and problems. *Archives of Toxicology*, Suppl. 14, 254–8.

Tsuchida, S., Maki, T. & Sato, K. (1990). Purification and characterization of glutathione transferases with an activity toward nitroglycerin from human aorta and heart. *Journal of Biological Chemistry*, **265**, 7150–7.

Van Bladeren, P. J. (1988). Formation of toxic metabolites from drugs and other xenobiotics by glutathione conjugation. *Trends in Pharmacological Sciences*, **9**, 295–8.

Van Bladeren, P. & Van Ommen, B. (1991). The inhibition of glutathione S-transferases: mechanisms, toxic consequences and therapeutic benefits. *Pharmacology and Therapeutics*, **51**, 35–46.

Vandenberghe, Y., Tee, L., Morel, F., Rogiers, V., Guilloiuzo, A. & Yeoh, G. (1991). Regulation of glutathione S-transferase gene expression by phenobarbital in adult rat hepatocytes. *FEBS Letters*, **284**, 103–8.

Van Ommen, B., Bogaards, J. J. P., Peters, W. H. M., Blaauboer, B. & Van Bladeren, P. J. (1990). Quantification of human hepatic glutathione S-transferase. *Biochemical Journal*, **269**, 609–13.

Van Poppel, G., de Vogel, N., Van Bladeren, P. J. & Kok, F. J. (1992). Increased cytogenetic damage in smokers deficient in glutathione S-transferase isozyme µ. *Carcinogenesis*, **13**, 303–5.

Vos, R. M. E. & Van Bladeren, P. J. (1990). Glutathione S-transferases in relation to their role in the biotransformation of xenobiotics. *Chemico-Biological Interactions*, **75**, 241–65.

Vos, R. M. E., Van Welie, R. T. H., Peters, W. H. M., Evelo, C. J. A., Boogaards, J. J. P., Vermeulen, N. P. E. & Van Bladeren, P.J. (1991). Genetic deficiency of human class mu glutathione-S-transferase isoenzymes in relation to the urinary excretion of the mercapturic acids of Z-and E-1,3-dichloropropene. *Archives of Toxicology*, **65**, 95–9.

Warholm, M., Guthenberg, C., Mannervik, B. & von Bahr, C. (1981). Purification of a new glutathione S-transferase (transferase µ) from human liver having high activity with benzo(α)pyrene-4,5 oxide. *Biochemical and Biophysical Research Communications*, **98**, 512–19.

Warholm, M., Guthenberg, C., Mannervik, B., Von Bahr, C. & Glaumann, H. (1980). Identification of a new glutathione S-transferase in human liver. *Acta Chemica Scandinavica B*, **34**, 607–10.

Wiencke, J. K., Kelsey, K. T., Lamela, R. A. & Toscano, Jr. W. A. (1990). Human glutathione S-transferase deficiency as a marker of susceptibility to epoxide-induced cytogenetic damage. *Cancer Research*, **50**, 1585–90.

Williams, R. T. (1959). *Detoxication Mechanisms*, pp. 237–50. London: Chapman & Hall.

Wong, E. L., Kandpal, G. & Bale, A. E. (1990). Two RFLPs at the glutathione S-transferase 3 gene. *Nucleic Acids Research*, **18**, 4964.

Woolf, B. (1954). On estimating the relation between blood group and disease. *Annals of Human Genetics (London)*, **19**, 251–3.

Yang, W. Z., Begleiter, A., Johnston, J. B., Israels, L. G. & Mowat, M. R. A. (1992). Role of glutathione and glutamine S-transferase in chlorambucil resistance. *Molecular Pharmacology*, **41**, 625–30.

Zhong, S., Howie, A. F., Ketterer, B., Taylor, J., Hayes, J. D., Beckett, G. J., Wathen, G., Wolf, C. R. & Spurr, N. K. (1991). Glutathione S-transferase mu locus: use of genotyping and phenotyping assays to assess association with lung cancer susceptibility. *Carcinogenesis*, **12**, 1533–7.

20 Methylation reactions

INTRODUCTION

THIS group of reactions involves the enzymic methylation of a variety of endogenous and exogenous substrates. Different substrates are methylated by different enzymes, each of which is controlled by alleles at different loci. The pharmacogenetics of the methylation reactions has been advanced principally by Dr Weinshilboum of the Mayo Medical School, Rochester, Minnesota from whose laboratory a large number of publications has been produced over the last 14 years.

The key to making progress in the study of the genetics of these enzymes was the development of sensitive assay methods, and applying them to measure the activities in a most accessible cell, namely, the erythrocyte. For all the enzymes the assay reaction consists of the donation of a radioactive methyl group from the donor [^{14}C]methyl-S-adenosyl-L-methionine to the specific substrate. The radioactive product is separated by organic solvent extraction and measured in a scintillation counter. The donor becomes S-adenosyl-homocysteine.

Of course, the red cells themselves would not contribute greatly to the body's capacity to metabolize drugs. However, in several instances it has been shown that there is an identity of genetic control of enzymes in red cells and metabolically active organs like the liver. Therefore studying what happens in the red cell mirrors what happens in the way of drug metabolism in the body generally. The individual enzyme systems will now be discussed.

THIOPURINE METHYLTRANSFERASE

The enzyme thiopurine methyltransferase (TPMT) catalyses the 5-methylation of a variety of potentially toxic thiopurine drugs including 6-mercaptopurine, 6-thioguanine and azathioprine (Table 20.1).

Assay and genetics

The assay consists of the formation of radioactive 6-methyl-mercaptopurine from 6-mercaptopurine after incubating a red cell homogenate with the radioactive methyl donor (Weinshilboum *et al.* 1978).

The application of this assay to a population survey of 298 unrelated adult subjects yielded a clearly trimodal frequency distribution histogram (Fig. 20.1). One individual was found to have virtually undetectable activity whilst about 33 were in the intermediate mode (the overlap with the high activity mode meant the enumeration was approximate). A further 373 samples from blood donors revealed one more individual with undetectable activity. These results suggested strongly that TPMT activity could be under the control of two co-dominant autosomal alleles (Weinshilboum & Sladek 1980) and the proportions of the proposed genotypes were in accordance with the Hardy–Weinberg equilibrium.

Therefore 215 first-degree relatives in 50

Table 20.1. *Pharmacogenetic aspects of methyltransferases*

Name and abbreviation	Atom to which methyl group is attached	Location of the enzyme within the cell	Tissue in which genetic studies performed	Drug substrates	Inhibitors	Perceived nature of inheritance	Allele frequencies	Other tissues with the same genetic control of the enzyme activity
Thiopurine methyl-transferase (TPMT) EC 2.1.1.67	S	Cytoplasmic	Erythrocyte	6-mercaptopurine azathioprine sulphydryl metabolites of cephalosporins 6-thioguanine	benzoic acid derivatives e.g. salicylic acid	Balanced polymorphism, phenotypes clearly separate in frequency distribution	high activity 0.94 low activity 0.06	lymphocyte kidney liver platelets
Thiol methyl-transferases (TMT) EC 2.1.1.9	S	Membrane	Erythrocyte	captopril D-penicillamine N-acetylcysteine 7-α-thiospironolactone	SKF 525A	Segregation analysis shows polygenic heritability 0.75 plus a Mendelian major gene	0.42 and 0.58	–
Catechol-O-methyl-transferase (COMT) EC 2.1.1.6	O	Cytoplasmic	Erythrocyte	L-dopa alpha-methyldopa	tropolone benzoic acid derivatives calcium	Phenotypes clearly separate in plots of activity versus thermal lability. Also segregation analysis of family data of activity revealed polymorphism	0.5	lymphocyte lung kidney liver
Histamine-N-methyltransferase (HNMT) EC 2.1.1.8	N	Cytoplasmic	Erythrocyte	histamine	–	polygenic $h^2 = 0.7$ to 0.9	–	–

h^2, heritability (the proportion of the population variance ascribable to the effects of inheritance).
Data derived from: Weinshilboum, 1988, 1989; Price *et al.* 1989.

Table 20.2. *Analysis of family data on red cell TPMT activity*

Mating type	Number expected[a]	Number observed	Number of offspring	$TPMT^L\ TPMT^L$ Exp.	Obs.	$TPMT^L\ TPMT^H$ Exp.	Obs.	$TPMT^H\ TPMT^H$ Exp.	Obs.
$TPMT^H\ TPMT^H \times TPMT^H\ TPMT^H$	39.240	40	93	–	–	–	–	93	93
$TPMT^H\ TPMT^H \times TPMT^H\ TPMT^L$	9.805	8	17	–	–	8.5	8	8.5	9
$TPMT^H\ TPMT^L \times TPMT^H\ TPMT^L$	0.610	1	3	0.75	–	1.5	–	0.75	3
$TPMT^H\ TPMT^H \times TPMT^L\ TPMT^L$	0.305	1	2	–	–	2	2	–	–

(Genotypes of offspring)

[a]Computed on the basis of the allele frequencies hypothesized from the population survey, i.e. $TPMT^H = \sqrt{\frac{264}{298}} = 0.9412$, $TPMT^L = 0.0588$.
Data from: Weinshilboum & Sladek 1980.

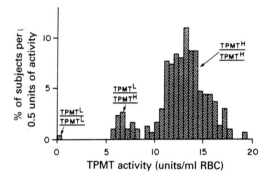

Fig. 20.1. Frequency distribution of erythrocyte TPMT activity in blood samples from 298 unrelated adult subjects. The distributions of genotypes at locus *TPMT* are indicated. (Modified from Fig. 2 of Weinshilboum & Sladek 1980.)

randomly selected families had their erythrocytic TPMT activity assayed. A similar trimodal frequency distribution to that yielded by the population study was obtained and a third individual with undetectable activity identified. The frequencies of the mating types were not significantly different from those predicted by the genotypic frequencies obtained from the population survey (Table 20.2). The numbers of offspring produced by the different mating types were also not significantly different from those expected (Weinshilboum & Sladek 1980).

A survey of erythrocytic TPMT activity in 303 unrelated healthy white French blood donors who were not taking any drugs was conducted by Tinel *et al.* (1991). They did not find any example of the nil activity phenotype. Their frequency distribution histogram did not reveal a clear bimodality, but on the basis of a change in slope on a probit plot they defined two phenotypes. The less common phenotype was 11% of the population, a frequency which agreed with that for heterozygotes in the study of Weinshilboum & Sladek (1980).

Inter-ethnic variability

A sample of 36 Saami Lapps investigated by Klemetsdal *et al.* (1992) showed that the *TPMT* gene frequencies were similar to that of Caucasians but the heterozygotes had about 65% more activity and the homozygotes about 84% more activity. This might have therapeutic implications (see below).

TPMT in other cells and tissues

A series of studies was then conducted to find out whether the genetic polymorphism of TPMT activity in the erythrocyte mirrored the same phenomenon in other cells and tissues. This proved to be the case as demonstrated in lymphocytes (Van Loon & Weinshilboum 1982) liver and (Fig. 20.2) kidney (Woodson *et al.* 1982; Van Loon & Weinshilboum 1990).

Immunoprecipitation studies with rabbit polyclonal antibodies raised against partially purified kidney TPMT have produced an interesting result. The zero activity $TPMT^L\ TPMT^L$ individuals had lower levels of TPMT protein in red cells and renal tissue than the other genotypes.

The molecular basis of the TPMT polymorphism remains unknown.

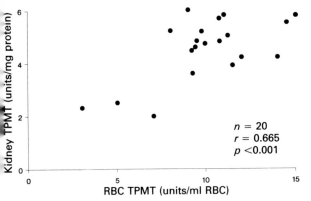

Fig. 20.2. Correlation of erythrocytic with kidney TPMT activity in samples from 20 patients who underwent clinically indicated nephrectomies. (From Woodson *et al.* 1982.)

Examination of the kidney tissue revealed an unexpected finding. Two isozymes of TPMT, which did not differ in other regards, could be separated by ion-exchange chromatography. However, these two isozymes did not appear to be related to the molecular basis for the genetic polymorphism which regulates both TPMT enzymic activity and the level of TPMT protein in human tissues (Van Loon & Weinshilboum 1990).

Samples from second trimester fetal livers were shown by Pacifici *et al.* (1991a) to have about one third of the activity of adult human livers.

In vitro substrates and inhibitors

The structure–activity relationships of substrates and inhibitors were studied by Ames *et al.* (1986). A series of 14 thiophenols with various substituent groups was tested. Many had low K_m values (0.8 to 7.8 μM), as compared with 550 and 2000 μM for 6-mercaptopurine and 2-thiouracil (methyl- and propylthiouracil do not appear to have been tested). Glutathione was found not to be a substrate for TPMT (Loo & Smith 1985).

A range of 27 benzoic acid derivatives was tested by Ames *et al.* (1986) for their ability to inhibit TPMT, and were found to be predictable in this regard by virtue of their hydrophilicity. The results were consistent with the idea that the binding site for inhibitors on the enzyme includes a hydrophobic cleft.

It is thought likely that thiophenol substrates and benzoic acid inhibitors may interact with different sites on the TPMT molecule.

Clinical applications

1 The drugs relevant to a discussion of the clinical importance of TPMT are azathioprine (AZA) and 6-mercaptopurine (6-MP). The first is widely used as an immunosuppressant in conditions as diverse as systemic lupus erythematosus and organ transplantation. The second is largely reserved for the treatment of leukaemia. The metabolism of AZA is explained in Fig. 20.3 and it will be seen that it gives rise to 6-MP. This compound itself is inert and must be anabolized into its active forms which are thought to be chiefly 6-thioinosine, 6-thioxanthosine, 6-thioguanosine, 6-methyl thioinosine and their corresponding mono-, di- and triphosphates.

2 The way in which 6-MP derivatives work is not entirely clear and probably multifocal (Van Scoik *et al.* 1985). One or more metabolites of 6-MP have been shown to (1) inhibit *de novo* purine ribonucleotide synthesis, (2) inhibit purine ribonucleotide interconversion, (3) be incorporated into cellular RNA and (4) be incorporated into cellular DNA. The last mechanism is thought to be particularly important. The difference between 6-MP and AZA is that the methyl-nitro-imidazolyl moiety of the latter with a sulphydryl group attached may be partly responsible for the immunosuppressive activity of the compound. The dynamics of the interplay of 6-MP and AZA metabolites with naturally occurring purines is very complex and the clinical relevance of many of the processes is poorly understood (Van Scoik *et al.* 1985).

6-Thioguanine nucleotides (6TGN) are major metabolites of AZA and 6-MP in humans (the difference between 6TGN and 6-thioguanosine referred to earlier is that in the latter the purine is joined at the 9 position to ribose). A method has been developed to measure the 6TGN concentration within erythrocytes (Lennard & Maddocks 1983), and it has been found that these concentrations are correlated directly with the risk for the development of leucopenia in patients treated with thiopurine drugs.

For example, Lennard *et al.* (1984) described a 57 year old man who developed severe megaloblastic

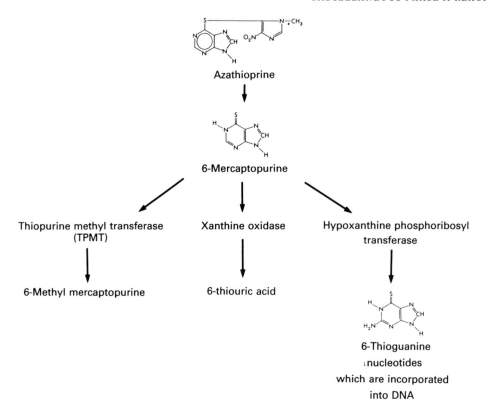

Fig. 20.3. Simplified scheme showing the metabolism and action of azathioprine and 6-mercaptopurine.

anaemia on azathioprine treatment. He was found to have very high red cell 6TGN levels. On stopping the azathioprine his blood became normal. Rechallenge with a single oral dose of azathioprine was followed by a climb of red cell 6TGN over a week to a level three times higher than in four patients taking 50 mg twice daily.

3 Examination of Fig. 20.3 will readily indicate that a deficiency of TPMT activity is likely to result in the production of more 6TGN (the pathway to thiouric acid shows little inter-individual variability). Because of this, studies were made by Lennard *et al.* (1987) to find out whether there was a relationship between the genetically controlled levels of erythrocyte TPMT activity and 6TGN concentrations. There was a negative correlation between these two vari-

ables in 40 children being treated with 6-MP for acute lymphatic leukaemia. This finding raised two points. (1) Were individuals with low TPMT activities (and hence high 6TGN concentrations) more liable to myelosuppression? (2) Were persons with high TPMT activities receiving inadequate therapy with thiopurine drugs?

To answer the first question, blood was obtained from six adult dermatology patients who had severe myelosuppression while being treated with AZA. 6TGN concentrations were measured in blood samples taken from them at diagnosis and in blood from 16 additional patients receiving chronic therapy with AZA for a wide variety of conditions without adverse effects (Fig. 20.4). The TMPT activities in the six probands 3 to 13 months after their myelosuppression ranged between 0.1 and 1.41 units TPMT per ml RBC, indicating the *TPMT*[L] *TPMT*[L] genotype. The 6TGN levels at the time of their illness had been very high compared with the 16 controls. One of these six patients was subsequently given a

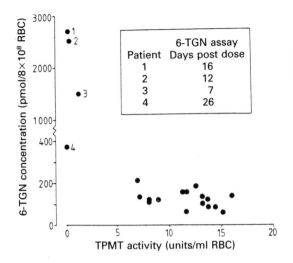

Fig. 20.4. Erythrocytic TPMT activity and 6-thioguanine nucleotide (6-TGN) concentrations in patients 1 to 4 compared with those in a group of 16 control patients who had no history of bone marrow failure. 6-TGN concentrations were measured 16, 12, 7 and 26 days after azathioprine withdrawal in patients 1, 2, 3 and 4, respectively. (From Lennard *et al.* 1987.)

single oral dose of AZA and this quickly gave a high erythrocytic 6TGN level, whereas in controls 6TGN became detectable only after 5 days of treatment (Lennard *et al.* 1989).

To find the answer to the second question has required a good deal of painstaking investigation. It was proposed by Lennard & Lilleyman (1987) that the failure to induce mild toxicity could lead to underdosing in some patients and enable residual leukaemic cells to survive and ultimately lead to relapse. A survey of 95 children with acute lymphoblastic leukaemia (ALL) was reported by Lennard *et al.* (1990). Erythrocytic TPMT activity once more showed a negative correlation with 6TGN concentrations. The PTMT activities were raised whilst the children were receiving treatment, presumably due to induction. Children with 6TGN concentrations below the median had significantly higher TPMT activities and a higher subsequent relapse rate with ALL during a period of over 50 months (as compared with those with 6TGN concentrations above the median). The upshot of all this has been the realization that (1) a more aggressive therapy of ALL with 6-MP producing a degree of marrow toxicity as

indicated by neutropenia leads to improved survival (Hale & Lilleyman 1991), and (2) there may be possible advantages of TPMT genotyping before therapy and 6TGN determinations during therapy for ALL. An HPLC method which rapidly measures plasma 6MP erthrocytic 6TGN and urinary 6-thiouric acid has been published (Bruunschuus & Schmiegelow 1989) which makes such a surveillance feasible. An alternative suggested by Lafolie *et al.* (1991) would be to monitor the levels of 6-MP in plasma and red cells at five times during the 4 hours after taking a dose to assess the area under the concentration/time curve, but this does seem rather cumbersome for routine use.

The paper of Evans *et al.* (1991) describes a patient who developed pancytopenia with red cell 6TGN levels of seven times the population median. She was found to have very low levels of red cell TPMT activity. Subsequently treatment with 6% of the usual dose of 6-MP led to a satisfactory response. This patient illustrates an important point which recurs in other sections of this book, namely, that the dose of a drug may have to be tailored to suit the individual metabolic capability of the patient.

4 In an attempt to develop an *in vitro* system which would show the *in vivo* effects of 6-MP, Van Loon & Weinshilboum (1987) cultured lymphocytes from persons of known *TPMT* genotypes with 6-MP, radioactive thymidine and the T-cell mitogen stimulants PHA (phytohaemagglutinin) and Con A (concanavalin A). Strangely, the results showed that *TPMT*^{L} *TPMT*^{L} lymphocytes were more resistant to 6-MP inhibition of thymidine incorporation than lymphocytes of the other two phenotypes. This result was contrary to the expectation based on the previously mentioned clinical findings. There is at present no satisfactory explanation.

5 It has been mentioned earlier that numerous benzoic acid derivatives were found to be inhibitors of TPMT activity. These benzoic acid derivatives include salicylic acid which is produced *in vivo* by the hydrolysis of acetylsalicylic acid. Plasma concentrations of salicylate of 1 to 2 mM are commonly produced by therapeutic doses, and these concentrations are inhibitory to TPMT. There is therefore a possibility that when aspirin is given with 6-MP or AZA, there may be a potentiation of the therapeutic

effects of these compounds (Woodson *et al.* 1983).

6 Paracetamol is in part excreted as an S-methyl derivative, and there is a possibility that TPMT may mediate this biotransformation (Woodson *et al.* 1983).

7 It has been observed that hypoprothrombinaemia occurs in occasional patients treated with cephalosporin antibiotics such as cephamandole (Hooper *et al.* 1980), cephazolin and moxolactam (Weitekamp & Aber 1983). The last has now been withdrawn (see British National Formulary 1990). This effect is not due to the action of the antibiotic in depressing the bacterial population of the bowel, because the effect does not occur with other antibiotics excreted through the bile, and menaquinone (bacterial vitamin K) is not absorbed in humans (Lipsky 1983).

These antibiotics contain heterocyclic side chains. In the case of moxolactam and cephamandole this is 1-methyltetrazole-5-thiol (MTT) and in the case of cephazolin it is 2-methyl-1,3,4-thiadiazole-5-thiol (MTD). It is known that MTT is split off in the human body and the same is probably true of MTD.

Carboxylation of glutamic acid residues as a mechanism of activating prothrombin is described in another chapter of this book. MTT was demonstrated by Lipsky (1983) to inhibit the γ-carboxylation of glutamic acid in a polypeptide by a rat microsomal liver preparation. Descarboxyprothrombin has been found in the blood of patients receiving MTT-containing antibiotics.

MTT and MTD were methylated by TPMT from human kidneys and by human liver microsomal thiol methyltransferase (see below) with K_m values similar to those of 6-mercaptopurine (TPMT) and captopril and D-penicillamine TMT (Kerremans *et al.* 1985).

The S-methylated MTD was shown to be an ineffective inhibitor of the carboxylation of glutamic acid residues in a polypeptide. The same is probably also true of S-methylated MTT.

So it appears quite possible (but it is not proven) that these methylation reactions are controlled by polymorphic methyltransferases, and that patients who develop hypoprothrombinaemia on the relevant cephalosporin antibiotics may be those genetically endowed with less active S-methylation enzymes.

THIOL METHYLTRANSFERASE

Introduction

The reaction catalysed by thiol methyltransferase (TMT) differs from TPMT in two ways; first the enzyme is 95% membrane-bound (Keith *et al.* 1984) and, secondly, the substrates are aliphatic sulphydryl compounds (Table 20.1). The suggestion was in fact made that TPMT should be named 'aryl thiol methyltransferase' and TMT 'alkyl thiol methyltransferase' (Keith *et al.* 1984) but this was not widely adopted.

The assay of the enzyme activity was conducted on erythrocyte membranes. A convenient substrate has been 2-mercaptoethanol. The compound S-adenosyl-L-[methyl-^{14}C] methionine was used as a methyl donor and the reaction was quantified by measuring radioactive S-methylmercaptoethanol following extraction with organic solvents. The loss of the methyl group converts the donor to S-adenosyl-L-homocysteine (Keith *et al.* 1984). As is very commonly the case with membrane-bound enzymes, TMT is inhibited by SF 525A.

Thiol methyltransferase activity was discovered in human renal cortex microsomes by Kerremans *et al.* (1984) and in foetal liver and placenta by Pacifici *et al.* (1991b). Captopril was shown to be metabolized by kidney and intestine TMT by Pacifici *et al.* (1991c). The levels of activity were lower in other tissues than in liver, and it is not clear if the activities in these internal organs correlated with the erythrocytic TMT activities.

Genetics

Red cell membrane TMT activity was investigated in 231 first-degree relatives in 47 randomly selected families by Keith *et al.* (1983a). The frequency distribution histograms for both sexes, and for parents and offspring, were unimodal and not significantly different from one another. Age did not influence the TMT activity. The correlation between spouses was not significant, indicating a lack of shared environmental influence. The midparent–mean offspring correlation was 0.69, indicating a high heritability.

The data of Keith *et al.* (1983), plus an extra two families, were analysed by Price *et al.* (1989) using commingling and segregation analyses. Transformed data removed the skewness in the data which had a unimodal distribution. Segregation analysis indicated the existence of a major gene polymorphism with allele frequencies as follows: low activity 0.58 and high activity 0.42, acting against a strong background influence from a polygenic phenotype. The authors mention that these findings will serve as a stimulus for future studies of the polymorphism with molecular techniques.

Drugs metabolized

A variety of drugs (Fig. 20.5) bearing a sulphydryl group were investigated by Keith *et al.* (1984) using the assay technique as described above. The activity of red cell membrane TMT against three drugs correlated excellently ($r > 0.96$) with 2-mercaptoethanol methylation. These three drugs were captopril, *N*-acetylcysteine and 7-α-thiospirolactone (the deacetyl metabolite of spironolactone). Another drug which might be a substrate for this enzymic system is D-penicillamine (Fig. 20.5) (Weinshil-

boum 1989). It is to be noted that there are as yet no data on the correlation of the whole-body metabolism of the drugs *in vivo* with the behaviour of erythrocytic membrane preparations *in vitro*.

Relation to spontaneous disease

The idea that Parkinson's disease could be due to the toxic effects of environmental chemicals provided the stimulus for Waring *et al.* (1989) to study the TMT activities in this condition. Three drug-free groups were studied for comparison, namely, normal controls, motor neurone disease and myasthenia gravis. The normal controls (NC) and myasthenia gravis (MG) populations gave very similar results. The erythrocyte TMT activities in Parkinson's disease were significantly lower and those in motor neurone disease were significantly higher than those in the NC plus MG groups (Fig. 20.6). This finding raises the possibility that there may be a predisposition to develop Parkinson's disease in persons who have a genetic endowment of low TMT activity. There is no clear view on how a raised TMT could operate in the aetiology of motor neurone disease.

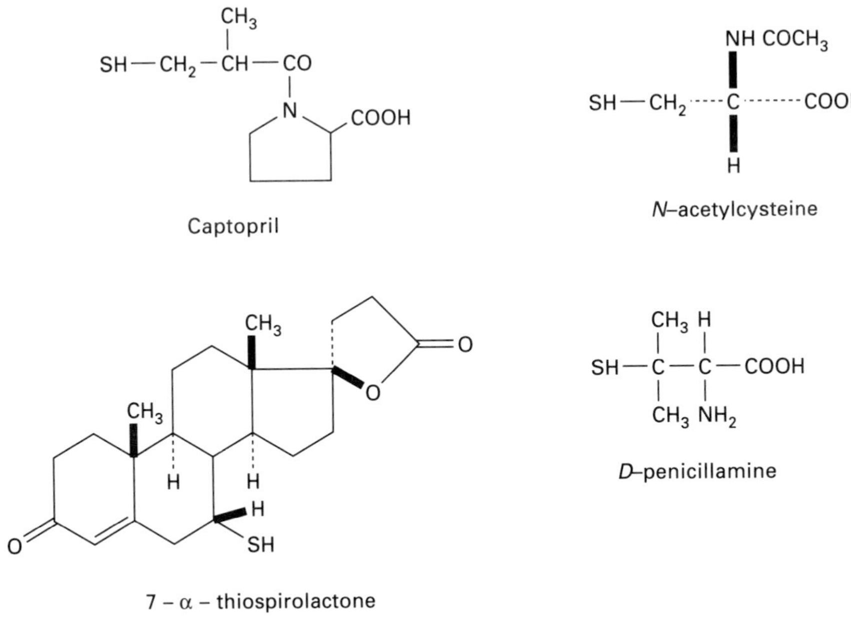

Fig. 20.5. Drugs methylated by thiol methyltransferase.

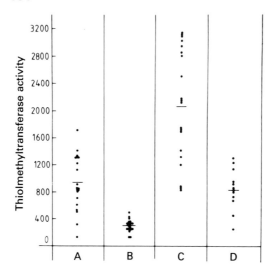

Fig. 20.6. Thiol methyltransferase activity in normal volunteers (A); patients with Parkinson's disease (B); motor neurone disease (C) and myasthenia gravis (D). (From Waring *et al.* 1989.)

A population of 120 rheumatoid arthritis (RA) patients were studied for their red cell membrane TMT activities by Bradley *et al.* (1991) and compared with 35 healthy volunteers. The TMT activity was not related to the acute phase response or to drug administration. There was a marked difference in TMT activity distributions between the two populations, in that only 36 RA patients had values in the normal range whilst the remainder had very low TMT activities.

In contrast, 39 systemic lupus erythematosus patients were examined the same way and compared with 47 healthy volunteer controls (Gordon *et al.* 1992). The distributions of TMT values in the two groups were almost exactly the same.

These results raise the possibility that a defect of methylation of thiol groups may be involved in the pathogenesis of RA. It may also provide the explanation why the thiol-containing drug penicillamine appears to give more adverse reactions in RA than in Wilson's disease.

CATECHOL-*O*-METHYLTRANSFERASE

The enzyme catechol-*O*-methyltransferase (COMT) is widely distributed in the body and is probably most well known for its activity in methylating adrenaline and noradrenaline following their release from nerve fibres. This is one component of the processes which limit adrenergic action. The enzyme can, however, catalyse the methylation of other catechol compounds. The assay of COMT activity in the erythrocyte is based upon the methylation of 3,4-dihydroxybenzoic acid.

Genetics

The population frequency distribution of erythrocyte COMT activities is strongly suggestive of a bimodal distribution (Weinshilboum & Raymond 1977; Fig. 20.7). Twin studies carried out by Grunhaus *et al.* (1976) and Winter *et al.* (1978) indicated a high heritability for red cell COMT activity. Complex segregation analyses of family data of COMT activity were performed by Flodereus *et al.* (1982), Siervogel *et al.* (1984) and Brahe *et al.* (1985). All these groups agreed that a Mendelian transmission of a major gene effect, with two alleles in Hardy–Weinberg equilibrium, could not be excluded. The first groups considered the allele giving low activity had a frequency of 0.46 with dominance 0.27, whilst the last group gave a value of 0.6 with dominance 0.5. Both groups found that a small polygenic effect was also present.

Heat inactivation of enzymes depends on their structure, and may differentiate between the products of allelic genes. With this in mind heat inactivation studies were carried out on erythrocyte lysates from individuals who were $COMT^L$ and $COMT^H$ homozygotes. The thermal stability (expressed as H/C, i.e. the ratio of activities after heating at 48 °C for 15 minutes divided by the control or preheating value) was lower in the $COMT^L$ homozygotes than in the $COMT^H$ homozygotes (Fig. 20.8). Following this pilot experiment a population of 316 unrelated white subjects was investigated and the results are shown in Fig. 20.8. The 25% of people who are $COMT^L$ $COMT^L$ have H/C ratios lower than others and form a separate cloud of dots (Scanlon *et al.* 1979). This would seem to be an attractive phenotyping procedure, and has been applied to a population study. However, it seems that it was not carried out on the samples from a large family survey, a fact that led to an unnecessarily complicated genetic analysis (Spielman & Weinshilboum 1981).

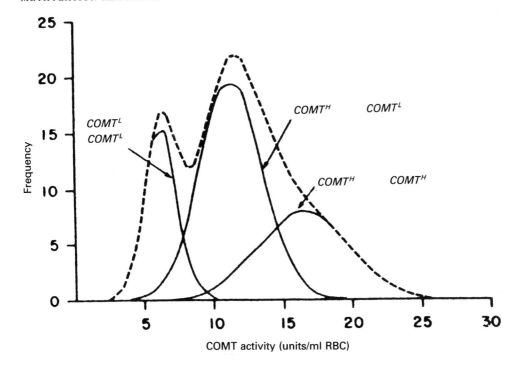

Fig. 20.7. Schematic representation of the frequency distribution of erythrocytic catechol-O-methyltransferase (COMT) and of *COMT* genotypes in a randomly selected population sample. The dashed line represents the distribution of levels of erythrocytic COMT activity in blood samples from 893 randomly selected subjects. The solid lines represent calculated distributions of genotypes at the locus *COMT*. Approximately 25% of the population sample is homozygous for the alleles *COMT^L* and *COMT^N* and approximately half is heterozygous. (From Spielman & Weinshilboum 1981.)

Detailed investigations with electrophoretic blotting and immune fixation following electrophoresis or isoelectric focusing by Grossman *et al.* (1992a) did not reveal a major structural alteration between the low and high activity forms of COMT in human erythrocytes. This led to the speculation that quite small changes may be responsible for the difference and these may be elucidated by molecular genetic techniques.

Linkage and gene localization

A study of 1189 individuals in five families by Wilson *et al.* (1984) included erythrocyte COMT activity and 25 marker loci. It ruled out linkage between COMT and 21 of the markers, and so ruled out the location of the *COMT* locus to 10 to 15% of the human gene map.

Brahe *et al.* (1986), using somatic cell hybrids, correlated the presence of COMT with the presence of chromosome 22. Later Grossman *et al.* (1992b), using rat COMT cDNA as a probe showed that it hybridized to 22q11.1 → q11.2, whilst Winqvist *et al.* (1992) using a human COMT cDNA probe showed that it hybridized to 22q11.2.

Identity of genetic control in erythrocytes and internal organs

Genetically determined levels of COMT activity in erythrocytes were shown to be correlated with the levels of the enzyme activity in human kidney, lung and lymphocyte. Therefore it was interesting to ascertain whether the major metabolic organ of the body, namely the liver, followed the same pattern. This problem was investigated by Boudikova *et al.* (1990), who found that liver COMT activity was higher in males than in females. The liver COMT H/C ratio was bimodally distributed, and when

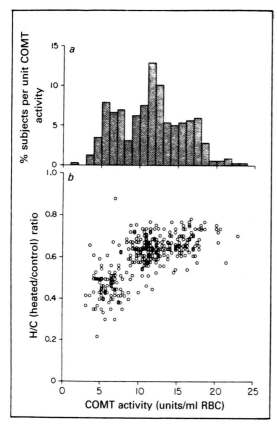

Fig. 20.8. Erythrocytic COMT activity and thermal stability in humans. (a) The frequency distribution histogram of erythrocytic COMT activity in blood samples from 316 randomly selected adult subjects. (b) The thermal stability of erythrocytic COMT as measured by heated/control ratio plotted against basal activity in the same subjects. (From Fig. 2 of Scanlon et al. 1979.)

plotted against red cell COMT activity gave two clouds of dots which were rather more distinct in females. There were positive highly significant correlations between erythrocyte and liver COMT activity and H/C ratios.

This study revealed that the same genes control COMT in both erythrocytes and liver, but rather unexpectedly, the level of liver COMT activity was one third higher in males than in females.

Clinical applications

1 The problem of the inter-individual variability in both the metabolism of, and the response to

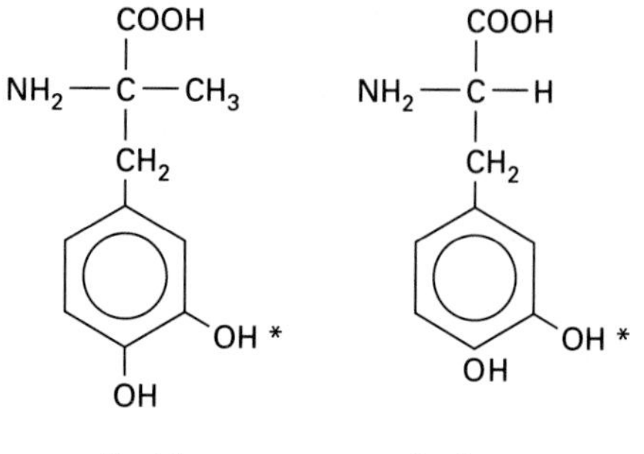

Fig. 20.9. Drugs methylated by catechol-O-methyl transferase. The site of methylation is indicated by an asterisk.

alphamethyl dopa (Fig. 20.9) was investigated by Campbell et al. (1984). This compound is subject to three independent biotransformations, i.e. sulphate conjugation, decarboxylation and O-methylation.

The formation of 3-O-methyl-α-methyldopa (3-OMAMD) was quantitatively less important in the metabolism of the drug than was the formation of the sulphate or alphamethyldopamine by decarboxylation. When the excreted drug and all its metabolites were considered, sulphate metabolites accounted for over half and 3-OMAMD for 6%. However, there was a correlation between the erythrocytic COMT activity and the proportion of methyldopa excreted as 3-OMAMD ($r = 0.485$, $p < 0.01$).

There does not seem to have been a systematic study correlating phenotype and alphamethyldopa metabolism with effect on blood pressure.

2. The anti-Parkinson's disease drug L-dopa (Fig. 20.9) is metabolized by O-methylation to 3-O-methyl-L-dopa (3OMLD) under the influence of COMT.

Three Parkinsonian patients who were non-responders to L-dopa (LD) were found by Rivera-Calimlim et al. (1977) not to improve when the L-dopa decarboxylase inhibitor carbidopa was added. Investigation revealed that these patients had high plasma 3OMLD levels on L-dopa alone, and these were increased still further after carbidopa was added. The plasma 3OMLD/LD ratios were >1, whereas in responding patients this ratio was <1. The metabolite 3OMLD has a long half-life and accumulates in the central nervous system.

The plasma 3OMLD/LD ratio was found by Reilly *et al.* (1980) to correlate with erythrocyte COMT activity, and the patients with higher COMT activities were those with less favourable clinical responses to L-dopa (Fig. 20.10).

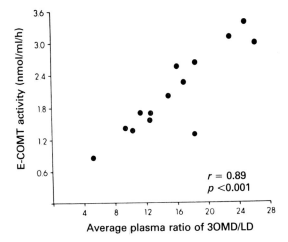

Fig. 20.10. Correlation between erythrocyte catechol-O-methyltransferase (E-COMT) activity and the average plasma concentraton ratio of 3-O-methyldopa to L-dopa (3OMD/LD). (From Reilly *et al.* 1980.)

A third study associating COMT activity with the response of Parkinson's disease to L-dopa was that of Reilly & Rivera-Calimlim (1979). They found that Filipino Parkinsonian patients did not tolerate the usual doses of L-dopa given to Americans. When 32 healthy Filipino and 29 healthy American subjects had their erythrocyte COMT activities determined, the values were higher in the former group, possibly suggesting the existence in Filipinos of a smaller proportion of 'poor methylators'.

This suggestion was followed by Rivera-Calimlim *et al.* (1984), who found that in a mixed group of 70 Oriental subjects the frequency distribution curve of erythrocyte COMT activities had a higher mean than the curve for 86 Caucasians. Also, the L-dopa responses of 52 Filipinos with Parkinsonism were compared with those of 66 Caucasians with Parkinsonism. There was a significantly greater incidence of dyskinesia from L-dopa in the former group, and this was not due to the body weights of Filipinos being lower. The authors also report in an addendum that a survey of erythrocyte COMT activities in

406 Thais showed a frequency distribution with 40% of the subjects having a value >5 units per ml (compared with about 25% in Caucasians).

The study of Feuerstein *et al.* (1977) was also in keeping with this general pattern. In 30 Parkinsonian French patients treated with L-dopa plus a peripheral decarboxylase inhibitor higher plasma *O*-methyldopa levels were found in those with dyskinesias than in patients who had no abnormal involuntary movements. The plasma dopa levels were not significantly different in the two groups.

So on this basis it is proposed that:

1 The $COMT^H COMT^H$ genotype may be more liable than the $COMT^L COMT^L$ genotype to develop dyskinesias on L-dopa because of their greater 3OMLD production;

2 There may be a lower $COMT^L$ allele frequency in Orientals as compared with Caucasians.

These matters do not appear to have been pursued any further. Thermal stability studies or erythrocyte COMT activity in different ethnic groups do not seem to have been reported.

3 In the course of extensive studies of various enzymes in alcoholics Agarwal *et al.* (1983) established that the erythrocytic COMT activity was not significantly different from the value in controls.

4 As a result of studying four large multigeneration old order Amish pedigrees which contained 11 individuals with bipolar and six individuals with unipolar affective disorders, Egeland *et al.* (1984) established that the erythrocyte COMT activities in them were not significantly different from the values in healthy members of these families.

HISTAMINE *N*-METHYLTRANSFERASE

The cytoplasmic enzyme histamine *N*-methyltransferase (EC 2.1.1.8) is present in the human erythrocyte as well as in other tissues. This enzyme catalyses the *N*τ-methylation of histamine and structurally related compounds (lower case Greek letters, tau in this instance, are used to designate atoms in organic molecules in relation to their nuclear magnetic resonance).

A survey of 241 individuals from 51 randomly selected families was carried out by Scott *et al.*

(1988a), and the histamine *N*-methyltransferase (HNMT) activity was determined in their erythrocytes. It was found that the activities were unimodally distributed and rose with age. Fathers, mothers, sons and daughters had age-corrected distributions that did not differ significantly. There was no significant correlation between spouses in 45 pairs, indicating a lack of effect of shared environment. There were highly significant correlations between parents and offspring (though, strangely, the midparent–mean offspring correlation was not given). These findings indicate a significant polygenic heritable control of the erythrocytic enzyme activity.

When 55 paired samples of both renal tissue and erythrocytes were obtained from the same persons, the HNMT activities did not correlate (Scott *et al.* 1988b). It remains to be determined whether the genetic regulation of erythrocytic HNMT activity gives information about the relative level of the enzyme in other tissues, and whether it can be correlated to individual differences in the *in vivo* *N*-methylation of histamine and structurally related compounds (Weinshilboum 1989). Future studies may be aided by the availability of a high performance liquid chromatographic method for histamine-*N*-methyltransferase activity (Fukuda *et al.* 1991).

Chloroquine was shown by Pacifici *et al.* (1992) to inhibit non-competitively histamine *N*-methyltransferase from various human tissues. This observation raises the possibility that some side effects of chloroquine may be due to inhibition of histamine *N*-methyltransferase. The facts that side effects occur only in some people, and that pruritis is a particular problem in Africans (see Chapter 36) raises the possibility of the existence of variant forms of the enzyme.

PHENOL METHYLTRANSFERASE

Phenol-*O*-methyltransferase (POMT, EC 2.1.1.25) is a membrane-bound enzyme that catalyses the *O*-methylation of phenolic but not of catechol compounds. Like most membrane-bound enzymes, it is inhibited by SKF 525A.

Keith *et al.* (1983b) investigated the activities of two forms of thiol methyltransferase namely those with high and low affinity for 2-mercaptoethanol, plus β-glucuronidase plus POMT in erythrocyte membranes from 22 individuals. The results showed

that β-glucuronidase activities did not correlate with the activities of any of the other three enzymes. However, highly significant correlations ($r > 0.95$) were present among all three methyltransferase activities which were unimodally distributed. These results were taken to mean that the three erythrocytic methyltransferase activities were either catalysed by the same enzyme or regulated in parallel. The three enzymes POMT and both TMT activities had similar subcellular distributions and similar responses to various ions and to enzyme inhibitors. The pharmacogenetics of POMT has not been further pursued (Weinshilboum 1989).

CONCLUSIONS

It has been fortunate that various methylation enzymes in erythrocytes have shown both genetic control and also correlation with the methylation activities in metabolically important organs like the liver and kidney. The erythrocytes themselves contribute very little to the metabolism of a therapeutic dose of a drug compound. However, they mirror the way the drug is metabolized in the body. So it has been possible to show that genetically determined variations in erythrocytic enzyme activity control the way a drug is metabolized. This has turned out to be clinically important in the cases of azathioprine and 6-mercaptopurine treatment as influenced by TPMT, and the treatment of Parkinson's disease with L-dopa. Other clinically significant aspects of genetically controlled methylation reactions may remain to be discovered.

The author would like to express his gratitude to Dr Peter R. H. Barbor, Department of Paediatrics, University of Nottingham, UK who made many helpful suggestions about the contents of this chapter.

Agarwal, D. P., Philippu, G., Milech, U., Ziemsen, B., Schrappe, O. & Goedde, H. W. (1983). Platelet monoamine oxidase and erythrocyte catechol-*O*-methyl transferase activity in alcoholism and controlled abstinence. *Drug and Alcohol Dependence*, **12**, 85–91.

Ames, M. M., Selassie, C. D., Woodson, L. C., Van Loon, J. A., Hansch, C. & Weinshilboum, R. M. (1986). Thiopurine methyl transferase: structure–activity relationships for benzoic acid inhibitors and thiophenol substrates. *Journal of Medicinal Chemistry*, **29**, 354–8.

Boudikova, B., Szumlanski, C., Maidak, B. & Weinshilboum, R. (1990). Human liver catechol-*O*-methyltransferase pharmacogenetics. *Clinical Pharmacology and Therapeutics*, **48**, 381–9.

Bradley, H., Waring, R. H. & Emery, P. (1991). Reduced thiol methyl transferase activity in red blood cell membranes from patients with rheumatoid arthritis. *Journal of Rheumatology*, **18**, 1787–9.

Brahe, C., Bannetta, P., Meera Khan, P., Arwert, F. & Serra, A. (1986). Assignment of the catechol *O*-methyltransferase gene to human chromosome 22 in somatic cell hybrids. *Human Genetics*, **74**, 230–4.

Brahe, C., Serra, A. & Morton, N. E. (1985). Erythrocyte catechol-*O*-methyltransferase activity: genetic analysis in nuclear families with one child affected by Down syndrome. *American Journal of Human Genetics*, **21**, 373–84.

British National Formulary (1990) **20**, xiii. London: British Medical Association and the Royal Pharmaceutical Society of Great Britain.

Bruunshuus, I. & Schmiegelow, K. (1989). Analysis of 6-mercaptopurine, 6-thioguanine nucleotides, and 6-thiouric acid in biological fluids by high-performance liquid chromatography. *Scandinavian Journal of Clinical and Laboratory Investigation*, **49**, 779–84.

Campbell, N. R. C., Dunnette, J. H., Mwaluko, G., Van Loon, J. & Weinshilboum, R. M. (1984). Platelet phenol sulphotransferase and erythrocyte catechol-*O*-methyl transferase activities: correlation with methyldopa metabolism. *Clinical Pharmacology and Therapeutics*, **35**, 55–63.

Egeland, J. A., Kidd, J. R., Frazer, A., Kidd, K. K. & Neuhauser, V. I. (1984). Amish Study V: Lithium–sodium counter transport and catechol-*O*-methyl transferase in pedigrees of bipolar probands. *American Journal of Psychiatry*, **141**, 1049–54.

Evans, W. E., Horner, M., Chu, Y. Q., Kalwinsky, D. & Roberts, W. M. (1991). Altered mercaptopurine metabolism, toxic effects, and dosage requirement in a thiopurine methyltransferase-deficient child with acute lymphocytic leukaemia. *Journal of Pediatrics*, **119**, 985–9.

Feuerstein, Cl., Tauche, M., Serre, F., Gavend, M., Pellat, J. & Perret, J. (1977). Does *O*-methyl-dopa play a role in levodopa-induced dyskinesias? *Acta Neurologica Scandinavica*, **56**, 79–82.

Floderus, Y., Iselius, L., Linsten, J. & Wetterberg, L. (1982). Evidence for a major locus as well as a multifactorial component in the regulation of human red blood cell catechol-*O*-methyl transferase activity. *Human Heredity*, **32**, 76–9.

Fukuda, H., Yamatodani, A., Imamura, I., Maeyama, K., Watanabe, T. & Wada, H. (1991). High-performance liquid chromatographic determination of histamine *N*-methyltransferase activity. *Journal of Chromatography*, **567**, 459–64.

Gordon, C., Bradley, H., Waring, R. H. & Emery, P. (1992). Abnormal sulphur oxidation in systemic lupus erythematosus. *Lancet*, **339**, 25–6.

Grossman, M. H., Emanuel, B. S. & Budarf, M. L. (1992b). Chromosomal mapping of the human catechol-*O*-methyltransferase to 22q 11.1→ q11.2. *Genomics*, **12**, 822–5.

Grossman, M. H., Szumlanski, C., Littrell, J. B., Weinstein, R. & Weinshilboum, R. M. (1992a). Electrophoretic analysis of low and high activity forms of catechol-*O*-methyltransferase in human erythrocytes. *Life Sciences*, **50**, 473–80.

Grunhaus, L., Ebstein, R., Belmaker, R., Sandler, S. G. & Jonas, W. (1976). A twin study of human red blood cell catechol-*O*-methyl transferase. *British Journal of Psychiatry*, **128**, 494–8.

Hale, J. P. & Lilleyman, J. A. (1991). Importance of 6-mercaptopurine dose in lymphoblastic leukaemia. *Archives of Disease in Childhood*, **66**, 462–6.

Hooper, C. A., Harvey, B. B. & Stone, H. H. (1980). Gastrointestinal bleeding due to vitamin K deficiency in patients on parenteral cefamandole. *Lancet*, **1**, 39–40.

Keith, R. A., Abraham, R. T., Pazmino, P. A. & Weinshilboum, R. M. (1983b). Correlation of low and high affinity thiol methyltransferase and phenol methyltransferase activities in human erythrocyte membranes. *Clinica Chimica Acta*, **131**, 257–72.

Keith, R. A., Jardine, I., Kerremans, A. & Weinshilboum, R. M. (1984). Human erythrocyte membrane thiol methyl transferase. *Drug Metabolism and Disposition*, **12**, 717–24.

Keith, R. A., Van Loon, J., Wussow, L. F. & Weinshilboum, R. M. (1983a). Thiol methylation pharmacogenetics: heritability of human erythrocyte thiol methyl transferase activity. *Clinical Pharmacology and Therapeutics*, **34**, 521–8.

Kerremans, A. L., Christensen, H. & Weinshilboum, R. M. (1984). Thiol methyl transferase (TMT) activity in human renal cortex microsomes. *Federation Proceedings*, **43**, 340 (Abstract 324).

Kerremans, A. L., Lipsky, J. J., Van Loon, J., Gallego, M. O. & Weinshilboum, R. M. (1985). Cephalosporin-induced hypoprothrombinaemia: possible role for thiol methylation of 1-methyltetrazole-5-thiol and 2-methyl 1,3,4-thiadiazole-5-thiol. *Journal of Pharmacology and Experimental Therapeutics*, **235**, 382–8.

Klemetsdal, B., Tollefsen, E., Loennechen, T., Johnsen, K., Utsi, E., Gisholt, K., Wist, E. & Aarbakke, J. (1992). Interethnic difference in thiopurine methyltransferase activity. *Clinical Pharmacology and Therapeutics*, **51**, 24–31.

Lafolie, P., Hayder, S., Björk, O. & Peterson, C. (1991). Intraindividual variation in 6-mercaptopurine pharmacokinetics during oral maintenance therapy of children with acute lymphoblastic leukaemia. *European Journal of Clinical Pharmacology*, **40**, 599–601.

Lennard, L. & Lilleyman, J. S. (1987). Are children with lymphoblastic leukaemia given enough 6-mercaptopurine? *Lancet*, **2**, 785–7.

Lennard, L., Lilleyman, J. S., Van Loon, J. & Weinshilboum, R. M. (1990). Genetic variation in response to 6-mercaptopurine for childhood acute lymphoblastic leukaemia. *Lancet*, **336**, 225–9.

Lennard, L. & Maddocks, J. L. (1983). Assay of 6-thioguanine nucleotide, a major metabolite of azathioprine, 6-mercaptopurine and 6-thioguanine in human red blood cells. *Journal of Pharmaceutical Pharmacology*, **35**, 15–18.

Lennard, L., Murphy, M. F. & Maddocks, J. L. (1984). Severe megaloblastic anaemia associated with abnormal azathioprine metabolism. *British Journal of Clinical Pharmacology*, **17**, 171–2.

Lennard, L., Van Loon, J. A., Lilleyman, J. S. & Weinshilboum, R. M. (1987). Thiopurine pharmacogenetics in leukaemia: correlation of erythrocyte thiopurine methyl transferase activity and 6-thioguanine nucleotide concentrations. *Clinical Pharmacology and Therapeutics*, **41**, 18–25.

Lennard, L., Van Loon, J. A. & Weinshilboum, R. M. (1989). Pharmacogenetics of acute azathioprine toxicity: relationship to thiopurine methyl transferase genetic polymorphism. *Clinical Pharmacology and Therapeutics*, **46**, 149–54.

Lipsky, J. J. (1983). *N*-methyl-thiotetrazole inhibition of the gamma carboxylation of glutamic acid: possible mechanism for antibiotic-associated hypoprothrombinaemia. *Lancet*, **2**, 192–3.

Loo, G. & Smith, J. T. (1985). Glutathione: an endogenous substrate for thiopurine methyl transferase? *Biochemical and Biophysical Research Communications*, **126**, 1201–7.

Pacifici, G. M., Danatelli, P. & Giuliani, L. (1992). Histamine *N*-methyltransferase: inhibition by drugs. *British Journal of Clinical Pharmacology*, **34**, 322–7.

Pacifici, G. M., Romiti, P., Giuliani, L. & Rane, A. (1991a). Thiopurine methyltransferase in humans – development and tissue distribution. *Developmental Pharmacology and Therapeutics*, **17**, 16–23.

Pacifici, G. M., Santerini, S. & Giuliani, L. (1991c). Methylation of captopril in human liver, kidney and intestine. *Xenobiotica*, **21**, 1107–12.

Pacifici, G. M., Santerini, S., Giuliani, L. & Rane, A. (1991b). Thiol methyl transferase in humans – development and tissue distribution. *Developmental Pharmacology and Therapeutics*, **17**, 8–15.

Price, R. A., Keith, R. A., Speilman, R. S. & Weinshilboum, R. M. (1989). Major gene polymorphism for human erythrocyte (RBC) thiol methyl transferase (TMT). *Genetic Epidemiology*, **6**, 651–62

Reilly, D. K. & Rivera-Calimlim, L. (1979). Racial difference in catechol-*O*-methyltransferase activity? A comparison of Filipinos with Caucasians in the United States. *Clinical Pharmacology and Therapeutics*, **25**, 244 (Abstract).

Reilly, D. K., Rivera-Calimlim, L. & Van Dyke, D. (1980). Catechol-*O*-methyltransferase activity: a determinant of levodopa response. *Clinical Pharmacology and Therapeutics*, **28**, 278–86.

Rivera-Calimlim, L. & Reilly, D. K. (1984). Difference in erythrocyte catechol-*O*-methyl transferase activity between Orientals and Caucasians: difference in levodopa tolerance. *Clinical Pharmacology and Therapeutics*, **35**, 804–9.

Rivera-Calimlim, L., Tandon, D., Anderson, F. & Joynt, R. (1977). The clinical picture and plasma levodopa metabolite profile of Parkinsonian non-responders. *Archives of Neurology*, **4**, 228–32.

Scanlon, P. D., Raymond, F. A. & Weinshilboum, R. M. (1979). Catechol-*O*-methyltransferase: thermolabile enzyme in erythrocytes of subjects homozygous for allele for low activity. *Science*, **203**, 63–5.

Scott, M. C., Szumlanski, C. L. & Weinshilboum, R. M. (1988a). Histamine *N*-methyltransferase (HNMT) pharmacogenetics: human kidney enzyme. *Clinical Pharmacology and Therapeutics*, **43**, 189.

Scott, M. C., Van Loon, J. A. & Weinshilboum, R. M. (1988b). Pharmacogenetics of *N*-methylation: heritability of human erythrocyte histamine *N*-methyltransferase activity. *Clinical Pharmacology and Therapeutics*, **43**, 256–62.

Siervogel, R. M., Weinshilboum, R., Wilson, A. F. & Elston, R. C. (1984). Major gene model for the inheritance of catechol-*O*-methyltransferase activity in five large families. *American Journal of Human Genetics*, **19**, 315–23.

Spielman, R. S. & Weinshilboum, R. M. (1981). Genetics of red cell COMT activity: analysis of thermal stability and family data. *American Journal of Medical Genetics*, **10**, 279–90.

Tinel, M., Berson, A., Pessayre, D., Letteron, P., Cattoni, M. P., Horsmans, Y. & Larrey, D. (1991). Pharmacogenetics of human erythrocyte thiopurine methyltransferase activity in a French population. *British Journal of Clinical Pharmacology*, **32**, 729–34.

Van Loon, J. A. & Weinshilboum, R. M. (1982). Thiopurine methyltransferase biochemical genetics: human lymphocyte activity. *Biochemical Genetics*, **20**, 637–58.

Van Loon, J. A. & Weinshilboum, R. M. (1987). Human lymphocyte thiopurine methyl transferase pharmacogenetics: Effect of phenotype on 6-mercaptopurine-induced inhibition of mitogen stimulation. *Journal of Pharmacology and Experimental Therapeutics*, **242**, 21–6.

Van Loon, J. A. & Weinshilboum, R. M. (1990). Thiopurine methyl transferase isozymes in human renal tissue. *Drug Metabolism and Disposition*, **18**, 632–8.

Van Scoik, K. G., Johnson, C. A. & Porter, W. R. (1985). The pharmacology and metabolism of the thiopurine drugs 6-mercaptopurine and azathiopurine. *Drug Metabolism Reviews*, **16**, 157–74.

Waring, R. H., Sturman, S. G., Smith, M. C. G., Steventon, G. B., Heafield, M. T. E. & Williams, A. C. (1989). S-methylation in motorneuron disease and Parkinson's disease. *Lancet*, **2**, 356–7.

Weinshilboum, R. M. (1988). Pharmacogenetics of methylation: relationship to drug metabolism. *Clinical Biochemistry*, **21**, 201–10.

Weinshilboum, R. M. (1989). Methyltransferase pharmacogenetics. *Pharmacology and Therapeutics*, **43**, 77–90.

Weinshilboum, R. M. & Raymond, F. A. (1977). Inheritance of low erythrocyte catechol-*O*-methyltransferase activity in man. *American Journal of Human Genetics*, **29**, 125–35.

Weinshilboum, R. M., Raymond, F. A. & Pazmino, P. A. (1978). Human erythrocyte thiopurine methyltransferase: radiochemical microassay and biochemical properties. *Clinica Chimica Acta*, **85**, 323–33.

Weinshilboum, R. M. & Sladek, S. L. (1980). Mercaptopurine pharmacogenetics: monogenic inheritance of erythrocyte thiopurine methyl transferase activity. *American Journal of Human Genetics*, **32**, 651–62.

Weitekamp, M. R. & Aber, R. C. (1983). Prolonged bleeding times and bleeding diathesis associated with moxalactam administration. *Journal of the American Medical Association*, **249**, 69–71.

Wilson, A. F., Elston, R. C., Siervogel, R. M., Weinshilboum, R. & Ward, L. J. (1984). Linkage relationships between a major gene for catechol-*O*-methyltransferase activity and 25 polymorphic marker systems. *American Journal of Human Genetics*, **19**, 525–32.

Winqvist, R., Lundström, K., Salminen, M., Laatikainen, M. & Ulmanen, I. (1992). The human catechol-*O*-methyltransferase (COMT) gene maps to band q 11.2 of chromosome 22 and shows a frequent RFLP with Bgl I. *Cytogenetics and Cell Genetics*, **59**, 253–7.

Winter, H., Herschel, M., Propping, P., Friedl, W. & Vogel, F. (1978). A twin study on three enzymes (DBH, COMT, MAO) of catecholamine metabolism. *Psychopharmacology*, **57**, 63–9.

Woodson, L. C., Ames, M. M., Selassie, C. D., Hansch, C. & Weinshilboum, R. M. (1983). Thiopurine methyl transferase: aromatic thiol substrates and inhibition by benzoic acid derivatives. *Molecular Pharmacology*, **24**, 471–8.

Woodson, L. C., Dunnette, J. H. & Weinshilboum, R. M. (1982). Pharmacogenetics of human thiopurine methyltransferase: kidney-erythrocyte correlation and immunotitration studies. *Journal of Pharmacology and Experimental Therapeutics*, **222**, 174–81.

21 Paraoxonase

INTRODUCTION

PARAOXON (0,0-diethyl-O-p-nitrophenyl phosphate) is an organophosphorus anticholinesterase compound. It has been used in man as a local preparation for the treatment of glaucoma (Fagerlind *et al.* 1952). It is produced in mammals by the oxidation of the insecticide parathion in the liver endoplasmic reticulum (Fukuto & Metcalf 1969). Parathion is inert until it is transformed into paraoxon, a highly toxic compound which can be absorbed even percutaneously.

Paraoxonase is an arylesterase (EC 3.1.1.2) which is capable of hydrolysing paraoxon to produce *p*-nitrophenol (Fig. 21.1) as first described by Aldridge (1953). It has no known natural substrate. The enzyme is widely represented in mammals and has been isolated and purified in sheep (Main 1960). It

was described in human plasma by Erdos & Boggs (1961) and characterized by Krisch (1968), who described a spectrophotometric method of determination.

GENETIC STUDIES

Pioneering work on the genetic aspects of serum paraoxonase in man was carried out by Geldmacher-v Mallinckrodt *et al.* (1969), who claimed that by incubating samples of serum from 75 subjects with paraoxon and determining the residual cholinesterase activity, a trimodal distribution due to different degrees of inhibition by paraoxon was obtained. In 1972 the same group showed that the degree of inhibition of cholinesterase correlated with the determination of serum arylesterase activity, as determined by the spectrophotometric method of Krisch (1968) ($r = 0.82$, significant at the 99% level).

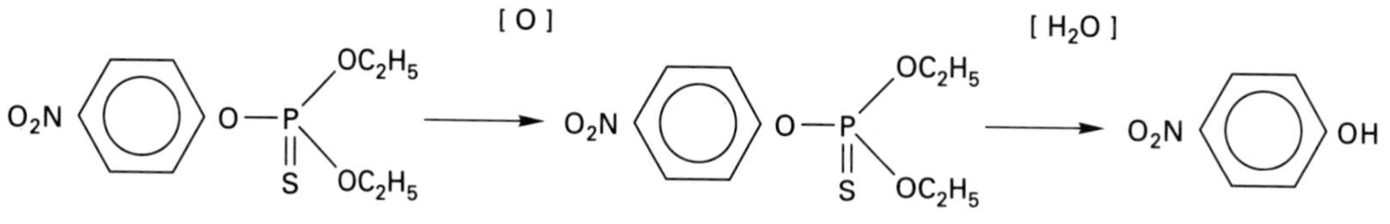

Fig. 21.1. Biotransformation of parathion and paraoxon. Parathion is converted to paraoxon by means of microsomal oxidation and paraoxon is hydrolysed to yield *p*-nitrophenol. The reaction is speeded by the plasma enzyme, paraoxonase.

346

In 1973 they claimed that using their anticholinesterase technique they were able to demonstrate a two-allele model controlling plasma arylesterase activity. Their evidence was, however, open to question as their family study contained only 52 offspring and they were unable to quote statistical significance for their results. They also had difficulty in defining their phenotypes as the overall distribution of results was not significantly different from unimodal.

Lauwerys & Murphy (1969) had compared the various methods available for studying the detoxification of paraoxon *in vitro*. They were concerned mainly with the detoxification of paraoxon in animals and compared spectrophotometric, anticholinesterase and manometric techniques. The first technique employed the measurement of paranitrophenol (PNP) released on hydrolysis of paraoxon. The anticholinesterase technique measured the loss of anticholinesterase activity after serum was incubated with paraoxon and was similar to that used by Geldmacher-v Mallinkrodt *et al.* (1969). The third technique measured carbon dioxide released into bicarbonate buffer. They found that the anticholinesterase method differed significantly from the spectrophotometric and the manometric methods. They suggested that the anticholinesterase technique measured other activities as well as the enzymatic

cleavage of the phosphorus-*p*-nitrophenol bond and was not specific for paraoxonase activity.

Krisch (1968), using a method whereby the *p*-nitrophenol released by the action of paraoxonase was measured, was able to define two activity groups. By adapting this approach to produce an autoanalyser method (Fig. 21.2) Playfer *et al.* (1976) showed a clear separation of 190 white British subjects into two phenotypes, with high and low enzyme activities (Fig. 21.3). Forty two-generation families which had 150 offspring were phenotyped. The evidence showed the low-activity phenotype to be an autosomal recessive Mendelian character (Table 21.1). Furthermore, inter-ethnic studies showed that the same clear bimodality as in Europeans could be shown in Indians but the gene frequencies were different. In Kenyans, Nigerians, Malays and Chinese clear bimodalities could not be found but there appeared to be rather small percentages of these populations with low enzyme activities.

An enormous family study (the largest in the whole field of pharmacogenetics) was published by Eiberg & Mohr (1981). Danish families comprising 1664 unrelated parents, 3169 children and 699 grandparents were studied, also by an autoanalyser method, but at pH 7.5 which gave an improved phenotypic separation. The main conclusion was

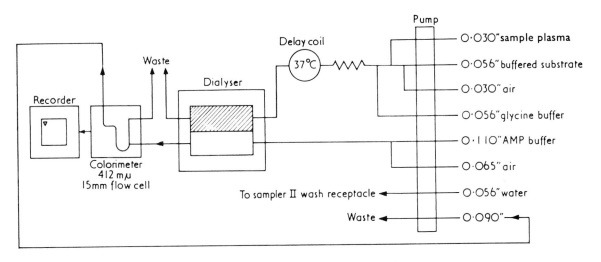

Fig. 21.2. Diagram of Technicon autoanalyser apparatus used to determine plasma paraoxonase activity. (From Playfer *et al.* 1976.)

Table 21.1. *Comparison of number of observed with number of expected phenotypes in offspring of 40 matings*

Matings male × female	Offspring				χ^2
	High activity		Low activity		
	Observed	Expected	Observed	Expected	
High activity × high activity	25	26.54	7	5.45	
Low activity × low activity	0	0	11	11	
Total	25	26.54	18	16.46	0.234
High activity × low activity	28	24.65	14	17.35	1.002
Low activity × high activity	11	12.90	11	9.10	0.677
					1.913

D.F. = 2; $p > 0.100$.   *From:* Playfer *et al.* 1976.

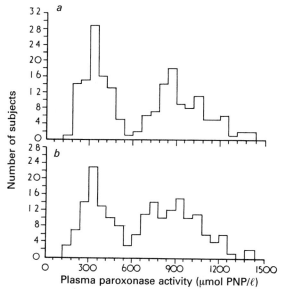

Fig. 21.3. Frequency distribution histograms of plasma paraoxonase activity in (a) 190 British blood donors, (b) British family members. (From Playfer *et al.* 1976.)

the same as that of Playfer *et al.* (1976), but the data were later subjected to more sophisticated analyses, which will be discussed below.

ADVANCES IN PHENOTYPING AND GENOTYPING TECHNIQUES

The family studies of Playfer *et al.* (1976) and Eiberg & Mohr (1981) were based upon measuring

the activity of paraoxonase in serum. Advances in phenotyping were then made by several groups based on either differential stimulation or inhibition of the enzymes categorizing the different phenotypes (or genotypes). These were qualitative differences as opposed to the previous quantitative methods. The principal techniques involved were:

1 addition of 1 M sodium chloride (Eckerson *et al.* 1983);
2 addition of 5×10^{-3} M calcium chloride (Carro-Ciampi *et al.* 1981);
3 addition of 10 mM EDTA (Mueller *et al.* 1983);
4 relative activity, namely, the ratio of paraoxonase activity to the hydrolysis of phenylacetate could be assessed with and without 0.1 mM chlorpromazine (La Du *et al.* 1986a).

Some of the results are illustrated in Figs. 21.4, 21.5 and 21.6 and all the available information is summarized in Table 21.2.

The genotypes could be clearly separated by some of the techniques.

Sera whose hydrolysing activities may have deteriorated somewhat during transportation or storage can still be phenotyped using qualitative methods (Brackley *et al.* 1983; Eckerson *et al.* 1983).

It should be possible to perform these qualitative methods using autoanalyser (e.g. Brackley *et al.* 1983) or other automated analytical techniques (e.g. Cobas Fara centrifugal analyser: Secchiero *et al.* 1989) by running aliquots of the same serum sample with and without the activator or inhibitor.

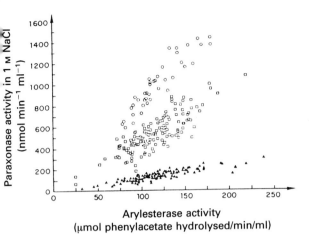

Fig. 21.4. Individual paraoxonase and arylesterase activities. A plot of individual paraoxonase activity with 1 M NaCl vs arylesterase activity with phenylacetate shows three groups of individuals, ▲, □, ○, corresponding to the three paraoxonase phenotypes, A, AB, and B. Results are from 348 individuals (unrelated and related). (From Eckerson *et al.* 1983.)

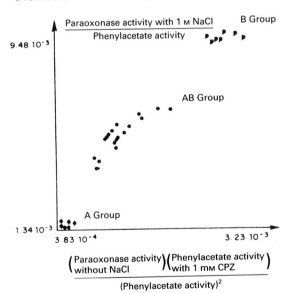

Fig. 21.5. A display of the distribution of Sudanese serum sample values using paraoxonase activity with or without 1 mM NaCl and arylesterase activity with or without 0.1 mM chlorpromazine. (From La Du *et al.* 1986.)

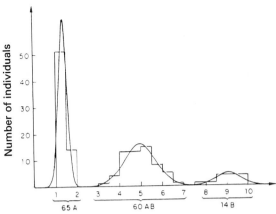

Fig. 21.6. The distribution of the ratio of the activity of paraoxonase stimulated by 1 M NaCl divided by the arylesterase activity, for 139 individuals. (From Vincent-Viry *et al.* 1986.)

It is clear that: (1) no amount of mathematical manipulation can replace an innovative biochemical and enzymological approach in order to define phenotypes (for example, compare Geldmacher-v Mallinckrodt *et al.* 1979; and Geldmacher-v Mallinckrodt 1983 with Diepgen *et al.* 1987); (2) it is essential to make maximal use of the phenotyping techniques available, e.g. the study of Ghanaians conducted by Williams *et al.* (1986) could have yielded interesting data if the paraoxonase had been measured with added salt and divided by the phenylacetate esterase activity.

INTER-ETHNIC VARIABILITY

The results of surveys in different ethnic groups are shown in Table 21.3 and Fig. 21.7. Thus, whilst over half of Caucasians are of the low activity group and not stimulated by sodium chloride and not inhibited by EDTA, only 6.7% of Indonesians, 9.6% of Ghanaians, 13.6% of Jamaicans, 17.0 to 19.6% of Koreans and 14.6% of Japanese have this genotype.

It can be speculated that in the event of accidental or occupational exposure to paraoxon, Caucasian populations would fare less well than others because over half the people involved would be relatively less able to detoxify the poison. Taylor *et al.* (1965) suggested that individuals with high enzyme activity would be at an advantage when

Table 21.2. *Compendium of family studies on serum paraoxonase*

Reference	Number of families and ethnic group	Number of offspring	Technique	Conclusion
Playfer et al. 1976	40 British white	107	Autoanalyser estimation of activity at pH 10.5	Low activity phenotype autosomal recessive
Geldmacher-v Mallinckrodt et al. 1979	99 German	180	Residual cholinesterase activity after incubating serum with paraoxonase	Inconclusive
Eiberg & Mohr 1981	832 Danish	3169	Autoanalyser estimation of activity at pH 7.5	Low activity phenotype autosomal recessive
Mueller et al. 1983	40 US Caucasians	58	Differential inhibition by EDTA	Two co-dominant alleles at an autosomal locus coding for high or low activity
Eckerson et al. 1983	38 US Caucasians	80	Percent stimulation of paraoxonase by molar NaCl divided by arylesterase activity	Two co-dominant alleles at an autosomal locus
Vincent-Viry et al. 1986	32 French	75	Same as Eckerson et al. 1983	Same as Eckerson et al. 1983
La Du et al. 1986b	22 Sudanese	85	Same as Eckerson et al. 1983	Same as Eckerson et al. 1983
Ishimoto et al. 1987	58 Japanese	79	Paraoxonase activity at pH 10.2	Suggests low activity is autosomal recessive

Table 21.3. *Inter-ethnic distribution of paraoxonase alleles*

Reference	Technique used	Ethnic group	Number of unrelated individuals examined	q (SE)	Comments on phenotype separation
Playfer et al. 1976	Paraoxonase activity using an autoanalyser method at pH 10.25	British white Indian	190 70	0.7034 (0.0258) 0.4629 (0.0530)	Good
Geldmacher-v Mallinckrodt et al. 1979	Residual cholinesterase activity after incubation of serum with paraoxon	Presumably German	799	0.7612 (0.0115)	Very indistinct
Eiberg & Mohr 1981	Paraoxonase activity using an autoanalyser method at pH 7.5	Danish	1664	0.7264 (0.0084)	Excellent
Carro-Ciampi et al. 1981	Paraoxon hydrolysis determined (a) at pH 10, (b) at pH 10 with 5×10^{-3} M $CaCl_2$ added, (c) as in b with 5×10^{-1} M NaCl added. Results expressed as c/b	Canadian Caucasians Orientals	82 9	0.7157 (0.0386) 0.3535 (0.1654)	Excellent separation of phenotypes
Carro-Ciampi et al. 1983	Same as Carro-Ciampi et al. 1981	Canadian Indians Inuit	57 67	0.2649 (0.0639) 0.2443 (0.0592)	Excellent separation of phenotypes
Eckerson et al. 1983	% stimulation of paraoxonase activity by M sodium chloride = x and ratio of x to arylesterase activity	US white Caucasians	219	0.6791 (0.0248)	Excellent separation of phenotypes. Also genotypes defined
Mueller et al. 1983 Goedde et al. 1984	Inhibition of paraoxonase activity by EDTA Technique of Krisch 1968. Paraoxonase activity at pH 11.2	US white Caucasians Atacameno Indians	531 171	0.6997 (0.0155) 0.8020 (0.0228)	Fair Good
La Du et al. 1986a	Plotting $\dfrac{\text{Paraoxonase activity with 1 M NaCl}}{\text{Phenylacetate hydrolysis activity}} = y$ against $\dfrac{\left\{\begin{array}{l}\text{Paraoxonase}\\ \text{activity}\\ \text{without NaCl}\end{array}\right\} - \left\{\begin{array}{l}\text{Phenylacetate}\\ \text{activity with}\\ \text{1 mM CPZ}\end{array}\right\}}{\text{[Phenylacetate activity]}^2} = x$	Sudanese	31	0.4399 (0.0806)	Excellent, and genotypes defined
La Du et al. 1986b	Hydrolysis ratio $\dfrac{\text{Paraoxonase with NaCl}}{\text{Arylesterase [phenylacetate]}}$	Sudanese	129	0.5134 (0.0378)	Genotypic separations clear

Table 21.3. (*cont.*)

Reference	Technique used	Ethnic group	Number of unrelated individuals examined	q (SE)	Comments on phenotype separation
Diepgen & Geldmacher-v Mallinckrodt 1987	Method of Krisch 1986	Europeans Indians	1231 306	0.7280 (0.0098) 0.6083 (0.0227)	Phenotype differentiation does not allow allele frequency to be calculated for Japanese, Nigerians, US American Negroes or Australian Aboriginals
Vincent-Viry et al. 1986	As Eckerson et al. 1983	French	139	0.6838 (0.0309)	Excellent genotype separation
Diepgen & Geldmacher-v Mallinckrodt 1987	Method of Carro-Ciampi 1981	Germans Italians Indonesians Koreans Ghanians Jamaicans	130 96 120 106 93 129	0.7570 (0.0286) 0.7791 (0.0320) 0.2588 (0.0441) 0.4427 (0.0435) 0.3098 (0.0493) 0.3688 (0.0409)	Excellent
Ishimoto et al. 1987	Method of Krisch 1968	Japanese	390	0.3823 (0.0234)	Considerable overlap between phenotypes
Rona et al. 1987	Residual cholinesterase activity after incubation with paraoxon	Hungarians	100	0.6300 (0.0388)	Considerable overlap between phenotypes
Szabo et al. 1987a	Salt activation of paraoxonase activity	Hungarians	176	0.6742 (0.0278)	Good separation between phenotypes
Paik et al. 1988	Method of Krisch 1968	Korean	534	0.4128 (0.0197)	Phenotype definition not clear
Furlong et al. 1988	Paraoxonase activity <u>Arylesterase activity</u> and Paraoxonase activity <u>Chlorpyrifos oxonase activity</u>	Random Caucasoids	320	0.6846 (0.0204)	Excellent discrimination between low activity homozygotes and the other two genotypes combined
Nogueira et al. 1988 Nogueira et al. 1992	Ratio of paraoxonase activity with salt to arylesterase	Saudi Arabians	248	0.7296 (0.0217)	Clear trimodality

Reference	Method	Population	n	q (SE)	Comments
Roy et al. 1991	Serum diluted in Tris buffer pH 7.6 in the presence of 10 mM Ca^{2+} ($CaCl_2$) as described by McElveen et al. (1986)	Chinese Filipinos Dravidian Indians	194 159 73	0.7680 (0.0173) 0.9245 (0.0109) 0.6712 (0.0336)	No figure presented in the article
Szabo et al. 1991[a]	Residual activity, paraoxonase activity determined in the presence of salt	Hungarians [a]adults children	100 102	0.4200 (0.0381) 0.1863 (0.0373)	Very blurred phenotype definition especially in children
Karakaya et al. 1991	Ratio of paraoxonase with salt to arylesterase	Turks	105	0.6324 (0.0378)	Very blurred phenotype definition

q, frequency of the allele governing the low activity, non-salt-responsive or A phenotype.
CPZ, chlorpromazine.
[a]A curious feature of this series was the sex difference in the frequency of the B phenotype.

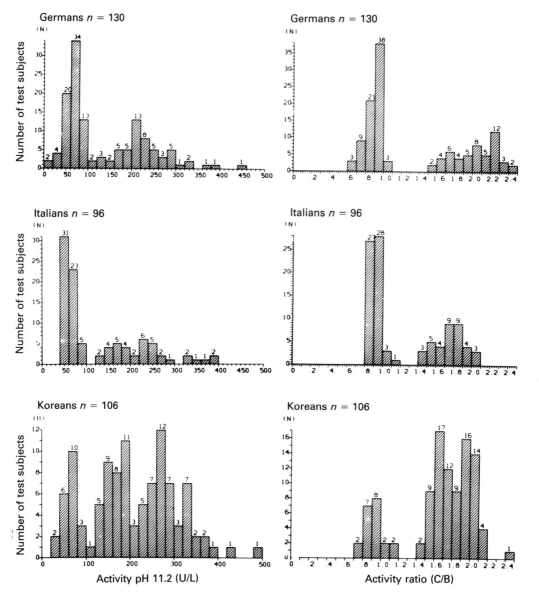

Fig. 21.7. Frequency distribution histograms of serum paraoxonase activity (pH = 11.2) and of serum paraoxonase activity ratio (c)/(b) (pH = 10.0) in different ethnic samples. (From Diepgen et al. 1987; and see Carro-Gampi et al. 1981, Table 21.3.)

poisoning occurs, an idea reiterated by Flugel et al. (1978). Model in vitro studies indicated that the catalytic hydrolysis by the serum esterase could provide some degree of protection during chronic expo-

sure to paraoxon (Eckerson & La Du 1984). There would be very little opportunity for the enzyme to act if individuals were exposed acutely to large concentrations of paraoxon (Geldmacher-v Mallinck-rodt, 1978).

Two animal experiments can be cited which are relevant in this context.

First, Main (1956) fed aldrin to rats and found that it raised the liver arylesterase activity and

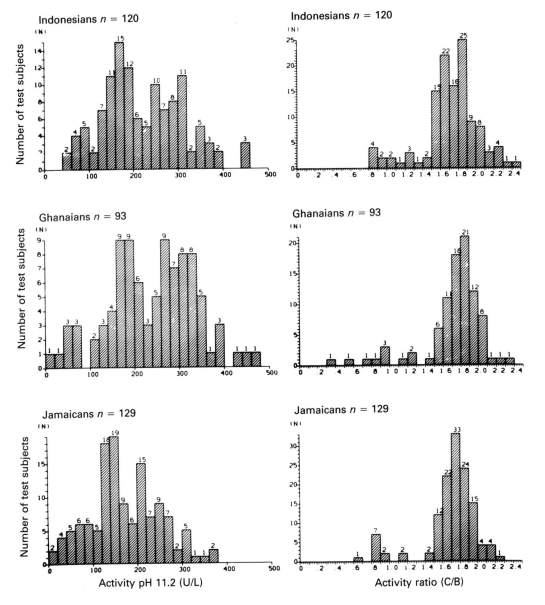

Fig. 21.7 (*cont.*).

lowered the serum activity. Rats so pretreated had a slight decrease in the LD_{50} of intravenous paraoxon. When the paraoxon was given orally the LD_{50} was three times larger in aldrin pretreated rats than in controls. The intravenous infusion of rabbit serum arylesterase into rats greatly reduced the mortality due to intravenously administered paraoxon.

Secondly Costa *et al* (1990) administered purified rabbit serum paraoxonase intravenously to rats. It was found that rats treated in this way were protected against paraoxon given intravenously but not against paraoxon given orally.

Since most humans are poisoned by paraoxon (or its precursor parathion) via the oral route, the significance of serum paraoxonase levels in providing protection remains at present unclear.

FURTHER GENETIC ANALYSES

Using the improved phenotyping and genotyping techniques referred to earlier, family studies have been conducted in different ethnic groups and are summarized in Table 21.2.

The extremely extensive Danish family material of Eiberg & Mohr (1981) was subjected to further genetic analysis.

Nielsen *et al.* (1986a) investigated (1) 416 matings with 1595 children where one parent had a high and the other low paraoxonase activity, (2) 185 matings with 684 children where both parents had high activity. Segregation of the offspring would be expected in these families. The plausibility of different genetic models was evaluated by means of a likelihood function constructed from a segregation analysis. The conclusion was that the inheritance of high and low activity of serum paraoxonase is due, with overwhelming probability, to a one-locus system with one or more alleles controlling the dominant character. If any secondary locus were involved its most common allele would probably have a frequency above 0.95.

In another paper Nielsen *et al.* (1986b) addressed the interesting possibility that there may be two or more alleles controlling high paraoxonase activity ('high genes'). Obviously, if that were so there would be two types of heterozygote, lh_1 and lh_2. Amongst other pieces of evidence extracted from their data the authors found that the distribution of paraoxonase activity amongst obligate heterozygotes was not normal and was in fact compatible with two overlapping normal distributions. The conclusion was that there seemed likely to be at least one allele for low activity and two alleles for high activity, all at the same locus. These hypothetical alleles were termed for convenience l, h_1 and h_2. The two alleles for high activity would be dominant to the one for low activity.

It will be interesting to see whether further enzymological and molecular biology techniques produce evidence to substantiate this possibility. A hint that this is so is given in the paper of Eiberg *et al.* (1985) where it is stated that $h_2 h_2$ individuals have the highest activity and are recognizable in some pedigrees, have their activities inhibited 30% by raising the pH of the incubate from 7.5 to 10.0 (with this change $h_1 h_2$ individuals are inhibited

by about 10%, the $h_1 h_1$ and $l h_2$ individuals are scarcely changed, while the $l h_1$ individuals are stimulated by about 20%).

The suspicion of multiple allelism has cropped up in other pharmacogenetic polymorphisms such as phenylthiourea (PTC) tasting. Actual multiple allelism has been found to occur in examples such as glucose-6-phosphate dehydrogenase deficiency, acute intermittent porphyria and N-acetyltransferase.

LINKAGE OF THE PARAOXONASE LOCUS WITH THE CYSTIC FIBROSIS LOCUS

Considerable interest was generated by the finding that the loci for paraoxonase and cystic fibrosis were linked (Eiberg *et al.* 1985).

The Danish pedigrees were examined for linkage between paraoxonase and 64 other polymorphic marker systems, and for linkage between paraoxonase and cystic fibrosis. There was no evidence for linkage of paraoxonase with the other 64 polymorphic marker systems. The linkage analysis between paraoxonase and cystic fibrosis was conducted in two ways: first, considering the paraoxonase polymorphism as a simple Mendelian dominant (i.e. two alleles) and second, in accordance with the hypothesis that there are three paraoxonase alleles, one for low and two for high activity. If the latter hypothesis were erroneous it would have tended to lower lod scores. In the event the highest lod score was obtained using the three allele model where $\hat{z} = 3.70$ at $\Theta = 0.09$ in males and $\Theta = 0.00$ in females. Statistical associations between paraoxonase and cystic fibrosis phenotypes were not found.

Later after a total of 41 informative families were analysed, a positive lod score of 3.46 at a recombination distance $\Theta = 0.07$ centiMorgan (cM) was found in males and 0.13 cM in females with the simple Mendelian two-allele model (one centiMorgan is approximately 1000 kilobases). Using the three allele model the combined lod score was $\hat{z} = 4.50$ at the same recombination distances (Schmiegelow *et al.* 1986).

In the event what happened very soon after this was the discovery of other markers in the vicinity of the cystic fibrosis gene (CF). One of these was the DNA marker 917 which was mapped to the long arm of chromosome 7 by the use of somatic cell hybrids and its locus named *D7S15*. Within a short time two other DNA segments on chromosome 7 were found closer to CF than either the paraoxonase gene locus or *D7S15*. The oncogene *met* and the anonymous DNA marker pJ3-11 (D7S8) were found to be within about 1% recombination either side of the CF gene (Buchwald *et al.* 1989) but still about 1600 kb apart.

The remainder of the story is one of the great achievements of molecular genetics. Lap-Chee Tsui and Francis Collins with their teams eventually found that the proteins produced by the normal and mutant (cystic fibrosis) genes differ by the deletion of one phenylalanine in the latter. This defect leads to defective chloride ion transport (Marx 1989).

ENZYMOLOGY

Paraoxonase is an A-esterase according to the terminology of Aldridge (1953). It differs from serine esterases such as cholinesterase, by being resistant to inhibitory compounds that react with serine groups such as di-isopropylfluorophosphate (DFP) and physostigmine (Eckerson *et al.* 1983). The enzyme is presumably manufactured in the liver (Whitehouse & Ecobichon 1975).

It seems likely that a single serum enzyme exists in two polymorphic forms. Both are equally able to hydrolyse phenylacetate so that this arylesterase activity is 'non-discriminating'. On the other hand, one is much superior to the other in hydrolysing paraoxon so this activity is 'discriminating'. The evidence in favour of this view is as follows (Eckerson *et al.* 1983).

1 Correlation of both basal paraoxonase and salt-stimulated paraoxonase with arylesterase activity in both paraoxonase phenotypes.
2 Cosegregation of the degree of stimulation of paraoxonase activity by salt and the paraoxonase/arylesterase activity ratio.
3 Phenylacetate inhibits paraoxonase of both phenotypes.

'Discriminating' ability may depend upon turnover numbers (Furlong *et al.* 1988).

It was originally pointed out by Erdos & Boggs (1961) that the activity of human serum in hydrolysing paraoxon was inhibited 86% by EDTA. A search for the origin of the remaining activity revealed that human albumin also hydrolysed paraoxon and that this hydrolysis could be inhibited by aurin tricarboxylic acid ammonium salt (aluminon) and this was not reversible by dialysis. This albumin-associated activity was not inhibited by oxalic acid or mercuric chloride but was inhibited by sodium, potassium or lithium chloride.

A return to this phenomenon was made by Ortigoza-Ferado *et al.* (1984), using gel filtration on Sephadex G-200 columns and monitoring the elution of proteins and paraoxonase activity. They showed that there were two distinct elution peaks, one fairly constant in the population which consisted of albumin with paraoxonase activity (but this was absent in the rare analbuminaemic individual) and the other elution peak of paraoxonase activity which was quite separate and which varied between individuals. The polymorphism resided in the latter peak (peak I), whose paraoxonase activity represented about 75% of the total serum activity in high, 56% in intermediate and 29% in the low activity phenotypes. In peak I the paraoxonase and arylesterase activities could not be dissociated and the activity was totally inhibited by 10 mM EDTA. On the other hand the peak I activities were increased and albumin-associated activities were decreased by the addition of 1 M NaCl.

The effect of pH on the serum paraoxonase activity of high and low activity phenotypes was clearly shown by Eiberg & Mohr (1981) and Ortigoza-Ferado *et al.* (1984). There was a much greater difference between the phenotypes at pH 7.5 to 8.0 as compared with that at 9.5 and above.

The effect of NaCl in separating the two phenotypes was shown by Eckerson *et al.* (1983) to increase up to about 1 M. On the other hand CaCl$_2$ at 1.0 M increased the non-enzymatic paraoxon hydrolysis to a rate exceeding enzymatic hydrolysis.

Mixing sera of the low and high activity (or non-salt responsive and salt-responsive) phenotypes had a purely additive effect. This was evidence against the presence of a diffusible stimulating agent whose effect was enhanced by salt.

The addition of NaCl to the salt-responsive (type B) phenotype produced no change in K_m but more than doubled V_{max}. This indicated an increase in the turnover number of active sites or an increase in the turnover number but not a change in the binding constant for paraoxon. Linear reaction rates with no lag phase were obtained when serum was added as the last reagent in the assays containing salt, indicating that the salt had an immediate effect.

Very similar results were obtained by Mueller *et al.* (1983), who also showed that the high activity sera were inhibited by EDTA at 10^{-4} to 10^{-2} M concentrations to a much greater degree than the low activity sera.

Ortigoza-Ferado *et al.* (1984) claimed that the K_m values for paraoxon for the albumin and non-albumin peaks were the same and that this explained the lack of biphasic kinetics in reciprocal plots of the substrate dependence of paraoxonase activity in whole serum.

Heat-inactivation studies conducted by Mueller *et al.* (1983) showed that the high-activity sera were more rapidly inactivated at 55 °C but there was a considerable overlap between the two groups. Heat inactivation at 37 °C and 55 °C revealed no differential features.

The kinetics of cholinesterase inhibition in human serum by paraoxon were explored in a mathematical model by Eckerson & La Du (1984). The motivation behind this work was the desire to separate the genotypes in the salt-responsive phenotype (type B) detected by the hydrolysis of paraoxon [there was a suggestion in the work of Geldmacher-v Mallinckrodt *et al.* (1973) that this might be possible]. The conclusion of Eckerson & La Du (1984) was that the percentage of initial activity remaining as residual activity depended primarily on the paraoxonase activity. So the residual cholinesterase activity test was an indirect measure of paraoxonase activity. The possibility was raised by this work that *in vivo* the paraoxonase phenotype may affect the clearance of paraoxon and hence affect its binding to target sites.

Human paraoxonase was purified (Gan *et al.* 1991) by a series of chromatographic steps in the presence of Ca $^{2+}$. The purified preparation gave a 43 kDa band on SDS-PAGE gels. The enzyme is a glycoprotein containing about 337 amino acids and 15.8% carbohydrate represented by up to three sugar chains per molecule.

Using purified enzyme samples of both phenotypes Smolen *et al.* (1991) compared the properties. The K_m values for both paraoxon and phenylacetate were slightly higher with the A type enzyme. The

type B enzyme showed a definite activity optimum at about pH 10 when stimulated by NaCl whereas the A type had an optimum at about pH 7.5 to 8.0. The turnover number (tn) (for paraoxon) was eight times higher with the B enzyme than with the A enzyme but the tn for arylesterase activity was very similar for both isozymes.

The two types of enzyme differ by one amino acid substitution (see p. 360).

The status of different substrates with regard to polymorphic and monomorphic paraoxonase activity is shown in Table 21.4. The natural substrates for the enzymes in this polymorphism remain unknown but a possible relation to lipid metabolism is discussed in the next section.

RELATIONSHIP OF PARAOXONASE TO MYOCARDIAL INFARCTION AND ASSOCIATION WITH HDL CHOLESTEROL

As has been pointed out earlier, a small fraction of serum paraoxonase activity resides in the albumin fraction (Erdos & Boggs 1961). The remainder of the activity was later found to be associated with high density lipoprotein (HDL). Because of the known protective effect of this lipoprotein against the development of atherosclerosis, McElveen *et al.* (1986) investigated the paraoxonase activities of sera from 88 patients of mixed age, race and sex who had suffered myocardial infarctions, as well as sera from 195 controls. The controls consisted of 52 patients who were suspected of having myocardial infarctions (MI) but who did not demonstrate the serum enzyme changes characteristic of an infarct, and the 143 others had various diagnoses. The results show a shift in the frequency distribution curve of paraoxonase activity in the MI patients but, oddly enough, also suggest relatively smaller proportion of them to have the low-activity phenotypes as compared with the controls. The authors do not state how long after the myocardial infarction they obtained their sera from the 88 patients and this should be considered in view of the known perturbations of serum lipids following the ictus.

The subject was reinvestigated by Secchiero *et al.* (1989) in 10 patients with acute myocardial infarctions. No significant variations of serum paraoxon-

Table 21.4. *Substrates for paraoxonase*

Compounds which are hydrolysed to different degrees by different phenotypes
paraoxon (the only 'discriminating' substrate)
ethylparaoxon
methylparaoxon
PO chlorothion
PO EPN
thiophenylacetate
p-nitrophenylacetate
O-nitrophenylacetate
2-naphthylacetate

Compounds which are monomorphically hydrolysed by paraoxonase
dicapthoxon
fenitroxin
phenylacetate
chlorpyrifos

Compounds which are hydrolysed by paraoxon but it is unclear whether they are polymorphic

Organophosphates
diisofluorophosphate
tabun
sarin
soman
aramine

Carbamates
carbaryl
3-isopropylphenyl-*N*-methylcarbamate

Aromatic carboxylic acid esters
4-nitrophenylacetate
2-naphthylacetate

Compounds which are not hydrolysed by paraoxonase
parathion
methylparathion
isopropylparaoxon
m-nitroparaoxon
o-nitroparaoxon
mono-desmethylparaoxon
di-desmethylparaoxon
chlorothion

Data obtained from: Eckerson, *et al.* 1983; Geldmacher-v Mallinckrodt *et al.* 1984; La Du *et al.* 1986a; Smolen *et al.* 1991.

ase activity were found following the ictus and so the authors concluded that this assay is not appropriate to monitor the clinical condition.

The controls included 25 with high, 10 with intermediate and 25 with low HDL cholesterol. The serum paraoxonase activity paralleled the HDL cholesterol levels. In the myocardial infarction patients the paraoxonase activities were similar to those found in the low HDL cholesterol controls.

It seems likely from the distribution histograms of paraoxonase activities shown in the paper of McElveen *et al.* (1986) that there may be an association between the low paraoxonase activity phenotype and myocardial infarction (or coronary artery atheroma).

The study by Szabo *et al.* (1987b) was meant to

shed light on this possibility. The 24 children of persons who had suffered a myocardial infarction below the age of 40 years were compared with 176 children of healthy parents. The serum paraoxonases were studied by the technique of Eckerson *et al.* (1983). Both groups were said to exhibit bimodal distributions (but the figures are not really convincing) and the first group had a lower mean value than the control. There were 80 individuals of low-activity, non-salt responsive phenotype in the control group and 14 such persons in the MI group so that χ_1^2 was 1.41 and hence not significant (Szabo *et al.* 1987a).

The matter has received further attention in the papers of Mackness *et al.* (1991) and Saha *et al.* (1991). The former studied three groups of patients: normal, familial hypercholesterolaemics and insulin-dependent diabetics (IDDM). The bimodality of activities was poor in the normals. Nevertheless there was a higher proportion of low paraoxonase activity individuals in the IDDM group. It was a pity they did not establish the phenotype with a technique such as paraoxonase activity/phenylacetate hydrolysis activity. As it was they made no assessment of the association between genetic constitution and disease. Saha *et al.* (1991) studied 163 healthy Chinese and determined the paraoxonase activity phenotypes (though unfortunately they do not show a figure on which the separation they achieved can be assessed). They found that the serum triglyceride level was significantly lower, the LDL cholesterol level higher and the ApoA-II and ApoB lower in individuals of both sexes with the low activity ('A') paraoxonase phenotype. In men only the A paraoxonase phenotype had a substantially higher serum total cholesterol concentration.

In an editorial comment La Du (1988) points out that it is possible that paraoxonase has an endogenous substrate related to lipoprotein metabolism and that this would explain its close association with the high density lipoprotein (HDL) complex. Alternatively, the enzyme may be unstable in serum without the HDL environment, and so the finding of low levels of paraoxonase activity in persons with Tangier disease or fish-eye disease (in which the HDL levels are very low) may be just a secondary effect. It would be of interest to see more studies where the enzyme phenotype (or genotype) as opposed to just the activity were available to study

assocations with diseases such as myocardial infarction.

In this context it is interesting to note that in their huge survey Eibert & Mohr (1981) came across five individuals who had almost complete absence of paraoxonase in their sera and they 'did not show any conspicuous disorder'. Two were children and three were grandparents. No lipid studies were incorporated in their survey. It is strange that whilst one would suspect some important biological function for an enzyme which is polymorphic and which has a different 'set' in different ethnic groups, some individuals appear to get along well with almost none of the enzymic activity under consideration. Thirty-one samples of umbilical cord bloods from newborn babies were found by Mueller *et al.* (1983) to have very low plasma paraoxonase activities.

MOLECULAR GENETICS

Two research groups have now produced information about the paraoxonase gene and enzyme and shed light on the basis for the genetic polymorphism.

A rabbit paraoxonase cDNA (rpcDNA) was isolated by Hassett *et al.* (1991) using oligonucleotide probes constructed as a result of studying the amino acid sequences of the enzyme. The rpcDNA was used as a hybridization probe to isolate human paraoxonase clones from a liver cDNA library. Three of the longest clones were sequenced.

One clone was of full length, containing an open reading frame of 1065 bases which predicted a 355 amino acid protein. Two clones predicted methionine (ATG) at position 55 and glutamine (CAA) at position 192, whilst the third predicted leucine (TTG) and arginine (CGA), respectively at these two positions. Presumably the person from whom the gene library was obtained was an AB heterozygote.

The Ann Arbor group sequenced tryptic digest peptides of human paraoxonase so that suitable oligonucleotide probes could be synthesized (Adkins *et al.* 1991). When the peptides were separated by high performance liquid chromatography one peptide was found to differ between the A and B isoenzymes. This observation led to the discovery that the thirtieth amino acid of the peptide was glutamine in the A isoenzyme and arginine in the B isoenzyme (Mody *et al.* 1992). Trypsin cleaves the B isoenzyme at this site but does not cleave the A isoenzyme. Studies of the DNA sequence of the coding region of the enzyme also revealed the same polymorphic site (Adkins *et al.* 1992).

So the basis for the polymorphism is most probably a single nucleotide substitution leading to a single amino acid difference.

Nothing is known as yet about the detailed organization of the gene.

Adkins, S., Gan, K. N., Mody, M. & La Du, B. N. (1991). Purification and cloning of human serum paraoxonase/arylesterase. *FASEB*, Abstract 648.

Adkins, S., Gan, K., Mody, M. & La Du, B. N. (1992). A point mutation appears to account for the human serum paraoxonase/arylesterase polymorphism. *FASEB*, Abstract 3742.

Aldridge, W. N. (1953). Serum esterases 2. An enzyme hydrolysing diethyl *p*-nitrophenyl phosphate (E600) and its identity with the A-esterase of mammalian serum. *Biochemical Journal*, **53**, 117–24.

Brackley, M., Carro-Giampi, G., Stewart, D. J., Lowden, A., Ray, A. K. & Kalow, W. (1983). Stability of the paraoxonase phenotyping ratio in collections of human sera with differing storage times. *Research Communications in Chemical Pathology and Pharmacology*, **41**, 65–78.

Buchwald, M., Tsui, L. C. & Riordan, J. R. (1989). The search for the cystic fibrosis gene. *American Journal of Physiology*, **257** (Lung Cell Mol Physiol 1): L47–52.

Carro-Ciampi, G., Gray, S. & Kalow, W. (1983). Paraoxonase phenotype distribution in Canadian Indian and Inuit populations. *Canadian Journal of Physiology and Pharmacology*, **61**, 336–40.

Carro-Ciampi, G., Kadar, D. & Kalow, W. (1981). Distribution of serum paraoxon hydrolyzing activities in a Canadian population. *Canadian Journal of Physiology and Pharmacology* **59**, 904–7.

Costa, L. G., McDonald, B. E., Murphy, S. D., Omenn, G. S., Richter, R. J., Motulsky, A,. G. & Furlong, C. E. (1960). Serum paraoxonase and its influence on paraxon and chloropyrifos-oxon toxicity in rate. *Toxicology and Applied Pharmacology*, **103**, 66–76.

Diepgen, T. L. & Geldmacher-v Mallinckrodt, M. (1986). Interethnic differences in the detoxification of organophosphates; the human serum paraoxonase polymorphism. *Archives of Toxicology*, Suppl. **9**, 154–8.

Diepgen, T. L., Geldmacher-v Mallinckrodt, M. & Goedde, H. W. (1987). The interethnic differences of the human serum paraoxonase polymorphism analysed by a quantitative and a qualitative method. *Toxicology and Environmental Chemistry*, **14**, 101–10.

Eckerson, H. W. & La Du, B. N. (1984). A mathematical model for evaluating the reaction of paraoxon with human serumcholinesterase and with polymorphic forms of paraoxonase. *Drug Metabolism and Disposition*, **12**, 57–62.

Eckerson, H. W., Wyte, C. M. & La Du, B. N. (1983). The human serum paraoxonase/arylesterase polymorphism. *American Journal of Human Genetics* **35**, 1126–38.

Eiberg, H. & Mohr, J. (1981). Genetics of paraoxonase.

American Journal of Human Genetics, **45**, 323–30.

Eiberg, H., Mohr, J., Schmiegelow, K., Nielsen, L. S. & Williamson, R. (1985). Linkage relationships of paraoxonase (PON) with other markers: indication of PON-cystic fibrosis synteny. *Clinical Genetics* **28**, 265–71.

Erdos, E. G. & Boggs, L. E. (1961). Hydrolysis of paraoxon in mammalian blood. *Nature* **190**, 716–17.

Fagerlind, L., Holmstedt, B. & Wallen, O. (1952). Preparation and determination of diethyl-*p*-nitrophenol (E 600) a drug used in the treatment of glaucoma. *Svensk farmaceutisk Tidskrift* **56**, 303–11.

Flügel, M. & Geldmacher-v Mallinckrodt, M. (1978). Zur kinetik des paraoxonspaltenden enzyms in menschlichen serum (EC 3,1,1,2). *Klinische Wochenschrift* **56**, 911–16.

Fukoto, T. R. & Metcalf, R. L. (1969). Metabolism of insecticides in plants and animals. *Annals of the New York Academy of Sciences* **160**, 97–113.

Furlong, C. E., Richter, R. J., Seidel, S. L. & Motulsky, A. G. (1988). Role of genetic polymorphism of human plasma paraoxonase/arylesterase in hydrolysis of the insecticide metabolites chlorpyrifos oxon and paraoxon. *American Journal of Human Genetics*, **43**, 230–8.

Gan, K. N., Smolen, A., Eckerson, H. W. & La Du, B. N. (1991). Purification of human serum paraoxonase/ arylesterase. *Drug Metabolism and Disposition*, **19**, 100–6.

Geldmacher-v Mallinckrodt, M. (1978). Polymorphism of human serum paraoxonase. *Human Genetics*, **1** [Suppl.], 65–8.

Geldmacher-v Mallinckrodt, M., Baumgartner, W., Petenyi, M., Burgis, H., Lindorf, H.H. & Metzner, H. (1972). Korrelation zwischen der unterschiedlichen Vergiftbarkeit der serum-cholinesterase durch E 600 und der Aktiv̈at des E600-spaltenden Enzym-Systems in menschlichen Seren. *Hoppe-Seylers Zeitschrift für Physiologische Chemie*, **353**, 217–20.

Geldmacher-v Mallinckrodt, M., Diepgen, T. L., Duhme, C. & Hommel, G. (1983). A study of the polymorphism and ethnic distribution differences of human serum paraoxonase. *American Journal of Physical Anthropology* **62**, 235–41.

Geldmacher-v Mallinckrodt, M., Diepgen, T. L. & Enders, P. W. (1984). Interethnic differences of human serum paraoxonase activity – relevance for the detoxification of organophosphorus compounds. *Archives Belges* Suppl.1, 243–51.

Geldmacher-v Mallinckrodt, M., Hommel, G. & Dumbach, J. (1979). On the genetics of the human serum paraoxonase. *Human Genetics*, **50**, 313–26.

Geldmacher-v Mallinckrodt, M., Lindorf, H. H., Petenyi, M., Flugel, M., Fischer, T. & Hiller, T. (1973). Genetisch determinierter polymorphismus de menschlichen serum-paraoxonase (EC 3,1,1,2). *Human Genetik* **17**, 331–5.

Geldmacher-v Mallinckrodt, M., Rabast, U. & Lindorf, H. H. (1969). Unterschidlische reaction menschlicher serum-cholinesterasen mit E 600 (00 Di-äthyl-*O*-(*p*-nitrophenyl)-phosphat). *Archives of Toxicology*, **25**, 223–8.

Goedde, H. W., Rothhammer, F., Benkmann, H. G. & Bogdanski, P. (1984). Ecogenetic studies in Atacameno Indians. *Human Genetics*, **67**, 343–6.

Hassettt, C., Richter, R. J., Humbert, R., Chapline, C., Crabb, J. W., Omiecinski, C. J. & Furlong, C. E. (1991).

Characterization of cDNA clones encoding rabbit and human serum paraoxonase: the mature protein retains its signal sequence. *Biochemistry*, **30**, 10149–51.

Ishimoto, G., Uchida, H. & Tsuge, A. (1987). Distribution of serum paraoxon hydrolysing activity in family and population samples. *Japanese Journal of Legal Medicine*, **41**, 347–50.

Karakaya, A., Suzen, S., Sardas, S., Karakaya, A. E. & Vural, N. (1991). Analysis of the serum paraoxonase/arylesterase ploymorphism in a Turkish population. *Pharmacogenetics*, **1**, 58–61.

Krisch, von K. (1968). Enzymatische Hydrolyse von diethyl-*p*-nitrophenol phosphat (E 600) durch menschliches Serum. *Zeitschrift für Klinische Chemie und Klinische Biochemie*, **6**, 41–5.

La Du, B. N. (1988). Invited editorial: The human serum paraoxonase/arylesterase polymorphism. *American Journal of Human Genetics*, **43**, 227–9.

La Du, B. N., Adkins, S. & Bayoumi, R. A.-L. (1986b). Analysis of the serum paraoxonase/arylesterase polymorphism in some Sudanese families. In *Ethnic Differences in Reactions to Drugs and Xenobiotics*, ed. W. Kalow, H. W. Geodde & D. P. Agarwal. Progress in Clinical and Biological Research, **214**, 87–98. New York: Alan R Liss.

La Du, B. N., Piko, J. I., Eckerson, H. W., Vincent-Viry, M. & Siest, G. (1986a). An improved method for phenotyping individuals for the human serum paraoxonase arylesterase polymorphism. *Annales de Biologie Clinique*, **44**, 369–72.

Lauwerys, R. R. & Murphy, S. D. (1969). Comparison of assay methods for studying 0,0-diethyl-*O-p*-nitrophenyl phosphate (paraoxon) detoxification *in vitro*. *Biochemical Pharmacology*, **18**, 789–800.

McElveen, J., Mackness, M. I., Colley, C. M., Peard, T., Warner, S. & Walker, C. H. (1986). Distribution of paraoxon hydrolytic activity in the serum of patients after myocardial infarction. *Clinical Chemistry* **32**, 671–3.

Mackness, M. I., Harty, D., Bhatnagar, D., Winocour, P. H., Arrol, S., Ishola, M. & Durrington, P. N. (1991). Serum paraoxonase activity in familial hypercholesterolaemia and insulin-dependent diabetes mellitus. *Atherosclerosis*, **86**, 193–9.

Main, A. R., (1956). The role of A-esterase in the acute toxicity of paraxon, TEPP and parathion. *Canadian Journal of Biochemistry and Physiology*, **34**, 197–216

Main, A. R. (1960). The purification of the enzyme hydrolysing diethyl-*p*-nitrophenyl phosphate (paraoxon) in sheep serum. *Biochemical Journal*, **74**, 10–20.

Marx, J. L. (1989). The cystic fibrosis gene is found. *Science*, **245**, 923–5.

Mody, M. Adkins, S., Gan, K. & La Du, B. (1992). Direct evidence from peptide sequencing for one amino acid difference in human serum paraoxonase/arylesterase A and B isozymes. *FASEB*, Abstract 3741.

Mueller, R. F., Hornung, S., Furlong, C. E., Anderson, J., Giblett, E. R. & Motulsky, A. G. (1983). Plasma paraoxonase polymorphism: A new enzyme assay, population, family, biochemical and linkage studies. *American Journal of Human Genetics*, **35**, 393–408.

Nielsen, A., Eibert, H., Fenger, K. & Mohr, J. (1986b). Number of 'high genes' involved in determining the activity of paraoxonase. *Clinical Genetics* **30**, 41–9.

Nielsen, A., Eibert, H. & Mohr, J. (1986a). Number of loci responsible for the inheritance of high and low activity of paraoxonase. *Clinical Genetics*, **29**, 216–21.

Nogueira, C. P., Evans, D. A. P. & La Du, B. N. (1988). The human paraoxonase/esterase in a sample population from Saudi Arabia. *Genome*, **30** (Suppl. 1), 362 (abstract).

Nogueria, C. P. Evans, D. A. P. & La Du, B. N. (1992). Study of the polymorphism of paraoxonase in a population sample from Saudi Arabia. *Pharmacogenetics* (in press).

Ortigoza-Ferado, J., Richter, R. J., Hornung, S. K., Motulsky, A. G. & Furlong, C. E. (1984). Paraoxon hydrolysis in human serum mediated by a genetically variable arylesterase and albumin. *American Journal of Human Genetics*, **36**, 295–305.

Paik, Y. K., Benkmann, H. G. & Goedde, H. W. (1988). Incidence of the homozygous phenotype for low activity serum paraoxonase in Korea. *Korean Journal of Genetics*, **10**, 261–4.

Playfer, J. R., Eze, L. C., Bullen, M. F. & Evans, D. A. P. (1976). Genetic polymorphism and inter-ethnic variability of plasma paraoxonase activity. *Journal of Medical Genetics*, **13**, 337–42.

Rona, K., Szabo, I., Gachalyi, B., Czinner, A. & Kaldor, A. (1987). A human szerum-paraoxonaz polimorfizmus. *Orvosi-Hetilap*, **126**, 2469–72.

Roy, A. C., Saha, N., Tay, J. S. H. & Ratnam, S. S. (1991). Serum paraoxonase polymorphism in three populations of South East Asia. *Human Heredity*, **41**, 265–9.

Saha, N., Roy, A. C., Teo, S. H., Tay, J. S. H. & Ratnam, S. S. (1991). Influence of serum paraoxonase polymorphism on serum lipids and apolipoproteins. *Clinical Genetics*, **40**, 277–82.

Schmiegelow, K., Eiberg, H., Tsui, L.-C., Buchwald, M., Phelan, P. D., Williamson, R., Warwick, W., Niebuhr, E., Mohr, J., Schwartz, M. & Koch, C. (1986). Linkage between the loci for cystic fibrosis and paraoxonase. *Clinical Genetics*, **29**, 374–7.

Secchiero, S., Mussap, M., Zaninotto, M., Bertorelle, R. & Burlina, A. (1989). Serum arylesterase (paraoxonase) activity following myocardial infarction. *Clinica Chimica Acta*, **183**, 71–6.

Smolen, A., Eckerson, H. W., Gan, K. N., Hailat, N. & La Du, B. N. (1991). Characteristics of the genetically determined allozymic forms of human serum paraoxonase/arylesterase. *Drug Metabolism and Disposition*, **19**, 107–12.

Szabo, I., Rona, K., Czinner, A. & Gachalyi, B. (1991). Human paraoxonase polymorphism: Hungarian population studies in children and adults. *International Journal of Clinical Pharmacology Therapy and Toxicology*, **29**, 238–41.

Szabo, I., Rona, K., Czinner, A., Gachalyi, B. & Kaldor, A. (1987a). A human szerum paraoxonaz-aktivitas polimorfmusanak vizsgalata gyermekekben. *Orvosi-Hetilap*, **128**, 631–3.

Szabo, I., Rona, K., Czinner, A., Gachalyi, B. & Kaldor, A. (1987b).Is paraoxon hydrolytic activity in serum predictive of myocardial infarction? *Clinical Chemistry*, **33**, 742–3.

Taylor, W. J. R., Kalow, W. & Sellers, E. A. (1965). Poisoning with organo-phosphorus insecticides. *Canadian Medical Association Journal*, **93**, 966–70.

Vincent-Viry, M., La Du, B. N., Lepage, L. & Mikstacki, T.

(1986). Distribution des differents phénotypes de la paraoxonase dans une population francaise. *Annales de Biologie Clinique*, **44**, 233–8.

Whitehouse, L. W. & Ecobichon, D. J. (1975). Paraoxon formation and hydrolysis by mammalian liver. *Pesticide Biochemistry and Physiology*, **5**, 314–22.

Williams, F. M., Nicholson, E. N., Woolhouse, N. W., Adjepon-Yamoah, K. K. & Rawlins, M. D. (1986). Activity of esterases in plasma from Ghanaian and British subjects. *European Journal of Clinical Pharmacology*, **31**, 485–9.

22 Sulphotransferases

INTRODUCTION

SULPHATE conjugation is a mechanism of detoxifying foreign compounds, especially phenols, which has been known for many years (see Williams 1959). The essential enzyme for this biotransformation is phenol-sulphotransferase (PST) (EC 2.8.2.1). The sulphate groups which are transferred are derived from 3'-phosphoadenosine-5'-phosphosulphate (PAPS: Fig. 22.1).

Fig. 22.1. 3'-phosphoadenosine-5'-phosphosulphate (PAPS). (From Williams 1959.)

The general setting for more recent studies was provided by Dodgson (1977), from which the following key points may be noted.

The sulphation pathway occurs in three steps:

ATP + SO$_4^-$ → APS + PPi (ATP-sulphate adenyltransferase)

APS + ATP → PAPS + ADP (ATP-adenylylsulphate 3'-phosphotransferase)

PAPS + acceptor → PAP + sulphated acceptor (sulphotransferase)

There was evidence for the supply of sulphate being limited. For example, increasing oral doses of salicylamide produced a decreasing fraction of the dose excreted as the sulphate – a phenomenon which was preventable by the concomitant consumption of L-cysteine.

Sulphotransferases were known to be cytosolic and also membrane-bound in the endoplasmic reticulum and Golgi apparatus. The former category sulphated small molecules including phenols, whilst the latter class sulphated larger molecules such as carbohydrates and tyrosine residues in polypeptides. The membrane-bound enzymes appeared early in embryogenesis whereas the cytosolic enzymes appeared just before birth. The enzymes were found to be difficult to purify, and because of this it was difficult to decide whether different cytosolic enzymes sulphated different substrates such as p-nitrophenol and tyramine.

Against this background a search was made to find how sulphotransferases could be examined easily in humans.

Platelets were found to contain two forms of PST that could be distinguished on the basis of differences in physical properties, substrate specificity and regulation. The two forms have been labelled TS (thermostable) and TL (thermolabile) by Weinshilboum's group (Reiter & Weinshilboum 1982) and P (specific for phenol) and M (specific for monoamines) by Bonham Carter et al. (1983). There is a fairly close identity between TS and P on the one hand and TL and M on the other. The substances metabolized at micromolar concentrations by the

Table 22.1. *The metabolism of drugs and other chemicals by the two forms of platelet sulphotransferase*

M-form thermolabile (TL)	P-form[a] thermostable (TS)
alphamethyldopa	phenol
dopamine	*p*-nitrophenol
m-tyramine	paracetamol
paracetamol[b]	salicylamide[c]
noradrenaline	*N*-oxide of minoxidil
adrenaline	tyrosines in peptides
5-hydroxytryptamine	tri-iodothyronine
p-hydroxyamphetamine	
isoprenaline	
salbutamol	
1-naphthol	
tri-iodothyronine	

[a] the P form is selectively inhibited by dichloronitrophenol.
[b] predominantly metabolized by the M form.
[c] at low concentrations, metabolized by the P form, but by the M form at higher concentrations.
Constructed from information given mainly in: Bonham Carter *et al.* 1983; Falany 1991.

two forms of enzyme are shown in Table 22.1. It seems likely that salbutamol, ritodrine and fenoterol are also metabolized by the M form because their sulphation was not inhibited by dichloronitrophenol (DCNP: Sodha & Schneider 1984).

Within the category of TS PST (usually determined using *p*-nitrophenol) the thermal stability at 44 °C for 15 minutes was found to exhibit interindividual variability. This was expressed as a ratio of heated/control activities (H/C). The frequency distribution of untransformed H/C ratios yielded a suggestion of an antimode at 0.33, and this gave rise to the curious designation of thermolabile TS PST in 13% of the population. This subgroup had low basal TS PST activities (Van Loon & Weinshilboum 1984).

Heroux & Roth (1988) found that PST P from platelets had a M_r of about 69 000 made up of subunits with M_r of about 34 000. It was found that PAPS protected the enzyme from the sulphydryl-modifying agent *N*-ethylmaleimide, and the suggestion was made that the active site contained at least one sulphydryl group. Heroux *et al.* (1989) raised antibodies to a purified preparation of the most electronegative form of the human platelet enzyme termed M_{II} PST. Two sizes of molecules reacted with these antibodies, namely, one of 34 kDa which had

dopamine sulphating activity and one of 32kDa which had phenol sulphating activity. So the evidence was strongly in favour of M(TL) PST being a homodimer of the 34 kDa units and the P(TS) PST being a homodimer of the 32 kDa units.

CORRELATION OF THE PHENOL SULPHOTRANSFERASE ACTIVITY OF PLATELETS WITH THAT OF OTHER CELLS AND TISSUES

Using dopamine sulphation as an index Anderson *et al.* (1991) found that 97% of whole blood TL PST activity was in platelets. Using *p*-nitrophenol as an index they found that 77% of whole blood TS PST activity was in platelets and 19% in granulocytes.

The idea behind investigating platelet PST activity was that this might mirror the activity in metabolically important internal organs. Therefore the enzyme has been investigated in various organs and then the activities in them correlated with that in the platelet. Thus a correlation has been found between the TS PST activities of platelets and those of cerebral cortex, liver and small intestinal mucosa. No such correlations were found for TL PST activities (Weinshilboum 1990).

In the course of this work some other interesting findings have emerged. In jejunal mucosa TL PST activity is much higher than elsewhere. In liver two types of TS PST could be separated using ion-exchange chromatography. Individual livers possessed one or other or both types (Table 22.2). Peak I had a specific activity $2\frac{1}{2}$ times that of Peak II. No information has yet been published correlating these individual liver TS PST phenotypes with platelet TS PST activities.

GENETIC STUDIES

An early twin study (Reveley *et al.* 1982/83) yielded high heritabilities for both TS PST and TL PST.

A study involving 231 first-degree relatives in 49 randomly selected families was carried out by Van Loon & Weinshilboum (1984) to find out the inheritance of 'thermolabile TS' PST. There were no significant differences between parents and children either in average basal enzymic activity levels or in average H/C ratios. It must be pointed out that the bimodality in the frequency distribution curve of the

Table 22.2. *Phenol sulphotransferase activities in various human tissues*

Reference	Tissue	Method of Assay	Conclusion
Campbell *et al.* 1987	Liver	Dopamine and *p*-nitrophenol sulphation estimated on fractions obtained from first ion-exchange and then gel-filtration chromatography	The two forms of PST i.e. TS and TL characterized. Correlation with individual platelet activity not made. Two peaks of TS PST found on ion-exchange chromatography. Individuals contained either one or the other or both peaks. These two peaks differed in thermal stability but were very similar for pH optima, lack of activity with dopamine, K_m for PAPS and *p*-nitrophenol
Sundaram *et al.* 1989a	Jejunal mucosa	Ditto	TS and TL forms of PST characterized, the latter activity being much higher than in other tissues
Sundaram *et al.* 1989b	Platelets and jejunal mucosa (per oral biopsy samples; 9 random & 5 because they had 'TL TS' PST in platelets)	Assays with dopamine and *p*-nitrophenol. Thermal stability experiments	Correlation between platelet and jejunal mucosa TS (*p*-nitrophenol) activity $r = 0.574$. Correlation between H/C TS activities ($r = 0.83$) in the two tissues. No correlation between platelet and jejunal mucosa TL (dopamine) activities $r = 0.265$.
Heroux *et al.* 1989	Various human tissues including platelets	Immuno-blotting techniques	Adrenal and liver showed the highest reactivity of P-PST with small amounts in placenta and platelets. M-PST activity ws detected in placenta and platelets only
Cappiello *et al.* 1990	Fetal and adult liver and placenta	Cytosolic fraction assayed with 2-naphthol	The placental concentration of PAPS was found to be about one-third of that in liver whereas the activity of PST was about one tenth. The activity of PST in fetal liver was lower than in adult liver

PST, phenolsulphotransferase; TS, thermostable approximately equivalent to P (phenolic); TL, thermolabile approximately equivalent to M (monoamine); PAPS, 3′-phosphoadenosine-5′-phosphosulphate; H/C, heated/control ratio of PST activity.

untransformed H/C ratio was not really striking. Probably because of this, the pedigree analysis was not presented in the manner customary for Mendelian characters. Nevertheless there was a significant aggregation of individuals with H/C < 0.33 ('thermolabile TS') in certain families.

Price *et al.* (1988) performed a sophisticated analysis on the TL PST activity (determined using dopamine as a substrate) in 232 individuals who comprised 49 nuclear families identified through randomly sampled individuals. Females had higher values than males, and there was a significant correlation of activity with age. Correcting for these variables and removing two extreme outlying values gave a frequency distribution curve with greatly reduced skewness but which was still significantly non-normal. The best fitting model for the untransformed data was one that included a dominantly expressed major gene with a frequency of 0.08 for the high activity allele and moderately heritable ($H = 0.49$) multifactorial background variation. A

polygenic model with high heritability (0.77) adequately accounted for the log transformed data. So the conclusions were that there was solid evidence for polygenic inheritance, and it was possible that there may have been in addition a major gene effect.

A similar paper (Price *et al.* 1989) dealing with TS PST yielded a heritability estimate of 0.81. In this case, however, there was also evidence for a single genetic locus with alleles for high and low activities with frequencies of 0.20 and 0.80, respectively (i.e. a genetic polymorphism).

THERMOSTABLE (P-FORM) HUMAN PHENOL SULPHOTRANSFERASE CLONED

Using a cDNA encoding phenol sulphotransferase (ST) from a rat as a probe Ozawa *et al.* (1992) isolated a human phenol cDNA from a human liver cDNA library. This human cDNA was inserted into

Table 22.3. *Ethnic comparisons of TS PST activities*

Ethnic group	Number	Total TS PST activity (u/10^8 platelets)[a]	H/C	Cut-off point (COP)	% of subjects below COP	Distribution of thermal ratio	TS PST activity	H/C
Black	104	0.59 ± 0.04	0.48 ± 0.02	0.32	13.5	< H/C 0.32 ($n=14$)	0.34 ± 0.06	0.22 ± 0.02
						> H/C 0.32 ($n=90$)	0.63 ± 0.05	0.52 ± 0.01
White	63	0.33 ± 0.02	0.40 ± 0.02	0.27	12.7	< H/C 0.27 ($n=8$)	0.19 ± 0.04	0.17 ± 0.02
						> H/C 0.27 ($n=55$)	0.35 ± 0.03	0.43 ± 0.01

TS, thermostable; PST, phenol sulphotransferase; H/C, heated/control.
[a] 1 unit = 1 nmol *p*-nitrophenol sulphated per hour of incubation at 37 °C.
Constructed from data in: Anderson *et al.* 1988.

Table 22.4. *Correlation of urinary excretion of paracetamol as sulphate with platelet PST activities in 29 individuals*

Method of estimating paracetamol excreted as sulphate	Compound used to assess platelet PST activity	r	p
% of dose ingested	*p*-nitrophenol	0.62	<0.001
	paracetamol	0.67	<0.001
	dopamine	0.46	<0.020
% of total of paracetamol and all metabolites excreted	*p*-nitrophenol	0.56	<0.002
	paracetamol	0.55	<0.002
	dopamine	0.32	>0.050

Data from: Reiter & Weinshilboum 1982.

an expression vector and transfected into *E. coli*. An immunoreactive ST was produced which catalysed the sulphation of minoxidil and *p*-nitrophenol.

INTER-ETHNIC COMPARISONS

Comparisons of TS PST activities in American blacks and whites were made by Anderson & Jackson (1984) and Anderson *et al.* (1988). The essential information from the latter study is condensed in Table 22.3 where it can be seen that the activity is higher in blacks than in whites. This finding was further confirmed by Anderson & Liebentritt (1990), who also studied seven American Indians who gave results closely similar to whites.

CORRELATIONS OF VARIABILITY IN PLATELET PST WITH DRUG METABOLISM

Paracetamol (acetaminophen) was shown to be a substrate for both platelet TS PST (assessed with

p-nitrophenol) and platelet TL PST. There was no correlation between these two activities.

Paracetamol 24 hour urinary excretion following a single oral dose of 10 mg per kg body weight was assessed as unchanged drug plus sulphate + glucuronide in 29 randomly selected subjects (14 white women, 14 white men and one black man) by Reiter & Weinshilboum (1982). The platelet PST activity as assessed with paracetamol correlated with the same as assessed using *p*-nitrophenol ($r = 0.78$) and dopamine ($r = 0.71$). There were significant correlations between the excretion of an oral dose of 10 mg paracetamol per kg body weight as the sulphate, and platelet PST activities (Table 22.4). The relative contributions of the TL and TS forms of the enzyme to the sulphation were estimated to vary over eight-fold between individuals. In view of the information already reviewed it is considered likely that the platelet enzyme activity mirrors the sulphotransferase activity in the internal organs. Other factors could affect the degree of sulphate conjugation of paracetamol, e.g. the availability of sulphate and

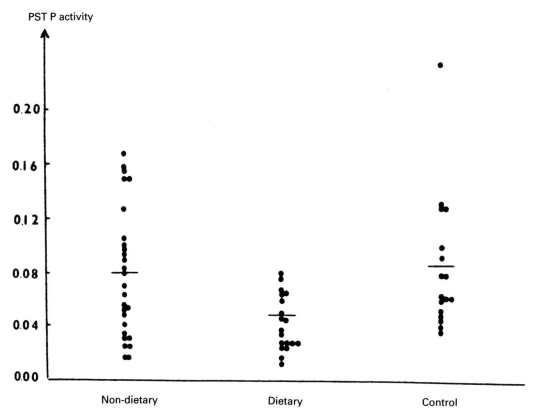

Fig. 22.2. PST-P activity values in migrainous patients and controls. Activity expressed as nmoles of phenol conjugated/mg protein/10 min. $p < 0.02$: dietary less than controls. $p < 0.01$: dietary less than non-dietary. $p < 0.01$: dietary less than non-dietary plus controls. (From Littlewood *et al.* 1982.)

glucuronide formation. The former was not thought to influence the result with the dose of paracetamol used. It was not possible fully to dissociate the variabilities in sulphate and glucuronide conjugation.

The amount of sulphate conjugate of paracetamol excreted after the ingestion of 1 g, was assessed for correlation with platelet PST activity using paracetamol, salicylamide, tyramine and phenol as substrates, by Bonham Carter *et al.* (1983). Only with the last compound was there a significant correlation ($r = 0.54$, $p < 0.05$) obtained. The reason for the disparity between the results of these two studies is unclear.

Another drug which is conjugated with sulphate in the body is the antihypertensive α-methyldopa. In order to assess the *in vivo/in vitro* correlation

Campbell *et al.* (1985) performed an experiment using 24 subjects who consumed 3.5 mg α-methyldopa per kg body weight. There was a significant positive correlation between platelet TL PST activity and the percentage of metabolites excreted as methyldopa sulphate ($r = 0.545$, $p < 0.01$), and a negative correlation with the proportion of the drug excreted as free methyldopa ($r = -0.624$, $p < 0.01$). These results could only be obtained in the presence of sulphate supplementation, suggesting that the enhanced supply of sulphate enabled the full potential of PST enzymes to be realized in the intestinal mucosa and/or liver.

It is strange that correlations of conjugation *in vivo* with platelet PST activities do not seem to have been assessed with other drugs.

RELATIONSHIP TO A SPONTANEOUS DISORDER

Classical migraine is well known to be precipitated in some patients by items of diet such as chocolate, cheese, citrus fruits, wines, etc. Sometimes the same individual gets migraine with more than one of these items.

Littlewood *et al.* (1982) investigated the possibility that a relative deficiency of PST might be a factor in the aetiology of 'dietary' migraine by measuring the platelet P PST (approximately equivalent to TS PST) and M PST (approximately equivalent to TL PST). They found that the P PST activity was significantly lower in 16 dietary migraine subjects (mean 0.043 nmol phenol conjugated/mg protein/10 minutes) than in 18 non-dietary migraine subjects (0.072) or in 17 non-migrainous controls (0.081) (Fig. 22.2). The M PST values (assessed with tyramine) were not significantly different between the groups.

A confirmatory study was carried out by Launay *et al.* (1988). They found that platelet P PST (using phenol) and M PST (using tyramine) were both significantly lower in 18 dietary migraine sufferers than in 13 non-dietary migraine sufferers in remission, 17 non-dietary migraine sufferers in an attack (including the preceding group) and 18 controls. The findings of Davis *et al.* (1987) were also confirmatory in that they found that the average TS PST for 19 unselected migrainous subjects was 70% that of controls.

So the postulated mechanism is that the dietary migraine subject may be, because of the genetic endowment of phenol sulphotransferase, relatively unable to detoxify by sulphation migraine-provoking substances occurring in the diet.

In this context it is difficult to evaluate the account given by Williams & Franklin (1989) of a 24 year old man who suffered from lymphoblastic leukaemia and received a successful bone marrow transplantation from his mother. Both the mother and her sister suffered from classical migraine. Within a month of receiving the transplanted marrow the patient started having severe classical migraine attacks without any identifiable dietary or other triggering factor. It is possible that he would have become migrainous without his transplant, or the illness with its associated drug therapy precipitated his migraine, or he may have acquired it along with his mother's marrow and platelets. The PST activities were unfortunately not studied in this patient. It seems in general that this pharmacogenetic system has been inadequately evaluated in clinical medicine.

Now that the gene for the thermostable (P-form) has been cloned the stage is set for an examination of inter-individual genetic variability at a molecular level. Then it may be possible to use restriction fragment length polymorphisms or allele-specific probes to investigate clinical phenomena more analytically.

N-SULPHOTRANSFERASE

The *N*-sulphotransferase activity of human tissues has hitherto received very little attention. Romiti *et al.* (1992) showed that using desipramine as a substrate there was a 27-fold variability in human liver and over 63-fold variation in platelets. The frequency distribution was markedly skewed. No genetic studies have yet been conducted on this enzymic activity.

Anderson, R. J., Garcia, M. J., Liebentritt, D. K. & Kay, H. D. (1991). Localization of human blood phenol sulfotransferase activities: novel detection of the thermostable enzyme in granulocytes. *Journal of Laboratory and Clinical Medicine*, **118**, 500–9.

Anderson, R. J. & Jackson, B. L. (1984). Human platelet phenol sulfo-transferase: stability of two forms of the enzyme with time and presence of a racial difference. *Clinica Chimica Acta*, **138**, 185–96.

Anderson, R. J., Jackson, B. L. & Liebentritt, D.K. (1988). Human platelet thermostable phenol sulfotransferase from blacks and whites: Biochemical properties and variations in thermal stability. *Journal of Laboratory and Clinical Medicine*, **112**, 773–83.

Anderson, R. J. & Liebentritt, D. K. (1990). Human platelet thermostable phenol sulfotransferase: assay of frozen samples and correlation between frozen and fresh activities. *Clinica Chimica Acta*, **189**, 221–30.

Bonham Carter, S. M., Rein, G., Glover, V. & Sandler, M. (1983). Human platelet phenol sulphotransferase M and P: substrate specificities and correlation with *in vivo* sulphoconjugation of paracetamol and salicylamide. *British Journal of Clinical Pharmacology*, **15**, 323–30.

Campbell, N. R. C., Sundaram, R. S., Werness, P. G., Van Loon, J. & Weinshilboum, R. M. (1985). Sulfate and methyldopa metabolism: Metabolite patterns and platelet phenol sulfotransferase activity. *Clinical Pharmacology and Therapeutics*, **37**, 308–15.

Campbell, N. R. C., Van Loon, J. A. & Weinshilboum, R. M. (1987). Human liver phenol sulfotransferase: assay conditions, biochemical properties and partial purification of isozymes of the thermostable form. *Biochemical Pharmacology*, **36**, 1435–46.

Cappiello, M., Franchi, M., Rane, A. & Pacifici, G. M. (1990). Sulphotransferase and its substrate. Adenosine-3'-phosphate-5'-phosphosulphate in human fetal liver and placenta. *Developmental Pharmacology and Therapeutics*, **14**, 62–5.

Davis, B. A., Dawson, B., Boulton, A. A., Yu, P. H. & Durden, D. A. (1987). Investigation of some biological trait markers in migraine. Deuterated tyramine challenge test, monoamine oxidase, phenol sulfotransferase, and plasma and urinary biogenic amine and acid metabolite levels. *Headache*, **27**, 384–9.

Dodgson, K. S. (1977). Conjugation with sulphate. In *Drug Metabolism from Microbe to Man*, ed. D. V. Parke & R. L. Smith, pp. 91–104. London: Taylor & Francis.

Falany, C. N. (1991). Molecular enzymology of human liver cytosolic sulfotransferases. *Trends in Pharmacological Sciences*, **12**, 255–9.

Heroux, J. A., Falany, C. N. & Roth, J. A. (1989). Immunological characterization of human phenol sulfotransferase. *Molecular Pharmacology*, **36**, 29–33.

Heroux, J. A. & Roth, J. A. (1988). Physical characterization of a monoamine-sulfating form of phenol sulfotransferase from human platelets. *Molecular Pharmacology*, **34**, 194–9.

Launay, J. M., Soliman, H., Pradalier, A., Dry, J. & Dreux, C. (1988). Activités PST plaquettaires, le 'trait' migraineaux? *Therapie*, **43**, 273–7.

Littlewood, J., Glover, V., Sandler, M., Petty, R., Peatfield, R. & Rose, F.C. (1982). Platelet phenolsulphotransferase deficiency in dietary migraine. *Lancet*, **1**, 983–6.

Ozawa, S., Nagata, K., Gong, D.-W., Yamazoe, Y. & Kato, R. (1992). Cloning expression and functional characterization of rat and human phenol sulfotransferases. *Journal of Pharmacobio-Dynamics*, **15**, 5–21.

Price, R. A., Cox, N. J., Spielman, R. S., Van Loon, J. A., Maidak, B. L. & Weinshilboum, R. M. (1988). Inheritance of human platelet thermolabile phenol sulfotransferase (TL PST) activity. *Genetic Epidemiology*, **5**, 1–15.

Price, R. A., Spielman, R. S., Lucena, A. L., Van Loon, J. A., Madik, B. L. & Weinshilboum, R. M. (1989). Genetic polymorphism for human platelet thermostable phenol sulfotransferase (TS PST) activity. *Genetics*, **122**, 905–14.

Reiter, C. & Weinshilboum, R. (1982). Platelet phenol sulfotransferase activity: correlation with sulfate conjugation of acetaminophen. *Clinical Pharmacology and Therapeutics*, **32**, 612–21.

Reveley, A. M., Carter, S. M. B., Reveley, M. A. & Sandler, M. (1982/3). A genetic study of platelet phenol sulfotransferase activity in normal and schizophrenic twins. *Journal of Psychiatric Research*, **17**, 303–7.

Romiti, P., Giuliani, L. & Pacifici, G. M. (1992). Interindividual variability in the *N*-sulphation of desipramine in human liver and platelets. *British Journal of Clinical Pharmacology*, **3**, 17–23.

Sodha, R. J. & Schneider, H. (1984). Sulphate conjugation of β_2-adrenoceptor stimulating drugs by platelet and placental phenol sulphotransferase. *British Journal of Clinical Pharmacology*, **17**, 106–8.

Sundaram, R. S., Szumlanski, C., Otterness, D., Van Loon, J. A. & Weinshilboum, R. M. (1989a). Human intestinal phenol sulfotransferase: assay conditions, activity levels and partial purification of the thermolabile form. *Drug Metabolism and Disposition*, **17**, 255–64.

Sundaram, R. S., Van Loon, J. A., Tucker, R. & Weinshilboum, R. M. (1989b). Sulfation pharmacogenetics: correlation of human platelet and small intestinal phenol sulfotransferase. *Clinical Pharmacology and Therapeutics*, **46**, 501–9.

Van Loon, J. & Weinshilboum, R. M. (1984). Human platelet phenol sulfotransferase: familial variation in thermal stability of the TS form. *Biochemical Genetics*, **22**, 997–1014.

Weinshilboum, R. M. (1990). Sulfotransferase pharmacogenetics. *Pharmacology and Therapeutics*, **45**, 93–107.

Williams, A. C. & Franklin, I. (1989). Migraine after bone-marrow transplantation. *Lancet*, **2**, 1286–7.

Williams, R. T. (1959). *Detoxication Mechanisms*, 2nd edn, pp. 79–82. London: Chapman & Hall.

23 Sulphoxidation deficiency

INTRODUCTION

THE DEFICIENCY of sulphoxidation has been studied in man principally using one compound, namely S-carboxymethyl-L-cysteine (SCMC: Fig. 23.1). This compound is marketed as a mucolytic agent taken orally, and a single dose can be regarded as innocuous for experimental purposes.

The metabolic fate of the compound was investigated by Waring (1978), who found that in humans the sulphoxide could be found in the urine. This finding was not reported by Turnbull *et al.* (1978). Later, Waring & Mitchell (1982) published a map showing the pathways of metabolism of SCMC, which indicated that four sulphoxides were produced in humans (Fig. 23.2).

For routine assessment of the metabolism of SCMC in individuals, descending paper chromatography of urine was carried out in four solvent systems. Different amounts of standards of known metabolites were added to control urine and chromatographed. The sulphur containing compounds were visualized as spots using a chloroplatinate reaction. The areas of the spots were measured by planimetric densitometry and the quantity of each metabolite determined by reference to the standard curve. The biological repeatability of the excretion pattern in 40 individuals on two occasions was high, and was almost identical in four individuals tested five times over a period of several months (Mitchell *et al.* 1984).

When the percentage of the drug which was excreted as sulphoxides (having been formed from

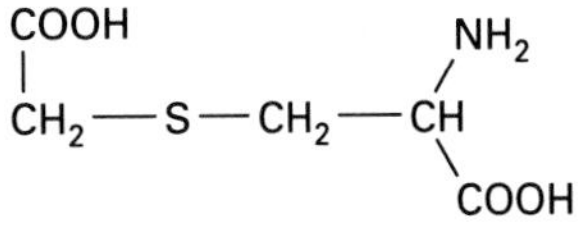

S–(carboxymethyl)–L–cysteine

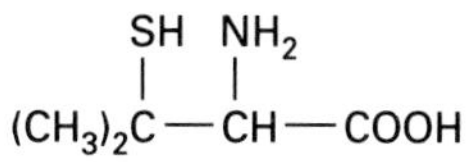

Penicillamine

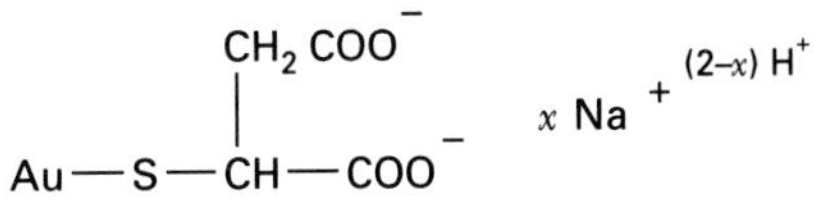

Sodium aureothiomalate

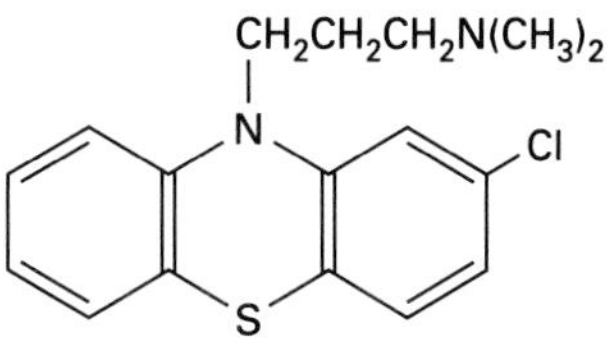

Chlorpromazine

Fig. 23.1. Structural formulae of some drugs discussed in connection with sulphoxidation.

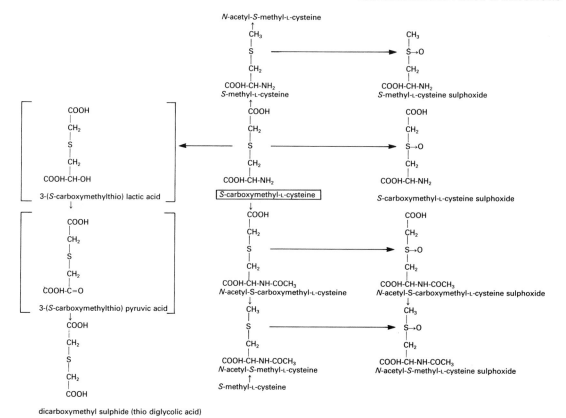

Fig. 23.2. Proposed pathways of metabolism of S-carboxymethyl-L-cysteine. (From Waring & Mitchell 1982.)

the original molecule directly or indirectly) was examined in 20 volunteer subjects, a very wide variability was found and there was a suggestion of a discontinuous frequency distribution (Waring 1980).

It was found that women on oral contraceptive steroids (OCS) excreted more sulphoxides than women not on OCS. Collection of the urine sample overnight for 8 hours following SCMC ingestion yielded less sulphoxides than daytime collection. The influence on the results of deliberately eating or not eating foods which are particularly rich in sulphur was not studied. This point is mentioned here because certain sulphur containing compounds are excreted in the sweat to a considerable degree after eating garlic, as mentioned by Harris et al. (1986). Preserved foods contain considerable amounts of sulphur dioxide and sulphites. Dried fruits are high in sulphur content as are shellfish, whilst meat,

chicken and fish have a moderately high content. It is possible, therefore, that variations in the diet might be capable of influencing the result of the SCMC test. Karim et al. (1989) investigating this possibility found that S-methyl-L-cysteine sulphoxide occurs in the urine after the ingestion of cauliflower, cabbage and leeks and calculations of the sulphoxidation index may be influenced by such dietary factors.

After this the story developed into two different aspects, which will now be briefly described.

GENETIC ASPECTS

Healthy persons were tested, first by Waring et al. (1982) and then by Mitchell et al. (1984), using a standard dose of SCMC and urine collected for 8 hours following ingestion. The percentage of the dose recovered in the urine as the sulphoxides was determined. The distribution of this parameter in 200 unrelated individuals showed significant deviation from normality as also did the distribution of the same data expressed as a 'sulphoxidation index' (SI) where

$$SI = \frac{100 - \% \text{ recovery as sulphoxides}}{\% \text{ recovery as sulphoxides}}$$

There was no clear bimodality of the former distribution curve on inspection but a maximum likelihood computer analysis showed that the best fit was given by a bimodal model which indicated the antimode to be at 14.3% recovery as sulphoxides (SI = 6). This finding gave rise to the concept that there were two metabolic phenotypes, with impaired and extensive sulphoxidation characteristics. Sex, age, and body weight had no correlation with SI. The authors point out that due to the overlap of the two curves, taking SI = 6 'as the cut off point will lead to a certain amount of misclassification with 1.3% of the impaired being misclassified as extensive and 12.3% of the extensives being misclassified as impaired' (Mitchell *et al.* 1984).

Despite this suggestion of bimodality a biometric (quantitative genetic) analysis was performed on pedigrees and yielded a marital correlation of 0.498 ($n = 12$) a parent–offspring correlation of 0.728 ($n = 44$) and a sib–sib correlation of 0.920 ($n = 12$). These findings suggested both genetic and environmental components of inter-individual variability.

A study of 22 sets of twins (11 sets monozygous) gave results pointing to a similar conclusion with a heritability estimate of 64.6% (Mitchell & Waring 1989).

A study of 39 two-generation family units possessed rather curious features. The frequency distribution of the percentage of the SCMS dose recovered in 0 to 8 hours after ingestion as sulphoxides in the parents was unimodal (Fig. 23.3) yet the cut-

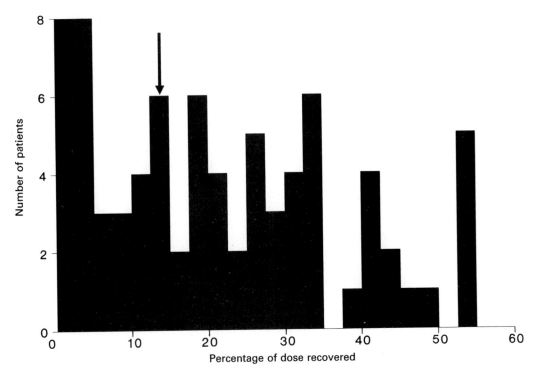

Fig. 23.3. The frequency distribution of the percentage of the dose of *S*-carboxymethyl-L-cysteine recovered in the urine in 0 to 8 hours as sulphoxide metabolites following ingestion of the drug in 78 parents. The arrow indicates the alleged antimodal point separating the phenotypes at 14.3%. (Drawn from data in Mitchell & Waring 1989.)

off point of 14.3% was employed. The proportions of impaired and extensive sulphoxidizers in the parents (30:48) was significantly different to that of the population study, i.e. 45:155 ($\chi_1^2 = 7.25$), yet the latter was taken for the gene frequency estimate on which to base the computations on the families. Although the misclassification estimates had been published earlier (as mentioned above) the frequencies of the phenotypes observed among the offspring of different mating types were amazingly close to expectations (Mitchell & Waring 1989).

RELATIONSHIP TO ESTABLISHED POLYMORPHISMS

There was found to be a lack of correlation between sulphoxidation status and the phenylthiocarbamide (PTC, phenylthiourea) taste-testing (Ayesh *et al.* 1988) and debrisoquine hydroxylation (Haley *et al.* 1985) polymorphisms.

SITE OF SULPHOXIDATION

Investigations carried out by Waring *et al.* (1986), using liver tissue from a variety of mammalian species including man, showed that the sulphoxidation enzymes were cytosolic; microsomal fractions had no activity. A huge improvement in sulphoxidation capacity following liver transplantation for various conditions was observed by Olomu *et al.* (1988).

A CURIOSITY – BLACK SPECKLED DOLLS

An interesting occupational hazard where the risk is to the product rather than to the operative was described by Harris *et al.* (1986). A healthy 16 year old girl made reproduction china dolls. Whenever she touched a doll's head when painting it, black speckles appeared at the next firing. Enquiry revealed that she ate a lot of garlic, and sulphur-containing compounds from this source were excreted in her sweat. The clay from which the dolls were made contained iron. So the likelihood was that the speckles were due to sulphides of iron. Their occurrence was prevented by the girl abstaining from garlic. Testing her with SCMC showed her to be an impaired sulphoxidizer.

CLINICAL STUDIES

A number of studies have been performed to discover whether there was a statistical association between either sulphoxidation phenotype (as defined earlier) and various clinical conditions.

The rationale for performing these association studies has been varied, and will be described before the results are presented.

Penicillamine was known to be extensively metabolized so that 4% of a dose was excreted as S-methyl-penicillamine, 25% as mixed disulphides and lesser amounts as intermediate oxidation products. There was also said to be some structural similarity between penicillamine and SCMC. Hence it was considered possible that sulphoxidation capacity might reflect the ability to eliminate penicillamine from the body, even though penicillamine is not itself sulphoxidized (Waring & Mitchell, 1988).

Some rheumatoid arthritis patients who develop adverse reactions to penicillamine are also prone to develop adverse reactions to aurothiomalate. Since it had been found that 'impaired sulphoxidizers' were more susceptible than 'extensive sulphoxidizers' to penicillamine adverse reactions, their relationship to aurothiomalate toxicity was also examined.

Patients with rheumatoid arthritis (of a fairly severe grade) were examined because of the above considerations.

The sulphoxide metabolites of chlorpromazine are known to be non-toxic, whereas the hydroxylated metabolites especially 7,8-dihydroxychlorpromazine are very toxic. Therefore the hypothesis was generated that chlorpromazine jaundice might be an adverse reaction to which extensive hydroxylators who were also impaired sulphoxidizers might be especially liable.

Since it is known that sometimes patients who have suffered chlorpromazine jaundice may proceed to develop a condition which resembles primary biliary cirrhosis, it was considered that a survey of the sulphoxidizer status of patients with the latter condition might be revealing.

The reasoning behind the examination of patients with food sensitivity was really tenuous. The diagnosis also was not precisely defined. The underlying idea was that there may be compounds in food which are detoxified by, and possibly eliminated

Table 23.1. *Sulphoxide phenotype distribution in rheumatoid arthritis*

Reference	Location of study	Rheumatoid arthritis patients sulphoxidation phenotype	
		Impaired	Extensive
Emery *et al.* 1984	London	37	29[a]
Ayesh *et al.* 1987	London	39	28
Madhok *et al.* 1987	Glasgow	21	9
Madhok *et al.* 1990	Glasgow	28	22
Total		125	88
Mitchell *et al.* 1984	London and	45	155
Healthy British white volunteers	Birmingham		
Emery *et al.* 1992	Birmingham		
Rheumatoid arthritis		82	32
Hospital controls		45	76
Normal controls		70	130
Aged controls		4	31

[a]The authors give results based on an antimode of $SI = 10$, but the figures shown here can be derived from their article using an antimode of $SI = 6$ the same as the other five series given in this table.

Note: The series of Panayi *et al.* (1983) had to be omitted because they only give information based on an antimode of $SI = 10$.

more speedily, following sulphoxidation. These compounds might be the triggers for food sensitivity. Therefore impaired sulphoxidation might be associated with food sensitivity.

With regard to motor neurone disease (MND), a case which occurred after asphyxiation with an insecticide suggested that detoxification mechanisms might be implicated in the aetiology of MND. Hence the sulphoxidation status of MND patients was surveyed. A similar philosophy lay behind the studies on Parkinson's disease and Alzheimer's disease patients.

Systemic lupus erythematosus was investigated because it is an autoimmune disorder the same as rheumatoid arthritis and primary biliary cirrhosis.

Now for a discussion of the results of these surveys.

Four series of rheumatoid arthritics are available which have been 'phenotyped' on the same criteria (Table 23.1). There is no heterogeneity ($\chi_3^2 = 1.92$, $p > 0.5$). When the pooled data are compared with the control series of Mitchell *et al.* (1984) which contains 45 impaired and 155 extensive sulphoxidizers,

the 'relative incidence' (computed by the method of Woolf 1954, modified by Haldane 1955) of rheumatoid arthritis in the impaired phenotype is 4.8. A high relative risk would also be given if the computation was made with other control series e.g. from Olomu *et al.* (1988) or Steventon *et al.* (1988a). A further series published by Emery *et al.* (1992) included 114 patients with rheumatoid arthritis and three different control groups. The proportion of poor sulphoxidiers in the rheumatoid arthritics was significantly higher than in the controls ($p > 0.001$). So there seems to be a definite association between 'impaired sulphoxidation' and rheumatoid arthritis *per se*.

A small study to see if there was genetic linkage between rheumatoid arthritis and sulphoxidation status (Deighton *et al.* 1990) gave negative results.

The results of studies seeking to associate adverse reactions to penicillamine and aurothiomalate to sulphoxidator status are shown in Table 23.2 and they indicate that the impaired sulphoxidizer is more prone than the extensive sulphoxidizer to toxicity with both compounds.

Table 23.2. *The relationship of sulphoxidation phenotype to drug toxicity in the treatment of rheumatoid arthritis*

| Reference | Patient status | Sulphoxidation phenotype | | χ_1^2 | | p |
		Impaired	Extensive			
Ayesh *et al.* 1987	with aurothiomalate toxicity	30	7	15.90		< 0.001
	without aurothiomalate toxicity	9	19			
Madhok *et al.* 1987	with aurothiomalate toxicity	13	1	4.64	Y	< 0.05
	without aurothiomalate toxicity	8	8			
Panayi *et al.* 1983	with penicillamine toxicity	5	1	8.65	Y	< 0.01
	without penicillamine toxicity	1	3			
Emery *et al.* 1984	with penicillamine toxicity	18	6	13.28		< 0.001
	without penicillamine toxicity	12	30			
Madhok *et al.* 1990	with penicillamine toxicity	15	3	8.52		< 0.01
	without penicillamine toxicity	13	19			

Y, with Yates' correction.

Table 23.3. *The association of impaired sulphoxidation status with miscellaneous disorders*

| Reference | Patient status and nature of control series | Sulphoxidation phenotype | | χ_1^2 | | p |
		Impaired	Extensive			
Olomu *et al.* 1988	Primary biliary cirrhosis (PBC)	40	4	24.91		< 0.001
	Non-PBC liver disease	29	37			
Scadding *et al.* 1988	Food sensitivity	58	16	43.85		< 0.001
	Normal controls	67	133			
Watson *et al.* 1988	Chlorpromazine jaundice	12	0	22.20	Y	< 0.001
	Mixed liver disorders	15	48			
Steventon *et al.* 1988b	Motor neurone disease (MND)	36	13	18.40		< 0.001
	Various non-MND neurologic disorders	45	76			
Steventon *et al.* 1989	Parkinson's disease (PD)	43	25	11.87		< 0.001
	Various non-MND and non-PD neurologic disorders	45	76			
Steventon *et al.* 1990	Alzheimer's disease	12	4	20.61		< 0.001
	Aged miscellaneous neurologic disorders	4	31			
Gordon *et al.* 1992	Systemic lupus erythematosus	25	10	9.98		< 0.010
	Healthy drug-free volunteers	17	30			

Y, with Yates' correction

Miscellaneous conditions studied for association with sulphoxidation status are shown in Table 23.3. They all, without exception, turned out to be highly significant.

The interpretation of all these results is made difficult by the fact that the natural substrates for this polymorphism are unknown. This criticism is the same as for many other association studies involving other polymorphisms which are described in this book.

It is somewhat disturbing that (1) no negative association studies involving sulphoxidation have been reported, and (2) all the analyses for all the association studies have been performed in only one laboratory.

Some other criticisms of the study design of the primary biliary cirrhosis survey were voiced by Scharschmidt & Lake (1989), particularly in relation to the detailed results in the 'other liver disorders' control patients.

A complication of these associations has arisen from the work of Kupfer & Idle (1990) who call attention to the fact that healthy individuals who have taken 750 mg SCMC by mouth excrete sulphoxidized metabolites over a variable period of time. The phenotyping tests referred to earlier were based on the excretion of these compounds in the first 8 hours after drug ingestion. Out of 40 healthy volunteers Kupfer & Idle (1990) found 19 impaired sulphoxidizers as assessed by the analysis of the 0 to 8 hour urine specimens. However the figure fell to four impaired sulphoxidizers when the 0 to 16 hour urine specimens were the basis of the phenotyping.

The relevance of this finding to the associations described above is obscure. It is possible that a disease, such as rheumatoid arthritis or primary biliary cirrhosis, for example, may delay the distribution of SCMC or impair its metabolism, or slow the excretion of metabolites as a secondary effect of the pathology.

THE STORY TAKES A NEW TURN

Using a battery of sophisticated techniques three research groups have re-evaluated the evidence concerning S-carboxymethyl-L-cysteine metabolism, especially its sulphoxidation. The evidence is condensed in Table 23.4. The amount of sulphoxidated metabolites produced is only a very small fraction of the ingested dose, so the original findings of Waring and her colleagues are not confirmed. Meese et al. (1990c).

In the course of these investigations, an additional novel metabolite was observed by thin layer chromatography (TLC) after sulphur-selective visualization. This metabolite of unknown structure was the only urinary component exhibiting a polymorphism in the population after the oral administration of S-carboxymethyl-L-cysteine. About 7.5 to 10% of the Swiss and British populations excreted only marginal amounts of this compound. After the administration of SCMC and its carbon-13 labelled analogue orally, the urines of two volunteers were extensively worked up with TLC, NMR, GCMS, etc. and the relevant compound was found to be

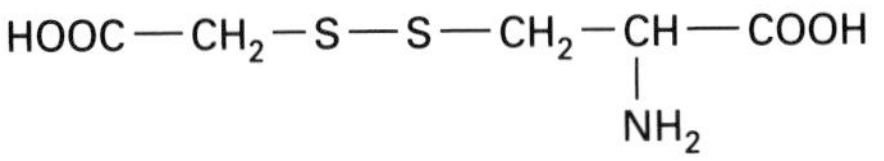

$$HOOC - CH_2 - S - S - CH_2 - CH - COOH$$
$$|$$
$$NH_2$$

Fig. 23.4. S-(carboxymethylthio)-L-cysteine.

S-(carboxymethylthio)-L-cysteine (Fig. 23.4). Meese et al. (1991).

In view of this evidence it seems very unlikely that the chromatographic spot (which was the basis of the polymorphism described by Waring and her colleagues) did really consist of SCMC sulphoxide. Despite this the statistical associations described above between putative phenotypes and clinical phenomena could be of considerable importance, still require explanation, and are worthy of reappraisal.

OTHER DRUGS WHICH ARE SULPHOXIDIZED

The most important group of drugs which are sulphoxidized are the phenothiazines (see chlorpromazine, Fig. 23.1). Examples of phenothiazines whose sulphoxidations have recently been studied in humans include promethazine (Taylor et al. 1983), fluphenazine (Hoffman et al. 1988) and thioridazine (Papadopoulos & Crammer 1986, Fig. 23.5). Enoximone, Fig. 23.6, which is a member of a new class of cardiotonic drugs, was shown to be eliminated primarily by sulphoxidation (Okerholm et al. 1987).

There are scientifically intriguing and clinically very important observations regarding thioridazine sulphoxidation published by Meyer et al. (1990). They observed a patient who had a relative inability to carry out this oxidation, with the result that he had high plasma levels of thioridazine (T) and low plasma levels of mesoridazine and sulphoridazine (Fig. 23.5) as compared with 24 other hospitalized schizophrenics even after his dosage of T had been reduced. Both phenotyping (dextromethorphan) and genotyping (XbaI endonuclease) tests showed this patient to be a poor metabolizer of the debrisoquine/sparteine polymorphism, whereas the other 24 patients were classified extensive metabolizers. Not surprisingly this patient suffered from marked oversedation on conventional doses. This observation is somewhat at variance with the results of the survey of Haley et al. (1985), who in 120 volunteers found no concordance between the 'sulphoxidation' and debrisoquine polymorphisms. Also Schulz & Schmoldt (1988) considered, after studying cimetidine metabolism by human liver microsomes, that no more than 40% of the total oxidation was accounted for by cytochrome P450-

Table 23.4. *Newer studies of S-carboxymethyl-L-cysteine metabolism*

Reference	Dose	Period for which urine collected	Number of subjects	Analytical technique	% of dose recovered	% of dose as SCMC sulphoxides	Evidence of sulphoxidation polymorphism
Woolfson et al. 1987	1.125 g	0–24 hours	3	HPLC after deriv. electrochemical detection	19% or less	0.17–1.03	NA
Brockmöller et al. 1988	1.125 g	0–8 hours	11	HPLC after deriv.	56% or less *	6% or less	NA
Karim et al. 1988	1.125 g	0–24 hours	8	HPLC after deriv. electrochemical detection	<31%	<2%	NA
Meese et al. 1990a	375 or 750 mg	0–8 hours	?	S-carboxyl [^{13}C] methyl-L-cysteine administered. ^{13}C-NMR HPLC after deriv. GC-MS	<53%	Nil	NA
Meese et al. 1990b	3.75 or 750 g	0–8 hours	15	ditto	?	<2%	NA
Specht et al. 1990	375 mg	0–24 hours	11	ditto	<2% CMC-SO 13–32% TDGA 8–19% TDGA-SO 6–22% unchanged drug	<2%	NA
Staffeldt et al. 1990	1.1 g	0–8 hours	30	HPLC after deriv.	10–30% unchanged drug 4–30% TDGA Others <2%	<1%	NA

SCMC, S-carboxymethyl-L-cysteine; HPLC, high performance liquid chromatography; deriv., derivatization; NA, none apparent; *, SCMC + SCMC sulphoxide; TDGA, thiodiglycolic acid; ?, information not given; NMR, nuclear magnetic resonance; GC-MS, gas chromatography–mass spectrometry; CMC-SO, S-carboxymethyl-L-cysteine sulphoxides; TDGA-SO, thiodiglycolic acid sulphoxide.
See also Gregory et al. 1992; Waring et al. 1992.

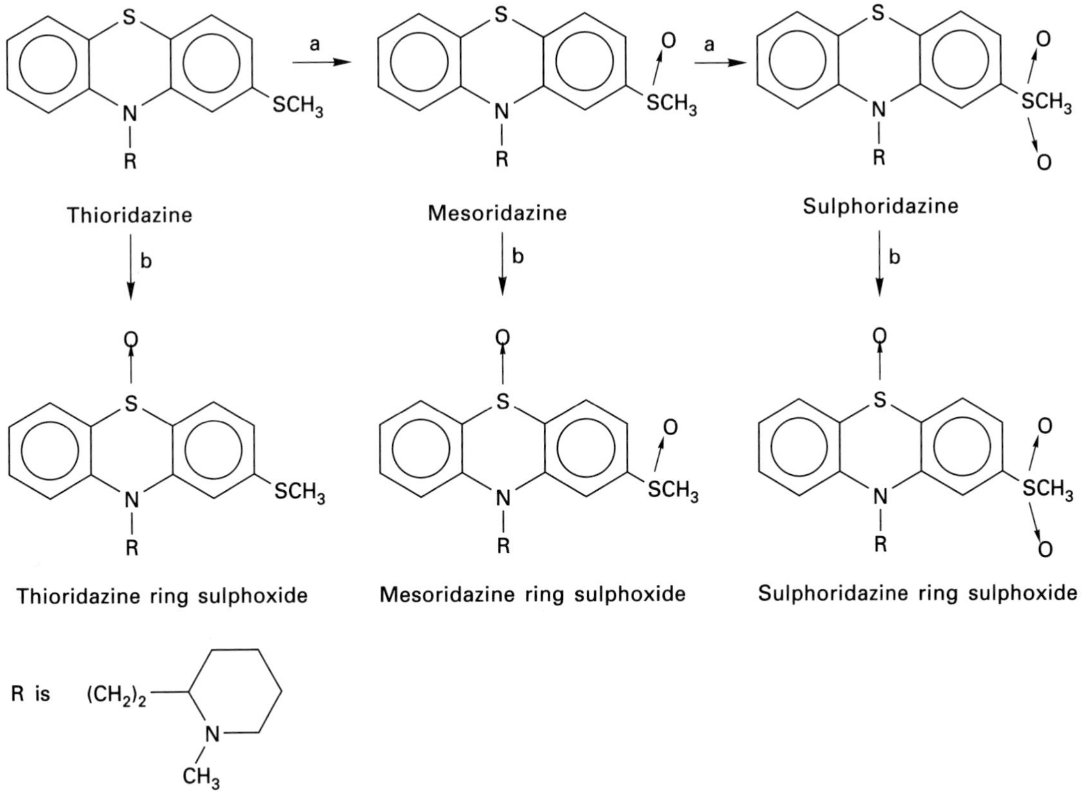

Fig. 23.5. Sulphoxides of thioridazine in man. **a**, Side-chain *S*-oxidation; **b**, ring *S*-oxidation. (From Papado-poulos & Crammer 1986.)

Enoximone

Cimetidine

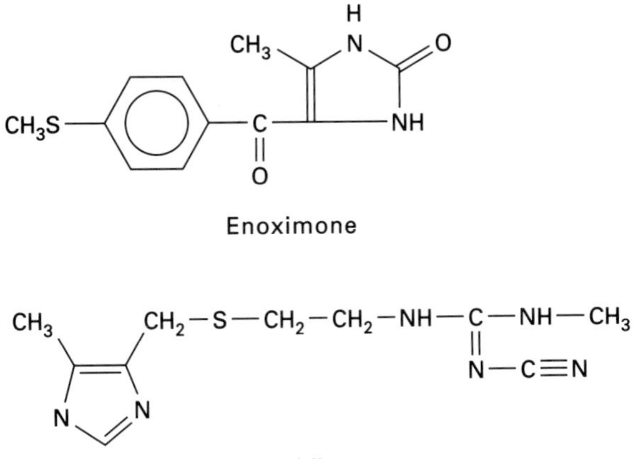

Fig. 23.6. The molecular structures of enoximone and cimetidine. (Enoximone from Okerholm *et al.* 1987.)

dependent sulphoxidation, and Waring *et al.* (1986) claimed that the sulphoxidation enzymes were cytosolic, not microsomal.

It seems clear that sulphoxidation is a biotransformation, which may well exhibit genetic variability that could be of considerable therapeutic significance.

Ayesh, R., Mitchell, S. C., Waring, R. H. & Smith, R. L. (1988). Taste sensitivity to phenylthiourea: lack of correlation with the debrisoquine and carboxymethylcysteine polymorphisms. *British Journal of Clinical Pharmacology*, **25**, 664P.

Ayesh, R., Mitchell, S. C., Waring, R. H., Withrington, R. H., Siefert, M. H. & Smith, R. L. (1987). Sodium aurothiomalate toxicity and sulphoxidation capacity in rheumatoid arthritic patients. *British Journal of Rheumatology*, **26**, 197–201.

Brockmöller, J., Simane, Z. J. & Roots, I. (1988). HPLC-analysis of S-carboxymethylcysteine and its sulphoxide metabolites. *Drug Metabolism and Drug Interactions*, **6**, 447–56.

Deighton, C. M., Ayesh, R., Walker, D. J. & Panayi, G. (1990). Linkage studies in sulfoxidation status, HLA and rheumatoid arthritis. *Journal of Rheumatology*, **17**, 1562–3.

Emery, P., Bradley, H., Gough, A., Arthur, V., Jubb, R. &

Waring, R. (1992). Increased prevalence of poor sulphoxidation in patients with rheumatiod arthritis: effect of changes in the acute phase response and second line drug treatment. *Annals of the Rheumatic Diseases*, **5**, 318–20.

Emery, P., Panayi, G. S., Huston, G., Welsh, K. I., Mitchell, S. C., Shah, R. R., Idle, J. R., Smith, R. L. & Waring, R. H. (1984). D-penicillamine induced toxicity in rheumatoid arthritis: the role of sulphoxidation status and HLA-DR3. *Journal of Rheumatology*, **11**, 626–32.

Gordon, C., Bradley, H., Waring, R. H. & Emergy, P. (1992). Abnormal sulphur oxidation in systemic lupus erythematosus. *Lancet*, **339**, 25–6.

Gregory, W. L., James, O. F. W. & Idle, J. R. (1992). Carbocisteine polymorphism and disease. *Lancet*, **339**, 616.

Haldane, J. B. S. (1955). The estimation and significance of the logarithm of a ratio of frequence. *Annals of Human Genetics (London)*, **20**, 309–11.

Haley, C. S., Waring, R. H., Mitchell, S. C., Shah, R. R., Idle, J. R. & Smith, R. L. (1985). Lack of congruence of S-carboxymethyl-L-cysteine sulphoxidation and debrisoquine 4-hydroxylation in a Caucasian population. *Xenobiotica*, **15**, 445–50.

Harris, C. M., Waring, R. H., Mitchell, S. C. & Hendry, G. L. (1986). The case of the black-speckled dolls: an occupational hazard of unusual sulphur metabolism. *Lancet*, **1**, 492–3.

Hoffman, D. W., Edkins, R. D. & Shillcutt, S. D. (1988). Human metabolism of phenothiazines to sulfoxides determined by a new high performance liquid chromatography-electrical detection method. *Biochemical Pharmacology*, **37**, 1773–7.

Karim, E. I. A., Mullership, J. S., Temple, D. J. & Woolfson, A. D. (1988). An investigation of the metabolism of S-carboxymethyl-L-cysteine in man using a novel HPLC-ECD method. *European Journal of Drug Metabolism and Pharmacokinetics*, **13**, 253–6.

Karim, E. F. I. A., Mullership, J. S., Temple, D. J. & Woolfson, A. D. (1989). The influence of diet on drug metabolism studies of S-carboxymethyl-L-cysteine. *International Journal of Pharmaceutics*, **52**, 155–8.

Küpfer, A. & Idle, J. R. (1990). False positives with current carbocisteine protocol for sulphoxidation phenotyping. *Lancet*, **335**, 1107.

Madhok, R., Capell, H. A. & Waring, R. (1987). Does sulphoxidation state predict gold toxicity in rheumatoid arthritis? *British Medical Journal*, **294**, 483.

Madhok, R., Zoma, A., Torley, H. I., Capell, H. A., Waring, R. & Hunter, J. A. (1990). The relationship of sulfoxidation status to efficacy and toxicity of penicillamine in the treatment of rheumatoid arthritis. *Arthritis and Rheumatism*, **33**, 574–7.

Meese, C. O., Fischer, C., Küfer, A., Wisser, H. & Eichelbaum, M. (1991). Identification of the 'major' polymorphic carbocysteine metabolite as S-(carboxymethylthio)-L-cysteine. *Biochemical Pharmacology*, **42**, R13–16.

Meese, C. O., Hofmann, U. & Eichelbaum, M. (1990c). Polymorphic sulphoxidation of carbocisteine. *Lancet*, **336**, 693–4.

Meese, C. O., Specht, D. & Fischer, P. (1990b). Revision of S-carboxymethyl-L-cysteine metabolism by ^{13}C-NMR spectroscopy. *Fresenius Journal of Analytical Chemistry*, **337**, 130–1.

Meese, C. O., Specht, D., Ratge, D., Wisser, H., Fischer, P., Oesselmann, J. & Gerding, A. (1990a) Reinvestigation of S-carboxymethyl-L-cysteine metabolism in humans by novel stable isotope tracer studies. *Naunyn-Schmeideberg's Archives of Pharmacology*, **341** (Suppl. R9), Abstract 34.

Meyer, J. W., Woggon, B., Baumann, P. & Meyer, U. A. (1990). Clinical implications of slow sulphoxidation of thioridazine in a poor metabolizer of the debrisoquine type. *European Journal of Clinical Pharmacology*, **39**, 613–14.

Mitchell, S. C. & Waring, R. H. (1989). The deficiency of sulfoxidation of S-carboxymethyl-L-cysteine. *Pharmacology and Therapeutics*, **43**, 237–49.

Mitchell, S. C., Waring, R. H., Haley, C. S., Idle, J. R. & Smith, R. L. (1984). Genetic aspects of the polymodally distributed sulphoxidation of S-carboxymethyl-L-cysteine in man. *British Journal of Clinical Pharmacology*, **18**, 507–21.

Okerholm, R. A., Chan, K. Y., Lang, J. F., Thompson, G. A. & Ruberg, S. J. (1987). Biotransformation and pharmacokinetic overview of enoximone and its sulfoxide metabolite. *American Journal of Cardiology*, **60**, 21C–6C.

Olomu, A. B., Vickers, C. R., Waring, R. H., Clements, D., Babbs, C., Warnes, T. W. & Elias, E. (1988). High incidence of poor sulfoxidation in patients with primary biliary cirrhosis. *New England Journal of Medicine*, **318**, 1089–92.

Panayi, G. S., Huston, G., Shah, R. R., Mitchell, S. C., Idle, J. R., Smith, R. L. & Waring, R. H. (1983). Deficient sulphoxidation status and D-penicillamine toxicity. *Lancet*, **1**, 414.

Papadopoulos, A. S. & Crammer, J. L. (1986). Sulphoxide metabolites of thioridazine in man. *Xenobiotica*, **16**, 1097–107.

Scadding, G. K., Ayesh, R., Brostoff, J., Mitchell, S. C., Waring, R. H. & Smith, R. L. (1988). Poor sulphoxidation ability in patients with food sensitivity. *British Medical Journal*, **297**, 105–7.

Scharschmidt, B. F. & Lake, J. R. (1989). Impaired sulfoxidation in patients with primary biliary cirrhosis. *Hepatology*, **9**, 654–8.

Schulz, M. & Schmoldt, A. (1988). On the sulphoxidation of cimetidine and etintidine by rat and human liver microsomes. *Xenobiotica*, **18**, 983–9.

Specht, D., Meese, C. O., Ratge, D., Eichelbaum, M. & Wisser, H. (1990). The metabolic pattern of S-carboxymethyl-L-cysteine. A new study with HPLC and a novel *ex vivo* carbon-13-NMR-method. *Fresenius Journal of Analytical Chemistry*, **337**, 63–4.

Staffeldt, B., Brockmöller, J. & Roots, I. (1990). Evaluation of possible polymorphisms in sulfoxidation of carbocystein analysed by HPLC-methods. *European Journal of Pharmacology*, **183**, 627–8.

Steventon, G. B., Heafield, M. T. E., Sturman, S., Waring, R. H. & Williams, A.C. (1988a). The metabolism of ^{35}S-D-penicillamine in man. *Xenobiotica*, **18**, 235–44.

Steventon, G. B., Heafield, M. T. E., Sturman, S., Waring, R. H. & Williams, A. C. (1990). Xenobiotic metabolism in Alzheimer's disease. *Neurology*, **40**, 1095–8.

Steventon, G. B., Heafield, M. T. E., Waring, R. H. & Williams, A. C. (1989). Xenobiotic metabolism in Parkinson's disease. *Neurology*, **39**, 883–7.

Steventon, G., Williams, A. C., Waring, R. H., Pall, H. S. & Adams, D. (1988b). Xenobiotic metabolism in motorneuron disease. *Lancet*, **2**, 644–7.

Taylor, G., Houston, J. B., Shaffer, J. & Mawer, G. (1983). Pharmacokinetics of promethazine and its sulphoxide metabolite after intravenous and oral administration to man. *British Journal of Clinical Pharmacology*, **15**, 287–93.

Turnbull, L. B., Teng, L., Kinzie, J. M., Pitts, J. E., Pinchbeck, F. M. & Bruce, R. B. (1978). Excretion and biotransformation of carboxymethyl-cysteine in rat, dog, monkey and man. *Xenobiotica*, **8**, 621–8.

Waring, R., Gordon, C. & Emery, P. (1992). Carbocisteine polymorphism and disease. *Lancet*, **339**, 616–17.

Waring, R. H. (1978). The metabolism of S-carboxymethylcysteine in rodents marmosets and humans. *Xenobiotica*, **8**, 265–70.

Waring, R. H. (1980). Variation in human metabolism of S-carboxymethylcysteine. *European Journal of Drug Metabolism and Pharmacokinetics*, **5**, 49–52.

Waring, R. H. & Mitchell, S. C. (1982). The metabolism and elimination of S-carboxymethyl-L-cysteine in man. *Drug Metabolism and Disposition*, **10**, 61–2.

Waring, R. H. & Mitchell, S.C. (1988). The metabolism of ³⁵S-D-penicillamine in man. *Xenobiotica*, **18**, 235–44.

Waring, R. H., Mitchell, S. C., O'Gorman, J. & Fraser, M. (1986). Cytosolic sulphoxidation of S-carboxymethyl-L-cysteine in mammals. *Biochemical Pharmacology*, **35**, 2999–3002.

Waring, R. H., Mitchell, S. C., Shah, R. R., Idle, J. R. & Smith, R. L. (1982). Polymorphic sulphoxidation of S-carboxymethyl-L-cysteine in man. *Biochemical Pharmacology*, **31**, 3151–4.

Watson, R. G. P., Olomu, A., Clements, D., Waring, R. H., Mitchell, S. & Elias, E. (1988). A proposed mechanism for chlorpromazine jaundice – defective hepatic sulphoxidation combined with rapid hydroxylation. *Journal of Hepatology*, **7**, 72–8.

Woolf, B. (1954). On estimating the relation between blood group and disease. *Annals of Human Genetics (London)*, **19**, 251–3.

Woolfson, A. D., Millership, J. S. & Karim, E. I. A. (1987). Determination of the sulphoxide metabolites of S-carboxymethyl-L-cysteine by high-performance liquid chromatography with electrochemical detection. *Analyst*, **112**, 1421–5.

24   Halothane hepatitis and other topics

HALOTHANE HEPATITIS

THE INCIDENCE of fatal hepatic necrosis following halothane anaesthesia was computed to be about 1 in 23 000. Severe liver dysfunction is thought to occur in 1 in 6000 to 1 in 20 000 (Ray & Drummond 1991). It is clear that the liver damage is more common after repeated exposure to halothane especially at short time intervals (Inman & Mushin 1974).

In addition to repeated exposure, the following factors have been observed to confer increased risk: middle age, obesity, female sex and possibly preceding use of agents such as phenobarbitone which can induce hepatic microsomal enzymes (Ray & Drummond 1991).

The possibility that there might be a genetic factor which confers susceptibility to halothane hepatitis was raised by Hoft et al. (1981), who described three pairs of closely related women of Mexican-Indian or Mexican-Spanish descent.

A test very similar to that used by Spielberg (1981), and described in the chapter on phenytoin, was used by Farrell et al. (1985) to assess capacity of lymphocytes to withstand phenytoin epoxide induced damage. In the absence of 1,1,1-trichloro-2-propene oxide (TCPO) there was no increase in cytotoxicity with concentrations of phenytoin up to 0.12 mM. With TCPO there was a slight increase in cytotoxicity in control cells (12% at 0.12 mM phenytoin), whereas people who had experienced halothane hepatitis (HH) gave a figure of 83% cytotoxicity at 0.12 mM phenytoin.

The families of four HH patients were studied including 15 first-degree relatives. Six of these 15 gave abnormal responses, and they included a mother, a daughter and four sons of three different probands.

So the suggestion was made that HH occurred in people who had an inadequate defence mechanism against an electrophilic halothane metabolite. Unlike phenytoin, halothane is not known to produce an epoxide. However, a study of 10 identical and 10 fraternal twinships (Cascorbi et al., 1971) showed that the urinary excretion of a halothane metabolite was under a considerable measure of genetic control. A range of oxidative and reductive metabolites is produced during halothane metabolism (Ray & Drummond, 1991) and the urinary metabolite is likely to be trifluoroacetic acid. However, there is a possibility that oxidative intermediates are produced. Whether this process varies between people and is under genetic control is unknown.

Recent experimental work on rats and also in human patients has shown that TFA produced from halothane binds to a number of hepatic proteins, some of which have been identified, e.g. carboxylesterase and disulphide isomerase. A series of neo-antigens is formed with molecular weights of 54, 57, 59, 76 and 100 kDa. Antibodies to the last two neo-antigens were found in the sera of patients who had developed halothane hepatitis (Kenna 1991).

Having reviewed the literature very thoroughly, Ray & Drummond (1991) were of the opinion that two probably distinct forms of liver damage occur with halothane. The first, relatively mild form may result from the reductive biotransformation of halothane, possibly influenced by genetic factors. The second, fulminant form is likely to be mediated by an immunological mechanism. It is, however, still unclear why only a rare person gets this illness.

METHOXYFLURANE

An intriguing observation was made by Wilson *et al.* (1972). They measured the 24 hour urine fluoride concentration and oxalic acid excretion in seven women undergoing caesarian section with light methoxyflurane anaesthesia. The interesting thing was that whilst all seven had a peak of increased fluoride excretion 2 to 5 days after drug exposure, only three of them had an increase in oxalic acid excretion of two or three times normal.

There have been subsequent surveys of methoxyflurane metabolism and its effects; for example Dahlgren (1977) showed that there was an early post-partum increase of serum creatinine concentration. However no attention has been paid to the possible polymorphism in oxalate excretion. Methoxyflurane is metabolized by cytochromes P450 in the liver and lung (Waskell *et al.* 1986) and can be induced by compounds such as phenytoin (Caughey *et al.* 1979). In view of the very considerable genetic diversity discovered in cytochromes P450 it might be interesting to re-examine the production of oxalic acid from methoxyflurane. This could be of clinical importance in view of the fact that both fluoride and oxalic acid are nephrotoxic, so individuals that produce more of the latter compound may be more prone to renal adverse effects.

CARBAMAZEPINE HYPERSENSITIVITY

Mild cutaneous reactions to carbamazepine (CBZ) are not uncommon, whereas severe reactions occur with a frequency of 1 in 5000 to 1 in 10 000 patients. These severe reactions are characterized by rashes, fever, arthralgia, jaundice and eosinophilia.

Experiments to find out whether phenytoin hypersensitivity was due to the formation of reactive intermediary metabolites have been described in the chapter which deals with that drug.

In order to find out whether a similar mechanism operated in the case of CBZ, Pirmohamed *et al.* (1991a) conducted a series of experiments with the help of seven patients who had sustained hypersensitivity reactions, five patients who had been treated chronically with the drug without developing adverse reactions, and healthy volunteer control subjects. The assessment of cytotoxicity was by means of the trypan blue exclusion of peripheral blood mononuclear cells (MNL).

It was found that microsomes prepared from human liver samples were capable of producing substances from CBZ which caused cytotoxicity. Human or mouse liver microsomes were incubated with CBZ, NADPH and MNL. The latter were then sedimented and incubated in a drug-free medium; after 16 hours they were assessed for cytotoxicity.

A large increase of cytotoxicity above basal was seen in the MNL of hypersensitive patients as compared with controls. This cytotoxicity was not produced when phenytoin was incubated with the same microsomal preparation. As a control measure it was observed that dapsone hydroxylamine and amodiaquine quinoneimine gave cytotoxicity which was not significantly different in hypersensitive patients and in controls.

While these results suggest that the hypersensitive patient's lymphocytes are unusually sensitive to the toxicity of CBZ metabolites they do not explain how the hypersensitivity phenomena are generated. A further patient, described by Pirmohamed *et al.* (1991b), may provide an important clue. This patient had suffered hypersensitivity to CBZ including jaundice. His MNL suffered enhanced cytotoxicity after incubation with the supernatant from microsomes which had been incubated with CBZ as described above. It was also found that he had an antibody which recognized a protein of 94 kDa in all nine samples of human liver microsomes tested but not in a variety of other tissues. Sera from healthy controls and other patients who had suffered CBZ-hepatitis did not contain this antibody.

The possibility was suggested that this antibody could combine with a reactive intermediary metabolite of CBZ which was inadequately detoxified by epoxide hydrolase (as shown by the cytotoxicity test) and attack a cellular protein giving rise to the hepatitis.

In a further paper Pirmohamed *et al.* (1992) showed that adding purified microsomal epoxide hydrolase to the microsomal-CBZ incubate significantly reduced the cytotoxicity of the supernatant.

ORAL CONTRACEPTIVE STEROIDS

The oral contraceptive steroids are interesting medications because they are consumed in standard amounts by more healthy persons than probably any other drug (if one does not count caffeine). Most of the research on the pharmacokinetics and biotransformation of these compounds has been carried out in the prestigious Department of Pharmacology and Therapeutics of the University of Liverpool (as was the work on proguanil and carbamazepine referred to elsewhere). A comprehensive account has been given by Orme *et al.* (1992). Some of the highlights appertaining to the variability in metabolism will be discussed here. Ethinyloestradiol is the steroid which has received most attention (Fig. 24.1).

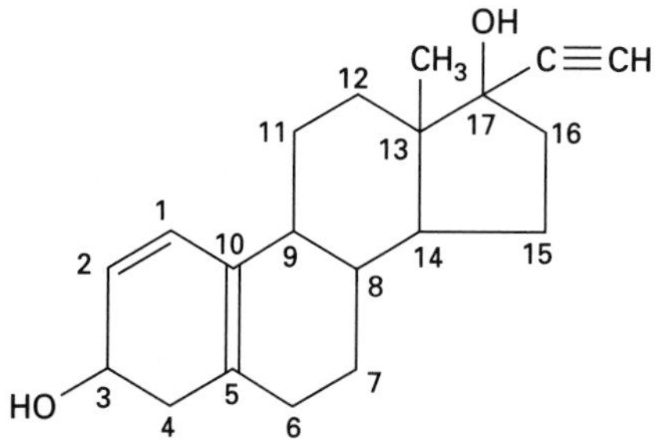

Fig. 24.1. The structure of ethinyloestradiol. (From Orme *et al.* 1992.)

Pharmacokinetics of ethinyloestradiol

The peak plasma concentration of ethinyloestradiol occurs 1.5 to 3 hours after a single oral dose and is followed by a biexponential curve. A secondary rise occurs at 12 to 14 hours after ingestion of the dose and is ascribed to enterohepatic recirculation. A very large variability in the kinetics was described both between series of subjects studied in different countries and within these series (Goldzieher *et al.* 1980; Fotherby *et al.* 1981). Absorption was fast in Bangkok and slow in Chandigarh, Singapore and Seoul as shown by the timing of the peak plasma concentration. At 24 hours after an oral dose of 50 µg ethinyloestradiol (EE) and 1 mg norethisterone, the mean plasma concentration of EE was 56 pg/ml in Alexandria and 135 pg/ml in Bangkok. The former figure was ascribed to poor absorption. Individual elimination half-life values varied from 2.5 hours to more than 30 hours. In Canada the mean was 8.9 hours and in Sydney it was 30.8 hours. As compared with an intravenous dose the bioavailability of the oral dose was 50%.

Both genetic and environmental factors could contribute to the observed variabilities in these pharmacokinetic parameters.

Environmental influences on the pharmacokinetics of oral contraceptive steroids

Multiple environmental factors can influence the plasma levels of oral contraceptive steroids and some of them are of clinical importance (see Table 24.1).

Biotransformation of ethinyloestradiol

The principal biotransformations which occur to the EE molecule are (1) sulphate conjugation at the 3 position which occurs in the intestinal mucosa, (2) hydroxylation which occurs principally at the 2 position and to a much lesser extent at positions 4, 6α and 16β, and (3) glucuronide conjugation of the hydroxyl groups at positions 2, 4, 6α, 16β and 17 (Orme *et al.* 1992).

About 10% of a single dose is excreted in the urine as EE sulphate (Kamyab *et al.* 1969; Kulkarni & Goldzieher 1970) and most of the excreted compound is in the form of glucuronides.

It has been observed that 2-hydroxylation of EE occurred to a much smaller extent in Nigerian women than in women in the USA, with Sri Lankan women in an intermediate position (Williams & Goldzieher 1980).

The human jejunal and ileal mucosa *in vitro* has been demonstrated to be the site of sulphate and glucuronide conjugation (Back *et al.* 1981). These reactions account for an average of 65% of the first pass effect of EE (Back *et al.* 1982). Human liver microsomes *in vitro* mediate 2-hydroxylation of EE and the resulting catechol undergoes further biotransformation to a material which is irreversibly bound to microsomal protein (Maggs *et al.* 1983a). *In vivo*, this process may be prevented by prompt glucuronidation.

Table 24.1. *Environmental factors influencing plasma concentrations of oral contraceptive steroids*

Factor	Mechanisms	Result
Diet Grapefruit juice	Inhibits hydroxylation	Higher plasma levels
Vitamin C	Competes for EE sulphate conjugation in gut wall	Higher plasma levels
Economic status	Norethisterone half-lives longer in women of high economic status possibly due to increased plasma protein binding	Higher plasma levels
Skin-fold thickness	Correlation between half-life of norgestrel and skin-fold thickness	Malnutrition may prolong half-life and give higher plasma levels
Drugs Phenobarbital, phenytoin, carbamazepine, primidone, rifampicin	Induce the metabolism of EE	Reduced plasma levels but the degree of reduction very variable between women
Antibiotics (ampicillin, amoxycillin, tetracycline, erythromycin, nitrofurantoin, cotrimoxazole)	Effect on gut flora reducing enterohepatic circulation	Reduced plasma levels variable between women
Other contraceptive steroids Desogestrel Gestodene	Possibly due to inhibition of metabolism	Increased plasma levels Greatly increased plasma levels
Gastrointestinal disorders Coeliac disease	Impaired gut wall conjugation	Higher plasma levels

EE, ethinyloestradiol.
Data from: Back & Orme 1984; Guengerich 1992; Orme *et al.* 1992.

Genetic control of the metabolism of ethinyloestradiol

Neither twin nor family studies of EE metabolism have been carried out. Consequently the evidence in favour of the genetic control of EE metabolism comes from two sources, namely (1) observation of the *in vivo* pattern of metabolism and the way it is influenced by other compounds and (2) observation *in vitro* of metabolism by liver microsomes and various preparations purified from them.

One of the most striking *in vivo* observations was made by Maggs *et al.* (1983b), who found an individual who was unable to hydroxylate EE at position 2, with the result that more unchanged EE was excreted as glucuronide and sulphate conjugates in the bile. This woman was an extensive metabolizer of sparteine. A family study was not performed. There has been no large population study carried

out to assess the frequency of this phenotype. A 'typed panel' study revealed that the sparteine (cytochrome P450 2D6) polymorphism did not influence the metabolism of EE, which means that enzyme is not responsible for its biotransformation (Back *et al.* 1984).

The formation of 2-hydroxy EE *in vitro* was not inhibited by phenytoin, mephenytoin, sparteine, antipyrine, chloroquine, or antipyrine, which suggests that it was not mediated by the cytochromes P450 responsible for the hydroxylations of these compounds (Purba *et al.* 1987; Ball *et al.* 1988). Also primaquine, previously shown to inhibit antipyrine metabolism *in vivo*, had no effect on the 2-hydroxylation of EE (Back *et al.* 1984).

Evidence has been produced that EE is hydroxylated by cytochrome P450 3A4 (Guengerich 1988). The administration of rifampicin and barbiturates, which are known to induce this enzyme, cause more rapid elimination of EE and loss of its contraceptive action. Thirty human liver microsomal preparations (Kerlan *et al.* 1992) showed inter-correlation of 2- and 4-hydroxylation of EE; the 2-hydroxylation correlated with nifedipine oxidation, erythromycin *N*-demethylation, testosterone 6β-hydroxylation and tamoxifen *N*-demethylation, all of which are known to be cytochrome P450 3A4/3A5 mediated reactions (see Table 4.1 and Chapter 8). It is possible that more than one cytochrome P450 mediates the hydroxylation of EE.

There do not appear to be any studies published to correlate EE metabolism with non-invasive assays of cytochrome P450 3A4 such as erythromycin *N*-demethylation and lidocaine *N*-deethylation.

Also, there have been no systematic studies of the variability of EE sulphation and gluronidation in the population as initial steps to try and assess what measure of genetic control there may be over these reactions.

It is not known what is the relevance of the observations cited above to the occurrence of jaundice on oral contraceptive steroids (Dalen & Westerholm 1974) in members of families in which idiopathic cholestasis of pregnancy is found (Kreek *et al.* 1967; Holzbach *et al.* 1983).

It would be of considerable interest and might be of clinical relevance to have a better understanding of the genetic aspects of the metabolism of oral contraceptive steroids.

ANTI-CANCER DRUGS

Problems arise because of the variability in the responses of patients with various types of cancer to chemotherapeutic regimens. Different mechanisms may be responsible, e.g. lack of bioavailability, the influence of concomitantly administered drugs and resistance on the part of the tumour cell itself (see the section on multidrug resistance).

One possibility which has not received much attention is that the patient may be metabolizing the active compound to an inactive metabolite, or have an inability to synthesize an active metabolite which is necessary to produce the desired clinical effect.

Unlike the situation with many other categories of drugs, the administration of anti-cancer drugs to normal healthy volunteers would be unethical. Consequently observations have to be made on

patients who have an illness requiring the treatment. This is usually cancer, and raises the possibility that the disease may be influencing the pharmacokinetics and biotransformation. The drug tamoxifen has been discussed in another section. Two other examples will be discussed briefly here.

Adriamycin is a naturally occurring antibiotic anti-cancer drug which is active against a whole range of solid tumours and leukaemias. One great drawback to the use of adriamycin is the occurrence of cardiotoxicity. This adverse effect can be avoided to a considerable degree by giving the drug as a continuous infusion, rather than in the form of bolus injections which give high peak levels (Eksborg *et al.* 1985). The anti-neoplastic activity is retained with the continuous infusion method of administration.

However there remains the problem of trying to relate blood levels of the drug and its metabolites with the clinical therapeutic effects. A contribution to this area was made by Cummings *et al.* (1986), who showed in 25 cancer patients that adriamycin (ADR) was biotransformed by three reactions. Seven metabolites were identified in plasma, namely, the alcoholic glycoside AOL, the 7-deoxyaglycone of ADR (ADR-DONE), the 7-deoxyaglycone of AOL (AOL-DONE) and four unidentified compounds. The three identified metabolites could also be quantified in urine.

The pharmacokinetics of the three identified metabolites were studied. The striking finding was that AOL-DONE was not detected in the serum of 12 patients, whereas it was a major metabolite in some of the others.

There is a speculation that adriamycinol 7-deoxyaglycone (AOL-DONE) may be formed in the heart and that it is cardiotoxic.

It is clearly desirable to find out more about the intra-individual variability in the metabolism of adriamycin. Obviously studies on healthy subjects and families would be inappropriate. Hence the *in vitro* methods using liver microsomes and known biotransformation genes expressed in cultured cells, yeasts or bacteria might be a feasible approach to the problem.

A similar situation has arisen in relation to cyclophosphamide (CP), which is a pro-drug requiring biotransformation to produce cytotoxic metabolites. It is considered that of these metabolites, phosphoramide mustard (PM), is the ultimate alkylating agent because it is the most reactive with DNA *in vitro* at a physiological pH. Oxidation of CP by a hepatic cytochrome P450 gives 4-hydroxy CP, from which PM is produced by spontaneous hydrolysis (Moore *et al.* 1988).

The metabolism of an intravenous injection of ^{14}C-cyclophosphamide was studied in 40 patients by Mouridsen *et al.* (1974). The unchanged drug and its metabolites were quantified sequentially in serum and urine. The usual pharmacokinetic parameters were investigated and they all exhibited very wide inter-individual variability. For example, the serum half-life of cyclophosphamide varied from 174 to 623 minutes and the percentage of the injected dose excreted in the urine as metabolites in 24 hours was 10 to 55.

In view of what we now know about the genetic variability in cytochrome P450 metabolism there are possibilities for such diversity to affect cyclophosphamide metabolism. Here again, this idea could be tested out using the recently developed *in vitro* techniques.

TRIMETHYLAMINE

This topic is mentioned briefly because of its potential importance in drug metabolism.

It has long been known (Humbert *et al.* 1970) that some individuals carry a smell which resembles that of rotting fish. This is due to the presence of trimethylamine (TMA) in the body liquids. The patient described by Humbert *et al.* (1970) was later reported to lack the liver enzyme required to convert TMA to its odourless N-oxide (TMAO) (Higgins *et al.* 1972). In this patient the urinary excretion of TMA was greatly increased after an oral load of TMA, whereas very little was excreted by normal persons.

An investigation of 169 healthy white volunteers (Al-Waiz *et al.* 1987a) with a TMA loading test disclosed two persons who converted less of it to TMAO than the others. The pedigrees of two patients with the fish-odour syndrome were also similarly investigated (Al-Waiz *et al.* 1988). These studies revealed that the affected patients were homozygous recessives and the two atypical individuals found in the population survey were heterozygotes (Al-Waiz *et al.* 1989).

The urinary excretion of TMAO is higher after consumption of marine fish (which are rich in TMAO) or other foodstuffs such as egg yolk (containing choline), liver (containing choline and lecithin) or soya beans (rich in lecithin), from which TMA can be produced in the body (Ayesh & Smith 1990).

In the normal person TMAO is to some extent reduced to TMA and subsequently oxidized again ('metabolic retroversion': Al-Waiz *et al.* 1987b). The former process is believed to be mediated by gut bacteria.

Secondary forms of fish-odour syndrome can result from the following: large doses of choline (8 to 20 g per day) used in certain treatment regimens, liver cirrhosis, renal failure and bacterial vaginosis (Ayesh & Smith 1990).

It is suspected that many secondary and tertiary amines and sulphur-containing compounds may be substrates for the enzyme responsible for TMA N-oxidation. Examples are chlorpromazine, guanethidine, morphine, nicotine (tertiary amines); propanolol, desipramine, nortriptyline, methamphetamine (secondary amines); methimazole, propylthiouracil, thioacetamide (sulphur compounds) (Ayesh & Smith 1990).

Nicotine N-oxidation was investigated by Ayesh *et al.* (1988) in two sisters with the fish-odour syndrome. They chewed a nicotine-containing gum and their urine was then found to contain much less nicotine N-oxide and more nicotine when compared with normal subjects. This constitutes persuasive evidence that the same alleles control TMA and nicotine N-oxidation, though it would be desirable to study the segregation within families.

Triethylamine (TEA) is used in industry in the vapour form as a curing agent for polyurethane. It is absorbed by inhalation and it has been recorded that resting subjects exposed to a concentration of 20 mg/m^3 for 8 hours developed visual symptoms termed 'foggy vision' or 'blue haze'. (Åkesson *et al.* 1988). More TEA would be inhaled by individuals doing moderately heavy industrial work, but they might be exposed only intermittently.

It is possible that TEA may be metabolized in the same way as TMA. If that turns out to be so, it might be a wise precaution that persons with the fish-odour syndrome should not be exposed to TEA as an occupational hazard.

Pinacidil N-oxidation (Ayesh *et al.* 1989) and verapamil N-dealkylation (Ayesh *et al.* 1991) did not co-segregate with trimethylamine oxidation.

Urine headspace

Urine

CH₃SH
Methanethiol

CH₃-S-CH₃
Dimethylsulphide

$$CH_2=CH-\overset{\overset{\text{O}}{\|}}{C}-SCH_3$$
S-methylthioacrylate

$$CH_3-S-CH_2-CH_2-\overset{\overset{\text{O}}{\|}}{C}-SCH_3$$
S-methyl-3-
(methylthio) thiopropionate

CH₃-SS-CH₃
Dimethyldisulphide

CH₃-S-CH₂-S-CH₃
Bis (methylthio) methane

Asparagus

CH₃-S-CH₃
Dimethylsulphone

$$CH_3-\overset{\overset{\text{O}}{\|}}{\underset{\underset{\text{O}}{\|}}{S}}-CH_3$$
Dimethylsulphoxide

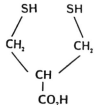

Dihydroasparagusic acid

Asparagusic acid

Fig. 24.2. Some sulphur-containing compounds found in asparagus, the urine of asparagus eaters, and urine headspace from asparagus eaters. (From Max 1989.)

ODORIFEROUS URINE AFTER ASPARAGUS INGESTION

It has been known for centuries that the urine of persons who have eaten asparagus has a peculiar smell.

The phenomenon was studied in a population of 115 persons by Allison & McWhirter (1956); they found that 46 of them were 'excretors' and suggested that this trait was an autosomal dominant Mendelian character.

The situation was complicated by the work of Lison *et al.* (1980), which was based on the idea that everyone who has eaten asparagus passes urine with the odour, but only some people can detect it. Support for this view was obtained by studying the 'smell detection threshold' by using doubling dilutions of a urine with the odour. It was noted that 'non-smellers' produced urine after eating asparagus, which was easily recognized as positive by 'smellers'. They held the view that everyone passes urine containing the smelly compounds after eating asparagus, an extrapolation which was not authenticated with suitable observations. Family studies to determine whether 'smelling' (versus 'non-smelling') were Mendelian characters were not reported.

As a result of studying 600 individuals, Mitchell *et*

al. (1987) found that 346 (43.25%) passed odorous urine after eating asparagus. The proportion was the same in both sexes. Twenty-five families were studied and the passing of odorous urine judged to be a Mendelian dominant character. The scoring of the urines was made by a panel of at least three 'smellers'.

Strangely, Richer *et al.* (1989) report that all 103 French citizens produced odorous urine after the ingestion of 60 g asparagus. This was a smaller 'dose' than used by others (450 g by Lison *et al.* 1980; and 250 to 300 g by Mitchell *et al.* 1987). It is not clearly stated who assessed the result, but presumably it was authenticated smellers.

This strange story may have relevance to pharmacogenetics because the biotransformation of sulphur-containing drugs may be mediated by the same processes as are involved in asparagus metabolism. The substances found in the urine after asparagus ingestion have included *S*-methylthioacrylate and *S*-methyl-3-(methylthio)thiopropionate. There is some dispute as to whether the addition of these compounds to urine reproduces the characteristic odour. The volatile compounds collected above the odorous urine include methanethiol, bis-(methylthio)methane, dimethyl sulphide, dimethyl-sulphoxide and dimethylsulphone (Fig. 24.2). It has been suggested that the reduced sulphur compounds (sulphides and disulphides) give the pungency to the aroma, whilst the partially oxidized sulphones and sulphoxides add a sweetness (Max 1989).

These sulphur-containing metabolites are believed to be produced from asparagusic acid, dihydro-asparagusic acid (2,2-dithiolisobutyric acid) and *S*-acetylhydroasparagusic acid, which are found in the vegetable.

Whether there are two traits involved – one metabolic and one olfactory – remains to be determined.

Åkesson, B., Skerfving, S. & Mattiasson, L. (1988). Experimental study on the metabolism of trimethylamine in man. *British Journal of Industrial Medicine*, **45**, 262–8.

Allison, A. C. & McWhirter, K. G. (1956). Two unifactorial characters for which man is polymorphic. *Nature*, **178**, 748–9.

Al-Waiz, M., Ayesh, R., Mitchell, S. C., Idle, J. R. & Smith, R. L. (1987a). A genetic polymorphism of the *N*-oxidation of trimethylamine in humans. *Clinical Pharmacology and Therapeutics*, **423**, 588–94.

Al-Waiz, M., Ayesh, R., Mitchell, S. C., Idle, J. R. & Smith, R. L. (1987b). Disclosure of the metabolic retroversion of trimethylamine *N*-oxide in humans: A pharmacogenetic approach. *Clinical Pharmacology and Therapeutics*, **42**, 608–12.

Al-Waiz, M., Ayesh, R., Mitchell, S. C., Idle, J. R. & Smith, R. L. (1988). Trimethylaminuria ('Fish-odour syndrome'): a study of an affected family. *Clinical Science*, **74**, 231–6.

Al-Waiz, M., Ayesh, R., Mitchell, S. C., Idle, J. R. & Smith, R. L. (1989). Trimethylaminuria: The detection of carriers using a trimethylamine load test. *Journal of Inherited Metabolic Disease*, **12**, 80–5.

Ayesh, R., Al-Waiz, M., Crothers, M. J., Cholerton, S., Mitchell, S. C., Idle, J. R. & Smith, R. L. (1988). Deficient nicotine *N*-oxidation in two sisters with trimethylaminuria. *British Journal of Clinical Pharmacology*, **25**, 664P – 5P.

Ayesh, R., Al-Waiz, M., McBurney, A., Mitchell, S. C., Idle, J. R., Ward, J. W. & Smith, R. L. (1989). Variable metabolism of pinacidil: lack of correlation with the debrisoquine and trimethylamine *C* -and *N*-oxidative polymorphisms. *British Journal of Clinical Pharmacology*, **27**, 423–8.

Ayesh, R., Kroemer, H., Eichelbaum, M. & Smith, R. L. (1991). Metabolism of verapamil in a family pedigree with deficient *N*-oxidation of methylamine. *British Journal of Clinical Pharmacology*, **31**, 693–6.

Ayesh, R. & Smith, R. L. (1990). Genetic polymorphism of trimethylamine *N*-oxidation. *Pharmacology and Therapeutics*, **45**, 387–401.

Back, D. J., Bates, M., Breckenridge, A. M., Ellis, A., MacIver, M., Orme, M. L'E. & Rowe, P.H. (1981). The *in vitro* metabolism of ethinyloestradiol, mestranol and levonorgestrel by human jejunal mucoasa. *British Journal of Clinical Pharmacology*, **11**, 275–8.

Back, D. J., Breckenridge, A. M., MacIver, M., Orme, M. L'E, Purba, H. S., Rowe, P. H. & Taylor, I. (1982). The gut wall metabolism of ethinyloestradiol and its contribution to the pre-systemic metabolism of ethinyloestradiol in humans. *British Journal of Clinical Pharmacology*, **13**, 525–30.

Back, D. J., Maggs, J. L., Purba, H. S., Newby, S. & Park, B. K. (1984). 2-hydroxylation of ethinyloestradiol in relation to the oxidation of sparteine and antipyrine. *British Journal of Clinical Pharmacology*, **18**, 603–7.

Back, D. J. & Orme, M. L'E. (1984). Interindividual variability in oral contraceptive disposition. *Trends in Pharmacological Sciences*, **5**, 480–3.

Ball, S., Back, D. J. & Orme, M. L'E. (1988). Characterisation and inhibition of oestrogen 2-hydroxylase activity in human liver microsomes. *British Journal of Clinical Pharmacology*, **25**, 643P–4P.

Cascorbi, H. F., Vesell, E. S., Blake, D. A. & Helrich, M. (1971). Genetic and environmental influence on halothane metabolism in twins. *Clinical Pharmacology and Therapeutics*, **12**, 50–5.

Caughey, G. H., Rice, S. A., Kosek, J. C. & Mazze, R. I. (1979). Effect of phenytoin (DPH) treatment on methoxyflurane metabolism in rats. *Journal of Pharmacology and Experimental Therapeutics*, **210**, 180–5.

Cummings, J., Milstead, R., Cunningham, D. & Kaye, S. (1986). Marked inter-patient variation in adriamycin biotransformation to 7-deoxyaglycones: evidence from metabolites identified in serum. *European Journal of Clinical Oncology*, **22**, 991–1001.

Dahlgren, B.-E. (1977). Influence of methoxyflurane–nitrous oxide analgesia during childbirth on renal and hepatic function. *British Journal of Anaesthesia*, **49**, 1271–7.

Dalen, E. & Westerholm, B. (1974). Occurrence of hepatic impairment in women jaundiced by oral contraceptives and their mothers and sisters. *Acta Medica Scandinavia*, **195**, 459–63.

Eskborg, S., Straudler, H.-S., Edsmyr, F., Ñaslund, I. & Tahanainen, P. (1985). Pharmacokinetic study of N infusions of adriamycin. *European Journal of Clinical Pharmacology*, **28**, 205–12.

Farrell, G., Prendergast, D. & Murray, M. (1985). Halothane hepatitis – detection of a constitutional susceptibility factor. *New England Journal of Medicine*, **313**, 1310–14.

Fotherby, K., Akpoviroro, J., Abdel-Rahman, H. A., Toppozada, H. K., de Souza, J. C., Coutinho, E. M., Koetsawang, S., Nukulkarn, P., Sheth, U. K., Mapa, M. K., Gopalan, S., Plunkett, E. R., Brenner, P. F., Hickey, M. V., Grech, E. S., Lichtenberg, R., Gual, C., Molina, R., Gomez-Rogers, C., Kwon, E., Kim, S. W., Chan, T., Ratnam, S. S., Landgren, B. M., Shearman, R. F. P., Goldzieher, J. W. & Dozier, T. S. (1981). Pharmacokinetics of ethynyloestradiol in women from different populations. *Contraception*, **23**, 487–96.

Goldzieher, J. W., Dozier, T. S. & de la Pena, A. (1980). Plasma levels and pharmacokinetics of ethynyl estrogens in various populations. *Contraception*, **21**, 1–16.

Guengerich, F. P. (1988). Oxidation of 17α-ethynylestradiol by human liver cytochrome P-450. *Molecular Pharmacology*, **33**, 500–8.

Guengerich, F. P. (1992). Human cytochrome P-450 enzymes. *Life Sciences*, **50**, 1471–8.

Higgins, T., Chaykin, S., Hammond, K. & Humbert, J. (1972). Trimethylamine *N*-oxide synthesis: a human variant. *Biochemical Medicine*, **6**, 392–6.

Hoft, H., Bunker, J. P., Goodman, H. I. & Gregory, P. B. (1981). Halothane hepatitis in three pairs of closely related women. *New England Journal of Medicine*, **304**, 1023–4.

Holzbach, R.T., Sivak, D.A. & Braun, W.E. (1983). Familial recurrent intrahepatic cholestasis of pregnancy: a genetic study providing evidence for transmission of a sex-limited dominant trait. *Gut*, **85**, 175–9.

Humbert, J. R., Hammond, K. B., Hathaway, W. E., Marcoux, J. G. & O'Brien, D. (1970). Trimethylaminuria: The fish-odour syndrome. *Lancet*, **2**, 770–1.

Inman, W. H.W. & Mushin, W. W. (1974). Jaundice after repeated exposure to halothane: An analysis of reports to the committee on Safety of Medicines. *British Medical Journal*, **1**, 5–10.

Kamyab, S., Fotherby, K. & Steele, S. J. (1969). Metabolism of [^{14}C]-ethynylestradiol in women. *Nature*, **221**, 360–1.

Kenna, J.G. (1991). The molecular basis of halothane-induced hepatitis. *Biochemical Society Transactions*, **19**, 191–5.

Kerlan, V., Dreano, Y., Bercovici, J.P., Beaune, P.H., Floch, H.H. & Berthou, F. (1992). Nature of cytochromes P450 involved in the 2-/4-hydroxylations of estradiol in human liver microsomes. *Biochemical Pharmacology*, **44**, 1745–56.

Kreek, M.J., Weser, E. Sleisenger, M.H. & Jeffries, G. H. (1967). Idiopathic cholestasis of pregnancy. *New England Journal of Medicine*, **277**, 1391–5.

Kulkarni, B. D. & Goldzieher, J. W. (1970). A preliminary report on urine excretion pattern and method of isolation of ^{14}C-ethynylestradiol metabolites in women. *Contraception*, **1**, 47–55.

Lison, M., Blondheim, S. H. & Melmed, R. N. (1980). A polymorphism of the ability to smell urinary metabolites of asparagus. *British Medical Journal*, **281**, 1676–8.

Maggs, J. L., Grabowski, P. S. & Park, B. K. (1983a). Drug protein conjugates II: An investigation of the irreversible binding and metabolism of 17α-ethinyloestradiol *in vivo*. *Biochemical Pharmacology*, **32**, 301–8.

Maggs, J. L., Grimmer, S. F. M,. Gilmore, I. T., Breckenridge, A. M., Orme, M. L'E. & Park, B. K. (1983b). The biliary and urinary metabolites in [^{3}H]17α-ethinyloestradiol in women. *Xenobiotica*, **13**, 421–31.

Max, B. (1989). This and That: chocolate addiction, the dual pharmacogenetics of asparagus eaters, and the arithmetic of freedom. *Trends in Pharmacological Sciences*, **10**, 390–4.

Mitchell, S. C., Waring, R. H., Land, D. & Thorpe, W. V. (1987). Odorous urine following asparagus ingestion in man. *Experientia*, **43**, 382–3.

Moore, M. J., Hardy, R. W., Thiessen, J. J., Soldin, S. & Erlichman, C. (1988). Rapid development of enhanced clearance after high-dose cyclophosophamide. *Clinical Pharmacology and Therapeutics*, **44**, 622–8.

Mouridsen, H. T., Faber, O. & Skovsted, L. (1974). The biotransformation of cyclophosphamide in man: analysis

of the variation in normal subjects. *Acta Pharmacologica et Toxicologica*, **35**, 98–106.

Orme, M. L'E., Back, D. J. & Ball, S. (1992). Interindividual variation in the metabolism of ethynylestradiol. In *Pharmacogenetics of Drug Metabolism*, ed. W. Kalow, pp. 757–67. New York: Pergamon.

Pirmohamed, M., Graham, A., Roberts, P., Smith, D., Chadwick, D., Breckenridge, A. M. & Park, B. K. (1991a). Carbamazepine-hypersensitivity: assessment of clinical and *in vitro* chemical cross-reactivity with phenytoin and oxcarbazepine. *British Journal of Clinical Pharmacology*, **32**, 741–9.

Pirmohamed, M., Kitteringham, N. R., Breckenridge, A. M. & Park, B. K. (1991b). Detection of an autoantibody directed against human liver microsomal protein in a patient with carbamazepine hypersensitivity. *British Journal of Clinical Pharmacology*, **33**, 183–6.

Pirmohamed, M., Kitteringham, N. R., Guenthner, T. M., Breckenridge, A. M. & Park, B. K. (1992). An investigation of the formation of cytotoxic, protein-reactive and stable metabolites from carbamazepine *in vitro*. *Biochemical Pharmacology*, **42**, 1675–82.

Purba, H., Maggs, J. L., Orme, M. L'E., Back, D. J, & Park, B. K. (1987). The metabolism of 17α-ethinyloestradiol by human liver microsomes in formation of catechol and chemically reactive metabolites. *British Journal of Clinical Pharmacology*, **23**, 447–53.

Ray, D. C. & Drummond, G. B. (1991). Halothane hepatitis. *British Journal of Anaesthesia*, **67**, 84–99.

Richer, C., Decker, N., Belin, J., Imbs, J. L., Montastrue, J. L. & Giudicelli, J. F. (1989). Odorous urine in man after asparagus. *British Journal of Clinical Pharmacology*, **27**, 640–1.

Speilberg, S. P., Gordon, G. B., Blake, D. A., Goldstein, D. A. & Herlong, H. F. (1981). Predisposition to phenytoin hepatotoxicity assessed *in vitro*. *New England Journal of Medicine*, **305**, 722–7.

Waskell, L., Canova-Davis, E., Philpot, R., Parandoush, L. & Chiang, J. Y. L. (1986). Identification of the enzymes catalyzing metabolism of methoxyflurane. *Drug Metabolism and Disposition*, **14**, 643–8.

Williams, M. C. & Goldzieher, J. W. (1980). Chromatographic patterns of urinary ethynyl estrogen metabolites in various populations. *Steroids*, **36**, 255–82.

Wilson, J., Marshall, R. W. & Hodgkinson, A. (1972). Excretion of methoxyflurane metabolites. *British Medical Journal*, **1**, 594.

25   Glucose-6-phosphate dehydrogenase deficiency

INTRODUCTION

GLUCOSE-6-PHOSPHATE dehydrogenase deficiency is the most common known enzymopathy and is probably the basis for the most common form of genetically determined adverse reaction to drugs. This is because the deficiency is (1) widespread throughout the world, (2) at a high prevalence in many populations, (3) the basis for haemolysis in response to a variety of drug chemicals.

The discovery of how a deficiency of the enzyme glucose-6-phosphate dehydrogenase (G6PD) can be the basis for a severe haemolytic episode, following the administration of the antimalarial primaquine, is a classic of medical detective work and scientific investigation (see Tarlov *et al.* 1962).

Haemolytic anaemia had been recognized as an occasional complication of pamaquin therapy when that drug was introduced in 1926 as an active agent against the exoerythrocytic forms of *Plasmodium vivax*. The phenomenon was suspected to be due to an immune mechanism but no antibody could be discovered in the blood. During the Second World War the closely similar drug primaquine was introduced on a large scale particularly to treat US servicemen who contracted malaria. Many more cases of haemolytic anaemia occurred following primaquine ingestion and this was the spur to intensive investigation (see Beutler 1959).

HAEMOLYTIC ANAEMIA AFTER PRIMAQUINE INGESTION

When a sensitive individual took 30 mg of primaquine daily a haemolytic anaemia developed after 2 or 3 days. His urine gradually turned brown, and muscular pains occurred followed by anaemia and sometimes jaundice. If the primaquine was discontinued the patient slowly returned to normal. If the symptoms were not too severe and the primaquine was continued the patient also gradually improved. This last observation turned out to be of great importance.

On investigation, the presence of a haemolytic anaemia was obvious with dark urine due to haemoglobinuria. There was no haemorrhage. The Coomb's test was negative, the erythrocyte fragility normal and there was no spherocytosis. The striking finding was the presence of Heinz bodies (denatured haemoglobin) in the red cells; after the condition had been present for some days a reticulocytosis occurred.

CROSS-TRANSFUSION EXPERIMENTS

Red cells labelled with ^{51}Cr were transfused from sensitive subjects into non-sensitive recipients. The survival of these cells was normal until primaquine was administered when they became lysed. On the other hand, when ^{51}Cr-labelled red cells were transfused from a non-sensitive donor to a sensitive individual they survived normally even when primaquine was administered, and even when the recipient's own red cells were lysed under the influence of the drug.

The observation that a sensitive individual recovered despite continued primaquine administration was similarly investigated. When red cells of a narrow age range were selectively labelled with [51]Fe, it was found that in a sensitive subject the red cells were lysed by primaquine when 63 to 76 days old but not when 8 to 21 days old. In this way it was established that it is the senescent erythrocyte which is lysed by primaquine. The reason for the spontaneous recovery during continued primaquine ingestion was shown to be the production of a new erythrocyte population with a low average age (Dern *et al.* 1954).

ENZYMIC BASIS

The normal red cell was known to possess enzymes concerned with glucose metabolism which proceeds by two routes, the Embden–Meyerhof pathway and the pentose monophosphate shunt (Fig. 25.1). The first enzyme (which is rate-controlling) in the second pathway is glucose-6-phosphate dehydrogen-

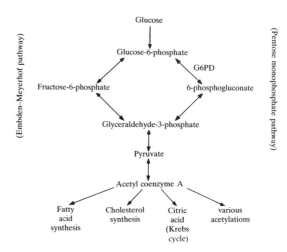

Fig. 25.1. Outline scheme of cellular glucose metabolism. One arrow may represent one or several enzyme reactions. (From Evans 1969.)

ase (Fig. 25.2) and its activity is diminished in primaquine-sensitive individuals. This discovery was made as a result of observations on reduced glutathione. It was found that when red cells from both sensitive and non-sensitive persons were incubated

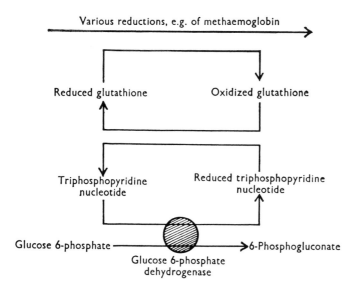

Fig. 25.2. The site of the metabolic defect in primaquine sensitivity is indicated by the shaded area. (From Evans & Clarke 1961.)

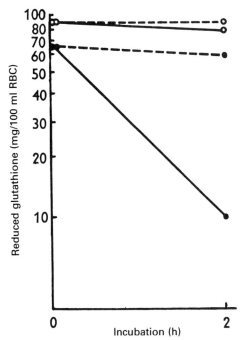

Fig. 25.3. Effect on reduced glutathione of incubating sensitive ● and non-sensitive ○ red cells with primaquine diphosphate (10 mg/ml) in the presence of glucose.
——, incubated with primaquine;
-------, incubated without primaquine.
(From Beutler 1960, by permission of McGraw Hill Book Co. Ltd.)

in vitro with primaquine but without glucose, the reduced glutathione content fell (Fig. 25.3). In the presence of glucose, however, only the glutathione content of the primaquine-sensitive cells fell (Beutler 1960). This observation suggested that the defect in the sensitive cell was a failure properly to metabolize glucose. This failure was tracked down to the enzyme glucose-6-phosphate dehydrogenase (G6PD) which converts glucose-6-phosphate (G6P) to 6-phosphoglucose-δ-lactone (Carson *et al.* 1956). This metabolic step generates NADPH from NADP, and the NADPH reduces glutathione. This is the key event concerning G6PD; when it is defective many diverse consequences (which will be described below) will follow. This reduced glutathione keeps haemoglobin from being denatured, probably by the reduction of hydrogen peroxide (see Liebowitz & Cohen 1968; Luzzatto 1986). Therefore deficiency of G6PD under conditions of stress leads to inefficient reduction of glutathione. Primaquine causes

the rapid loss of reduced glutathione from the older G6PD deficient cells. This in turn leads to the formation of denatured haemoglobin and to cell lysis (Carson 1968).

GENETIC STUDIES

Family studies by Childs *et al.* (1958) utilized a glutathione stability test similar to that described above but with acetylphenylhydrazine as the stressing chemical. A total of 16 Negro families involving 163 persons was tested and the results were very suggestive of sex-linkage, but a sex-limited autosomal character could not be excluded. Siniscalco *et al.* (1960) measured G6PD levels in 41 complete two-generation family units with 152 children and confirmed that G6PD deficiency is carried on the X chromosome and linked to colour blindness. Histograms showing the clear-cut bimodality of G6PD values in 104 men and the presence of an intermediate group in 113 women were published by Larizza *et al.* (1960). About 15% of American Negro males were found to be G6PD deficient.

Davidson *et al.* (1964) studied the non-G6PD-deficient male offspring of heterozygote mothers by measuring their erythrocyte G6PD activity. The variability between 32 sibships was found to be much greater than the variability within sibships. This finding suggested the existence of a number of 'normal' alleles controlling G6PD variants with differing enzymic activities in the population. Direct evidence for the existence of variants of 'normal' alleles was provided by Modiano *et al.* (1979), who demonstrated the existence of two types of G6PD B (called B1 and B2) separated by column chromatography on DEAE-Sephadex. They also demonstrated two types of G6PD A, and showed that these variants of both B and A had different kinetic properties.

It is to be noted that the work referred to above was based purely on quantitative variations in red cell enzyme activity.

VARIANT FORMS OF G6PD

Intensive study of G6PD, especially by electrophoresis, revealed variants in the population and it was also found that some of these variants had diminished activity.

When the enzyme was studied by starch gel

Table 25.1. *The characteristics of the main G6PD variants*

Variant	Population	% of normal RBC activity	Electophoretic mobility approx % of normal	K_m G6P (μM)	K_m NADP (μM)	2dG6P utilization	Heat stability	Population frequency
Normal B	Various	100	100	50–78	2.9–4.4	<4	Normal	Usual
A	Negro	88	110	Normal	Normal	<4	Normal	18%
A−	Negro	8–20	110	Normal	Normal	<4	Normal	10–15%
Mediterranean	Mediterranean peoples & Indians	0–7	Normal	19–26	1.2–1.6	23–37	Low	Common
Canton	Southern Chinese	4–24	105	20–36	2.0–2.4	4–15	Slightly reduced	Common

2dG6P, 2-deoxyglucose-6-phosphate.
Adapted from: Standardization of procedures for the study of glucose-6-phosphate dehydrogenase. Report of a WHO Scientific group (1967).

electrophoresis at pH 8.5 the usual type of G6PD migrated slowly toward the anode and so was called B. The common variant form in non-G6PD-deficient American negroes moved faster toward the anode and was called A (Boyer *et al.* 1962).

A technical report was published by the World Health Organization in 1967 which (1) summarized the position with regards to the clinical manifestations associated with variants of G6PD, (2) laid down criteria for characterizing a new variant, (3) introduced a standardized system for naming variants.

In order that putative new variants should be systematically compared with known variants it was suggested that the minimum characterization should be by means of:

- Red cell G6PD activity
- Electrophoretic migration
- Michaelis constants for G6P
- Relative rate of utilization of 2dG6P
- Thermal stability

Other desirable studies listed include, for example, the determination of pH optima.

Twenty-four variants (including the 'normal') were tabulated in the WHO report. The characteristics of the main variants are shown in Table 25.1.

The WHO group established a standardized nomenclature, as follows:

1 the already existing designations B, A and A- were retained;
2 variants should be given geographic or trivial names;
3 when referring to the enzyme itself it is appropriate to use the abbreviation G6PD, such as G6PD Mediterranean;
4 the phenotypic and genotypic symbol should be Gd;
5 in the case of the genotypic symbol the d should be italicized, the specific genetic designation being a superscript (e.g. Gd^B);
6 in the phenotypic characterization of a female heterozygote the actually observed phenotypic expression should be indicated not the phenotype of inference. An oblique line can be used to separate the two names in the genotypic designations (e.g. Gd^A/Gd^B).

The X-linked inheritance which was demonstrated using erythrocytic G6PD activity has also been confirmed by observing the disposition of several variants within pedigrees; for example in appropriate Negro families males are either (B) or (A)

whereas females can be (B) or (A) or (BA), (Boyer *et al.* 1962; Kirkman & Hendrickson 1963).

A recent, conveniently available compilation (Beutler & Yoshida 1988) listed over 370 variants, and as McKusick emphasized in a foreword to the article:

as indicated by the authors G6PD enjoys the distinction among enzymes of having the largest number of identified variant forms. Indeed, it is likely that it has the largest number of variants of any single polypeptide chain, and therefore the largest number of known mutations in one gene.

Similar tables were published by Luzzatto & Mehta (1989), Beutler (1990) and Vulliamy *et al.* (1993).

Variants have been found in all racial groups from Irish to Chinese, and geographically from Finland to New Guinea. Some variants (as Table 25.1 indicates) are very common, particularly in the tropics, subtropics and Mediterranean regions. Other variants (such as those causing hereditary non-spherocytic haemolytic anaemia – see below) are very rare and occur in all ethnic groups. Variants are divided into numbered classes according to the clinical manifestations which they cause, as indicated at the foot of Table 25.2.

ANALYSIS OF THE PROTEIN STRUCTURE

By means of classical amino acid fingerprinting methods Yoshida (1967) was able to demonstrate that the Negro variant A enzyme differed from the normal B enzyme by a change in one amino acid. Asparagine in the normal B enzyme was substituted by aspartic acid in the A Negro variant.

Despite the fact that such a large number of enzyme variants were described using the criteria mentioned above, no progress was made in elucidating the structures of the different forms until the advent of molecular genetics.

MOLECULAR GENETICS

The structure of the enzyme was worked out from cDNA clones isolated from a number of human tissues by Persico *et al.* (1986a, b). These clones enabled the entire coding region to be sequenced. The predicted polypeptide consisted of 515 amino acids with a molecular weight of 59 kDa. This is the subunit, and the whole enzyme exists as a homodimer or homotetramer.

Table 16.3. *Evidence for the polymorphic acetylation of drugs other than isoniazid*

Drug investigated	Pharmacological action	Parameter differentiating between phenotypes	Compound with which panel of volunteers phenotyped	Reference
SM	Antimicrobial	Percentage urinary SM acetylated	Isoniazid	Evans 1962
SM	Antimicrobial	Metabolism of SM by human liver homogenates		Evans & White 1964
SM	Antimicrobial	Percentage urinary SM acetylated		Peters et al. 1965
SM	Antimicrobial	As above plus percentage serum SM acetylated		Evans 1969
SM	Antimicrobial	As above plus percentage serum SM acetylated		Mattila et al. 1969a
SM	Antimicrobial	As above plus percentage serum SM acetylated		Rao et al. 1970
SM	Antimicrobial	As above plus percentage serum SM acetylated		Ellard & Gammon 1977
Sulphamerazine	Antimicrobial	Percentage urinary SM acetylated	Isoniazid	Mattila et al. 1969a
Sulphamerazine	Antimicrobial	Plasma and urinary half-lives	SM	Vree et al. 1983
Sulphadimethoxine	Antimicrobial	Plasma half-life and urinary excretion pattern	SM	Vree et al. 1990
SP	Antimicrobial	Percentage acetylation of SP in serum and urine	SM	Schröder & Evans 1972a
SP	Antimicrobial	Percentage acetylation of SP in serum and urine		Das & Eastwood 1975
Procainamide	Antiarrhythmic	Percentage acetylated procainamide in urine	Isoniazid	Karlsson et al. 1975
Procainamide	Antiarrhythmic	Percentage acetylated procainamide in urine	SP	Karlsson & Molin 1975
Procainamide	Antiarrhythmic	Percentage acetylated procainamide in urine	Isoniazid	Gibson et al. 1975
Procainamide	Antiarrhythmic	Percentage acetylated procainamide in plasma and urine	DDS	Reidenberg et al. 1975
Procainamide	Antiarrhythmic	Percentage acetylated procainamide in plasma and urine	SM	Frislid et al. 1976
Hydralazine	Antihypertensive	Metabolism of hydralazine in liver homogenates	SM	Evans & White 1964
Hydralazine	Antihypertensive	Plasma hydralazine concentrations following oral doses higher in S than in R	MADDS/DDS and isoniazid	Reidenberg et al. 1973
Hydralazine	Antihypertensive	Plasma hydralazine concentrations following oral doses higher in S than in R	SM	Zacest & Koch-Weser 1972
Hydralazine	Antihypertensive	Plasma hydralazine concentrations following oral doses higher in S than in R	SM	Talseth 1976
Hydralazine	Antihypertensive	Plasma hydralazine concentrations following oral doses higher in S than in R	SM	Jounela et al. 1975
Hydralazine	Antihypertensive	S excrete less NAc HPZ and TP than R but more PZ and HH	SM	Facchini & Timbrell 1981
Hydralazine	Antihypertensive	Bimodal distribution of OH MTP/HH	SM	Timbrell et al. 1980

No.	Name	Exon	Nucleotide	Nucleotide change	Codon change	Amino acid	Amino acid change	WHO class	Reference
39	Guadaljara	10	1159	C → T	CGC → TGC	387	Arg → Cys	I	Beutler et al. 1992a
40	Mt Sinai	10,5	1159	C → T	CGC → TGC	387	Arg → Cys	I	Vlachos et al. unpublished
			376	A → G	AAT → GAT	126	Asn → Asp		
41	Beverly Hills[k]	10	1160	G → A	CGC → CAC	387	Arg → His	I	Hirono et al. 1989
42	Nashville[l]	10	1178	G → A	CGC → CAC	393	Arg → His	I	Beutler et al. 1991b
43	Alhambra	10	1180	G → C	GTG → CTG	394	Val → Leu	I	Beutler et al. 1992a
44	Peurto Limon	10	1192	G → A	GAG → AAG	398	Glu → Lys	I	Beutler et al. 1991a
45	Riverside	10	1228	G → T	GGC → TGC	410	Gly → Cys	I	Hirono et al. 1989
46	Japan	10	1229	G → A	GGC → GAC	410	Gly → Asp	I	Beutler et al. 1992a
47	Tokyo[m]	10	1246	G → A	GAG → AAG	416	Glu → Lys	I	Hirono et al. 1992
48	Atlanta-1	10	1284	C → A	TAC → TAA	428	Tyr → Stop	I	Beutler et al. unpublished
49	Pawnee	10	1316	G → C	CGC → CCC	439	Artg → Pro	I	Beutler et al. 1992a
50	Telti	11	1318	C → T	CTC → TTC	440	Leu → Phe	I	Busutil et al. unpublished
51	Santiago de Cuba	11	1339	G → A	GGG → AGG	447	Gly → Arg	II	Vulliamy et al. 1988
52	Cassano	11	1347	G → C	CAG → CAC	449	Gln → His	II	Calabro et al. 1992
53	Chinese-2[n]	11	1360	C → T	CGC → TGC	454	Arg → Cys	I	Perng et al. 1992
54	Andalus	11	1361	G → A	CGC → CAC	454	Arg → His	II	Vives-Corrons et al. 1990
55	Canton[o]	12	1376	G → T	CGT → CTT	459	Arg → Leu	II	Stevens et al. 1991
56	Cosenza	12	1376	G → C	CGT → CCT	459	Arg → Pro	II	Calabro et al. 1992
57	Kaiping[p]	12	1388	G → A	CGT → CAT	463	Arg → His	II	Chiu et al. 1991b
58	Campinas	13	1463	G → T	GGC → GTC	488	Gly → Val	I	Baronciani et al. unpublished

Other variations listed with same mutation:

[a]Gaozhou, Ube, Bodia-like and Sapporo-like (Chao et al. 1991).

[b]Matera (Vulliamy et al. 1988), Betica (Beutler et al. 1989), Tepic, Distrito Federal and Castilla (Beutler et al. 1991d), Alabama (Beutler 1991), Kabyle and Laghouat (Nafa et al. 1993).

[c]Ube (Hinoro et al. 1992).

[d]Dallas and Birmingham (Beutler & Kuhl 1990), Cagliari and Sassari (DeVita et al. 1989), Panama (Beutler et al. unpublished).

[e]Marion and Gastonia (Beutler et al. 1991b), Le Jeune (Beutler et al. 1991c).

[f]Modena (Fiorelli et al. 1990), Lodi (Ninfali et al. 1991).

[g]Jammu (Beutler et al. 1991c), Mahidol (Vulliamy, unpublished).

[h]Kerala (Ahluwalia et al. 1992).

[i]Selma and Betica (Betler et al. 1989), Guantanemo (Mason et al. unpublished).

[j]Walter Reed, Iowa City and Springfield (Hirono et al. 1989).

[k]Genoa (Argusti et al. unpublished), Worcester (Beutler et al. unpublished).

[l]Anaheim (Beutler et al. 1991b), Portici (Filosa et al. 1992), Calgary (Beutler et al. unpublished).

[m]Dundee (Stevens et al. unpublished).

[n]Maewo (Town et al. unpublished).

[o]Taiwan-Hakka, Gifu and Agrigento-like (Chiu et al. 1991b).

[p]Anant, Dhon, Petrich-like and Sapporo-like (Chiu et al. 1991b).

Only nucleotide changes which cause amino acid changes are shown.
WHO class I, non-sphaerocytic haemolytic anaemia; II, severe deficiency; III, moderate deficiency; IV, no deficiency.
A, adenine; G, guanine; T, thymine; C, cytosine.
Ala, Alanine; Arg, arginine; Asp, aspartic acid; Asn, asparagine; Cys, cysteine; Gln, glutamine; Glu, glutamic acid; Gly, glycine; His, histidine; Ile, isoleucine; Leu, leucine; Lys, Lysine; Met, methionine; Phe, phenylalanine; Pro, proline; Ser, serine; Thr, threonine; Trp, tryptophan; Tyr, tyrosine; Val, valine.
Reproduced with permission from: Vulliamy et al. 1993.

This work was amplified by Martini et al. (1986) who demonstrated that the gene was 18 kb long with 13 exons; the protein-coding region was divided into 12 segments ranging in size from 12 to 236 base pairs.

Following these developments progress could then be made in working out the nucleotide sequence changes in variants (Table 25.2).

It was shown by Takizawa et al. (1987) that the change from G6PD B to G6PD A was 376 A→ G which matched the deduction made by Yoshida 20 years earlier, namely, that 126 asparagine (coded by AAT) was substituted by aspartic acid (coded by GAT).

Twenty-nine males with the G6PD A− phenotype were investigated by Beutler et al. (1989). They all had the A → G transition at nucleotide 376 which was found in G6PD A. In addition three other base changes at different positions were found as shown in Table 25.2. These men were mainly American blacks but two Mexicans, two Puerto Ricans, four Spanish and one white American were included.

The great benefit of having the DNA structure of a given variant determined (as the authors point out) is unequivocal recognition. Also, it is technically easier to determine the base sequence and then work out the amino acid pattern from it than to work in the reverse direction.

With precise molecular identification, G6PD molecules which were previously thought (because of biochemical behaviour) to be different have turned out to be the same (e.g. A− is present not only in Africans but in Europeans; also, supposedly different Mediterranean G6PD enzymes turn out to be all of the 563 C → T nucleotide mutation type). Most G6PD mutants are due to a 3 bp deletion in exon 2 causing the loss of an isoleucine. The diversity of molecular forms of G6PD is further expanded by the mechanism discovered by Hirono & Beutler (1989). It was already known that different forms of G6PD were present in different tissues. These authors discovered that a novel human cDNA having an extra 138 bases encoding 46 amino acids was isolated from a lymphoblastoid cell library. This extra sequence was found to be derived from the 3'-end of intron 7 by alternative splicing. The long form of mRNA or cDNA was also present in granulocytes and sperm of a normal male.

It is thought that the region around lysine 205 is the G6P binding site and the NADP binding site between 363 Asn and 416 Glu.

The way in which a charge difference created by an amino acid substitution changes electrophoretic mobility is clear, but exactly how the structural changes are responsible for the changes in the other physico-chemical properties of enzyme variants and the clinical consequences remains at present to some extent obscure. As more molecular variants become identified and their enzymological characteristics are correlated with their structures it will be possible to see more clearly which parts of the G6PD interact with the substrate and cofactor. An advance in understanding would result from knowing the three dimensional structure in the same way as has been done, for example, in the case of P450$_{cam}$ which is described in another chapter. This goal is now definitely within sight since Bautista et al. (1992) have been able to express the cDNA for human G6PD in E. coli, and purify it to homogeneity. It is interesting to note that the enzyme so produced was much more stable during storage than enzyme prepared from red cells. The way is now open for crystallographic observations to be made on the purified enzyme. Also site directed mutagenesis techniques (see Chapter 38, Common Themes) will be able to produce mutants whose biochemical properties and 3D structures can be examined.

AN EVOLUTIONARY PERSPECTIVE

The main G6PD variants have been put into an evolutionary perspective by means of two studies. Vulliamy et al. (1991) analysed 54 male African subjects for seven polymorphic sites within the G6PD gene and determined the presence of linkage disequilibrium. Only seven of the 128 possible different haplotypes were observed, indicating marked disequilibrium. The most economical pattern of evolution, assuming each mutation to have arisen only once and that A− was the most recent allele, indicated that B was the primordial allele and that A arose from it, and A− from A. Presumably A− became widespread because it conferred in the heterozygous state resistance against malaria (see below). Why A became widespread at the expense of B is unclear. This evolutionary scheme is supported by the finding that the G6PD of the chimpanzee is B-like and its nucleotide 376 is adenine.

A very similar investigation on 54 American black

males (Kay *et al.* 1992) produced the same general conclusion. Also on a set of arbitrary, but reasonable, assumptions these workers calculate that the 202 G → A mutation giving rise to G6PD A− could have arisen as recently as 10 000 years ago.

GENETIC LINKAGE

Since G6PD deficiency was recognized to be sex-linked by means of family studies it was a natural step to see if it was also linked to colour blindness. This was investigated by Porter *et al.* (1962) who found that in the American Negro the maximum likelihood estimate of the recombination fraction for deutan colour blindness and G6PD deficiency was 0.05 with 90% confidence limits of 0.009 and 0.18. For protan colour blindness and G6PD deficiency the estimated recombination fraction was zero with 90% confidence limits of <0.26. As a result of studying a Sardinian family Siniscalco *et al.* (1964) confirmed that recombination occurred between deutan and protan genes showing that they were sited at different loci. They found the linkage between G6PD and deutan to be very close and that between G6PD and protan to be somewhat looser. Hence the conclusion was that the sequence of the three loci was Deutan − − − − − G6PD − − − − − Protan.

Boyer & Graham (1965) showed that the G6PD electrophoretic B/A polymorphism was closely linked to classical haemophilia (haemophilia A). Recombination was absent in 17 opportunities in the three pedigrees studied.

Another marker which invited study was the Xg blood group. No evidence of direct measurable linkage was found between the locus and G6PD by Siniscalco *et al.* (1966) and Adam *et al.* (1967).

GENE LOCALIZATION

The precise point at which the G6PD genes are located on the X chromosome was established by the study of somatic cell hybrids using human cells carrying various X rearrangements (McKusick 1987). For example, Pai *et al.* (1980) studied a black girl with mental retardation and a complex karyotypic rearrangement. They were able to assign the G6PD locus to band Xq28.

Much of this work has now been superseded by newer methods. Kenwrick & Gitschier (1989) used pulsed-field gel electrophoresis to produce a phys-

Table 25.3. *G6PD activity in different cells and tissues of persons with G6PD deficient red cells*

Cells or tissues	Negro	Caucasian	Chinese
White cells	Normal or slightly decreased	Low	Severe deficiency
Liver			
Platelet	Low	Low	
Lens			
Skin	−	Low	
Saliva			
Adrenal	−	−	
Kidney			

From: Chan *et al.* 1965; Justice *et al.* 1966; Bonsignore *et al.* 1966.

ical map of the Xq28 region and, using RFLPs, derived the following order of the loci of the genes mentioned above protan–deutan colour blindness − − − − − G6PD − − − − − Factor VIII deficiency. A similar result was found by Trask *et al.* (1991) using *in situ* hybridization with fluorescent probes in interphase nuclei which gave centromere − − − − − Factor VIII deficiency − − − − − G6PD − − − − − protan/deutan colour blindness − − − − − telomere. The discrepancy between the previous data suggesting that the protan and deutan loci were on opposite sides of G6PD and the newer findings, remains unexplained.

G6PD IN CELLS AND TISSUES OTHER THAN ERYTHROCYTES

On electrophoretic analysis of G6PD from Negro leucocytes Boyer *et al.* (1962) found patterns similar to those found in red cells. However, the situation with regard to enzymic activity varies in different tissues in different ethnic groups as summarized in Table 25.3.

X-INACTIVATION IN THE FEMALE

The wide variation of G6PD activity in the red cells of heterozygous females was recognized in some of the earliest investigations (see, for example, Larizza *et al.* 1960). Some individuals had normal activities whilst others had activities like those of severely

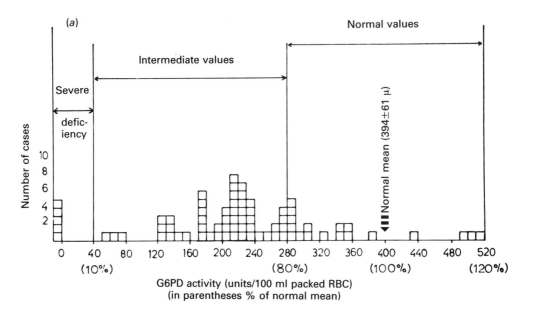

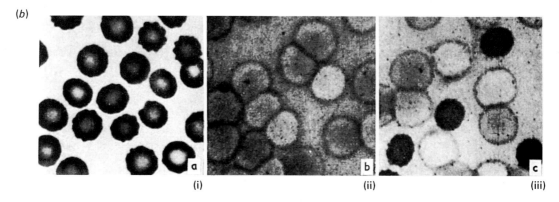

Fig. 25.4.(a) Red cell G6PD activity in 75 female hetero-zygotes detected by pedigree analysis. (b) Results of the cyanmethaemoglobin elution technique in three heterozygotes who were sisters. (i) Stained cells with normal activity (388 units); (ii) unstained (ghost) cells with total absence of activity; (iii) two populations of normal and deficient cells in a heterozygote with an intermediate level of activity (208 units). (From Kattamis 1967.)

deficient males and others had intermediate values. The X-inactivation hypothesis of Lyon (1962) offered an explanation for these findings. Essentially the hypothesis stated that of the two X chromo-somes in any cell, a random one of them became inactive at an early stage of development. Further-more, the progeny of a cell in which this event had occurred would maintain the same pattern (i.e. an X once inactivated would not thereafter be reactivated). This matter was investigated by Kat-tamis (1967) using 75 female heterozygotes detected by pedigree analysis (Fig. 25.4a). The cyan-methaemoglobin elution technique enabled differ-ent cells to be recognized microscopically (Fig. 25.4b). The frequency distribution histogram sug-gested the existence of three types of females: (1) those in whom X inactivation had occurred in such a way that normal G6PD activities were found, (2) those in whom the normal and deficient X chromosomes had been inactivated to an equal extent so that the enzyme activity was intermediate, (3) those in whom the deficient X was preserved and so the G6PD level was very low. Examination of the individual red cells of heterozygotes showed cells showing G6PD activity or cells not showing G6PD activity with no intermediates.

An elegant application of microspectrophotometry of individual erythrocytes by Ashmun et al. (1986) showed that in a female heterozygous for G6PD deficiency there were two types of cells with different rates of reaction for methaemoglobin reduction.

Another way of testing the applicability of the Lyon hypothesis to red cell G6PD was provided by Yoshida et al. (1967). Partially purified enzyme preparations were made of B, the common Negro variant A with normal activity, and the rare low activity Welsh–Scottish variant 'Seattle'. The activities were 0.4 to 0.6 for the first two and 0.1 to 0.2 units/mg protein for the last. Hybridization of (A and B) and of (A and Seattle) was performed by chemical means and proved by two techniques. Column chromatography showed that a hybrid molecule had been produced eluting between A and B. Starch gel electrophoresis showed that a hybrid molecule migrated between A and Seattle. No such hybrid molecules were found on examining the blood cells of appropriate heterozygous females, which suggested that only the product of one X-carried G6PD gene is formed in vivo in any one cell.

THE CLINICAL EFFECTS OF G6PD VARIANTS

The clinical effects caused by G6PD variants are very different depending on the properties of the mutant enzyme. With some variants it would appear that the structure and function of the enzyme is not greatly affected and there are no clinical consequences. In other instances (fairly rare) the enzyme is changed to give rise to a chronic nonspherocytic haemolytic anaemia in the absence of any chemical or other stress. Some variants produce severe haemolysis only under the influence of oxidative drugs and fava beans. Neonatal jaundice and malaria are other clinical events of great importance influenced by G6PD phenotypes. The presence of severe grades of G6PD deficiency leads to a much more serious course of the illness in certain infec-

tions. Rickettsial disorders (e.g. Raoult et al. 1986) and hepatitis (e.g. Agarwal et al. 1985) are typical examples. Other illnesses such as poorly controlled diabetes can cause haemolytic episodes (Burka et al. 1966).

The biochemical basis of the clinical effects of G6PD variants was discussed in detail by Rattazzi et al. (1971), and Luzzatto & Afolayan (1971). In normal erythrocytes only 7% of the glucose metabolized passes through the pentose shunt and it has been calculated from data such as the concentration of NADP which is 1 μM that G6PD is working at less than 0.1% of its potential activity. In Gd Mediterranean erythrocytes glucose utilization is normal but only 1.5% is shunted through the pentose pathway, therefore although potential G6PD activity is less than 1% of normal, actual function of this pathway is 20% of normal. Thus these erythrocytes might usually be capable of sustaining NADPH levels above a threshold below which chronic haemolysis ensues but fail to increase NADPH regeneration in situations where the concentration of intracellular NADP rises.

There is a fundamental difference between the A– variants on the one hand and the Mediterranean and Oriental variants on the other. In the former case, when the red cells are young their content of G6PD is almost normal and then falls off with age. In the latter case even the young cells have G6PD deficiency. So the A– person can compensate for haemolysis by reticulocytosis (as noted in the early primaquine experiments on American negroes) but the Mediterranean and Oriental G6PD deficiency persons cannot.

Malaria

Undoubtedly the most important ecological and medical aspect of G6PD deficiency is its relationship to malaria, a major killing disease.

Early on in the history of the investigation of G6PD deficiency it was observed that there is in general a low frequency of G6PD deficiency in populations where the incidence of malaria is low, and a high frequency of the deficiency in malarious areas (and areas which have been malarious until recently). This observation led to the thought that G6PD deficiency might (like haemoglobin S whose geographic distribution is similar) be protective against malaria.

Table 25.4. *The effect of G6PD genotype on* $\log_{10}$ *P.* falciparum *ring count: children, 4 months to 3 years of age*

Enzyme activity	Number examined	Mean $\log_{10}$ ring count
Normal	148	1.7187
Deficient	53	1.2758
Total	201	–

$d = 2.281$ $(0.03 > p > 0.02)$, taking d to be an approximately standard normal variate.
From: Harris & Gilles 1961.

In support of this view it was found that in an untreated population, parasite rates and densities of *Plasmodium falciparum* in the blood were significantly lower in young male Tanganyikan children with erythrocyte G6PD deficiency than in male children with normal enzymic activity (Allison & Clyde 1961). Likewise in untreated young Nigerian children lower *P. falciparum* ring counts were found in G6PD-deficient than in non-deficient individuals by Harris & Gilles (1961) (Table 25.4).

However, a disappointingly low correlation was found between the frequency of G6PD deficiency and past malarial morbidity in two different districts of Italy (Bottini *et al.* 1978). Also, Kruatrachue *et al.* (1962) could not find any protection against *P. falciparum* in hemizygous males between 1 and 3 years of age in Thailand. However as Harris (1962) observed only nine G6PD deficient children who were 'falciparum positive' were observed, and it seemed that these (unlike some of the G6PD normals with infection) did not need antimalarials, so the information from Thailand does not seem to negate the African findings. More objections to the 'protection' theory were raised by Kidson & Gorman (1962), principally on the grounds that G6PD deficiency and malaria do not invariably coexist. They cite Malays, Indonesians, Armenians and some Melanesians as being large population groups with low frequencies of G6PD deficiency which inhabit malarious areas.

Nevertheless, the positive evidence in favour of the theory that the heterozygous female is at an advantage is very convincing. Bienzle *et al.* (1972) studied 700 Nigerian children from a rural area of holo-endemic *P. falciparum* malaria who presented to hospital with fever. There was no evidence that G6PD-deficient males had any greater resistance to malaria than normal individuals, but amongst non-deficient males those with the A variant had significantly lower counts than those with the B variant. Females heterozygous for G6PD deficiency (specifically individuals of Gd^{A-}/Gd^{B} genotype) had significantly lower parasite counts than any other group of either sex. In an extension of this work Bienzle *et al.* (1979) studied 337 children aged between 1 and 6 years in Abeokuta, Nigeria, who were homozygous for haemoglobin A (so the antimalarial effect of HbS was eliminated). Thirty subjects typed as Gd^{A-}/Gd^{B} showed the lowest median, lowest 90th percentile and lowest 'maximum parasite density'. Statistical comparisons revealed that whilst the difference in parasitaemia between normal and deficient G6PD subjects was not significant, there *was* a significant difference between normal and heterozygous Gd^{A-}/Gd^{B} individuals.

The suggestion was made by Kosower & Kosower (1970) that G6PD deficiency might protect against malaria by virtue of the fact that it raises the level of oxidized glutathione (GSSG) inside the erythrocyte. They found that the rate of protein synthesis in different systems is lowered by GSSG. Since the malaria parasite was synthesizing protein very actively it would be deleteriously affected by a modest rise in GSSG concentration, and this would be to the host's advantage.

The ability to grow *P. falciparum* in red cells in culture opened the door to many interesting experiments. One novel finding has been that the parasite itself is capable of manufacturing G6PD which is electrophoretically slow moving due to its large size (about 450 kDa) rather than to its charge (Ling & Wilson 1988) and distinct from the mammalian host's G6PD (Kurdi-Haidar & Luzzatto 1990) assessed by various biochemical characteristics such as K_m^{G6P}.

The natural selective advantage of this adaptive parasitic G6PD was revealed by the experiments of Usanga & Luzzatto (1985). Parasites previously grown in normal cells were introduced to normal and A− erythrocytes, and their proliferation was much greater in the former. After four cycles, however, the rate of proliferation was the same in both types of cell. The parasite made its own G6PD but only in G6PD-deficient erythrocytes. This finding, according to the authors, explains why hemizygous

G6PD-deficient males are not protected whereas heterozygous females are protected. The reasoning is thus. In the heterozygous females, *P. falciparum* merozoites have an even chance of infecting a normal or a G6PD-deficient cell. In the latter case the chance to complete successfully the next schizogonic cycle is reduced by about 50%, thus justifying the reduced parasitaemia observed. The chance to build up a population of parasites with an adaptive increase of G6PD is much less that in the normal G6PD B person. On the other hand, in the hemizygous G6PD-deficient male all the parasites in all the red cells produce their own G6PD after four cycles so that afterwards their proliferation is the same as in normal cells.

There is some clash of evidence between the findings of Roth & Schulman (1988) and those of Usanga & Luzzatto (1985). The former showed that the low parasite proliferation on first introduction occurs only in G6PD Mediterranean deficient cells (and not in A−). Roth & Schulman (1988) also showed increased resistance to oxidative stress by acetylphenylhydrazine in G6PD deficient adapted parasites (compared with unadapted) when they were growing in G6PD Mediterranean red cells. This phenomenon did not occur in G6PD A− red cells. The authors suggest that the adaptive G6PD produced by the parasite may have some function other than enhancing the ability to withstand oxidative stress.

Favism

Favism is a condition known since antiquity in Mediterranean countries and in its severe form is characterized by a life-threatening haemolysis following the ingestion of the bean *Vicia faba* or the inhalation of its pollen. The condition also occurs in Chinese. It is predominantly a disease of children. Males who are G6PD deficient are particularly liable to the condition.

However, the relationship between G6PD deficiency and favism is not straightforward. Favism occurs in some G6PD deficient families and not in others, and the disorder can be common in areas where the frequency of G6PD deficiency is low and vice versa. Some G6PD deficient subjects tolerate *V. faba* well, even though their relatives have suffered from favism.

According to Sartori (1971), females who suffer severe favism have very low red cell G6PD levels and have a high proportion of their erythrocytes deficient. American Negroes with G6PD deficiency were thought not suffer from favism and this was the basis for the idea that individuals with the G6PD A− variant were not prone to the disease. Galiano *et al.* (1990) described three patients, which showed that this concept is incorrect. It is not clear whether the lack of favism reports from Africa is due to the absence of the bean or to some unknown protective factor.

The hypothesis has been advanced by Sartori (1971) that there is an autosomally determined predisposition to favism *per se* and that severe haemolytic favism is due to a superadded Mediterranean type G6PD deficiency.

The levels of acid phosphatase in favic red cells was shown to be lower than normal by Kattamis & Zannos-Mariolea (1965), and also evidence has been produced by Bottini (1973) that the P^B allele controlling red cell acid phosphatase is protective against the occurrence of haemolytic favism in the presence of G6PD deficiency. Thalassaemia is also claimed to be protective (Bottini *et al.* 1978).

There are also variable factors in the beans themselves which influence the incidence of haemolytic favism. Some varieties are more potent than others (Vural & Sardas 1984). Likewise beans eaten fresh (as opposed to stored or cooked), grown during a sunny dry spring, grown in the north of Sardinia (compared with the south), below 250 m altitude (as opposed to above 250 m) and gathered after sunshine (as opposed to gathered after rain), are more prone to cause haemolytic favism.

Efforts to determine the substances in the beans which are responsible for the toxic effects have focused on the ability of extracts to reduce the GSH levels when incubated with erythrocytes, as well as to cause haemolysis *in vitro*.

The substances vicine and convicine (Fig. 25.5) have been investigated and there is evidence in favour of them being the haemolytic agents. The content of these agents differs markedly between varieties and according to the conditions of cultivation of the beans. Both chemicals reduced GSH levels more in red cells from favism-prone than from normal subjects. Vicine was more potent than convicine (Vural & Sardas 1984).

Vegetables other than *V. faba* can cause favism (Bottini 1973), and in this context a well-studied

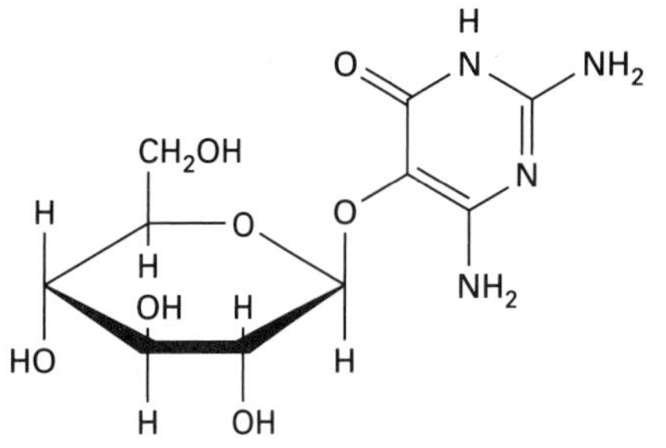

Fig. 25.5. The structures of vicine and convicine. Vicine: When the sugar moiety is removed by glucosidase the aglycone divicine (2,6-diamino-4,5-dihydroxy-pyrimidine) is formed. Convicine: When the sugar moiety is removed by glucosidase the aglycone isouramil (2,4,5-trihydroxy-6-amino-pyrimidine) is formed. (From The Merck Index, 1976.)

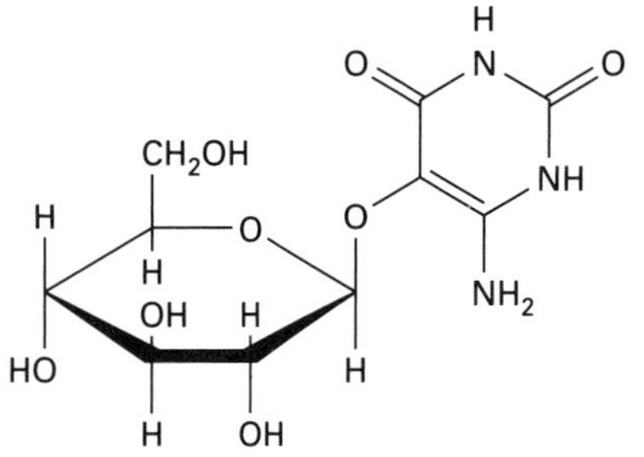

case described by Goblerman *et al.* (1984) is of interest. A 4 year old boy developed a severe haemolytic episode after eating unripe peaches. An extract of unripe peaches was shown to exert an oxidative challenge on normal and asymptomatic G6PD-deficient erythrocytes. However, neither isouramil nor divicine could be identified in the extract. So presumably other constituents of vegetables can have a similar oxidative effect.

The enzymes superoxide dismutase (EC 1.15.1.1) and glutathione peroxidase (EC 1.11.1.9) were studied by Mavelli *et al.* (1984) in the red blood cells of favism patients (1) during a haemolytic crisis, (2) during remissions, and (3) in normal controls and G6PD-deficient individuals who had never experienced haemolysis. In the first group there was more superoxide dismutase and less glutathione peroxidase activity than in the other three groups, and this change was not due to an increased reticulocyte population. The same changes could be produced in normal cells by high concentrations of divicine and ascorbate. Haemolysis occurred when the cells were resuspended in homologous plasma. It was postulated that hydrogen peroxide production by a redox cycle lowered the reduced glutathione and NADPH contents of the erythrocytes, then some factor in the plasma finally precipitated the haemolysis.

The compound L-dopa occurs in *Vicia faba* and it was thought that this might be a haemolytic agent. However, there are two pieces of evidence which make this unlikely. First, large numbers of patients with Parkinsonism (doubtless including some with severe Mediterranean G6PD deficiency) have been given substantial amounts of L-dopa regularly and no haemolysis has been reported. Secondly, Gaetani *et al.* (1970) placed ^{51}Cr-tagged red cells which were severely G6PD deficient into normal volunteer recipients. The administration of intravenous L-dopa to these persons did not speed the destruction of the tagged red cells.

The possibility of a triple interaction between malaria, G6PD deficiency and fava beans was raised by the studies of Golenser *et al.* (1983) and Clarke *et al.* (1984). The former group showed that untreated G6PD deficient and normal erythrocytes supported the *in vitro* growth of *P. falciparum* equally well. Pre-treatment with isouramil led to a difference. The G6PD deficient cells no longer supported parasite growth whereas the normal cells were unaffected. When parasitized cells were exposed to isouramil, the parasites in both types of cells were destroyed. Isouramil is a powerful reducing agent and is known to exert a massive oxidant stress on the erythrocytes, which makes the environment inside the cell less favourable to the growth of the parasite. The direct effect of isouramil on the parasite itself is unclear. The authors suggest their findings may indicate that the normal individual may be partially protected and G6PD-deficient individuals more completely protected against malaria by eating fava beans.

Along similar lines, Clark *et al.* (1984) showed that divicine injected intravenously into mice infected with *Plasmodium vinckei* rapidly killed the parasites and caused haemolysis. Degenerating parasites were seen inside intact erythrocytes, indicating that their death was not a passive consequence of haemolysis. It is not clear if the dose of divicine (25 mg/kg) was equivalent to the amount that would enter the systemic circulation after eating suitable beans. The authors suggest that eating beans may control the parasite sufficiently for the host to acquire immunity and could have also influenced the selection of genes for G6PD deficiency.

Both studies imply the possibility of a new approach to antimalarial chemotherapy.

There are obviously still some facets of favism which warrant further investigation.

A marked reduction in the incidence of favism was observed in a district of Sardinia by Meloni *et al.* (1992), following systematic neonatal screening for G6PD deficiency and health education programmes. This success was more marked in boys than in girls, possibly because of a failure of the screening method to detect heterozygotes for G6PD deficiency.

Neonatal jaundice

Soon after the phenomenon of G6PD deficiency had been discovered it was found that it was present in male children who suffered severe jaundice leading to kernicterus starting about 2 days after birth. These cases were observed in ethnic groups in which Rhesus haemolytic disease did not occur, for example in Malays as described by Weatherall (1960). In connection with this report Pitcher (1960) suggested the possibility that the G6PD deficiency involved was one which led to congenital non-spherocytic anaemia, rather than the primaquine-sensitive variety.

An extensive analysis of neonatal jaundice in Athens was made by Doxiadis *et al.* (1961). In an unselected series collected over 6 months they excluded haemolytic disease due to Rhesus and ABO incompatibility, and to 'physiological jaundice'. The remainder constituted a group of 'unknown aetiology' in which there were 13 males and four females: 10 of the males and none of the females were G6PD-deficient. The parents were also investigated and two mothers of male patients were 'intermediate' on the G6PD test whilst three fathers of the female patients were G6PD deficient. Similar results (i.e. indicating a high frequency of persons with G6PD deficiency) were found in the families

of a separate group ascertained in a different way, namely, by means of a history of severe neonatal jaundice of unknown cause. With regard to the question of non-spherocytic anaemia, this condition was not observed in any of the babies.

The authors commented that it was unknown why the erythrocytes of the susceptible individuals were particularly prone to spontaneous haemolysis at this period of life. The importance was stressed, of being alert to the importance in ethnic groups with a high incidence of G6PD deficiency of a history of a previously affected infant or favism or drug-induced haemolysis in the family. The presence of such a history should trigger the avoidance of vitamin K analogues, the performance of G6PD assays, frequent observations of serum bilirubin levels and prompt exchange transfusion when indicated (which may be as late as the second week of life, as emphasized by Doxiadis & Valaes 1964).

The same group (Fessas *et al.* 1962) published further information on the topic. They found that only one of 21 unselected newborn males with G6PD deficiency and no other cause of haemolysis showed any marked hyperbilirubinaemia. Why only a few G6PD deficient babies develop severe jaundice generated the following possible explanations:

known extrinsic factors (e.g. Vitamin K analogues and naphthalene) – these were absent;
unsuspected extrinsic factor – these were eliminated in the patients born in hospital;
additional endogenous factor – e.g. hypoglycaemia, anoxia, immaturity of the liver enzyme systems, etc.

The last explanation was attractive because the siblings of the index cases had an unexpectedly high frequency of severe neonatal jaundice. The possibility of an additional genetic factor might explain (1) why some females with almost normal G6PD activity develop severe neonatal jaundice and (2) why severe neonatal jaundice is uncommon in some racial groups with a high incidence of G6PD deficiency.

A similar clinical picture was reported in Chinese male infants in Hong Kong by Yue & Strickland (1965). Amongst G6PD-deficient babies 27% developed serum bilirubin levels over 15 mg/100 ml (256.5 mM). Likewise, Wong (1986) reported the Singapore experience and identified indigenous herbs along with conventional pharmaceuticals and naphthalene as significant triggers.

Cases of neonatal jaundice associated with G6PD deficiency have also been described in Latin Americans (Boada 1967; Lopez & Cooperman 1971), in Indians (Madan & Sood 1987) and in Sephardic Jews (Kaplan & Abramor 1992).

Neonatal jaundice in G6PD deficient babies was observed to occur in Nigeria by Gilles & Taylor (1961) and Bienzle et al. (1976) as a result of a large survey in Ibadan which concluded that G6PD deficiency of type A− was the single most important factor in the pathogenesis of severe neonatal jaundice in that population. Owa (1989) highlighted the importance of naphthalene and menthol in causing the haemolysis.

Curiously, the condition has not been described in full term babies in American Negroes. However, a survey of 87 premature American Negro babies (Eshaghpour et al. 1967) revealed 10 who were G6PD-deficient, and serum bilirubin levels of 20 mg/100 ml (342 mm) occurred in six of these ten, five of whom required exchange transfusions. Only eight of the remaining 77 infants required exchange transfusions. The authors listed the following factors as likely to be responsible for the increased susceptibility to haemolysis of G6PD-deficient erythrocytes in the newborn: acidosis, high serum ascorbic acid concentrations, and decreased intra-erythrocytic activities of catalase and glutathione peroxidase.

Meloni et al. (1987) made an analytical study of 100 G6PD deficient male babies born in Northern Sardinia, 26 of whom developed neonatal jaundice. There were no significant differences between those who did or who did not develop neonatal jaundice with regard to mean birth weights, haemoglobin levels or cord blood G6PD activity. Four possibilities to explain why only some G6PD-deficient babies developed jaundice were considered:

1 environmental influences – unlikely, as they were all born and cared for under standardized conditions;
2 effect of an additional genetic or environmental deficiency – glutathione reductase and glutathione peroxidase activities did not reveal any differences;
3 heterogeneity in G6PD activity – disproven by the data;
4 since the jaundice was largely non-haemolytic, it seemed possible that the difference might be due to the expression of G6PD deficiency within hepatocytes.

(Oluboyede et al. (1979) had previously shown in adults that the enzyme activity in liver biopsy tissue was lower in persons with G6PD-deficient erythrocytes than in normals.)

Reporting 69 babies with severe jaundice from Malacca, Malaysia, Singh (1986) described an informational campaign. Parents were advised to avoid Chinese herbal medicines (e.g. San Chi and Chuan Lian), conventional medicines (he gave a list of 35), naphthalene and ginger. The result was a drop in the number of exchange transfusions required (1982: 77; 1983: 46; 1984: 23). Hence public awareness, avoidance of triggering factors and early detection can prevent the sequelae of kernicterus, i.e. mental retardation and cerebral palsy. A similar experience in Hong Kong was recounted by Fok & Lau (1986) and in Greece by Missiou-Tsagaraki (1992).

The ability to make a prenatal diagnosis of G6PD deficiency using molecular genetic techniques after amniocentesis was demonstrated by Beutler et al. (1992c). This test could be of value in high risk groups.

Hereditary non-spherocytic haemolytic anaemia

This category of anaemia is heterogeneous. It is differentiated clinically from hereditary spherocytosis by the fact that the red cells are not spherocytes. The osmotic fragility is normal and splenectomy is usually not beneficial. The condition can be due to various causes but G6PD deficiency is very commonly the basis. Other biochemical abnormalities which may be responsible are disorders in the activity of pyruvate kinase, diphosphoglycerate mutase and triose phosphate isomerase.

Hereditary non-spherocytic haemolytic anaemia (HNSHA) occurs rarely in all ethnic groups all over the world and is due to a large number of different G6PD variants as delineated by the WHO (1967) criteria.

An early definitive paper on the topic was that of Beutler et al. (1968). It is interesting to note that several of his patients had been subjected (apparently erroneously) to splenectomy for supposed hereditary spherocytosis. (However, it appears that the differentiation between the two conditions can be difficult. Benbassat & Ben-Ishay (1969) report a father and son who had spherocytosis, increased osmotic fragility and a satisfactory response to splenectomy and both possessed the common Mediterranean variant of G6PD.)

The clinical features of HNSHA in remission in the patients of Beutler *et al.* (1968) were variably low haemoglobin with normochromia and variable reticulocytosis. The half life of ^{51}Cr-tagged red cells was reduced. A number of the patients gave a history of neonatal jaundice. Haemolysis and jaundice became pronounced, with a variety of stresses including infection such as pneumonia and drugs such as sulphonamides and chloramphenicol. Aplastic crises also occurred in response to infection.

It was pointed out by Ravindranath & Beutler (1987) that the understanding of this condition would be put on a sound footing by determining the cDNA structure of the G6PD variant responsible in an individual patient, in addition to determining the biochemical characteristics. Subsequent work along these lines has revealed that what were considered to be different variants turned out to be the same (Beutler 1991). Nevertheless the mutations in many Class I (non-spherocytic haemolytic anaemia) G6PD variants have now been worked out. Seventeen are in the region of amino acids 363–454 (see Table 25.2). This is the part of the molecule thought to be the NADP binding site. However although $K_{\mathrm{m}}^{\mathrm{NADP}}$ is raised above normal, the elevation of $K_{\mathrm{m}}^{\mathrm{G6P}}$ is very much greater for Anaheim Nashville and Portici (Beutler *et al.* 1991b; Filosa *et al.* 1992). It is thought that these effects are brought about because the enzyme molecule may be folded in such a way that the NADP and G6P sites are close to each other. The mutations in three Class I variants which have been sequenced are sited in the vicinity of the G6P binding site (Table 25.2).

An interesting speculation concerns the very variable severity of the condition. Possible explanations given by Beutler *et al.* (1968) were as follows.

1 Different G6PD variants give different clinical pictures. In this context it is to be noted that the clinical picture may vary with the same G6PD variant, for example within families.
2 Undiscovered environmental agents such as drugs.
3 Different genetic backgrounds accompanying the abnormal G6PD. These authors had studied catalase, glutathione reductase, pyruvate kinase and hexokinase activities in the proposita of their study and had found no abnormality. However, as they point out,

Table 25.5. *Drugs and chemicals which have clearly been shown to cause clinically significant haemolytic anaemia in G6PD deficiency.*

Acetanilid	Pamaquine
Dapsone	Pentaquine
Doxorubicin	Phenazopyridine
Methylene blue	Sulphanilamide
Nalidixic acid	Sulphacetamide
Naphthalene	Sulphapyridine
Niridazole	Sulphamethoxazole
Nitrofurantoin	Thiazolesulphone
Phenylhydrazine	Toluidine blue
Primaquine	Trinitrotoluene

Reproduced with permission from: Beutler 1984, with some additions.

a large number of other factors – enzymatic or structural – can influence the life span of the G6PD-deficient red cell.

Chemicals causing haemolysis in G6PD deficient subjects

A number of chemicals can cause haemolysis and amongst these are various drugs (Table 25.5). The clinical effect depends on the nature of the drug, the dose the patient absorbs and also on the exact defect of the G6PD enzyme molecule which is present. The disease for which the patient is being treated can also play a part in causing haemolysis – important examples being pyrexia from any cause, a wide variety of infections, hypoglycaemia (Shalev *et al.* 1985) or the stress of the neonatal period. The role of diabetic keto-acidosis as a precipitating cause has been disputed (Shalev *et al.* 1984). The problems of anaesthesia in G6PD-deficient individuals have been discussed by Smith & Snowdon (1987), who concluded that haemolysis should not occur if known oxidant drugs are avoided and patients with infections are observed carefully.

Different drugs oxidize different target molecules. For example, methylene blue oxidizes NADPH directly; ascorbic acid, nitrofurantoin and doxorubicin oxidize reduced glutathione. Primaquine, on the other hand, oxidizes both target molecules and in addition consumes NADPH for the detoxification of itself and its hydroxylated metabolites which produce peroxides (Hohl *et al.* 1991).

Of equal relevance to practical medicine is a list of drugs which do *not* cause haemolysis in G6PD-deficient subjects who do not have non-spherocytic haemolytic anaemia (Table 25.6).

The status of aspirin deserves a comment. It is true that haemolysis may occur in patients with a common G6PD variant who are given aspirin (e.g. Meloni *et al.* 1989). However, there is a possibility that the haemolysis may have been due to infection and fever, rather than to the G6PD deficiency.

Drugs that did not aggravate haemolysis in individuals having G6PD deficiency with Chinese variants are also important (Table 25.7). A possible caveat must be entered regarding chloroquine in view of the report of 50 cases of haemolysis following malaria prophylaxis with this drug in Laotian soldiers (Sicard *et al.* 1978). Possibly some particular southeast Asian G6PD variant is sensitive to chloroquine.

Table 25.6. *Drugs likely to be safe when given in therapeutic doses to G6PD deficient subjects who do not also have non-spherocytic haemolytic anaemia.*

Acetaminophen (Paracetamol, hydroxyacetanilid)	*p*-Aminobenzoic acid
	Phenylbutazone
Acetophenetidine (phenacetin)	Phenytoin
Acetylsalicylic acid	Probenecid
(aspirin)	Procainamide hydrochloride
Aminopyrine	Pyrimethamine
Antazoline	Quinidine
Antipyrine	Quinine
Ascorbic acid	Streptomycin
Benzhexol	Sulphcytine
Chloramphenicol	Sulphadiazine
Chlorguanidine (proguanil)	Sulphaquanidine
Chloroquine	Sulphamerazine
Colchicine	Sulphamethoxypyriadazine
Diphenylhydramine	Sulphisoxazole
Isoniazid	Trimethoprim
L-Dopa	Tripelennamine
Menadione sodium bisulphite	Vitamin K
Menaphthone	

Reproduced with permission from: Beutler 1984.

Table 25.7. *Drugs that did not aggravate haemolysis in G6PD deficiency in Chinese*

Drug	Daily dose	Number of studies	G6PD variant[a]
Antimalarials			
Chloroquine	20 mg/kg	1	Canton
Proguanil	300 mg	1	
Pyrimethamine	25 mg/week		
Analgesics:			
Paracetamol	2 g →	1	
Phenylbutazone	600 mg	2	
Others			
Colchicine	1.5 mg ⎫	2	Canton
Probenecid	1.5 mg ⎭		
Chloramphenicol	50 mg/kg	5	{ Canton (3) { B(−) Chinese (2)
Streptomycin	1 g	3	{ Canton (1) { B(−) Chinese (1)
Isoniazid	300 mg		
PAS	10 g		
Menaphthone sodium bisulphite	40 mg	2	Canton
Trimethoprim	18 mg/kg	8	{ Canton (5) { Hong Kong-Pokfulam (1)
Levodopa	2–3 g		{ Canton (8) { B(−) Chinese (1)
Benzhezol	6 mg	1	Canton
Phenytoin	300 mg	2	Canton

[a]Numbers of donors are given in parentheses.
Reproduced with permission from: Chan *et al.* 1976.

The exact type of the individual patient's G6PD variant has a great influence on determining the clinical outcome. The Mediterranean variants are associated with more severe reactions that the Negro A− variant. The variants associated with hereditary non-spherocytic haemolytic anaemia are associated with particularly serious red cell destruction. The same drug can have different effects on different variants; for example chloramphenicol does not shorten the survival of red cells in individuals with G6PD Canton, 'G6PD B− Chinese' or G6PD A−, but it has been reported to do so in subjects with G6PD Mediterranean (McCaffrey et al. 1971).

Apparently, some children and adults (including pregnant women) chew and ingest mothballs containing naphthalene as a perversion of appetite. It has been found that this chemical produces a haemolytic anaemia associated with low glutathione concentrations in the erythrocytes (Zinkham & Childs 1958), the most likely cause of which is G6PD deficiency. This chemical exposure still continues on a wide scale, 2300 ingestions of naphthalene having been reported in the USA in 1989, and G6PD-deficient children with haemolysis due to this cause continue to require hospitalization (Todisco et al. 1991).

Bacterial and viral infections

There are two aspects to the inter-relationship of infections and G6PD deficiency. First, are deficient individuals more prone to develop infections? Secondly, when infection occurs do deficient individuals suffer a more severe illness?

The answer to the first question appears to be dependent upon the geographic location in which the phenomenon is studied. In a number of Asiatic sites it appears that infections occur more commonly in G6PD-deficient children than in the general population. However, in the well-studied population of Northern Sardinia, Meloni et al. (1991) found otherwise. Possibly different types of G6PD deficiency may give different effects.

More solid information is available on the second point. In southern Turkey, Kilinc & Kümi (1990) found that of 83 G6PD deficient patients admitted to hospital with a haemolytic episode, 30 (36%) had infections (especially upper respiratory) as the precipitating cause, whereas 40 (48%) had a drug-precipitated episode. The more serious clinical illnesses due to rickettsial infections and hepatitis in G6PD deficiency have been referred to earlier.

METHODS OF DETECTING G6PD DEFICIENCY

There are a number of methods available to detect the G6PD deficiency phenotype in a population or family study. The enzymic activity can be estimated spectrophotometrically by the change in optical density produced by the reduction of NADP to NADPH. This technique, when used to make one test on each subject, gave a complete separation of two modes in American negro males (Porter et al. 1962).

For many practical purposes, however, a simple screening test is highly desirable. The International Committee for Standardisation in Haematology recommended the fluorescent spot test (which relies on the fact that NADPH but not NADP is fluorescent). The test requires a longwave ultraviolet light (365 nm), 10 μl of whole blood and the following reagent mixture:

Glucose-6-P sodium salt 10 mM	200 μl
β-NADP 7.5 mM	100 μl
Saponin (sigma) 10 g/l	200 μl
Tris–HCl buffer 750 mM (pH 7.8)	300 μl
Oxidized glutathione 8 mM	100 μl
Water	100 μl

This reaction mixture is stable at +4 °C for 2 months and at −20 °C for 2 years. Normal blood samples fluoresce brightly whilst deficient samples show little or no fluorescence (Beutler et al. 1979). An improved version of this test was published by Solem et al. (1985).

MISCELLANEOUS OBSERVATIONS

(a) Glucose tolerance

The red cells of G6PD-deficient Negro men have a general depression of glucose metabolism and this is a similar abnormality, though less severe, to that found in diabetes. Because of these considerations, Eppes et al. (1969) investigated the results of glucose tolerance tests in normal and G6PD-deficient Negro men. A standard oral glucose tolerance test showed no differences between the groups. However, in both standard intravenous and cortisone-modified intravenous glucose tolerance tests the glucose levels were higher at all time points in the G6PD-deficient men. Despite the higher blood glucose levels the mean serum immunoreactive insulin levels were not significantly different in the two groups.

The authors speculated that their results might be due to a deficiency in the active pentose pathway inside the beta cells of the pancreatic islets. This might be linked to deficiencies of glutathione, glutathione reductase and 6-phosphogluconic dehydrogenase, which are integrally related in the oxidative metabolism of glucose and are associated with primaquine sensitivity. A possible reason why the impaired glucose tolerance was shown only with the intravenous test might be the absence of the influence of intestinal hormones which play a part in the oral test.

The subject was re-investigated in 318 Iraqi diabetics by Saeed et al. (1985). A strong association between diabetes mellitus and G6PD deficiency was found. These authors pose the question, 'Are those with G6PD deficiency genetically deficient, through bearing an abnormal allele at the G6PD locus, or is the deficiency acquired through abnormal glucose metabolism?' The latter explanation was favoured by the higher frequency of G6PD deficiency in the younger diabetics, 90% of whom were insulin-dependent, than in the older patients. This is in keeping with the fact that the hexose monophosphate shunt is stimulated by insulin.

Either a molecular genetic approach, or studies to see whether there is an association between G6PD deficiency and diabetes within families, might be ways to try and resolve this puzzle.

(b) Hypertension, pulse rate and serum creatinine

Data acquired from a screening clinic were utilized by Wiesenfeld et al. (1970) to compare 55 G6PD-deficient and 1154 non-deficient Negro men. A large number of measured variables were not significantly different between the groups. However systolic blood pressure was 7 mm Hg higher, diastolic blood pressure 8 mm Hg higher, pulse rate four beats per minute higher and serum creatinine 0.12 mg/100 ml higher in G6PD-deficient persons, all being significant ($p < 0.05$) differences.

The pathophysiologic bases and clinical implica-

tions of these observations remain obscure. Interestingly, G6PD deficiency, apparently secondary to renal stasis during decompensated cardiac failure with raised plasma creatinine concentrations, was reported by Salageanu et al. (1968).

(c) Cancer

The possibility of a relationship between a decrease in cancer incidence and G6PD deficiency was posed by Kessler (1970). His suggestion was based partly on the fact that cancer incidence has been found to be low in diabetics in whom the activity of the hexosemonophosphate shunt is depressed. There was also some support for the idea in the fact that G6PD activity is raised in some neoplasms.

The association between various types of cancers in 241 consecutive admissions, and G6PD deficiency in American negroes was studied by Naik & Anderson (1971). Their control groups were 266 healthy negro male blood donors from a jail and 142 negro females attending the planned parenthood and maternity clinics of the city of Houston. They found that the frequency of G6PD deficiency was less in both male and female cancer subjects than in the controls. The authors point out that the number of male cancer patients (66) was small and that the disease itself might have an influence on the G6PD test. Drugs known to cause haemolysis in G6PD-deficient persons had been excluded as a cause of producing a younger cell population with higher (normal) enzyme values. Hence their evidence made a *prima facie* case that G6PD deficiency might be protective against cancer. Some support for their idea was provided by very preliminary Sardinian data (Sulis 1972).

The idea was evaluated in a variety of haematological malignancies in Sardinians by Ferraris et al. (1988). This group found the same incidence of G6PD deficiency in 481 male patients and 16 219 controls. Likewise, the same conclusion was reached by comparing the frequency of expression of the Gd^B gene in 23 heterozygous women having a clonal haematological disease and a control group of 37 healthy heterozygotes. So the conclusion was that in this Mediterranean population G6PD deficiency did not confer protection against developing haematological malignancy.

The blood mononuclear cell G6PD activity of 150 Sardinian women with breast cancer was determined and 23 were found to be deficient (21 heterozygous and 2 homozygous). These frequencies were not different from those expected based on the known gene frequencies in the relevant population. Red blood cell G6PD activity was assessed in 156 Sardinian male patients with lung cancer by Pisano *et al.* (1991); 27 were deficient, a result not significantly different from 13 out of 79 controls.

Likewise, Cocco *et al.* (1989) studied 187 patients (19 with leukaemia, 57 with lymphomas and 111 with a variety of non-haematological malignancies) also in Sardinia. The G6PD activity was significantly higher in these patients than in 186 selected patient controls, and the proportion of G6PD-deficient individuals was similar in both groups. Due to confounding factors this result could not definitely reject the hypothesis of a lower cancer risk in G6PD-deficient subjects, but nevertheless was weighty contrary evidence. In a review of the previously available evidence Cocco (1987) had concluded that there was no proof or disproof that G6PD deficiency protected against cancer.

(d) Clonal origin of tumours

It is believed that in some types of neoplasm all the abnormal cells arise from a single precursor cell, and so represent a 'clone'. This idea became testable when the phenomenon of X-inactivation (or 'Lyonization') became understood.

The first study (Linder & Gartler 1965) concerned 27 uterine leiomyomas from G6PD heterozygous AB women, and 86 samples of normal myometrium. Extracts of all samples were subjected to electrophoresis. In only one instance did the normal myometrium fail to show both bands, but in all the leiomyomas only one band occurred: either A or B but never both. In a single patient both A type tumours and B type tumours were observed. The likely explanation is that these tumours each arise from only one cell. A number of other possibilities considered by the authors were less tenable.

Another simple tumour, namely hereditary trichoepithelioma (epithelioma adenoides cysticum), which is a skin tumour inherited as a Mendelian autosomal dominant (McKusick MIM No. 132700), gave a different result. Gartler *et al.* (1966) studied this condition in a Jewish Yemeni family which also had the Mediterranean form of G6PD deficiency. The G6PD activity in both normal skin and tumours from a heterozygous female gave values intermediate between those of a normal hemizygote male

and those of a hemizygous deficient male. This information suggests that each tumour arises from more than one cell and so contains cells in which both X chromosomes are active.

Attention then turned to malignant tumours, two of which were studied by Beutler *et al.* (1967). In a heterozygous AB woman who died of chronic lymphatic leukaemia the tumour masses from various sites showed predominantly the A enzyme in all instances. The very small amount of B enzyme present was thought to come from blood and supporting tissues. A single clone of cells accounted for all the tumours in the body.

However, in a heterozygous AB woman who died of a metastatic cancer of the colon, multiple tumour nodules were studied and some contained predominantly the A isozyme whilst others contained predominantly B. Erythrocytes, stomach, kidney and myocardium contained A and B enzymes in approximately equal intensity. (Curiously, normal liver showed a marked disparity between the intensity of the two electrophoretic bands – type B enzyme being present in concentrations several times higher than type A. This was an unexplained finding). Though supporting tissue contributed A and B enzymes to the homogenate it seems likely that the predominance of either A or B in individual tumour masses indicated a multifocal origin of this neoplasm.

It would seem, however, that this colonic cancer is the exception. Fialkow (1976) presented a table of results incorporating many haematological and non-haematological malignancies (e.g. chronic myeloid leukaemia, polycythaemia, rubra vera idiopathic myelofibrosis, paroxysmal nocturnal haemoglobinuria, Burkitt's lymphoma, breast carcinoma) and most of them, on the basis of G6PD evidence, would appear to have a monoclonal origin. Apart from colonic cancer and trichoepithelioma which have been mentioned, neurofibroma, venereal warts and some invasive cervical carcinomas appear, on G6PD evidence, to have a multifocal origin.

(e) Oestrogen receptors in breast cancer

It has been known for some years that breast cancers which have oestradiol receptors are more likely to respond to hormonal therapy than those which do not possess such receptors. Because glucose-6-phosphate dehydrogenase in rat tumours had been found to be induced by oestrogens the relationship between G6PD activity and oestrogen receptors (ER) in human breast cancer was studied by Messeri *et al.* (1983). A total of 143 tumours were analysed and 71% were ER positive. G6PD activity was higher in the ER positive group than in the ER negative group. The frequency distribution of G6PD values in the former group was suggestive of bimodality. The possibility is raised that ER positive, high G6PD activity tumours may be those most responsive to oestrogen therapy.

(f)   Thyrotoxicosis and erythrocytic G6PD activity

It is known that erythrocytic G6PD activity is elevated in hyperthyroidism, and investigations to find out the mechanism were carried out by Dada *et al.* (1983). They studied G6PD B, G6PD A and G6PD A− activities with the substrates NADP and G6P, under the influence of T4, T3 and cAMP. They found that the thyroid hormones *inhibited* the activity of the enzyme *in vitro* and this rules out the possibility of a direct activation as an explanation of the clinical finding. The authors make the following suggestion. Divalent metals like Cu^{2+} and Co^{2+} are inhibitors of G6PD and also are bound as complexes by T4. It seems possible that inhibitory metal ions which normally restrain G6PD activity are complexed and sequestered by the increased amount of T4 and T3 in hyperthyroidism hence causing an increased enzyme activity.

(g)   Interactions between G6PD deficiency and sickle haemoglobin

A number of investigations have been made to find out if there exists some phenotypic interaction between these two genetic phenomena. The results differ in different locations.

Luzzatto & Allan (1968) found no difference in Nigerian males of the distribution of the B, A and A− variants of G6PD in persons who have the haemoglobin *AA, AS* and *SS* genotypes. These workers point out that in SS homozygotes the red cell population is younger than normal so their G6PD level will be higher with consequent risk of misclassification. The G6PD genotypes of 100 homozygous Nigerian male sicklers were determined by Bienzle *et al.* (1975). They used a combination of quantitative

assays, cytochemical testing and starch-gel electrophoresis. The distribution of G6PD genotypes did not differ significantly between the sicklers and normal subjects.

Niewenhuis *et al.* (1986), in males of Bantu origin in Mozambique, found no statistical association between Gd− and haemoglobin AS.

A very careful study of 801 male sicklers derived from different locations in the USA by Steinberg *et al.* (1988), which included 85 Gd^{A-} individuals, showed the following:

1 There was no difference in the prevalence of G6PD deficiency in different age groups (2 to < 40 years), suggesting that G6PD was not a selective factor for longevity or mortality.
2 Haematologic parameters were not significantly different between Gd^{A-}, Gd^{A+} and Gd^{B} individuals.
3 No differences were found in the incidence of painful episodes, sepsis and acute anaemic events in patients classified as G6PD-deficient as compared with normal activity.

Similarly, Saad & Costa (1992) found in Brazilians that the frequency of G6PD deficiency in sicklers was not different from that observed in the general population. Compared with patients who were not G6PD-deficient there were no significant differences in the haemoglobin concentration and reticulocyte counts in patients with sickle cell disorders who were deficient.

On the other hand in Saudi Arabia the study of Samuel *et al.* (1986) conducted in Jeddah on randomly selected Saudi Arabs gave different results (see Table 25.8), indicating a significant association between G6PD deficiency and the possession of a sickle haemoglobin allele. It is possible that this result may have been produced by stratification. In other words, the AS individuals might be from a stratum within the population sampled in which G6PD deficiency was more common than it was in the AA individuals. In the case of the Nigerian samples, for example, it was known that the population was genetically homogeneous. In Saudi Arabia, on the other hand, it is known that the frequencies of both sickle and G6PD vary greatly between fairly small populations in different locations. These populations have become more mobile (especially to big cities like Jeddah where the study was carried out) and mixed since 1950.

It is known that sickle cell anaemia (SCA) occurs in two different forms in Saudi Arabia, a mild form

Table 25.8. *G6PD deficiency in heterozygous sickle cell trait in Jeddah Arab males*

	AA	AS
Gd^{B+}	537	35
Gd^-	33	13
%$Gd-$	5.8	27.1

χ_1^2 (with Yates' correction) = 26.1.
Compiled from data in: Samuel *et al.* 1986.

in the eastern province (EP) and a severe form in the southwestern province (SWP). The relationship between G6PD deficiency and both types of SCA was studied in various regions of the country by El Hazmi & Warsy (1984, 1989) and El Hazmi *et al.* (1990, 1991). In the northwest there was a statistical association in males between possession of a sickle gene and G6PD deficiency. The clinical features of the sickle cell disease (SCD) were not different between G6PD-deficient and normal individuals in the southwest. This was contrary to the experience of these workers in the eastern province, where it seemed that the possession of G6PD deficiency ameliorated the clinical features of SCD (e.g. haemoglobin levels high and less bone pains, hepatomegaly, jaundice, etc.). It is possible that the heterogeneity in these observations may arise from the fact that the nature of the sickle cell disease is different in different areas of Saudi Arabia (El Hazmi 1989).

(h)   Cataracts

It is known that the ocular lens contains G6PD and the activity of this enzyme in the lens is reduced in individuals with primaquine-sensitive erythrocytes (Tanaka 1971). The decline in G6PD activity with advancing age and at successive stages of lens development was studied by van Heyningen (1971). No clear evidence could be found that G6PD deficiency had any bearing on cataract development, but it appears that the erythrocytic G6PD activity was not studied in the individuals from whom the lens specimens were derived.

A survey of the G6PD and reduced glutathione contents of lenses was made by Vanella *et al.* (1987). Males who were G6PD-deficient as assessed on their red cells had undetectable G6PD and almost no

reduced glutathione in their lenses, compared with non-G6PD-deficient males and females and G6PD deficient females (presumed heterozygotes). All these patients were non-diabetic.

The subject was investigated by El Fakhri *et al.* (1987) with the following facts in mind: (1) diminished concentrations of reduced glutathione (GSH) are associated with cataract formation in diabetics, (2) glucose-6-phosphate dehydrogenase deficiency gives low GSH concentrations, (3) cataract was thought to be more common in G6PD-deficient subjects. They therefore studied erythrocytic GSH concentrations in eight groups of male subjects. Unfortunately they missed the opportunity to do a proper factorial experiment. Nevertheless, it seemed that erythrocyte GSH was markedly lower as compared with normal subjects in diabetics with cataracts, particularly if they had low G6PD levels or G6PD deficiency. Individuals with senile cataracts (presumably without diabetes) and individuals with G6PD deficiency (and presumably no cataracts) had intermediate erythrocyte GSH values.

Yüregir *et al.* (1989) in southern Turkey found a much higher frequency of erythrocytic G6PD deficiency in both male and female patients coming for cataract surgery than in controls. In about half the red blood cell G6PD-deficient patients, the lenses were also deficient in G6PD. However, Meloni *et al.* (1990), in a well-organized survey of 467 cataract patients in Northern Sardinia, found the G6PD deficiency frequency to be not significantly different from that in the general population. Furthermore, the age of development of cataract was not different in G6PD-deficient and normal patients, even though the enzyme activity within the lens was markedly diminished in the former group.

So it seems likely that G6PD-deficient persons are not more prone to develop cataracts than normal persons. It is possible that series showing a positive association may have suffered from some bias of ascertainment.

(i)   Apparent severe deficiency of leucocyte glucose-6-phosphate dehydrogenase

Patients have been described by Cooper *et al.* (1972), Gray *et al.* (1973) and Fite *et al.* (1983) who were Caucasians with apparently absent leucocytic G6PD activity. It must be observed that the apparent absence might be due to the fact that G6PD was undetectable in crude lysates. Purified preparations might have revealed G6PD activity. So it might be more accurate to describe patients of this type as having greatly reduced levels of G6PD activity. With some degree of purification and modern molecular biological techniques the G6PD structures might be determinable.

The patient described by Cooper *et al.* (1972) presented at the age of 30 years with a non-spherocytic haemolytic anaemia with a moderate reduction of red cell G6PD. The patient died aged 52 years, of *Escherichia coli* and *Klebsiella pneumoniae* sepsis.

The leucocytes from this patient failed to reduce nitroblue tetrazolium (NBT) *in vitro* until NADPH or NADH was added to the sonicates. The phagocytosing activity of the leucocytes was normal. Allowing the intact leucocytes to phagocytose polystyrene particles did not cause any reduction of NBT. Methylene blue (MB) failed to stimulate hexose monophosphate shunt activity in the leucocytes (leucocytes from patients with chronic granulomatous disease respond to MB with increased shunt activity). Hydrogen peroxide production was very low both in the resting and phagocytosing states.

A number of hypotheses were considered to explain the defect in this patient. She was not homozygous for any known G6PD deficiency allele because her son, four brothers and two sisters had normal G6PD levels. There was no evidence to suggest the existence of a G6PD-destroying enzyme. She might have had two genetic abnormalities coincidentally. Yet another possible explanation was that she might be heterozygous for a known X-linked gene for G6PD and X-inactivation might have occurred in such a way in the single leucocyte precursor cell as to inactivate the normal X in all progeny white cells.

The basic defect in the patient's leucocytes was an inability to produce hydrogen peroxide (H_2O_2) and this led to the fatal absence of bactericidal activity. A bacterium which produced H_2O_2, namely *Streptococcus faecalis*, was killed normally, but bacteria which failed to produce H_2O_2, namely *Staphylococcus aureus*, *E. coli* and *Serratia marcescens* were not killed by the patient's leucocytes, and survived within the cells after phagocytosis.

A similar 31 year old Spanish man, who presented with pneumonia due to an unidentified organism, was described by Fite *et al.* (1983).

Three brothers described by Gray *et al.* (1973) had complete absence of erythrocytic and leucocyte G6PD activity with chronic non-spherocytic haemolytic anaemia and impaired leucocytic bactericidal and metabolic activity. Two of the brothers had cervical lymphadenitis. The features revealed by *in vitro* testing of leucocytes were similar to those of the patient described by Cooper *et al.* (1972). For example, *Strep. faecalis* was killed at a normal speed, but *Staph. aureus* was killed more slowly than normal by the patient's leucocytes. The patient's mother was demonstrated to be heterozygous for G6PD, as shown by the possession of red cells of two different sorts – normal and G6PD defective.

The leucocytes from these patients have some resemblance to those found in chronic granulomatous disease (CGD), though the metabolic defects are different. In the case of G6PD deficiency the addition of methylene blue does not stimulate the hexose monophosphate shunt. In at least some patients with CGD the G6PD levels are normal, but there is possibly a deficiency of NADH oxidase and the addition of methylene blue stimulates the shunt producing an increase in H_2O_2. The clinical presentation is at a much later age and with milder features in the leucocyte G6PD deficiency than in classical CGD.

(j) Serum lipids

In a large Sardinian population survey it was observed that G6PD-deficient males had lower serum levels of total cholesterol, low density lipoprotein cholesterol (LDL-C), high density lipoprotein cholesterol (HDL-C) and apolipoprotein B, compared with normals. There was evidence that dietary habits and lifestyle were not different between the two groups. The deficiency of G6PD, though usually assessed in red cells, is known to be manifested in the liver in Sardinians (<60% of normal values) and the liver is the most important site of cholesterol synthesis. It was suspected that the low serum levels of cholesterol might be due to increased expression of LDL receptors. This idea was tested on monocytes by Muntoni *et al.* (1992) with inconclusive results, but a decreased synthesis of cholesterol was definitely demonstrated when they were G6PD-deficient. So it appears that G6PD-deficient Sardinian males have a serum lipoprotein pattern of reduced atherogenicity, whatever the mechanism. An epidemiologic evaluation of whether this leads to a lower incidence of clinically manifested coronary arterial disease is awaited.

PREDICTIONS OF HAEMOLYSIS *IN VIVO* FROM LABORATORY DATA

As more variants of G6PD became available for study it was clear that they varied greatly both in their propensity for causing haemolysis *in vivo* and with regard to their biochemical behaviour *in vitro*. Therefore attention was given to the possibility that the *in vitro* behaviour might be used to predict the haemolytic risk when the patient was exposed to an oxidative stress. The ratio

$$\frac{\text{Relative } V_{\text{max}} \, (\%)}{K_{\text{m}} \, \text{G6P} \, (\mu\text{M})}$$

was shown to be a useful predictor by Kirkman (1968). This worker stressed the importance of using physiological concentrations of substrates and showed that the values of this ratio were six times higher in persons not liable to haemolysis (possessing G6PD B and G6PD A) than in individuals susceptible to drug-induced haemolytic anaemia. Red cells from persons with hereditary non-spherocytic haemolytic anaemia had greatly reduced values.

The topic was re-examined by Vergnes *et al.* (1982). They showed, using 19 variants of G6PD, that scattergrams of (1) V_{max} G6PD versus glutathione reductase activity, and (2) glutathione regeneration ability versus Kirkman's ratio, were able to separate the variants into three groups, namely, those with severe, moderate and nil liability to intravascular haemolysis.

As Luzzatto (1986) pointed out, opinion has swung very much against doing *in vivo* tests such as those carried out with ^{51}Cr-labelled cells by Dern *et al.* (1954). On the other hand, the biochemical characteristics of the enzyme *in vitro* do not take account of all the factors which may be present in a patient after he has taken the drug – the biotransformation of the drug being one obvious example. Because of these considerations 'semi-*in vivo*' tests were designed.

In the first version red cells and serum were obtained from a person who was G6PD-normal. Then the person took the drug which was being tested, and a few hours later serum containing the drug plus its metabolites was obtained. By examining the behaviour of this volunteer person's red cells in the two samples of serum the effect of the drug plus metabolites on the pentose monophosphate shunt was assessed. Most drugs that are haemolytic stimulate this pathway.

Another test published by Magon *et al.* (1981) was as follows. Liver microsomes were prepared from mice which had been induced by phenobarbital. Then an incubate was prepared consisting of (1) red cells, (2) mouse liver microsomes, (3) an NADPH-generating system, (4) the drug being tested and (5) glucose. Normal and G6PD-deficient red cells could be tested in different incubates. Reduced glutathione was assayed before and after incubation.

According to Luzzatto (1986), 'both these techniques have given results which largely and rather satisfactorily correlate with the *in vivo* haemolytic potential of numerous drugs'. The suggestion is made that tests of this type should be carried out before a drug is introduced for use in areas where G6PD deficiency is common.

CONCLUSION

The study of G6PD deficiency was initiated by an adverse effect to a drug, and in the more than 30 years since then a wealth of biological and clinical information has been gleaned. Light has been shed on the mechanism of evolution of the enzyme. Because of increased understanding very simple measures have led to sharp decreases in the incidences of three important illnesses – neonatal jaundice, favism and drug-induced haemolysis.

With the advances now taking place it is likely that further insight will be gained into the disorders associated with G6PD variants.

The author would like to express his gratitude to Professor Lucio Luzzatto, FRS, Department of Haematology, Royal Postgraduate Medical School, London, UK who made many helpful suggestions about the contents of this chapter.

Adam, A, Tippett, P., Gavin, J., Noades, J., Sanger, R. & Race, R. R. (1967). The linkage relation of Xg to G-6-PD in Israelis: the evidence of a second series of families. *Annals of Human Genetics (London)*, **30**, 211–16.

Agarwal, R. K., Moudgil, A., Kishore, K., Srivastava, R. N. & Tandon, R. K. (1985). Acute viral hepatitis, intravascular haemolysis, severe hyperbilirubinaemia and renal failure in glucose-6-phosphate dehydrogenase deficient patients. *Postgraduate Medical Journal*, **61**, 971–5.

Ahluwalia, A., Corcoran, C. M., Vulliamy, T. J., Ishwad, C. S., Naidu, J. M., Argusti, A., Stevens, D. J., Mason, P. J. & Luzzatto, L. (1992). G6PD Kalyan and G6PD Kerala: two deficient variants in India caused by the same 317 Glu→, Lys mutation. *Human Molecular Genetics*, **1**, 209–10.

Allison, A. C. & Clyde, D. F. (1961). Malaria in African children with deficient erythrocyte glucose-6-phosphate dehydrogenase. *British Medical Journal*, **1**, 1346–9.

Ashmun, R. A., Hultquist, D. E. & Schultz, J. S. (1986). Kinetic analysis in single intact cells by microspectrophotometry: Evidence for two populations of erythrocytes in an individual heterozygous for glucose-6-phosphate dehydrogenase deficiency. *American Journal of Haematology*, **23**, 311–16.

Bautista, J. M., Mason, P. J. & Luzzatto, L. (1992). Purification and properties of human glucose-6-phosphate dehydrogenase in *E. coli. Biochimica et Biophysica Acta*, **1119**, 74–80.

Ben Bassat, J. & Ben-Ishay, D. (1969). Hereditary hemolytic anemia associated with glucose-6-phosphate dehydrogenase deficiency (Mediterranean type). *Israel Journal of Medical Sciences*, **5**, 1053–9.

Beutler, E. (1959). The hemolytic effect of primaquine and related compounds: a review. *Blood*, **14**, 103–39.

Beutler, E. (1960). Glucose-6-phosphate dehydrogenase deficiency. In *The metabolic basis of inherited disease*, 1st edn, ed. J. B. Stanbury, J. B. Wyngaarden & D. S. Fredrickson, pp. 1031–37. New York: McGraw-Hill.

Beutler, E. (1984). Sensitivity to drug-induced haemolytic anaemia in glucose-6-phosphate dehydrogenase deficiency. In *Genetic variability in responses to chemical exposure*, ed. G. S. Omenn & H. V. Gelboin, pp. 205–11. Banbury Report 16, Cold Spring Harbor Laboratory.

Beutler, E. (1990). The genetics of glucose-6-phosphate dehydrogenase deficiency. *Seminars in Haematology*, **27**, 137–64.

Beutler, E. (1991). Glucose-6-phosphate dehydrogenase deficiency. *New England Journal of Medicine*, **324**, 169–74.

Beutler, E., Blume, K. G., Kaplan, J. C., Löhr, G. W., Ramot, B. & Valentine, W. N. (1979). International Committee for standardization in haematology: recommended screening test for glucose-6-phosphate dehydrogenase (G-6-PD) deficiency. *British Journal of Haematology*, **43**, 469–77.

Beutler, E., Collins, Z. & Irwin, L. E. (1967). Value of genetic variants of glucose-6-phosphate dehydrogenase in tracing the origin of malignant tumors. *New England Journal of Medicine*, **276**, 389–91.

Beutler, E. & Kuhl, W. (1990). The NT 1311 polymorphism of G6PD: G6PD Mediterranean mutation may have originated independently in Europe and Asia. *American Journal of Human Genetics*, **47**, 1008–12.

Beutler, E., Kuhl, W., Fox, M., Tabsh, K. & Crandall, B. F. (1992c). Prenatal diagnosis of glucose-6-phosphate dehydrogenase deficiency. *Acta Haematologica (Basel)*, **87**, 103–4

Beutler, E., Kuhl, W., Gelbart, T. & Forman, L. (1991b). DNA sequence abnormalities of human glucose-6-phosphate dehydrogenase variants. *Journal of Biological Chemistry*, **266**, 4145–50.

Beutler, E., Kuhl, W., Ramirez, E. & Lisker, R. (1991d). Some Mexican glucose-6-phosphate dehydrogenase (G-6-PD) variants revisited. *Human Genetics*, **86**, 371–4.

Beutler, E., Kuhl, W., Saenz, G. F. & Rodriguez, W. (1991a). Mutation analysis of G6PD variants in Costa Rica. *Human Genetics*, **87**, 462–4.

Beutler, E., Kuhl, W., Vives-Corrons, J.-L. & Prchal, J. T. (1989). Molecular heterogeneity of glucose-6-phosphate dehydrogenase A−. *Blood*, **74**, 2550–5.

Beutler, E., Lisker, R. & Kuhl, W. (1990). Molecular biology of G6PD variants. *Biomedica Biochimica Acta*, **49**, S236–41.

Beutler, E., Mathai, C. K. & Smith, J. E. (1968). Biochemical variants of glucose-6-phosphate dehydrogenase giving rise to congenital non-spherocytic hemolytic disease. *Blood*, **31**, 131–50.

Beutler, E., Westwood, B. & Kuhl, W. (1991c). Definition of the mutations of G6PD Wayne, G6PD Viangchan, G6PD Jammu and G6PD 'LeJeune'. *Acta Haematologica (Basel)*, **86**, 179–82.

Beutler, E., Westwood, B., Kuhl, W. & Hsia, Y. E. (1992b). Glucose-6-phosphate dehydrogenase variants in Hawaii. *Human Heredity*, **42**, 327–9.

Beutler, E., Westwood, B., Prchal, J. T., Vaca, C. S., Bartsocas, C. S. & Baronciani, L. (1992a). New glucose-6-phosphate dehydrogenase mutations from various ethnic groups. *Blood*, **80**, 255–6.

Beutler, E. & Yoshida, A. (1988). Genetic variation of glucose-6-phosphate dehydrogenase: a catalog and future prospects. *Medicine (Baltimore)*, **67**, 311–34.

Bienzle, U., Ayeni, O., Lucas, A. O. & Luzzatto, L. (1972). Glucose-6-phosphate dehydrogenase and malaria: greater resistance of females heterozygous for enzyme deficiency and of males with non-deficient variant. *Lancet*, **1**, 107–10.

Bienzle, U., Effiong, C. & Luzzatto, L. (1976). Erythrocyte glucose 6-phosphate dehydrogenase deficiency (G6PD type A⁻) and neonatal jaundice. *Acta Paediatrica Scandinavica*, **65**, 701–3.

Bienzle, U., Guggenmoos-Holzmann, I. & Luzzatto, L. (1979). Malaria and erythrocyte-6-phosphate dehydrogenase variants in West Africa. *American Journal of Tropical Medicine and Hygiene*, **28**, 619–21.

Bienzle, U., Sodeinde, O., Effiong, C. E. & Luzzatto, L. (1975). Glucose 6-phosphate dehydrogenase deficiency and sickle cell anaemia: frequency and features of the association in an African community. *Blood*, **46**, 591–7.

Boada, J. J. B. (1967). Glucosa-6-fosfato deshidrogenasa: Incidencia e importancia en la ictericia neonatal. *Acta Científica Venezolana*, **18**, 41–3.

Bonsignore, A., Fornaini, G., Leoncini, G., Fantoni, A. & Segni, P. (1966). Characterization of leukocyte glucose 6 phosphate dehydrogenase in Sardinian mutants. *Journal of Clinical Investigation*, **45**, 1865–74.

Bottini, E. (1973). Favism: current problems and investigations. *Journal of Medical Genetics*, **10**, 154–7.

Bottini, E., Gloria-Bottini, F. & Maggioni, G. (1978). On the relation between malaria and G6PD deficiency. *Journal of Medical Genetics*, **15**, 363–5.

Boyer, S. H. & Graham, J. B. (1965). Linkage between the X chromosome loci for glucose-6-phosphate dehydrogenase electrophoretic variation and hemophilia A. *American Journal of Human Genetics*, **17**, 320–4.

Boyer, S. H., Porter, I. H. & Weilbacher, R. G. (1962). Electrophoretic heterogeneity of glucose-6-phosphate dehydrogenase and its relationship to enzyme deficiency in man. *Proceedings of the National Academy of Sciences (USA)*, **48**, 1868–76.

Burka, E. R., Weaver, Z. III. & Marks, P. A. (1966). Clinical spectrum of hemolytic anaemia associated with glucose-6-phosphate dehydrogenase deficiency. *Annals of Internal Medicine*, **64**, 817–25.

Calabro, V., Mason, P., Civitelli, D., Citadella, R, Filosa, S., Tagarelli, A., Martini, G., Brancati, C. & Luzatto, L. (1992). Genetic heterogeneity at the glucose-6-phosphate dehydrogenase locus in southern Italy: a study on a population from the Counza district. *American Journal of Human Genetics*, **52**, 527–36.

Carson, P. E. (1968). Hemolysis due to inherited erythrocyte enzyme deficiencies. *Annals of the New York Academy of Sciences*, **151**, 765–76.

Carson, P. E., Flanagan, C. L., Ickes, C. E. & Alving, A. S. (1956). Enzymatic deficiency in primaquine-sensitive erythrocytes. *Science*, **124**, 484–5.

Chan, T. K., Todd, D. & Tso, S. C. (1976). Drug-induced haemolysis in glucose-6-phosphate dehydrogenase deficiency. *British Medical Journal*, **2**, 1227–9.

Chan, T. K., Todd, D. & Wong, C. C. (1965). Tissue enzyme levels in erythrocyte glucose-6-phosphate dehydrogenase deficiency. *Journal of Laboratory and Clinical Medicine*, **66**, 937–42.

Chao, L., Du, C.-S., Louie, E., Zuo, L., Chen, E., Lubin, B. & Chiu, T. Y. (1991). A to G substitution identified in exon 2 of the G6PD gene among G6PD deficient Chinese. *Nucleic Acids Research*, **19**, 6056.

Childs, B., Zinkham, W., Browne, E. A., Kimbro, E. L. & Torbert, J. C. (1958). A genetic study of a defect in glutathione metabolism in the erythrocyte. *Bulletin Johns Hopkins Hospital*, **102**, 21–37.

Chiu, D. T. Y., Zuo, L., Chen, E., Chao, L. T., Louie, E., Lubin, B. H. & Du, C. S. (1991a). DNA sequence abnormalities in Chinese glucose-6-phosphate dehydrogenase (G6PD) variants. *Blood*, **78**, 252a.

Chiu, D. T. Y., Zuo, L., Chen, E., Chao, L. T., Louie, E., Lubin, B. H., Liu, T. Z. & Du, C. S. (1991b). Two commonly occurring nucleotide base substitutions in Chinese G6PD variants. *Biochemical and Biophysical Research Communications*, **180**, 988–93.

Clark, I. A., Cowden, W. B., Hunt, N. H., Maxwell, L. E. & Mackie, E. J. (1984). Activity of divicine in *Plasmodium vinckei*-infected mice has implications for treatment of favism and epidemiology of G-6-PD deficiency. *British Journal of Haematology*, **57**, 479–87.

Cocco, P. (1987). Does G6PD deficiency protect against cancer? A critical review. *Journal of Epidemiology and Community Health*, **41**, 89–93.

Cocco, P., Dessi, S., Avataneo, G., Picchiri, G. & Heinemann, E. (1989). Glucose-6-phosphate dehydrogenase deficiency and cancer in a Sardinian male population: a case-control study. *Carcinogenesis*, **10**, 813–16.

Cooper, M. R., De Chatelet, L. R., McCall, C. E., La Via, M. F., Spurr, C. L. & Bachner, R. L. (1972). Complete deficiency of leucocyte glucose-6-phosphate dehydrogenase with defective bactericidal activity. *Journal of Clinical Investigation*, **51**, 769–78.

Corcoran, C. M., Calabro, V., Tamagnini, G., Town, M., Haidar, B., Vulliamy, T. J., Mason, P. J. & Luzzatto, L. (1992). Molecular heterogeneity underlying the G6PD Mediterranean phenotype. *Human Genetics*, **88**, 688–90.

Dada, O. A., Abugo, O. & Ogunmola, G. B. (1983). Thyroid hormones and the reactivities of genetic variants of human erythrocytic glucose-6-phosphate dehydrogenase. *Enzyme*, **30**, 217–22.

Davidson, R. G., Childs, B. & Siniscalco, M. (1964). Genetic variations in the quantitative control of erythrocyte glucose-6-phosphate dehydrogenase activity. *Annals of Human Genetics*, **28**, 61–70.

De Vita, G., Alcalay, M., Sampietro, M., Cappelini, M. D., Fiorelli, G. & Toniolo, D. (1989). Two point mutations are responsible for G6PD polymorphism in Sardinia. *American Journal of Human Genetics*, **44**, 233–40.

Dern, R., Weinstein, I. M., Le Roy, G. V., Talmadge, D. W. & Alving, A. S. (1954). The hemolytic effect of primaquine I. The localization of the drug-induced hemolytic defect in primaquine-sensitive individuals. *Journal of Laboratory and Clinical Medicine*, **43**, 303–9.

Doxiadis, S. A., Fessas, Ph. & Valaes, T. (1961). Glucose-6-phosphate dehydrogenase deficiency. *Lancet*, **1**, 297–301.

Doxiadis, S. A. & Valaes, T. (1964). The clinical picture of glucose-6-phosphate dehydrogenase deficiency in early infancy. *Archives of Disease in Childhood*, **39**, 545–53.

El Fakhri, M., Sheriff, D. S., Chandrasena, L., Gupta, J. D., Rai, S. T. & Qureshi, M. S. (1987). Erythrocyte glutathione concentrations in diabetics with cataracts with and without glucose-6-phosphate dehydrogenase deficiency. *Clinical Chemistry*, **33**, 1936–7.

El-Hazmi, M. A. F. (1989). Sickle cell anaemia patients and sickle cell trait cases in Saudi Arabia. *Saudi Medical Journal*, **10**, 78–9.

El-Hazmi, M. A. F., Al-Swailem, A. R., Bahakim, H. M., Al-Faleh, F. Z. & Warsy, A. S. (1990). Effect of alpha-thalassaemia, G6PD deficiency and HbF on the nature of sickle cell anaemia in South-Western Saudi Arabia. *Tropical and Geographical Medicine*, **42**, 241–7.

El-Hazmi, M. A. F., Al-Swailem, A. R., Bahakim, H. M., Al-Faleh, F. Z. & Warsy, A. S. (1991). Patterns of sickle cell, thalassemia and glucose-6-phosphate dehydrogenase deficiency genes in north-western Saudi Arabia. *Human Heredity*, **41**, 26–34.

El-Hazmi, M. A. F. & Warsy, A. S. (1984). Aspects of sickle cell gene in Saudi Arabia -interaction with glucose-6-phosphate dehydrogenase deficiency. *Human Genetics*, **68**, 320–3.

El-Hazmi, M. A. F. & Warsy, A. S. (1989). The effects of glucose-6-phosphate dehydrogenase deficiency on the haematological parameters and clinical manifestations in patients with sickle cell anaemia. *Tropical and Geographical Medicine*, **41**, 52–6.

Eppes, R. B., Lawrence, A. M., McNamara, J. V., Powell, R. D. & Carson, P. E. (1969). Intravenous glucose tolerance in Negro men deficient in glucose-6-phosphate dehydrogenase. *New England Journal of Medicine*, **281**, 60–3.

Eshaghpour, E., Oski, F. A. & Williams, M. (1967). The relationships of erythrocyte glucose-6-phosphate dehydrogenase deficiency to hyperbilirubinemia in Negro premature infants. *Journal of Pediatrics*, **70**, 595–601.

Evans, D. A. P. (1969). Pharmacogenetics. In *Selected Topics in Medical Genetics*, ed. C. A. Clarke, p. 86. London: Oxford University Press.

Evans, D. A. P. & Clarke, C. A. (1961). Pharmacogenetics. *British Medical Bulletin*, **17**, 234–40

Ferraris, A. M., Broccia, G., Meloni, T., Forteleoni, G. &
  Gaetani, G. F. (1988). Glucose-6-phosphate
  dehydrogenase deficiency and incidence of hematologic
  malignancy. *American Journal of Human Genetics*, **42**, 516–
  20.

Fessas, Ph., Doxiadis, S. A. & Valaes, T. (1962). Neonatal
  jaundice in glucose-6-phosphate dehydrogenase deficient
  infants. *British Medical Journal*, **2**, 1359–62.

Fialkow, P. J. (1976). Clonal origin of human tumors.
  Biochimica et Biophysica Acta, **458**, 283–321.

Filosa, S., Calabro, V., Dallone, D., Poggi, V., Mason, P.,
  Pagnini, D., Alfinito, F., Rotoli, B., Martini, G., Luzzatto,
  L. & Battistuzzi, G. (1992). Molecular basis of chronic
  non-spherocytic haemolytic anaemia: a new G6PD variant
  (393 Arg→His) with abnormal K_m^{G6P} and marked *in vivo*
  instability. *British Journal of Haematology*, **80**, 111–16.

Fiorelli, G., Anghinelli, L., Carandina, G., Toniolo, D.,
  Sampietro, M., Capelloni, M. D. & Pareti, F. I. (1990).
  Point mutations in two G6PD variants previously
  described in Italy. *Blood*, **76** (Suppl.), 7a.

Fite, E., Morell, F., Zuazu, J., Julia, A. & Morera, J. (1983).
  Leucocyte glucose-6-phosphate dehydrogenase deficiency
  and necrotizing pneumonia. *European Journal of
  Respiratory Diseases*, **64**, 150–4.

Fok, T.-F. & Lau, S.-P. (1986). Glucose-6-phosphate
  dehydrogenase deficiency: a preventable cause of mental
  retardation. *British Medical Journal*, **1**, 829.

Gaetani, G., Salvidio, E., Panacciulli, I., Ajmar, F. &
  Paravidino, G. (1970). Absence of haemolytic effects of L-
  Dopa on transfused G6PD-deficient erythrocytes.
  Experientia, **26**, 785–6.

Galiano, S., Gaetani, G. F., Barabino, A., Cottafava, F.,
  Zeitlin, H., Town, M. & Luzzatto, L. (1990). Favism in the
  African type of glucose-6-phosphate dehydrogenase
  deficiency (A⁻). *British Medical Journal*, **300**, 236.

Gartler, S. M., Ziprkowski, L., Krakowski, A., Ezra, R.,
  Szeinberg, A. & Adam, A. (1966). Glucose-6-phosphate
  dehydrogenase mosaicism as a tracer in the study of
  hereditary multiple trichoepithelioma. *American Journal of
  Human Genetics*, **18**, 282–7.

Gilles, H. M. & Taylor, B. G. (1961). The existence of the
  glucose-6-phosphate dehydrogenase deficiency trait in
  Nigeria and its clinical implications. *Annals of Tropical
  Medicine and Parasitology*, **55**, 64–9.

Globerman, H., Navok, T. & Chevion, M. (1984).
  Haemolysis in a G6PD-deficient child induced by eating
  unripe peaches. *Scandinavian Journal of Haematology*, **33**,
  337–41.

Golenser, J., Miller, J., Spira, D. T., Navok, T. & Chevion,
  M. (1983). Inhibitory effect of a Fava bean component on
  the *in vitro* development of *Plasmodium falciparum* in
  normal and glucose-6-phosphate dehydrogenase deficient
  erythrocytes. *Blood*, **61**, 507–10.

Gray, G. R., Stamatoyannopoulos, G., Naiman, S. C.,
  Kliman, M. R., Klebanoff, S. J., Austin, T., Yoshida, A. &
  Robinson, G. C.-F. (1973). Neutrophil dysfunction,
  chronic granulomatous disease and non-spherocytic
  haemolytic anaemia caused by complete deficiency of
  glucose-6-phosphate dehydrogenase. *Lancet*, **2**, 530–4.

Harris, R. (1962). Erythrocyte glucose-6-phosphate
  dehydrogenase and malaria in Thailand. *Lancet*, **2**, 1378–
  9.

Harris, R. & Gilles, H. M. (1961). Glucose-6-phosphate
  dehydrogenase deficiency in the peoples of the Niger
  delta. *Annals of Human Genetics (London)*, **25**, 199–206.

Hirono, A. & Beutler, E. (1988). Molecular cloning and
  nucleotide sequence of cDNA for human
  glucose-6-phosphate dehydrogenase variant (A-).
  Proceedings of the National Academy of Sciences (USA), **85**,
  3951–4.

Hirono, A. & Beutler, E. (1989). Alternative splicing of
  human glucose-6-phosphate dehydrogenase messenger
  RNA in different tissues. *Journal of Clinical Investigation*, **83**,
  343–6.

Hirono, A., Fujü, H., Hirono, K., Kanno, H. & Miwa, S.
  (1992). Molecular abnormality of a Japanese
  glucose-6-phosphate dehydrogenase variant (G6PD
  Tokyo) associated with hereditary non-spherocytic
  hemolytic anemia, *Human Genetics*, **88**, 347–8.

Hirono, A., Kuhl, W., Gelbart, T., Forman, L., Fairbanks, V.
  F. & Beutler, E. (1989). Identification of the binding
  domain for NADP⁺ of human glucose-6-phosphate
  dehydrogenase by sequence analysis of mutants.
  Proceedings of the National Academy of Sciences (USA), **86**,
  10015–17.

Hohl, R. J., Kennedy, E. J. & Frischler, H. (1991). Defenses
  against oxidation in human erythrocytes: role of
  glutathione reductase in the activation of glucose
  decarboxylation by hemolytic drugs. *Journal of Laboratory
  and Clinical Medicine*, **117**, 325–31.

Justice, P., Shih, L.-Y., Gordon, J., Grossman, A. & Hsia, D.
  Y.-Y. (1966). Characterization of leukocyte
  glucose-6-phosphate dehydrogenase in normal and
  mutant human subjects. *Journal of Laboratory and Clinical
  Medicine*, **68**, 552–9.

Kaplan, M. & Abramov, A. (1992). Neonatal
  hyperbilirubinemia associated with glucose-6-phosphate
  dehydrogenase deficiency in Sephardic Jewish neonates:
  incidence, severity and the effect of phototherapy.
  Pediatrics, **90**, 401–5.

Kattamis, C. A. (1967). Glucose-6-phosphate dehydrogenase
  deficiency in female heterozygotes and the X-inactivation
  hypothesis. *Acta Paediatrica Scandinavica*, Suppl. 172, 103–9.

Kattamis, ChA. & Zannos-Mariolea, L. (1965). Acid
  phosphatase activity in glucose-6-phosphate
  dehydrogenase (G-6-PD) deficient Greeks. *Proceedings 10th
  Congress (1964) International Society Blood Transfusion
  Stockholm*, pp. 603–6.

Kay, A. C., Kuhl, W., Prchal, J. & Beutler, E. (1992). The
  origin of glucose-6-phosphate-dehydrogenase (G6PD)
  polymorphisms in African-Americans. *American Journal of
  Human Genetics*, **50**, 394–8.

Kenwrick, S. & Gitshier, J. (1989). A contiguous, 3-Mb
  physical map of Xq28 extending from the colourblindness
  locus to DXS15. *American Journal of Human Genetics*, **45**,
  873–82.

Kessler, II. (1970). A genetic relationship between diabetes
  and cancer. *Lancet*, **1**, 218–220.

Kidson, C. & Gorman, J. G. (1962). A challenge to the
  concept of selection by malaria in glucose-6-phosphate
  dehydrogenase deficiency. *Nature*, **196**, 49–51.

Kilinc, Y. & Kümi, M. (1990). Haemolytic crises due to
  glucose-6-phosphate dehydrogenase deficiency in the
  mid-southern region of Turkey. *Acta Paediatrica
  Scandinavica*, **79**, 1075–9.

Kirkman, H. N. (1968). Glucose-6-phosphate dehydrogenase
  variants and drug-induced hemolysis. *Annals of the New
  York Academy of Sciences*, **151**, 753–64.

Kirkman, H. N. & Hendrickson, E. M. (1963). Sex-linked
  electrophoretic difference in glucose 6-phosphate

dehydrogenase. *American Journal of Human Genetics*, **15**, 241–58.

Kosower, N. S. & Kosower, E. M. (1970). Molecular basis for selective advantage of glucose-6-phosphate dehydrogenase deficient individuals exposed to malaria. *Lancet*, **2**, 1343–5.

Kruatrachue, M., Charoenlarp, P., Chongsuphajaisiddhi, T. & Harinasuta, C. (1962). Erythrocyte glucose-6-phosphate dehydrogenase and malaria in Thailand. *Lancet*, **2**, 1183–6.

Kurdi-Haidar, B. & Luzzatto, L. (1990). Expression and characterization of glucose-6-phosphate dehydrogenase of *Plasmodium falciparum*. *Molecular and Biochemical Parasitology*, **41**, 83–92.

Larizza, P., Brunetti, P. & Grignani, F. (1960). Anemic emolitiche enzimopeniche. *Haematologica Archivio*, **45**, 123–210.

Liebowitz, J. & Cohen, G.. (1968). Increased hydrogen peroxide levels in glucose-6-phosphate dehydrogenase deficient erythrocytes exposed to acetylphenylhydrazine. *Biochemical Pharmacology*, **17**, 983–8.

Linder, D. & Gartler, S. M. (1965). Glucose-6-phosphate dehydrogenase mosaicism: utilization as a cell marker in the study of leiomyomas. *Science*, **150**, 67–9.

Ling, I. T. & Wilson, R. J. M. (1988). Glucose-6-phosphate dehydrogenase activity of the malaria parasite *Plasmodium falciparum*. *Molecular and Biochemical Parasitology*, **31**, 47–56.

Lopez, R. & Cooperman, J. M. (1971). Glucose-6-phosphate dehydrogenase deficiency and hyperbilirubinaemia in the newborn. *American Journal of Diseases of Children*, **122**, 66–70.

Luzzatto, L. (1986). Glucose-6-phosphate dehydrogenase and other genetic factors interacting with drugs. In *Ethnic Differences in Reactions to Drugs and Xenobiotics. Progress in Clinical and Biological Research*, ed. W. Kalow, H. W. Goedde & D. P. Agarwal, **214**, 385–99.

Luzzatto, L. & Afolayan, A. (1971). Genetic variants of human erythrocyte glucose-6-phosphate dehydrogenase II. *In vitro* and *in vivo* function of the A⁻ variant. *Biochemistry*, **10**, 420–3.

Luzzatto, L. & Allan, N. C. (1968). Relationship between the genes for glucose-6-phosphate dehydrogenase and for haemoglobin in a Nigerian population. *Nature*, **219**, 1041–2.

Luzzatto, L. & Mehta, A. (1989). Glucose-6-phosphate dehydrogenase deficiency. In *The Metabolic Basis of Inherited Disease*, 6th edn, ed. C. R. Scriver, A. L. Beaudet, W. S. Sly & D. Vale, Chapter 91. New York: McGraw-Hill.

Lyon, M. F. (1962). Sex chromatin and gene action in the mammalian X-chromosome. *American Journal of Human Genetics*, **14**, 135–48.

McCaffrey, R. P., Halsted, C. H., Wahab, M. F. A. W. & Robertson, R. P. (1971). Chloramphenicol-induced hemolysis in Caucasian glucose-6-phosphate dehydrogenase deficiency. *Annals of Internal Medicine*, **74**, 722–6.

MacDonald, D., Town, M., Mason, P., Vulliamy, T., Luzzatto, L. & Goff, D. K. (1991). Deficiency in red blood cells. *Nature*, **350**, 115.

McKusick, V. A. (1987). The morbid anatomy of the human genome. A review of gene mapping in clinical medicine. (Third of four parts). *Medicine (Baltimore)*, **66**, 237–96.

Madan, N. & Sood, S. K. (1987). Role of G6PD, ABO incompatibility, low birth weight and infection in neonatal hyper-bilirubinaemia. *Tropical and Geographical Medicine*, **39**, 163–8.

Maeda, M., Constantoulakis, P., Chen, C.-S., Stomatoyannopoulos, G. & Yoshida, A. (1992) Molecular abnormalities of a human glucose-6-phosphate dehydrogenase variant associated with undetectable enzyme activity and immunologically cross-reacting material. *American Journal of Human Genetics*, **51**, 386–95.

Magon, A. M., Leipzig, R. M., Zannoni, V. G. & Brewer, G. J. (1981). Interactions of glucose-6-phosphate dehydrogenase deficiency with drug acetylation and hydroxylation reactions. *Journal of Laboratory and Clinical Medicine*, **97**, 764–70.

Martini, G., Toniolo, D., Vulliamy, T., Luzzatto, L., Dono, R., Viglietto, G., Paonessa, G., D'Urso, M. & Persico, M. G. (1986). Structural analysis of the X-linked gene encoding human glucose-6-phosphate dehydrogenase. *EMBO Journal*, **5**, 1849–55.

Mavelli, I., Cirolo, M. R., Rossi, L., Meloni, T., Forteleoni, G., de Flora, A., Benatti, U., Morelli, A. & Rotilio, G. (1984). Favism: a hemolytic disease associated with increased superoxide dismutase and decreased glutathione peroxidase activities in red blood cells. *European Journal of Biochemistry*, **139**, 13–18.

Meloni, T., Carta, F., Forteleoni, G., Carta, A., Ena, F. & Meloni, G. F. (1990). Glucose-6-phosphate dehydrogenase deficiency and cataract of patients in northern Sardinia. *American Journal of Ophthalmology*, **110**, 661–4.

Meloni, T., Cutillo, S., Testa, U. & Luzzatto, L. (1987). Neonatal jaundice and severity of glucose-6-phosphate dehydrogenase deficiency in Sardinian babies. *Early Human Development*, **15**, 317–22.

Meloni, T., Forteleoni, G., Ena, F. & Meloni, G. F. (1991). Glucose-6-phosphate dehydrogenase deficiency and bacterial infections in northern Sardinia. *Journal of Pediatrics*, **118**, 909–11.

Meloni, T., Forteleoni, G. & Meloni, G. F. (1992). Marked decline of favism after neonatal glucose-6-phosphate dehydrogenase screening and health education. The Northern Sardinian experience. *Acta Haematologica*, **87**, 29–31.

Meloni, T., Forteleoni, G., Ogana, A. & Franca, V. (1989). Aspirin-induced acute haemolytic anaemia in glucose-6-phosphate dehydrogenase-deficient children with systemic arthritis. *Acta Haematologica*, **81**, 208–9.

Messeri, G., Tozzi, P., Boddi, V. & Ciatto, S. (1983). Glucose-6-phosphate dehydrogenase activity and estrogen receptors in human breast cancer. *Journal of Steroid Biochemistry*, **19**, 1647–50.

Missiou-Tsagaraki, S. (1992). Screening for glucose-6-phosphate dehydrogenase deficiency. *Journal of Pediatrics*, **121**, 166.

Modiano, G., Battistuzzi, G., Esan, G. J. F., Test, U. & Luzzatto, L. (1979). Genetic heterogeneity of 'normal' human erythrocyte glucose-6-phosphate dehydrogenase: An isoelectrophoretic polymorphism. *Proceedings of the National Academy of Sciences (USA)*, **76**, 852–6.

Muntoni, S., Beretta, B., Dessi, S., Muntoni, Sa. & Pani, P. (1992). Serum lipoprotein profile in Mediterranean variant of glucose-6-phosphate dehydrogenase deficiency. *European Journal of Epidemiology*, **8** (Suppl. to No. 2), 48–53.

Nafa, K., Reghis, A., Osmani, N., Baghli, L., Benabadji, M., Vulliamy, T. & Luzzatto, L. (1992). G6PD Aures: a new mutation 48 Ile → Thr causing mild G6PD is associated with favism. *Human Molecular Genetics*, **2**, 81–2.

Naik, S. N. & Anderson, D. E. (1971). The association between glucose-6-phosphate dehydrogenase deficiency and cancer in American Negroes. *Oncology*, **25**, 356–64.

Niewenhuis, F., Wolf, B., Bomba, A. & de Graaf, P. (1986). Haematological study in Cabo Delgado province Mozambique, sickle cell trait and G6PD deficiency. *Tropical and Geographical Medicine*, **38**, 183–7.

Ninfali, P., Bresolin, N., Baronciani, L., Fotunato, F., Comi, G., Magnani, M. & Scarlato, G. (1991). Glucose-6-phosphate dehydrogenase Lodi 844C: a study on its expression in blood cells and muscle. *Enzyme*, **45**, 180–7.

Oluboyede, O. A., Esan, G. J. F., Francis, T. L. & Luzzatto, L. (1979). Genetically determined deficiency of glucose 6-phosphate dehydrogenase (type A⁻) is expressed in the liver. *Journal of Laboratory and Clinical Medicine*, **93**, 783–9.

Owa, J. A. (1989). Relationship between exposure to icterogenic agents, glucose-6-phosphate dehydrogenase deficiency and neonatal jaundice in Nigeria. *Acta Paediatrica Scandinavica*, **78**, 848–52.

Pai, G. S., Sprenkle, J. A., Do, T. T., Mareni, C. E. & Migeon, B. R. (1980). Localization of loci for hypoxanthine phosphoribosyltransferase and glucose-6-phosphate dehydrogenase and biochemical evidence of non-random X chromosome expression from studies of a human X-autosome translocation. *Proceedings of the National Academy of Sciences (USA)*, **77**, 2810–13.

Perng, L., Chiou, S.-S., Liu, T.-C. & Chang, J.-G. (1992). A novel C to T substitution at nucleotide 1360 of cDNA which abolishes a natural HhaI site accounts for a new G6PD deficiency gene in China. *Human Molecular Genetics*, **1**, 205.

Persico, M. G., Viglietto, G., Martini, G., Toniolo, D., Paonessa, G., Moscatelli, C., Dono, R., Vulliamy, T., Luzzatto, L, & D'Urso, M. (1986a). Isolation of human glucose-6-dehydrogenase (G6PD) cDNA clones: primary structure of the protein and unusual 5′ non-coding region. *Nucleic Acids Research*, **14**, 2511–22.

Persico, M. G., Viglietto, G., Martini, G., Toniolo, D., Paonessa, G., Moscatelli, C., Dono, R., Vulliamy, T., Luzzatto, L. & D'Urso, M. (1986b). *Corrigendum*: Isolation of human glucose-6-dehydrogenase (G6PD) cDNA clones: primary structure of the protein and unusual 5′ non-coding region. *Nucleic Acids Research*, **14**, 7822.

Pisano, M., Cocco, P., Cherechi, R., Onnis, R. & Cherihi, P. (1991). Glucose-6-phosphate dehydrogenase deficiency and lung cancer: a hospital based case-control study. *Tumori*, **77**, 12–15.

Pitcher, C. S. (1960). Enzyme deficiency in haemolytic disease of the newborn. *Lancet*, **2**, 979–980.

Poggi, V., Town, M., Foulkes, N. S. & Luzzatto, L. (1990). Identification of a single base change in a new human mutant glucose-6-phosphate dehydrogenase gene by polymerase-chain-reaction amplification of the entire coding region from genomic DNA. *Biochemical Journal*, **271**, 157–60.

Porter, I.H., Schulze, J. & McKusick, V. A. (1962). Genetical linkage between the loci for glucose-6-phosphate dehydrogenase deficiency and colour-blindness in American Negroes. *Annals of Human Genetics (London)*, **26**, 107–22.

Raoult, D., Lena, D., Perrimont, H., Gallais, H., Walker, D. H. & Casanova, P. (1986). Haemolysis with Mediterranean

spotted fever and glucose-6-phosphate dehydrogenase deficiency. *Transactions of the Royal Society of Tropical Medicine and Hygiene*, **80**, 961–2.

Rattazzi, M. C., Corash, L. M., Van Zanen, G. E., Jaffe, E. R. & Piomelli, S. (1971). G6PD deficiency and chronic hemolysis: four new mutants – relationships between clinical syndrome and enzyme kinetics. *Blood*, **38**, 205–18.

Ravindranath, Y. & Beutler, E. (1987). Two new variants of glucose-6-phosphate dehydrogenase associated with hereditary non- spherocytic hemolytic anemia. *American Journal of Haematology*, **24**, 357–63.

Roth, Jr. E. & Schulman, S. (1988). The adaptation of Plasmodium falciparum to oxidative stress in G6PD deficient human erythrocytes. *British Journal of Haematology*, **70**, 363–7.

Saad, S. T. O. & Costa, F. F. (1992). Glucose-6-phosphate dehydrogenase deficiency and sickle cell disease in Brazil. *Human Heredity*, **42**, 125–8.

Saeed, Th. Kh., Hamamy, H. A. & Alwan, A. A. S. (1985). Association of glucose-6-phosphate dehydrogenase deficiency with diabetes mellitus. *Diabetic Medicine*, **2**, 110–12.

Salageanu, D., Ilie, M. & Teitel, P. (1968). Erythrocyte G6PD and renal stasis. *Lancet*, **1**, 753.

Samuel, A.P. W., Saha, N., Acquaye, J. K., Omer, A., Ganeshaguru, K. & Hassounh, E. (1986). Association of red cell glucose-6-phosphate dehydrogenase with haemoglobinopathies. *Human Heredity*, **36**, 107–12.

Sartori, E. (1971). On the pathogenesis of favism. *Journal of Medical Genetics*, **8**, 462–7.

Shalev, O., Ehakim, R., Lugassy, G. Z. & Menczel, J. (1985). Hypoglycaemia-induced hemolysis in glucose-6-phosphate dehydrogenase deficiency. *Acta Haematologica*, **74**, 227–9.

Shalev, O., Wollner, A. & Menczel, J. (1984). Diabetic ketoacidosis does not precipitate haemolysis in patients with the Mediterranean variant of glucose-6-phosphate dehydrogenase deficiency. *British Medical Journal*, **288**, 179–80.

Sicard, D., Kaplan, J.-C. & Labie, D. (1978). Haemoglobin-opathies and G-6-PD deficiency in Laos. *Lancet*, **2**, 571–2.

Singh, H. (1986). Glucose-6-phosphate dehydrogenase deficiency: a preventable cause of mental retardation. *British Medical Journal*, **1**, 397–8.

Siniscalco, M., Filippi, G. & Latte, B. (1964). Recombination between protan and deutan genes; data on their relative positions in respect of the G6PD locus. *Nature*, **204**, 1062–4.

Siniscalco, M., Filippi, G., Latte, B., Piomelli, S., Rattazzi, M., Gavin, J., Sanger, R. & Race, R. R. (1966). Failure to detect linkage between Xg and other X borne loci in Sardinians. *Annals of Human Genetics (London)*, **29**, 231–52.

Siniscalco, M., Motulsky, A. G., Latte, B. & Bernini, L. (1960). Gentica-Indagini genetiche sulla predisposizione al favismo. II Dati familiari. Associazione genica con il daltonismo. *Atti della Accademia Nazionale dei Lincei*, **28**, 903–9.

Smith, C. L. & Snowdon, S. L. (1987). Anaesthesia and glucose-6-phosphate dehydrogenase deficiency. *Anaesthesia*, **42**, 281–8.

Solem, E., Pirzer, C., Siege, M., Kollmann, F., Romero-Saravia, O., Bartsch-Trefs, O. & Kornhuber, B. (1985). Mass screening for glucose-6-phosphate dehydrogenase deficiency: improved fluorescent spot test. *Clinica Chimica Acta*, **152**, 135–42.

Steinberg, M. H., West, M. S., Gallagher, D., Mentzer, W. and the cooperative study of sickle cell disease (1988). Effects of glucose-6-phosphate dehydrogenase deficiency upon sickle cell anaemia. *Blood*, **71**, 748–52.

Stevens, D. J., Wanachiwanawin, W., Mason, P. J., Vulliamy, T. J. & Luzzatto. L. (1991). G6PD Canton a common variant in South East Asia caused by a 459 Arg → Leu mutation. *Nucleic Acids Research*, **18**, 7190.

Sulis, E. (1972). G6PD deficiency and cancer. *Lancet*, **1**, 1185.

Takizawa, T., Yoneyama, Y., Miwa, S. & Yoshida, A. (1987). A single nucleotide base transition is the basis of the common human glucose-6-phosphatase variant A (+). *Genomics*, **1**, 228–31.

Tanaka, K. R. (1971). Introduction to discussion of glucose-6-phosphate dehydrogenase deficiency. *Experimental Eye Research*, **11**, 396–401.

Tang, T. K., Huang, C.-S., Huang, M.-J., Tam, K.-B., Yeh, C.- H. & Tang, C.-J. C. (1992). Diverse point mutations result in glucose-6-phosphate dehydrogenase (G6PD) polymorphism in Taiwan. *Blood*, **79**, 2135–40.

Tarlov, A. R., Brewer, G. J., Carson, P. E. & Alving, A. S. (1962). Primaquine sensitivity. *Archives of Internal Medicine*, **109**, 209–34.

Todisco, V., Lamour, J. & Finberg, L. (1991). Hemolysis from exposure to naphthalene moth balls. *New England Journal of Medicine*, **325**, 1660.

Trask, B. J., Massa, H., Kenwrick, S. & Gitschier, J. (1991). Mapping of human chromosome Xq28 by two-color fluorescence *in situ* hybridization of DNA sequences to interphase cell nuclei. *American Journal of Human Genetics*, **48**, 1–15.

Usanga, E. A. & Luzzatto, L. (1985). Adaptation of *Plasmodium falciparum* to glucose-6-phosphate dehydrogenase deficient host red cells by production of parasite-encoded enzyme. *Nature*, **313**, 793–5.

Vanella, A., Gorgone, G., Cavallaro, N., Castorina, C., Campisi, A., Di Giacomo, C., Bousquet, E., Li Violti, S. & Mollica, F. (1987). Superoxide dismutase activity and reduced glutathione content in cataractous lens of patients with glucose-6-phosphate dehydrogenase deficiency. *Ophthalmic Paediatrics and Genetics*, **8**, 191–5.

Van Heyningen, R. (1971). Contribution to the discussion of the paper of Tanaka, K. R. (1971). *Experimental Eye Research*, **11**, 398.

Vergnes, H., Sevin, A. & Brun, H. (1982). Kinetic characteristics of different glucose-6-phosphate dehydrogenase variants and their hemolytic incidence in man. *Enzyme*, **27**, 204–14.

Viglietto, G., Montanaro, V., Calabro, V., Vallone, D., D'Urso, M., Persico, M. G. & Battistuzzi, G. (1990). Common glucose-6-phosphate dehydrogenase (G6PD) variants from the Italian population: Biochemical and molecular characterization. *Annals of Human Genetics (London)*, **54**, 1–15.

Vives-Corrons, J.-L., Kuhl, W., Pujades, M. A. & Beutler, E. (1990). Molecular genetics of the glucose-6-phosphate dehydrogenase (G6PD) Mediterranean variant and description of a new G6PD mutant – G6PD Andalus. *American Journal of Human Genetics*, **47**, 575–9.

Vulliamy, T., Beutler, E. & Luzzatto, L. (1993). Variants of glucose-6-phosphate dehydrogenase are due to missense mutations spread throughout the coding region of the gene *Human Mutation*, **2** (in press).

Vulliamy, T. J., D'Urso, M., Battistuzzi, G., Estrada, M., Foulkes, N. S., Martini, G., Calabro, V., Poggi, V., Giordano, R., Town, M., Luzzatto, L. & Persico, M.G. (1988). Diverse point mutations in the human glucose-6-phosphate dehydrogenase gene cause enzyme deficiency and mild or severe hemolytic anaemia. *Proceedings of the National Academy of Sciences (USA)*, **85**, 5171–5.

Vulliamy, T. J., Othman, A., Town, M., Nathwani, A., Falusi, A. G., Mason, P. J. & Luzzatto, L. (1991). Polymorphic sites in the African population detected by sequence analysis of the glucose-6- phosphate dehydrogenase gene outline the evolution of variants A and A−. *Proceedings of the National Academy of Sciences (USA)*, **88**, 8568–71.

Vulliamy, T. J., Wanachiwanawin, W., Mason, P. J. & Luzzatto, L. (1989). G6PD Mahidol, a common deficient variant in South East Asia is caused by a (163) glycine→serine mutation. *Nucleic Acids Research*, **17**, 5868.

Vural, N. & Sardas, S. (1984). Biological activities of broad bean (*Vicia faba* L.) extracts cultivated in South Anatolia in favism sensitive subjects. *Toxicology*, **31**, 175–9.

Weatherall, D. J. (1960). Enzyme deficiency in haemolytic disease of the newborn. *Lancet*, **2**, 835–7.

Wiesenfeld, S. L., Petrakis, N. L., Sams, B. J., Cullen, M. F. & Cutler, J. L. (1970). Elevated blood pressure, pulse rate and serum creatinine in Negro males deficient in glucose-6-phosphate dehydrogenase. *New England Journal of Medicine*, **282**, 1001–2.

Wong, H. B. (1986). Erythrocyte G6PD deficiency and its significance with special emphasis on malaria. *Journal of the Singapore Paediatric Society*, **28**, 35–44.

World Health Organisation (1967). Standardization of procedures for the study of glucose-6-phosphate dehydrogenase. *World Health Organisation Technical Report Series*, **366**, 18–19.

Yoshida, A. (1967). A single amino acid substitution (Asparagine to aspartic acid) between normal (B+) and the common Negro variant (A+) of human glucose-6-phosphate dehydrogenase. *Proceedings of the National Academy of Sciences (USA)*, **57**, 835–40.

Yoshida, A., Steinmann, L. & Harbert, P. (1967). In vitro hybridization of normal and variant human glucose-6-phosphate dehydrogenase. *Nature*, **216**, 275–6.

Yue, P. C. K. & Strickland, M. (1965). Glucose-6-phosphate dehydrogenase deficiency and neonatal jaundice in Chinese male infants in Hong Kong. *Lancet*, **1**, 350–1.

Yüregir, G., Varinli, I. & Donma, O. (1989). Glucose-6-phosphate dehydrogenase deficiency both in red blood cells and lenses of the normal and cataractous native population of Cukurova the southern part of Turkey. *Ophthalmic Research*, **21**, 155–7.

Zinkham, W. H. & Childs, B. (1958). A defect of glutathione metabolism in erythrocytes from patients with a naphthalene-induced hemolytic anaemia. *Pediatrics*, **22**, 461–71.

Zuo, L., Chen, E., Du, C. S., Chang, C. N. & Chiu, D. T. Y. (1990). Genetic study of Chinese G6PD variants by direct PCR sequencing. *Blood*, **76** (Suppl.), 51a.

PART VIII   The hepatic porphyrias

26   The hepatic porphyrias

INTRODUCTION

THESE disorders may be considered to be the prototypes of pharmacogenetic clinical disorders. It is a century since some individuals were observed with massive 'haematoporphyria' due to chronic sulphonal poisoning. The hepatic porphyrias represent a group of metabolic disorders which, though individually rare, are of considerable practical as well as theoretical importance. Every year in a general hospital of, say, 600 beds it can be expected that several new patients will present with one of these disorders. Often such patients attend for a while before they are diagnosed. Unrecognized the hepatic porphyrias can be lethal, whereas with proper management the recovery from acute attacks is usually excellent. The members of this group of disorders show how a drug, given for therapeutic purposes, can precipitate a serious illness in a person possessing a specific metabolic abnormality. Recognition of the susceptible phenotype beforehand can prevent such an iatrogenic illness from occurring.

Comprehensive accounts of the porphyria group of disorders are readily available, e.g. Brodie & Goldberg (1980), Kappas *et al.* (1983), Hindmarsh (1986), Desnick *et al.* (1990) and Moore *et al.* (1990). The laboratory investigations of the porphyrias have recently been reviewed by Elder *et al.* (1990). An interesting survey incorporating 50 years' experience in the field has been provided by Rimington (1989). The purpose of including a chapter on the hepatic porphyrias in this book is to point out how genetically determined variants of enzymes in the biosynthetic pathway result in different responses when the individuals concerned are exposed to drugs and similar chemicals.

HAEM SYNTHESIS

The basic building materials for porphyrin synthesis are molecules of 5-aminolaevulinic acid (ALA) which are themselves made from glycine and succinate under the influence of the enzyme ALA synthetase. This enzyme has been mapped to 3p21 (Astrin *et al.* 1988) and the cDNA sequenced (Bawden *et al.* 1987); no genetic variants have been discovered. Two ALA molecules condense to form one porphobilinogen (PBG) molecule the characteristic feature of which is a pyrrole ring (Fig. 26.1).

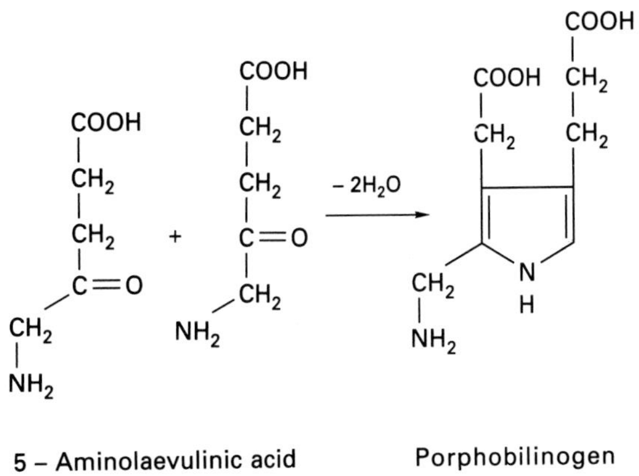

Fig. 26.1. The condensation of two molecules of 5-aminolaevulinic acid to form porphobilinogen.

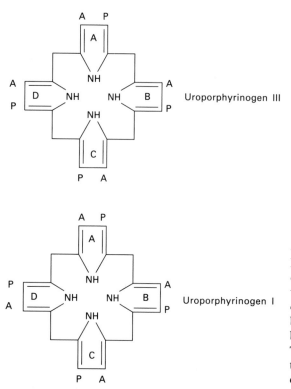

Uroporphyrinogen III

Uroporphyrinogen I

Fig. 26.2. Uroporphyrinogen of the type III and type I isomer series. In porphyrins of type III the sequence of the side chains of pyrrole ring D is reversed. P, propionic acid; A, acetic acid.

This chemical reaction occurs under the influence of the enzyme PBG synthase otherwise known as ALA dehydratase.

The next step is the assembly of the first compound which contains the characteristic 4-pyrrole ring porphyrin structure. This is uroporphyrinogen which is a colourless compound and possesses eight carboxyl groups. Two successive steps are governed by two different enzymes. First, PBG is deaminated by PBG deaminase, and then the four pyrrole rings are joined together in a linear chain as hydroxymethylbilane (Rimington 1989). Then cyclic uroporphyrinogen I is formed from this compound rather slowly and non-enzymatically, whilst uroporphyrinogen III (which requires a reversal of the last pyrrole ring which has been added) is formed more quickly by the action of the enzyme uroporphyrinogen synthase. At this point it is necessary to make a digression to explain some points that cause much confusion.

The first point concerns the nomenclature of the porphyrins, whose complexity was most lucidly explained by Meyer & Schmid (1978) from whose account the following description has been adapted.

The classification of porphyrin isomers is based on the four synthetically prepared isomers of etioporphyrin designated as I, II, III and IV. Only porphyrins belonging to the isomer series I and III have been identified in nature. The protoporphyrin of haemoglobin and all other haem proteins have the basic structure of a porphyrin type III isomer (Fig. 26.2). It has been pointed out that there are 60 theoretically possible positional isomers of protoporphyrin depending on the sequence of the pyrrole substituents about the porphyrin ring. However, in all naturally occurring porphyrins each pyrrole ring carries a pair of non-identical substituents, and this limits the number of theoretically possible isomers of naturally occurring protoporphyrin isomers to 15, which have been arbitrarily designated I to XV. Only one of these 15 possible protoporphyrin isomers has been found in nature, namely number IX which is by definition a type III porphyrin isomer (Fig. 26.2). The protoporphyrin isomers that would fall into the type I porphyrin category do not exist in nature, even though other porphyrins of the type I isomer series do occur.

The second point is also related to series I and series III isomers. Both types of uroporphyrinogen, i.e. series I type and series III type, are formed from deaminated PBG and subsequently decarboxylated step-wise to the respective coproporphyrinogens. However, the series I compounds apparently serve no useful purpose, and only the series III compounds are used eventually to produce haem.

The third point is that the oxidized coloured compounds uroporphyrin III and coproporphyrin III are side products made from colourless uroporphyrinogen and coproporphyrinogen, and they appear to serve no useful purpose. All the enzymic steps from uroporphyrinogen III to protoporphyrinogen IX serve to modify six of the eight carboxylic side chains derived from the four PBG molecules.

Protoporphyrinogen IX is oxidized to protoporphyrin IX by protoporphyrinogen oxidase (Fig. 26.3) and when an iron atom is inserted into this compound by the enzyme ferrochelatase then haem is formed.

The whole scheme of haem synthesis is shown in Fig. 26.4, and the relevant enzymes and the disorders associated with them in Table 26.1.

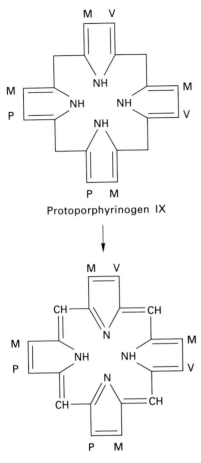

Protoporphyrinogen IX

Protoporphyrin IX

Fig. 26.3. Under the influence of protoporphyrinogen oxidase, protoporphyrinogen IX is oxidized to protoporphyrin IX. M, methyl; V, vinyl; P, propionic acid.

As the number of carboxylic acid-containing side chains are progressively reduced in number the physico-chemical characteristics of the porphyrin compounds are changed, becoming less water-soluble. For this reason their disposition in body liquids and excretion patterns are altered – hence, for example, the names uroporphyrin and coproporphyrin.

Table 26.2 summarizes the disturbances of haem synthesis pathway metabolites found in the conditions to be discussed in this chapter. Tables showing the normal values of these metabolites in urine, faeces and red cells have been published by Goldberg *et al.* (1987) and Elder (1990).

The ways in which the symptoms and signs of each individual porphyria disorder are produced are partially understood. To some extent the clinical phenomena are determined by the physico-chemical characteristics of the compound whose biotransformation is impaired and which consequently is produced in excess. The exact way other features are produced, notably the neurological aspects of, for example, acute intermittent porphyria, remain a matter for conjecture but seem related to the accumulation of ALA and/or deficiency of cytochromes P450.

Haem is a constituent of many compounds other than haemoglobin. Another section in this book deals with cytochrome P450 – an integral part of whose molecule is a haem moiety. Enzymes such as catalase and peroxidase also have haem as part of their structures. Haem is formed in many cells of the body but the principal sites of synthesis are the marrow and the liver.

Strangely enough, only exceptional examples of the hepatic porphyria disorders have been shown to be characterized by a deficient production of haemoglobin.

CLASSIFICATION OF PORPHYRIA DISORDERS

The porphyrias are traditionally classified into two groups, hepatic and erythropoietic, and as Hindmarsh (1986) pointed out this approach has the merit of simplicity.

It is in the hepatic porphyrias that clinical manifestations are 'induced' by the consumption of drugs and other chemical compounds in persons who are genetically predisposed. This account will be limited to a discussion of those disorders.

The hepatic porphyrias are themselves divided into two groups: (a) acute porphyrias, (b) porphyria cutanea tarda. The acute porphyrias are four namely:

1. porphobilinogen synthase deficiency (ALA dehydratase deficiency, plumboporphyria);
2. acute intermittent porphyria ('Swedish' porphyria);
3. hereditary coproporphyria (with also harderoporphyria);
4. porphyria variegata ('South African' porphyria).

The first named occurs as an autosomal recessive condition. The other three diseases occur in some persons who are heterozygous for the biochemical

Table 26.1. *Enzymes of the haem synthesis pathway and the disorders associated with them*

Enzyme	EC number	Chromosomal location	Disorder caused by deficiency of the enzyme	Inheritance of the disorder	McKusick (MIM) reference number
1 ALA synthase (hepatic)	2.3.1.37	3p21	–	–	125290
2 PBG synthase (ALA dehydratase)	4.2.1.24	9q34	PBG synthase deficiency (plumboporphyria)	autosomal recessive	125270
3 PBG deaminase	4.3.1.8	11q23.2–11qter	Acute intermittent porphyria	autosomal dominant	176000
4 Uroporphyrinogen III synthase (or co-synthase)	4.2.1.75	10q25.2–q26.3	Congenital erythropoietic porphyria	autosomal recessive	263700
5 Uroporphyrinogen decarboxylase	4.1.1.37	1p34	Porphyria cutanea tarda	autosomal dominant	176100
6 Coproporphyrinogen oxidase	1.3.3.3	9	Hereditary coproporphyria	autosomal dominant	121300
7 Protoporphyrinogen oxidase	1.3.3.4	14q32 18q22[a]	Porphyria variegata	autosomal dominant	176200
8 Ferrochetalase	4.99.1.1	18q21.3[b]	Erythropoietic protoporphyria	autosomal dominant	177000

The enzymes are numbered in the sequence indicated in Fig. 26.4.
Step 6 may be composed of two sequential reactions in the first of which the propionate side chain of pyrrole ring A is oxidized to a vinyl group to form harderoporphyrinogen, to be followed by a second step in which a similar biotransformation occurs to pyrrole ring B.
Only the familial form of porphyria cutanea tarda (type II) is represented in this table. The sporadic form has MIM No. 176090 (McKusick 1992).
[a]Whitcombe *et al.* 1991.
[b]Taketani *et al.* 1992.

Table 26.2. *Changes in porphyrins in the porphyrias and porphyrinurias*

	Urine ALA	PBG	URO	COPRO	Faeces COPRO	PROTO	Blood PROTO
Acute porphyrias							
Plumboporphyria	Raised in attacks	Normal	Raised in attacks	Greatly raised in attacks	Normal	Normal	Slight increase
Acute intermittent porphyria	Raised very high in attack	Raised very high in attack	Usually raised	Sometimes raised	Sometimes raised	Sometimes raised	Normal
Variegate porphyria	Raised in attack	Raised in attack	Usually raised	Usually raised	Raised	Raised	Normal
Hereditary coproporphyria	Raised in attack	Raised in attack	Sometimes raised in attack	Usually raised – always in attack	Raised	Usually normal	Normal
Non-acute porphyrias							
Porphyria cutanea cutanea	Normal	Normal	Very raised	Slightly raised	Raised in remission	Raised in remission	Normal
Other conditions							
Lead poisoning	Raised	Normal	Normal	Sometimes raised	Normal	Normal	Raised where blood lead > 2 μmol/l
Iron deficiency anaemia	Normal	Normal	Normal	Normal	Normal	Normal	Raised

Adapted from: Moore *et al.* 1990.

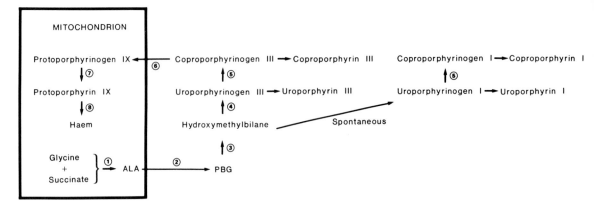

Fig. 26.4. Scheme of haem synthesis. See Table 26.1 for details of the enzymes catalysing the numbered chemical reactions. ALA, 5-aminolaevulinate; PBG, porphobilinogen.

disorder, but in several instances very rare examples of a much more severe disease have been recognized due to the existence of the abnormal homozygote.

THE ACUTE PORPHYRIAS

The principal clinical manifestations of the acute porphyrias are neurological in origin, and have been described in detail by most of the large porphyria units whose accounts are closely similar.

The experience of the Glasgow porphyria unit as shown in Fig. 26.5 is representative and shows that the symptoms of abdominal pain and vomiting are the most common, whereas hypertension and tachycardia are the most common signs.

However, it is worth noting that in some special clinical environments the clinical presentation may be atypical and unexpectedly frequent. This is emphasized in the psychiatric field by the experience of Tishler *et al.* (1985), who surveyed 3867 psychiatric inpatients for acute intermittent porphyria by means of a spot test carried out on the blood for porphobilinogen deaminase deficiency. They found eight cases, a frequency of 0.21% which is higher than the general adult prevalence figures available of 0.001 to 0.008%. Other psychiatric surveys producing similar results to theirs are reviewed by Tishler *et al.* (1985). Their patients had axis I DSM-III diagnoses of atypical psychosis and schizo-

affective disorder, and only one had abdominal pain.

Another atypical presentation was emphasized by Laiwah *et al.* (1983), who found a highly significant association between proven acute intermittent porphyria (AIP) and early onset chronic renal failure. They considered three aetiologic mechanisms, namely analgesic nephropathy, porphyria-induced hypertension and the nephrotoxic effects of porphyrins and their precursors as being potentially responsible for the renal damage.

It was formerly considered that pregnancy in a porphyric woman carried a poor prognosis. This view was shown to be incorrect by Brodie *et al.* (1976), who analysed the features of 87 pregnancies in 35 women with hereditary hepatic porphyrias.

The mechanism of production of the acute porphyrias

There is considerable evidence in experimental systems that the agents which precipitate attacks of porphyria are inducers of ALA synthase. Many of these agents are also inducers of hepatic cytochromes P450. It is thought that the massive induction of cytochromes P450 synthesis depletes the intracellular haem pool. As a result ALA synthase, which is the rate-limiting step in the haem synthesis pathway is de-repressed. As a consequence much more ALA is produced than normal and is fed into the subsequent enzymic steps. A normal individual has enzymes along the pathway which can handle this increased molecular traffic. However, an individual who only has half the

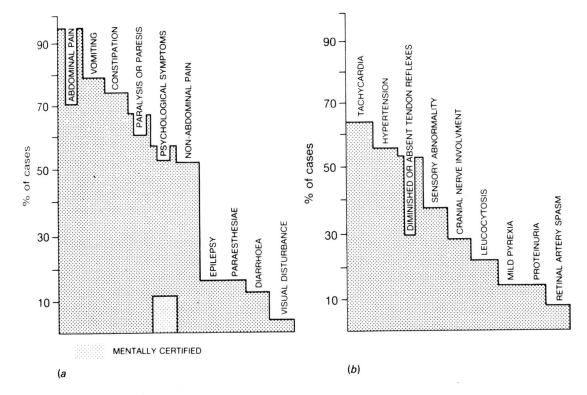

Fig. 26.5. (a) Incidence of symptoms, and (b) incidence of physical signs, blood, and urine findings in 50 cases of acute intermittent porphyria. (From Goldberg et al. 1987.)

normal enzymic capacity or less at any individual step cannot do this and so precursors accumulate, while at the same time there is curtailment in haem formation.

The molecular mechanisms responsible for the neurological features of the acute porphyrias are not fully understood. However, it is believed they are mediated to some extent by 5-aminolaevulinic acid (ALA). This view is supported by the fact that they occur in homozygous PBG synthase deficiency and in lead poisoning. The most popular views are: (1) ALA acts as a neurotoxin, causing haem deficiency within neurones, (2) ALA is structurally similar to 4-aminobutyric acid, which is the major inhibitory transmitter in the vertebrate central nervous system, and so it may have the ability to disturb neurophysiological mechanisms (Straka et al. 1990). In

severe attacks of porphyria structural damage to the neurones occurs.

Having demonstrated an impaired aminopyrine demethylation breath test in 42% and increased postprandial serum bile acid concentration in 75% of porphyrics in remission, Ostrowski et al. (1983) suggested that there may be defective hepatic cytochromes P450 production in these patients (most of whom had acute intermittent porphyria).

Similar results were obtained using antipyrine kinetics (Birnie et al. 1987). Half-lives were prolonged and plasma clearance reduced in patients with acute porphyria attacks. There was a negative correlation between weight-adjusted antipyrine clearance and the urinary excretion of ALA and PBG. These data suggested that the more severe the porphyric attack the greater the impairment of hepatic mono-oxygenase activity.

Although haem production inside the cerebral neurones is much less than in the liver, the essential mechanism is the same. There is suggestive evidence that in acute porphyria there is diminished haem production in the neurones leading to haem deficiency and de-repression of ALA synthase. Lack of haem presumably leads to a deficiency of cytochromes P450 (as in the liver) and cytochrome c oxidase (as has been demonstrated in muscle) (Moore *et al.* 1987).

In hereditary coproporphyria and more particularly porphyria variegata there are increased quantities of porphyrins in the body. The presence of these porphyrins in the skin sets the scene for the occurrence of photochemical damage in the presence of sunlight. Solar energy is absorbed at about 400 nm (depending on the particular porphyrin involved), and light at 615 nm is emitted. The energy difference produces a transient excited electronic state of the porphyric molecule which can react with molecular oxygen, causing the production of singlet state excited oxygen which in turn can damage various structures such as cell membranes (see Poh-Fitzpatrick 1982).

The therapy of the acute porphyrias

The acute attacks of porphyrias are serious illnesses carrying a mortality of up to 10%. It is obvious, therefore, that all attempts should be made to prevent their occurrence, diagnose them correctly with minimal delay and treat them effectively.

This topic has recently been reviewed by Moore & McColl (1989) and the reader is referred to their article for detailed information. (See also Kauppinen & Mustajoki 1992 for a discussion of features precipitating acute attacks.)

Undoubtedly the major effort should be preventative. Susceptible individuals should be identified; these include patients who have previously experienced an acute attack of porphyria and their relatives. The screening of relatives of such patients to recognize latent cases is an important public health preventative measure.

Effective communication is of the utmost importance. The susceptible individual must be clearly informed about the risks, and understand that she must inform any doctor that she consults of the fact that she is at risk. The possession of an information bracelet (e.g. Medic Alert) or necklace or card giving a warning regarding the dangers of drug administration (including anaesthetics) is advantageous.

Some drugs are known to have precipitated attacks of acute porphyria in patients, whilst others have been shown to be porphyrinogenic in animals

or with *in vitro* systems and they are listed in Table 26.3.

Equally important are drugs which are known to be safe for use in porphyric subjects and they are listed in Table 26.4.

Often oral contraceptives and alcohol are not considered to be drugs by lay persons, and so it must be explained and stressed that these agents should also be avoided.

Other precipitants which should be recognized and dealt with in an appropriate manner include infections and operations.

Since a full account of the management of the acute attacks has been provided by Moore & McColl (1989), only a few remarks on some selected aspects are included here.

Because the first and rate-controlling enzyme of the haem synthesis pathway is ALA synthase, which is subject to negative feed-back inhibition by haem, it is a logical approach to try and diminish the activity of this enzyme in the acute attack by the administration of haem (Mustajoki *et al.* 1989). Over the years there has been a lot of difficulty in producing a stable, well tolerated haem preparation for clinical use. Haem forms a highly soluble compound with arginine, which is stable after the addition of 1,2-propanediol and alcohol. This compound haem arginate can be infused intravenously undiluted, or diluted with physiological saline, and seems to produce far fewer side effects than previously available haem medications.

The administration of haem to patients with acute attacks of porphyria causes a marked reduction in urinary ALA and PBG excretion in acute intermittent porphyria and also of urinary and faecal porphyrins in porphyria variegata and hereditary coproporphyria. The former occurs within about one week and the latter more slowly, presumably due to a wash-out lag interval.

In addition to inhibiting the activity of the haem-synthesis pathway, haem administration improves liver cytochrome P450 function, as shown by antipyrine clearance (Mustajoki *et al.* 1992).

The clinical evidence indicates that haem (3 to 4 mg per kg body weight intravenously every 12 or 24 hours) is highly efficacious in controlling the acute attacks. Usually clinical improvement is seen within 3 days. Haem infusions seem superior to glucose and Mustajoki *et al.* (1989) recommends that they should be used as initial therapy.

Carbohydrate is known to have the ability in

Table 26.3. Drugs unsafe for use in acute porphyria

These drugs have been classified as 'unsafe' because all have been shown to be porphyrinogenic in animals or *in vitro* systems, or to have been associated with acute attacks in humans [ ] Bracketed drugs are those in which there is conflicting experimental evidence of porphyrinogenicity – some positive – some negative.
*Those marked in bold with an asterisk have been associated with acute attacks of porphyria.

A:
Alcohol
Alcuronium
Allyloxy-3-methyl benzamide
*Alphaxalone:Alphadolone
Aluminium preparations
Aminoglutethimide
Amidopyrine
Amiodarone
[Amitriptyline]
[Amphetamines]
Amylobarbitone
Anabolic steroids
Antidepressants
Antihistamines
Antipyrine
Apronalide
Auranofin
Azapropazone

B:
Baclofen
*Barbiturates
*Bemegride
Bendrofluazide
Benzodiazepines
Benoxaprofen
Bromocriptine
Busulphan

C:
Captopril
*Carbamazepine
*Carbromal
*Carisoprodol
[Cefuroxime]
[Cephalexin]
[Cephalosporins]
[Cephradine]
[Clorambucil]
*Chloramphenicol
*Chlordiazepoxide
Chlormezanone
Chloroform
*Chlorpropamide
Chlorzoxazone
Cimetidine
Cinnarizine
Clemastine
[Clobazam]
Clomipramine
[Clonazepam]
Clonidine HCl
Clorazepate
Cocaine
Colistin
Contraceptive steroids
Cotrimoxazole

D:
Danazol
Dapsone
Dextropropoxyphene

[Diazepam]
*Dichloralphenazone
Diclofenac Na
Diethylpropion
*Dihydroergotamine
Diltiazem
*Dimenhydrinate
Diphenhydramine
Dipyrone
Dixyrazine
Doxycycline
Drotaverine
[Dydrogesterone]

E:
Econazole
Enalapril
Enflurane
*Ergot compounds
Ergotamine maleate
Erythromycin
Ethamsylate
*Ethanol
*Ethchlorvynol
Ethinamate
Ethionamide
Ethosuximide
Ethotoin
Etidocaine
Etomidate

F:
[Flucloxacillin]
*Flufenamic acid
Flunitrazepam
Flupenthixol
Flurazepam
Fluroxene
[Frusemide]

G:
*Glutethimide
Glymidine
Gold Salts
Gramicidin
*Griseofulvin
Guaiphenesin

H:
*Halothane
*Hydantoins
Hydralazine
[Hydrochlorothiazide]
Hydroxyzine
*Hyoscine butylbromide

I:
*Imipramine
Iproniazid
Isometheptene mucate
[Isoniazid]
Isopropyl antipyrine

K:
Ketoconazole

L:
Lignocaine
Lofepramine
Loprazolam
Loxapine
Lysuride maleate

M:
Mebeverine
[Mefanamic acid]
Megestrol acetate
Menopausal steroids
Mephenesin
Mepivacaine
*Meprobamate
Mercaptopurine
Mercury compounds
Mestranol
Methamphetamine
Methohexitone
Methotrexate
Methoxyflurane
Methsuximide
*Methyl dopa
*Methyl sulphonal
*Methyprylone
[Metoclopramide]
Metronidazole
Metyrapone
Miconazole
Minoxidil

N:
Nalidixic acid
Nifedipine
*Nikethamide
Nitrazepam
[Nitrofurantoin]
Norethynodrel
Nortriptyline
Novobiocin

O:
*Oral contraceptives
*Orphenadrine
Oxanamide
[Oxazepam]
Oxycodone
Oxymetazoline
Oxyphenbutazone
Oxytetracycline

P:
Paramethadione
Pargyline
*Pentazocine
*Pentylenetetrazol
Phenacetin
Phenelzine
*Phenobarbitone

Phenoxybenzamide
Phensuximide
[Phenylbutazone]
Phenylhydrazine
*Phenytoin
Pitramide
Piroxicam
*Pivampicillin
Prazepam
Prenylamine
[Prilocaine]
*Primidone
[Probenecid]
*Progesterone
Promethazine
[Propanidid]
*Pyrazinamide
Pyrrocaine

Q:
Quinalbarbitone

R:
Rifampicin

S:
Simvastatin
Sodium aurothiomalate
Sodium oxybate
[Sodium valproate]
Spironolactone
Stanozolol
Succinimides
*Sulphadimidine
*Sulphasalazine
Sulphinpyrazone
Sulphonylureas
Sulpride
Sulthiame

T:
Tamoxifen
Terfenadine
[Tetracyclines]
*Theophylline
*Thiopentone Sodium
Thioridazine
Tilidate
Tinidazole
Tolazamide
Tolbutamide
Tranylcypromine
Trazodone HCl
Trimethoprim
Trimipramine
Troxidone

V:
Valproate
Verapamil
Viloxazine HCl

Z:
Zuclopenthixol

Note: While very great care has been taken in the compilation of this table and the drug information is given in the belief that it is correct at the time of publication, all information herein and opinions expressed must be taken as information and opinions given for general guidance only.

Medical practitioners and patients must make their own decisions in the circumstances of the particular case about therapy appropriate in any case of acute porphyria.

Adapted from: Moore & McColl 1989 and British National Formulary No. 21 (March 1991).

Table 26.4. *Drugs thought to be* safe *for use in acute porphyria*

Each bracketed drug [ ] has had conflicting evidence of experimental porphyrinogenicity. Occasionally positive, but mainly negative – none of the drugs in this entire list has been associated with human porphyric attacks.

A:	D:	L:	Procaine
Acetaminophen	Danthron	Labetalol	Prochlorperazine
Acetazolamide	Demerol	LHRH	Proguanil HCl
Acetylcholine	Desferrioxamine	Liquorice	Promazine
Acetylsalicylic acid	Dexamethasone	Lithium salts	Propantheline Br
Acyclovir	[Dextromoramide]	[Loperamide]	Propofol
Adenosine monophosphate	Diamorphine	[Lorazepam]	Propranolol
Adrenaline	Diazoxide		Propylthiouracil
Alclofenac	Dicyclomine HCl	M:	[Proxymetacaine]
Allopurinol	Diflunisal	Magnesium sulphate	Pseudoephedrine HCl
Alpha tocopheryl acetate	Digoxin	[Mebendazole]	Pyridoxine
Amethocaine	Dihydrocodeine	Mecamylamine	[Pyrimethamine]
Amiloride	Dimercaprol	Meclozine	
Aminocaproic acid	Dimethicone	[Melphalan]	Q:
Amoxycillin	Diphenoxylate HCl	Mequitazine	Quinine
Amphotericin	[Disopyramide]	Metformin	
Ampicillin	Domperidone	Methadone	R:
Ascorbic acid	Dothiepin HCl	[Methotrimeprazine]	[Ranitidine]
Aspirin	Doxorubicin HCl	Methylphenidate	Reserpine
Atenolol	Droperidol	Methyluracil	Resorcinol
Atropine		Metipropranolol	
Azathioprine	E:	Metoprolol	S:
	Ethacrynic acid	Mianserin	Salbutamol
B:	Ethambutol	[Midazolam]	Senna
Beclomethasone	[Ethinyl Oestradiol]	Minaxolone	Sodium bromide
Beta-carotene	Ethoheptazine citrate	Morphine	Sodium Ca EDTA
Biguanides			Sodium fusidate
[Bromazepam]	F:	N:	Streptomycin
Bromides	Fenbrufen	Nadolol	Sulindac
Bumetanide	Fenoprofen	Naftidrofuryl oxalate	Sulphadoxine
Bupivacaine	Fentanyl	Naproxen Sodium	Suxamethonium
Buprenorphine	[Flucytosine]	Natamycin	
Buserelin	Flurbiprofen	Nefopam HCl	T:
Butacaine	Folic acid	Neostigmine	Talampicillin
	FSH	Nitrous oxide	Temazepam
C:			Tetracaine
Canthanxanthin	G:	O:	[Tetracyclines]
Carbimazole	Gentamicin	Oxybuprocaine	Thiouracils
Chloral hydrate	Glafenine	[Oxyphenbutazone]	Thyroxine
[Chlormethiazole]	Glipizide	Oxytocin	Tiaprofenic acid
[Chloroquine]	Glucagon		Timolol maleate
[Chlorothiazide	Glycerol trinitrate	P:	Tolazoline
Chlorpheniramine	Guanethidine	[Pancuronium bromide]	Tranexamic acid
Chlorpromazine		Paracetamol	Triamterene
Cisplatin	H:	Paraldehyde	Triazolam
Clofibrate	Haem arginate	Penicillamine	[Trichlormethiazide]
Clomiphene citrate	Heparin	Penicillin	Trifluoperazine
Cloxacillin	Hexamine	Pentolinium	Tripelennamine
[Cocaine]	[Hydrocortisone]	Pethidine	Tubocurarine
Co-codamol		Phenformin	
Codeine phosphate	I:	Phenoperidine	V:
Colchicine	Ibuprofen	Phentolamine mesylate	[Vincristine]
[Corticosteroids]	Indomethacin	Pipothiazine palmitate	
Corticotrophin [ACTH]	Insulin	Pirbuterol	W:
[Co-trimoxazole]	Iron	Pirenzepine	Warfarin sodium
Coumarins		[Prazosin]	
Cyclizine	K:	[Prednisolone]	Z:
Cyclopropane	[Ketamine]	Primaquine	Zinc preparations (topical)
[Cyproterone acetate]	Ketoprofen	Probucol	
	[Ketotifen]		

Note: While very great care has been taken in the compilation of this table and the drug information is given in the belief that it is correct at the time of publication, all information contained herin and opinions expressed must be taken as information and opinions given for general guidance only.

The authors hereby disclaim for themselves, the Porphyrias Service, the University of Glasgow and the Greater Glasgow Health Board, all responsibility for any mis-statement or for the consequences to any person acting in reliance on any statement or opinion contained herein.

Medical practitioners and patients must make their own decisions in the circumstances of the particular case about therapy appropriate in any case of acute porphyria.

From: Moore & McColl 1989.

experimental systems of preventing the induction of ALA synthase by porphyrinogenic drugs. It is therefore logical to ensure that there is an adequate supply of carbohydrate to the liver cells to diminish ALA production as much as possible. If it is not possible to supply an adequate amount of carbohydrate by mouth then it has to be administered intravenously through a central venous line.

Paralyses are a feature of acute porphyria and the most serious form is paralysis of the respiratory muscles. The patients have to be carefully monitored. It is better to put the patient on assisted ventilation earlier rather than later.

Luckily, drugs required to control pain appear in the list of 'safe' drugs (Table 26.2). Acetaminophen (paracetamol) and aspirin will suffice for mild pain. More severe pain merits pethidine, morphine or buprenorphine. There is a very considerable danger of drug addiction in porphyrics.

Epilepsy in porphyrics presents a difficult therapeutic problem since most of the customary antiepileptic drugs are porphyria- provoking. Moore & McColl (1989) advocate the use of intravenous diazepam for the control of status epilepticus. They also state that 'seizure prophylaxis can be undertaken as a calculated risk with clonazepam or sodium valproate if this is essential, although sporadic clinical reports of porphyrinogenicity do exist'.

PORPHOBILINOGEN SYNTHASE DEFICIENCY

This condition is concerned with the cytosolic enzyme porphobilinogen synthase (PBG-S) formerly called ALA dehydratase (ALA-D) which is the second in the haem synthesis pathway. This enzyme is not known to have genetic variants differentially influenced by drugs. Nevertheless, it is included in this book for two reasons: (1) acute porphyria has occurred with genetic variants of PBG-S and this indicates strongly that it is ALA and not PBG which is responsible for the features of that syndrome though it must be emphasized that ALA on its own will not produce the features – another factor, most probably haem deficiency (as explained above) is also involved; (2) it appears likely that enzyme variants are differentially affected by lead. This latter aspect indicates that porphobilinogen synthase (PBG-S) is important in the field of ecogenetics – a discipline whose ideas are very similar to those of pharmacogenetics.

Enzyme polymorphisms

The first polymorphism of porphobilinogen synthase (PBG-S) was found by Bird et al. (1979), who surveyed a student population for the activity of the enzyme in red cells. One 16 year old healthy female was found with a level at about 22% of normal. The 21 members of her family showed a bimodality with 11 showing low levels and 10 showing normal levels of enzymic activity. The pattern of inheritance of the low activity appeared (strangely) to be that of an autosomal dominant. There was no history of attacks of clinical features of porphyria in the family. The authors speculate that the low activity phenotype might be especially sensitive to environmental lead exposure.

A starch gel electrophoresis polymorphism for PBG-S was described by Battistuzzi et al. (1981). Three phenotypes were displayed (1-1, 1-2 and 2-2) which were shown by family studies to be due to two co-dominant autosomal alleles. The enzymic activity was the same in all three phenotypes. From this study and subsequent surveys by Petrucci et al. (1982) and Benkman et al. (1983), the allele frequencies for *ALA-D1* were Italy 0.90, Germany 0.889, Japan 0.942 and Liberia 1.000. The allele frequency for *ALA-D1* in Koreans was shown to be 0.958 by Pak et al. (1988), who also produced a comprehensive table of allele distributions in different populations. The lowest fequency of *ALA-D1* was 0.7979 in Ashkenazi Jews.

This polymorphism of normal people was re-examined using the techniques of molecular biology by Wetmur et al. (1991). Total RNA from a 2-2 homozygote was reverse transcribed and the *ALA-D2* cDNA amplified, subcloned and sequenced. Compared with the *ALA-D1* sequence the only difference in the *ALA-D2* cDNA was a 177G → C transversion creating an *Msp*I restriction site and an amino acid change 59 lysine → asparagine which lost a positive charge (thus accounting for the electrophoretic difference). An independent *Rsa*I polymorphism at nucleotide 168 could also be detected by the same technique.

A type of acute porphyria

Several patients have been described as presenting with acute porphyria which has been shown to be due to gross PBG-S deficiency. Doss et al. (1982) described two young men who had classical acute porphyria attacks with greatly increased ALA and porphyrin excretion (mainly coproporphyrin isomer III). There was no exposure to drugs, lead or alcohol abuse. Tyrosinaemia was excluded (PBG-S is inhibited by succinylacetone which accumulates in hereditary tyrosinaemia: Straka *et al.* 1990). Their red cell PBG-S activity levels were shown to be extremely low. The influence of an inhibitor substance was disproved. A crossreactive immunologic material corresponding to 20 and 30% of the control level was demonstrated in these two patients by de Verneuil *et al.* (1985), indicating the existence of a structurally altered enzyme (Fig. 26.6). Family surveys showed that these two patients were homozygotes. Nine heterozygotes were identified with

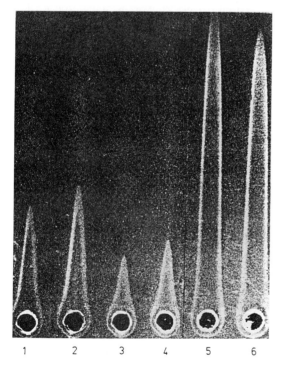

Fig. 26.6. Rocket immunoelectrophoresis of ALA-D in haemolysates from patients and from two normal controls. ALA-D was partially purified from 0.25 ml of packed erythrocytes by CM-Sepharose chromatography followed by ammonium sulphate precipitation (50% saturation). The enzyme was resuspended in 0.1 ml of barbital buffer (pH 8.6) used for electrophoresis. Three microlitre samples were added to each well. 1 and 2, Patient B; 3 and 4, Patient H; 5 and 6, two controls. (From de Verneueil *et al.* 1985.)

activities between normals and the probands. Starch gel electrophoresis displayed no activity of PBG-S from red cell preparations from the probands. The electrophoretic bands from the other family members did not correlate with their red cell PBG-S activities (Doss *et al.* 1986).

A further patient with acute hepatic porphyria and red cell PBG-S activity at 2% of normal was described by Fujita *et al.* (1987); using immunochemical methods a crossreactive material to the extent of 28% of the normal enzyme could be demonstrated in the erythrocytes of the proband. The same group (Sassa *et al.* 1991) showed extremely low levels of PBG-S activity in EB-virus transformed lymphocytes from two probands. Other porphyrin synthesis enzymes were normal. Heterozygote members of the two families had PBG-S activities of a little less than half normal.

PBG-S is the enzyme which normally has the highest activity among all the enzymes of the haem synthesis pathway. There is a huge excess of this enzyme in the marrow. This is a possible reason why these probands with only 2% of normal activity did not develop anaemia. Alternatively, the marrow may not suffer the same deficiency as the red cells.

Two previously healthy men in their twenties presented within 10 days of each other, with acute porphyria, to Wolff *et al.* (1991). Their red cell PBG-S activities were very low and remained so months later when they had recovered. There was neither a history nor analytical evidence of lead exposure.

Molecular biology

The PBG-S gene has been mapped to chromosome 9 by Wang *et al.* (1984) and Beaumont *et al.* (1984) and to 9q34 by Potluri *et al.* (1987) by *in situ* hybridization. The cDNA sequence has been elucidated by Wetmur *et al.* (1986a, b), revealing an open reading frame of 990 bases.

PBG-S has eight identical subunits each with a molecular mass of 31 kDa and containing a zinc atom. Each zinc atom is bound to a subunit by a 'zinc finger' domain consisting of four cysteine and two histidine residues. The zinc atoms protect essential sulphydryl groups and are displaced by lead and other metals. The catalytically active centre is thought to be lysine at position 252.

Advances have now been made in understanding the molecular biology of the low PBG-S type of porphyria. The patient described by Fujita *et al.* (1987) was reinvestigated by Plewinska *et al.* (1991). He was shown to be heteroallelic for an *Rsa*I polymorphic site in the coding region of the PBG-S gene. This heteroallelism was found by subjecting a 704 bp polymerase chain reaction product to the action of *Rsa*I; when the restriction site was present fragments of 579 and 125 bp were produced. The maternal *Rsa*I-positive allele had a nucleotide transition 397G → A (the last nucleotide in exon 6), giving 133 glycine → arginine. The paternal *Rsa*I-negative allele had an 823G → A transition giving 275 valine → methionine. Both changes markedly affected the enzyme's catalytic function and possibly the latter rendered the protein unable to form the normally occurring multimers.

Similarly, a patient originally described by Doss *et al.* (1986) was shown by Ishida *et al.* (1992) to have two mutations in the *PBG-S* genes, namely 718 C → T causing 240 arginine → tryptophan, and 820 G → A causing 274 alanine → threonine. The two mutant genes were individually expressed in Chinese hamster ovary cells. The 718 mutant produced an enzyme with a normal half-life whilst the enzyme produced by the 820 mutant had a markedly decreased half-life.

Lead toxicity

The evidence for the relationship between genetic variation in *PBG-S* and lead toxicity will now be briefly reviewed.

A 30 year old painter was described by Doss *et al.* (1984). He presented with an acute porphyria syndrome and anaemia. His blood lead concentration was elevated up to 414 µg/l (normal up to 290 µg/l) and the urinary lead concentration was raised. His red cell PBG-S activity was low on presentation and remained low 4 years later when his lead levels had fallen to within the normal range. His mother also showed PBG-S red cell activities of half-normal. It is suggested that the patient and his mother were heterozygotes for a low PBG-S activity allele which conferred undue susceptibility to lead toxicity.

The relationships between blood lead concentration, red blood cell PBG-S activity and the PBG-S electrophoretic phenotype were examined in a group of 202 male lead-exposed workers by Ziemsen *et al.* (1986). Their conclusion was that the response of PBG-S activity to a given blood lead concentration was independent of the PBG-S electrophoretic phenotype (but see below).

Children living in New York City neighbourhoods at high risk of lead exposure were studied by Astrin *et al.* (1987). PBG-S electrophoretic polymorphism and blood lead concentrations were determined. The 1-2 phenotype was significantly associated with a raised blood level in the whole sample of 1051 persons and in a subsample of 345 blacks (but, oddly, not in a subsample of 259 Hispanics). The idea was put forward that the *ALA-D2* allele was able more firmly to bind lead than the *ALA-D1* allele.

More sophisticated statistical analyses of both the above studies were carried out by Wetmur *et al.* (1991), and they showed convincingly that homozygotes and heterozygotes for the *ALA-D2* allele who expressed the 2-2 or 1-2 isozyme phenotype had median blood lead levels which were about 9 to 11 µg/l greater than similarly exposed individuals who were homozygous for the *ALA-D1* allele.

It must be emphasized that although PBG-S, ferrochetalase and coproporphyrinogen oxidase activities are all markedly depressed by lead (Moore *et al.* 1987), PBG-S is the enzyme along the haem synthesis pathway which is inhibited by the lowest concentrations of lead. Porphyric patients suffer depression of their PBG-S activity relatively more than normal people at a given blood lead level (Batlle *et al.* 1987). However, that is not really the point upon which this section focuses. It is the differential liability of ALA-D phenotypes (arising because of the different enzymic structures dictated by the two alleles) to the toxic effects of lead exposure which is of eco-genetic interest.

ACUTE INTERMITTENT PORPHYRIA

Clinical features

The clinical features of acute intermittent porphyria (AIP) are the occurrence of attacks as described under 'acute porphyria' (see above). These attacks virtually never occur before puberty and there are no disorders of the skin. In an attack the urine, when passed, may be a normal colour or slightly brownish and becomes dark on standing, especially if the urine is acid and is exposed to ultraviolet light. This colour change is due to porphobilinogen (PBG) polymerizing to uroporphyrin and a brownish-red pigment, porphobilin.

Interest has been aroused recently in the development of hepatocellular carcinoma (HCC) in AIP patients. The frequency appears to be greater than that which would be due to coincidence. How the metabolic disturbances of AIP might lead to HCC is unclear (Lithner & Wetterberg 1984; Gubler et al. 1990; Kauppinen & Mustajoki 1992).

Diagnosis and biochemical investigations

The key to diagnosis is to think of the possibility of AIP as an explanation of a clinical picture. The proof of the diagnosis has hitherto been the examination of body liquids for intermediates in the haem synthesis pathway and of appropriate enzymes.

There is a marked difference between the results of biochemical investigations which are seen in an exacerbation, and those which are seen in remissions.

The key investigation is the examination of urine for excess PBG. For a screening 'bedside' test the detection and measurement of PBG is based on its reaction with p-dimethylaminobenzaldehyde in hydrochloric acid (Ehrlich's reagent), which gives a red compound. Saturated sodium acetate is mixed vigorously with the red solution. Then butanol or amyl alcohol is mixed vigorously and removed. This last step is repeated until the organic phase is colourless. If the aqueous phase had any red colour remaining in it, this qualitative test is positive for PBG (modified Watson–Schwartz test: see Elder et al. 1990). Positive tests should be confirmed by specific quantitative measurement of urinary PBG. If the clinical picture is convincing the laboratory diagnosis should still be pursued with other investigations even if the screening test is negative because the reliability is not high (Buttery et al. 1990).

Porphyrins in urine arise mainly in vitro from PBG. There may be a slight increase in faecal coproporphyrin and protoporphyrin.

In remissions urinary PBG excretion falls markedly but very rarely to normal. Hence, in a suspected latent patient, if the urinary ALA, urinary PBG excretion, total urinary porphyrins and total faecal porphyrins are all normal, then the diagnosis is excluded for all practical purposes (Elder et al. 1990).

The estimation of erythrocytic PBG-D activity may be useful as an aid to diagnosis of latent cases (Pierach et al. 1987), particularly when combined with estimates of ALA-S as emphasized by McColl et al. (1982). However, in a minority of pedigrees red cell PBG-D may be normal, as explained below.

The situation has now changed with the advent of specific probes by which the precise defect can be identified in DNA obtained from peripheral blood leucocytes amplified by the use of the polymerase chain reaction (see below). The availability of this technique of direct examination of the genome may solve puzzles like the one posed by Herrick et al. (1989). They described two patients on antiepileptic therapy who developed an AIP illness, but their red cell PBG-D activities were normal and family histories negative. (A number of explanations were advanced by the authors, including the possibility that the patients represented the variant of AIP described by Mustajoki & Tenhunen (1985) – see below).

It is to be noted that the biochemical abnormality is inherited as an autosomal dominant Mendelian character. Only a minority of persons possessing the biochemical defect actually develop the clinical illness of AIP and females are significantly more likely to do so than males due to the influence of endogenous oestrogens.

Identification of the enzymic defect

Building on the knowledge that there was a defective production of porphyrins from PBG in AIP, it was shown by Meyer et al. (1972) that there was a genetic defect in erythrocytic porphobilinogen deaminase (PBG-D). This enzyme joins up four PBG molecules one at a time to make hydroxymethylbilane, as explained above. The defect of PBG-D has also been shown to be present in other tissues, such as liver, cultured skin fibroblasts, amniotic cells and cultured lymphoblasts (see Anderson et al. 1981). Comparison of the physical and kinetic properties of the PBG-D activity in erythrocyte lysates from heterozygotes for AIP and normal individuals showed essentially identical electrophoretic abilities, apparent Michaelis constant (K_m) values and heat-denaturation profiles. When lymphocytes from AIP

Table 26.5. *Different types of heterozygotes who have suffered attacks of acute intermittent porphyria*

Mutant type	Red cell lysate PBG-D activity	Amount of material in red cell lysate cross-reacting with antibody for normal PBG-D (per unit enzymic activity)
CRIM-negative type 1	About 50% of normal	1.0
CRIM-negative type 2	normal	1.0
CRIM-positive type 1	About 50% of normal	1.7
CRIM-positive type 2	About 50% of normal	5.7

Adapted from: Table III of Desnick *et al.* 1985.

heterozygotes were induced with mitogens, only 50% of the PBG-D activity seen in normal individuals was produced. It remained unclear whether the defect responsible for AIP was a regulatory or a structural gene defect.

A considerable advance in understanding was made by the study of Anderson *et al.* (1981), who used two techniques. In the first, an IgG rabbit antibody to purified human PBG-D was prepared and used in sensitive immunotitration and rocket immunoelectrophoretic studies. Equal PBG-D activities from 25 AIP heterozygotes from 21 unrelated families were studied and no differences in rocket peak heights of immunoreactive enzyme were seen as compared with normals (CRIM-activity ratio = 1.0). This type of result was designated 'cross-reacting immunologic material negative' (CRIM-negative), since it was considered that the defective allele was neither producing an active enzyme nor a molecule which was recognizable by the antibody. In contradistinction, in seven AIP heterozygotes from a family of Basque ancestry, rocket peak heights for equal enzymic activity were 1.6 times greater than normal (CRIM-positive). PBG-D enzyme–substrate intermediates could be separated from red cell lysates by anion-exchange chromatography. These represented compounds formed by the sequential addition of single pyrrole rings building up hydroxymethylbilane which was eventually released. These intermediates were further studied by iso-electric focusing and crossed immunoelectrophoresis. No evidence of structural variants could be obtained in either CRIM-negative or CRIM-positive categories by these techniques. The authors speculated that structural variants of PBG-D were

present which did not possess a charge difference but might have altered catalytic or substrate-binding sites.

Further evidence for genetic heterogeneity of the PBG-D gene was provided by Desnick *et al.* (1985), Mustajoki & Tenhunen (1985) and Mustajoki & Desnick (1985). These workers advanced the work published by Anderson *et al.* (1981) by studying 165 AIP heterozygotes from 92 unrelated families derived from different ethnic and geographical backgrounds. The new findings were essentially two.

1 Typical cases of AIP were recognized in whom raised δ-ALA, PBG and coproporphyrin were found in the urine but in whom the erythrocytic URO-S, PBG-D, coproporphyrinogen oxidase and haem synthase were normal. These fell into the CRIM-negative category described earlier.
2 Patients with AIP who yielded red cell lysates in which the amount of CRIM-positive material was about 5.7-fold that in normal lysates as shown by immunotitration and quantitative rocket immunoelectrophoresis.

Following this work it became clear that there existed four enzymic types of heterozygotes liable to attacks of AIP (Table 26.5). Their existence was not explained by any haematological disorders or differential mean erythrocytic age. Lannfelt *et al.* (1989), employing an ELISA technique showed that the erythrocyte PBG-D specific activity (i.e. per gram protein) was about 83% of normal in CRIM-negative type I and about 31% in CRIM-positive mutants, also indicating that they were different mutations. The CRIM-positive type 2 enzyme was most resistant to heat denaturation. It was suggested that the CRIM-negative type 2 had a defect of

PBG-D activity in the liver, even though the enzyme was normal in the red cells. There was no convincing evidence that there was any difference in liability to acute attacks between the four types.

Molecular genetics

The chromosomal assignment of the human PBG-D structural gene was made to the distal portion of the long arm of chromosome 11 (11q23 → 11qter) by Wang *et al.* (1981) and 11q24.1 → q24.2 by Namba *et al.* (1991). The cDNA for human erythrocyte PBG-D was cloned and sequenced by Raich *et al.* (1986). The reading frame of 1032 bp encoded for 344 amino acids, and there was a 5′ non-coding region of 81 bp and a complete 3′ non-coding region of 266 bp excluding the poly(A) tail. The gene was encoded by one copy per haploid genome.

The structural gene for PBG-D was found to be 10 kb long and to contain 15 exons. The interesting feature was the possession of two promoters. A promoter is a region of the gene which contains special sequences of DNA separated by nucleotides which have no particular meaning. The enzyme RNA polymerase binds to the promoter, and the tighter the binding the more mRNA is made per unit time. In the case of PBG-D the ubiquitous upstream promoter which is active in all cells is located 3 kb of DNA upstream from the erythroid cell promoter.

The consequence of this arrangement is that the ubiquitous mRNA is transcribed from exons 1 and 3 (omitting exon 2), whereas the erythroid mRNA is transcribed from exons 2 and 3 (omitting exon 1). The structure of the mRNA governed by exons 3 to 15 is the same in both types. The ubiquitous PBG-D is 17 amino acids longer at the 5′ end than the erythroid PBG-D.

A series of ingenious experiments was carried out by Beaupain *et al.* (1990) in which they prepared various structural modifications of fragments of the PBG-D gene. The function of these fragments was examined with *in vitro* transcription assays and *in vivo* in cultured cells. A 15 bp element which extended 1 bp 5′ and 14 bp 3′ from the initiation site was identified as being necessary and sufficient for accurate initiation of transcription *in vitro*. Other elements lying upstream at around −70 were required for accurate transcription *in vivo*.

The promoter for the erythroid type of PBG-D is very similar to that for human β-globin, which suggests the possibility of a common control of different genes active in erythroid cells (Grandchamp *et al.* 1987; Chretien *et al.* 1988).

Restriction fragment length polymorphisms (RFLP) have been investigated in acute intermittent porphyria with the idea of using them as diagnostic tools which might be simple to use and more reliable for the detection of latent cases than assays of excretion products and red cell PBG-D activity.

Informative restriction endonucleases (RE) have been *Msp*I, *Pst*I, *Bst*NI, *Apa*LI and *Nhe*I. Various fragments of the cDNA of *PBG-D* have been used as probes (e.g. Llewellyn *et al.* 1987; Lee *et al.* 1988).

Two interesting findings have resulted from this work. First, there was marked linkage disequilibrium between the haplotypes in both normal individuals and patients with AIP, and the significance of this finding is at present obscure. Secondly, the individual RFLPs and the haplotype information can both be successfully used to detect AIP heterozygote latent carriers (Fig. 26.7) but only in informative families where sufficient relatives are available (Lee *et al.* 1988, 1990; Kauppinen *et al.* 1990; Scobie *et al.* 1990a).

Several mutations have been described in the PBG-D gene as shown in Table 26.6. The first two occur in the 3 kb portion of the gene which lies upstream of the erythroid form of the gene. The consequence of this is that the function of the gene in the liver and other tissues is abnormal, but the erythroid gene works normally and so red cell PBG-D activity is normal. This explains the existence of the CRIM negative type 2 form of AIP.

A CRIM-positive form of the disease is explained by the penultimate entry in Table 26.6. Here the enzyme, although it is missing 40 amino acids, is stable and is recognized as the normal structure by an antibody: nevertheless, it is catalytically inactive.

One practical application of this information is shown in Figs. 26.8 and 26.9. The mutant allele was cloned from a patient with AIP and with normal red cell PBG-D activity. Sequencing the portion of the gene which is important for its expression in non-erythroid cells, namely the 5′ promoter, the first exon and the 5′ portion of the first intron revealed a G → T change at the last position of the first exon modifying the normal sequence of splicing CGGTGAGT to CTGTGAGT (second row of Table 26.6). This base change does not modify the amino acid specified by the last codon of the exon

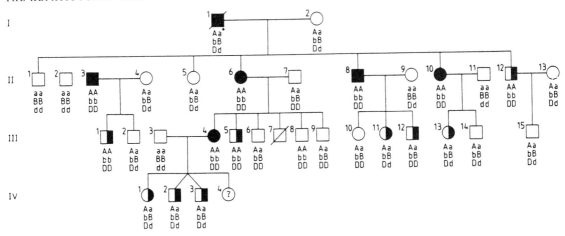

Fig. 26.7. Pedigree of family with acute intermittent porphyria. Black symbols indicate patients, half shaded symbols carriers, dashed subjects deceased (?) not tested (*) predicted haplotype.

Fragments: BstNI   D 0.8 kb   d 0.5 kb
                MspI   A 3.0 kb   a 1.9 kb
                PstI   B 2.2 kb   b 1.4 kb

(From Lee et al. 1988.)

(arginine). As will be seen in Fig. 26.8, probes were constructed to detect both the normal and mutated sequences; Fig. 26.9 shows how these successfully identified heterozygous AIP-prone individuals within a pedigree (Grandchamp et al. 1989a). Similar studies using specific probes were carried out with the other mutations listed in Table 26.6. However, as Scobie et al. (1990a) point out many mutations that are responsible for AIP have yet to be identified, so the true extent of heterogeneity in this disorder remains to be defined.

It is known that there is genetic heterogeneity of the PBG-D gene in Sweden (Lee et al. 1991a). However, in their discussion of the most common mutation causing AIP in Sweden, Lee et al. (1991b) point out that it can easily be detected by restriction enzyme digestion of amplified DNA products. This allows a clinical diagnosis to be made within a day without access to other biochemical or pedigree data, which is a great practical achievement.

Homozygous AIP

Since the gene for AIP is rare in the population, it is obvious that homozygosity is likely to be very rare. Cousin marriage and assortative mating (e.g.

of patients attending a special clinic) would raise the chances greatly above random.

Beukeveld et al. (1990) describe a girl who was noted to have peculiar red staining of her diapers; she later showed mental retardation and eventually died aged 8 years. She excreted large amounts of ALA, PBG and uroporphyrin. Her teeth showed red fluorescence as did her liver at postmortem. The brain showed severe abnormalities. The parents and the patient's brother were shown to be AIP heterozygotes. Using in vitro amplification of cDNA from lymphoblastoid cells followed by hybridization with allele-specific oligonucleotides it was shown that the father had 500 G → A and the mother 518 G → A mutations (numbering according to the coding sequence of the non-erythroid mRNA). The CRIM ratios were 3.2 and 1.5 in the red cells of the father and mother, respectively (Picat et al. 1990). So it appears likely that the patient was a compound heterozygote with sufficient residual enzymic activity to enable her to survive for 8 years.

A similar situation was described in a brother and sister born of unrelated parents by Llewellyn et al (1992). They inherited a mutant gene 499 C → T changing arginine to tryptophan and the mutant gene 500 G → A. Each parent was heterozygous for one of these mutations.

HEREDITARY COPROPORPHYRIA

Hereditary coproporphyria (HC) was first identified by Berger & Goldberg (1956), and arises because of a genetically determined deficiency of the enzyme

Table 26.6. *Molecular variants of porphobilinogen deaminase*

Reference	Nucleotide mutation	Location	Amino acid change	Crim	Details of effect on the enzyme
Picat et al. 1991	C/T polymorphism – 64 relative to the initiation translational codon	Exon 1			
Grandchamp et al. 1989a	G→T	Within the 5'-splice donor sequence of intron 1 at the last position of exon 1		Neg	Interrupts the sequence coding for the non-erythroid form of PBG-D
Grandchamp et al. 1989b	G→A	First position of first intron		Neg	Interrupts the sequence coding for the non-erythroid form of PBG-D
Lee et al. 1990	C→T	Exon 8	arginine → tryptophan	Neg	
Nordmann et al. 1990	G→A	Exon 9	arginine → glutamine	Neg	
Scobie et al. 1990b	412 C→T (a)	Changes codon CAG to TAG (coding STOP) in Exon 9	glutamine → STOP at 138 (erythroid) (b)	Neg	Catalytically defective PBG-D
Gu et al. 1992	499 C→T	Exon 10	arginine → tryptophan	Pos	4% of normal activity
Delfau et al. 1990	500 G→A (c)	Exon 10	167 arginine → glutamine (d)	Pos	Specific activity c. 0.7% of normal, pH optimum greatly decreased
Delfau et al. 1990	518 G→A (e)	Exon 10	173 arginine → glutamine (f)	Pos	Specific activity 0.6% of normal
Lee 1991	517 C→T	Exon 10 CGG → TGG	173 arginine → tryptophan	Neg	Truncated inactive protein easily degraded
Lee & Anvert 1991	G→A	Exon 10 TGG → TAG	198 tryptophan → STOP codon	Neg	Truncated protein
Nordmann et al. 1990	G→T	Exon 10 deletion of 9 bases of cDNA	3 amino acids deleted	Neg	Truncated protein
Nordmann et al. 1990	T→G	Exon 12	leucine → arginine	Neg	
Grandchamp et al. 1989c	G→A	Last position (i.e. within donor splicing site) of exon 12 which is thereby excluded	40 amino acids encoded by exon 12 are missing	Pos	Stable but catalytically inactive
Nordmann et al. 1990	T deleted	Frameshift of a STOP codon in exon 13		Neg	Truncated protein

Discrepancies between some of the numbers shown above and those published by Raich *et al.* (1986) are due to the fact that they gave the erythroid cDNA and isoform of porphobilinogen deaminase. (a) and (b) are in the same numbering as Raich *et al.* (1986). Most of the numbers in the table belong to the ubiquitous protein and mRNA. Equivalent numbers in Raich *et al.* (1986) are (c) 530, (d) 150, (e) 548, (f) 156.

5' GCAACGGCGGTGAGTGCTG 3'
3' <u>CGTTGCCGCCACTCACGAC</u> 5'

Normal sequence

5' <u>GCAACGGCT$\overset{*}{G}$TGAGTGCTG</u> 3'
3' CGTTGCCGCTACTCACGAC 5'

Mutated sequence

Fig. 26.8. Probes used for hybridization of amplified genomic DNA. The sequence of the two oligonucleotides is underlined. The asterisk indicates the position of the base change. (From Grandchamp *et al.* 1989.)

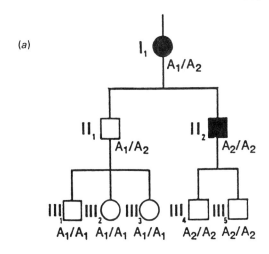

(a)

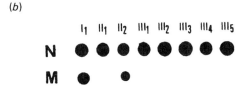

(b)

Fig. 26.9. Detection of gene carriers among family members. (a) Pedigree of a section from a Finnish family investigated. Solid circles and squares represent individuals with clinical or biological abnormalities (increased PBG level in urine). A_1 denotes the presence of an allele without the Msp_1 polymorphic site, A_2 with the Msp_1 site. (b) Dot-blot analysis of amplified DNA using allele-specific oligonucleotides. The amplified fragment from each genomic DNA was hybridized in duplicate with a probe corresponding to the normal sequence (N) and with a probe matching the mutated sequence (M). (From Grandchamp *et al.* 1989.)

coproporphyrinogen oxidase (Elder *et al.* 1976; Brodie *et al.* 1977) which biotransforms coproporphyrinogen III to protoporphyrinogen IX (Fig. 26.10). This leads to a deficient throughput of molecules when only one defective allele is present, and so the biochemical abnormality is inherited as an autosomal Mendelian dominant character. In the same way as with acute intermittent porphyria, only a minority of persons who have the biochemical abnormality actually develop the clinical illness and the attacks almost never occur before puberty. A very informative pedigree published by Andrews *et al.* (1984) illustrates these points. Of 135 members screened for faecal porphyrins 27 were found to have inherited the gene, as well as the proband. Seven (six female and one male) were considered to have suffered attacks of acute porphyria. The attacks were almost always precipitated by drugs the same as with AIP.

The clinical illness has the same neurological and other features as the other acute porphyrias which have been described in a previous section. Also some individuals with HC develop skin fragility and blistering on light-exposed areas.

Biochemically the principal abnormalities found at the time of the clinical illness are:

1 increased urinary ALA excretion;
2 marked increase in PBG excretion;
3 increased urinary coproporphyrin III excretion;
4 greatly increased faecal coproporphyrin III excretion;

5 diminished mitochondrial coproporphyrinogen oxidase activity in nucleated cells (Elder *et al.* 1990).

When the clinical condition of the patient reverts towards normal the first four biochemical abnormalities become far less pronounced and after prolonged remission all haem precursor studies may become normal. This may create difficulties in family studies and might constitute an indication for the difficult, and specialized cellular enzyme studies.

Up until the present time knowledge of the molecular genetics has not made progress though

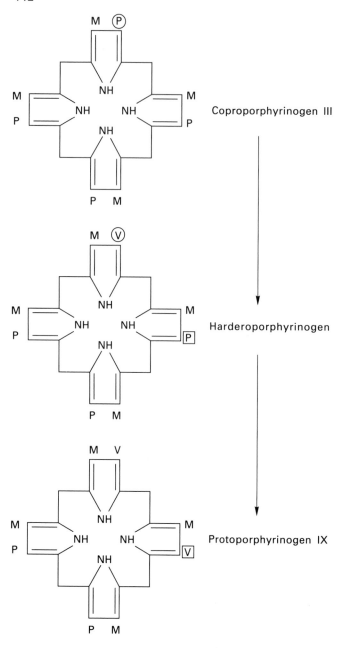

Coproporphyrinogen III

Harderoporphyrinogen

Protoporphyrinogen IX

Fig. 26.10. Biotransformations catalysed by copropor-phyrinogen oxidase. M, methyl; V, vinyl; P, propionic acid.

the gene has been localized to chromosome 9 (Grandchamp *et al.* 1983). However, information of importance has emerged from the study of patients with harderoporphyria and patients homozygous for HC.

Harderoporphyrin is so named because it was first found in the Harderian glands of rodents. The Harderian glands are accessory lacrimal glands at the inner corner of the eye in animals that possess nictitating membranes. These glands are so named because they were discovered by Johann Jacob Harder (1656–1711), a Swiss anatomist. This intermediary compound in haem synthesis is also discussed in connection with the biochemical abnormalities in PCT (see Fig. 26.11).

Four patients excreting harderoporphyrin had intense jaundice and haemolytic anaemia at birth. They excreted a high level of coproporphyrin in the urine and faeces. The major faecal porphyrin was harderoporphyrin. Both sets of parents were cousins and had lymphocyte coproporphyrinogen III oxidase activities of 50% of normal, whereas the patients had < 10% of normal. In these patients K_m was 5 to 20 times normal with a V_{max} of half the normal value and marked sensitivity to thermal denaturation (Nordmann *et al.* 1983; Doss *et al.* 1984).

Patients with homozygous HC have also been described. Grandchamp *et al.* (1977) described a patient who suffered attacks of acute porphyria with hypertrichosis and skin pigmentation. The urine and faeces contained large amounts of coproporphyrin together with raised ALA PBG and uroporphyrin. The parents were cousins and their lymphocyte coproporphyrinogen III oxidase activity was half normal.

The clinical and biochemical differences between harderoporphyria and homozygous HC suggest the existence of heterogeneous abnormalities in the coproporphyrinogen oxidase gene.

PORPHYRIA VARIEGATA

Porphyria variegata (PV) came into prominence particularly through the work of Dean and his collaborators. Dean's account in his monograph of his personal discovery of the porphyria problem in South African medicine makes fascinating reading (Dean 1963). Since Dean's work in South Africa the condition has been recognized and studied in many other lands but appears to be quite rare (Mustajoki 1980 gives an estimate of 1.3 per 100 000 for Finland).

Clinical features

The features of acute porphyria (see above) which usually develop after puberty are the most important part of the clinical picture of PV. In the attacks the urine develops a red (port-wine) discoloration. The precipitants of the acute attacks are the same as described previously. Recovery from the acute attacks can be very protracted.

The great clinical point of differentiation between PV and the other acute porphyrias is the high incidence of skin abnormalities. Dean (1963) gives a dramatic account of how he became acquainted with the skin abnormalities of PV in an interview with the father of a young nurse who had just died in an acute porphyric attack. The condition was locally known as 'van Rooyen's skin', as persons possessing the abnormality were descendants of a man of that name who was born in 1814. The skin is sensitive, abrades easily when knocked and blisters in sunlight. When healing occurs scars are formed and the hands of affected subjects usually show pigmentation.

Mustajoki (1980) described 57 Finnish patients with PV and 17 of them provided information about seasonal variation; eight reported more severe skin fragility in summertime, especially late summer, one patient suffered more in winter and the other patients had not noted any seasonal variation. Of the 15 patients who had suffered acute porphyria attacks seven had skin symptoms and eight did not. The skin and neurological disturbances can occur together or separately (hence the name 'variegata').

Biochemical abnormalities

The biochemical basis of PV lies in a defective protoporphyrinogen oxidase (see Fig. 26.3) which was demonstrated in skin fibroblast cultures by Brenner & Bloomer (1980). They showed that ferrochetalase activity (which is defective in protoporphyria) was normal in these cultures but protoporphyrinogen oxidase was reduced to 43% of normal.

In the acute attacks the urine shows increased quantities of PBG and coproporphyrin III. The faeces show increased coproporphyrin and protoporphyrin (with a preponderance of the latter) and also porphyrin-X which refers to a mixture of porphyrin-peptide conjugates not soluble in ether/acetic acid but which can be extracted by urea–Triton

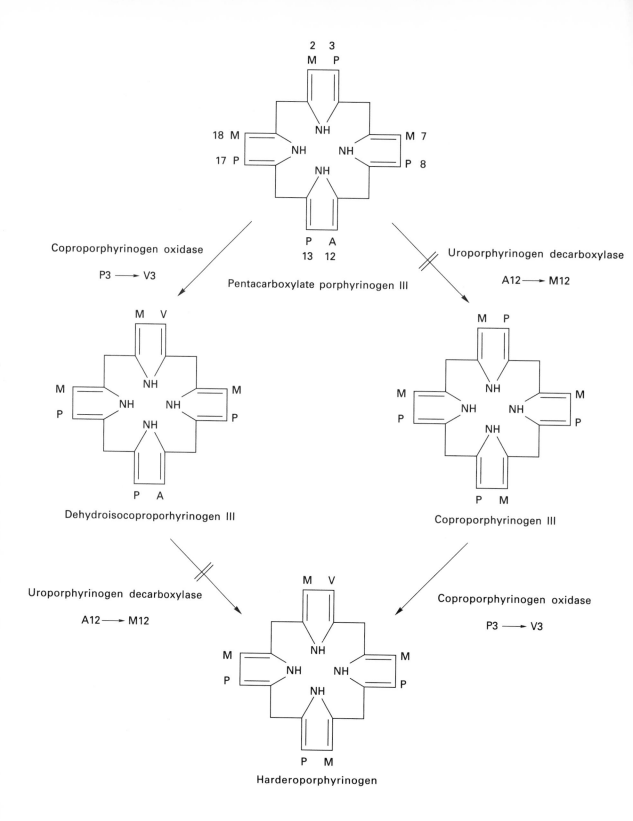

Coproporphyrinogen oxidase

P3 ⟶ V3

Uroporphyrinogen decarboxylase

A12 ⟶ M12

Pentacarboxylate porphyrinogen III

Dehydroisocoproporhyrinogen III

Coproporphyrinogen III

Uroporphyrinogen decarboxylase

A12 ⟶ M12

Coproporphyrinogen oxidase

P3 ⟶ V3

Harderoporphyrinogen

(Rimington *et al.* 1968). The urinary and faecal porphyrins are mainly type III. The plasma also contains porphyrins and is fluorescent.

Genetics

The enzymic deficiency of protoporphyrinogen oxidase (PO) deficiency is inherited as an autosomal dominant character. A linkage has been reported between PV and the α-1-antitrypsin genes on chromosome 14 (Bissbort *et al.* 1988). The localization of PO at 14q32 is not yet confirmed.

A remarkable example of genetic drift was recorded by Dean (1963), who traced most South African cases of PV to a common ancestral mating. Gerrit Jansz emigrated from Holland to the Cape in South Africa in 1685. He was one of the first free burghers and was given a grant of land in the Stellenbosch district. At this time he was unmarried. In order to provide the settlers with wives the Dutch East India company sent eight orphan girls from Rotterdam out to the Cape in 1688. Ariaantje Jacobs (or Ariaantje Adriaanse, or Arijaentgen Jacobs van den Berg) married Gerrit Jansz within a month of her arrival at the Cape. Dean (1963) states 'every single family group that I have succeeded in tracing in detail leads back to Gerrit and Ariaantje'. It appears therefore that the thousands who have inherited the PV gene in South Africa are members of one huge family. Dean (1971) stated that three out of every 1000 Caucasians in South Africa had inherited PV. The condition does not appear to be more common in Holland than in other European populations.

Hitherto neither the cDNA nor the structural gene for protoporphyrinogen oxidase have been cloned and no linked restriction fragment length polymorphism described.

Homozygous porphyria variegata

Homozygous PV (HPV) was reported by Korda *et al.* (1984) in two siblings who had serious photoderm-

Fig. 26.11. The origin of dehydroisocoproporphyrinogen and reactions which are defective in porphyria cutanea tarda. (The position numbering is according to the IUPAC/IUB system.) M, methyl; V, vinyl; P, propionic acid; A, acetic acid. [The decarboxylation of the pentacarboxylate is the last and fastest step catalysed by uroporphyrinogen decarboxylase. It is used in *in vitro* tests (Kappas *et al.* 1989.]

atosis and severe neurological symptoms (with mental retardation) starting in the first few days of life. The activity of lymphocytic protoporphyrinogen oxidase was very low in both probands and typical of PV in both parents. The faecal porphyrin excretion was abnormal in the father and paternal grandmother but normal in the mother of the probands. A further proven and a suspected patient with HPV were recorded by Murphy *et al.* (1986) and another well-documented patient by Mustajoki *et al.* (1987); they too had the skin manifestations from an early age but without neurological abnormalities. Three patients published by Norris *et al.* (1990), Coakley *et al.* (1990) and D'Alessandro Gandolfo *et al.* (1991) again showed the same skin features but with mental retardation. It is interesting to note that in one of Korda's patients a haematological abnormality is mentioned: 'at 6 months bone marrow examination revealed dyserythropoietic anaemia without changes in peripheral blood picture'; and all the published patients had elevated erythrocytic protoporphyrin concentrations, otherwise they were haematologically normal. This suggests that the structure or control of coproporphyrinogen oxidase may be different in the marrow and liver.

PORPHYRIA CUTANEA TARDA

This condition, which is the most common form of porphyria with a frequency said to be 1 in 25 000 in the USA, is a disorder of adults characterized by cutaneous lesions on areas of the skin exposed to sunlight, such as the forehead and backs of the hands and forearms. Lesions may be seen in women on the legs and dorsal aspects of the feet.

Small white lesions called milia precede the formation of blisters after sun-exposure. Minor trauma may also lead to the formation of bullae. The bullous lesions become crusts and heal slowly usually leaving atrophic scars. A violaceous or erythematous colour of the face may be accompanied by increased facial hair in some patients. An onset before the age of 20 years is characteristic of the familial type. There is a definite association with excessive alcohol consumption.

The urine may be dark after drinking bouts and this is a particular feature of porphyria cutanea tarda (PCT), as seen in the South African Bantu (Dean 1963).

The liver function tests are frequently abnormal

and liver biopsy may reveal cirrhosis but gross clinical signs of liver damage, such as spider naevi, portal hypertension (splenomegaly and ascites) and encephalopathy (confusion, flapping tremor, etc) are uncommon in Caucasian patients (Waldenstrom & Haeger-Aronsen 1967).

Metabolic abnormalities

A widespread and complex disturbance of porphyrin metabolism and excretion is seen in PCT. Only the main features will be described here, as derived principally from Kappas *et al.* (1983) and the useful article of Elder *et al.* (1990).

In a patient with PCT skin lesions (i.e. in an exacerbation) the urine contains increased total porphyrins. The increase is mainly of uroporphyrin types I and III; heptacarboxylic porphyrin (principally type III) is raised to a lesser extent. In the faeces the increased porphyrin excretion is mainly type III isocoproporphyrin and to a lesser extent heptacarboxylic porphyrin. (Isocoproporphyrin, oxidized form of isocoproporphyrinogen, is normally only formed in very small amounts in the body. However, since the enzymic insufficiency is distal to it, large amounts are formed in PCT: see Fig. 26.11.)

The plasma may show the typical fluorescence of porphyrins. The liver fluoresces red in the presence of ultraviolet light (405 nm). The skin shows an increased porphyrin content in areas which are not exposed to sunlight (presumably the porphyrins are destroyed when subjected to ultraviolet light).

Hepatocellular carcinoma occurs more frequently than random in PCT and should be excluded by a suitable liver scan and serum α-fetoprotein estimation (Rank *et al.* 1990).

On entering remission the total urinary and faecal porphyrin excretion may be normal, but the proportions of the individual porphyrins may be abnormal as demonstrated by high pressure liquid chromatography or thin layer chromatography.

Enzymological and genetic studies

The basis of PCT was recognized as a defect in liver uroporphyrinogen decarboxylase (URO-D) by Kushner *et al.* (1976), Elder *et al.* (1978) and Felsher *et al.* (1978). This enzyme URO-D successively removes four carboxyl groups from uroporphyrin-

ogen III, one at a time, to produce coproporphyrinogen III (see Figs 26.10 and 26.11; Lash 1991; Luo & Lim 1991). The enzyme was also found to be defective in other tissues. In PCT patients who had affected relatives, URO-D activity was defective in erythrocytes, and when pedigrees were studied this character was an autosomal dominant (Kushner *et al.* 1976).

The subject was further investigated in 27 PCT patients by Elder *et al.* (1980). Erythrocytic URO-D was found to be about 50% of normal in eight PCT patients from six different families in which this biochemical abnormality behaved as an autosomal dominant. However erythrocytic URO-D was normal in another 19 PCT patients, five of whom had a positive family history. On the other hand, Felsher *et al.* (1982) found that hepatic URO-D activity was lowered to about half the normal level in all of 17 PCT patients except one who had an alcohol-induced fatty liver. Felsher *et al.* (1982) found that the hepatic URO-D activity was lowered in four PCT patients both before and after treatment with phlebotomy sufficient to induce a mild anaemia and a normal or nearly normal urinary uroporphyrin excretion. Neither the hepatic iron, nor porphyrin (which can lower enzyme activity) were reported. This finding of a lowered hepatic URO-D activity after treatment has been disputed (see below) but was advanced as evidence against a direct toxic effect of iron to lower enzyme activity.

An advance was made by Elder *et al.* (1983), who showed that in familial PCT the immunoreactive URO-D, measured by rocket electrophoresis of red cell haemolysates, was reduced to half the normal level – the same as the catalytic activity (signifying the lack of a cross-reactive immunological material, i.e. a CRIM-negative mutation). In sporadic PCT both measurements were normal. It was proposed that this simple immunological test could replace the more difficult enzymologic assay.

The progress of PCT abnormalities in the liver during exacerbations and remissions was assessed by Elder *et al.* (1985). Patients with skin lesions had lowered hepatic URO-D catalytic activity, increased hepatic immunoelectrophoretic enzyme (especially in sporadic cases) and the specific activity (catalytic activity/concentration of immunoreactive enzyme) was decreased. In all patients that had been adequately treated by venesection these abnormalities tended to normalize along with hepatic porphyrin concentration (a different result from that of Felsher *et al.* 1982). In four sporadic cases which had been in remission for over 4 years normal specific activities were observed whereas in a familial case in remission catalytic and immunoreactive enzyme measurements were 59% and 55% of mean control values, respectively. The view was advanced that familial cases were heterozygous for a defective enzyme, but that the molecular pathology in sporadic cases was more enigmatic. There was no proof that sporadic PCT was an inherited disorder of URO-D. It seems likely, from experimental work in animals (Elder *et al.* 1989), that in the truly sporadic case of PCT, a normal URO-D is inhibited by iron overload and requires induction of a P450 isoenzyme. Why only a few people develop PCT in response to common hepatotoxic agents is unclear.

The same research group investigated red cells from 17 patients with PCT from 10 families, from 74 of their relatives and from 47 control subjects. These families were found to be of two types: A, with normal red cell URO-D (the same as sporadic PCT), and B, those with decreased red cell URO-D segregating as an autosomal dominant character. The PCT in patients in group A was regarded as familial on the ground that at least two individuals in each family had overt PCT. Hence familial PCT is a heterogenous disorder and only in some families can red cell URO-D be taken as an indicator of what is going on in the liver (Roberts *et al.* 1988). Similar findings were published by Held *et al.* (1989).

The kinetic properties of red cell URO-D were found by Mukerji & Pimstone (1985) to fit in with the above ideas. Using both pentacarboxylic porphyrinogen I and uroporphyrinogen I as substrates these authors found that K_m and V_{max} for sporadic PCT were not significantly different from normal. In two patients with familial PCT the K_m was significantly raised and the V_{max} significantly reduced. The significance to PCT of their later finding, that there are two distinct types of red cell URO-D enzymes with molecular masses of *c.* 52 kDa and *c.* 35 kDa, remains to be determined (Mukerji & Primstone 1992).

Porphobilinogen deaminase (PBG-D) activity was first found to be elevated in the red cells of patients with PCT by Brodie *et al.* (1976). Others have confirmed this finding and Siersema *et al.* (1990) found

the activity to be raised in PCT both familial and sporadic, in exacerbation and in remission. The authors suggest that this finding may arise from diminished degradation of the enzyme, which could arise as follows. There is evidence for a slight increase of PBG production in PCT possibly due to a reduction of ALA-S inhibition by haem. The presence of PBG stabilizes PBG-D. Since PBG-D has the next lowest endogenous activity to ALA-S of the enzymes of the haem pathway, it may constitute a second control step. The increased level of PBG-D could account both for URO accumulation and for the absence of acute attacks in PCT.

Hepato-erythropoietic porphyria

Hepato-erythropoietic porphyria (HEP) is an extremely rare disorder, first described in 1975, in which the patient exhibits severe photosensitivity in the first year of life, leading to scarring, anaemia, hypertrichosis and evidence of liver disease. Czarnecki (1980) called attention to the fact that the disturbance of porphyrin metabolism in this condition was the same as that found in PCT. The possibility that HEP might be the homozygous form of PCT was raised by Elder *et al.* (1980), who described three HEP patients whose URO-D activities in red cells and fibroblasts were 7 and 8% of those of normal subjects. One of the patients was Czarnecki's and her father's fibroblast URO-D activity was 62% of normal value which was characteristic of familial PCT.

Proof of the homozygous nature of HEP was also provided by de Verneuil *et al.* (1984), Lazaro *et al.* (1984) and Toback *et al.* (1987), who described further patients with HEP whose parents fulfilled all the criteria for familial PCT including reduced red cell URO-D activities. The condition occurs in siblings and parent-to-child transmission of HEP has not been described.

A further HEP patient was described by Koszo *et al.* (1990), who also provided an analysis of all the previously published cases. They point out that there is heterogeneity between these patients on two counts. First, though the red cell URO-D activity was usually 3 to 13% of that of controls, in two patients it was 27 and 24%. Secondly, some patients were cross-reactive immunological material (CRIM) negative and some were CRIM-positive.

Enzyme–environment interaction

The features of the disorder of porphyria cutanea tarda arise because of a relative insufficiency of URO-D in the liver, and in hepato-erythropoietic porphyria the disease is much more marked.

As has been explained above PCT patients fall into different categories, as follows.

I   Sporadic PCT with normal red cell URO-D activity and no family history.
II(a) Familial PCT in which red cell URO-D activities are normal. This variety is similar to the sporadic form except that there is familial aggregation of cases.
II(b) Familial PCT in which the red cell URO-D activity is diminished, and this biochemical character is inherited as an autosomal dominant Mendelian character.
III Toxic PCT which is due to poisoning by compounds such as hexachlorobenzene, and which does not appear to have a genetic predisposition as its basis.

Only a minority of persons with the biochemical abnormality in Types II(a) and II(b) actively develop overt clinical PCT. So it may be supposed that some environmental factor or additional genetic factor is required to produce the illness in a person who is genetically predisposed.

Type I PCT is significantly associated with alcohol overindulgence as one environmental precipitant (49 out of 62 patients in the series of Koszo *et al.* 1991). Yet only a minority of persons who overindulge in alcohol develop this illness, a fact which suggests that a genetic predisposition may be present. It is clear that increased liver iron content is a standard feature of sporadic PCT, which goes into remission when the excess iron is removed and URO-D activity returns towards normal.

As Kushner (1982) emphasized, the cause of the hepatic siderosis required for the clinical expression of an intrinsic URO-D abnormality is an important aspect. The demonstration of increased iron absorption and high plasma iron turnover in PCT raises the possibility that these patients may be heterozygous for a haemochromatosis gene as well as having genetically defective URO-D.

Some support for this suggestion was provided in an interesting pedigree published by Kushner *et al.* (1985), in which eight individuals were heterozygous for an HLA-linked haemochromatosis gene and one of whom had sporadic PCT. The proband's mother, sister and three sons had normal urinary porphyrin excretion and hepatic URO-D activity. The suggestion was made that the proband might have a recessive form of URO-D abnormality, which in the presence of siderosis caused the enzymic activity to be insufficient, resulting in PCT. It is known that iron can inhibit URO-D *in vitro*. An interesting patient in whom long-continued iron ingestion was followed by PCT was described by Ginsburg *et al.* (1990).

It is not clear how the common precipitant of alcohol overindulgence is related to the occurrence of the hepatic siderosis.

Other factors implicated in the pathogenesis of overt PCT are oestrogens and halogenated aromatic hydrocarbons. An unfortunate example of the latter was the basis of 'Turkish porphyria', which came to prominence when seed wheat treated with hexachlorobenzene was used to make bread. The hydrocarbon was concentrated in breast milk and many children were affected with severe blistering, scarring, hypertrichosis and deformities. Whether there was a genetic susceptibility to the effects of this mass poisoning is doubtful.

All the compounds implicated in PCT causation are cytochrome P450 inducers and it is possible that they may influence URO-D via a cytochrome P450-mediated mechanism. At present however this remains a speculation (see Sweeney 1986).

Attention was called to a PCT-like distribution of porphyrins in the body liquids of patients on chronic haemodialysis for renal failure by Seubert *et al.* (1985). They grade the patients into three groups: I – no blisters but mildly elevated plasma porphyrins (mainly uroporphyrin and heptacarboxylic porphyrin): II – blisters and plasma porphyrins the same as the first group: III – blisters and strongly elevated plasma porphyrins – considered to have PCT in addition to their renal failure and dialysis.

The occurrence of PCT in men with human immunodeficiency virus infections is difficult to evaluate. This may be due to coincidence, but if it is not, it represents another precipitating agent whose manner of action is unknown (Cohen *et al.* 1990; Tebas *et al* 1992).

Molecular genetics

The gene governing URO-D was mapped to 1p34 by de Verneuil *et al.* (1984) and Mattei *et al.* (1985) and the complete cDNA was published by Romeo *et al.* (1986) along with the deduced amino acid sequence, which agreed with information already determined from direct protein sequencing. Subsequent cloning and sequencing of the human *URO-D* gene demonstrated that it had 10 exons spread over 3 kb (Grandchamp & Nordmann 1988).

Almost immediately after the structure of the cDNA was worked out, four point mutations were described at nucleotide positions 87, 325, 860 and 931 in a lymphoblastoid cell line from a patient with hepato-erythropoietic porphyria (HEP) (de Verneuil *et al.* 1986). An *in vitro* transcription–translation system in rabbit reticulocytes allowed the enzyme proteins elaborated from the normal and abnormal alleles to be studied. The mutant enzyme was rapidly degraded whereas the normal enzyme showed no significant degradation over 8 hours at 37 °C.

Later, a different mutation at nucleotide 860 and a splice site mutation were both shown to account for the production of a short-lived URO-D in familial PCT (Table 26.7). Exactly why a nucleotide change at the 5'-end of intron 6 causes exon 6 to be deleted is obscure (Garey *et al.* 1990).

Thus different mutations, all producing incompetent *URO-D*, can cause familial PCT (Type IIb) and HEP. The rare condition HEP can be explained by the possession of two alleles causing PCT, but it is not clear yet whether these alleles need be the same or whether they can be different.

No light has been shed yet by molecular genetics on the basis for sporadic PCT or on persons who have developed the very severe and prolonged illness which follows the ingestion of hexachlorobenzene.

A search made by Hansen *et al.* (1988) for restriction fragment length polymorphisms within the URO-D gene proved unsuccessful.

Management

There are four main lines of treatment available.

1 Stop exposure to any environmental agent which may be responsible
2 Remove excess iron from the body
3 A much more controversial measure is the administration of chloroquine
4 Topical

In the first category are included persuading the patient to stop drinking alcohol, discontinuing oral contraceptive steroids and therapeutically prescribed oestrogens, and stopping iron supplements (including iron incorporated in multi-vitamin preparations).

Venesection to remove iron is the mainstay of treatment. It is the simplest and cheapest method and a clinical response usually occurs after the removal of 8 to 20 units of blood. The alternative of using subcutaneous desferrioxamine is cumbersome, expensive, and not so effective.

Controversy surrounds the use of chloroquine. The action of this drug seems to be to flush uroporphyrin out of sick liver cells as shown by a sharp rise in urinary porphyrin excretion. An accompaniment to this event is the occurrence of a temporary rise of serum transaminase levels. There is a definite risk that some liver cells necrose as a result of chloroquine administration. Nevertheless, chloroquine can sometimes produce a remission when venesection alone seems to be ineffective (Sweeney 1986).

Topical measures include avoidance of the sun, wearing photoprotective clothing such as a hat, long sleeves and gloves, and a topical sunscreen with a protection factor of 15.

DUAL PORPHYRIA AND CHESTER PORPHYRIA

This small section deals with two different phenomena. First, examples have come to light where genes for two different types of porphyria are segregating independently in the same pedigree and consequently some individuals suffer from both disorders. Secondly, there is a pedigree where PBG-D and protoporphyrinogen oxidase deficiencies seem to be consistently associated in the same individuals.

As has already been explained, in PV elevated levels of faecal protoporphyrin and usually coproporphyrin are diagnostic; the urinary levels of coproporphyrin and uroporphyrin are sometimes raised in an acute attack together with PBG. Dual porphyria was first detected when a patient with PV was found to have increased amounts of heptacarboxyporphyrin in his urine, and both heptacarboxyporphyrin and isocoproporphyrin in his faeces. These latter abnormalities are typical of PCT. Following this discovery Day *et al.* (1982) investigated 106 patients with PV and found 25 of them to have the additional excretion pattern of PCT. No factor known to precipitate PCT was responsible and no clear genetic pattern emerged. The relevant haem

Table 26.7. *Molecular variants of uroporphyrinogen decarboxylase*

Reference	Mutation	Amino acid change	Enzymic change	Clinical correlation
de Verneuil *et al.* 1986; de Verneuil *et al.* 1988; Garey *et al.* 1989	860 ↓ GGG → GAG	281 Gly → Glu	Produces an enzyme with a half-life of 15 hours (normal 102 hours)	Present in members of 2 Spanish families affected with HEP Absent in an Italian patient with HEP Absent in a Portuguese patient with HEP Absent in 13 unrelated patients with familial PCT
Garey *et al.* 1989	860 ↓ GGG → GTG	281 Gly → Val	Produces an enzyme with a half-life of 12 hours (normal 102 hours)[a]	A probe constructed to detect the mutant sequence hybridized to DNA from affected individuals within one familial PCT pedigree, but not to DNA from affected individuals from 4 other familial PCT pedigrees
de Verneuil *et al.* 1986	87 ↓ GCT → GCC	23 Ala → Ala	Nil. Silent mutation	
Garey *et al.* 1989	931 ↓ TTG → CTG	305 Leu → Leu	Nil. Silent mutation	
	1027 ↓ TTG → CTG	337 Leu → Leu	Nil. Silent mutation	
	325 ↓ AGC GGC	103 Ser → Gly	Nil. Does not affect the stability or function	
Garey *et al.* 1990	Splice site mutation ↓ G → C at the first position of the 5'-end of intron 6. Exon 6 consisting of 162 bases between 491 and 655 deleted	54 amino acids missing	Lacks catalytic activity and is rapidly degraded with a half-life of 19 hours (normal 69 hours)[b]	Present in 5 of 22 unrelated familial PCT pedigrees tested
Romana *et al.* 1991	517G → A	167 Glu → Lys	Enzyme degradation was twice as rapid as normal in the presence of cell lysate	Found in patient with HEP
de Verneuil *et al.* 1992	892C → G	292 Arg → Gly	–	Found in 2 sisters with HEP. Not present in 13 unrelated patients with familial PCT
	Large deletion (> 3 kb) as yet unidentified	–	Probably the whole gene is deleted so that no enzyme is formed	Found in 2 sisters with HEP

HEP hepato-erythropoietic porphyria; PCT, porphyria cutanea tarda; other abbreviations for bases and amino acids as in Table 25.2.

[a]The ^{35}S-methionine labelled URO-D enzyme was translated from the RNA in a rabbit reticulocyte lysate system and exposed to a lysate prepared from cultured lymphoblasts. The amount of URO-D remaining was determined by densitometry of autoradiograms made from SDS gels.

[b]The URO-D half-life was estimated by the same technique as in (*a*). It is not clear why the two estimates of the half-life of the normal enzyme should differ so much.

synthesis pathway enzymes were studied by Sturrock *et al.* (1989) in haemolysates and lymphoblasts from 10 similar patients. The mean protoporphyrinogen oxidase (PO) activity was decreased by 45% and the mean URO-D reduced by 33% in lymphoblasts and 27% in haemolysates. The clinical presentation was such that it might easily be diagnosed as either PV or PCT and in the latter case attacks of acute porphyria might not be recognized. Two similar patients were recorded by Chan (1987).

Another puzzling observation was reported by Meissner *et al.* (1986). They studied the red cells and cultured transformed lymphoblasts of 27 patients with PV. In both types of cell the PBG-D activity was reduced from normal by 28 and 24%, respectively. In the cultures PO activity was reduced by 52% and in one three-generation family in which 14 individuals were studied six persons possessed both enzymic defects. It is likely that PBG-D activity is inhibited by protoporphyrinogen.

Another form of dual porphyria was reported by Doss (1989a, b), in which there were features coexisting of AIP and PCT. In two patients suspected clinically of having AIP, high levels of heptacarboxyporphyrin and faecal isocoproporphyrin were found which are typical of PCT. In two patients clinically diagnosed as PCT raised urinary levels of ALA and PBG were found which are indicative of an acute hepatic porphyria and not seen in PCT. Measurements of the erythrocytic enzymes PBG-D and URO-D showed about a 50% reduction in both. In one pedigree ascertained by a dual porphyria proband the two abnormalities were shown to segregate independently, indicating the likelihood that these four individuals were double heterozygotes arising by chance.

A patient with a severe porphyric disease was described by Nordmann *et al.* (1990). She was found to be heterozygous for hereditary coproporphyria, having inherited this gene from her mother. She was also found to be homozygous for congenital erythropoietic porphyria, a condition for which both parents (first cousins) were heterozygous.

Chester porphyria was named after a city in the UK where a seemingly unique porphyric family was studied by McColl *et al.* (1985). The proposita was a 21 year old girl who had suffered neuro-visceral dysfunction with greatly raised urinary PBG and was diagnosed as having acute intermittent porphyria. Investigation of her family, however, showed that the excretion pattern of haem synthesis pathway intermediates was very variable between individuals. Some had raised urinary PBG and to a lesser extent ALA with normal faecal porphyrin excretion (AIP pattern); others had increase faecal porphyrin excretion – mainly protoporphyrin with normal urinary excretion of porphyrin precursors (PV pattern), and yet others showed raised urinary PBG and faecal protoporphyrin (intermediate, mixed pattern). Enzymic studies showed a consistent pattern, i.e. raised white blood cell ALA-S, (mean × 6 control) reduced red blood cell PBG-D (58% of control) and reduced white blood cell PO (23% of control). This dual enzyme deficiency was present in all the persons with abnormal excretion patterns and clinical presentation whether of the AIP or PV type. The genetic explanation of this pedigree is unclear. If there is double heterozygosity for independent genes they should segregate unless tightly linked. It is accepted that PBG-D is on chromosome 11 whilst preliminary evidence has mapped PO to chromosome 14. The latest evidence (Norton 1992) is that the Chester porphyria gene is localized at chromosome 11q. There has hitherto been no evidence to suggest common control of PBG-D and PO, and how a gene on chromosome 11 might influence PO is at present a mystery.

PSEUDOPORPHYRIA

This condition gets its name (Harber & Bickers 1984) purely from the fact that it has a morphological resemblance to PCT (Ramsay 1991) in that blisters appear on the skin, sometimes on exposure of white-skinned people to strong Australian sunshine (Howard *et al.* 1985) or after the use of a sunbed (Bilsland & Douglas 1990), but sometimes with no particular actinic exposure (Mayon & Black 1986). The blood, urine and faeces are consistently negative to porphyrin investigations. The condition is brought on by the ingestion of a variety of drugs including nalidixic acid, naproxen, tetracycline, frusemide, oral contraceptives and ibuprofen. The last three are known to be potential photosensitizers. Skin biopsy shows subepidermal bullae with IgA and IgM at the dermo–epidermal junction, IgG and IgM in the basement membrane and IgG and C3 in the walls of the dermal vessels. The principal differential diagnosis is epidermolysis bullosa acquisitiva (Mayon & Black 1986) but is distinguished by the presence of IgG in the upper dermis (below the basal lamina-anchoring fibril zone) and absence of IgM in the basement membrane in the latter (Yaoita *et al.* 1981).

Interestingly, Wilson & Mendelsohn (1992) report the condition in monozygotic 22 year old twin sisters who lived at a distance from each other. Both had used oral contraceptive steroids and UVA sunbeds. This observation raises the possibility of a genetic predisposition to this condition.

CONCLUSIONS

Considerable advances have been made in understanding the enzymology of the porphyria group of disorders. The techniques of molecular biology promise to shed further light on various aspects which are at present ill understood. The introduction of cloned human cDNA for the haem synthesis pathway enzymes into expression vectors *in vitro* will enable large amounts of pure enzymes to become available. As a result (as has been stated in this book in discussion of other enzymes), the exact three-dimensional structures can be studied and then it will be better understood how different genetic variants produce their biochemical and clinical effects.

The techniques of molecular genetics may also offer a way of finding out more about haem synthesis in the marrow and other sites which hitherto have been studied very little, particularly the central nervous system. It should be possible to find out how the constituent steps of the whole pathway are coordinated and controlled.

This chapter has shown how genetic variants can interact with environmental factors, principally drugs, to give rise to clinically important disorders.

In the case of PBG-D and URO-D considerable diversity of genetic mechanisms which produce abnormal forms of the enzymes are already apparent. Doubtless more mechanisms remain to be discovered, and similar diversities can be anticipated for porphobilinogen synthase, coproporphyrinogen oxidase and protoporphyrinogen oxidase. Areas of uncertainty like dual porphyria and Chester porphyria will also probably be clarified.

Much of the information now available has been focused on the acute hepatic porphyrias. This is of great practical importance because more precise phenotyping tests, e.g. using gene probes and restriction fragment length polymorphism linkages

can enable improved detection of latent carriers of the acute porphyrias. These potential sufferers can consequently receive more accurate counselling and this will constitute a significant contribution to preventive medicine.

The author would like to express his gratitude to Emeritus Professor Sir Abraham Goldberg, FRTS Ed and Dr Michael R. Moore, Department of Medicine, University of Glasgow, UK, and Dr Paul-Henri Romeo, Unite de Recherche en Génétique, Moleculaire et en Haematologie, Inserm U-91-CNRS UA 607, Hôpital Henri Mondor, Cretail, 94010, France who made many helpful suggestions about the contents of this chapter.

Anderson, P. M., Reddy, R. M., Anderson, K. E. & Desnick, R. J. (1981). Characterization of the porphobilinogen deaminase deficiency in acute intermittent porphyria. *Journal of Clinical Investigation*, **68**, 1–12.

Andrews, J., Erdjument, H. & Nicolson, D.C. (1984). Hereditary coproporphyria: incidence in a large English family. *Journal of Medical Genetics*, **21**, 341–9.

Astrin, K. H., Bishop, D. F., Wetmur, J. G., Kaul, B. Davidow, B. & Desnick, R. J. (1987). δ-aminolevulinic acid dehydratase isozymes and lead toxicity. *Annals of the New York Academy of Sciences*, **514**, 23–9.

Astrin, K. H., Desnick, R. J. & Bishop, D. F. (1988). Assignment of human (d)-aminolevulinate synthase (ALAS) to chromosome 3. *Cytogenetics and Cell Genetics*, **46**, 573.

Baccino, E., Lan Cheong Wah, L. S. H., Bressollette, L. & Mottier, D. (1989). Cimetidine in the treatment of acute intermittent porphyria. *Journal of the American Medical Association*, **262**, 3000.

Batlle, A. M. del C., Fakuda, H., Parera, V. E., Wider, E. & Stella, A. M. (1987). In inherited porphyrias, lead intoxication is a toxogenetic disorder. *International Journal of Biochemistry*, **19**, 717–20.

Battistuzzi, G., Petrucci, R., Silvagni, L., Urbani, F. R. & Caiola, S. (1981). δ-aminolevulinate dehydrase: a new genetic polymorphism in man. *Annals of Human Genetics (London)*, **45**, 223–9.

Bawden, M. J., Borthwick, I. A., Healy, H. M., Morris, C. P., May, B. K. & Elliott, W. H. (1987). Sequence of human δ-aminolevulinate synthase cDNA. *Nucleic Acids Research*, **20**, 8563.

Beaumont, C., Foubert, C., Grandchamp, B., Weil, D., N'Guyen, V. C., Gross, M. S. & Nordmann, Y. (1984). Assignment of the human gene for δ-aminolevulinate dehydrase to chromosome 9 by somatic cell hybridization and specific enzyme immunoassay. *Annals of Human Genetics (London)*, **48**, 153–9.

Beaupain, D., Eleouet, J. F. & Romeo, P. H. (1990). Initiation of transcription of the erythroid promoter of the porphobilinogen deaminase gene is regulated by a cis-acting sequence around the cap site. *Nucleic Acids Research*, **18**, 6509–15.

Benkmann, H.-G., Bogdanski, P. & Goedde, H. W. (1983). Polymorphism of delta-aminolevulinic acid dehydratase in various populations. *Human Heredity*, **33**, 62–4.

Berger, H. & Goldberg, A. (1955). Hereditary copro-porphyria. *British Medical Journal*, **2**, 85–8.

Beukeveld, G. J. J., Walthers, B. G., Nordmann, Y., Deybach, J. C., Grandchamp, B. & Wadman, S. K. (1990). A retrospective study of a patient with homozygous form of acute intermittent porphyria. *Journal of Inherited Metabolic Disease*, **13**, 673–83.

Bilsland, D. & Douglas, W. S. (1990). Sunbed pseudo-porphyria induced by nalidixic acid. *British Journal of Dermatology*, **123**, 547.

Bird, T. D., Hamernyik, P., Nutter, J. Y. & Labbe, R. (1979). Inherited deficiency of delta-aminolevulinic acid dehydratase. *American Journal of Human Genetics*, **31**, 662–8.

Birnie, G. G., McColl, K. E. L., Thompson, G. G., Moore, M. R., Goldberg, A. & Brodie, M. J. (1987). Antipyrine metabolism in acute hepatic porphyria in relapse and remission. *British Journal of Clinical Pharmacology*, **23**, 358–61.

Bissbort, S., Hitzeroth, H. W. & du Wertzel, D. P. (1988). Linkage between the variegate porphyria (VP) and the α-1-antitrypsin (PI) genes on chromosome 14. *Human Genetics*, **79**, 289–90.

Bremner, D. A. & Bloomer, J. R. (1980). The enzymatic defect in variegate porphyria. Studies with human cultured skin fibroblasts. *New England Journal of Medicine*, **302**, 765–9.

British National Formulary (1991), No. 21. London: British Medical Association and Royal Pharmaceutical Society of Great Britain.

Brodie, M. J., Beattie, A. D., Moore, M. R. & Goldberg, A. (1976). Pregnancy and hereditary hepatic porphyria. In *Porphyrins in Human Diseases*. First International Porphyrin meeting, Freiburg, pp. 251–4. Basel: Karger.

Brodie, M. J. & Goldberg, A. (1980). Acute hepatic porphyrias. *Clinical Haematology*, **9**, 253–72.

Brodie, M. J., Thompson, G. G., Moore, M. R., Beattie, A. D. & Goldberg, A. (1977). Hereditary coproporphyria – demonstration of the abnormalities in haem biosynthesis in peripheral blood. *Quarterly Journal of Medicine, New Series*, **46**, 229–41.

Buttery, J. E., Carrera, A.-M. & Paunall, P. R. (1990). Reliability of the porphobilinogen screening assay. *Pathology*, **22**, 197–8.

Chan, K.-M., Ladenson, J. H., Valdya, H. C. & Kanan, R. (1987). Dual porphyria – an underdiagnosed entity? *Clinical Chemistry*, **33**, 1190–3.

Chretien, S., Dubart, A., Beaupain, D., Raich, N., Grandchamp, B., Rosa, J., Goossens, M. & Romeo, P.-H. (1988). Alternative transcription and splicing of the human porphobilinogen deaminase gene result in either tissue-specific or in housekeeping expression. *Proceedings of the National Academy of Sciences (USA)*, **85**, 6–10.

Coakley, J., Hawkins, R., Crinis, N., McManus, J., Blake, D., Nordmann, Y., Sloan, L. & Connelly, J. (1990). An unusual case of variegate porphyria with possible homozygous inheritance. *Australia and New Zealand Journal of Medicine*, **20**, 587–9.

Cohen, P. R., Suarez, S. M. & de Leo, V. A. (1990). Porphyria cutanea tarda in human immunodeficiency virus-infected patients. *Journal of the American Medical Association*, **264**, 1315–16.

Czarnecki, D. B. (1980). Hepatoerythropoietic porphyria. *Archives of Dermatology*, **116**, 307–11.

D'Alessandro Gandolfo, L., Macri, A., Biolcati, G., Griso, D., Phung, L. N., Deybach, J. C., Da Silva, V., Nordmann, Y. & Topi, G. C. (1991). Homozygous variegate porphyria: revision of a diagnostic error. *British Journal of Dermatology*, **124**, 211.

Day, R. S., Eales, L. & Meissner, D. (1982). Co-existent variegate porphyria and porphyria cutanea tarda. *New England Journal of Medicine*, **307**, 36–41.

de Verneuil, H., Beaumont, C., Deybach, J.-C., Nordmann, Y., Sfar, Z. & Kastally, R. (1984). Enzymatic and immunological studies of uroporphyrinogen decarboxylase in familial cutanea tarda and hepatoerythropoietic porphyria. *American Journal of Human Genetics*, **36**, 613–22.

de Verneuil, H., Bourgeois, F., de Rooij, F., Siersema, P. D., Wilson, J. H. P., Grandchamp, B. & Nordmann, Y. (1992). Characterization of a new mutation (R292G) and a deletion at the human uroporphyrinogen decarboxylase locus in two patients with hepatoerythropoietic porphyria. *Human Genetics*, **89**, 548–52.

de Verneuil, H., Doss, M., Brusco, N., Beaumont, C. & Nordmann, Y. (1985). Hereditary hepatic porphyria with delta-aminolevulinate dehydrase deficiency: Immunologic characterization of the non-catalytic enzyme. *Human Genetics*, **69**, 174–7.

de Verneuil, H., Grandchamp, B., Beaumont, C., Picat, C. & Nordmann, Y. (1986). Uroporphyrinogen decarboxylase structural mutant (Gly $^{281}\rightarrow$ Glu) in a case of porphyria. *Science*, **234**, 732–4.

de Verneuil, H., Grandchamp, B., Foubert, C., Weil, D., N'Guyen, V. C. Gross, M.-S., Sassa, S. & Nordmann, Y. (1984). Assignment of the gene for uroporphyrinogen decarboxylase to human chromosome 1 by somatic cell hybridization and specific immunoassay. *Human Genetics*, **66**, 202–5.

de Verneuil, H., Hansen, J., Picat, C., Grandchamp, B., Kushner. J., Roberts, A., Elder, G. & Nordmann, Y. (1988). Prevalence of the 281 (Gly→ Glu) mutation in hepatoerythropoietic porphyria and porphyria cutanea tarda. *Human Genetics*, **78**, 101–2.

Dean, G. (1963). *The Porphyrias: A Story of Inheritance and Environment*. London: Pitman Medical.

Dean, G. (1971). *The Porphyrias: A Story of Inheritance and Environment*, 2nd edn. London: Pitman Medical.

Delfau, M. H., Picat, C., de Rooji, F. W. M., Hamer, K., Bogard, M., Wilson, J. H .P., Deybach, J. C., Nordmann, Y. & Grandchamp, B. (1990). Two different point G to A mutations in exon 10 of the porphobilinogen deaminase gene are responsible for acute intermittent porphyria. *Journal of Clinical Investigation*, **86**, 1511–16.

Desnick, R. J., Ostasiewicz, L. T., Tishler, P. A. & Mustajoki, P. (1985). Acute intermittent porphyria: characterization of a novel mutation in the structural gene for porphobilinogen deaminase. *Journal of Clinical Investigation*, **76**, 865–74.

Desnick, R. J., Roberts, A. G. & Anderson, K. (1990). The inherited porphyrias. In *Principles and Practice of Medical Genetics*, 2nd edn, ed. A. E. H. Emery & D. L.Rimoin. pp. 1474–70. Edinburgh: Churchill Livingstone.

Doss, M., Benkmann, H.-G. & Goedde, H.-W. (1986). δ-aminolevulinic acid dehydrase (porphobilinogen synthase) in two families with inherited enzyme deficiency. *Clinical Genetics*, **30**, 191–8.

Doss, M., Laubenthal, F. & Stoeppler, M. (1984). Lead poisoning in inherited δ-aminolevulinic acid dehydratase deficiency. *International Archives of Occupational and Environmental Health*, **54**, 55–63.

Doss, M., Schneider, J., von Tiepermann, R. & Brandt, A. (1982). New type of acute porphyria with porphobilinogen synthase (δ-aminolevulinic acid dehydratase) defect in the homozygous state. *Clinical Biochemistry*, **15**, 52–5.

Doss, M. O. (1989). New form of dual porphyria: co-existent acute intermittent porphyria and porphyria cutanea tarda. *European Journal of Clinical Investigation*, **19**, 20–5.

Doss, M. O. (1989). Dual porphyria in double heterozygotes with porphobilinogen deaminase and uroporphyrinogen decarboxylase deficiencies. *Clinical Genetics*, **35**, 146–51.

Elder, G. H., de Salamanca, R. E., Urquhart, A. J., Munoz, J. J. & Bonkovsky, H. L. (1985). Immunoreactive uro-porphyrinogen decarboxylase in the liver in porphyria cutanea tarda. *Lancet*, **2**, 229–33.

Elder, G. H., Evans, J. O., Cox, R., Brodie, M. J., Moore, M. R., Goldberg, A. & Nicholson, D. C. (1976). The primary enzyme defect in hereditary coproporphyria. *Lancet*, **2**, 1217–19.

Elder, G. H., Lee, G. B. & Tovey, J. A. (1978). Decreased activity of hepatic uroporphyrinogen decarboxylase in sporadic porphyria cutanea tarda. *New England Journal of Medicine*, **299**, 274–8.

Elder, G. H., Roberts, A. G. & de Salamanca, R. E. (1989). Genetics and pathogenesis of human uroporphyrinogen decarboxylase defects. *Clinical Biochemistry*, **22**, 163–8.

Elder, G. H., Sheppard, D. M., de Salamanca, R. E. & Olmos, A. (1980). Identification of two types of porphyria cutanea tarda by measurement of erythrocyte uroporphyrinogen decarboxylase. *Clinical Science*, **58**, 477–84.

Elder, G. H., Smith, S. G., Herrero, C., Mascaro, J. M., Lecha, M., Muniesa, A. M., Czarnecki, D. B., Brenan, J., Poulos, V. & de Salamanca, R. E. (1981). Hepato-erythropoeitic porphyria: a new uroporphobilinogen defect or homozygous porphyria tarda? *Lancet*, **1**, 916–19.

Elder, G. H., Smith, S. G. & Smyth, S. J. (1990). Laboratory investigation of the porphyrias. *Annals of Clinical Biochemistry*, **27**, 395–412.

Elder, G. H., Tovey, J. A., Sheppard, D. M. & Urquhart, A. J. (1983). Immunoreactive uroporphyrinogen decarboxylase in porphyria cutanea tarda. *Lancet*, **1**, 1301–4.

Felsher, B. F., Carpio, N. M., Engleking, D. W. & Nunn, A. T. (1982). Decreased hepatic uroporphyrinogen decarboxylase activity in porphyria cutanea tarda. *New England Journal of Medicine*, **306**, 766–9.

Felsher, B. F., Norris, M. E. & Shih, J. C. (1978). Red cell uroporphyrinogen decarboxylase activity in porphyria cutanea tarda and in other forms of porphyria. *New England Journal of Medicine*, **299**, 1095–8.

Fujita, H., Sassa, S., Lundgren, J., Holmberg, L., Thunell, S. & Kappas, A. (1987). Enzymatic defect in a child with hereditary hepatic porphyria due to homozygous δ-aminolevulinic acid dehydratase deficiency: immunochemical studies. *Pediatrics*, **80**, 880–5.

Garey, J. R., Hansen, J. L., Harrison, L. M., Kennedy, J. B. & Kushner, J. P. (1989). A point mutation in the coding region of uroporphyrinogen decarboxylase associated with familial porphyria cutanea tarda. *Blood*, **73**, 892–5.

Garey, J. R., Harrison, L. M., Franklin, K. F., Metcalf, K. M., Radisky, E. S. & Kushner, J. P. (1990). Uroporphyrinogen decarboxylase: A splice site mutation causes the deletion

of exon 6 in multiple families with porphyria cutanea tarda. *Journal of Clinical Investigation*, **86**, 1416–22.

Ginsburg, A. D., Margesson, L. J. & Feleki, K. (1990). Porphyria cutanea tarda due to ferrous gluconate. *Canadian Medical Association Journal*, **143**, 747–9.

Goedde, H. W., Rothhammer, F., Benkmann, H. G. & Bogdanski, P. (1984). Ecogenetic studies in Atacameno Indians. *Human Genetics*, **67**, 343–6.

Goldberg, A., Moore, M. R., McColl, K. E. L. & Brodie, M. J. (1987). Porphyrin metabolism and the porphyrias. In *Oxford Textbook of Medicine*, 2nd edn, ed. D. J. Weatherall, J. G. G. Ledingham & D. A. Warrell, pp. 9.136–9.145. Oxford: Oxford University Press.

Grandchamp, B., de Verneuil, H., Beaumont, C., Chretien, S., Walter, O. & Nordmann, Y. (1987). Tissue-specific expression of porphobilinogen deaminase. Two isoenzymes from a single gene. *European Journal of Biochemistry*, **162**, 105–10.

Grandchamp, B. & Nordmann, Y. (1988). Enzymes of the heme biosynthesis pathway: recent advances in molecular genetics. *Seminars in Haematology*, **25**, 303–11.

Grandchamp, B., Phung, N. N. & Nordmann, Y. (1977). Homozygous case of hereditary coproporphyria. *Lancet*, **2**, 1348–9.

Grandchamp, B., Picat, C., de Rooji, F., Beaumont, C., Wilson, P., Deybach, J. C. & Nordmann, Y. (1989c). A point mutation G→ A in exon 12 of the porphobilinogen deaminase gene results in exon skipping and is responsible for acute intermittent porphyria. *Nucleic Acids Research*, **17**, 6637–49.

Grandchamp, B., Picat, C., Kauppinen, R., Mignotte, V., Peltonen, L., Mustajoki, P., Romeo, P.-H., Goosens, M. & Nordmann, Y. (1989a). Molecular analysis of acute intermittent porphyria in a Finnish family with normal erythrocyte porphobilinogen deaminase. *European Journal of Clinical Investigation*, **19**, 415–18.

Grandchamp, B., Picat, C., Mignotte, V., Wilson, J. H. P., Te Velde, K., Sandkuyl, L., Romeo, P. H., Goossens, M. & Nordmann, Y. (1989b). Tissue specific splicing mutation in acute intermittent porphyria. *Proceedings of the National Academy of Sciences (USA)*, **86**, 661–4.

Grandchamp, B., Weil, D., Nordmann, Y., Van Cong, N., de Verneuil, H., Foubert, C. & Gross, M. S. (1983). Assignment of the human coproporphyrinogen oxidase gene to chromosome 9. *Human Genetics*, **64**, 180–3.

Gu, X.-F., de Rooij, F., Voortman, G., Velde, K. T., Nordman, Y. & Grandchmap, B. (1992). High frequency of mutations in exon 10 of the porphobilinogen deaminase gene in patients with a CRIM-positive sub-type of acute intermittent porphyria. *American Journal of Human Genetics*, **51**, 660–5.

Gubler, J. G., Bargetzi, M. J. & Meyer, U.A. (1990). Primary liver carcinoma in two sisters with acute intermittent porphyria. *American Journal of Medicine*, **89**, 540–1.

Hansen, J. L., O'Connell, P., Romana, M., Romeo, P.-H. & Kushner, J. P. (1988). Familial porphyria cutanea tarda: hybridization analysis of the uroporphyrinogen decarboxylase locus. *Human Heredity*, **38**, 283–6.

Harber, L. C. & Bickers, D. R. (1984). Porphyria and pseudoporphyria. *Journal of Investigative Dermatology*, **82**, 207–9.

Held, J. L., Sassa, S., Kappas, A. & Harber, L. C. (1989). Erythrocyte uroporphyrinogen decarboxylase activity in porphyria cutanea tarda: a study of 40 consecutive patients. *Journal of Investigative Dermatology*, **93**, 332–4.

Herrick, A. L., McColl, K. E. L., Moore, M. R., Brodie, M. J., Adamson, A. R. & Goldberg, A. (1989). Acute intermittent porphyria in two patients on anticonvulsant therapy and with normal erythrocyte porphobilinogen deaminase activity. *British Journal of Clinical Pharmacology*, **27**, 491–7.

Hindmarsh, J. T. (1986). The porphyrias: recent advances. *Clinical Chemistry*, **32**, 1255–63.

Howard, A. M., Dowling, J. & Varigos, G. (1985). Pseudoporphyria due to naproxen. *Lancet*, **1**, 819–20.

Ishida, N., Fujita, H., Fukuda, Y., Noguchi, T., Doss, M., Kappas, A. & Sassa S. (1992). Cloning and expression of the defective genes from a patient with S-aminolevulinate dehydratase porphyria. *Journal of Clinical Investigation*, **89**, 1431–7.

Kappas, A., Sassa, S. & Anderson, K. E. (1983). The porphyrias. In *The Metabolic Basis of Inherited Disease*, 5th edn, ed. J. B. Stanbury, J. B. Wyngaarden, D. S. Fredrickson, J. L. Goldstein & M. S. Brown, pp. 1301–84. New York: McGraw-Hill.

Kappas, A., Sassa, S., Galbraith, R. A. & Nordmann, Y. (1989). The porphyrias. In *The Metabolic Basis of Inherited Disease*, ed. C. R. Scriver, A.L. Beaudet, W. S. Sly & D. Valle, pp. 1305–65. New York: McGraw-Hill.

Kauppinen, R. & Mustajoki, P. (1992). Prognosis of acute porphyria: occurrence of acute attacks precipitating factors, and associated disease. *Medicine*, **7**, 1–13.

Kauppinen, R., Peltonen, L., Palotie, A. & Mustajoki, P. (1990). RFLP analysis of three different types of acute intermittent porphyria. *Human Genetics*, **85**, 160–4.

Korda, V., Deybach, J. Ch., Maretasek, P., Zeman, J., da Silva, V., Nordmann, Y., Houstkova, H., Rubin, A. & Holub, J. (1984). Homozygous variegate porphyria. *Lancet*, **1**, 851.

Koszo, F., Elder, G. H., Roberts, A. & Simon, N. (1990). Uroporphyrinogen decarboxylase deficiency in hepato-erythropoietic porphyria: further evidence for genetic heterogeneity. *British Journal of Dermatology*, **122**, 365–70.

Koszo, F., Morvay, M., Dobozy, A. & Simon, N. (1992). Erythrocyte uroporphyrinogen decarboxylase activity in 80 unrelated patients with porphyria cutanea tarda. *British Journal of Dermatology*, **126**, 446–9.

Kushner, J. P. (1982). The enzymatic defect in porphyria cutanea tarda. *New England Journal of Medicine*, **306**, 799–800.

Kushner, J. P., Barbito, A. J. & Lee, G. R. (1976). An inherited enzymatic defect in porphyria cutanea tarda – decreased uroporphyrinogen decarboxylase activity. *Journal of Clinical Investigation*, **58**, 1089–97.

Kushner, J. P., Edwards, C. Q., Dadone, M. M. & Skolnick, M. H. (1985). Heterozygosity for HLA-linked haemochromatosis as a likely cause of the hepatic siderosis associated with sporadic porphyria cutanea tarda. *Gastroenterology*, **88**, 1232–8.

Laiwah, A. A. C. Y., Mactier, R., McColl, K. E. L., Moore, M. R. & Goldberg, A. (1983). Early-onset chronic renal failure as a complication of acute intermittent porphyria. *Quarterly Journal of Medicine, New Series*, **II**, 92–8.

Lannfelt, L., Wetterberg, L., Gellefors, P., Lilius, L., Floderus, Y. & Thunell, S. (1989). Mutations in acute intermittent porphyria detected by ELISA measurement of porphobilinogen deaminase. *Journal of Clinical Chemistry and Clinical Biochemistry*, **27**, 857–62.

Lash, T. D. (1991). Action of uroporphyrinogen decarboxylase on uroporphyrinogen III: a reassessment of the clockwise decarboxylation hypothesis. *Biochemical Journal*, **278**, 901–3.

Lazaro, P., de Salamanca, R. E., Elder, G. H., Villaseca, M. L., Chinarro, S. & Jaqueti, G. (1984). Is hepatoerythropoietic porphyria a homozygous form of porphyria cutanea tarda? Inheritance of uroporphyrinogen decarboxylase deficiency in a Spanish family. *British Journal of Dermatology*, **110**, 613–17.

Lee, J.-S. (1991). Molecular genetic investigation of the human porphobilinogen deaminase gene in acute intermittent porphyria. MD thesis, Karolinska Institute, Stockholm.

Lee, J.-S. & Anvert, M. (1991b). Identification of the most common mutation within the porphobilinogen deaminase gene in Swedish patients with acute intermittent porphyria. *Proceedings of the National Academy of Sciences (USA)*, **88**, 10912–15.

Lee, J.-S., Anvert, M., Lindsten, J., Lannfelt, L., Gellefors, P., Wetterberg, L., Floderus, Y. & Thunell, S. (1988). DNA polymorphisms within the porphobilinogen deaminase gene in two Swedish families with acute intermittent porphyria. *Human Genetics*, **79**, 379–81.

Lee, J.-S., Grandchamp, B. & Anvert, M. (1990). A point mutation of the human porphobilinogen deaminase gene in a Swedish family with acute intermittent porphyria. *American Journal of Human Genetics*, **47** (Suppl.), A162.

Lee, J.-S., Lindsten, J. & Anvret, M. (1990). Haplotyping of the human porphobilinogen deaminase gene in acute intermittent porphyria by polymerase chain reaction. *Human Genetics*, **84**, 241–3.

Lee, J.-S. Lundin, G., Lannfelt, L., Forsell, L., Picat, C., Grandchamp, B. & Anvert, M. (1991a). Genetic heterogeneity of the porphobilinogen deaminase gene in Swedish families with acute intermittent porphyria. *Human Genetics* **87**, 484–8.

Lithner, F. & Wetterberg, L. (1984). Hepatocellular carcinoma in patients with acute intermittent porphyria. *Acta Medica Scandinavica*, **215**, 271–4.

Llewellyn, D. H., Elder, G. H., Kalsheker, N. A., Marsh, O. W. M., Harrison, P. R., Grandchamp, B., Picat, C., Nordmann, Y., Romeo, P.H. & Goossens, M. (1987). DNA polymorphism of human porphobilinogen deaminase gene in acute intermittent porphyria. *Lancet*, **2**, 706–8.

Llewellyn, D. H. Smyth, S. J. Elder, G. H., Hutchesson, A. C. Rattenbury, J. M. & Smith, M. F. (1992). Homozygous acute intermittent porphyria: compound heterozygosity for adjacent base transitions in the same codon of the porphobilinogen deaminase gene *Human Genetics*, **89**, 97–8.

Luo, J. & Lim, C. K. (1991). Action of uroporphyrinogen decarboxylase on uroporphyrinogen III. *Biochemical Journal*, **278**, 903.

McColl, K. E. L., Moore, M. R., Thompson, G. G. & Goldberg, A. (1982). Screening for latent acute intermittent porphyria: the value of measuring both leucocyte δ-aminolaevulinic acid synthase and erythrocyte uroporphyrinogen-1-synthase activities. *Journal of Medical Genetics*, **19**, 271–6.

McColl, K. E. L., Thompson, G. G., Moor, M. R., Goldberg, A., Church, S. E., Qadiri, M. R. & Youngs, G. R. (1985).

Chester porphyria: biochemical studies of a new form of acute porphyria. *Lancet*, **2**, 796–9.

McKusick, V. A. (1992). *Mendelian Inheritance in Man*, 10th edn. Baltimore: Johns Hopkins University Press.

Marcus, D. L., Nadel, H., Lew, G. & Freedman, M. L. (1990). Cimetidine suppresses chemically induced experimental hepatic porphyia. *American Journal of Medical Science*, **300**, 214–17.

Mattei, M. G., Dubart, D., Goossens, M. & Mattei, J. F. (1985). Localization of the uroporphyrinogen decarboxylase gene to 1p34 band by *in situ* hybridization. *Cytogenetics and Cell Genetics*, **40**, 692 (Abstract).

Mayun, S. & Black, M. M. (1986). Pseudoporphyria due to naproxen. *British Journal of Dermatology*, **114**, 519–20.

Meissner, P. N., Day, R. S., Moore, M. R., Disler, P. B. & Harley, E. (1986). Protoporphyrinogen oxidase and porphobilinogen deaminase in variegate porphyria. *European Journal of Clinical Investigation*, **16**, 257–61.

Meyer, U. A. & Schmid, R. (1978). The porphyrias. In *The Metabolic Basis of Inherited Disease*, 4th edn, ed. J. B. Stanbury, J. B. Wyngaarden & D. S. Fredrickson, pp. 1165–220. New York: McGraw-Hill.

Meyer, U. A., Strand, J., Doss, M., Rees, A. C. & Marver, H. S. (1972). Intermittent acute porphyria – demonstration of a genetic defect in porphobilinogen metabolism. *New England Journal of Medicine*, **286**, 1277–82.

Moore, M. R., Goldberg, A. & Yeung-Laiwah, A. A. C. (1987). Lead effects on the heme biosynthetic pathway. *Annals of the New York Academy of Sciences*, **514**, 191–203.

Moore, M. R. & McColl, K. E. L. (1989). Therapy of the acute porphyrias. *Clinical Biochemistry*, **22**, 181–8.

Moore, M. R., McColl, K. E. L., Fitzsimons, E. J. & Goldberg, A. (1990). The porphyrias. *Blood Reviews*, **4**, 88–96.

Mukerji, S. K. & Pimstone, N. R. (1985). Reduced substrate affinity for human erythrocyte uroporphyrinogen decarboxylase constitutes the inherent biochemical defect in porphyria cutanea tarda. *Biochemical and Biophysical Research Communications*, **127**, 517–25.

Mukerji, S. K. & Pimstone, N. R. (1992). Uroporphyrinogen decarboxylases from human erythrocytes: purification, complete separation and partial characterization of two isoenzymes. *International Journal of Biochemistry*, **24**, 105–19

Murphy, G. M., Hawk, J. L. M., Magnus, I. A., Barrett, D. F., Elder, G. H. & Smith, S. G. (1986). Homozygous variegate porphyria: two similar cases in unrelated families. *Journal of the Royal Society of Medicine*, **79**, 361–3.

Mustajoki, P. (1980). Variegate porphyria. Twelve years experience in Finland. *Quarterly Journal of Medicine, NS*, **49**, 191–203.

Mustajoki, P. & Desnick, R. J. (1985). Genetic heterogeneity in acute intermittent porphyria: characterisation and frequency of porphobilinogen deaminase mutations in Finland. *British Medical Journal*, **291**, 505–9.

Mustajoki, P., Himberg, J. J., Tokola, O. & Tenhunen, R. (1992). Rapid normalization of antipyrine oxidation by heme in variegate porphyria. *Clinical Pharmacology and Therapeutics*, **51**, 320–4.

Mustajoki, P. & Tenhunen, R. (1985). Variant of acute intermittent porphyria with normal erythrocyte uroporphyrinogen-1-synthase activity. *European Journal of Clinical Investigation*, **15**, 281–4.

Mustajoki, P., Tenhunen, R., Niemi, K. M., Nordmann, Y., Kaariainen, H. & Norio, R. (1987). Homozygous variegate

porphyria. A severe skin disease of infancy. *Clinical Genetics*, **32**, 300–5.

Mustajoki, P., Tenhunen, R., Pierach, C. & Volin, L. (1989). Heme in the treatment of porphyrias and hematological disorders. *Seminars in Hematology*, **26**, 1–9.

Namba, H., Narahara, K., Tsuji, K., Yokoyama, Y. & Seino, Y. (1991). Assignment of human porphobilinogen deaminase to 11q 24.1→q 24.2 by in situ hybridization and gene dosage studies. *Cytogenetics and Cell Genetics*, **57**, 105–8.

Nordmann, Y., Amram, D., Deybach, J. C., Phung, L. N. & Lesbros, D. (1990). Coexistent hereditary coproporphyria and congenital erythropoietic porphyria (Günther disease). *Journal of Inherited Metabolic Disease*, **13**, 687–91.

Nordmann, Y., de Verneuil, H., Deybach, J.-C., Delfau, M.-H. & Grandchamp, B. (1990). Molecular genetics of porphyrias. *Annals of Medicine*, **22**, 383–91.

Nordmann, Y., Grandchamp, B., de Verneuil, H., & Phung, L. (1983). Harderoporphyria: a variant hereditary copro-porphyria. *Journal of Clinical Investigation*, **72**, 1139–49.

Norris, P. G., Elder, G. H. & Hawk, J. L. M. (1990). Homozygous variegate porphyria: a case report. *British Journal of Dermatology*, **122**, 253–7.

Norton, B., Lanyon, W. G., Moore, M. R., Youngs, G. R. & Connor J. M. (1992). Evidence for the localisation of the Chester poprhyria gene to chromosome 11 q. *Demonstration 78 at the Annual Meeting of the Association of Physicians of Great Britain and Ireland*, Liverpool, April 1992.

Ostrowski, J., Kostrzewska, E., Michalak, T., Zawirska, B., Medrzejewsk, W. & Gregor, A. (1983). Abnormalities in liver function and morphology and impaired aminopyrine metabolism in hereditary hepatic porphyrias. *Gastroenterology*, **85**, 1131–7.

Paik, Y. K., Lee, C. C., Benkmann, H. G. & Goedde, H. W. (1988). Genetic polymorphism of δ-aminolevulinate dehydrase in several population groups in Korea. *Korean Journal of Genetics*, **10**, 123–6.

Petrucci, R., Leonardi, A. &, Battistuzzi, G. (1982). The genetic polymorphism of Δ-aminolevulinate dehydrase in Italy. *Human Genetics*, **60**, 289–90.

Picat, C., Bourgeois, F. & Grandchamp, B. (1991). PCR detection of a C/T polymorphism in exon 1 of the porphobilinogen deaminase gene (PBGD). *Nucleic Acids Research*, **19**, 5099.

Picat, C., Delfau, M. H., de Rooij, F. W. M., Beukeveld, G. J. J., Wolthers, B. G., Wadman, S. K., Nordmann, Y. & Grandchamp, B. (1990). Identification of the mutations in the parents of a patient with a putative compound heterozygosity for acute intermittent porphyria. *Journal of Inherited Metabolic Diseases*, **13**, 684–6.

Pierach, C. A., Weimer, M. K., Cardinal, R. A., Bossenmaier, I. C. & Blommer, J. R. (1987). Red blood cell porphobilinogen deaminase in the evaluation of acute intermittent porphyria. *Journal of the American Medical Association*, **257**, 60–1.

Plewinska, M., Thunell, S., Holmberg, L., Wetmur, J. G. & Desnick, R. J. (1991). δ-aminolevulinate dehydratase deficiency porphyria: identification of the molecular lesions in a severely affected homozygote. *American Journal of Human Genetics*, **49**, 167–74.

Poh-Fitzpatrick, M. B. (1982). Pathogenesis and treatment of the photocutaneous manifestations of the porphyrias. *Seminars in Liver Disease*, **2**, 164–76.

Potluri, V. R., Astrin, K. H., Wetmur, J. B., Bishop, D. F. &
Desnick, R. J. (1987). Chromosomal localization of the
structural gene for human ALA-dehydratase to 9q34 by in
situ hybridization. *Human Genetics*, **76**, 236–9.

Raich, N., Romeo, P. H., Dubart, A., Beaupain, D., Cohen-
Solal, M. & Goossens, M. (1986). Molecular cloning and
complete primary sequence of human erythrocyte
porphobilinogen deaminase. *Nucleic Acids Research*, **14**,
5955–68.

Ramsay, C. A. (1991). Drug induced pseudoporphyria.
Journal of Rheumatology, **18**, 799–800.

Rank, J. M., Straka, J. C. & Bloomer, J. R. (1990). Liver in
disorders of porphyrin metabolism. *Journal of
Gastroenterology and Hepatology*, **5**, 573–85.

Rimington, C. (1989). Haem biosynthesis and porphyrias; 50
years in retrospect. *Journal of Clinical Chemistry and Clinical
Biochemistry*, **27**, 473–86.

Rimington, C., Lockwood, W. H. & Belcher, R. V. (1968).
The excretion of porphyrin-peptide conjugates in
porphyria variegata. *Clinical Science*, **35**, 211–47.

Roberts, A. G., Elder, G. H., Newcombe, R. G., de
Salamanca, R. E. & Munoz, J. J. (1988). Heterogeneity of
familial porphyria cutanea tarda. *Journal of Medical
Genetics*, **25**, 669–76.

Romana, M., Grandchamp, B., Dubart, A., Amselen, S.,
Chabret, C., Nordmann, Y., Goossens, M. & Romes, P. H.
(1991). Identification of a new mutation responsible for
hepato-erythropoietic porphyria. *European Journal of
Clinical Investigation*, **21**, 225–9.

Romeo, P.-H., Raich, N., Dubart, A., Beaupain, D., Pryor,
M., Kushner, J., Cohen-Solal, M. & Goossens, M. (1986).
Molecular cloning and nucleotide sequence of a complete
human uroporphyrinogen decarboxylase cDNA. *Journal of
Biological Chemistry*, **261**, 9825–31.

Sassa, S., Fujita, H., Doss, M., Hassoun, A., Verstraeten, L.,
Mercelis, R. & Kappas, A. (1991). Hereditary hepatic
porphyria due to homozygous δ-aminolevulinic acid
dehydratase deficiency: studies in lymphocytes and
erythrocytes. *European Journal of Clinical Investigation*, **21**,
244–8.

Scobie, G. A., Llewellyn, D. H., Urquhart, A. J., Smyth, S. J.,
Kalsheker, N. A., Harrison, P. R. & Elder, G. H. (1990b).
Acute intermittent porphyria caused by a C→ T mutation
that produces a stop codon in the porphobilinogen
deaminase gene. *Human Genetics*, **85**, 631–4.

Scobie, G. A., Urquhart, A. J., Elder, G. H., Kalsheker, N. A.,
Llewellyn, D. H., Smyth, J. & Harrison, P. R. (1990a).
Linkage disequilibrium between DNA polymorphisms
within the porphobilinogen deaminase gene. *Human
Genetics*, **85**, 157–9.

Seubert, S., Seubert, A., Rumpf, K. W. & Kiffe, K. (1985). A
porphyria cutanea tarda-like distribution pattern of
porphyrins in plasma, hemodialysate, hemofiltrate and
urine of patients on chronic dialysis. *Journal of Investigative
Dermatology*, **85**, 107–9.

Siersema, P. D., de Rooij, F. W. M., Edixhoven-Bosdijk,
A. & Wilson, J. H. P. (1990). Erythrocyte porphobilinogen
deaminase activity in porphyria cutanea tarda. *Clinical
Chemistry*, **36**, 1779–83.

Straka, J. G., Rank, J. M. & Bloomer, J. R. (1990).
Porphyria and porphyrin metabolism. *Annual Review of
Medicine*, **41**, 457–69.

Sturrock, E. D., Meissner, P. N., Maeder, D. L. & Kirsch, R.
E. (1989). Uroporphyrinogen decarboxylase and

protoporphyrinogen oxidase in dual porphyria. *South
African Medical Journal*, **76**, 405–8.

Sweeney, G. D. (1986). Porphyria cutanea tarda or the
uroporphyrinogen decarboxylase deficiency diseases.
Clinical Biochemistry, **19**, 3–15.

Taketani, S., Inazawa, J., Nakahashi, Y., Abe, T. &
Tokunaga, R. (1991). Structure of the human
ferrochelatase gene. Exon/intron gene organization and
location of the gene to chromosome 18. *European Journal
of Biochemistry*, **205**, 217–22.

Tebas, P., Arzauga, J. A., Roman, F., Maetsu, R. P. & de
Letona, J. M. L. (1992). Association between porphyria
cutanea tarda and human immunodeficiency virus
infection. *Archives of Internal Medicine*, **152**,
1726.

Tishler, P. V., Woodward, B., O'Connor, J., Holbrook, D. A.,
Seidman, L. J,. Hallett, M. & Knighton, D. J. (1985). High
prevalence of intermittent acute porphyria in a psychiatric
patient population. *American Journal of Psychiatry*, **142**,
1430–6.

Toback, A. C., Sassa, S., Poh-Fitzpatrick, M. B., Schechter,
J., Zaider, E., Harber, L. C. & Kappas, A. (1987).
Hepatoerythropoeitic porphyria: clinical, biochemical and
enzymatic studies in a three-generation family lineage.
New England Journal of Medicine, **316**, 645–50.

Waldenström, J. & Haeger-Aronsen, B. (1967). The
porphyrias: a genetic problem. In *Progress in Medical
Genetics*, Vol. 5, ed. A. G Steinberg & A. G. Bearn, pp. 58–
101.

Wang, A.-L., Arredondo-Vega, F. X., Giampietro, P. F.,
Smith, M., Anderson, W. F. & Desnick, R. J. (1981).
Regional gene assignment of human porphobilinogen
deaminase and esterase A4 to chromosome 11q23 –
11qter. *Proceedings of the National Academy of Sciences (USA)*,
78, 5734–8.

Wang, A.-L., Smith, M., Astrin, K. H. & Desnick, K. J.
(1984). Assignment of the structural gene for human δ-
aminolevulinate dehydratase (ALAD) to human
chromosome 9 (9q11→ qter). *American Journal of Human
Genetics*, **36**, 208S (Abstract).

Wetmur, J. B., Bishop, D. F., Cantelmo, C. & Desnick, R. J.
(1986b). Human δ-aminolevulinate dehydratase:
nucleotide sequence of a full-length cDNA clone.
Proceedings of the National Academy of Sciences (USA), **83**,
7703–7.

Wetmur, J. B., Bishop, D. F., Ostasiewicz, L. & Desnick, R.
J. (1986a). Molecular cloning of a cDNA for human δ-
aminolevulinate dehydratase. *Gene*, **43**, 123–30.

Wetmur, J. G., Kaya, A. H., Plewinska, M. & Desnick, R. J.
(1991). Molecular characterization of the human δ-
aminolevulinate dehydratase 2 (ALAD²) allele:
implications for molecular screening of individuals for
genetic susceptibility to lead poisoning. *Americal Journal of
Human Genetics*, **49**, 757–63.

Wetmur, J. G., Lehnert, G. & Desnick, R. J. (1991). The
δ-aminolevulinate dehydratase polymorphism: higher
blood lead levels in lead workers and environmentally
exposed children with the 1-2 and 2-2 isozymes.
Environmental Research, **56**, 109–19.

Whitcombe, D. M., Carter, N. P., Albertson, D. G., Smith, S.
J., Rhodes, D. H. & Cox, T. M. (1991). Assignment of the
human ferrochelatase gene (*FECH*) and a locus for
protoporphyria to chromosome 18q 22. *Genomics*, **11**,
1152–4.

Wilson, C. L. & Mendelsohn, S. S. (1992). Identical twins with sunbed-induced pseudoporphyria. *Journal of the Royal Society of Mediicne*, **85**, 45–6.

Wolff, C., Piderit, F. & Armas-Merino, R. (1991). Deficiency of porphobilinogen synthase associated with acute crisis. *European Journal of Clinical Chemistry and Clinical Biochemistry*, **29**, 313–15.

Yaoita, H., Briggman, R. A., Lawley, T. J., Provost, T. T. &

Katz, S. I. (1981). Epidermolysis bullosa acquisita: ultrastructural and immunological studies. *Journal of Investigative Dermatology*, **76**, 288–92.

Ziemsen, B., Angerer, J., Lehnert, G., Benkmann, H. G. & Goedde, H. W. (1986). Polymorphism of delta-aminolevulinic acid dehydratase in lead-exposed workers. *International Archives of Occupational and Environmental Health*, **58**, 245–7.

PART IX   Malignant hyperthermia

27   Malignant hyperthermia

CLINICAL DESCRIPTION

THE SYNDROME of malignant hyperthermia (syn: malignant hyperpyrexia) was first described by Denborough & Lovell (1960) in a young man with a broken leg who was concerned about his anaesthetic risk because 10 of his 24 relatives had died under general anaesthesia. He also developed the disease under general anaesthesia but survived. It seems quite probable that the event occurred from time to time before then but was unrecognized (see, for example, Harrison & Isaacs 1992). Malignant hyperthermia (MH) is an uncommon complication of general anaesthesia or emergency intubation which used to carry a very high mortality. Inhalational agents such as halothane, enflurane, isoflurane, methoxyflurane, diethyl ether, trichloroethylene, cyclopropane and ethylene have been incriminated as precipitating the event. So also have the muscle relaxants succinylcholine, D-tubocurarine and decamethonium. Halothane and succinylcholine used to be the most common triggering drugs, probably because their use was so widespread (Galloway & Denborough 1986). The syndrome may, however, be precipitated by stress, severe exercise and other drugs (see below).

The disorder develops during triggering agent medication. An early sign may be failure of the muscles of the jaw to relax, i.e. severe masseter muscle spasm, following the administration of succinylcholine (see Ellis *et al.* 1992). Other early signs include tachycardia, hypercarbia and generalized muscular rigidity. Later the soda lime canister may be noticed to be hot. The other clinical features were succinctly summarized by Ellis (1984a) as follows. There is

a potentially fatal rise in body temperature which occurs during certain types of anaesthesia in genetically susceptible individuals. The rise in body core temperature may be at an alarming rate of greater than 5 °C per hour and indicates the presence of an appreciable and inappropriate metabolic stimulation. If left untreated the temperature will rise progressively towards 43 °C to 45 °C at which death occurs. The pyrexia is accompanied by a tachycardia, a progressive rise in oxygen consumption with cyanosis, and a rise in carbon dioxide production with respiratory acidosis.

The sinus tachycardia may switch to a ventricular dysrhythmia.

The foregoing is a description of a florid case. Nowadays the 'abortive case' is the commonest presentation.

One feature of MH is muscle spasm, as mentioned earlier. It may occur at induction following the administration of succinylcholine, or it may occur more gradually following the administration of inhalational anaesthetics. The muscle spasm may become generalized (in about 80% of cases there is muscular rigidity in the limbs) and the contracted muscle liberates potassium, causing hyperkalaemia which may be fatal. Creatine kinase is released from the muscles and the activity of this enzyme in the serum reaches very high levels. Likewise myoglobin is released which may cause tubular obstruction leading to renal failure. Lactic acid from the muscles

459

causes metabolic acidosis with the blood pH falling to 7.0 or below.

A consumptive coagulopathy may complicate the clinical picture with bleeding from mucous membranes and into surgical wounds.

Death used to occur in about two thirds of the patients who experienced these adverse reactions, but it is thought that the mortality has fallen in the last decade, presumably because the condition is now well known to anaesthetists and specific therapy with dantrolene (see below) is now available. A mortality of 20 to 40% in the United Kingdom was given by Ellis (1984a) but now the mortality is less than 1%.

INCIDENCE

It is clearly difficult to determine precise incidence figures. In l969 the incidence at the Hospital for Sick Children in Toronto was estimated to be 1 in 10 000 with a range of 1 in 5000 to 1 in 70 000 (Britt *et al.* 1969). The incidence in North America as given by Britt (1985) was 1 in 15 000 to 1 in 150 000.

MH is most common in children, adolescents and young adults.

ETHNIC DISTRIBUTION

Large numbers of patients and families have been recorded in Caucasians from many countries. Negro patients have been described (Britt *et al.* 1969) but are still uncommon enough to arouse comment; for example, Lombard & Couper (1988) reported the fourth case of MH in a South African black patient, and they cite hospital statistics of 1 in 170 000 and 1 in 250 000 anaesthetics in blacks.

It has been reported that MH occurs in all major racial groups (Cantin *et al.* 1986). According to Britt (1985) the incidence in Japan is 1 in 7000 to 1 in 110 000.

So, on the rather scanty evidence now available it may be said that the reported frequency of the alleles responsible for MH is lower in Negroes and possibly in Chinese than in Caucasians. Racial, climatic or reporting variations could be responsible.

PREVENTING MH

The first and most obvious thing to point out is that, like many situations in clinical medicine, there is no substitute for a good history, and listening to the patient. There is an instance on record of a patient who pointed out to the doctors that a close relative had died of MH. The patient was reassured that all would be well, but very soon died under the anaesthetic. Ellis (1992) also states, 'From our own work we know of two British families in which a second proband was discovered and both died of malignant hyperthermia.' However, it must be pointed out that many MH patients did not have a positive personal or family history of MH prior to their event.

The next requirement is to conduct a careful and thoughtful physical examination. Minor signs of muscle abnormality should be sought, though the significance of such findings to the existence of MH is now very doubtful, with some rare exceptions which will be discussed below.

If there is suggestive previous history or family history predictive tests should then be performed and these will be discussed below.

If anaesthesia is to be performed then safe and appropriate drugs should be selected. Larach *et al.* (1987) state that 'thiopental, nitrous oxide/oxygen, a narcotic, pancuronium, neostigmine, atropine and/or glycopyrrolate appears to be a safe anesthetic regimen for MH susceptible children'. Gallen (1991) and Allen (1991) drew attention to the fact that propofol is safe for use in malignant hyperpyrexia-prone individuals.

The equipment used to administer the anaesthesia must be free of contamination with the known triggering agents. Contraindicated drugs include all potent inhalational anaesthetics, depolarizing muscle relaxants, succinylcholine and decamethonium (Cantin *et al.* 1986).

WHEN MH OCCURS

The first sign of onset of MH during anaesthesia may be masseter rigidity or spasm. This commonly follows succinylcholine administration (Allen & Rosenberg 1990).

With modern monitoring methods (infra-red detection) a rise in end-tidal CO_2 concentration in the presence of adequate minute ventilation may be observed before much rise in temperature has occurred and before the soda lime canister has become hot (Neubauer & Kaufman 1985).

As soon as a provisional diagnosis of MH is made

the anaesthesia must be stopped if possible. If the condition for which the surgery is being performed is life-threatening (e.g. peritonitis from a ruptured appendix: Neubauer & Kaufman 1985), then the procedure can be completed with 'safe' anaesthesia.

General management includes monitoring the temperature, electrocardiogram and blood chemistry (blood gases, pH, K^+, CPK) repeatedly, and appropriate measures should be taken to remedy any abnormalities. An adequate urinary volume should be maintained to avoid acute tubular necrosis.

The specific drug which must be given intravenously without delay is dantrolene (Fig. 27.1). Dantrolene acts by reducing the ionized calcium concentration in muscles by an effect either on the sarcolemma or on the sarcoplasmic reticulum. It increases the contraction activation threshold. In addition, dantrolene has a primary anti-arrhythmic effect (Sessler 1986).

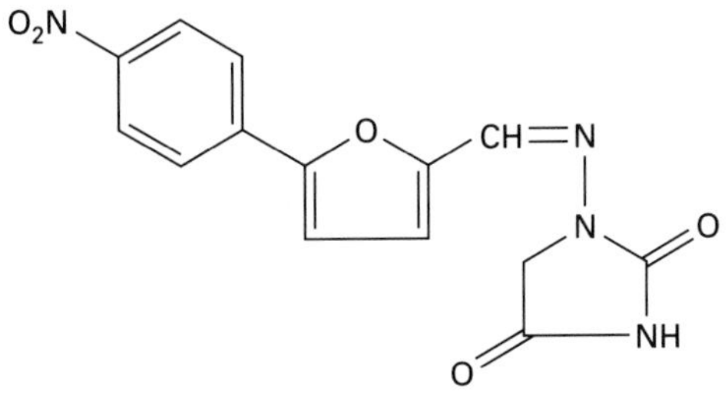

Fig. 27.1. Dantrolene [1–{[5-(*p*-nitro-phenyl)furfurylidine]amino}hydantoin]. (From *The Merck Index*, 1983.)

Flewellen *et al.* (1983) made pharmacokinetic observations on dantrolene and correlated them with the effects on muscular strength, heart rate and respiratory ventilation. Their conclusion was that an intravenous dose of 2.4 mg per kg body weight would be appropriate for the initial treatment of MH. An immediate dose of 2.5 mg/kg is advocated by Sessler (1986) and if the signs of MH, such as rigidity, acidosis and tachycardia, persist after 45 minutes a further intravenous dose of 7.5 mg/kg dantrolene should be administered. Then 2.5 mg/kg dantrolene should be given every 6 hours until the crisis resolves. The exhaled CO_2 should be observed to diminish and the muscular rigidity to relax.

Cooling the body is imperative. The most effective way is to spray ice-water on the torso, or place crushed ice on the torso and blow air longitudinally. Other methods include irrigating the stomach with cold solutions, and to give cool liquids intravenously (but never centrally). The one peril is to induce shivering which would jeopardize the recovery.

High doses of glucocorticoids may be helpful because they are positively inotropic, induce peripheral vasodilatation and stabilize membranes (Ellis 1984a).

The use of dantrolene prior to the operation as a precautionary measure in MH-susceptible individuals is contentious. As reported by Watson *et al.* (1986), it can cause clinically significant muscle weakness in patients with underlying myopathies.

The occurrence of post-operative pyrexia (POP) is not indicative of MH, according to the investigations of Halsall & Ellis (1992). They performed *in vitro* muscle contracture tests on 30 patients with a history of POP and they were all negative.

Comprehensive practical guidelines for the management of an episode of MH were provided by Krivosic-Horber (1988).

THE MH PHENOTYPE – A POSSIBLE OCCUPATIONAL HAZARD

An interesting patient was described by Denborough *et al.* (1988). This man was the father of a 12 year old girl who had survived an episode of MH. *In vitro* testing of muscle from the father with halothane and caffeine (see below) showed that he too was susceptible to MH.

This man moved to a job which involved discharging bromochlorodifluoromethane (BCDF) from fire extinguishers before refilling them. Some of the gas was inhaled in the process. He complained of malaise and of stiffness and weakness in his forearms and hands whilst he had been working at this job. The symptoms became worse as the week progressed and he improved at weekends. Serum creatine kinase activity was 1056 iu/l on a Saturday and 544 iu/l the following Monday. BCDF produced the same contracture as halothane on human and porcine MHS muscle *in vitro*. The patient followed advice to change his job and his symptoms immediately improved.

Table 27.1. *Responses of normal muscle and muscle from malignant hyperthermia-susceptible individuals to various chemicals*

Chemical	Normal muscle	Muscle from MH-susceptible individuals
Halothane	Small contracture or none	Large contracture
Caffeine	Small slow contracture	Much larger and rapid contracture
Succinylcholine	No contracture	Large, long and sustained contracture
Potassium chloride 80 mM	No contracture	Large contracture
Procaine	–	Inhibited halothane and succinylcholine contractures

Data from: Moulds & Denborough 1974a.

TESTS WHICH IDENTIFY THE MH-SUSCEPTIBLE PHENOTYPE

The muscle contracture test

The test which has established itself as much more reliable and important than all others is the muscle contracture test. The muscle test is the standard against which all other predictive tests should be judged, and is hitherto the basis on which genetic counselling is most soundly based.

Caffeine had long been known to cause contracture of frog skeletal muscle, principally by causing a release of calcium into the myoplasm from the sarcoplasmic reticulum. With remarkable foresight Kalow *et al.* (1970) proposed that caffeine contracture could be used as a model for studying MH. They showed that muscle from patients susceptible to MH showed an increased susceptibility to undergo contracture under the influence of caffeine. A greater potentiating effect of halothane was also observed. Halothane also lowered the calcium content of sarcoplasmic reticulum from MH patients but did not do so in sarcoplasmic reticulum from controls.

A similar approach was taken by Ellis *et al.* (1972) who performed a biopsy on the vastus medialis muscle under local anaesthesia, identified the motor end point by electrical stimulation and took a specimen to include the motor innervation. Each muscle specimen was exposed *in vitro* to halothane alone and also to halothane plus succinylcholine (H + S). Seven subjects were investigated from four different families in each of which there had been a patient with MH. The muscle specimens from four individuals produced contractures with halothane alone, and the muscle from one additional individual showed contracture with H + S.

In a survey of 20 individuals from six families known to include survivors from MH, Moulds & Denborough (1974a, b) investigated muscle biopsy behaviour in 15 subjects.

The essential results are condensed in Table 27.1. The influence of extracellular calcium is worth elaborating. Malignant hyperpyrexia muscle gave a contracture when first exposed to halothane in the absence of extracellular calcium ions, but was then unable to give a further contracture on re-exposure to halothane. When calcium ions in their normal concentration were added to the bath solution the muscle again gave a contracture on exposure to halothane. Similar results were obtained with caffeine (Moulds & Denborough 1974a). A contracture was defined as a sustained increase of at least 0.2 g in baseline tension.

With this solid background an important step was taken in April 1983, when physicians from eight European countries (Austria, Denmark, Eire, France, Holland, Sweden, United Kingdom, West Germany) met in Lund, Sweden. There they established an European Malignant Hyperpyrexia Group with the following aims:

- to provide a forum for discussion between the various European centres;
- to standardize the investigation of MH subjects to allow comparisons between centres;
- to establish a common data bank;
- to allow for combined research facilities.

The full protocol for muscle testing was published (The European Malignant Hyperpyrexia Group 1984) and is reproduced in Table 27.2 and Fig. 27.2.

The same group re-convened in Leeds, United Kingdom in December 1983 and assessed the results from 200 investigations. It was found that the persons tested could be divided into three groups:

Table 27.2. *Protocol for caffeine halothane muscle contracture test according to the European Malignant Hyperpyrexia Group*

1. The biopsy should be performed on the quadriceps muscle and the samples taken from the region of the muscle which includes the motor point.
2. Biopsy specimens suitable for *in vitro* investigation should measure 15–25 mm in length with a thickness of 2–3 mm.
3. The muscle should be placed immediately in carboxygenated Krebs–Ringer solution with a composition of:

NaCl	118.1 mM
KCl	3.4 mM
$MgSO_4$	0.8 mM
KH_2PO_4	1.2 mM
Glucose	11.1 mM
$NaHCO_3$	25.0 mM
$CaCl_2 \cdot 6H_2O$	2.5 mM
pH	7.4

4. The muscle should be transported to the laboratory in Krebs–Ringer solution at ambient temperature. In the laboratory it should be kept at room temperature and carboxygenated.
5. The time from biopsy to the completion of the tests should not exceed 5 h.
6. The tests should be performed at 37 °C in a tissue bath perfused either intermittently or continuously with Krebs–Ringer solution and oxygenated continuously with carbogen.
7. The muscle specimen should be electrically stimulated with a 1 ms supramaximal stimulus at a frequency of 0.2 Hz.
8. Three tests should be performed, each on a fresh specimen. The tests include: a static caffeine test, a static halothane test and a dynamic halothane test.

9. For the static tests the muscle tension should be gradually increased to produce a reasonable twitch height; this will usually occur with 2 g preload.
10. *The static cumulative caffeine test and measurement of the caffeine threshold.* The concentration of caffeine in the tissue bath should be increased step-wise as follows: 0.25, 0.5, 1.0, 1.5, 2.0, 3.0 and 4.0 mM.
Each successive concentration of caffeine should be administered as soon as the maximum contracture plateau, induced by the previous concentration of caffeine, has been reached, or after exposure to the caffeine concentration for 3 min if no contracture occurs. The muscle is not washed with Krebs solution in between successive concentrations of caffeine.
The result of this test will be reported as a caffeine threshold which is defined as the lowest concentration of caffeine which produces a sustained increase of at least 0.2 g in baseline tension.
11. *The static halothane test and measurement of static halothane threshold.* The halothane threshold is obtained using the nominal halothane concentrations 0.5, 1.0, 2.0 and 3.0% v/v. The measurement of the threshold is similar to (10) above.
12. *The dynamic halothane test and measurement of dynamic halothane threshold.* After 3 min exposure to halothane, the muscle is stretched at a constant rate of 4mm/min for 1.5 min and held at this new length for 1 min. The stretching process is then reversed. At each cycle the halothane concentration is increased from 0.5, 1.0, 2.0, to 3.0% v/v. The dynamic halothane threshold is defined as the concentration of halothane which produces a sustained increase of at least 0.2 g in the muscle tension compared with a pre-halothane control measured at the point shown in Fig. 27.2.

From: The European Malignant Hyperthermia Group, 1984.

MHS – indicating a definite susceptibility to MH
MHN – indicating an insusceptible subject from a proven MH pedigree
MHE – indicating an equivocal result (which for the sake of safety will often be reported to the patient and referring doctor as synonymous with MHS).

(Ellis 1984b; The European Malignant Hyperpyrexia Group 1984).

When experience with 349 patients had accumulated, the criteria defining the above three categories were changed a little with the effect of halving the number of persons classed as MHE (Figs. 27.3 and 27.4).

These new criteria were as follows.

MHS – a halothane contracture at 2% v/v or less and a caffeine contracture at 2 mmol/l or less
MHN – no halothane contracture at 2% v/v or less and no caffeine contracture at 2 mmol/l or less
MHE – all other results

(European MH group 1985).

It has subsequently been pointed out that the halothane concentration should be measured in the bath liquid, and only free caffeine base should be used since benzoate and citrate ions depress muscle contracture (Heytens *et al.* 1991).

In November 1987 in Lake Bluff, Illinois 47 representatives from 24 North American MH centres met to discuss the development of a standardized muscle contracture testing using caffeine and

(a) **MHN**

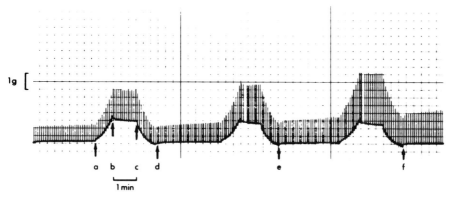

(b) **MHS**

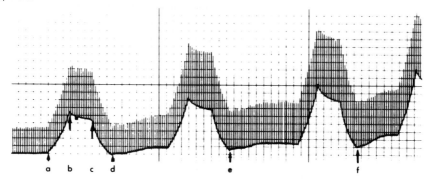

Fig. 27.2.(a) MHN: The dynamic test is performed by stretching the muscle specimen at a rate of 4 mm/min for 1.5 min (a–b). The muscle is held at this new length for 1 min (b–c) and then released at the same rate (c–d). After three control cycles, halothane 0.5% v/v is administered (d) and 3 min later a cycle is performed. The halothane concentration is then changed (e) according to the protocol. The halothane threshold is assessed by comparing the muscle baseline tension at point c in successive cycles. The figure shows a muscle stimulated electrically at a frequency of 0.2 Hz to produce mechanical twitches, thus demonstrating good viability. This result is part of a recording of a patient classified as MHN. (b) MHS: This result is part of a recording of a patient classified as MHS. (From The European Malignant Hyperpyrexia Group, 1984.)

the diagnostic muscle biopsy was not addressed in the report of the European group. On this point the North American group said, 'patients undergoing MH muscle biopsy may receive any non-triggering anaesthetic agent as long as the anaesthetic is not preceded by dantrolene administration' (Larach et al. 1989).

The North American guidelines for an abnormal (MHS) response were as shown in Table 27.3. The results of Larach et al. (1992) suggest that the thresholds for the diagnosis of MHS have been set too low in that 25% of presumed MHN individuals had a positive halothane contracture test (≥ 0.2 g at 3%) and 15% had a positive caffeine test (≥ 0.2 g at 2 mM).

The requirement for positive contractures on both caffeine and halothane tests as set out by the European criteria appears to be more reliable.

Age and muscle fibre type composition were found to have no influence on in vitro muscle halo-

halothane. There were minor differences between the recommended North American protocol and the European protocol, principally that the muscle should be exposed to 3% v/v halothane rather than 2% v/v halothane. The question of anaesthetic for

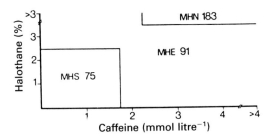

Fig. 27.3. Protocol for caffeine–halothane muscle contracture test. Diagnostic grouping of 349 patients according to original criteria. (From European Malignant Hyperpyrexia Group, 1985.)

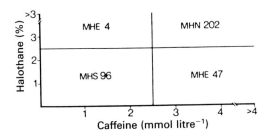

Fig. 27.4. Protocol for caffeine–halothane muscle contracture test. Re-grouping of the 349 patients according to new diagnostic limits. (From European Malignant Hyperpyrexia Group, 1985.)

thane caffeine contracture testing by Ørding *et al.* (1988).

The usefulness of a negative contracture test was demonstrated by Allen *et al.* (1990), who found that no MH events occurred in patients who had been shown to be MHN and who had been exposed to known MH-triggering anaesthetic agents. Similarly, Ørding *et al.* (1991) followed up 371 patients from 142 families who had been tested for MH susceptibility on the Danish MH register. Thirty-six MHS patients had been anaesthetised 52 times (without dantrolene) with no MH events. Thirty-five MHN patients had been anaesthetized 64 times, and 13 of them had received triggering agents 26 times without any signs of MH.

The results of muscle contracture testing were correlated with the clinical events which led to 402 probands being referred to the Leeds MH Unit (Ellis *et al.* 1990). Classical signs of MH – masseter spasm with raised creatine kinase (CK) levels, myoglobinuria, raised core temperature and cardiac

Table 27.3. *The proposed guidelines for an abnormal contracture test according to the North America Malignant Hyperthermia Group*

For purposes of clinical diagnoses, a patient shall be considered to be MH susceptible even if only one of his viable muscle strips demonstrates an abnormal contracture response after exposure to either 3% halothane alone, caffeine alone, or for those laboratories performing this test, the joint halothane and caffeine assay.

- A positive halothane contracture test is defined as a > 0.2–0.7 g contracture after exposure to 3% halothane for 10 min. The exact value of this range of abnormal shall be determined by each testing laboratory after the evaluation of at least 30 normal control muscle biopsies.
- A positive caffeine contracture test is defined as the observation of either (1) the development of ⩾ 0.2 g tension at 2 mM caffeine or (2) a caffeine specific concentration (CSC) at < 4 mM caffeine or (3) the percentage of maximal tension is > 7% change above the baseline at 2 mM caffeine.
- A positive joint halothane and caffeine contracture assay is defined as the development of a 1 g contracture after exposure to a concentration of 1 mM or less caffeine in the presence of 1% halothane. These are suggested values and must be modified by each laboratory.

From: Larach, M. G. for the North America Malignant Hyperthermia Group, 1989.

arrhythmias – were associated with the highest frequencies of MHS phenotyping.

Drugs and the *in vitro* muscle contracture test

Details of the administration of drugs in relation to *in vitro* contracture testing were discussed by Ørding (1988).

It would seem wise that the patient should avoid taking the following medications prior to the muscle biopsy because they can interfere with the result of the test.

dantrolene
verapamil
diltiazem
procaine
propanolol

Ørding (1989) investigated the influence of propanolol on muscle contracture testing *in vitro* and found that it significantly increased the caffeine threshold in the MHS group but not the normal group; the halothane responses were unaffected. The author concluded that β-blockers should be discontinued before muscle tests are carried out for MH susceptibility.

Creatine phosphokinase

Elevation of creatine phosphokinase (CPK) activity in serum is an indicator of muscle damage. It was found in some susceptible individuals in MH families and up to the early 1970s it was the only marker available. Britt & Kalow (1968) were of the opinion that MH cases could be divided into those characterized by the presence of rigidity and those in which rigidity was absent. In the former group the authors found there was not infrequently pre-existing musculoskeletal disease and raised serum CPK activities, amongst other abnormalities. Hence the serum CPK activity was used for family studies and as a predictive test for susceptibility to MH (see, for example, Britt *et al.* 1976). After the papers of Moulds & Denborough (1974a, b) appeared, however, the emphasis shifted from CPK testing, to muscle testing which despite its invasive and cumbersome nature was much more reliable and specific. As is well known the CPK measurements may be raised in many conditions unassociated with malignant hyperpyrexia. The level can be raised by strenuous exercise and intramuscular injections and there is considerable intra-individual variability. As Moulds & Denborough (1974b) pointed out, there was no direct evidence that persons with high CPK activity who were related to patients who had suffered MH were themselves susceptible.

The definitive evaluation of CPK level as a screening test for susceptibility to MH was published by Paasuke & Brownell (1986). *In vitro* muscle contracture tests were performed on 121 persons suspected of being liable to MH. The pre-biopsy serum CPK levels of 87 non-MHS patients were all in the normal range (<225 units/l), whereas the CPK levels of 34 MHS patients without other muscle disease were also in the normal range. The overlap was great; although the mean CPK level was slightly higher in the MHS group the test was completely non-diagnostic for an individual.

Prediction of MH susceptibility by means of clinical signs

This topic was investigated in relation to muscle contracture test results by Larach *et al.* (1987). Forty-two patients (mainly children) were biopsied because of a previous adverse reaction to anaesthesia that was clinically equivocal for MH. Patients with clear-cut MH were not biopsied. The results showed 17 positive biopsies (MHS), 24 negative and one equivocal.

The data were then examined for correlations between the clinical abnormal findings made before the biopsy was performed and the result of the biopsy. Neither formal neurological examination, serum CPK activity nor electromyography were predictive of the biopsy outcome. The only predictor of MH susceptibility was generalized muscle rigidity during the initial adverse anaesthetic.

Similarly, Hackl *et al.* (1990) studied 61 patients (mainly adults) who had experienced adverse reactions *thought* to be MH. *In vitro* contracture tests (European protocol) showed 38 to be MHS. Generalized rigidity, ventricular arrhythmias, cyanosis and post-operative myoglobinuria were observed significantly more often in the MHS patients.

Muscle abnormalities to be found in the MHS phenotype

In the early days of the investigation of the MH syndrome the idea was generated that some patients were characterized by a sudden development of rigidity whilst others developed rigidity more gradually. It seemed that musculoskeletal disorders (kyphoscoliosis, herniated nucleus pulposus, arthrogryposis, equinovarus, pes excavatum, umbilical hernia, strabismus and polymyositis) were present in the swift rigidity group (Britt & Kalow 1968).

Then a lot of work was done on the plasma creatine kinase activity (CPK) of MHS individuals and it was found to be elevated in them when they were investigated at a time quite separate from clinical illnesses and anaesthesia. Since CPK elevation is associated with muscle damage this finding focused attention on the fact that there was an abnormality of the muscles in at least some MHS patients.

However, a balanced view could be obtained only when the halothane/caffeine contracture test was established as a definitive diagnostic procedure to identify the MHS subject. A most extensive experience in this context was reported by Harriman (1988), who had the opportunity of studying the histology of 1400 biopsies made in the Leeds Malignant Hyperpyrexia Investigation Unit. He emphasized the point that sizeable numbers of biopsies from normal muscles are not available for comparison. However, the conclusion from a great deal of work and a lot of confusing evidence is that the majority of MHS patients have normal muscle histology. A small number of characteristic changes (internal nuclei, cores and moth-eaten fibres, i.e. type 1 fibres altered by one or more areas of pallor due to loss of mitochondria, of irregular outline and soft edge) are seen in a minority of MHS subjects.

So the conclusion is that with a standardized muscle contracture test being applied to large numbers of people the idea of a specific MH myopathy has lost its popularity. The muscle may be somehow abnormal in MH and may sometimes leak CPK, but in most MHS persons there is no clinically detectable myopathy.

Other predictive tests

A comprehensive compendium of tests which have been deployed to diagnose the susceptibility to malignant hyperthermia in man was published by Ørding (1988). The muscle contracture test has already been described earlier in this chapter. Many proposed tests have proved valueless. Three new tests have promise and are worth discussing.

Magnetic resonance spectroscopy, detecting ^{31}P, has been proposed as a means of performing a non-invasive test for MHS muscles. Using this technique the intracellular inorganic phosphate (Pi) and phosphocreatine (PCr) concentrations can be determined. Olgin et al. (1991) found that MHS individuals had higher resting forearm muscle Pi/PCr values than MHN individuals. Also MHS individuals had a significantly slower recovery rate of PCr/Pi after exercise, compared with MHN individuals. Interestingly, the MHS group as a whole was heterogenous with regard to these two parameters (i.e. some individuals exhibited one abnormality whilst some other individuals showed the other abnormality), but within a single family the MHS subjects all exhibited the same abnormality. This

was suggested to be evidence in favour of genetic heterogeneity. Payen et al. (1991) using the same technique for calf muscle found a significantly larger peak for phosphodiesters in MHS subjects over the age of 35 years, compared with MHN subjects of the same age. For reasons which were unclear the difference was not apparent below 25 years of age.

Cell membranes are suspected to be abnormal in MHS individuals. This aspect was investigated in red cell membranes by Ohnishi et al. (1988) and by Ohnishi & Ohnishi (1988), who used 16-doxyl stearic acid as a spin-label. The results indicated that the membranes from MHS subjects were fluidized by halothane to a greater degree than those from MHN subjects.

Similar results were obtained in sarcolemmal membranes from pigs by Thomas et al. (1991). The mobility of the labels (two oxazolidine nitroxide stearates) was higher in MHS than in MHN preparations.

The relaxation rate of the adductor pollicis muscle following tetanic stimulation was found to be higher on average in MHS than in MHN human subjects by Lennmarken et al. (1987) and Urwyler et al. (1990). However, there was a very substantial overlap between the groups which meant that this simple non-invasive test could not be used diagnostically for MH screening.

COUNSELLING AND INFORMATION

It will be appreciated that a condition such as MH, which can often be fatal and which is hereditary, causes a great deal of anxiety in affected families. The way in which an interested doctor can help with this problem is described by Mulrooney (1988). He described meetings at which families can be informed, and he advocates keeping general practitioners supplied with correct information, and encouraging diagnostic tests (especially muscle testing: see below) in individuals who may have inherited the susceptibility. Persons who have been identified as susceptibles were advised by Mulrooney to register with Medic Alert, always to wear their Medic Alert disc, to carry written counselling instructions with them at all times, and inform any new doctor whom they might consult of their susceptibility.

There is a British Malignant Hyperpyrexia Newsletter which is extremely valuable in the promotion of knowledge and mutual support to concerned relatives in MH-afflicted families (Mulrooney 1988). Similarly, 'The Communicator' is published by the Malignant Hyperthermia Association of the United States.

Details of information centres which can be contacted by telephone are given at the end of this chapter.

REACTIONS OF THE MH TYPE OCCURRING IN OTHER DISORDERS

This topic was extensively reviewed by Brownell (1988) who identified three fundamental questions (1) A decision has to be made on the criteria that must exist before one will accept that MH has in fact occurred. (2) If there has not been a clinical MH reaction, what evidence is there that the MH gene exists in a particular individual? (3) The diagnostic criteria for the proposed associated disorder must be defined.

The first two considerations are largely met by the *in vitro* contracture test described above. The third point, namely the diagnostic criteria for the proposed associated disorder, must be reviewed in each individual example.

Central core disease

Brownell (1988) was of the opinion that central core disease (CCD) was almost certainly related to MH. The essential diagnostic feature of CCD is the appearance of unstained cores within a significant number of muscle fibres when oxidative enzyme histochemistry is applied to fresh frozen sections of biopsied skeletal muscle. The condition is inherited as an autosomal dominant (McKusick No. 117000); persons who have this abnormality may be severely disabled or asymptomatic (Shuaib *et al.* 1987).

Biopsied muscle from CCD patients which has been submitted to the *in vitro* contracture test has almost always shown a positive response.

Therefore asymptomatic relatives of patients diagnosed as having CCD should be regarded as being at risk of developing MH when they are given an anaesthetic. The probability is that the two disorders are independent genetic entities, but for this idea to be proved the molecular genetics of CDD will have to be elucidated.

Duchenne muscular dystrophy

There have been a number of reports of clinical MH occurring in patients with Duchenne muscular dystrophy (DMD). When the *in vitro* contracture test became available Paasuke & Brownell (1986) described a positive result in a patient with DMD who had suffered clinical MH under anaesthesia. Brownell *et al.* (1985) reported that in the family of such a child investigation of other family members proved that the traits for DMD and MH were independent. It was clear anyway that this deduction was correct because DMD is an X-linked disorder and MH is autosomal. Now in addition to this we know that in DMD dystrophin is missing whilst the defect in some examples of MH may be in the ryanodine receptor of the sarcoplasmic reticulum (see below). On this point it is of considerable interest as made clear by Duncan (1989) that the biochemical disturbance in the two conditions is very similar, namely an elevation of $[Ca^{2+}]$ within the muscle cell.

The King–Denborough syndrome

In 1973 King and Denborough described the occurrence of MH in four white male patients who exhibited anomalies which included small stature, delayed motor development, thoracic kyphosis, lumbar lordosis, pectus carinatum, hypognathia, low-set ears, webbed necks, anti-mongoloid slant of the palpebral fissures and cryptorchidism. It mainly occurs in whites but a black patient with the syndrome was described by Pippin *et al.* (1988) and this boy died after MH. A white patient was described by Heiman-Patterson *et al.* (1986), who suffered MH and who subsequently was shown to have a positive halothane contracture test. His mother, who had had three previous anaesthesias without incident and whose only complaint was of leg cramps also had a positive halothane contracture test.

As pointed out by Brownell (1988), the position is unclear because the specific abnormality in the King–Denborough syndrome has not been defined.

Myoadenylate deaminase deficiency

This is a fairly common biochemical abnormality which may be accompanied by exercise fatigue and muscle cramps. An interesting family was described by Fishbein *et al.* (1985) in which MH apparently was inherited from the paternal side and myo-adenylate deaminase deficiency (MDD) from the maternal side. So this association between MH and MDD appeared to be due to coincidence.

Myotonia

Events similar to MH have been observed in patients with myotonia when they have been given triggering anaesthetic agents.

The relationship between the two conditions was explored by Lehmann-Horn & Iaizzo (1990), who carried out standard *in vitro* contracture tests (European protocol) on 44 patients with various disorders including six recessive generalized myotonia, six myotonia congenita and 17 myotonic dystrophy patients. Only four positive results were obtained and they were in patients with myotonic dystrophy. Although (as the authors point out) both diseases are characterized by abnormalities of muscle calcium metabolism they are controlled by genes widely distanced on chromosome 19, and they really are quite separate disorders. This finding of Lehmann-Horn & Iaizzo (1990) points out that the *in vitro* MH contracture test lacks specificity. Even though MH may not occur when myotonic patients are anaesthetized, the authors advocate the use of non-triggering agents.

Two sisters with myotonia congenita (Thomsen's disease, McKusick 160800) were described as having positive *in vitro* contracture tests by Heiman-Patterson *et al.* (1988); an unaffected third sister had a negative contracture test. This evidence again may possibly demonstrate the non-specificity of the contracture test.

Other conditions

A condition in which the occurrence of MH is difficult to evaluate is the new form of arthrogryposis reported by Froster-Iskenius *et al.* (1988). Muscle halothane contracture tests were not carried out on the probands and so one is left with some uncertainty.

An interesting possibility was suggested by Isaacs & Gericke (1990), namely that the occurrence of a non-fatal rise of temperature in an MH offspring *in utero* might be responsible for the production of developmental abnormalities. This idea was based on finding positive *in vitro* contracture tests in two pairs of mothers and offspring where the latter had various deformities. Evidence against this idea is that the phenomenon has not been described more frequently in the large number of MH families which have been studied.

Brownell (1988) listed the following conditions, with regard to which the evidence as to whether they were associated more than just coincidentally with MH was inconclusive.

Schwartz–Jampel syndrome
Fukuyama type of congenital muscular dystrophy
Becker muscular dystrophy
hyperkalaemic periodic paralysis (but see p. 479)
sarcoplasmic reticulum adenosine triphosphatase
    deficiency syndrome
mitochondrial myopathy

to which list could be added

glucose-6-phosphate dehydrogenase deficiency

(Younker *et al.* 1984).

The putative association between the Wolf–Hirschhorn syndrome and MH (Ginsburg & Purcell-Jones 1988) was refuted by Ellis & Halsall (1989).

When exercise-induced myolysis patients were investigated with a muscle contracture test only a minority of them were discovered to be of the MHS phenotype (Hackl *et al.* 1991; Krivosic-Horber *et al.* 1991).

POSSIBLE ASSOCIATIONS BETWEEN MH AND OTHER CONDITIONS

Sudden infant death syndrome (cot death)

The idea that the sudden infant death syndrome (SIDS) might be a manifestation of or in close association with MH (Denborough *et al.* 1982) was investigated by Ellis *et al.* (1988) by means of three studies.

1 A questionnaire to 195 MHS patients (as proven by muscle contracture test) to find out if they had SIDS offspring. Three such offspring were found: an incidence which does not differ from the general population.
2 A questionnaire to 106 SIDS parents to find out if there was any history of MH. No convincing case was found.
3 Fourteen SIDS parents had halothane/caffeine contracture tests. All were normal.

Similar results were obtained by Brownell (1986), so the hypothesis is most likely disproved.

Neuroleptic malignant syndrome

This is a syndrome which occurs in patients who have been given psychiatric drugs such as phenothiazines, butyrophenones and thioxanthines, and is characterized by hyperthermia, hypertonicity of skeletal muscles, fluctuating consciousness, and instability of the autonomic nervous system. These disturbances are mediated by the effects of the drugs on the central nervous system.

In vitro muscle contracture tests in patients who have experienced the neuroleptic malignant syndrome have mainly been negative, but some have been positive (Caroff *et al.* 1987; Adnet & Krivosic-Horber 1990). The same patients who developed the neuroleptic malignant syndrome have been given anaesthesia for electroconvulsive therapy with no ill effect (Brownell 1988). The relationship between the neuroleptic malignant syndrome and MH is unclear.

ABERRANT PHYSIOLOGY

Normal muscle contraction

In order to understand what goes wrong in malignant hyperthermia it is first necessary to review the steps which take place to cause mammalian striated muscle to contract and relax under normal circumstances.

When the nerve impulse reaches the motor endplate, acetylcholine is released which binds with receptors on the muscle cell membrane. This process initiates an action potential which not only spreads over the surface of the muscle cell but also spreads into the inside of the cell along the transverse tubules (T-tubules).

What happens next is the subject of some dispute (Caswell & Brandt 1989). There are two main hypotheses.

1 Depolarization of the T-tubule causes the release of a transmitter into the junctional space which binds to a receptor and causes the opening of the calcium channel in the sarcoplasmic reticulum.
2 There is a direct mechanical communication between the T-tubule and the terminal cisternae of the sarcoplasmic reticulum (SR), in which depolarization of the T-tubule causes a conformational alteration of the spanning structure thus opening the calcium channel of the SR.

The T-tubule is held in immediate juxtaposition to the SR by electron-dense protrusions called junctional feet. Calcium release is associated predominantly with the terminal cisternae portion of the SR which is the domain held in apposition to the transverse tubule. The T-tubules have been shown to be an extremely rich source of dihydropyridine receptor which is the putative calcium channel. It is possible that this molecule may be the voltage sensor for muscle excitation, and that calcium release from the T-tubule triggers calcium release from the SR, but the speed with which the former process occurs appears to be too slow to account for subsequent events (Caswell & Brandt 1989). There is another calcium channel in the SR which has been shown to be identical with the protein previously identified as junctional feet. Whatever the mechanism by which the process is initiated, calcium ions rapidly flood out of the sarcoplasmic reticulum whose terminal cisternae are in close apposition to the muscle fibres which contain the contractile elements (Fig. 27.5).

The muscle fibres themselves are complex structures consisting of thick and thin fibres which slide past each other to produce the contraction. The thin filament is formed from actin (A), tropomyosin (TM) and three troponins (TN) (Fig. 27.6). F-actin, which is a helical two-stranded filament of G-actin, is the backbone of the thin filament. Troponin binds periodically along the TM filament and is a complex of three polypeptides, TN-C (calcium binding), TN-I (inhibitory) and TN-T (TM binding). The TN-TM proteins form the calcium-binding regulatory complex of vertebrate striated muscle (Payne & Rudnick (1989).

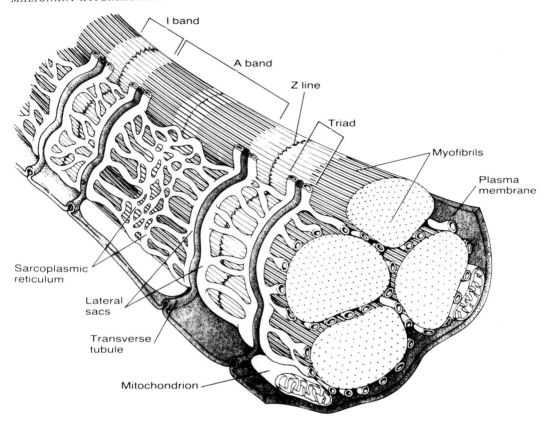

Fig. 27.5. Transverse tubules and sarcoplasmic reticulum of a skeletal muscle fibre. The transverse (T) tubule is a protrusion of the cell membrane into the cell. The sarcoplasmic reticulum (SR) spreads around and between the muscle fibres. The T-tubule is held in immediate juxtaposition to the SR by protrusions called junctional feet. (From Mason 1983.)

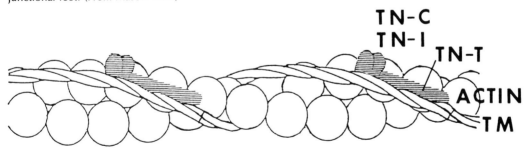

Fig. 27.6. Structure of the thin filament in vertebrate striated muscle. The TN complex consists of globular TN-C and TN-I and an elongated TN-T. (From Payne & Rudnick 1989.)

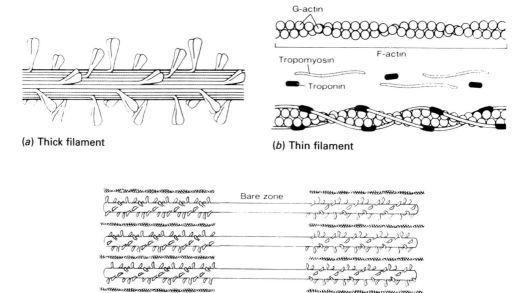

(a) Thick filament   (b) Thin filament

(c) Longitudinal section of filaments

Fig. 27.7. Composition of the myofilaments. (a) The thick filament consists mainly of golf-club-shaped molecules of myosin bundled together so that the heads of the molecules project from the shaft of the filament and spiral around the shaft. (b) The thin filament. Individual G-actin subunits link into a double chain of F-actin. In a single thin filament, two chains of G-actin subunits twist around one another. Along the surface of each chain lie threadlike tropomyosin molecules that each cover seven G-actin subunits. Each tropomyosin molecule is attached to a molecule of troponin. Troponin is also attached to actin. (c) Longitudinal view of thick and thin filaments as arranged in a sarcomere. Note that the myosin molecules project in opposite directions on either side of the bare zone. The thin filaments slide in relation to the thick filaments. (From Mason 1983.)

When calcium floods out of the terminal cisternae of the SR it binds to TN-C and this is an essential step towards causing muscle contraction, since it overcomes the inhibitory effect of TN-I. The morphology of the thin fibre is altered because following the changes in the TNs the TM moves into a groove which lies along the thin filament. This change allows the G-actin part of the thin filament to be exposed for interaction with myosin.

The thick filaments consist of myosin molecules, which are shaped like golf clubs bound together in pairs. There are about 200 myosin molecules in every thick filament (Dowben 1980) and the twin heads protrude outwards (Fig. 27.7). Myosin heads possess ATPase activity which in the resting state is inhibited by TM. When Ca^{2+} binds to TN-C this inhibition of ATPase by TM ceases. Actin, on the other hand, activates myosin ATPase. The effect of the activated myosin ATPase is to produce activated myosin and ADP. In activated myosin the head is at right angles to the stem (Mason 1983).

With the TM out of the way the myosin heads become attached to G-actin. The energy is then discharged from the myosin and the head returns to an angulated position relative to the stem. This causes the thin filament to slide relative to the thick filament, and this is the reason why the muscle contracts (Fig. 27.8).

This process is cyclical in that the bent myosin head is re-charged with another molecule of ATP, which is hydrolysed, giving again activated myosin with its head at right angles to the shaft, attached to actin etc.

What brings muscle contraction to an end? When the nerve impulses cease the whole process goes into reverse and a key step is the gathering back of the calcium ions into the SR. This is an active-transport, energy-requiring process. Much of the calcium is gradually transported to the extracellular

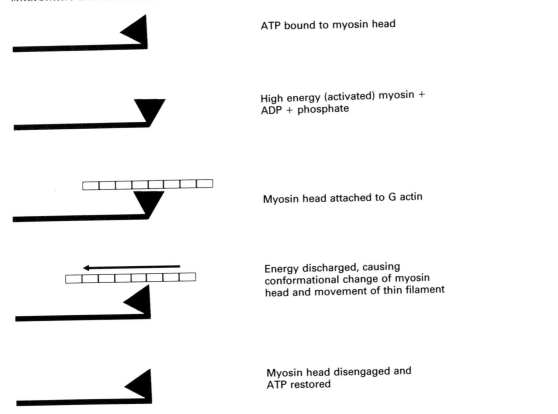

ATP bound to myosin head

High energy (activated) myosin +
ADP + phosphate

Myosin head attached to G actin

Energy discharged, causing
conformational change of myosin
head and movement of thin filament

Myosin head disengaged and
ATP restored

Fig. 27.8. The mechanism whereby the myosin head of the thick filament causes the thin filament to slide.

liquid. With the removal of the calcium from TN-C, the TN-I molecule exerts its effects and TM moves out of the thin filament groove to interpose itself between the myosin heads and the actin molecule, and so contraction ceases.

The MH muscle

The very complicated processes controlling calcium metabolism in the muscle cell, and their disturbances in MH, were reviewed by Foster (1990). Here the discussion is focused on one particular aspect, namely the studies of the calcium channel of SR which have been carried out using the plant alkaloid ryanodine (Fig. 27.9), which has been used as an insecticide. The ryanodine receptor (RYR) molecular mass > 300 kDa (Mickelson *et al.* 1988) or about 400 kDa (Lai *et al.* 1988) is identical with the protein which forms the feet between the transverse tubule

and the SR terminal cisternae. The close association between RYR and the SR calcium release channel has been demonstrated by the binding of [^{3}H]ryanodine to its receptor which is (1) stimulated by agents which stimulate Ca^{2+}-induced calcium release (micromolar Ca^{2+} and ATP), (2) inhibited by agents which inhibit Ca^{2+} release (millimolar Ca^{2+}, Mg^{2+} and ruthenium red). Also, RYR incorporated into lipid bilayers shows calcium channel behaviour similar to that of the calcium channel of isolated terminal cisternae (Mickelson *et al.* 1988).

Considerable light has been shed on the abnormal properties of MH muscle by making vesicles of sarcoplasmic reticulum (SR) *in vitro* and studying the behaviour of the calcium channel which they contain. These experiments have been carried out with porcine SR. It has been shown that the rate constant of Ca^{2+}-induced calcium release from MHS SR was significantly greater than from normal SR at three different Ca^{2+} concentrations. Higher Ca^{2+} concentrations were required to inhibit ryanodine binding to MHS SR than to normal SR.

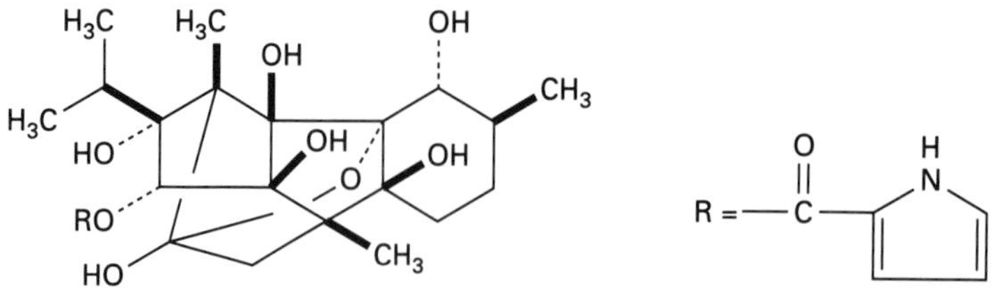

Fig. 27.9. Ryanodine. (From *The Merck Index*, 1983.)

RYR of the SR of MHS muscle, at the optimal calcium concentration of 6 μM, had a higher affinity for ryanodine than its normal counterpart ($K_d = 92$ vs 265 nM, $p < 0.001$).

Both MHS and normal intact muscle bundles responded to increasing ryanodine concentrations with diminishing twitch and tetanic force production accompanied by contractures. However, MHS muscle required significantly lower ryanodine concentrations for these effects than did normal muscle.

The evidence is compatible with the view that (1) there is an abnormality in the MHS muscle RYR, (2) the RYR is the calcium channel of SR and (3) the Ca^{2+}-dependent gating mechanism(s) of the SR calcium release channel is abnormal in MHS muscle. The end result is probably an abnormally high calcium release accounting for the increased twitch tension of MHS muscle fibre bundles (Mickelson *et al.* 1988; Joffe *et al.* 1992).

It is thought that the abnormal calcium release first activates metabolic processes, perhaps by an action on phosphorylase increasing oxygen consumption and causing the production of abnormal amounts of heat, CO_2 and lactic acid. More calcium ions activate myosin ATPase, liberating more heat by hydrolysis of ATP and causing muscular contraction (Britt 1985).

It was demonstrated by Allsop *et al.* (1991) that after a short period of intensive exercise the pH inside the human vastus lateralis muscle falls lower in MHS individuals than in normals, and recovers much more slowly. This was a direct *in vivo* demonstration of disturbed biochemistry (Ellis *et al.* 1991).

Malignant hyperthermia in pigs

The syndrome of malignant hyperthermia has been described in a number of animals including dogs, cats, horses and pigs (Denborough 1980). The phenomenon has been most intensively studied in the pig.

There was a commercial interest in investigating two conditions affecting pig meat production. These were called porcine stress syndrome (PSS) and pale soft exudative pork syndrome (PSEPS). The former was a type of shock which occurred in susceptible animals as a result of transportation, exercise or fighting, and consisted of dyspnoea, hyperthermia, cyanosis, collapse and death. Rigor mortis developed swiftly. PSEPS was a term referring to poor quality meat produced as a result of a very quick fall in pH after slaughter before chilling and processing could take place (Denborough 1980).

Eventually it turned out that PSS, PSEPS and malignant hyperthermia (MH) are all manifestations of the same condition. The breeds of pigs affected include Landrace, Large White (Okumura *et al.* 1979), Poland China (Gronert *et al.* 1976) and French Pietrain (Smith & Bampton 1977). It is of interest to note that it seems to have been selective breeding for heavily muscled animals that has brought this genetic condition into prominence.

The availability of MH susceptible pigs has been valuable in researches on the syndrome because the physiological and biochemical abnormalities seem to be the same as in affected humans. Hence, for example, drugs have been tested using muscle preparations, the properties of the sarcoplasmic reticulum have been investigated, and genetic linkage elucidated using the pig model (see below).

GENETIC ASPECTS

Soon after the syndrome of MH became recognized it was clear that there was a familial aggregation of cases, suggesting the possibility that there might be a genetic basis (Britt & Kalow 1968). Nevertheless, since anaesthesia is a fairly uncommon event in a person's lifetime and given for different types of operation, and not all anaesthetics include MH trig-

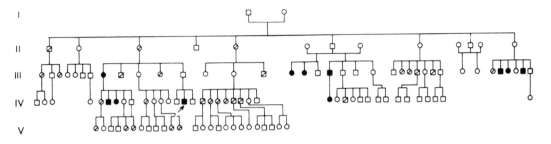

Fig. 27.10. Pedigree indicating fatal reaction (hyperthermia) to general anaesthesia. Squares, males; circles, females; ■, ●, fatal reaction; ▨, ⊘, normal reaction; □, ○, not exposed, i.e. no anaesthetic received. (From Denborough *et al.* 1962.)

gering agents, it was not surprising that sufficient pedigree information gathered retrospectively to work out the pattern of inheritance was rather slow in being accumulated.

The subject was critically surveyed by Britt *et al.* (1969). Previously, Denborough had reported a large Australian kindred in which there were 11 (6 female) affected individuals and 27 individuals who had received anaesthetics without reactions (Fig. 27.10). This pedigree showed female-to-male, female-to-female and male-to-female transmission. An autosomal dominant character seemed likely. [An autosomal recessive would most likely require inbreeding, which was not present; a sex-linked recessive was unlikely as females account for half the affected cases, a sex-linked dominant could not be excluded.] Another large pedigree from Wausau, Wisconsin studied by Britt *et al.* (1969) showed male-to-male transmission, which ruled out sex-linked dominant inheritance (Fig. 27.11). The intermarriage in this second pedigree still left a doubt about an autosomal recessive character masquerading as an autosomal dominant but parental consanguinity was neither a feature of many isolated cases nor a feature of other pedigrees wherein only two or three cases had occurred. For an autosomal recessive explanation to be tenable the persons marrying into the pedigree and producing an affected offspring would have to be heterozygotes, which

seemed very unlikely. Polygenic inheritance was unlikely since offspring and parents seemed about equally severely affected and about half the offspring in a sibship were affected.

Since some instances of apparent 'skipping' a generation were present, some explanation had to be adduced. 'Reduced penetrance' might have been due to the anaesthetic being very brief or noxious agents not used, or there may have been the modifying effect of some other gene.

In a later paper Britt *et al.* (1976) examined 1802 individuals from 56 families. MH crises had occurred in 124 patients of whom 72 were available for testing. By then, the assessment of each individual was not based solely on the account of what happened under anaesthesia but was supplemented by the serum creatine phosphokinase measurement and muscle biopsy testing. Using these extra items of information the susceptibility to MH (i.e. MHS) was clearly shown in sizeable pedigrees to be an autosomal dominant character.

The question of heterogeneity in MH was explored by McPherson & Taylor (1982), who pointed out that about half the patients were shown to be autosomal dominants. About 20% of cases were sporadic and in a few instances recessive inheritance could not be excluded. These authors pointed out that genes for other well-known conditions may contribute to MH susceptibility, and that it is possible that not all cases of MH necessarily share a common cause. It is possible that MH might be a symptom-complex due to a variety of genetic and environmental factors.

An interesting family, in which both parents of three probands had positive *in vitro* contracture

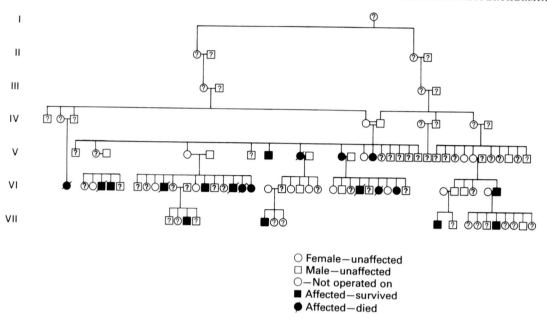

○ Female—unaffected
□ Male—unaffected
◐—Not operated on
■ Affected—survived
⬤ Affected—died

Fig. 27.11. Malignant hyperthermia – pedigree 'CW'. (From Britt *et al.* 1969.)

tests, was described by Mauritz *et al.* (1988). This finding could be explained by a high incidence of the abnormal gene in a genetic isolate with inbreeding in Vorarlberg, Austria.

So the standard situation is for the susceptibility to MH to be an autosomal dominant character and for MH to follow the administration of anaesthetic agents. However, atypical cases with regard to their pedigree pattern and precipitating causes occur from time to time. The topic of other pre-existing disorders predisposing to the development of MH has been discussed in another section.

Linkage

The occurrence of MH in pigs was known since the early days of the investigation of the disorder and has proven of great value in elucidating its basis in humans. It will be observed that this combined approach, namely studying an animal model in conjunction with a human disease condition, has led to advances in knowledge in several pharmacogenetic conditions.

In pigs MH is inherited as an autosomal recessive character (Smith & Bampton 1977), and has been

investigated for genetic linkage. Using a cloned porcine glucose phosphate isomerase (GPI) cDNA a close linkage was found between the locus for MH (termed *HAL*) and the locus for GPI on the pig's chromosome number 4.

In the human genome *GPI* had been shown to be located on chromosome 19 at q12–q13.2 (McMorris *et al.* 1973). Since there is a tendency for genes in mammals to have stayed together during evolution it seemed likely that *HAL* was also on chromosome 19. Another gene known to be located on chromosome 19 at 19p13.2–p13.1 was the complement component C3 (McKusick *et al.* 1987).

A linkage study with 19 markers was conducted using five German families segregating for MH (Bender *et al.* 1990). The markers were on many different chromosomes but LE (Lewis blood group) and C3 (complement component-3) were on number 19. Positive lod scores were obtained with C3 ($z = 0.72$, Θ 0.11) indicating that *HAL* was in the region 19p13.2–p13.1.

Quite a lot was already known about the region q12–q13.2 of chromosome 19 because of the interest in myotonic dystrophy which had been found to be at q12, as well as a number of polymorphic loci including an apolipoprotein gene cluster (*APOC1*, *APOC2*, *APOE*) BCL3 (B-cell chronic lymphatic leukaemia/lymphoma-3), *CYP 2A* and the DNA marker *D19S9*. The order of 14 markers spanning 63 cM on 19q had been determined (Fig. 27.12).

In three large Irish families in which MH cases had occurred, McCarthy *et al.* (1990) sought linkage between *MHS* (as defined by an *in vitro* muscle contracture test using European MH Group criteria) and the 14 polymorphic loci. The discovery was made that the *MHS* locus was linked to *CYP 2A* (Fig. 27.13) and the data indicated that *D19S9* and *APOC2* flanked the *MHS* locus.

In the same issue of the journal *Nature*, MacLennan *et al.* (1990) published another linkage

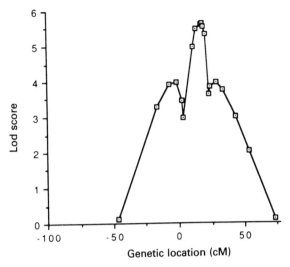

Fig. 27.13. Location map summarizing location scores (log$_{10}$ likelihood difference) calculated for *MHS* at various map positions in a fixed marker map. Joint likelihoods were calculated for the six loci simultaneously. Here the support for linkage of MHS is calculated at various map locations in a fixed map of polymorphic markers. The most likely location for *MHS* is at *CYP 2A* with a lod score of 5.65. On the x-axis *APOC2* is arbitrarily set at 0 cM, *D19S9* is at +20 cM and *CYP 2A* at +15 cM, based on linkage maps published for this region. (From McCarthy *et al.* 1990.)

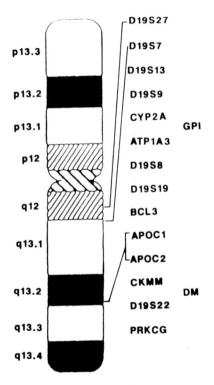

Fig. 27.12. Linkage map of 14 markers on chromosome 19q. *MHS*, malignant hyperthermia susceptibility locus; *GPI*, glucose phosphate isomerase locus; *DM*, myotonic dystrophy locus.
CYP2A, cytochrome P450 subfamily 2A locus; *ATP1A3*, sodium–potassium–ATPase, alpha-3 polypeptide locus; *BCL3*, B-cell chronic lymphatic leukaemia/lymphoma-3 locus; *APOC1*, apolipoprotein C-I locus; *APOC2*, apolipoprotein C-II locus; *CKMM*, creatine kinase, muscle type locus; *PRKCG*, protein kinase C, gamma polypeptide locus; plus loci for 7 DNA markers (*D19S27*, etc.). (From McCarthy *et al.* 1990.)

study. The background to their work was that they had been able to clone the complementary DNA and genomic DNA encoding the human ryanodine receptor (*RYR*). They then mapped *RYR* to q13.1 of human chromosome 19. Linkage studies were carried out in MH-containing families, whose ethnic origin was not specified, using markers on chromosome 19 including some within *RYR*. Seventeen out of 21 families were informative. The MH status was determined by means of an *in vitro* muscle contracture test using the North American criteria (Hopkins *et al.* 1992 criticized the study on this account because of the high false positivity rate). The results indicated a close linkage between the *RYR* and *MH* gene loci. Illustrative families are shown in Fig. 27.14.

A single point mutation

An investigation of porcine *RYR* cDNA from animals shown to be MHS and MHN revealed an 1843C → T substitution causing an amino acid change 615

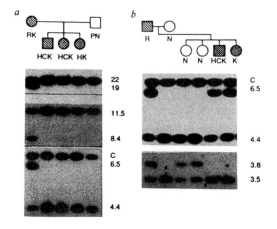

Fig. 27.14. Segregation of *RYR* gene markers and flanking markers in families 5 and 12. Diagnosis of MH status was carried out using the caffeine-halothane contracture test described previously. Family members are labelled with an R if they have had an MH reaction and with H, C, or K if they tested positive for the halothane test, the caffeine test or the halothane + caffeine test, respectively. Individuals labelled N tested normal in the contracture tests; PN is presumed normal. Southern blot autoradiographs for selected informative markers are shown with the DNA tracks aligned below the corresponding family member. In family 5 (a), the three informative markers were HRR3 (*Hind*III alleles of 19 and 22 kb); HRR4 (*Bcl*I alleles of 11.5 kb and 8.4 + 2.9 kb; the 2.9 kb band is not shown) and HRR3 (*Pvu*II alleles of 6.5 kb and 4.4 + 1.9 kb; the 1.9 kb band is not shown). In family 12 (b), two informative markers are HRR3 (*Pvu*II alleles of 6.5 kb and 4.4 + 1.9 kb; the 1.9 kb band is not shown) and ApoCII (*Taq*I alleles of 3.8 and 3.5 kb). (From MacLennan *et al.* 1990.)

arginine → cysteine (Fuji *et al.* 1991). Following on from this study Gillard *et al.* (1991) screened 35 Canadian MH families with (1) an *in vitro* muscle contracture test, (2) DNA analysis using specially made oligonucleotide probes, one with 1840C and the other with 1840T, (3) restriction endonuclease analysis since the nucleotide change 1840C → T deletes an *Rsa*I site, (4) direct sequencing. In only one family three individuals were found to have both the MHS phenotype on muscle testing and the base substitution. This work was confirmed by Hogan *et al.* (1992), who found that one MHS individual out of 62 possessed the 1840 deletion, and that this segregated with the MHS phenotype in the pedigree.

Three MHS individuals were investigated very thoroughly by Gillard *et al.* (1992). Twenty-one mutations were found in *RYR1*, four of which led to a change in an amino acid. Out of 45 families tested, a single family showed co-segregation of a 248 Arg for Gly mutation with the MHS phenotype. The other three amino acid changes thus appeared to be polymorphisms and not candidate mutations causing MHS. These authors point out the availability of some 32 polymorphisms in the *RYR1* gene, 24 of which are detected as RFLPs which can be used for analysis of the inheritance of specific *RYR1* haplotypes informative in most MH families.

Central core disease, which (as discussed earlier) is associated with the MHS phenotype, has been shown to be linked to *RYR1*. It is therefore possible that an abnormality in *RYR1* may give rise to both the MHS status and the spontaneous disorder (Maclennan 1992).

A survey of three unrelated families was made by Levitt *et al.* (1991). The individuals were tested by an *in vitro* muscle contracture test and their DNA was investigated with 14 probes. These included *RYR* and detected loci at which polymorphisms could occur both sides of *RYR*. In their paper (Fig. 27.15) it is shown that *RYR* could be excluded as a candidate gene for MH in these families. The data suggest that there is at least a second locus in addition to RYR involved in the production of MH and that clinical variability in expression may be associated with molecular heterogeneity.

Similarly, Fagerlund *et al.* (1992) investigated eight Swedish MH families and found three of them informative with respect to genetic linkage between *MHS* and *RYR*. In one of these families no recombination was found, but two recombinants were found in one family and 1 in another. Also Deufel *et al.* (1992) investigated two Bavarian MHS families and demonstrated a lack of linkage between the MHS phenotype and *RYR1*. So these studies confirm the existence of genetic heterogeneity.

It would seem, therefore, that a mutation in the *RYR* gene can account for some but not all human MH patients. So as forecast by Davies (1990) a small structural change in this large (564 kDa) protein renders it functionally insufficient in the presence of a greatly increased metabolic load or stress.

Twelve of the 16 MHS families investigated by Olkers *et al.* (1992) were unlinked to chromosome 19q. In seven of these families MHS was linked to

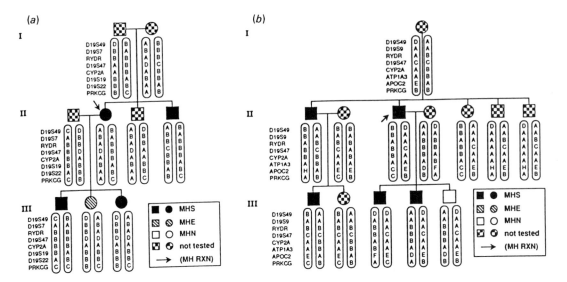

Fig. 27.15. Segregation data for selected informative polymorphisms within genes and anonymous DNA markers in the 19q12–q13.3 linkage groups. Genes and markers are placed in the order that the literature suggests they occur. Markers that have not yet been accurately mapped were placed in the order suggested by these three families. This is purely for purposes of illustration since only two-point analyses of MHS with each marker were performed.

(a), Segregation data for Family 1. The diagnosis of MHS was established in the proband (II-2) from this family by her clinical response to anaesthesia. Anaesthesia was induced with halothane and nitrous oxide. Muscle rigidity and an irregular heart rhythm were observed following the administration of succinylcholine. Postoperative muscle soreness was noted and CPK levels rose to 3132 on the evening of surgery. The grandparents (I-1, I-2) were not tested for MHS; however, both of their affected children (II-2, II-4) inherited the same chromosome 19 from their father (I-1) but different chromosomes 19 from their mother (I-2). In the second generation, the proband (II-2) transmitted this same chromosome 19 haplotype to her affected son (III-1). However, individual III-3 was found to be MHS by contracture testing, and inherited only a portion of this maternal haplotype demonstrating recombination between MHS and D19S49, D19S7, RYDR, D19S47, CYP2A and D19S19. Individuals II-3 and III-2 also demonstrate recombination on this same chromosome between D19S19 and D19S22. These represent the minimum number of crossovers that have occurred and suggest that in this family the gene responsible for MHS is located distal to D19S19, or elsewhere in the genome.

(b), Segregation data from Family 2. The proband in this family experienced an increase in exhaled CO_2, an elevated temperature, and a decreased serum pH during anesthesia. His CPK rose to over 87 000 postoperatively, and he noted significant muscle weakness and soreness for several weeks. The maximum contracture response was 2.2 g to 3% halothane and 0.2 g to 2 mM caffeine. Affected individuals II-1 and III-1 share a chromosome 19 haplotype inherited from individual I-1. The proband (II-3) and his affected sons (III-3, III-4) inherited in common a different chromosome 19 haplotype from individual I-1. However, an unaffected son (III-5) also inherited this same chromosome 19 haplotype, thus excluding it as carrying the defective gene producing MHS. Therefore, recombination between MHS and D19S49, D19S9, RYDR, D19S47, CYP2A, ATP1A3, APOC2 and PRKCG has occurred; the most likely explanation for these data is that the markers in the 19q12–13.3 linkage groups do not co-segregate with MHS in this family. (From Levitt et al. 1991.)

markers on chromosome 17q11.2–q24. There is a strong possibility that a mutation in the adult muscle sodium channel α-subunit (SCN4A) located at 17q23.1–q25.3 may be responsible for MHS. A single amino acid substitution in the sodium channel alters it so that it functions largely as a calcium channel. Paramyotonia congenita (MIM 168300) and hyperkalemic periodic paralysis (MIM 170500) are thought to arise from mutations in SCN4A, so an explanation may thus be provided for the association between these disorders and MHS.

There is also a possibility that there are different types of MHS linked to different genes on chromosome 17q, and obviously in some families MHS is linked neither to chromosome 19q nor to chromosome 17q.

Looking to the future, it seems likely that a variety of allele-specific probes will be developed (Levitt 1992). These can be used to screen family members of MH probands to determine MH susceptibility status and so it should be possible eventually to do away with the *in vitro* muscle contracture test.

The author would like to express his gratitude to Professor Francis G. Ellis, Department of Anaesthesia, University of Leeds, UK, Dr Marilyn Larach, Department of Anaesthesia, Pennsylvania State University, College of Medicine, Hershey, PA, USA and Dr H. Ørding, Department of Anaesthesia, Herlev University Hospital, Denmark who made many helpful suggestions about the contents of this chapter.

Appendix 27.1
An international registry of reported cases was established by Britt & Kalow (1970). The North American Malignant Hyperthermia Registry Inc. is located at the Department of Anaesthesia of the Pennsylvania State University College of Medicine (Larach 1989; Rosenberg 1989).

The Malignant Hyperthermia Association of the United States operates an MH hotline to answer the questions of physicians concerning the management of MH and MH-susceptible patients (Tel: 209-634-4917).

Informative pamphlets on MH are available from the Malignant Hyperthermia Association of the United States (MHAUS), Box 191, Westport, CT 06881-0191, USA. Tel: 203-655-3007. A periodical for the layman entitled *The Communicator* is published five times a year by MHAUS at the same address.

A booklet for patients, entitled *A guide to Malignant Hyperthermia* is available for purchase from the Malignant Hyperthermia Association, 2 Bloor Street West, Box 144, Toronto, Ontario M4W 3EZ, Canada. Tel: 416-447-0052 (Britt 1985).

Information regarding 'Medic Alert' discs and the British Malignant Hyperpyrexia Newsletter can be obtained from Dr P. L. Mulrooney, Mansfield and District General Hospital, Mansfield, NG18 1PH, UK.

Information can be obtained in Germany from Klinikum Charlottenburg der Freien Universität, Berlin, set up in an Information service for Malignant Hyperthermia emergencies. 030/3035 504 (daytime) or 030/3035 1 (outside regular office hours), where expert staff may be contacted and a consultation service in available. (Schulte-Sasse & Eberlein (1987).

Appendix 27.2 *Diagnostic centre directory*

USA and Canada
Dr Glenn E. DeBoer, MD
The Division of Anesthesiology
Cleveland Clinic Foundation
9500 Euclid Avenue
Cleveland, OH 44195
USA

Tel. 216-444-6331
Fax. 216-444-9248

Dr Henry Rosenberg MD
Department of Anesthesiology
Mail Stop 310
Hahnemann University Hospital
Broad and Vine Streets
Philadelphia, PA 19102
USA

Tel. 215-448-7960
Fax. 215-448-8656

Dr Denise J. Wedel, MD
Department of Anesthesiology
Mayo Clinic
200 First Street SW
Rochester, MN 55905
USA

Tel. 507-255-4236
Fax. 507-255-6463

Dr Gregory Allen, MD
Department of Anesthesia
Main Division
Ottawa Civic Hospital
1053 Carling Avenue
Ottawa, Ontario K1Y 4E9
Canada

Tel. 613-761-4169
Fax. 613-725-2909

Dr Marshall Millman, MD PhD
Department of Anesthesiology
Presbyterian University Hospital Room 2405
Pittsburgh, PA 15213
USA

Tel. 412-647-3260

Dr Beverley A. Britt, MD
Malignant Hyperthermia Investigation Unit
Toronto General Hospital
200 Elizabeth Street
Room CCRW2-834
Toronto, Ontario M5G 2C4
Canada

Tel. 416-340-3128
Fax. 416-340-4706

Dr Jordan D. Miller, MD
Department of Anesthesiology
Center for Health Sciences
UCLA School of Medicine
10833 LeConte Avenue
Los Angeles, CA 90024-1778
USA

Tel. 213-825-9198

Dr Sheila M. Muldoon, MD
Department of Anesthesiology
**Uniformed Services University of the Health
Services**
4301 Jones Bridge Road
Bethesda, MD 20815
USA

Tel. 301-295-3140
Fax. 301-295-3586

Dr Gerald A. Gronert, MD
Department of Anesthesiology
School of Medicine, TB 170
University of California
Davis, CA 95616
USA

Tel. 916-752-7805
Fax. 916-752-6363

Dr Leena Patel, MD
Department of Anesthesia
Children's Hospital
University of Manitoba
Room AE203
840 Sherbrook Street
Winnipeg, Manitoba R3A 1S1
Canada
Tel. 204-787-2560

Dr Barbara E. Waud, MD
Department of Anesthesiology
University of Massachusetts Medical Center
55 Lake Ave N
Worcester, MA 01655
USA
Tel. 508-856-3160
Fax. 508-856-5911

Dr Dennis F. Landers, MD PhD
Anesthesiology Department
S. Lab
University of Nebraska Medical Center
42nd and Dewey Avenue
Omaha, NE 68105
USA
Tel. 402-559-7405
Fax. 402-559-7372

Dr Dan R. Richards, MD
Department of Anesthesiology
University of South Florida
Medical Center, PO Box 59
12901 Bruce B. Downs Blvd
Tampa, FL 33612-4799
USA
Tel. 813-251-7438
Fax. 813-251-7418

Dr Thomas E. Nelson, PhD
Department of Anesthesiology
University of Texas Health Science Center
6431 Fannin MSB 5.020
Houston, TX 77030
USA
Tel. 713-792-5566
Fax. 713-794-4157

Dr John F. Kreul, MD
Department of Anesthesiology
University of Wisconsin Hospital and Clinics,
B6/387
CSC 600 Highland Avenue
Madison, WI 53792
USA

Tel. 608-263-8100
Fax. 608-263-0575

Dr Paul A. Iaizzo, PhD
University of Minnesota,
Minneapolis, MN 55455,
USA

Tel. 612-624-7912
Fax. 612-626-2363

Australia
Dr M. A. Denborough
John Curtin School of Medical Research,
Australian National University
Canberra, ACT 2601
Australia

Tel. 06-249-2207
Fax. 06-249-0415

Dr R. F. W. Moulds
Department of Clinical Pharmacology
Royal Melbourne Hospital PO
Victoria 3050
Australia

Tel. 03-342-7137
Fax. 03-342-7940

New Zealand
Dr Neil Pollock
Dept of Anaesthesia and Intensive Care
Palmerston North Hospital
Palmerston North
New Zealand.

Tel. 06-350-8821
Fax. 06-351-6669

Europe
Austria
Dr Werner Hackl
Klinik für Anaesthesie
Spitalgasse 23
A-1090 Wien

Tel. 43-140-4000 Ext 2251
Fax. 43-140-400 4519

Belgium
Dr Luc Heytens
Dept. of Intensive Care
Universitair Ziekenhuis Antwerpen
Wilrijkstraat 10
B-2520 Edegem

Tel. 32-3-829-1111 Ext 51 639
Fax. 32-3-829-05-20

Denmark
Dr Helle Ørding
The Danish Malignant Hyperthermia Register
Dept of Anaesthesia
Herlev University Hospital
DK-2730 Herlev

Tel. 45-44-53-53-00 Ext 3578
Fax. 45-44-53-53-32

United Kingdom
Professor F. Richard Ellis
MH Investigation Unit
Clinical Sciences Building
St. James' University Hospital
Leeds LS9 7TF
UK

Tel. 44-532-43-31-44 Ext 5274
Fax. 44-532-42-64-96

Germany
Dr Edmund Hartung
Dept. of Anaesthesia
University Hospital Würzburg
Josef Schneider Strasse 2
D-8700 Würzburg

Tel. 49-931-20-11
Fax. 49-931-201-34-44

Dr Frank Lehmann-Horn
Dept of Neurology
Technical University of Munich
Möhlstrasse 28
D-8000 München 80.
Tel. 49-89-41-40-46-70 or 4635
Fax. 49-89-91-77-45

Professor W. Mortier
Kinderklinik Wuppertal
Heusnerstrasse 40
D-5600 Wuppertal
Tel. 49-20-25-66-441

Dr Norbert Roewer
Dept of Anesthesiology
University Hospital Eppendorf
Martinistrasse 52
D-2000 Hamburg 20

France
Professor Renée Krivosic-Horber
Départementd'Anesthésie-Réanimation
Hopital B
**Centre Hospitalier Régional
Universitaire de Lille**
Bd. du Professeur J. Lerclercq
F-59037 Lille
Tel. 33-20-44-62-70

Dr Geneviève Kozak Ribbens
CRMBM Faculté de Médecine la Timone
27 Bd. Jean Moulin
F-13005 Marseille
Tel. 33-91-25-50-90

Professor Paul Stieglitz
Département d'Anesthésie-Réanima
Chirurgicale
**Centre Hospitalier Régional
Universitaire de Grenoble**
F-38700 La Tronche
Tel. 33-76-42-33-86
Fax. 33-76-42-46-21

Holland
Dr Mathieu Gielen
Dept of Anaesthesia
University Hospital
Geert Grooteplein 10
NL-6525 GA Nijmegen
Tel. 31-80-51-44-06

Iceland
Dr Stefan B. Sigurdsson
Dept. of Physiology
Vatnsmyrarvegir 16
IS-101 Reykjavik
Tel. 354-1-69-48-31
Fax. 354-1-69-48-84

Ireland
Professor James J. A. Heffron
Dept of Biochemistry
University College
Cork
Eire
Tel. 353-21-27-68-71 Ext 2208
Fax. 353-21-27-40-34

Italy
Dr Amalia Bellugi
Ospedale Bentivoglio
Via Marconi 35
I-40010 Bentivoglio
Bologna
Tel. 39-51-66-44-11
Fax. 39-51-66-40-634

Dr Virginia Brancadoro
**Instituto di Anestesia e Rianimazione
Facolta de Medicina**
Via S. Pansini 5
I-80131 Napoli

Dr Santolo Cozzolino
Presidio Multizonale di Prevenzione
USL 40 Via S. Giacomo dei Capri 66
I-80131 Napoli
Tel. 39-81-54-52-788, 39-81-54-62-262
Fax. 39-81-54-63-838

Dr Vincenzo E. Tegazzin
Dept of Anesthesiology and Critical Care Medicine
Traumatologic-orthopedic Hospital
Via Facciolati 71
I-35126 Padova
Tel. 39-49-821-6511 or 6522
Fax. 39-49-821-6631

Norway
Dr Stefan Mohr
Dept of Anaesthesia
Telemark Sentralsjukehus
N-3700 Skien
Tel. 47-035-25-000

Sweden
Dr Eva Ranklev
Dept of Anesthesia
Lasarettet University Hospital
S-221 85 Lund
Tel. 46-46-17-19-49
Fax. 46-46-14-23-13

Switzerland
Dr Albert Urwyler
Dept of Anaesthesia
University Hospital Kantonsspital
CH-4031 Basel
Tel. 41-61-25-25-25
Fax. 41-61-26-60-22

Adnet, P. J. & Krivosic-Horber, R. M. (1990). Neuroleptic malignant syndrome and malignant hyperthermia susceptibility (letter). *Acta Anaesthesiologica Scandinavica*, **34**, 605.

Allen, G. (1991). Propofol and malignant hyperthermia. *Anesthesia and Analgesia*, **73**, 359.

Allen, G. C. & Rosenberg, H. (1990). Malignant hyperthermia susceptibility in adult patients with masseter muscle rigidity. *Canadian Journal of Anaesthesia*, **37**, 31–5.

Allsop, P., Jorfeldt, L., Rutberg, H., Lennmarken, C. & Hall, G. M. (1991). Delayed recovery of muscle pH after short duration, high intensity exercise in malignant hyperthermia susceptible subjects. *British Journal of Anaesthesia*, **66**, 541–5.

Bender, K., Senff, H., Wienker, T. F., Speiss-Kiefer, C. & Lehmann-Horn, F. (1990). A linkage study of malignant hyperthermia (MH). *Clinical Genetics*, **37**, 221–5.

Britt, B. A. (1985). Malignant hyperthermia. *Canadian Anaesthetists Society Journal*, **32**, 666–77.

Britt, B. A., Endrenyi, L., Peters, P. L., Kwong, F. H.-F. & Kadijevic, L. (1976). Screening of malignant hyperthermia susceptible families by creatine phosphokinase measurement and other clinical investigations. *Canadian Anaesthetists Society Journal*, **23**, 263–84.

Britt, B. A. & Kalow, W. (1968). Hyper-rigidity and hyperthermia associated with anaesthesia. *Annals of the New York Academy of Sciences*, **151**, 947–58.

Britt, B. A. & Kalow, W. (1970). Malignant hyperthermia: a statistical review. *Canadian Anaesthetists Society Journal*, **17**, 293–315.

Britt, B. A., Locher, W. G. & Kalow, W. (1969). Hereditary aspects of malignant hyperthermia. *Canadian Anaesthetists Society Journal*, **16**, 89–98.

Brownell, A. K. W. (1988). Malignant hyperthermia: relationship to other diseases. *British Journal of Anaesthesia*, **60**, 303–8.

Brownell, A. K. W., Fowlow, S. B. & Paasuke, R. T. (1985). Coexistence of malignant hyperthermia and Duchenne muscular dystrophy in the same pedigree. *Neurology*, **35**, (Suppl. 1), 195.

Cantin, R. Y., Poole, A. & Ryan, J. F. (1986). Malignant hyperthermia. *Oral Surgery, Oral Medicine, Oral Pathology*, **62**, 389–92.

Caroff, S. N., Rosenberg, H., Fletcher, J. E., Heiman-Patterson, T. D. & Mann, S. C. (1987). Malignant hyperthermia susceptibility in neuroleptic malignant syndrome. *Anesthesiology*, **67**, 20–5.

Caswell, A. H. & Brandt, N. R. (1989). Does muscle activation occur by direct mechanical coupling of transverse tubules to sarcoplasmic reticulum? *Trends in Biochemical Sciences*, **14**, 161–5.

Davies, K. (1990). Malignant hyperthermia may be due to a defect in a large Ca^{2+} release channel protein. *Trends in Genetics*, **6**, 171–2.

Denborough, M. A. (1980). The pathopharmacology of malignant hyperpyrexia. *Pharmacology and Therapeutics*[B], **9**, 357–65.

Denborough, M. A., Forster, J. F. A., Lovell, R. R. H., Maplestone, P. A. & Villiers, J. D. (1962). Anaesthetic deaths in a family. *British Journal of Anaesthesia*, **34**, 395–6.

Denborough, M. A., Galloway, G. J. & Hopkinson, K. C. (1982). Malignant hyperpyrexia and sudden infant death syndrome. *Lancet*, **2**, 1068–9.

Denborough, M. A., Hopkinson, K. C. & Banney, D. G. (1988). Firefighting and malignant hyperthermia. *British Medical Journal*, **296**, 1442–3.

Denborough, M. A. & Lovell, R. R. H. (1960). Anaesthetic deaths in a family. *Lancet*, **2**, 45.

Deufel, T. Golla, A., Iles, D., Meinal, A., Meitinger, T., Schindelhauer, D., DeVries, A., Pongratz, D., Maclennan, D. H., Johnson, K. J. & Lehmann-Horn, F. (1992). Evidence for genetic heterogeneity of malignant hyperthermia susceptibility. *American Journal of Human Genetics*, **50**, 1151–61.

Dowben, R. B. (1980). Contractility with special reference to skeletal muscle. In *Medical Physiology*, Vol. 1, ed. V. B. Mountcastle. pp. 82–119. St. Louis: Mosby.

Duncan, C. J. (1989). Dystrophin and the integrity of the sarcolemma in Duchenne muscular dystrophy. *Experientia*, **45**, 175–7.

Ellis, F. R. (1984a). Malignant hyperpyrexia. *Archives of Disease in Childhood*, **59**, 1013–15.

Ellis, F. R. (1984b). European Malignant Hyperpyrexia Group (Editorial). *British Journal of Anaesthesia*, **56**, 1181–2.

Ellis, F. R. (1992). Detecting susceptibility to malignant hyperthermia. *British Medical Journal*, **304**, 791–2.

Ellis, F. R., Green, J. H. & Campbell, I. T. (1991). Muscle activity pH and malignant hyperthermia. *British Journal of Anaesthesia*, **66**, 535–7.

Ellis, F. R. & Halsall, P. J. (1989). Malignant hyperthermia in the Wolf–Hirschhorn syndrome (letter). *Anaesthesia*, **44**, 519.

Ellis, F. R., Halsall, P. J. & Christian, A. S. (1990). Clinical presentation of suspected malignant hyperthermia during anaesthesia in 402 probands. *Anaesthesia*, **45**, 838–41.

Ellis, F. R., Halsall, P. J. & Harriman, D. G. F. (1988). Malignant hyperpyrexia and sudden infant death syndrome. *British Journal of Anaesthesia*, **60**, 28–30.

Ellis, F. R., Hopkins, P. M. Halsall, P. J. & Christian, A. S. (1992). Masseter muscle spasm and the diagnosis of malignant hyperthermia susceptibility. *Anesthesia and Analgesia*, **75**, 143.

Ellis, F. R., Keaney, N. P., Harriman, D. G. F., Sumner, D. W., Kyei-Mensah, K., Tyrrell, J. H., Hargreaves, J. B., Parikh, R. K. & Mulrooney, P. L. (1972). Screening for malignant hyperpyrexia. *British Medical Journal*, **3**, 559–61.

European Malignant Hyperpyrexia Group (1984). A protocol for the investigation of malignant hyperpyrexia susceptibility. *British Journal of Anaesthesia*, **56**, 1267–9.

European Malignant Hyperpyrexia Group (1988). Laboratory diagnosis of malignant hyperpyrexia susceptibility (MHS). *British Journal of Anaesthesia*, **57**, 1038–46.

Fagerlund, T., Islander, G., Ranklev, E., Harbitz, I., Hauge, J. B., Møokleby, E. & Berg, K. (1992). Genetic recombination between malignant hyperthermia and calcium release channel in skeletal muscle. *Clinical Genetics*, **41**, 270–2.

Fishbein, W. N., Muldoon, S. M., Deuster, P. A. & Armbrustmacher, V. W. (1985). Myoadenylate deaminase deficiency and malignant hyperthermia susceptibility: Is there a relationship? *Biochemical Medicine*, **34**, 344–54.

Flewellen, E. H., Nelson, T. E., Jones, W. P., Arens, J. F. & Wagner, D. L. (1983). Dantrolene dose response in awake man: implications for management of malignant hyperthermia. *Anesthesiology*, **59**, 275–80.

Foster, P. S. (1990). Malignant hyperpyrexia. *International Journal of Biochemistry*, **22**, 1217–22.

Froster-Iskenius, U. G., Waterson, J. R. & Hall, J. G. (1988). A recessive form of congenital contractures and torticollis associated with malignant hyperthermia. *Journal of Medical Genetics*, **25**, 104–12.

Fuji, J., Otsu, K., Zorzato, F., DeLeon, S., Khanna, V. K., Weiler, J. E., O'Brien, P. J. & MacLennan, D. H. (1991). Identification of a mutation in porcine ryanodine receptor associated with malignant hyperthermia. *Science*, **253**, 448–51.

Gallen, J. S. (1991). Propofol does not trigger malignant hyperthermia. *Anesthesia and Analgesia*, **72**, 413.

Galloway, G. J. & Denborough, M.A. (1986). Suxamethonium chloride and malignant hyperpyrexia. *British Journal of Anaesthesia*, **58**, 447–50.

Gillard, E. F., Otsu, K. Fujii, J., Duff, C., deLeon, S., Khanna, V. K., Britt, B. A., Worton, R. G. & MacLennan, D. H. (1992). Polymorphisms and deduced amino acid substitutes in the coding sequence of the ryanodine receptor (RYR1) gene in individuals with malignant hyperthermia. *Genomics*, **13**, 1247–54.

Gillard, E. F., Otsu, K., Fuji, J., Khanna, V. K., deLeon, S.,

Derdemezi, J., Britt, B. A., Duff, C. L., Worton, R. G. & MacLennan, D. H. (1991). A substitution of cysteine for arginine 614 in the ryanodine receptor is potentially causative of human malignant hyperthermia. *Genomics*, **11**, 751–5.

Ginsburg, R. & Purcell-Jones, G. (1988). Malignant hyperthermia in the Wolf–Hirschhorn syndrome. *Anaesthesia*, **43**, 386–8.

Gronert, G. A., Milde, J. H. & Theye, R. A. (1976). Porcine malignant hyperthermia induced by halothane and succinylcholine. *Anesthesiology*, **44**, 124–32.

Hackl, W., Mauritz, W., Schemper, M., Winkler, M., Sporn, P. & Steinbereithner, K. (1990). Prediction of malignant hyperthermia susceptibility: statistical evaluation of clinical signs. *British Journal of Anaesthesia*, **64**, 425–9.

Hackl, W., Winkler, M., Mauritz, W., Sporn, P. & Steinbereithner, K. (1991). Muscle biopsy for diagnosis of malignant hyperthermia susceptibility in two patients with severe exercise-induced myolysis. *British Journal of Anaesthesia*, **66**, 138–40.

Halsall, P.J. & Ellis, F. R. (1992). Does postoperative pyrexia indicate malignant hyperthermia susceptibility? *British Journal of Anaesthesia*, **68**, 209–10.

Harriman, D. G.F. (1988). Malignant hyperthermia myopathy – a critical review. *British Journal of Anaesthesia*, **60**, 309–16.

Harrison, G. G. & Isaacs, H. (1992). Malignant hyperthermia – An historial vignette. *Anaesthesia*, **47**, 54–6.

Heiman-Patterson, T., Martino, C., Rosenberg, H., Fletcher, J. & Tahmoush, A. (1988). Malignant hyperthermia in myotonia congenita. *Neurology*, **38**, 810–12.

Heiman-Patterson, T. D., Rosenberg, H. R., Binning, C. P. S. & Tahmoush, A. J. (1986). King–Denborough syndrome: contracture testing and literature review. *Pediatric Neurology*, **2**, 175–7.

Heytens, L., Heffron, J. J. A. & Camu, F. (1991). The caffeine contracture test for malignant hyperthermia: caffeine citrate, caffeine benzoate or caffeine free base? *Acta Anaesthesiologica Scandinavica*, **35**, 541–4.

Hogan, K., Couch, F., Powers, P. A. & Gregg, R. G. (1992). A cysteine-for-arginine substitution (R614C) in the human muscle calcium release channel cosegregates with malignant hyperthermia. *Anesthesia and Analgesia*, **75**, 441–8.

Hopkins, P. M., Ellis, F. R. & Halsall, P. J. (1992). Inconsistency of data linking the ryanodine receptor and malignant hyperthermia genes. *Anesthesiology*, **76**, 659.

Isaacs, H. & Gericke, G. (1990). Concurrence of malignant hyperthermia and congenital abnormalities. *Muscle and Nerve*, **13**, 915–17.

Joffe, M., Savage, N. & Silove, M. (1992). The biochemistry of malignant hyperthermia: recent concepts. *International Journal of Biochemistry*, **24**, 387–98.

Kalow, W., Britt, B. A., Terreau, M. E. & Haist, C. (1970). Metabolic error of muscle metabolism after recovery from malignant hyperthermia. *Lancet*, **2**, 895–8.

King, J. D. & Denborough, M. A. (1973). Anesthetic-induced malignant hyperpyrexia in children. *Journal of Pediatrics*, **83**, 37–40.

Krivosic-Horber, R. (1988). Optimal treatment for malignant hyperthermia today. *Acta Anaesthesiologica Belgica*, **39** (Suppl. 2), 255–9.

Krovosic-Horber, R., Adnet, P. & Reyford, H. (1991). Relationship between exercise-induced myolysis and malignant hyperthermia. *British Journal of Anaesthesia*, **67**, 221–8.

Lai, F. A., Erickson, H. P., Rousseau, E., Liu, Q.-Y. & Meissner, G. (1988). Purification and reconstitution of the calcium release channel from skeletal muscle. *Nature*, **331**, 315–19.

Larach, M. G., (1989), for the North American Malignant Hyperthermia Group. Standardization of the caffeine halothane muscle contracture test. *Anesthesia and Analgesia*, **69**, 511–15.

Larach, M. G., Landis, J. R., Bunn, J. S. & Diaz, M. (1992). The North American Hyperthermia Registry Prediction of malignant hyperthermia susceptibility in low-risk subjects. *Anesthesiology*, **76**, 16–27.

Larach, M. G., Rosenberg, H., Larach, D. R. & Broennle, A. M. (1987). Prediction of malignant hyperthermia susceptibility by clinical signs. *Anesthesiology*, **66**, 547–50.

Lehmann-Horn, F. & Iaizzo, P. A. (1990). Are myotonias and periodic paralysis associated with susceptibility to malignant hyperthermia? *British Journal of Anaesthesia*, **65**, 692–7.

Lennmarken, C., Rutberg, H. & Henriksson, K. G. (1987). Abnormal relaxation rates in subjects susceptible to malignant hyperthermia. *Acta Neurologica Scandinavica*, **75**, 81–3.

Levitt, R. C. (1992). Prospects for the diagnosis of malignant hyperthermia susceptibility using molecular genetic approaches. *Anesthesiology*, **76**, 1039–48.

Levitt, R. C., Nouri, N., Jedlicka, A. E., McKusick, V. A., Marks, A. R., Shutack, J. G., Fletcher, J. E., Rosenberg, H. & Meyers, D. A. (1991). Evidence for genetic heterogeneity in malignant hyperthermia susceptibility. *Genomics*, **11**, 543–7.

Lombard, T. P. & Couper, J. L. (1988). Malignant hyperthermia in a black adolescent. *South African Medical Journal*, **73**, 726–9.

McCarthy, T. V., Healy, J. M. S., Heffron, J. J. A., Lehane, M., Deufel, T., Lehmann-Horn, F., Farall, M. & Johnson, K. (1990). Localization of the malignant hyperthermia susceptibility locus to human chromosome 19q 12–13.2. *Nature*, **343**, 562–4.

McKusick, V. A. (1987). The morbid anatomy of the human genome: a review of gene mapping in clinical medicine [third of four parts]. *Medicine*, **66**, 237–96.

MacLennan, D. H. (1992). The genetic basis of malignant hyperthermia. *Trends in Pharmacological Sciences*, **13**, 330–4.

MacLennan, D. H., Duff, C., Zorzato, F., Fujii, J., Phillips, M., Korneluk, R. G., Fordis, W., Britt, B. A. & Worton, R. G. (1990). Ryanodine receptor gene is a candidate for predisposition to malignant hyperthermia. *Nature*, **343**, 559–61.

McMorris, F. A., Chen, T. R., Ricciuti, F., Tischfield, J., Creagan, R. & Ruddle, F. (1973). Chromosome assignment in man of the genes for two hexosephosphate isomerases. *Science*, **179**, 1129–31.

McPherson, E. & Taylor, Jr. C. A. (1982). The genetics of malignant hyperthermia: evidence for heterogeneity. *American Journal of Medical Genetics*, **11**, 273–85.

Mason, E. B. (1983). *Human Physiology*, pp. 121–33. Menlo Park CA: The Benjamin/Cummings Publishing Co. Inc.

Mauritz, W., Sporin, P. & Steinbereithner, K. (1988). Malignant hyperthermia susceptibility confirmed in both parents and probands. A report of three Austrian families. *Acta Anaesthesiologica Scandinavica*, **32**, 24–6.

Mickelson, J. R., Gallant, E. M., Litterer, L. A., Johnson, K. M., Rampel, W. E. & Louis, C. F. (1988). Abnormal sarcoplasmic reticulum ryanodine receptor in malignant hyperthermia. *Journal of Biological Chemistry*, **263**, 9310–15.

Moulds, R. F. W. & Denborough, M. A. (1974a). Biochemical basis of malignant hyperpyrexia. *British Medical Journal*, **2**, 241–4.

Moulds, R. F. W. & Denborough, M. A. (1974b). Identification of susceptibility to malignant hyperpyrexia. *British Medical Journal*, **2**, 245–7.

Mulrooney, L. (1988). Counselling on Malignant Hyperpyrexia (Editorial). *Anaesthesia*, **43**, 727–8.

Neubauer, K. R. & Kaufman, R.D. (1985). Another use for mass spectrometry: detection and monitoring of malignant hyperthermia. *Anesthesia and Analgesia*, **64**, 837–9.

Ohnishi, S. T., Katagi, H., Ohnishi, T. & Brownell, A. K. W. (1988). Detection of malignant hyperthermia susceptibility using a spin label technique on red blood cells. *British Journal of Anaesthesia*, **61**, 565–8.

Ohnishi, S. T. & Ohnishi, T. (1988). Halothane induced disorder of red cell membranes of subjects susceptible to malignant hyperthermia. *Cell Biochemistry and Function*, **6**, 257–61.

Okumura, F., Crocker, B. D. & Denborough, M.A. (1979). Identification of susceptibility to malignant hyperpyrexia in swine. *British Journal of Anaesthesia*, **51**, 171–6.

Olgin, J., Rosenberg, H., Allen, G., Seestedt, R. & Chance, B. (1991). A blinded comparison of non-invasive, *in vivo* phosphorus nuclear magnetic resonance spectroscopy and the in vitro halothane/caffeine contracture test in the evaluation of malignant hyperthermia susceptibility. *Anaesthesia and Analgesia*, **72**, 36–47.

Olkers, A., Meyers, D. A., Meyers, S., Taylor, E. W. Fletcher, J. E., Rosenberg, H. Isaacs, H. & Levitt, R. C. (1992). Adult muscle sodium channel α-subunit is a gene candidate for malignant hyperthermia susceptibility. *Genomics*, **14**, 829–31.

Ørding, H. (1988). Diagnosis of susceptibility to malignant hyperthermia in man. *British Journal of Anaesthesia*, **60**, 287–302.

Ørding, H. (1989). Influence of propanolol on the *in vitro* response to caffeine and halothane in malignant hyperthermia-susceptible muscle. *Acta Anaesthesiologica Scandinavica*, **33**, 405–8.

Ørding, H, Hedengran A. M. & Skovgaard L. T. (1991). Evaluation of 119 anaesthetics received after investigation for susceptibility to malignant hyperthermia. *Acta Anaesthesiologica Scandinavica*, **35**, 711–16.

Otsu, K., Khanna, V. K., Archibald, A. L. & MacLennan, D. H. (1991). Cosegregation of porcine malignant hyperthermia and a probably causal mutation in the skeletal muscle ryanodine receptor gene in backcross families. *Genomics*, **11**, 744–50.

Paasuke, R. T. & Brownell, A. K. W. (1986). Serum creatine kinase level as a screening test for susceptibility to malignant hyperthermia. *Journal of the American Medical Association*, **255**, 769–71.

Payen, J.-F., Bourdon, L., Mezin, P., Jacquot, C., le Bas, J.-F., Streglitz, P. & Benabid, A. L. (1991). Susceptibility to malignant hyperthermia detected non-invasively. *Lancet*, **337**, 1550–1.

Payne, M. R. & Rudnick, S. E. (1989). Regulation of vertebrate striated muscle contraction. *Trends in Biochemical Sciences*, **14**, 357–9.

Pippin, L. K., Armstrong, J. & Schreiber, T. (1988). Malignant hyperthermia in a patient with King syndrome. *Journal of the American Association of Nurse Anesthesia*, **56**, 234–7.

Rosenberg, H. (1989). Standards for halothane/caffeine contracture test. *Anesthesia and Analgesia*, **69**, 429–30.

Schulte-Sasse, U. & Eberlein, H. J. (1987). Informationsdienst für Maligne-Hyperthermie-Notfalle. *Deutsche Medizinische Wochenschrift*, **112**, 614.

Sessler, D. I. Malignant hyperthermia. (1986). *Journal of Pediatrics*, **109**, 9–14.

Shuaib, A., Paasuke, K. T. & Brownell, A. K. W. (1987). Central core disease, clinical features in 13 patients. *Medicine*, **66**, 389–96.

Smith, C. & Bampton, P. R. (1977). Inheritance of reaction to halothane anaesthesia in pigs. *Genetical Research Cambridge*, **29**, 287–92.

Thomas, M. A., Rock, E. & Viret, J. (1991). Membrane properties of the sarcolemma and sarcoplasmic reticulum of pigs susceptible to malignant hyperthermia. Action of halothane. *Clinica Chimica Acta*, **200**, 201–10.

Urwyler, A., Ellis, F. R., Halsall, P. J. & Hopkins, P. M. (1990). Muscle relaxation rates in individuals susceptible to malignant hyperthermia. *British Journal of Anaesthesia*, **65**, 421–3.

Watson, C. B., Reierson, N. & Norfleet, E.A. (1986). Clinically significant muscle weakness induced by oral dantrolene sodium prophylaxis for malignant hyperthermia. *Anesthesiology*, **65**, 312–14.

Windholz, M. (ed.) (1983). *The Merck Index*, 10th edn. Rahway, NJ: Merk.

Younker, D., De Vore, M. & Hartlage, P. (1984). Malignant hyperthermia and glucose-6-phosphate dehydrogenase deficiency. *Anesthesiology*, **60**, 601–3.

PART X   Miscellaneous systems showing genetic variability in responses to drugs

28   Chlorpropamide–alcohol flushing

INTRODUCTION

WHEN some diabetics who are on treatment with chlorpropamide consume ethanol they are aware of a flushing of the face and sometimes of the neck, most intense over the malar region and around the eyes where it may be accompanied by conjunctival suffusion (Johnston *et al*. 1984). This reaction may be seen by observers. In a minority of patients exhibiting chlorpropamide–alcohol flushing (CPAF) there is also breathlessness and wheezing.

CPAF was described very soon after chlorpropamide was introduced into clinical practice. However, it was only later that it became the subject of close and critical study (Bertram *et al*. 1956).

DIFFERENTIATION FROM FLUSHING ON ETHANOL ALONE

It is well known that some persons flush after consuming ethanol alone. There are two points that differentiate this phenomenon from CPAF, namely:

1 Many CPAF positive individuals do not flush with ethanol alone.
2 The ethanol-alone flush is more pronounced with increasing doses, whereas CPAF seems to be more of a threshold phenomenon occurring after a relatively small dose (e.g. 8 g) of ethanol (Johnston *et al*. 1984).

INHERITANCE

In families with Mason-type diabetes (mild familial diabetes with dominant inheritance) an autosomal

manner of inheritance of chlorpropamide–alcohol flushing was described by Leslie & Pyke (1978). In their researches the test was carried out with a single 250 mg dose of chlorpropamide followed by 20 ml sherry at 12 and also at 36 hours later. The results were recorded as subjective assessments. It is unclear how many of the subjects may have already been taking chlorpropamide regularly as therapy. Other families with diabetes of maturity-onset type in young persons failed to show an autosomal dominant inheritance of CPAF (Dreyer *et al*. 1980; Panzram & Adolph 1982).

Subsequent studies mounted to check the original observation of the pattern of inheritance of CPAF have been small and the results they have given have been contradictory (Hillson & Hockaday 1984; Wiles & Pyke 1984).

There does not appear to be published a family study to elucidate the genetics of CPAF using a rigorously standardized test procedure.

ASSOCIATIONS WITH DIABETES

Two sets of associations have been described: first, an association of CPAF with diabetes, and secondly within populations of diabetics an association of CPAF with the absence of complications.

The original accounts of these associations were based on surveys performed with a dose of sherry given either to persons who were already being treated with chlorpropamide (CPAF positives 86%) or to persons who had been given one oral dose of chlorpropamide before the test (CPAF positives

Table 28.1. *Prevalence of chlorpropamide–alcohol flush (CPAF) in 71 patients by type of diabetes and by chlorpropamide (CP) treatment category*

	Number of patients		CPAF+ (%)
	Total	CPAF+	
NIDD	53	34	64
CP+	14	12	86
CP−	39	22	56
IDD	18	5	28
Total	71	39	55

CPAF+, CPAF positive; NIDD, non-insulin dependent diabetes: IDD, insulin dependent diabetes; CP+, NIDD patients on CP therapy; CP−, NIDD patients not on CP therapy. *From:* Segal *et al.* 1985.

Table 28.2. *Serum chlorpropamide (CP) concentrations (μg/ml) in CPAF-positive and -negative patients, by type of diabetes and by CP treatment category*

	Total group	CPAF+	CPAF−
NIDD			
CP +	143 ± 68	147 ± 70	122 ± 52
	(14)	(12)	(2)
CP −	17 ± 7	17 ± 8	17 ± 5
	(34)	(18)	(16)
IDD	18 ± 9	15 ± 5	19 ± 10
	(18)	(5)	(13)

Values are means ± SD for the number of determinations in parentheses.
NIDD, non-insulin dependent diabetes; IDD, insulin dependent diabetes. *From:* Segal *et al.* 1985.

14%). No baseline observations with ethanol alone had been performed (Hillson & Hockaday 1984).

It is these associations which make CPAF really of potential importance in clinical medicine. The factors which determine which diabetic develops complications and which does not have been almost a complete mystery, so anything which sheds light on the problem would be a substantial step forward in knowledge.

It has been stated that the association of CPAF positivity with a family history of non-insulin dependent diabetes is dependent on age. There is, however, no significant difference in the CPAF positivity frequency in propositi or first-degree relatives when individuals below and above 30 years of age are contrasted (Hillson & Hockaday 1984).

Studies of non-insulin dependent diabetics (NIDD) with most of the subjects taking chlorpropamide long-term showed CPAF frequencies of about 65% (Hillson & Hockaday 1984; Segal *et al.* 1985). In NIDD frequencies have been found of 30% of CPAF at 12 hours after a single 250 mg tablet of chlorpropamide and 38.5% (F 5%, M 19.6%) after four tablets of chlorpropamide by Bonisolli *et al.* (1985) and 73% after 250 mg chlorpropamide for 14 days (Wiles & Pyke 1984) (see Tables 28.1, 28.2 and 28.3).

In insulin-dependent diabetes (IDD) a single tablet test revealed a frequency of CPAF of 5 to 28% (Leslie & Pyke 1978; Pontiroli *et al.* 1983; Barnett *et al.* 1981a; Segal *et al.* 1985). In IDD Bonisolli *et*

al. (1985) found 36.5% CPAF (F 64.7, M 12.5%) after four tablets of chlorpropamide. Using a 7 day test (which gives plasma chlorpropamide levels approaching steady state concentrations) a CPAF positivity rate of 40% was found (Wiles & Pyke 1984).

It would appear, therefore, that at similar chlorpropamide plasma concentrations the CPAF positive response is more frequent in NIDD than in IDD but is more frequent in both types than in normal controls (Bonisolli *et al.* 1985).

Köbberling *et al.* (1980), who used the same test as Leslie & Pyke (1978), found that it was poorly reproducible, and likewise with a test using a skin temperature probe. There was no statistically significant association of positive responses with any type of diabetes.

Flushers and non-flushers seem to be very similar as regards their insulin production following oral doses of glucose, naloxone or salicylate (Hershon *et al.* 1982). Groop *et al.* (1984a) found that the basal and glucagon-stimulated serum C-peptide concentrations were higher and the insulin binding to erythrocytes lower in CPAF positive than in CPAF negative diabetics. The two phenotypes were not significantly different as regards the concentrations of their plasma lipids or haemostatic factors (Micossi *et al.* 1982).

The frequency of CPAF positivity in non-diabetics has been investigated with the single tablet test and showed rates of less than 10% (Leslie & Pyke 1978;

Table 28.3. Frequency of CPAF (assessed by agreement of subject and observer as 'flusher' or 'non-flusher', and as 'intermediate' if disagreed), and plasma chlorpropamide levels in 76 NIDDs after 250 mg of chlorpropamide daily for 1, 7 or 14 days

	Day 1 (48)			Day 7 (16)			Day 14 (56)		
	Non-flushers	Intermediate	Flushers	Non-flushers	Intermediate	Flushers	Non-flushers	Intermediate	Flushers
Number of subjects	29 (60%)	4(8%)	15(31%)	8(50%)	0	8(50%)	11 (20%)	7 12%)	38 (68%) *
Chlorpropamide (mg/l)	22.7±1.0	18.2±0.6	23.4±1.9	74.8±10.3	–	72.4±8.4	66.2±8.7	68.2±8.8	70.1±3.7

Mean values ± SEM are shown. * p<0.001 compared with day 1.
From: Wiles & Pyke 1984.

Leslie *et al.* 1979). When a four-tablet test (to give a higher plasma chlorpropamide level) was used 26 of 32 young normal subjects gave a positive response and six a partial response (Hoskins *et al.* 1987).

ASSOCIATIONS WITH THE COMPLICATIONS OF DIABETES

Non-insulin dependent diabetics who were CPAF positive had a lower frequency of proteinuria (Barnett *et al.* 1981b), retinopathy (Leslie *et al.* 1979) and large vessel disease (Barnett & Pyke 1980) than CPAF negative persons who had been diabetic for a similar length of time. Likewise, amongst IDD the CPAF positives had a lower frequency of retinopathy and proteinuria (Barnett *et al.* 1981a).

The freedom of CPAF-positive diabetics from retinopathy has been both confirmed (Micossi *et al.* 1981) and denied (Carducci *et al.* 1981; Groop *et al.* 1984a), as also has been their comparative freedom from large vessel disease (Jentorp & Almer 1981; Laakso *et al.* 1983).

Hitherto it seems that no study has been published which reveals the results of a prospective survey of previously phenotyped patients to see what becomes of them over a period of years.

ASSOCIATION WITH ACETYLATOR PHENOTYPE

Bonisolli *et al.* (1985) found two associations:

1 fast acetylators were more frequently CPAF-positive than slow acetylators;
2 the percentage of sulphadimidine acetylated showed a positive correlation with speed of increase of skin temperature.

The meanings of these associations are at present obscure.

THE POSSIBILITY OF AN *IN VITRO* TEST

The features of CPAF are very similar to the reaction experienced by individuals who are consuming disulfiram when they ingest ethanol, a reaction which is believed to be mediated by acetaldehyde. Ethanol is oxidized to acetaldehyde by alcohol dehydro-genase and then to acetate by aldehyde dehydrogenase which is inhibited by chlorpropamide. Accurate assays of plasma acetaldehyde concentrations have revealed a rise which is greater in CPAF positive 'flushers' than in 'non-flushers' (Jerntorp *et al.* 1980; Barnett *et al.* 1981c; Jerntorp 1983).

It has been shown that dialysed haemolysates of human erythrocytes with added NAD can metabolize acetaldehyde (Inoue *et al.* 1978). Disulfiram is a powerful inhibitor. The erythrocyte aldehyde dehydrogenase resembles the high K_m acetaldehyde dehydrogenase of liver (which is strongly inhibited by disulfiram). There is also a second acetaldehyde dehydrogenase in liver which is only weakly inhibited by disulfiram.

Flushers are more sensitive to disulfiram than non-flushers and this may indicate that their erythrocytic aldehyde dehydrogenase is different (Johnston *et al.* 1984). However, no evidence of any electrophoretic difference between the red cell aldehyde dehydrogenase of flushers and non-flushers could be revealed under various conditions by Johnston *et al.* (1986).

Acetaldehyde was found to be metabolized more slowly *in vitro* by erythrocyte homogenates from flushers than from non-flushers (Ohlin *et al.* 1982) and erythrocyte aldehyde dehydrogenase (ALDH) was diminished in activity *in vivo* by chlorpropamide in flushers but not in non-flushers. Hillson *et al.* (1987), however, measured RBC ALDH activity in 21 diabetics on long-term chlorpropamide therapy and found it to be no different in flushers and non-flushers and not correlated with chlorpropamide concentration.

CIRCULATING METENKEPHALIN IN CPAF

It has been found that CPAF can be imitated by the administration of the metenkephalin analogue DAMME [(D-Ala^2, MePhe^4, MNet (*O*)-ol) enkephalin] and blocked by naloxone (Medbak *et al.* 1981). A similar rise of circulating metenkephalin concentration occurs after chlorpropamide and ethanol in diabetics and non-diabetics and in flushers and non-flushers. Intravenous naloxone does not prevent the metenkephalin rise even when it blocks the flush. Intravenous ethanol administration which is followed by CPAF is not followed by a rise in metenkephalin concentration (Wiles & Pyke 1984).

In view of the foregoing it seems unlikely that met-enkephalins mediate CPAF.

Ethanol intoxication (as assessed by errors made when typing a simple piece of text with an electric typewriter) was significantly greater in CPA flushers than non-flushers in the survey of Baraniuk *et al.* (1987). This effect could be reversed by naloxone in the flushers but not in the non-flushers. The suggestion was made that acetaldehyde condensation products or other ethanol–opioid interactions were important only in the flushers and antagonized by naloxone.

PROSTAGLANDIN SYNTHETASE INHIBITORS

The prostaglandin synthetase inhibitors aspirin (Strakosch *et al.* 1980), naproxen (Jerntorp *et al.* 1981) and indomethacin (Barnett *et al.* 1980) can block CPAF, suggesting that prostaglandins may be involved in producing the flush. There is, however, no rigorous experimental proof of this idea.

THE PHENOTYPING TEST

Much of the controversy concerning CPAF arises because the details of the way in which the test has been performed vary between investigators. A casual clinical observation like CPAF needs critical examination before it can be accepted as a reliable phenotyping test. The account of the event may be a subjective one from the patient or the flushing may be witnessed by an observer. In a series of 120 tests the subjects and observers agreed on the results in 109 (91%) but of course there may be observer bias in assessing the presence or absence of a flush (Wiles & Pyke 1984). The repeatability of the subjectively assessed CPAF has been estimated as about 80% (Hillson & Hockaday 1984).

Another way of assessing the result is by measuring the skin temperature. A rise in skin temperature of 1 to 2 °C has been used by different workers as indicating the presence of a flush (see, for example, Fig. 28.1).

Two techniques have been employed to assess

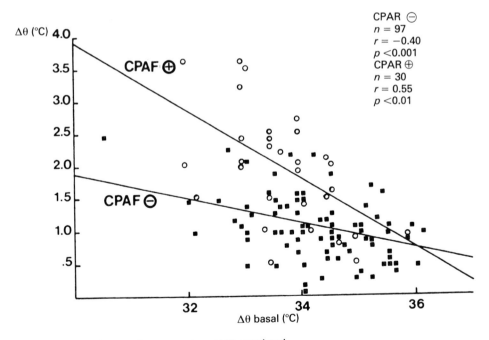

Fig. 28.1. The elevation in temperature ($\Delta\theta$) correlated with the basal temperature in individuals showing clinically positive (CPAF+; ○) and clinically negative (CPAF−; ■) responses. (From Guillausseau *et al.* 1984.)

skin temperature rise, namely thermography and a thermocouple. With the former there is no overlap between flushers and non-flushers whereas an overlap was found using a thermocouple (Wiles & Pyke 1984).

The rise of skin temperature produced in the test is higher the lower the basal temperature and the separation between flushers and non-flushers is greater at lower basal skin temperatures of 32 °C and below (Hillson & Hockaday 1984; Wiles & Pyke 1984). In order to ensure this a room with a controlled stable temperature of 20.0 ± SD 0.3 °C (Hillson *et al.* 1987) or 20 to 22 °C (Groop *et al.* 1984a) is required (see Fig. 28.2).

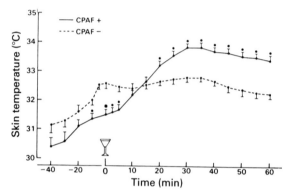

Fig. 28.2. Changes in facial skin temperature after intake of alcohol and chlorpropamide in 160 patients (mean ± SEM). *$p < 0.001$, significance of differences from placebo. (From Groop *et al.* 1984a.)

A weak correlation was found between plasma chlorpropamide concentration (up to 40 mg/l) and rise in facial temperature by Groop *et al.* (1984b). However, Groop *et al.* (1984c) found that 'flushers' (determined subjectively and objectively) had significantly higher blood acetaldehyde and chlorpropamide concentrations than 'non-flushers'. They suggested that CPAF is caused by the inhibition of aldehyde dehydrogenase by chlorpropamide and emphasize that its plasma concentration should, like alcohol, be as standardized as possible.

Segal *et al.* (1985) found no significant difference in plasma chlorpropamide concentrations between flushers and non-flushers who were on long-term treatment with chlorpropamide at the time of testing. The pharmacokinetics of chlorpropamide

showed no significant differences between flushers and non-flushers (Wiles & Pyke 1984).

The effect of prolonged chlorpropamide treatment on facial temperature rise was assessed by Fiu *et al.* (1983); they found that out of 20 patients who had been negative flushers on a single dose test, 15 became positive after 7 days' treatment which brought them close to a steady-state plasma concentration. It is interesting to note that (1) there appeared to be an excellent separation in the facial temperature rise between the two groups on the second test, (2) the plasma chlorpropamide concentrations were not significantly different between flushers and non-flushers on either occasion.

Cheek temperature rises were measured after alcohol by Hillson *et al.* (1983) in 43 diabetics receiving maintenance chlorpropamide therapy. They recorded whether these patients had experienced flushing sensations after alcohol at home. There was no correlation between the two observations. Unfortunately, many of these details about the factors which influence the test were not known when the early surveys were made.

It is still not clear which is the better for phenotyping, a low chlorpropamide plasma concentration or a high one. No very sophisticated examination of the kinetics, inhibition, etc. of erythrocyte aldehyde dehydrogenase in relation to chlorpropamide appears to have been made. So the most suitable dosage schedule of chlorpropamide to detect the phenotype remains in doubt.

A dose of 8 g of ethanol given in 100 ml of fruit juice is sufficient to produce the response, though a dose computed according to body weight has been advocated by Guillausseau *et al.* (1984).

As implied above an ambient temperature of about 20 °C seems essential to conduct the test so as to lower the facial skin temperature to 32 °C or below (Wiles & Pyke 1984; Groop *et al.* 1984a). Thermography may be a superior technique to assess facial skin temperature and this needs to be observed for a sufficient time before and after ethanol ingestion (Leslie *et al.* 1979).

A baseline test with ethanol alone prior to which the subjects should not have been exposed to any drugs is perhaps an Utopian ideal, but it does allow non-specific (i.e. ethanol only) flushers to be identified (Hillson & Hockaday 1984).

The features of some seemingly successful testing procedures are detailed in Table 28.4; it is a pity

Table 28.4. *Some successful chlorpropamide–alcohol flushing surveys*

Reference	Location of study	Number and type of patient or volunteer	Chlorpropamide ingestion prior to test	Alcohol dose	Temperature of room in which test conducted	Method of assessing facial skin temperature	Criteria for positive temperature response	Subjective sensations recorded also?	Objectively visible phenomena recorded also?	Percentage exhibiting positive CPAF response
Micossi *et al.* 1982	Milan	108 type II diabetics	250 mg the evening before the test	40 ml sherry (Tío Pepe)	17 °C	Sensor probes readings before ethanol and 20 min later	1.4 ± SD 0.85 °C in positives; 0.4 ± SD 0.15 °C in negatives	Yes	Yes	17 (non specific flushers excluded)
Fui *et al.* 1983	London	20 diabetics (10 type I and 10 type II) with negative responses to standard placebo-controlled CPAF tests (The type II diabetics had been treated with glibenclamide & metformin)	250 mg chlorpropamide every morning for 7 days	40 ml sherry	21 ± 1 °C	Thermocouples applied to both cheeks. The temp. was observed to stabilize before the test	Observed for 45 min after alcohol ingestion	Yes	Yes	15 had flush - subjectively and objectively. Their increase in skin temp. plotted against basal temp. gave a quite different curve to the 5 negatives
Groop *et al.* 1984a	Helsinki	21 non-diabetic controls 160 type II diabetics	Regular treatment and diet 250 mg chlorpropamide the previous evening	60 ml vinum medicale	20 to 22 °C	Skin thermometer reading every 5 min for 1 h before and 1 h after the alcohol dose	Peak rise 2.8 ± 0.1 °C in positives and 0.9 ± 0.1 °C in negatives. Separation point 1.5 °C rise	Not clear	Yes	27.5 in patients on diet or oral anti-diabetic drugs
Guillauseau *et al.* 1984	Paris	41 non-diabetics 30 type I diabetics 56 type II diabetics	250 mg the evening before	40 ml sherry	20 ± 1 °C	Electric skin thermometer resolution 0.1 °C observed to be stable for 20 min before alcohol and measured every 5 min afterwards for 1 h	Wilkin's index (I)[a]	Yes	Yes	28.7 overall

Table 28.4. (*cont.*)

Reference	Location of study	Number and type of patient or volunteer	Chloropropamide ingestion prior to test	Alcohol dose	Temperature of room in which test conducted	Method of assessing facial skin temperature	Criteria for positive temperature response	Subjective sensations recorded also?	Objectively visible phenomena recorded also?	Percentage exhibiting positive CPAF response
Bonisolli et al. 1985	Milan	15 controls 74 type I diabetics 109 type II diabetics	Insulin not withdrawn None on chlor-propamide treatment before testing for CPAF. Oral hypo-glycaemics (but not insulin) withdrawn 72 h before testing for CPAF	40 ml Martini vermouth (a) 12 h after placebo and (b) after 4 doses of CP 250 mg BD for 2 days	23 °C and skin temp. observed to be steady 30 min before test	Thermocouple probe discrimination 0.01 °C with chart recorder	2 °C, or for differential speed of ascent of temperature 9° angle	Yes	Yes	Controls 20 type I 36.5 type II 38.5 (non-specific flushers excluded)
Segal et al. 1985	Tel-Hashomer	18 type I diabetics 53 type II diabetics	250 mg 12 h before the test On regular CP. 250 mg 12 h before the test	40 ml dry vermouth 18% ethanol	24 °C	Skin thermometer measured every 5 min until stabilization	Peak temp. rise above basal more or less than 1.2 °C	Yes	Yes	See Table 28.2
Hoskins et al. 1987	London	23 young healthy volunteers	250 mg chlorpropamide BID for 2 days before test which occurred 2 h after last tablet	9 ml 90% ethanol in 100 ml lemon squash	Not clear 'maintained at 0.3 °C of starting temp.'	Thermocouple recorded every 5 min until stable and for 30 min after alcohol	$\geqslant 35\%$ of possible rise regarded as positive (assuming 36.5 °C to be the maximum)	Yes	Yes	18 positive 5 intermediate none negative

[a] $I = \dfrac{\Theta max - 20}{37 - \Theta max} \left| \dfrac{\Theta B - 20}{37 - \Theta B} \right.$

where ΘB = basal temperature, Θmax = temperature at 30 minutes after alcohol; the assumptions are made that the ambient temperature is 20 °C and the core temperature of the body is 37 °C.

CP, chlorpropamide; CPAF, chlorpropamide–alcohol flush; BID, twice daily.

that none of these workers provide a frequency distribution of the temperature change recorded. If such a histogram were clearly bimodal and the readings repeatable in individuals it would form a solid basis on which to establish a Mendelian character.

The whole situation has been made more complex by the findings of Hoskins *et al.* (1987) that most healthy young persons are CPAF positive with their four tablet test. This might indicate that CPAF negativity is a phenomenon that develops with age. There is a suggestion in the results of Groop *et al.* (1984a) and Guillausseau *et al.* (1984) that the basal skin temperature (i.e. before ethanol) is lower in CPAF positive persons than in non-flushers. This raises the possibility that vasomotor tone might differ between flushers and non-flushers after taking chlorpropamide but before taking ethanol.

CONCLUSION

Any test which promises to explain why some individuals become diabetic and why some diabetics develop serious complications is worthy of a lot of attention.

The chlorpropamide-flushing test has been the subject of a great deal of disagreement. The causes of the confusion have been enumerated by Hillson & Hockaday (1984). However, it does seem to be fairly universally agreed that:

1 some individuals are flushers whilst others are non-flushers (even though there might be some lack of repeatability);
2 the frequency of flushers is higher in NIDD than in IDD.

There does not seem to have been published any account of experiments to evaluate the influence of the known variability in aldehyde dehydrogenase (discussed in another chapter) on the chlorpropamide–alcohol flush phenomenon. This seems a pity because chlorpropamide is an inhibitor of aldehyde dehydrogenase (Medbak *et al.* 1981).

Further efforts to evaluate this phenomenon and its underlying mechanisms in healthy persons and in diabetics would seem warranted.

The author would like to express his gratitude to Dr David Pyke, Royal College of Physicians, London, UK who made many helpful suggestions about the contents of this chapter.

Baraniuk, J. N., Murray, R. B. & Mabbee, W. G. (1987). Naloxone, ethanol and the chlorpropamide alcohol flush. *Alcoholism: Clinical and Experimental Research*, **11**, 518–20.

Barnett, A., Gonzalez-Auvert, C., Pyke, D. A., Saunders, J. B., Williams, R., Dickinson, C. J. & Rawlins, M. D. (1981c). Blood levels of acetaldehyde during the chlorpropamide alcohol flush. *British Medical Journal*, **283**, 939–41.

Barnett, A. H., Mace, P. J. E. & Pyke, D. A. (1981a). Chlorpropamide–alcohol flushing and microangiopathy in insulin-dependent diabetes. *British Medical Journal*, **282**, 523.

Barnett, A. H., Leslie, R. D. G. & Pyke, D. A. (1981b). Chlorpropamide–alcohol flushing and proteinuria in non-insulin dependent diabetics. *British Medical Journal*, **1**, 522–3.

Barnett, A. H. & Pyke, D. A. (1980). Chlorpropamide–alcohol flushing and large-vessel disease in non-insulin dependent diabetics. *British Medical Journal*, **281**, 261–2.

Barnett, A. H., Spiliopoulos, A. J. & Pyke, D. A. (1980). Blockade of chlorpropamide–alcohol flushing by indomethacin suggests an association between prostaglandins and diabetic vascular complications. *Lancet*, **2**, 164–6.

Bertram, F., Berfelt, E. & Otto, H. (1956). Indikationen und Erfeolge der Peroralen Behandlung des Diabetes Mellitus mit einem sulphonylharnstoffderivat. *Deutsche Medizinische Wochenschrift*, **81**, 274–8. (Cited by Jerntorp 1983.)

Bonisolli, L., Pontiroli, A. E., De Pasqua, A., Calderara, A., Maffi, P., Gallus, G., Radaelli, G. & Pozza, G. (1985). Association between chlorpropamide–alcohol flushing and fast acetylator phenotype in type I and type II diabetes. *Acta Diabetologica Latina*, **22**, 305–15.

Carducci Artensio, S., Ragonese, F., Forte, F., Guerrisi, O., Catalano, O. & Consolo, F. (1981). Chlorpropamide alcohol flushing in diabetics. *Diabetologia*, **21**, 81–2.

Dreyer, M., Kuhnau, J. & Rudiger, H. W. (1980). Chlorpropamide–alcohol flushing is not useful for individual genetic counselling of diabetic patients. *Clinical Genetics*, **18**, 189–90.

Fui, S. N. T., Keen, H., Jarrett, J., Gossain, V. & Marsden, P. (1983). Test for chlorpropamide–alcohol flush becomes positive after prolonged chlorpropamide treatment in insulin- dependent and non-insulin-dependent diabetics. *New England Journal of Medicine*, **309**, 93–6.

Groop, L., Eriksson, C. J. P., Huupponen, R., Ylikahri, R. & Pelkonen, R. (1984c). Roles of chlorpropamide, alcohol and acetaldehyde in determining the chlorpropamide – alcohol flush. *Diabetologia*, **26**, 34–8.

Groop, L., Eriksson, C. J. P., Wahlin-Boll, E. & Melander, A. (1984b). Chlorpropamide–alcohol flush: Significance of body weight, sex and serum chlorpropamide level. *European Journal of Clinical Pharmacology*, **26**, 723–5.

Groop, L., Koskimies, S. & Tolppanen, E. M. (1984a). Characterisation of patients with chlorpropamide–alcohol flush. *Acta Medica Scandinavica*, **215**, 141–9.

Guillausseau, P. J., Kkoka, C. & Lubetzki, J. (1984). Test a l'alcool-chlorpropamide. Etude et valeur diagnostique des variations de la temperature cutanée. *La Presse Medicale*, **13**, 1249–51.

Hershon, K. S., Bierman, E. L., Bruzzone, C. M. & Ensinck, J. W. (1982). Insulin responses to glucose in non-insulin dependent diabetic subjects with and without the chlorpropamide–alcohol flush: effect of salicylate and naloxone. *Diabetes Care*, **5**, 404–8.

Hillson, R. M. & Hockaday, T. D. R. (1984). Chlorporpamide–alcohol flush: a critical reappraisal. *Diabetologia*, **26**, 6–11.

Hillson, R. M., Ring, H. H., Smith, R. F., Yajnik, C. S., Crabbe, J. & Hockaday, T. D. R. (1987). Erythrocyte aldehyde dehydrogenase, plasma chlorpropamide concentrations and the chlorpropamide alcohol flush. *Diabete et Metabolisme (Paris)*, **13**, 23–6.

Hillson, R. M., Smith, R. F., Dhar, H., Moore, R. A. & Hockaday, T. D. R. (1983). Chlorpropamide–alcohol flushing and plasma chlorpropamide concentrations in diabetic patients on maintenance chlorpropamide therapy. *Diabetologia*, **24**, 210–12.

Hoskins, P. J., Wiles, P. G., Volkmann, H. P. & Pyke, D. A. (1987). Chlorpropamide alcohol flushing: a normal response? *Clinical Science*, **73**, 77–80.

Inoue, K., Ohbora, Y. & Yamasawa, K. (1978). Metabolism of acetaldehyde by human erythrocytes. *Life Sciences*, **23**, 179–84.

Jerntorp, P. (1983). The chlorpropamide alcohol flush test in diabetes mellitus: methods for objective evaluation. *Scandinavian Journal of Clinical and Laboratory Investigation*, **43**, 249–54.

Jerntorp, P. & Almer, L. O. (1981). Chlorpropamide-alcohol flushing in relation to macro-angiopathy and peripheral neuropathy in non-insulin dependent diabetes. *Acta Medica Scandinavica*, Suppl. 656, 33–6.

Jerntorp, P., Ohlin, H., Bergstrom, B. & Almer, L. O. (1980). Elevation of plasma acetaldehyde – the first metabolic step in CPAF? (abstract). *Diabetologia*, **19**, 296.

Jerntorp, P., Ohlin, H., Bergstrom, B. & Almer, L. O. (1981). Increase of plasma acetaldehyde – an objective indicator of the chlorpropamide alcohol flush. *Diabetes*, **30**, 788–91.

Johnston, C., Saunders, J. B., Barnett, A. H., Ricciardi, B. R., Hopkinson, D. A. & Pyke, D. A. (1986). Chlorpropamide–alcohol flush reaction and isoenzyme profiles of alcohol dehydrogenase and aldehyde dehydrogenase. *Clinical Science*, **71**, 513–17.

Johnston, C., Wiles, P. G. & Pyke, D. A. (1984). Chlorpropamide–alcohol flush: the case in favour. *Diabetologia*, **26**, 1–5.

Köbberling, J., Bengsch, N., Brüggeboes, B., Schwarck, H., Tillil, H. & Weber, M. (1980). The chlorpropamide alcohol flush. Lack of specificity for familial non-insulin dependent diabetes. *Diabetologia*, **19**, 359–63.

Laakso, M., Nourva, K., Aro, A., Uusitupa, M., Siitonen, O. & Huupponen, R. (1983). Chlorpropamide alcohol flushing and coronary heart disease in non-insulin diabetics. *British Medical Journal*, **286**, 1317–18.

Leslie, R. D. G., Barnett, A. H. & Pyke, D. A. (1979). Chlorpropamide alcohol flushing and diabetic retinopathy. *Lancet*, **1**, 997–9.

Leslie, R. D. G. & Pyke, D. A. (1978). Chlorpropamide-alcohol flushing (1) A dominantly inherited trait associated with diabetes. *British Medical Journal*, **2**, 1519–21.

Medbak, S., Wass, J. A. H., Clement-Jones, V., Cooke, E. D., Bowcock, S. A., Cudworth, A. G. & Rees, L. H. (1981). Chlorpropamide alcohol flush and circulating metenkephalin. A positive link. *British Medical Journal*, **283**, 837–9.

Micossi, P., Mannucci, P. M., Librenti, M., Raggi, U., D'Angelo, A., Corallo, S., Garimberti, B., Bozzini, S. & Malacco, E. (1982). Chlorpropamide–alcohol flushing in non-insulin dependent diabetes: prevalence of small and large vessel disease and of risk factors for angiopathy. *Acta Diabetologica Latina*, **19**, 141–9.

Ohlin, H., Jerntorp, P., Bergstrom, B. & Almer, L. O. (1982). Chlorpropamide alcohol flushing, aldehyde dehydrogenase activity and diabetic complications. *British Medical Journal*, **285**, 838–40.

Panzram, G. & Adolph, W. (1982). Chlorpropamide alcohol flush test in non-insulin dependent diabetes in young age (MODY type). *Endokrinologie*, **79**, 221–6.

Pontirolli, A. E., de Pasqua, A., Colombo, R., Ricordi, C. & Pozza, G. (1983). Characterisation of the chlorpropamide-alcohol flush in patients with type I and type II diabetes. *Acta Diabetologica Latina*, **20**, 117–23.

Segal, P., Brazo-Albu, J., Almog, S. & Berezin, M. (1985). Prevalence of chlorpropamide alcohol flush in Jewish Israeli diabetics. *Israel Journal of Medical Sciences*, **21**, 98–101.

Strakosch, C. R., Jeffreys, D. B. & Keen, H. (1980). Block of chlorpropamide alcohol flush by aspirin. *Lancet*, **1**, 394–6.

Wiles, P. G. & Pyke, D. A. (1984). The chlorpropamide alcohol flush. *Clinical Science*, **67**, 375–81.

29 Glucocorticosteroids and intraocular pressure

AN ADVERSE REACTION

THE INTRODUCTION of corticosteroids into ophthalmological practice caused a considerable step forward in the treatment of a number of eye disorders, for example, iritis. However, it soon became apparent that the same corticosteroids could have deleterious effects such as the production of subcapsular cataracts, activation of herpetic keratitis and other corneal infections.

Some cases of raised intraocular pressure caused by corticosteroids were described as early as 1953 (Stern 1953) and others followed (Francois 1961; Goldmann 1962). These papers indicated that raised intraocular pressure in patients on corticosteroids occurred more frequently than had been suspected and that it could on occasion be severe enough to impair vision.

The intraocular pressure rose only in some subjects on the administration of topical corticosteroids and this seemed to occur more commonly in glaucomatous individuals.

It was already known that glaucoma itself exhibits familial aggregation, indicating the possibility that genetic factors are of importance in its causation.

Because of the foregoing it was a natural development that interest should be taken in the possible genetic aspects of the response of intraocular pressure following the administration of topical corticosteroids.

POPULATION SURVEYS

Detailed surveys of the effects of topical corticosteroids on intraocular pressure and fluid dynamics were undertaken (Armaly 1963a; Becker & Mills 1963). These surveys showed that application of dexamethasone eye drops in one normal eye consistently resulted in an increase in intraocular pressure and a diminished outflow facility in the population tested. The magnitude of the effects was greater in subjects aged over 40 years than in persons under this age and the effects were also greater in glaucomatous than in normal eyes but were similar in both low and high tension open angle glaucoma patients.

Thirty completely normal volunteers had topical corticosteroids instilled daily into one eye only in each subject for 4 weeks (Becker & Mills 1963). The change in ocular pressure resulting appeared to separate these subjects into two populations: those responding with a considerable rise of pressure and those with only a small rise (Fig. 29.1).

Furthermore, the effect of dexamethasone in producing hypertension in the clinically normal eye was shown to be proportional to the concentration of the dexamethasone drops instilled and to be consistent in an individual on different occasions (Armaly 1966a). Small changes were found to occur in the untreated eye paralleling those in the eye into which the drops had been instilled. These contralateral changes were ascribed to the absorption of corticosteroid from the conjunctival sac into the bloodstream as well as from the eye into which the drug had penetrated by diffusion.

Table 29.1. *Population surveys of ocular pressure responses to topical corticosteroids*

Reference	Parameter of response	Number of subjects	Distribution of steroid response (mm Hg)		
Becker & Kolker 1966	Final pressure in eye medicated 6 weeks with 0.1% betamethasone 4 times daily	50	≤ 19	20–31	≥ 32
			35	13	2
			70%	26%	4%
Armaly 1965	Change in pressure in eye medicated 4 weeks with 0.1% dexamethaxone 3 times daily	80	≤ 5	6–15	≥ 16
			53 (66%)	23 (29%)	4 (5%)
Godel *et al.* 1972	Change in pressure in eye medicated 4 weeks with 0.1% dexamethaxone 3 times daily	59	≤ 5	6–15	≥ 16
			39 (66%)	18 (30%)	2 (3%)

From: Evans 1977.

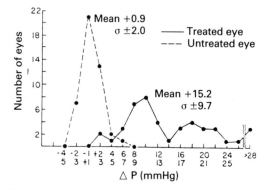

Fig. 29.1. The effect of topical betamethasone on intra-ocular pressure in open-angle glaucoma. The change in application pressure (ΔP) in mm Hg is demonstrated for the treated (solid line) and untreated (interrupted line) eyes of the same 44 patients after up to two months of betamethasone therapy. The untreated eyes showed no significant change in pressure and a reasonably normal distribution of ΔP around the point ΔP= 0; the treated eyes demonstrated a marked increase in intraocular pressure, averaging 15.2 mm Hg. (From Becker & Mills 1963.)

Three independent research groups conducted careful population surveys. Two of the groups used identical methods and came up with almost identical results (Armaly 1965; Godel *et al.* 1972). The third group used a slightly different procedure but their results were very similar to those obtained by the other two groups (Becker & Kolker 1966).

In the frequency distribution histograms three separate modes were found. In each of the three series the numbers of persons were in the ratios predicted by the Hardy–Weinberg equilibrium for two alleles at one autosomal locus (Table 29.1). Hence the evidence was strongly in favour of the existence of a polymorphism.

FAMILY STUDIES

Family studies were performed to test the hypothesis that the intraocular pressure response to the steroid was controlled by two allelic genes at one autosomal locus. These alleles were termed P^L (determining the low pressure response) and P^H (determining the high pressure response). Consequently the three hypothetical genotypes were $P^L P^L$, $P^L P^H$ and $P^H P^H$. Moderately large families were sought in which both parents and all their offspring could reliably participate in the study and had normal eyes (Armaly 1968). The phenotyping criteria were those shown in Table 29.1 (Armaly 1965). The offspring resulting from the various mating types are shown in Table 29.2.

Similar results were obtained by a second group using the same methodology (Feiler-Ofry *et al.* 1972). A third group (Becker & Kolker 1966) also investigated families using different phenotyping criteria as shown in Table 29.1.

As might be expected from the overlap of the

Table 29.2. *Family data to investigate genetic control of the response of intraocular pressure to topical corticosteroids*

Reference	Genotype mating type[a]	Number of matings	Number of offspring	Genotypes of offspring and distributions observed		
				nn	ng	gg
Becker & Kolker 1966	$nn \times nn$	–	21	95%	5%	–
	$nn \times ng$	–	42	48%	52%	–
	$ng \times ng$	–	25	20%	56%	24%
	$gg \times gg$	–	12	–	–	100%
				$P^L P^L$	$P^L P^H$	$P^H P^H$
Armaly 1968	$P^L P^L \times P^L P^L$	7	41	40	1	–
	$P^L P^L \times P^L P^H$	7	33	18	13	2
	$P^L P^L \times P^H P^H$	3	14	1	11	2
	$P^L P^H \times P^L P^H$	7	27	6	16	5
	$P^L P^H \times P^H P^H$	4	18	1	8	9
Feiler Ofry *et al.* 1972	$P^L P^L \times P^L P^L$	4	13	13	–	–
	$P^L P^L \times P^L P^H$	6	13	7	6	–
	$P^L P^H \times P^L P^H$	1	6	1	5	–
	$P^H P^H \times P^L P^H$	1	1	–	–	1

[a]Definition of proposed genotypes from ocular pressure responses are described in text and Table 29.1.
From: Evans 1977.

modes in the population frequency distributions, results in the offspring (Table 29.2) are not in perfect agreement with what would be expected from the parental mating types. However, taken as a whole the results are in keeping with the genetic hypothesis.

FURTHER GENETIC STUDIES – CONFLICTING EVIDENCE

The genetics of the response to topical cortico-steroids were examined afresh by an independent research group (Schwartz *et al.* 1972; Schwartz *et al.* 1973a, b). These workers used an identical medication schedule and examination technique to that used by Armaly (1966b). Sixty-three pairs of twins (37 monozygotic and 26 like-sexed dizygotic) were investigated. The change of pressure during steroid medication and also the final intraocular pressure were both considered. The results indicated that (1) the frequency distribution histograms did not deviate significantly from normal, (2) concordance in monozygous twins was low and it should have been complete on the monogenic hypothesis, (3) 'heritability' computations revealed that the genetic component of variance was small. Hence the view taken

by the authors was that the intraocular pressure response to local corticosteroids is multifactorial with a small 'polygenic component'.

As far as the frequency distribution of intraocular pressure after 3 weeks' local dexamethasone is concerned the result obtained by Francois *et al.* (1966) seems to indicate the existence of at least two modes (see Figs. 29.2 and 29.3).

Why different research groups came up with widely different results remains an unresolved mystery. It must be pointed out that the twin data of Schwartz and co-workers are not as extensive as the family studies mentioned earlier nor the population surveys of Francois *et al.* (1966).

THE CONTRIBUTION OF THE P^H AND P^L ALLELES TO THE CONTROL OF THE BASAL PRESSURE OF THE HEALTHY EYE

The approximately normal unimodal distribution curve of intraocular pressure in the healthy eye before the instillation of steroid eyedrops was investigated in families by Armaly (1967a). A correlation was found between mean-offspring pressure and mid-parent pressure, whereas there was

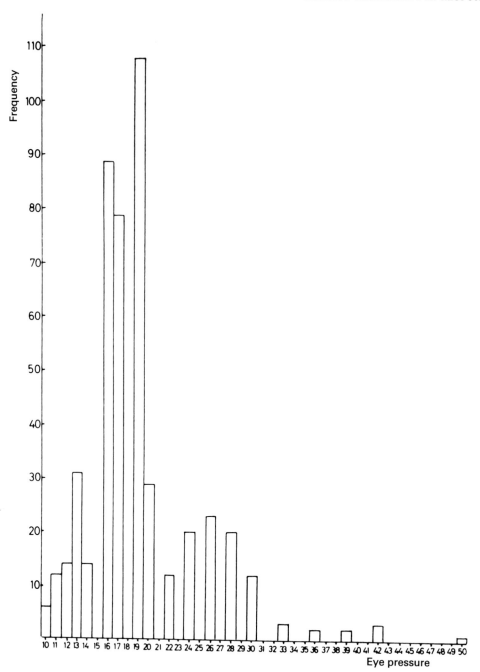

Fig. 29.2. Histogram. Normal subjects from families
free from glaucoma. Intraocular pressure after a three-
week corticosteroid test. (From François *et al.* 1966.)

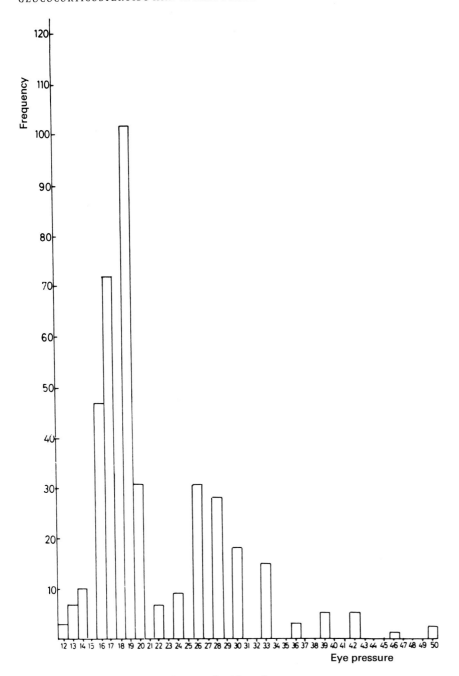

Fig. 29.3. Histogram. Apparently normal subjects from glaucomatous families. Intraocular pressure after a three-week corticosteroid test. (From François *et al.* 1966.)

an absence of significant correlation between the pressures of spouses. These findings were strongly suggestive of polygenic control.

An investigation was therefore made to see whether the P^L and P^H alleles made any significant contribution to the determination of the polygenically controlled basal intraocular pressure. It was found that the applanation pressure corrected for age was significantly higher in the $P^H P^H$ homozygote than in the $P^L P^L$ homozygote and the pressures of $P^L P^H$ heterozygotes were intermediate (Armaly *et al.* 1968). These results indicated that these two alleles were involved in determining the ocular pressure in the clinically normal eye. When the environment was changed by the instillation of corticosteroid eyedrops the effects of these alleles became much more obvious – that is to say the variability due to this allele pair became very large relative to the variability due to other factors and the phenomenon of polymorphism was displayed.

PREDISPOSITION TO PRIMARY GLAUCOMA DETECTED BY OCULAR CORTICOSTEROID TEST?

Two different hypotheses have been advanced: (1) by Becker & Hahn (1964), that the individual who is highly responsive to local steroids producing considerable elevations of intraocular pressure is constitutionally predisposed naturally to become glaucomatous later in life; (2) by Armaly (1967b) which suggested that glaucoma is polygenically determined and that the P^H allele was an important contributant to develop the condition. In other words the condition could develop without the possession of a P^H allele but it was more likely to develop in the presence of a P^H allele and even more so with two such alleles. The possession of one or even two P^H alleles did not signify that glaucoma would inevitably develop but did make it more likely. The 'relative risks' of the three genotypes to develop glaucoma were suggested by Armaly (1967b) to be $P^L P^L = 1$, $P^L P^H = 18$ and $P^H P^H = 101$.

In order to study the first hypothesis an extensive investigation was undertaken by Francois *et al.* (1966). One drop of either 0.1% betamethasone or 0.1% dexamethasone was ordered to be instilled into one eye four times daily for 3 weeks, in (a) 480 subjects with normal eyes who

Table 29.3. *The development of glaucoma in persons who were normotensive at the time of the phenotyping test*

Phenotype (corticosteroid response)[a]	Number who did not develop glaucoma	Number who did develop glaucoma
High	111	6
Intermediate	199	2
Low	250	0

[a]According to the Becker criteria.
From data in the text in: Lewis et al. 1988.

did not have a family history of glaucoma and (b) 396 subjects with apparently normal eyes who were relatives of glaucoma patients. The question of compliance obviously arose and the authors state 'we have every reason to believe that the instillations were done regularly particularly since in nearly 50% of cases the pupil was more dilated on the side treated'.

Two definite results emerged from this study. First, there was a clear deviation from normality in the frequency distributions after 3 weeks' treatment in that at least two modes were discernible in both groups. Furthermore, high pressure responders constituted a significantly larger proportion of the population made up of relatives of the glaucomatous patients than in the control group (Figs 29.2 and 29.3).

Secondly, there was a test of the hypothesis that (1) high pressure response indicated a heterozygous state, and (2) glaucoma indicated the 'abnormal' homozygous state. According to this theory all parents and children of glaucoma patients should be high pressure responders. This was found not to be the case. The evidence against this view was subsequently marshalled in detail by Francois (1978).

Nevertheless, the results of this large survey (provided one believes in the compliance) did indicate the existence of different phenotypes in the population and more high level responders in the relatives of glaucoma patients than in the control group. These findings are in keeping with the idea that high pressure responders might be more prone in later life to the development of glaucoma.

The whole idea was re-examined in retrospect by Lewis *et al.* (1988). They traced 788 individuals who had been years previously tested with dexamethasone as described above. There was an association between being a high level responder and developing glaucoma in individuals whose basal ocular tensions were normal at the time of the original test (Table 29.3). The result of the phenotyping test to predict the development of glaucomatous visual field loss was not as good as the predictive power of a multivariate model that included patient age, race, baseline intraocular pressure, baseline outflow facility, baseline cup/disk ratio and systemic hypertension.

SECONDARY GLAUCOMA

A group of 28 patients with various types of secondary glaucoma (following cataract surgery or trauma or angle closure) was found to resemble normal volunteers without a family history of glaucoma in that 32% of both groups responded to betamethasone with a raised intraocular pressure (Becker 1964). This pharmacological effect was thus different from that in the primary glaucoma population in which there were 92% responders (Armaly *et al.* 1968). This result was in keeping with the idea that high pressure responders might be predisposed to primary glaucoma.

TWO TESTS INFLUENCED BY THE ALLELIC GENES P^L AND P^H

(a)   Glucose tolerance

The finding that ocular hypertension induced by dexamethasone was a genetically determined response encouraged the search for other glucocorticoid responses in extraocular systems that might also be influenced by the same alleles.

A population of 55 subjects (aged 20 to 41 years, median 25 years) with clinically normal eyes and no history of diabetes was subjected to a dexamethasone test and the genotype of each individual for P^L and P^H was determined. On a separate occasion each subject had an oral glucose tolerance test (75 g glucose; blood taken fasting and at 30 minute intervals for 2 hours). The results are shown in Table 29.4 and they suggested strongly that an impaired glucose tolerance was associated with the P^H allele (Armaly 1967c).

There is known to be a clinical association between diabetes and glaucoma. Also, a raised intraocular pressure has been demonstrated in dia-

Table 29.4. *The results of oral glucose tolerance tests in relation to the alleles P^L and P^H*

Genotype	Sum of glucose concentrations (mg/100 ml) at 30, 60 and 90 min following oral ingestion of 75 g glucose		
	200–249	250–399	>400
$P^L P^L$	5	9	0
$P^L P^H$	4	20	1
$P^H P^H$	0	9	7

From: Armaly 1967c.

betic patients (Armstrong *et al.* 1960; Safir *et al.* 1964; Becker *et al.* 1966). Evidence has been produced to show that the frequency of high responders to topical corticosteroids is greater in diabetics than in non-diabetics (Becker & Kolker 1966).

(b)   The plasma cortisol suppression test

This test is based upon the fact that the pituitary production of ACTH is suppressed by a small dose of dexamethasone, therefore the adrenals whose stimulation is withdrawn will produce less cortisol and the plasma concentration will fall below the level at the start of the test.

A negative correlation was found between the suppression of plasma cortisol by dexamethasone and the rise in intraocular pressure in response to topical corticosteroids (Levene & Schwartz 1968; Rosenbaum *et al.* 1970; Becker & Ramsey 1970). This finding suggests that the possession of the P^H allele leads to an enhanced suppression of the pituitary by dexamethasone.

CONCLUSION

A disagreement was noted above about the genetics of the control of intraocular pressure responses to topical corticosteroids. Nevertheless, the weight of evidence from independent groups favours the existence of a genetic polymorphism in the population.

The problems of diabetes and associated eye problems, especially glaucoma, are clinically so important that this work should not be neglected. Not much work has been done in this area in the last few years. The *in vivo* testing on which all the work described above was based carries a definite hazard. For example, in the study of Schwartz *et al.* (1973a) six previously normal subjects among the glaucoma relatives became frankly glaucomatous with visual field defects during the course of the test procedure. In view of this unacceptable risk an *in vitro* test has obvious appeal. Attempts to develop tests based on lymphocyte responses (eg, Palmberg *et al.* 1977; Sowell *et al.* 1977) have been disappointing.

Armaly, M. F. (1963a). Effect of corticosteroids on intraocular pressure and fluid dynamics. I The effect of dexamethasone in the normal eye. *Archives of Ophthalmology (New York)*, **70**, 482–91.

Armaly, M. F. (1963b). Effect of corticosteroids on intraocular pressure and fluid dynamics. II. The effect of dexamethasone in the glaucomatous eye. *Archives of Ophthalmology (New York)*, **70**, 492–9.

Armaly, F. M. (1965) Statistical attributes of the steroid hypertensive response in the clinically normal eye. I. The demonstration of three levels of response. *Investigative Ophthalmology*, **4**, 187–97.

Armaly, M. F. (1966a) Dexamethasone ocular hypertension in the clinically normal eye. II. The untreated eye outflow facility and concentration. *Archives of Ophthalmology (New York)*, **75**, 776–82.

Armaly, M. F. (1966b). The heritable nature of dexamethasone-induced ocular hypertension. *Archives of Ophthalmology*, **75**, 32–5.

Armaly, M. F. (1967a). The genetic determination of ocular pressure in the normal eye. *Archives of Ophthalmology (New York)*, **78**, 1867–92.

Armaly, M. F. (1967b). Inheritance of dexamethasone. Hypertension and glaucoma. *Archives of Ophthalmology (New York)*, **77**, 747–61.

Armaly, M. F. (1967c). Dexamethasone ocular hypertension and eosinopenia and glucose tolerance test. *Archives of Ophthalmology (New York)*, **78**, 193–7.

Armaly, M. F. (1968). Genetic factors related to glaucoma. *Annals of the New York Academy of Sciences*, **151**, 861–75.

Armaly, M. F., Montstavicius, B. F. & Sayegh, R. E. (1968). Ocular pressure and aqueous outflow facility in siblings. *Archives of Ophthalmology (New York)*, **80**, 350–60.

Armstrong, J. R., Daily, R. K., Dobson, H. H. & Girard, L. J. (1960). The incidence of glaucoma in diabetes mellitus. *American Journal of Ophthalmology*, **50**, 55–63.

Becker, B. (1964). The effect of topical corticosteroids in secondary glaucomas. *Archives of Ophthalmology (New York)*, **72**, 769–71.

Becker, B., Bresnick, G., Chevrette, L., Kolker, A. E., Oaks, M. & Cibis, M. (1966). Intraocular pressure and its response to topical corticosteroids in diabetics. *Archives of Ophthalmology (New York)*, **76**, 477–83.

Becker, B. & Hahn, K. A. (1964). Topical corticosteroids and heredity in primary open-angle glaucoma. *American Journal of Ophthalmology*, **57**, 543–51.

Becker, B. & Kolker, A. E. (1966). Topical corticosteroid testing in conditions related to glaucoma. In *Corticosteroids and the Eye*. Vol. 6 of International Ophthalmology Clinics, ed. B. Schwartz, pp. 1005–15. Boston: Little Brown.

Becker, B. & Mills, D. W., (1963). Corticosteroids and intraocular pressure. *Archives of Ophthalmology (New York)* **70**, 500–7.

Becker, B. & Ramsey, C. K. (1970). Plasma cortisol and the intraocular pressure response to topical corticosteroids. *American Journal of Ophthalmology*, **69**, 999–1002.

Evans, D. A. P. (1977). Human pharmacogenetics. In *Drug Metabolism from Microbe to Man*, ed. D. V. Parke & R. L. Smith, pp. 369–91. London: Taylor & Francis.

Feiler-Ofry, V., Godel, V. & Stein, R. (1972). Systemic steroids and ocular fluid dynamics. III. The genetic nature of the ocular response and its different levels. *Acta Ophthalmologica*, **50**, 699–706.

Francois, J. (1961). Glaucome apparemment simple secondaire a la cortisono-therapie locale. *Ophthalmologica, (Basel)*, **142**, 517–23.

Francois, J. (1978). Corticosteroid glaucoma. *Metabolic Ophthalmology*, **2**, 3–11.

Francois, J., Heintz-De Bree, C. & Tripathi, R. C. (1966). The cortisone test and the heredity of primary open-angle glaucoma. *American Journal of Ophthalmology*, **62**, 844–52.

Godel, V., Feiler-Ofry, V. & Stein, R. (1972). Systemic steroids and ocular fluid dynamics. II. Systemic versus topical steroids. *Acta Ophthalmologica*, **50**, 664–76.

Goldmann, H. (1962). Cortisone glaucoma. *Archives of Ophthalmology (New York)*, **68**, 621–6.

Levene, R. Z. & Schwartz, B. (1968). Depression of plasma cortisol and the steroid ocular pressure response. *Archives of Ophthalmology (New York)*, **80**, 461–6.

Lewis, J. M., Priddy, T., Judd, J., Gordon, M. O., Kass, M. A., Kolker, A. E. & Becker, B. (1988). Intraocular pressure response to topical dexamethasone as a predictor for the development of primary open angle glaucoma. *American Journal of Ophthalmology*, **106**, 607–12.

Palmberg, P. F., Hajek, S., Cooper, D. & Becker, B. (1977). Increased cellular responsiveness to epinephrine in primary open-angle glaucoma. *Archives of Ophthalmology (New York)*, **95**, 855–6.

Rosenbaum, L. J., Alton, E. & Becker, B. (1970). Dexamethasone testing in South-Western Indians. *Investigative Ophthalmology*, **9**, 325–30.

Safir, A., Paulsen, E. P. & Klayman, J. (1964). Elevated intraocular pressure in diabetic children. *Diabetes*, **13**, 161–3.

Schwartz, J. T., Reuling, F. J., Feinleib, M., Garrison, R. J. & Collie, D. J. (1972). Twin heritability study of the effect of corticosteroids on intraocular pressure. *Journal of Medical Genetics*, **9**, 137–43.

Schwartz, J. T., Reuling, F. H., Feinleib, M., Garrison, R. J. & Collie, D. J. (1973a). Twin study on ocular pressure after topical dexamethasone. I. Frequency distribution of pressure response. *American Journal of Ophthalmology*, **76**, 126–36.

Schwartz, J. T., Reuling, F. H., Feinleib, M., Garrison, R. J. & Collie, D. J. (1973b). Twin study on ocular pressure following topically applied dexamethasone. II. Inheritance of variation in pressure response. *Archives of Ophthalmology (New York)*, **90**, 281–6.

Sowell, J. F., Levene, R. Z., Bloom, J. & Bernstein, M. (1977). Primary open-angle glaucoma and sensitivity to corticosteroids *in vitro*. *American Journal of Ophthalmology*, **84**, 715–20.

Stern, J. J. (1953). Acute glaucoma during cortisone therapy. *American Journal of Ophthalmology*, **36**, 389–90.

30   Unstable haemoglobins

CLINICAL OBSERVATIONS

THE OCCURRENCE of haemolytic anaemia after the ingestion of sulphonamides in persons with unstable haemoglobin variants was first recognized in the case of haemoglobin Zürich (Hitzig *et al.* 1960; Huisman *et al.* 1960).

The clinical story which started the investigation was that of a small girl and her father. The girl had suffered haemolysis after ingestion of sulphisomidine and on another occasion after sulphadimethoxine. The father, a 27 year old Swiss, had a serious haemolysis following a 4 day course of sulphamethoxypyridazine. His history disclosed that since childhood he had experienced occasional mild episodes of jaundice with dark urine. One such episode was caused by [8-(dimethylaminoantipyrin)] oxyquinoline sulphonic acid ('Causyth'). These events were not necessarily related to the intake of medications. The patient noticed, however, that after taking certain drugs for colds and other minor ailments he was frequently tired and pale for a few weeks. Otherwise he was well (Frick *et al.* 1962).

Following haemolysis the blood of both these patients showed a low haemoglobin with anisocytosis and fragmentation of erythrocytes on the blood film. Over 80% of red cells contained inclusion bodies which in the father's blood were unusually large and only one of them was present in each cell. They were negative for iron by Prussian blue stain. A leucocytosis was present. The marrow showed moderately increased erythropoiesis. Direct and indirect Coombs tests were negative as also were screening tests for warm and cold agglutinins. The plasma and urine were dark brown and contained methaemoglobin.

Both patients needed blood transfusions in these severe acute episodes, following which they exhibited a dramatic reticulocytosis and returned to their normal health. The girl normally had a haemoglobin of 11.2 g/100 ml with a reticulocyte count of 5.4%, whilst the father had a haemoglobin of 14.7 g/100 ml with reticulocyte counts varying between 2.4 and 7.8%. Inclusion bodies were absent.

LABORATORY INVESTIGATIONS

Haemoglobin electrophoresis showed the presence of two haemoglobins, namely A and another with a slower mobility intermediate between A and sickle (S) haemoglobin (Fig. 30.1). The abnormal haemoglobin was named haemoglobin Zürich after the city where the patients were described (the patients actually came from Attinghausen).

Various other haematological parameters estimated after recovery were normal, e.g. catalase, methaemoglobin reductase, glutathione concentration and glutathione stability in the presence of acetylphenylhydrazine. The glucose-6-phosphate dehydrogenase activity was raised in keeping with the reticulocytosis. The male patient's ^{51}Cr half-life of red cells was 12 days (normal 30 ± 3 days) when infused into himself and when infused into a normal recipient. Normal erythrocytes survived a normal length of time in the haemoglobin Zürich patient. Ferrokinetic studies revealed a very rapid uptake

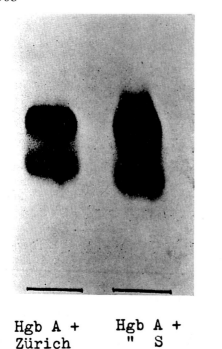

Hgb A +   Hgb A +
Zürich   " S

Fig. 30.1. Haemoglobin electrophoresis. (From Frick *et al.* 1962.)

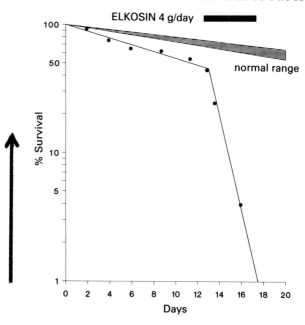

Fig. 30.2. Effect of Elkosin (sulphisomidine) on survival of labelled cells from Case 2 in normal recipient. (From Frick *et al.* 1962.)

into the marrow reaching a maximum in 2 days. The percentage of ^{59}Fe present in the circulating red cells attained only 45% (normal range 77 to 94%).

Some of the patients' red cells were labelled with ^{51}Cr and infused into normal recipients who then ingested a variety of drugs, one at a time. An accelerated disappearance of these cells from the circulation was caused by five different sulphonamides (Fig. 30.2) plus primaquine and [8-(dimethyl-aminoantipyrin)] oxyquinoline sulphonic acid.

GENETIC STUDIES

The pedigree ascertained by means of the two probands was published by Hitzig *et al.* (1960). Fifteen persons were recognized as having the two haemoglobins A plus Zürich out of the 65 related persons examined (Fig. 30.3). The two haemoglobins were controlled by co-dominant autosomal alleles. Some heterozygotes had histories of anaemia and episodes of slight jaundice but none had suffered severe episodes of haemolysis other than the two probands – probably because they had not sustained the relevant drug exposure.

It was interesting that the illness produced by a short-acting sulphonamide was much less severe than that produced by long acting sulphonamides. The exact mechanism of action of the sulphonamides on the haemoglobin Zürich was unknown but it was speculated that the inclusion body within erythrocytes, and later extruded, consisted of denatured haemoglobin.

The properties of haemoglobin Zürich

The physico-chemical properties of haemoglobin Zürich were extensively examined by Bachmann & Marti (1962). The heat stability in the cyanmethaemoglobin form showed that the haemoglobin Zürich was destroyed three times faster than haemoglobin A. The erythrocytes and haemolysates of haemoglobin Zürich carriers showed an increased tendency to form methaemoglobin. When incubated with acetylphenylhydrazine the erythrocytes behaved like glucose-6-phosphate dehydrogenase-deficient red cells. It was thought probable that red cells containing the same number of molecules of haemoglobin A and haemoglobin Zürich were made in the marrow but selective loss led to only 25% of the

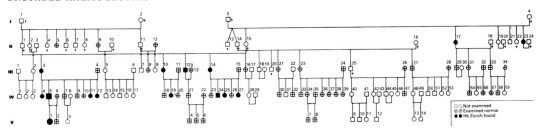

Fig. 30.3. The pedigree of family S. The probands were IV.5 and V.1. (From Hitzig *et al.* 1960.)

haemoglobin in the peripheral blood being of the latter type (Stauffer 1961). The abnormality in the structure of haemoglobin Zürich as compared with haemoglobin A was found to be the substitution of arginine for histidine in position 63 of the β chain.

A second haemoglobin Zürich family

A second family, in which six members in three generations had haemoglobin A plus haemoglobin Zürich in the red blood cells, was described by Rieder *et al.* (1965). This family living in Maryland, USA was also thought to be of Northern European extraction. The clinical features were very similar to those recorded in the Swiss cases as detailed above. Two patients had suffered haemolyses after the ingestion of sulphonamides. One patient had suffered life-threatening haemolysis after 'triple sulfa' (sulphamethazine, sulphadiazine and sulphamerazine) which was prescribed for otitis media. Another had a relatively milder haemolysis following sulphacetamide given for an urinary tract infection. On the other hand a 41 year old female with bronchiectasis who had haemoglobin Zürich took sulphisoxazole for 5 months without any ill effect. Four of the six haemoglobin Zürich individuals were prone to jaundice but two had no icteric episodes. Zinkham *et al.* (1979) showed that incubation of blood *in vitro* at 37 °C for 6 hours or 41 °C for 3 hours caused the appearance of inclusion bodies in the red cells containing haemoglobin Zürich but none in normal red cells. They suggest that this mechanism may be the basis of the fever-induced haemolysis.

Phenazopyridine and carbon monoxide

A further, unrelated patient with haemoglobin Zürich was described by Virshup *et al.* (1963). This 35 year old white woman had previously developed a severe anaemia with reticulocytosis after consuming a sulphonamide preparation. When observed she had another severe haemolysis after consuming phenazopyridine (PAP) for persistent post-operative urinary retention. This clinical observation led to an *in vitro* investigation of the effects of PAP on red cells containing haemoglobin Zürich from three different donors. The fall in glutathione concentration and percentage of cells containing Heinz bodies were both very much less in one of the three subjects who was a smoker with carboxyhaemoglobin (HbCO)) levels of 15 to 18%, than in the other two subjects who were non-smokers with HbCO levels of 4 to 6%. It was already known that haemoglobin Zürich had an affinity for carbon monoxide many times greater than haemoglobin A. It was also shown *in vitro* that converting the haemoglobin Zürich into the carboxy form prevented methaemoglobin and Heinz body formation under the influence of PAP. This is an interesting example of a protective effect of one foreign chemical against the deleterious effect of another.

THE MOLECULAR BASIS OF THE INTERACTION OF SULPHONAMIDES WITH HAEMOGLOBIN ŽURICH

The histidine in position β63 of haemoglobin A participates in haem–ligand binding. When arginine is substituted for histidine the structural conformation and the ligand-binding properties of the haemoglobin are altered. Tucker *et al.* (1978) as a result of X-ray analysis and infra-red absorption studies have shown that the replacement of histidine by arginine leaves a gap at the entrance to the haem pocket which allows sulphanilamide and other small reactive compounds easy access to the haem iron. It is suggested that the amide group of the drug could donate one electron to the bound oxygen. The donation of a second electron by the iron atom

Table 30.1. *Haemoglobins other than Zurich shown to produce adverse reactions with sulphonamides*

Reference	Haemoglobin (Hb)	Structural difference from haemoglobin A	Clinical and *in vitro* observations
Rigas & Koler 1961	H	β_4 instead of $\alpha_2\beta_2$	Drop in erythrocytic survival curve and decreased Hb values to 8 gm% observed after sulphisoxazole. *In vitro* sulphisoxazole caused methaemoglo-
bin			
Beretta *et al.* 1968	Torino	α43 Phe → Val	formation and precipitation of Hb H[a] Haemolytic crisis following treatment with a 'sulphonamide derivative'
White *et al.* 1970	Shepherd's Bush	β74 Gly → Asp	Haemoglobinuria after sulphonamides
King *et al.* 1972	Peterborough	β111 Val → Phe	Haemolysis after sulphonamides

[a]Amyl nitrate had the same effect as sulphisoxazole but not sulphanilamide, chloramphenicol, tetracycline, acetanilide, sodium ascorbate, meprobamate, mandelamine, acetophenetidine, sodium salicylate and sodium acetyl salicylate.

would cause oxygen to be reduced to peroxide. The oxidation of the haem would form methaemoglo- bin, resulting in the production of Heinz bodies and haemolysis. The binding of carbon monoxide to the molecule prevents this train of events because unlike molecular oxygen it cannot act as an electron acceptor. The conformational change in the haemo- globin molecule also explains why carbon monox- ide is displaced more slowly by oxygen than is the case in haemoglobin A.

OTHER UNSTABLE HAEMOGLOBINS AFFECTED BY SULPHONAMIDES

Examples of other unstable haemoglobins which are deleteriously influenced by sulphonamides are shown in Table 30.1.

The common feature of these unstable haemo- globins is distortion of the architecture of the haem pocket. For example, in haemoglobin Shepherds Bush (White *et al.* 1970) the introduction of the aspartic acid side chain interferes with the side chains of neighbouring amino acids. The effect of this is to weaken the hydrophobic forces which hold the haem pocket together thus allowing access to the haem for a sulphonamide molecule.

CONCLUSION

The detailed structures of haemoglobin variants are better known than is the case for many macromol-

ecules. Therefore the examples given above serve as models of how small drug molecules can interact with genetic variants of macromolecules to produce clinical effects.

Bachmann, F. & Marti, H. R. (1962). Hemoglobin Zürich II. Physicochemical properties of the abnormal hemoglobin. *Blood*, **20**, 272–86.

Beretta, V., Prato, V., Gallo, E. & Lehmann, H. (1968). Haemoglobin Torino-α43(CD1) Phenylalanine→Valine. *Nature*, **217**, 1016–18.

Frick, P. G., Hitzig, W. H. & Betke, K. (1962). Hemoglobin Zürich I. A new hemoglobin anomaly associated with acute hemolytic episodes with inclusion bodies after sulfonamide therapy. *Blood*, **20**, 261–71.

Huisman, T. H. J., Horton, B., Bridges, M. T., Betke, K. & Hitzig, W. H. (1961). A new abnormal hemoglobin. Hb: Zürich. *Clinica Chimica Acta*, **6**, 347–55.

King, M. A. R., Wiltshire, B. G., Lehmann, H. & Morimoto, H. (1972). An unstable haemoglobin with reduced oxygen affinity: haemoglobin Peterborough, β111 (G13) Valine→Phenylalanine, its interaction with normal haemoglobin and with haemoglobin Lepore. *British Journal of Hematology*, **22**, 125–34.

Reider, R. F., Zinkham, W. H. & Holtzmann, N. A. (1965). Hemoglobin Zürich. Clinical, chemical and kinetic studies. *American Journal of Medicine*, **39**, 4–20.

Rigas, D. A. & Koler, R. D. (1961). Decreased erythrocyte survival in Hemoglobin H disease as a result of the abnormal properties of Hemoglobin H: the benefit of splenectomy. *Blood*, **18**, 1–17.

Stauffer, U. G. (1961). Familienuntersuchung der hämoglobin-Zürich-Sippe. *Helvetica Paediatrica Acta*, **16**, 226–43.

Tucker, P. W., Phillips, S. E. V., Perutz, M. F., Houtchens, R. & Caughey, W. S. (1978). Structure of hemoglobins Zürich (His E7(63)β→Arg) and Sydney (Val E11(67)β→Ala) and role of the distal residues in ligand binding. *Proceedings of the National Academy of Sciences (USA)*, **75**, 1076–80.

Virshup, D. M., Zinkham, W. H., Sirota, R. L. & Caughey, W. S. (1983). Unique sensitivity of Hb Zürich to oxidative injury by phenazopyridine: reversal of the effects by elevating carboxyhemoglobin levels *in vivo* and *in vitro*. *American Journal of Hematology*, **14**, 315–24.

Von Hitzig, W. H., Frick, P. G., Betke, K. & Huisman, T. H. J. (1960). Hamoglobin Zürich: Eine neue Hamoglobinanomalie mit sulfonamidinduzierter Innenkörperañamie. *Helvetica Paediatrica Acta*, **15**, 499–514.

White, J. M., Brain, M. C., Lorkin, P. A., Lehmann, H. & Smith, M. (1970). Mild 'unstable haemoglobin haemolytic anaemia' caused by haemoglobin Shepherds Bush (B74(E18)Gly→Asp). *Nature*, **225**, 939–41.

Zinkham, W. H., Liljestrand, J. D., Dixon, S. M. & Hutchison, J. L. (1979). Observations on the rate and mechanism of haemolysis in individuals with Hb Zürich [His E7(63)β→Arg]. II Thermal denaturation of hemoglobin as a cause of anaemia during fever. *The Johns Hopkins Medical Journal*, **144**, 109–16.

31 Human lymphocyte antigens and adverse reactions to drugs

INTRODUCTION

HUMAN lymphocyte antigens (HLA) are the most polymorphic systems known in man, and different HLA types have been shown to be associated with many disorders, the most well known being HLA B27 with ankylosing spondylitis. It seems very likely that these genetically controlled factors are relevant in determining which patients develop adverse reactions to drug medications. This seems to be a relatively unresearched area of clinical medicine.

The most common class of adverse reactions to drugs includes those clinical phenomena such as rashes, proteinuria and haematological reactions which appear to have a basis of hypersensitivity. In only a few instances, however, has a really convincing immunologic mechanism been demonstrated, examples being 'Sedormid' and quinine purpuras.

A small subsection of pharmacogenetics has shed a light on these common events in clinical medicine. In a few instances associations have been found between an HLA phenotype and adverse reactions.

REACTIONS TO THE TREATMENT OF RHEUMATOID ARTHRITIS

Gold preparations are amongst the most toxic non-cancer medicines used clinically. Because of the interest in the HLA status of rheumatological conditions a considerable amount of attention has been paid to the HLA antigens possessed by patients who have developed adverse reactions to treatment for their rheumatoid arthritis The bulk of the evidence is condensed in Table 31.1.

It will be seen that 12 series present evidence for an association between DR3 and adverse reactions to gold salts (principally sodium aurothiomalate) and D-penicillamine, principally in Northern Europeans. Bardin *et al.* (1982) also found associations between adverse reactions to gold salts and A1, B8 and Cw7 antigens. They also performed family studies and found a significant correlation ($\chi_1^2 = 8.4$) between gold salt intolerance and the haplotype A1 Cw7 B8 DR3. They also noted that three out of four patients with renal intolerance as a result of D-penicillamine were of the Cw7 B8 DR3 haplotype.

Adachi *et al.* (1984) described three patients who developed thrombocytopenia while taking gold therapy and all three possessed the antigens HLA-B8 and DR3.

Attempts have been made to discover whether the HLA associations are different with the various types of adverse reactions. The most analytical of these studies was that of Nüsslein *et al.* (1984), who concluded that three types of associations could be found.

1 A significantly positive association with HLA-Bw35 was seen exclusively with mucocutaneous lesions but not with nephropathy. In addition, neither a positive association with HLA-DR3 or the phenotypic combination HLA-A1 B8 DR3, nor a significant negative association with HLA-DR2 was observed in this group.
2 There was no HLA-Bw35 association in patients with nephropathy, but a significant positive association with HLA-DR3, the phenotypic combination HLA-A1 B8 DR3 and a significant negative association with HLA-DR2.

Table 31.1. *Associations of HLA antigens with adverse reactions to the treatment of rheumatoid arthritis with gold salts and D-penicillamine*

Reference	Frequency of relevant HLA associated with the disorder	Frequency of relevant HLA in control group	χ_1^2	p
Mielants & Vey 1978	7 out of 9 patients with HLA-B27 developed adverse reactions (mainly haematological) to levamisole			
Panayi et al. 1978	7 out of 8 patients with DRW2, and 14 out of 18 with DRW3 developed adverse reactions to SA or DP	16 out of 33 patients without either DRW2 or DRW3 developed adverse reactions to SA or DP	6.48	<0.020
Wooley et al. 1980	19 of 24 patients developing proteinuria with SA &/or DP were B8 DRW3	18 of 77 patients without proteinuria had DRW3	24.53	<0.001
	14 out of 15 patients with SA-induced proteinuria were DRW3 positive	22 out of 72 patients without proteinuria on SA were DRW3 positive		
	9 out of 13 patients with DP-induced proteinuria were DRW3 positive	12 out of 36 patients without proteinuria on DP were DRW3 positive		
	5 out of 16 with mouth ulcers on SA &/or DP were DRW2 positive	6 out of 75 patients without mouth ulcers on SA &/or DP were DW2 positive	4.70 with Yates	<0.050
Latts et al. 1980	Adverse reactions to SA occurred in 9 out of 13 patients with HLA B12	Adverse reactions to SA occurred in 5 out of 19 without HLA B12	5.78	<0.020
Swiss Federal Commission 1981	6 patients who developed proteinuria on SA &/or DP were all DR3	DRW3 present in 12.6% of healthy controls	25.46	<0.001
Coblyn et al. 1981	12 out of 15 patients who developed thrombocytopenia on SA possessed DR3	26 out of 84 patients who did not develop thrombocytopenia possessed DR3	12.95	<0.001
Bardin et al. 1982	30 patients with side effects to aurothiopropanol, 14DR3	37 patients with no side effects, 5DR3	8.96	<0.001
Gran et al. 1983	15 out of 16 patients who possessed DR3 developed adverse reactions mainly rashes and proteinuria on SA	71 out of 116 patients who did not possess DR3 developed adverse reactions on SA	6.56	<0.020
Vischer 1983	5 out of 16 patients who developed albuminuria after SA or DP were DR3 positive			
Nüsslein et al. 1984	16 patients developed renal and 33 developed mucocutaneous lesions, both adverse reactions were seen in 2 patients. All treated with SA. 64.7% of patients with renal and 23.5% of patients with mucocutaneous adverse reactions possessed DR3	25 patients without adverse reactions on SA. 12% of these patients had DR3	2P$_{corr}$ for renal adverse reactions	<0.050

Table 31.1. (*cont.*)

Reference	Frequency of relevant HLA associated with the disorder	Frequency of relevant HLA in control group	χ_1^2	p
Alarcon *et al.* 1985	Out of 12 patients who developed renal side effects on 'chrysotherapy', 4 had DR3	9.5% of 105 patients who did not exhibit side effects had DR3	3.75 with Yates	>0.050
Delamere *et al.* 1983	DP-induced myasthenia in 16 patients with rheumatoid arthritis; 10 of them had DR1	'local' control population of 59 subjects, 10 of whom had DR1		<0.005
Majoos *et al.* 1981	'no association between the development of side effects to SA and the HLA DRW2 or DRW3 antigen or between HLA B8 and proteinuria' (complete data not presented)			
Karr *et al.* 1980	'patients with DRW2 or DRW3 were not more likely to have toxic reactions to gold or DP therapy than patients with other antigens (blacks χ^2 1.78, whites χ^2 0.12)'			
Dequeker *et al.* 1984	96 patients treated with DP and 123 patients treated with aurothiopropanolol sulphate. The only significant HLA association with side effects was an increased frequency of B8 in D-penicillamine-induced proteinuria			<0.001
Bensen *et al.* 1984	Out of 19 patients with side effects to SA 13 had DR3 and 12 had B8	out of 38 patients without side effects 4 had DR3 and 5 had B8	both highly significant	
Van Riel *et al.* 1983	Out of 25 RA patients treated with aurothioglucose 14 developed adverse reactions and 5 of them had DR3	11 patients did not develop side effects and of them 1 had DR3		NS
Tishler *et al.* 1988	60% of 20 RA patients who had mucocutaneous side effects on aurothioglucose therapy had B35 (DR3 not associated with side effects)	31.5% of 40 RA patients who had no side effects had B35		p_c<0.050
Barger *et al.* 1984	21.1% of 39 RA patients who developed toxicity treated with either SA or aurothioglucose possessed DR3	8.2% of 110 RA patients who did not develop toxicity when treated with gold possessed DR3		p<0.05
Scherak *et al.* 1984	SA treatment of RA 13 patients with more than 2 side effects (A) 69% B8 54% DR3	76 patients had no side effects (C) 25% B8 13% DR3	A–B p<0.0005 A–C p<0.0050	
	44 patients with 1 side effect (B) 14% B8 7% DR3 DP treatment of RA 33 with side effects DR2 and/ or DR3 55%	44 without side effects DR2 and/or DR3 25%		p<0.010
Salvarani *et al.* 1990	DR3 occurred in 50% of RA patients. 40 out of 102 patients developed side effects on gold thiosulphate treatment and these included only one patient who had proteinuria. That patient had DR3	DR3 in 22.3% normal controls		

Table 31.1. (*cont.*)

Reference	Frequency of relevant HLA associated with the disorder	Frequency of relevant HLA in control group	χ_1^2	p
Cohen *et al.* 1991	6% of Hong Kong Chinese with RA had DR3, 4 patients stopped treatment due to toxicity to SA. Only one with proteinuria had DR3	6% of healthy control Hong Kong Chinese had DR3		

RA, rheumatoid arthritis; SA, sodium aurothiomalate; DP, D-penicillamine.

3 There were common associations for both types of adverse reactions during gold therapy: a significant increase of HLA-A1 and HLA-B8 as well as a significant decrease of HLA-B7 was seen in the frequency of these determinants in patients with nephropathy as well as in those with mucocutaneous lesions.

In a Greek series (Pachoula-Papasteriades *et al.* 1986) 50 patients with rheumatoid arthritis were treated with sodium aurothiomalate (SA), 19 with D-penicillamine (DP) and 26 with both drugs. Severe adverse reactions (skin, stomatitis, proteinuria or haematuria and leukopenia) were seen in 30, 4 and 9 of these three groups of patients respectively. This study confirmed that patients possessing DR3 were at great risk of developing these adverse reactions to SA and PD, but it was also found that HLA-DRw6 had nearly as great a risk as DR3. Possibly this new feature, as compared with the other studies, might be due to an ethnic factor.

An ethnic factor seems almost certain in the series of Cohen *et al.* (1991), who point out the low incidence of toxicity to sodium aurothiomalate in Hong Kong Chinese who also have a low frequency of DR3. Whether the latter fact accounts for the former observation is of course conjectural.

It has been suggested that HLA typing might be considered before starting aurothiomalate treatment for rheumatoid arthritis. This does not seem a practical proposition because non-DR3 persons are also at an appreciable risk and all careful doctors make a clinical check, test the urine and obtain a blood count prior to each injection.

SYSTEMIC LUPUS ERYTHEMATOSUS-LIKE SYNDROME (PSEUDOLUPUS)

The condition of pseudolupus is a faithful mimic of the spontaneous disorder with clinical features of arthralgia, arthritis, myalgia, pleurisy, myocarditis, liver involvement, rashes and raised ESR. This illness develops after a few months of treatment.

The most well known pseudolupus syndrome occurs during the treatment of hypertension with hydralazine. This condition is discussed in another chapter where it is pointed out that it is almost exclusively a disorder of slow acetylators. Batchelor *et al.* (1980) found that 73% of 26 patients with this syndrome possessed HLA-DR4 antigen, compared with four out of 16 patients treated with hydralazine for more than 1 year who had not developed the syndrome ($\chi_1^2 = 9.24$, $p < 0.01$). The HLA-DR4 frequency in 113 healthy subjects was 33%, and in 20 patients with idiopathic systemic lupus was 25%. Brand *et al.* (1984), however, could not confirm this pseudolupus/HLA-DR4 association in 15 patients (5% of whom had DR4) compared with 140 normal Melbourne residents (29% of whom had DR4). It must be commented that the controls of Batchelor *et al.* (1980) were more appropriate than those of Brand *et al.* (1984).

Other pseudolupus conditions produced by drugs which have been associated with HLA antigens include procainamide-induced lupus and HLA-DR6Y (Whiteside *et al.* 1982), and autoantibody formation in chlorpromazine-treated patients and HLA-B44 (Canoso *et al.* 1982).

Fifty-six patients who had developed a pseudolupus syndrome produced by 'Venopyronum dragées' (a phenopyrazone-containing compound used to treat varicose veins and superficial thrombophlebitis) were studied by Grosse-Wilde *et al.* (1987). Healthy white blood donors ($n = 582$) served as controls. A significant increase of HLA-DR4 (57.1% vs 26.5%, relative risk 3.7) and a decrease of HLA-DR3 were found in the patient group. They also found the haplotype Gm1;21 and phenotype Gm1,3;5,21 significantly increased and associated with HLA-DR4 in the pseudolupus patients but not in the controls.

MECHANISM

Presumably some HLA antigens play a part in producing hypersensitivity phenomena. How some HLA antigens interact with foreign chemicals to produce hypersensitivity reactions, whilst other HLA antigens do not do so, is at present unclear. Whatever the mechanism, it seems to be distinct and separate from that causing the disease being treated.

Adachi, J. D., Bensen, W. G., Singal, D. P. & Powers, P. J. (1984). Gold induced thrombocytopenia: platelet associated IgG and HLA typing in three patients. *Journal of Rheumatology*, **11**, 355–7.

Alarcon, G. S., Koopman, W. J., Acton, R. T. & Barger, B. O. (1985). HLA-Bw35 and gold toxicity in rheumatoid arthritis. *Arthritis and Rheumatism*, **288**, 236–7.

Bardin, T., Dryll, A., Bebeyre, N., Ryckewaert, A., Legrand, L., Markelli, M. & Dausset, J. (1982). HLA system and side-effects of gold salts and D-penicillamine treatment of rheumatoid arthritis. *Annals of the Rheumatic Diseases*, **41**, 599–601.

Barger, B. O., Acton, R. T., Koopman, W. J. & Alarcon, G. S. (1984). DR antigens and gold toxicity in white rheumatoid arthritis patients. *Arthritis and Rheumatism*, **27**, 601–5.

Batchelor, J. R., Welsh, K. I., Mansilla-Tinoco, R., Dollery, C. T., Hughes, G. R. V., Bernstein, R., Ryan, P., Naish, P. F., Aber, G. M., Bing, R. F. & Russell, G. I. (1980). Hydralazine-induced systemic lupus erythematosus: influence of HLA-DR and sex on susceptibility. *Lancet*, **2**, 1107–9.

Bensen, W. G., Moore, N., Tugwell, P., D-Souza, M. & Singal, D. P. (1984). HLA antigens and toxic reactions to sodium aurothiomalate in patients with rheumatoid arthritis. *Journal of Rheumatology*, **11**, 358–61.

Brand, C., Davidson, A., Littlejohn, G. & Ryan, P. (1984). Hydralazine-induced lupus: no association with HLA-DR4. *Lancet*, **1**, 462.

Canoso, R. T., Lewis, M. E. & Yunis, E. J. (1982). Association of HLA-Bw44 with chlorpromazine-induced autoantibodies. *Clinical Immunology and Immunopathology*, **25**, 278–82.

Coblyn, J. S., Weinblatt, M., Holdsworth, D. & Glass, D. (1981). Gold-induced thrombocytopenia. *Annals of Internal Medicine*, **95**, 178–81.

Cohen, M. G., Ng, P. Y., Chan, K. A. L. & Li, E. K. (1991). Low incidence of toxicity from gold thiomalate in Hong Kong Chinese patients with rheumatoid arthritis. *Journal of Rheumatology*, **18**, 630–1.

Delamere, J. P., Jobson, S., Mackintosh, L. P., Wells, L. & Walton, K. W. (1983). Penicillamine-induced myasthenia in rheumatoid arthritis: its clinical and genetic features. *Annals of the Rheumatic Diseases*, **42**, 500–4.

Dequeker, J., van Wanghe, P. & Verdickt, W. (1984). A systematic survey of HLA-A, B, C and D antigens and drug toxicity in rheumatoid arthritis. *Journal of Rheumatology*, **11**, 282–6.

Gran, J. T., Husby, G. & Thorsby, E. (1983). HLA DR antigens and gold toxicity. *Annals of the Rheumatic Diseases*, **42**, 63–6.

Grosse-Wilde, H., Genth, E., Grevesmühl, A., Vögeler, U., Zarnowski, H., Mierau, R., Doxiadis, G., Doxiadis, I. & Maas, D. (1987). HLA-DR4 and Gm 1;21 haplotypes are associated with pseudolupus induced by Venopyronum dragées. *Arthritis and Rheumatism*, **30**, 878–83.

Karr, R. W., Rodey, G. E., Lee, T. & Schwartz, B. D. (1980). Association of HLA-DRw4 with rheumatoid arthritis in black and white patients. *Arthritis and Rheumatism*, **23**, 1241–5.

Latts, J. R., Antel, J. P., Levinson, D. J., Arnason, B. G. W. & Medof, M. E. (1980). Histocompatibility antigens and gold toxicity. A preliminary report. *Journal of Clinical Pharmacology*, **20**, 206–9.

Majoos, F. L., Klemp, P., Meyers, O. L. & Briggs, B. (1981). Gold therapy in rheumatoid arthritis. *South African Medical Journal*, **59**, 971–4.

Mielants, H. & Vey, E. M. (1978). A study of the haematological side effects of levamisole in rheumatoid arthritis with recommendations. *Journal of Rheumatology*, **5** (Suppl. 4), 77–83.

Nüsslein, H. G., Jahn, H., Lösch, G., Guggenmoos-Holzmann, I., Leibold, W. & Kalden, J. R. (1984). Association of HLA-Bw35 with mucocutaneous lesions in rheumatoid arthritis patients undergoing sodium aurothiomalate therapy. *Arthritis and Rheumatism*, **27**, 833–6.

Pachoula-Papasteriades, C., Boki, K., Varia-Leftherioti, M., Kappos-Rigatou, I., Fostiropoulos, G. & Economidou, J. (1986). HLA-A, -B, and -DR antigens in relation to gold and D-penicillamine toxicity in Greek patients with RA. *Disease Markers*, **4**, 35–41.

Panayi, G. S., Wooley, P. & Batchelor, J. R. (1978). Genetic basis of rheumatoid disease: HLA antigens disease manifestations and toxic reactions to drugs. *British Medical Journal*, **2**, 1326–8.

Salvarani, C., Macchioni, P., Zizzi, F., Rossi, F., Baricchi, R., Mantovani, W., Ghirelli, L., Capozzoli, N., Frizziero, L. & Portioli, I. (1990). Low incidence of proteinuria in RA after gold thiosulfate treatment. *Journal of Rheumatology*, **17**, 271–2.

Scherak, O., Smolen, J. S., Mayr, W. R., Mayrhofer, F., Kolarz, G. & Thumb, N. J. (1984). HLA antigens and toxicity to gold and penicillamine in rheumatoid arthritis. *Journal of Rheumatology*, **11**, 610–4.

Swiss Federal Commission for the Rheumatic Diseases, Subcommission for Research. (1981). HLA-DR antigens in rheumatoid arthritis. *Rheumatology International*, **1**, 111–13.

Tishler, M., Caspi, D., Gazit, E. & Yaron, M. (1988). Association of HLA-B35 with mucocutaneous lesions in Israeli patients with rheumatoid arthritis receiving gold treatment. *Annals of Rheumatic Diseases*, **47**, 215–17.

Van Riel, P. L. C. M., Reekers, P., van de Putte, L. B. A. & Gribnan, F. W. J. (1983). Association of HLA antigens, toxic reactions and therapeutic response to auranofin and aurothioglucose in patients with rheumatoid arthritis. *Tissue Antigens*, **22**, 194–9.

Vischer, T. L. (1983). Pharmacogenetics in therapy with gold and other slow-acting anti-rheumatic drugs. *Rheumatology*, **8**, 220–4.

Whiteside, T., Mulhern, L., Buckingham, R. & Luksick, J. (1982). Procainamide-induced lupus is associated with an increased frequency of HLA-DR 6y. *Arthritis and Rheumatism*, **25** (Suppl.), S41 (Abstract).

Wooley, P. H., Griffin, M. B., Panayi, G. S., Batchelor, J. R., Welsh, K. I. & Gibson, T. J. (1980). HLA-DR antigens and toxicity to sodium aurothiomalate and D-penicillamine in rheumatoid arthritis. *New England Journal of Medicine*, **303**, 300–2.

32 The polymorphism for tasting phenylthiocarbamide (PTC *syn* phenylthiourea)

PROLOGUE

THIS chapter is included in this book for the following reasons. The PTC tasting polymorphism can be detected by a number of commonly employed drug compounds. The polymorphism has been shown to be genetic in nature, and the frequencies of the different phenotypes vary considerably between ethnic groups.

Associations have been shown to exist between the tasting phenotypes and some clinical disorders, and these associations may well be of considerable importance in elucidating aetiology and pathogenesis. As far as the author is aware there are no data on associations between PTC taste phenotypes and adverse reactions to drugs.

The alternative names for the same molecule, namely phenylthiourea and phenylthiocarbamide (PTC), have been used in the literature since 1931. Since the abbreviation PTC is commonly employed it will be used in this chapter.

DISCOVERY

A short anonymous note in *Science* in 1931 reported the discovery of what is now known as the PTC taste-testing polymorphism thus:

Tasteblindness is the only term that can be found to describe the reaction of those who can not taste para-ethoxy-phenyl-thio-urea, for those who can taste it find it intensely bitter. This curious difference in perception has been discovered by Dr Arthur L. Fox of the laboratories of EI duPont de Nemours and Company.

He has tried this very complex organic compound on every one who would volunteer to taste it and has found that approximately three fifths of his 'victims' declared it intensely bitter, while the rest say that it 'has no more taste than sand'.

Fox's own account is somewhat more graphic:

Some time ago the author had occasion to prepare a quantity of phenyl-thio-carbamide, and while placing it in a bottle the dust flew around in the air. Another occupant of the laboratory, Dr. C. R. Noller, complained of the bitter taste of the dust, but the author, who was much closer, observed no taste and so stated. He even tasted some of the crystals and assured Dr. Noller they were tasteless but Dr. Noller was equally certain it was the dust he tasted. He tried some of the crystals and found them extremely bitter. With these two diverse observations as a starting point, a large number of people were investigated and it was established that this peculiarity was not connected with age, race or sex. Men, women, elderly persons, children, negroes, Chinese, Germans and Italians were all shown to have in their ranks both tasters and non-tasters.   (*Fox 1932*)

THE TECHNIQUE OF DETECTING THE PTC TASTE POLYMORPHISM

The technique of determining the PTC tasting phenotype employed by Fox (1932) and other earlier workers was to place the crystals directly upon the tongue. A variant of this procedure, which has been used occasionally by quite recent workers (e.g. Whittmore 1986), was to use filter paper impregnated with PTC.

However, it was realized that this simple subdivision of people into tasters and non-tasters did not really represent the true situation. The employment of serial dilutions, first introduced by Blakeslee & Salmon (1935), allowed the concentration threshold at which the bitter taste of PTC was detectable to be determined for each individual.

The whole subject was critically and exhaustively re-examined by Harris & Kalmus (1949a) and the method developed by them has remained the standard way of determining the phenotypes ever since. The details of their method were described as follows:

A stock solution containing 0.13% of phenylthiourea (PTC) is made up in boiled tap water and serial dilutions are made up as given in Table 32.1. The test proper consists of two stages:

(1) Starting from the higher dilutions and working down, the subject is given a few cc in a tumbler till he first says that he perceives a definite taste. This gives an approximate value for the threshold.
(2) The subject is now presented with eight tumblers, four of which contain a few cc of water and four containing a few cc of the solution determined in stage (1). The glasses are arranged at random. The subject is told that four of them contain the substance and four contain water, and he is asked to taste them all and to separate them into the two groups of four. The quantity of fluid is not limited and tumblers are refilled during the test if desired. If the two groups of four are correctly separated the test is repeated with the next lower concentration and so on, until the subject can no longer discriminate correctly. The lowest concentration at which a completely correct answer is given is taken as the threshold. If, on the other hand, the subject is unable to separate the two groups accurately, the test is repeated in the same manner with increasing concentrations till a concentration is reached where a completely correct answer is given.

Boiled tap water was used both for making up the solutions and for controls. It was stored in bottles, care being taken to ensure that all solutions were at the same temperature. This procedure was adopted because preliminary experiments had shown that fresh tap water was easily distinguished by some individuals from stale tap water. Distilled water was ruled out because of its unaccustomed taste and the inconvenience of preparing large quantities for routine testing. (*Harris and Kalmus 1949a*).

Table 32.1. *Concentration of PTC solutions used for taste-testing*

Solution no.	PTC (mg/l)
1	1300.00
2	650.00
3	325.00
4	162.50
5	81.25
6	40.63
7	20.31
8	10.16
9	5.08
10	2.54
11	1.27
12	0.63
13	0.32
14	0.16

From: Harris & Kalmus 1949a.

The results obtained by this method (see Fig. 32.1) have been found to be highly repeatable by many workers (see, for example, Li *et al.* 1990).

Fischer *et al.* (1961) and Fischer *et al.* (1965) claimed that:

1 it was better to use distilled water rather than tap water because the latter has a variable composition and may have a taste or smell of its own;
2 the compound 6-*n*-propylthiouracil (PROP) may be a better discriminator between phenotypes than PTC, because the differentiation relies entirely on taste whereas with PTC there may be an element of smell involved as well.

[However, the results given by these authors of testing 66 persons with both compounds did not show the PROP results to be superior.]

It is known that PTC has definite toxicity for rodents, and is possibly toxic to humans, but just how toxic is unknown. However as Wheatcroft & Thornburn (1972) point out, it is a wise precaution for subjects being tested to spit out the test solutions after tasting them.

Further work to try and improve the classification of the PTC taster phenotypes and genotypes was undertaken by Kalmus (1958). This was based on the fact, which was already known, that there is a considerable variability in the ability to taste quinine. A population of individuals was tested to determine for each person both the PTC threshold and the quinine threshold. It was found that the quinine

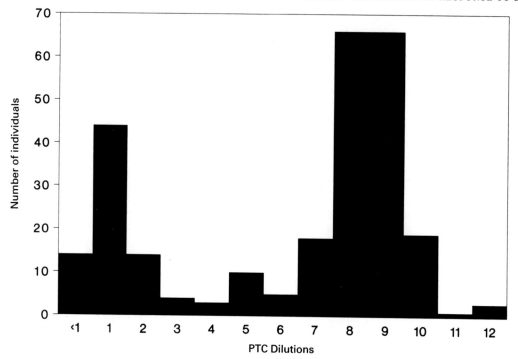

Fig. 32.1. Bimodal distribution of PTC taste thresholds. (From Fig. 4 Control Group; 265 individuals, Kitchin *et al*. 1959.)

thresholds appeared to have a normal distribution in the PTC non-tasters and another similar normal distribution in the PTC tasters but with a slightly higher mean threshold value in the latter. Further, there was a significant correlation within each phenotype of the thresholds for the two compounds (Fig. 32.2). After calculating a discriminant function it was used to make a small correction to the PTC threshold value for each person. This resulted in making the bimodality of the frequency distribution histogram a little more pronounced (Figs 32.3). Whether the additional quinine tests are worth the extra time involved to produce the slight improvement in the PTC frequency distribution histogram is very much a matter for the individual investigator to decide.

Extensive experiments of the same type involving *N*-propylthiouracil thresholds and quinine thresholds (Table 32.2) were published by Fischer & Griffin (1964) and Fischer *et al*. (1966). They advanced the possibly useful concept of 'bimodal

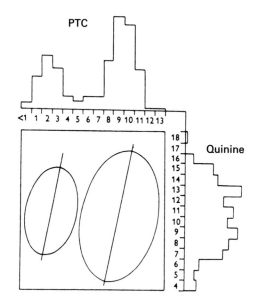

Fig. 32.2. Illustration of the hypothesis that the quinine thresholds of PTC tasters and non-tasters vary around the same mean value. (From Kalmus 1958.)

Table 32.2. *Frequency distribution of taste thresholds for quinine and 6-N-propylthiouracil (PROP) (n = 228).* Brackets include subjects with taste thresholds for PROP at the antimode

Quinine solution no.	PROP solution no.												Number of subjects	
	3	4	5	6	7	8	9	10	11	12	13	14		
0	–	–	1	–	–	–	–	–	–	–	–	–	1	
1	–	–	–	2	2	–	–	–	–	–	–	–	4	
2	1	–	–	1	2	–	[1]	1	1	–	–	–	6	[7]
3	–	–	1	6	3	7	–	–	5	9	2	–	33	
4	–	2	–	6	8	11	[6]	4	7	5	2	–	45	[51]
5	–	–	2	2	10	10	[7]	1	10	6	–	–	40	[47]
6	–	–	–	–	7	6	[4]	6	3	7	4	–	33	[37]
7	–	–	–	3	2	3	5	[2]	2	2	7	4	28	[30]
8	–	–	–	–	3	3	[2]	[2]	–	2	1	1	13	[15]
9	–	–	–	–	–	–	–	[1]	–	–	1	1	2	[3]
Number of subjects	1	2	4	20	34	40	8 [26]	12 [17]	28	31	17	8	205 [228]	

From: Fischer & Griffin 1964.

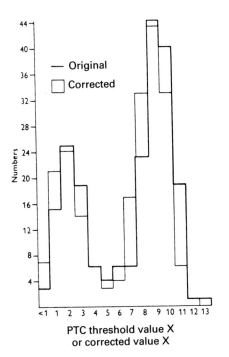

PTC threshold value X
or corrected value X

Fig. 32.3. The frequency of PTC thresholds among 212 students and the frequency of individuals in arbitrary classes after taking their quinine threshold into account. (From Kalmus 1958.)

receptors' (PTC) and 'unimodal receptors' (quinine) – referring to the shapes of the population frequency distribution histograms.

It was shown by Kalmus (1958) that brucine solution thresholds were also correlated with the PTC taste thresholds in 'tasters'. By using this information also a 'corrected' PTC distribution histogram could be produced with an improved bimodality. However, since brucine is a dangerous poison Kalmus (1958) advised that the use of this compound could not be recommended for routine testing.

There is a large body of information on taste physiology (Beidler 1961) which is outside the scope of this book. However, it should be mentioned that there appear to be different mechanisms to detect salt, sweet, sour and bitter tastes. The PTC taste polymorphism represents a special subset of the bitter taste perception. It is of some interest that in the irradiated patient of Kalmus & Farnsworth (1959) the abilities to taste salt, sucrose, PTC, quinine and picric acid were all severely affected but the ability to taste hydrochloric acid was unaffected indicating that it has a different physico-chemical mechanism from the remainder.

Kalmus (1958) points out an important fact, namely that a person who has a very high threshold for both PTC and quinine should be suspected of having ageusia, i.e. a generalized pathological impairment of taste.

GENETICS

The inheritance of the ability to taste para-ethoxyphenylthiourea (PEPT) and PTC was very swiftly investigated. After Fox's discovery was announced and also in 1931, Snyder presented a 'preliminary report of the occurrence of the condition in one hundred families', and concluded that the character was neither sex-linked nor sex-influenced. He characterized 'the taste deficiency as a unit-factor recessive'. Snyder (1931) did not give the exact details of his method but presumably used crystals of PEPT placed on the tongue. Also in 1931, Blakeslee and Salmon reported their findings which included 283 persons tested with PTC crystals and tests with four different aqueous dilutions of the compound on 166 of these persons who were unable to taste the crystals. They found 25.2% non-tasters in females and 38.2% in males. A total of 47 families including 88 children revealed the non-tasters to be autosomal recessives. There was a suggestion that children may have had higher tasting scores than adults. In none of the 25 offspring of 12 matings of non-tasters in these two first studies were there any taster offspring. The authors do not say so but presumably all the subjects were white American Caucasians.

In 1932 Snyder reported his expanded data on 800 families with 2043 offspring tested by the PTC crystal technique (Table 32.3). Five taster and 218 non-taster offspring were produced by 86 matings of non-tasters. There was no really satisfactory explanation for this anomaly. In the same year Blakeslee presented his results on 103 families using his dilutions method. In addition to confirming the main finding with regard to inheritance, he suggested that the acuteness of taste among the taster children might increase in line with the increase in taste acuity in one of the parents.

The inheritance of PTC tasting in 20 monozygous twinships was reported by Rife (1933). All but one showed concordance, and the exceptional individual had a general inability to taste following poliomyelitis. A sample of 3156 American Negroes was investigated by Lee (1934) and 291 (9.2%) were found to be non-tasters of PTC by the 'crystals' method; also 265 offspring of 124 Negro families showed the same inheritance pattern as in whites. The authors also gave data indicating the percentage

Table 32.3. *Summary of 800 families studied for inheritance of taste deficiency for phenylthiocarbamide, showing observed and calculated proportions of tasters and non-tasters in the offspring of the various types of matings. Total for 3643 parents and children: tasters, 70.2%; non-tasters, 29.8%*

	Children	
Matings	Tasters	Non-tasters
Taste × Taste 425	929	130
	obs. 0.877 ± 0.007	0.123 ± 0.007
	calc. 0.876 ± 0.001	0.124 ± 0.001
	dev. 0.001 ± 0.007	0.001 ± 0.007
Taste × Taste deficient 289	483	278
	obs. 0.634 ± 0.012	0.366 ± 0.012
	calc. 0.646 ± 0.002	0.354 ± 0.002
	dev. 0.012 ± 0.012	0.012 ± 0.012
Taste deficient × Taste deficient 86	5	218
	obs. 0.021	0.979
	calc. 0.000	1.000
	dev. 0.021	0.021

From: Snyder 1932.

of non-tasters amongst other ethnic groups: American Indians 6.0%, Kenyans 8.1%, Sudanese 9.6%.

An experiment carried out by Setterfield *et al.* (1936) set out to categorize 477 white Americans by means of their PTC tasting thresholds (i.e. using serial dilutions) and the result is shown in Fig. 32.4. The bimodality is obvious and in keeping with the family studies mentioned earlier. However, the authors also say 'The continuous occurrence of individuals tasting the solutions throughout the series of dilutions would suggest that there are modifying factors that are operating on the postulated simple pair of allelomorphs . . .'

In a study of 145 twin pairs and 78 non-twin sibling pairs, Kaplan *et al.* (1967) note that 'the intra-pair differences observed in our sample of monozygotic twins indicate that non-genetic factors also influence taste thresholds.'

Doubts were expressed regarding the adequacy of the two-allele explanation of the PTC tasting polymorphism by Boyd (1950a). In an attempt to shed light on the problem Harris & Kalmus (1951) studied 384 sib-pairs and 'failed to confirm in detail the genetical hypothesis postulated for the observed dimorphism in taste thresholds'. Then, using the

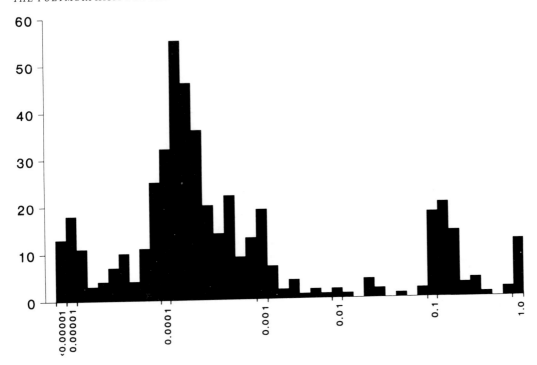

Fig. 32.4. Frequencies of tasters and non-tasters in white persons with the scale of dilutions of PTC given in fractions of a 1% solution. (Constructed from data in Table 1 of Setterfield *et al.* 1936.)

technique of Harris & Kalmus (1949a) the problem was addressed again by Das (1956), who studied 845 sib-pairs. The data were tested for conformity with two hypotheses: (A) recessive inheritance of the non-taster phenotype; (B) chance combination of pairs without any influence of heredity. Neither of the two hypotheses agreed with the mass of data but (A) was much closer than (B). When the phenotypes, well away from the antimode, were tested hypothesis (A) agreed very well with the data. Around the antimode hypothesis (B) agreed slightly better with the data than hypothesis (A).

A very careful analysis was performed by Merton (1958) on 60 Norwegian families with 176 children. In the 11 families where both parents were non-tasters there were 21 non-taster and five taster offspring, confirmed by re-testing. However overall the family data showed a satisfactory agreement with the genetic hypothesis, namely that non-tasting was

an autosomal recessive phenotype. A sib-pair analysis arrived at discordant conclusions, but the author comments 'The reason is probably of statistical rather than biological nature, the sib-pair method being not strictly correct except for sib-pairs of only two sibs'.

An interesting mathematical technique, based on the assumption that the frequency distribution curves of all three genotypes are normal, was developed by Kalmus & Maynard Smith (1965). This technique was applied to several sets of data and successfully revealed the distributions of the homozygotes and heterozygotes within the dominant mode.

More recently, the newer technique of segregation analysis has been applied to family data. Rao & Morton (1977) tested 272 Brazilian parents and their 282 offspring using serial dilutions of PTC in the vicinity of the antimode only. Complex segregation analysis showed the existence of a major locus with no evidence for any other cause of family resemblance. So this study supported the original monogenic hypothesis.

Using the complete sorting test of Harris &

Kalmus (1949a) modified by Mohr (1951), Indian families were tested by Reddy & Rao (1989), yielding 178 parents and their 257 children. Complex segregation analysis showed that the dominance of tasters was incomplete and that there were additional multifactorial effects influencing the extent of taste sensitivity. They speculated that the ability to taste PTC is determined by a nearly-dominant major locus, while quantitative variation in the thresholds is controlled by a multifactorial component.

In the same journal issue Olson *et al.* (1989) reported pedigree segregation analysis of 1152 individuals from 120 Ohio families who were tested using the Harris & Kalmus (1949a) dilutions method. They found that several two-locus models and two one-locus, three-allele models each provided a substantially better fit to the PTC data than the traditional one-locus recessive model. The best fit was obtained by a two-locus model which predicted two types of non-tasters (PTC non-tasters, and general non-tasters). This model allows for apparent PTC non-taster × PTC non-taster matings to produce PTC taster offspring; there were 11 such offspring in the data of Olson *et al.*

Pointers to the complexity of genetic control for the PTC tasting polymorphism have also arisen from surveys of the PTC tasting polymorphism in different populations. Observations were made by Lugg (1966a, b, 1970) which indicated that there was a polymodal distribution of PTC taste thresholds in the Ainu of Northern Japan, and very sensitive individuals were found among the Ami and Atayal aborigines of Taiwan. Multiple allelism was suggested as an explanation. A very interesting survey was conducted in Kirghizia by Ibraimov & Mirrakhimov (1979) in which Kirghiz schoolchildren and students could taste dilution number 29 on the scale of Harris & Kalmus (1949a), as compared with Russian students examined by the same test procedure in the same location in whom dilution 16 was the limit of detection (Fig. 32.5). In the Kirghiz families this 'supertaster' phenotype appeared to be genetically determined.

These observations, together with the most modern genetic analyses of Caucasian families which indicate that a simple two-allele model does not provide a fully satisfactory explanation of family data, suggest strongly that either alleles at more than one locus, or more than two alleles at one locus, control the PTC taste threshold.

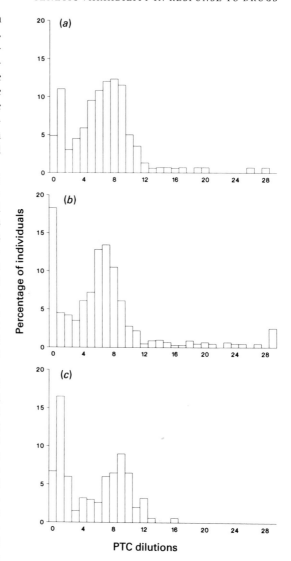

Fig. 32.5. Total histogram, not taking into account sex and age. (a) Kirghiz students (640 subjects); non-tasters (NT) = 19.6%; hypersensitive (HS) = 1.2%; gene frequency = 0.44; (b) Kirghiz children from Kyzyl-Dzhar schools (734 subjects): NT = 29.1%; HS = 4.2%; t = 0.54; (c) Russian students (245 subjects): NT = 31.9%; HS = 0; t = 0.56. (From Ibraimov & Mirrakhimov 1979.)

It seems quite possible that in the future the techniques of molecular biology may reveal a complex genetic structure for the PTC tasting polymorphism in a manner similar to that found in the case of the acetylation polymorphism which is described in another chapter.

LINKAGE

Slight evidence for linkage between the PTC and Kell blood group loci had been found by Chautard-Freire-Maia (1974), who analysed data on 22 autosomal polymorphic loci in a Brazilian population.

The subject was re-examined by Conneally *et al.* (1976) who added some Indiana pedigrees to the Brazilian data. Forty sibships with 157 offspring were informative for Kell:PTC linkage and a further four sibships with 13 offspring were informative for Sutter:PTC linkage (Sutter blood group is part of the Kell blood group system). The combined maximum likelihood estimate for Θ for both sexes was 0.047 with a lod score of 10.778, which leaves little doubt that the Kell and PTC loci are linked.

The Kell blood group locus – and therefore the PTC locus also – have recently been mapped to the short arm of chromosome 7 (McKusick 1992; Appendix IV).

FACTORS INFLUENCING THE PTC TASTE-TITRE

Age

The influence of age upon the PTC taste threshold was examined thoroughly by Harris & Kalmus (1949a). They studied schoolboys, male university students and staff, and Chelsea Pensioners (veterans, most of whom were aged over 65 years), a total of 441 individuals. It was clearly demonstrated that the taste sensitivity diminished with age in both phenotypes (about 1 dilution step every 20 years: Kalmus 1958) and so the position of the antimode between the phenotypes moved to a higher concentration (Fig. 32.6). The implication of this is that the dividing point between phenotypes appropriate for college students would not be appropriate to categorize an older population. For the classification of any individual as a 'taster' or 'non-taster' reference should be made to the threshold distribution of his age group. However, in addition to a shift in the antimode there was also clearly a diminution in the proportion of really sensitive individuals able to detect PTC in solution 11 to 14. The findings of Akcasu & Özalp (1977) who studied 684 Turks, and Leguebe (1960) who studied 225 Belgian men and 200 Belgian women, were very similar.

It is of relevance that Harris & Kalmus (1949a)

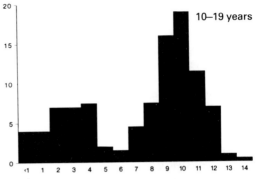
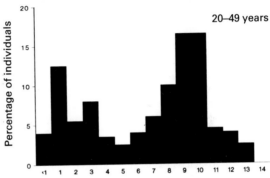
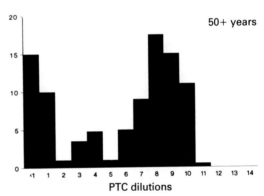

Fig. 32.6. Distribution of taste thresholds for PTC of three age groups of males. (From Harris & Kalmus 1949a.)

found that the relative proportions of the two phenotypes showed no significant change with age, suggesting (1) no change of phenotype from taster to non-taster due to deterioration of the taste mechanism, and (2) no differential viability.

Kalmus & Trotter (1962) re-tested 110 individuals after a lapse of 10 to 15 years. The individual PTC sensitivity of adults (presumably Caucasians) was found to decline by about 0.05 threshold units (approx 3%) annually. Age, thyroid condition and taster status did not affect the rate of decline.

The determination of the PTC taste phenotypes of young infants was demonstrated to be feasible by Kalmus (1976), showing that the character is established soon after birth.

Sex

Almost all investigators have found that females are more sensitive than males, the estimated differences varying between 0.3 and 0.79 of a dilution step. For example, Harris & Kalmus (1951) and Das (1956) found differences of 0.79 and 0.69 dilution steps, respectively, though the relative proportions of tasters and non-tasters were the same in the two sexes. Kaplan *et al.* (1964) stated that the sex difference in *n*-propylthiouracil sensitivity equals approximately one threshold by the time the population reaches the age of 50 years.

Smoking

The influence of smoking on taste threshold of *n*-propylthiouracil was studied by Kaplan *et al.* (1967), who tested 145 twin pairs and 78 non-twin sibling pairs. Their conclusions were that threshold differences were significantly associated with smoking habits: specifically, heavy smoking over a period of years tended to increase the taste threshold, while smoking habits apparently had no significant effects on the taste thresholds of subjects aged 20 years or less.

THE MECHANISM WHICH IS RESPONSIBLE FOR THE TASTE-TESTING POLYMORPHISM

There has been considerable speculation about what exactly is the difference between tasters and non-tasters. There have been two main ideas, namely (1) a difference in the properties of the saliva, (2) a difference in the property of the receptor presumably sited in the taste buds.

Pursuing the first idea, Cohen & Ogdon (1949) phenotyped college students into 26 tasters and seven non-tasters. Then the following three solutions were prepared:

saturated solution of PTC in tap water and placed on a dry tongue;
PTC in non-taster's saliva;
PTC in taster's saliva;

With none of these was any person able to taste PTC. So the authors suggested that, in order to taste PTC as bitter, a person must have both the correct 'taste apparatus' and his own saliva.

Then results of Cohen & Ogdon (1949) were confirmed by Fischer & Griffin (1964), using 6-propylthiouracil, and they also found that when a taster's saliva was briefly boiled it was then rendered unsuitable for tasting. However, Kalmus (1959) cast doubt upon this finding.

A physico-chemical difference between the salivas of tasters and non-tasters was described by Fischer & Griffin (1960). When propylthiouracil (PROP) was incubated with the saliva a decrease in optical density between 276 and 284 mμ was observed to occur over 8 minutes at a significantly faster rate in non-tasters' than in tasters' salivas. This difference between the phenotypes was annulled by cellulose and a silica lattice of glass with electrolytic desalting. The difference was enhanced by polyvinylpyrrolidone, by cupric chloride and even more so by a combination of cupric chloride and sodium thiocyanate. Though a similar reaction could be observed by the action of hydrogen peroxide on PROP, the dialysed saliva of a non-taster remained more active than that of a taster (Fischer *et al.* 1961).

These observations led the authors to study salivary catalase activity and, according to Fischer & Griffin (1964) a typical taster saliva decomposes 0.134 μM hydrogen peroxide per second whereas a typical non-taster saliva decomposes 0.038 μM per second. The compound 2,4-dichlorophenol was found to be a stronger inhibitor of salivary peroxide decomposition in 'tasters' than in 'non-tasters' of propylthiouracil.

A similar optical density effect to that with propylthiouracil was observed by Griffin & Fischer (1960a) using 2-mercapto-imidazole, 1-methyl-2-mercapto-imidazole, 2-mercapto-4 (or 5)-imidazole carboxylic acid, 1-methyl-2-mercapto-5-imidazole carboxylic acid (the first two of which are compounds capable of differentiating taster phenotypes), and by Fischer *et al.* (1962), using chlorpromazine.

THE PHYSICO-CHEMICAL INVESTIGATION OF TASTE THRESHOLDS

An interesting idea was explored by Rubin *et al.* (1962). This was a development of the finding (which had been previously made by others, e.g. Kalmus 1958: see above) that whereas taste thresholds for PTC and propylthiouracil are bimodal, the taste thresholds for quinine are unimodal. Furthermore, there is a relationship between the two as shown in Table 32.2, in that although the quinine thresholds are unimodally distributed their mean levels are different for the two propylthiouracil phenotypes. [It is to be noted that in the Harris & Kalmus (1949) test the most concentrated solution is No. 1. However in all the work of Fischer & Griffin the most dilute solution is called zero.]

The solution in the saliva and the solute molecules on receptors were considered to be two phases. When a mixture of the two compounds was tasted it was assumed that at the taste threshold all available sites of a receptor 'phase' were occupied by Np molecules of propylthiouracil and Nq molecules of quinine. 'Isothermal' taste diagrams for the binary mixtures were produced from the taste or no-taste data, indicating areas of synergism and antagonism. This application of adsorption theory does not seem to have led to any deeper understanding of the taste-testing polymorphism.

The physico-chemical characteristics of solutes were investigated in relation to taste modalities by Shamil & Birch (1990). They found that the apparent specific volume correlated with the type of sensation. Specific volume ($m^{-1} l^3$) is the reciprocal of density ($m l^{-3}$) and is denoted by $^\Phi V$. Apparent specific volume (ASV) is $^\Phi V$ divided by the molecular weight, and as it increases it indicates decreasing water-compatibility and penetrating power of the material whose taste is being investigated. Salty substances had low ASV values and bitter substances high ASV values. The authors propose that bitter substances exert their effects in the superficial layers of the taste epithelium. These observations may have some relationship to the results of Frank & Korchmar (1985), who assessed the intensity judgement reaction times for taste in persons phenotyped with PTC. Non-tasters of PTC were consistently slower than tasters about making intensity judge-

ments with regard to the concentrations of sucrose, sodium chloride, quinine and hydrochloric acid. It was proposed that there may be two types of non-taster as assessed by their reaction times. In view of these findings the topology of taste receptors in relation to the PTC phenotype might merit investigation.

EFFECT OF THYROXINE PRECURSORS ON TASTE-TESTING

According to Griffin & Fischer (1960b) and Fischer *et al.* (1961), the presence of 3×10^{-3} M 3-mono-iodotyrosine and 7.5×10^{-4} M tyrosine or 3,5-di-iodotyrosine, when used as solvents for either PTC or propylthiouracil taste-testing, markedly lower the sensitivity of tasters to detect these compounds. They also lower the sensitivity to detect the taste of quinine.

These various pieces of information were thought by Fischer and Griffin to indicate an increased salivary metabolite formation through the action of peroxidase on thyroid precursors in 'non-tasters' as compared with 'tasters'. These authors did not, however, produce direct proof of this proposition by measuring the products of such an enzymic reaction in the salivas of persons of the two phenotypes.

An enzymic activity also investigated, with the idea that it is present in both thyroid tissue and saliva, was thiourea desulphuration. No difference in salivary activity between the taster phenotypes was found by Shepard *et al.* (1963).

NEUROLOGICAL CONSIDERATIONS

It has always been thought that the receptors influenced by PTC were on the taste buds, but exactly which ones are involved in perceiving the bitter sensation remains a matter of some dispute. It was formerly thought that the circumvallate papillae, on the posterior third of the tongue and innervated by the glossopharyngeal nerve, were responsible. However, it turns out that in lesions of this nerve the tasting ability is not lost. Also, three patients who had suffered chorda tympani resections (so denervating the anterior two-thirds of the tongue) showed no subsequent loss of taste thresholds (Fischer *et al.* 1966).

Some interesting evidence on this point has also emerged from the study of patients with familial dysautonomia (Riley–Day syndrome: MIM 223900) which is a rare autosomal recessive disorder principally occurring in Ashkenazi Jews and characterized by lack of tear formation, emotional lability, paroxysmal hypertension, increased sweating, cold extremities, corneal anaesthesia, orthostatic hypotension, erythematous blotching of the skin, pain and temperature insensitivity and drooling. As a part of this widespread disorder of neurological function due to aplasia of peripheral autonomic neurones, there is an abnormally high taste threshold. Henkin & Kopin (1964) studied six patients with this disorder, in whom neither fungiform nor circumvallate papillae could be found on the tongue (but filiform papillae were present in all patients). Three of the six were able to detect or recognize a saturated solution of PTC whereas two were unable, and one patient was not tested. According to Fischer *et al.* (1966), the high thresholds in such patients were restored to normal by the systemic administration of methacholine. It was suggested by these authors that since the taste buds are absent in such patients they may be able to detect taste using free nerve endings.

The results of irradiating the oropharynx for the treatment of metastatic squamous carcinoma of the tongue are described by Kalmus & Farnsworth (1959). The threshold for PTC was raised from solution No. 10 (a 'taster' level) to solution No. 2 (a 'non-taster' level). No recovery was observed over 6 weeks of observation.

The observations on the familial dysautonomia patients indicate that PTC tasting depends on the integrity of the taste buds but does not contribute to the understanding of the way the polymorphism is determined. Irradiation might damage both the taste buds and salivary glands, so again gives no helpful information. With regard to the manner of operation of the polymorphism, the deleterious influence of age and smoking might be considered to lower the sensitivity of the taste bud apparatus, but this again does not shed light on the polymorphic physiology.

SUBSTANCES OTHER THAN PTC WHICH DETECT THE TASTING POLYMORPHISM

Dr Fox, being a chemist, was naturally interested in the relationship between molecular structure and the polymorphism which he had discovered (Fox 1932). Phenylthiocarbamide is an arylthiocarbamide (Fig. 32.7) and so a wide variety of other arylthiocarbamides were prepared, and they were all capable of detecting the tasting polymorphism. For example, several symmetrical diarylthiocarbamides such as di-(2-methoxy-5- methylphenyl) thiocarbamide were prepared and they retained the ability to detect the polymorphism as also did asymmetrical diarylthiocarbamides, e.g. *N*-para-ethoxy-*N'*-phenylthiocarbamide. Some aralkyl- and alkylthiocarbamides were also investigated and, for example, the compound dibenzylthiocarbamide was shown to have a similar property. The aliphatic dicrotylthiocarbamide (Fig. 32.7) was found to have a slightly bitter taste to PTC non-tasters but an extremely bitter taste to PTC tasters.

On the other hand, tetramethylthiocarbamide (Fig. 32.8) was shown to have a sour but not lasting taste to both phenotypes and dibutylthiocarbamide was somewhat bitter to both classes. Thiocarbamide itself was found to have a nauseating taste, not bitter but sour to both PTC tasters and non-tasters alike using the method employed by Fox, i.e. placing crystals on the tongue.

So the conclusion from all this was that the polymorphic tasting of the bitterness of PTC had something to do with the $>C=S$ structure in the molecule.

The compound para-ethoxy-phenylcarbamide (Fig. 32.8) tasted 300 times sweeter than sugar and did not differentiate between phenotypes. However, when the oxygen atom was replaced by a sulphur atom to make para-ethoxy-phenylthiocarbamide, then a bitter taste was perceived by 'tasters' and 'non-tasters', but the phenotypes were differentiated.

Fox (1932) speculated on various explanations for the existence of the polymorphism, including:

differential solubilities in the salivas of the two phenotypes,
the presence of a precipitating agent in the saliva of non-tasters.

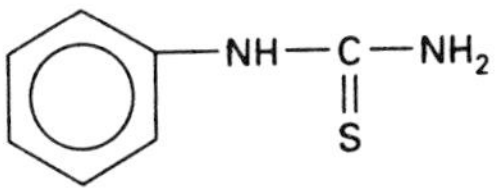

Phenylthiocarbamide (PTC syn. phenylthiourea)

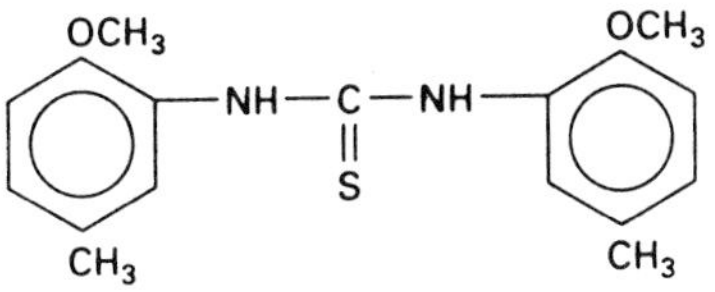

Di (2–methoxy–5–methyl–phenyl) thiocarbamide

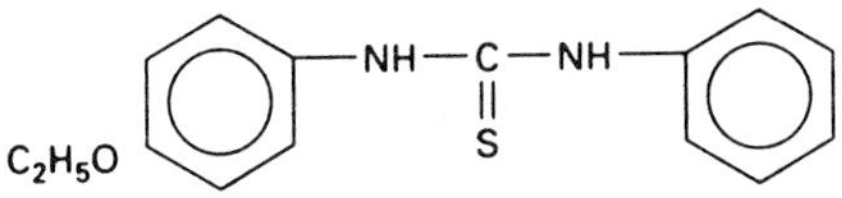

N–para–ethoxyphenyl–N'–phenyl thiocarbamide

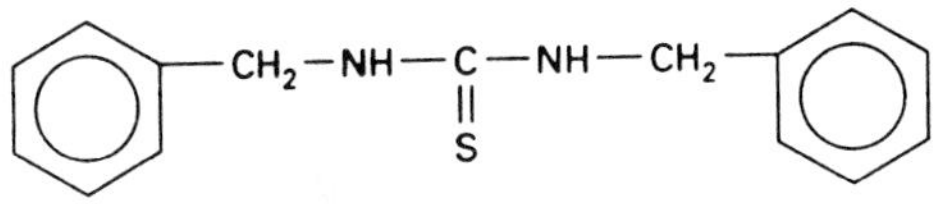

Dibenzyl thiocarbamide

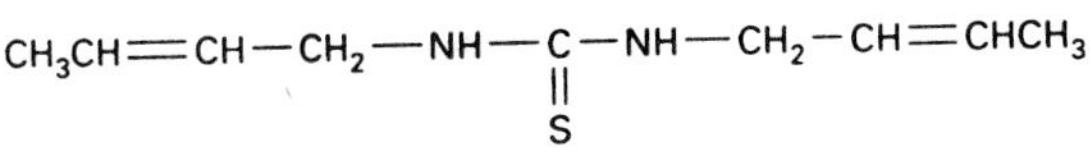

Dicrotyl thiocarbamide

Fig. 32.7. Structural formulae of compounds which can detect the PTC tasting polymorphism. (From Fox 1932.)

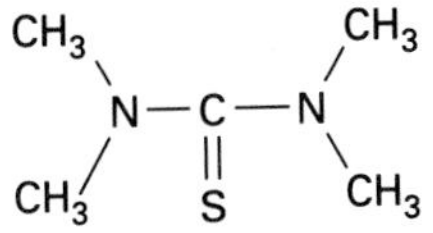

Tetramethyl thiocarbamide

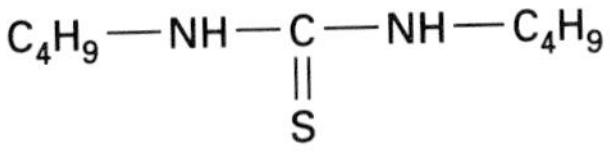

Dibutyl thiocarbamide

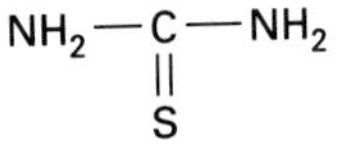

Thiocarbamide

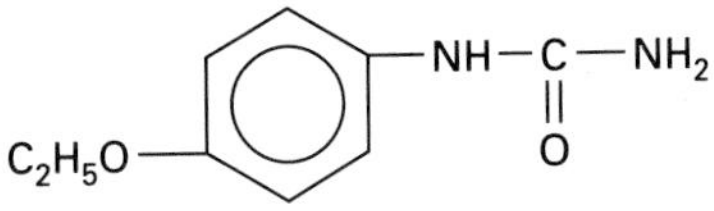

Para-ethoxyphenyl carbamide

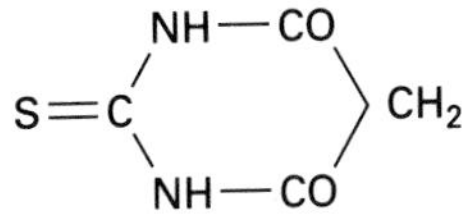

Thiobarbituric acid

Fig. 32.8. Structural formulae of compounds which are unable to detect the PTC tasting polymorphism. (Mainly from Fox 1932.)

The subject was further investigated by Hopkins (1938), who extracted and purified the chemical substance responsible for the bitter taste of *Conringia orientalis* L. (Dumort), or hare's ear mustard, which is a common weed in the wheat fields of western Canada. The relevant compound was found to be 2-mercapto-5,5-dimethyloxazoline and it was taste-less to some persons (including Hopkins himself), whilst others (including Hopkins's co-worker Mr D. C. Caplan) found it intensely bitter. Hopkins (1942) established that the new compound was detecting the same polymorphism as PTC and that it was the first instance of a nitrogen ring compound to do so.

He then proceeded to investigate a number of thiazo and oxazo compounds and sulphur-containing compounds on 'a group of individuals some of whom were tasters and some non-tasters as deter-mined by their reaction to phenylthiourea'. The results are incorporated into Tables 32.4 and 32.5. Hopkins concluded that the grouping

$$=N-\underset{\underset{S}{\|}}{C}-$$

was responsible for the dual taste reaction, but noted that there were some exceptions the most outstanding of which was thiobarbituric acid.

Table 32.4. *Compounds which are able to detect the PTC taste-testing polymorphism*

Compound	Method of testing	Number of individuals tested	Correlation of threshold with that of PTC (or alternative expression of result)	Reference
para-ethoxyphenyl thiocarbamide	Crystals	Not stated	Stated to correlate well	Fox 1932
ortho-tolyl thiocarbamide				
meta-tolylthiocarbamide				
para-tolylthiocarbamide				
para-nitrophenyl thiocarbamide				
2,5-dichlorophenylthiocarbamide				
para-methoxyphenylthiocarbamide				
para-fluorophenylthiocarbamide				
para-chlorophenylthiocarbamide				
para-bromophenyl thiocarbamide				
β-naphthylthiocarbamide				
α-naphthylthiocarbamide				
para-β-hydroxyethoxyphenyl-thiocarbamide				
sym-diphenyl thiocarbamide (thiocarbanilide)				
sym-di-ortho-tolylthiocarbamide				
sym-di-meta-tolylthiocarbamide				
sym-di-para-tolylthiocarbamide				
sym-di-(2-methoxy-5-methylphenyl) thiocarbamide				
N-meta-tolyl-N'-phenyl-thiocarbamide				
N-para-ethoxyphenyl-N'-phenyl-thiocarbamide				
sym-dibenzyl thiocarbamide				
dicrotyl thiocarbamide				
thiouracil	Powder	60	Complete correlation	Riddle & Wybar 1944
5,5-dimethyl-2-thio-oxazolidine	Crystals	Not stated	Complete correlation	Hopkins 1942
2-thio-5,5-dimethyl-thiazolidine				
2-thio-5-methyl-oxazolidine				
2-thio-5-methyl-thiazolidine				
2-thio-thiazolidine				
2-thio-4,5-dimethyl-thiazoline				
thioacetamide				
thioacetanilide				
iso-dithiocyanic acid				
thiourea	Serial dilutions	37	0.886	Harris & Kalmus 1949b
diphenylthiourea		18	0.821	
thioglyoxaline		21	0.740	
methylthiouracil		22	0.757	
acetylthiourea		18	0.950	
diacetyl thiourea		19	0.942	
thiomethyl hydantoin		19	0.892	
para-chlorophenylthiourea	Serial dilutions	20	0.966	Barnicot et al. 1951
allylthiourea		20	0.904	
ethylene thiourea		19	0.745	
1,3-diethyl thiourea		19	0.671	
tetramethyl thiourea		19	0.830	
thiouracil		22	0.745	

Table 32.4. (*cont.*)

Compound	Method of testing	Number of individuals tested	Correlation of threshold with that of PTC (or alternative expression of result)	Reference
propylthiouracil		16	0.915	
thioacetamide		17	0.824	
mercaptobenzothiazole		13	0.974	
pentothal		19	0.789	
2-mercapto-5,5-dimethyl-thiazolidine		22	0.913	
4-methyl-2-thioimidazole		14	0.933	
thiourea	Serial dilutions	22	High correlation	Shephard 1961
propylthiouracil		19 }	Complete	
5-vinyl-2-thio-oxazolidone (goitrin)		24 }	correspondence	
anetholtrithione	Serial dilutions	95	0.875	Dawson *et al.* 1967

Data derived from: Barnicot *et al.* 1951; Fox 1932; Harris & Kalmus 1949b; Hopkins 1942; Shephard 1961.

Harris & Kalmus (1949b) and Barnicot *et al.* (1951) re-investigated the subject using serial dilutions of the compounds being tested. An important difference from Fox (1932) was the finding that thiourea (syn. thiocarbamide) *did* detect the polymorphism. The results were summarized as correlations between the detection thresholds for the compound under investigation and PTC. An example, namely propylthiouracil, is shown in Table 32.6, and the results are condensed in Tables 32.4 and 32.5. It is to be noted that the taste thresholds for 34 compounds in tasters and non-tasters of 6-N-propylthiouracil are listed by Fischer & Griffin (1964).

The hypothesis that the chemical configuration

$$=N-\underset{\underset{S}{\|}}{C}-$$

was solely responsible for differentiating between tasters and non-tasters of PTC was upset by the following pieces of evidence, in addition to the thiobarbituric acid example given above.

1 Acetalyl-phenylthiourea, di-*O*-tolylthiourea and 4-methyl-2-imidazylbenzyl sulphide contain the grouping and do not differentiate between the phenotypes.
2 A further striking example of a relevant compound which does not contain the NC=S group was dis-

covered by Goedde & Ohligmacher (1965) and further investigated by Dawson *et al.* (1967), who introduced some refinements in the technique. There is no nitrogen in the molecule of anetholtrithione (Fig. 32.9) but its taste thresholds are highly repeatable in the individual and highly correlated with PTC thresholds (Dawson *et al.* 1967).

So after a large amount of work over many years, the result is inconclusive. Nearly all compounds which detect the 'PTC' taste-testing polymorphism contain the N–C=S grouping, but not all compounds containing this grouping do so. Anetholtrithione, which does not contain the N–C=S group, has the ability to detect the two phenotypes. This seems to reduce the necessary structure to the $>$C=S grouping, which is what Fox (1932) originally suggested. It would be interesting to investigate some further examples containing the grouping

$$-S-\underset{\underset{S}{\|}}{C}-$$

like anetholtrithione.

A quotation from Snyder (1932) concerning one of the compounds investigated by Fox (see Table 32.5) is also of interest to round off this discussion.

A word may be added as to the inheritance of taste deficiency to di-ortho-tolyl-thio-carbamide, another compound investigated. Approximately 35% of the

Table 32.5. *Compounds of interest which are not able to detect the PTC taste-testing polymorphism*

Compound	Method of testing	Number of individuals tested	Correlation of threshold with that of PTC (or alternative expression of result)	Reference
tetra-methylthiocarbamide	Crystals	Not stated	Sour but not lasting taste to both T & N	Fox 1932
sym-dibutylthiocarbamide			Somewhat bitter to both T & N	
thiocarbamide			Nauseating taste, not bitter, not sour to both T & N	
N-3-β-hydroxyethoxy-*N'*-3-ethoxyphenylthiocarbamide			Tasteless to both T & N	
thiobarbituric acid	Crystals	Not stated	Faint but not bitter taste to both T & N	Hopkins 1942
urea	Serial dilutions	20	−0.103	Harris & Kalmus (1949b)
uracil		19	−0.269	
aminothiouracil			Completely tasteless to all subjects	
allylisothiocyanate			Strong smell, little taste to all subjects	
methylisothiocyanate			Strong smell, little taste to all subjects	
sodium diethyl dithiocarbamate			Variable irritating peppery sting not correlated with PTC phenotype	
S-methyl-pseudothiourea			Smell of rotten cabbages. No clear difference between PTC phenotypes	
quinine		38	+0.062 (NS)	
phenylurea		19	−0.052	
acetalylphenylthiourea	Serial dilutions	13	−0.004	Barnicot *et al.* 1951
di-*O*-tolylthiourea		20	+0.239 (NS)	
diphenylguanidine hydrobromide		11	−0.034	
nembutal		20	No duality of taste thresholds	
4-methyl-2-imidazylbenzyl-sulphide		14	−0.036	
brucine	Serial solutions	109	Mean threshold value the same for both PTC phenotypes	Kalmus 1958

T, taster of PTC; N, non-taster of PTC; NS, not significant.
Data derived from: Barnicot *et al.* 1951; Fox 1932; Harris & Kalmus 1949b; Hopkins 1942; Kalmus 1958.

Table 32.6. *Distribution of taste thresholds of 16 individuals for propylthiouracil and phenylthiouracil*

Propylthiouracil solution no.	Phenylthiourea solution no.													
	<1	1	2	3	4	5	6	7	8	9	10	11	12	13
9	.	.	.	.	.	.	.	.	.	.	.	.	1	.
8	.	.	.	.	.	.	.	.	.	1	1	.	.	.
7	.	.	.	.	.	.	.	.	.	.	1	.	.	.
6	.	.	.	.	.	.	.	.	.	3	.	.	.	.
5	.	.	.	.	.	.	.	.	1	.	.	.	.	.
4	.	.	.	.	.	.	.	.	.	.	.	.	.	.
3	.	1	.	.	.	.	.	.	.	.	.	.	.	.
2	1	3	.	.	.	.	1	.	.	.	.	.	.	.
1	1	1	.	.	.	.	.	.	.	.	.	.	.	.

The solution numbers of propylthiouracil represent serial dilutions by $\frac{1}{2}$ of a solution containing 0.1 g/100 ml (solution 1).

The solution numbers of phenylthiourea represent serial dilutions by $\frac{1}{2}$ of a solution containing 0.13 g/100 ml. Solution 1 is 0.13 g/100 ml. Solution 2 is 0.065 g/100 ml, etc.

From: Barnicott *et al.* 1951.

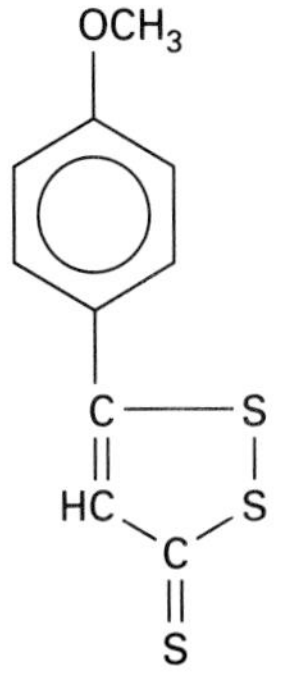

Fig. 32.9. Anethoaltrithione. (From Dawson *et al.* 1967.)

individuals tested could taste both compounds, an equal number tasted only phenylthiocarbamide, and about 30% could not taste either compound. Moreover, in many families where neither parent tasted the second compound, some of the offspring did. This indicates an epistatic relationship of the two factors concerned.

ANOTHER SIMILAR TASTE-TESTING POLYMORPHISM

The substance diphenylguanidine (Fig. 32.10) was found by Snyder & Davidson (1937) to divide people into two classes, namely tasters and non-

Table 32.7. *Reaction of 442 individuals to PTC and diphenylguanidine (DPG)*

Reaction	Number	Proportion
Taste both compounds	227	0.5136
Taste PTC only	87	0.1968
Taste DPG only	106	0.2398
Taste neither compound	22	0.0498

From: Snyder & Davidson 1937.

tasters. This polymorphism was shown by them to be independent of the PTC taste-testing polymorphism (Table 32.7). Family studies gave results compatible with control of this tasting polymorphism by two alleles at an autosomal locus (Table 32.8). Diphenylguanidine was confirmed not to detect the PTC taste-testing polymorphism by Barnicot *et al.*

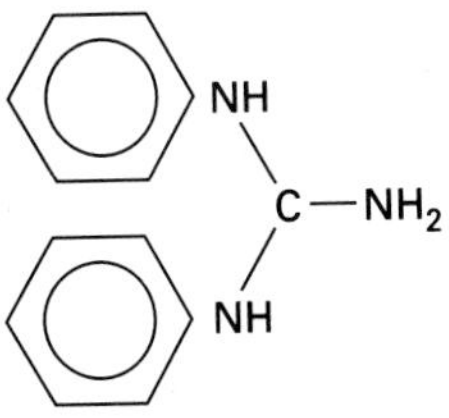

Fig. 32.10. Diphenylguanidine.

Table 32.8. *Genetic analysis of 100 families comprising 442 individuals studied for taste deficiency to diphenyl-quanidine on the hypothesis that non-tasters are Mendelian autosomal recessives*

| Mating | Number of matings | | Phenotypes of Offspring | | | | χ^2 | Degrees of freedom | p |
| | Observed | Expected | Tasters | | Non-tasters | | | | |
			Observed	Expected	Observed	Expected			
T × T	59	56.8	128	122.6	22	15.1	3.39	1	
T × N	32	37.2	52	60.1	29	29.8	1.11	1	
N × N	9	6.1	0	0	11	11	0	0	
							4.50	2	>0.05

T, taster; N, non-taster.
The expected figures have been computed using $q = \sqrt{\frac{109}{442}} = 0.4966$ from Table 32.7.
Adapted from: Snyder & Davidson 1937.

(1951) (see Table 32.5); otherwise, not much attention seems to have been paid to this potentially interesting tasting polymorphism.

INTER-ETHNIC VARIABILITY

In the remarkable compilation of Mourant *et al.* (1976) on the distribution of the human blood groups and other polymorphisms, the PTC taste testing polymorphism was included and received detailed attention as what Sir Ronald Fisher used to call an 'honorary blood group'. Their Table 65 is 13 pages long, containing the results of nearly 400 population samples, the most recent of which were published in 1971. As Mourant *et al.* (1976) stated:

Throughout Europe and Asia the frequency of tasters is not far from 70 per cent corresponding to a frequency of the taster gene of a little under 50 per cent. The relatively few results from other regions show that there are significantly fewer non-tasters among Africans than among Europeans and that a very large proportion of American Indians are tasters.

Some surveys which have appeared since Mourant's book was published are shown in Table 32.9. The frequency of the allele responsible for the recessive character is shown to vary between 0.43 and 0.59 in Europe. The Pacific, Turkish and South American series give lower values, and the African series a mixed picture.

A useful compilation, including a lot of Indian data, was published by Das (1966).

ASSOCIATIONS OF PTC PHENOTYPES WITH SPONTANEOUS DISORDERS
Thyroid disorders

The most important studies are those which show an association between PTC phenotypes and thyroid disorders. This body of knowledge came into being as a result of the convergence of two lines of investigation, as fully explained by Mourant *et al.* (1976, 1978).

First, it was found that compounds which occur naturally in plants can cause goitres in animals. Some of these compounds contained the =N—C=S grouping. A line of research initiated by this finding led eventually to the discovery of thiouracil and later other compounds such as methylthiouracil and propylthiouracil as drugs which reduce the production of thyroxine. The successful introduction of these therapeutic agents into clinical practice to treat hyperthyroidism was described by Astwood *et al.* (1945).

The second line of research was that into the elucidation of the PTC tasting polymorphism, which has been described above.

The two lines of research converged in the experiment of Riddle & Wybar (1944), who demonstrated in 60 persons a correlation between the abilities to taste PTC and thiouracil.

The compound 5,5-dimethyl-2-thio-oxazolidine, found by Hopkins (1938) in a weed, was shown by Hopkins (1942) to detect the PTC tasting polymorphism and was found to have anti-thyroid properties by Astwood *et al.* (1945).

Table 32.9. *Ethnic distribution of the PTC polymorphism*

Reference	Location	Method of testing	Population		Total number	Number of non-tasters	Frequency of the allele t responsible for the recessive character	± SE
	Europe							
Mitchell et al. 1977	Cumbria, UK	Harris & Kalmus 1949a	British children	male	518	97	0.4327	0.0198
				female	336	72	0.4629	0.0242
	Isle of Man[a]	Harris & Kalmus 1949a	Manx children	male	175	54	0.5555	0.0314
				female	218	63	0.5376	0.0286
		Harris & Kalmus 1949a	Manx adults	male	168	44	0.5118	0.0331
				female	138	33	0.4890	0.0371
Forrai & Bankovi 1981	Budapest	Harris & Kalmus 1949a	School children		436	140	0.5667	0.0197
Pentzos-Daponte & Grefen-Peters 1983	Thessalonika[b]	PTC-impregnated filter paper	Adults 20 to 50 years	male	3743	1080	0.5372	0.0069
				female	3790	907	0.4892	0.0071
Panayotou et al. 1983	Salmis Island, Greece	Harris & Kalmus 1949a	Native islanders	male	63	18	0.5345	0.0532
				female	120	41	0.5845	0.0370
Facchini et al. 1990	Emilia, Italy	Harris & Kalmus 1949a	Healthy adults	male	196	39	0.4461	0.0320
				female	115	17	0.3845	0.0430
	Pacific							
Kang & Cho 1968	Hong-do & Huksan-do islands, Korea	Harris & Kalmus 1949a	Native islanders	male	602 }	121	0.3437	0.0147
				female	422 }			
Boyce et al. 1976	Karkar Island, Papua New Guinea	Harris & Kalmus 1949a	School children		48	2	0.2041	0.0706
de Villiers 1976	Johannesburg	Harris & Kalmus 1949a	Chinese school children	male	156	3	0.1387	0.0376
				female	128	5	0.1976	0.0410
	Indian subcontinent							
Rastogi & Tyagi 1975	Uttar Pradesh[c]	Harris & Kalmus 1949a	Rastogis	male	150	31	0.4546	0.0364
				female	150	20	0.3651	0.0380
Bhatia et al. 1979	Delhi	Harris & Kalmus 1949a	University medical students	male	102	30	0.5423	0.0416
Mathur et al. 1983	Hyderabad AP[d]	Harris & Kalmus 1949a as modified by Das 1956	Presumably adults	male	178	108	0.7789[h]	0.0235
				female	244	136	0.7466	0.0213

Table 32.9. (cont.)

Reference	Location	Method of testing	Population		Total number	Number of non-tasters	Frequency of the allele t responsible for the recessive character	± SE
Akcasu & Özalp 1977	Istanbul & Resadiye (Eastern Turkey)[e]	Harris & Kalmus 1949a	Turks	male	447	20	0.2115	0.0231
				female	237	8	0.1837	0.0319
	Remainder of Asia							
Ibraimov & Mirrakhimov 1979	Frunze, Kirghizia[f]	Harris & Kalmus 1949a with the successive dilutions increased to 29	Russian students	male	45 }	78	0.5642	0.0264
				female	200 }			
			Kirghiz students	male	320 }	125	0.4419	0.0177
				female	320 }			
			Kirghiz school children	male	361 }	214	0.5400	0.0155
				female	373 }			
Ben-David et al. 1983	South Sinai peninsula	Harris & Kalmus 1949a	Tribal Bedouin from 6 Bedouin tribes	Jebalia	92	27	0.5417	0.0436
				Ulad-Said	23	6	0.5108	0.0894
				Imzine	170	71	0.6463	0.0293
				Hamada	23	13	0.7518	0.0686
				Alikat	46	26	0.7518	0.0490
				Krarshe	68	46	0.8225	0.0346
Kusenov 1984	Aktyubinsk	Harris & Kalmus 1949a	Kazakh students	male } female	405	97	0.4894	0.0217
			Russian students	male } female	161	46	0.5345	0.0333
	South America							
Mendez de Araujo et al. 1972	Porto Alegre, Brazil	Harris & Kalmus 1949a	Caucasoid		192	42	0.4677	0.0319
			Negroid		60	12	0.4472	0.0577
de Stefano & Molieri 1976	Nicaragua	Harris & Kalmus 1949a	Miskito	male	43	10	0.4823	0.0668
				female	53	10	0.4344	0.0619
			Sumo	male	40	3	0.2739	0.0760
				female	45	4	0.2982	0.0711
			Rama	male	35	0	0.0000	–
				female	44	1	0.1507	0.0706
Frisancho et al. 1977	Peru Central Highlands	Harris & Kalmus 1949a	Quechua	male	167	5	0.1730	0.0381
				female	162	5	0.1757	0.0387
	Eastern Lowlands		Quechua	male	442	28	0.2517	0.0230
				female	278	20	0.2682	0.0289
	Eastern Lowlands		Mestizo	male	436	32	0.2709	0.0230
				female	428	27	0.2512	0.0234

Study	Region	Method	Group	Sex				
Scott-Emuakpor et al. 1975	Africa Nigeria[g]	Harris & Kalmus 1949a modified, and impregnated paper strips (cross-correlated)	Eastern group	male	151	32	0.4603	0.0361
				female	114	10	0.2962	0.0447
			Mid Western group	male	259	39	0.3895	0.0286
				female	147	19	0.3595	0.0385
			Western group	male	773	98	0.1268	0.0183
				female	552	53	0.3099	0.0202
Aquaron et al. 1984	Cameroon	Harris & Kalmus 1949a	Bamileke melanoderms	male	59	21	0.5966	0.0522
				female	65	7	0.3282	0.0586
			Bamilekes albinos	male	65	15	0.4804	0.0544
				female	35	4	0.3381	0.0795
			Bamilekes melanoderms	male	44	12	0.5222	0.0643
				female	77	27	0.5922	0.0459

[a]Cites other data in Britain and Ireland.
[b]Cites other European series.
[c]Cites other Uttar Pradesh series.
[d]Cites other Indian series.
[e]Includes data on age.
[f]Includes some family data.
[g]Contains genetic analysis of 21 families.
[h]These results are so much out of line showing over half the population to be non-tasters, that a technical error in the phenotyping procedure must be suspected.

Table 32.10. *Test of the association between PTC non-tasting and polynodular goitre*

Reference	Location	Polynodular goitre		Controls		Relative incidence (x)	$\log_e x$ (y)	Sampling variance (V)	weight $\left(\frac{1}{v}=w\right)$	(wy)	(wy^2)
		Taster	Non-Taster	Taster	Non-Taster						
Harris *et al.* 1949	London, UK	79	55	372	169	1.5342	0.4280	0.0389	25.6937	10.9972	4.7069
Kitchin *et al.* 1959	Liverpool, UK	149	97	187	78	1.5577	0.4432	0.0348	28.6960	12.7191	5.6376
Hollingsworth 1963	Hiroshima, Japan	43	11	129	34	0.9923	−0.0077	0.1423	7.0263	−0.0540	0.0004
Brand 1963	U. Galilee, Israel	228	60	642	32	5.2343	1.6552	0.0526	19.0049	31.4576	52.0693
Azevedo *et al.* 1965	São Paolo, Brazil	34	12	3422	566	2.1889	0.7834	0.1075	9.2980	7.2842	5.7066
Covarrubias *et al.* 1965	Pedregoso Valley, Chile	70	3	25	1	0.8439	−0.1696	0.8025	1.2460	−0.2114	0.0359
DeLuca & Cramarossa 1965	Frosinone, Italy	25	6	364	87	1.0618	0.0600	0.1954	5.1171	0.3071	0.0184
Mendez de Araujo *et al.* 1972 (A)	Porto Alegre, Brazil	58	22	150	42	1.3620	0.3089	0.0903	11.0736	3.4212	1.0570
Mendez de Araujo *et al.* 1972 (B)	Porto Alegre, Brazil	15	5	48	12	1.3768	0.3197	0.3265	3.0628	0.9793	0.3131
Facchini *et al.* 1990	Bologna, Italy	32	19	255	56	2.7133	0.9982	0.4048	2.4705	2.4659	2.4614
								Totals	112.6890	69.3661	72.0068

A, Caucasoids; B, Negroids.

Weighted mean value of $y = Y = \frac{\Sigma wy}{\Sigma w} = 0.61555$; SE $(Y) = \sqrt{\frac{1}{\Sigma w}} = 0.0942$.

95% fiducial limits of $Y = Y \pm t_{9,\ 0.05}$ $(\Sigma w)^{-\frac{1}{2}} = 0.8286$ and 0.4025.

Antilog of $Y = X = $ combined estimates of $x = 1.8507$.

The equivalent X values to the 95% fiducial limits of $Y = 2.2902$ and 1.4955.

Significance of X from unity $= X_1^2 = \frac{(\Sigma wy)^2}{\Sigma w} = 42.6986$ $(p < 0.001)$.

Heterogeneity estimate $X_9^2 = \Sigma wy^2 - \frac{(\Sigma wy)^2}{\Sigma w} = 72.0068 - 42.6986 = 29.3083$ $(p < 0.001)$.

The calculations have been carried out to six places of decimals but the figures have been rounded off to four places of decimals for presentation in this table.
Source: Method of Woolf (1954) as modified by Haldane (1955).

The above lines of thought were also captured in the paper of Boyd (1950b), who pointed out that L-5-vinyl-2-thio-oxazolidone (later known as goitrin: Fig. 32.11) occurred in nature particularly in turnips and cabbages. Furthermore, the ability to taste this compound exactly paralleled the ability to taste PTC, and it was known to have anti-thyroid properties. This researcher planned to phenotype persons with thyroid disorders and further speculated on the nature of heterozygote advantage in the PTC tasting polymorphism.

$$CH_2 = CH - CH - CH_2$$

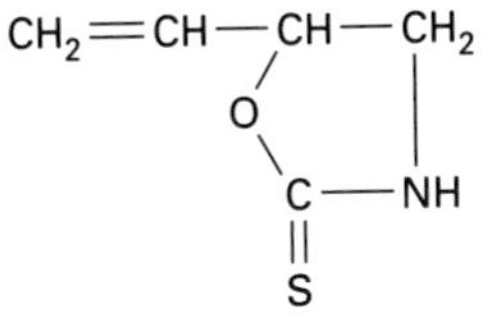

Fig. 32.11. 5-Vinyl-2-thio-oxazolidone (goitrin). (From Shepard 1961.)

Later, Shepard (1961) also showed that goitrin could detect the PTC polymorphism in man.

Stimulated by the researches summarized above, Harris *et al.* (1949) investigated the possibility that non-tasters might be more susceptible to develop thyroid disorders than PTC tasters. The results as far as polynodular goitre is concerned are summarized in Table 32.10. Though there is very significant heterogeneity between the series (some in fact did not find any association), taking the data overall non-tasters are associated with the disease 1.85 times more frequently than they should be. On the other hand, for diffuse goitre there is no positive association (Table 32.11).

The study of Boyce *et al.* (1976) could not be included in the analyses shown in Tables 32.10 and 32.11 because the authors do not specify the type of goitre they investigated. However, their result shows that goitre was significantly commoner in non-tasters than in tasters when they investigated the population of a village in Papua New Guinea for both phenomena.

Negoescu *et al.* (1980) studied goitre occurrence and PTC non-tasting in children in the endemic goitre areas of Cimpa and Cimulung in Romania. The non-taster frequency was rather higher in the goitre bearing children than in those without goitres.

Another example where there seems to be a strong association between PTC non-tasting and thyroid disease is athyreotic cretinism (Table 32.12). It must be noted, however, that there are difficulties in testing such patients and neither worker used a solution such as brucine (which gives a pronounced bitter taste in both tasters and non-tasters of PTC: see Widstrom & Henschen 1963) to check that the tasting mechanism in general was functioning. However, both groups tested the relatives of the patients and found an excess of non-tasters (Table 32.13). It is assumed that Fraser's subjects were white British; Shepard & Gartler (1960) stated that 95% of their subjects were of European ancestry, so the expected frequency of non-tasters would be about 30%. The fact that PTC non-tasters were not unduly common among metabolic cretins suggested that defects in thyroid synthesis were not responsible for the finding. So the possibility exists that in PTC non-tasting mothers, more goitrogenic substances (like goitrin itself) may be consumed during pregnancy and so may prevent thyroid development in the fetus. Obviously some other factor must also be present to cause the disease because the probands had normally-developed non-taster siblings. Shepard (1961) found no evidence that the mothers of athyreotic cretins consumed more goitrogenous foods than a control group but he did not report the data on the subsets of PTC non-taster mothers.

The relationship between the PTC taste response and thyroid function was explored by Widström & Henschen (1963) who measured the protein-bound iodine (PBI) levels in 509 subjects whose PTC taste thresholds were determined by the method of Harris & Kalmus (1949a). The non-tasters tended to have low PBI levels whilst higher levels were found in tasters (Table 32.14). The exact physiological interpretation of this finding is obscure except that it suggests the PTC tasting polymorphism might have some effect on thyroid function.

Food dislikes and preferences

The associations between various thyroid disorders and PTC taste-testing phenotypes gave rise to the idea that 'non-tasters' might consume more naturally occurring goitrogenic compounds in their food than tasters. Pursuing this idea, Fischer & Griffin (1961, 1964) presented a list of 118 foodstuffs to

Table 32.11. *Test of the association between PTC non-tasting and diffuse goitre*

Reference	Location	Diffuse goitre		Controls		Relative incidence (x)	$Log_e x$ (y)	Sampling variance (V)	weight $\left(\frac{1}{v}=w\right)$	(wy)	(wy²)
		Taster	Non-Taster	Taster	Non-Taster						
Harris et al. 1949	London, UK	151	67	372	169	0.9791	−0.0211	0.0298	33.5031	−0.7060	0.0149
Kitchin et al. 1959	Liverpool, UK	116	24	187	78	0.5023	−0.6885	0.0665	15.0322	−10.3502	7.1265
Hollingsworth 1963	Hiroshima, Japan	64	21	129	34	1.2512	0.2241	0.0971	10.2984	2.3080	0.5172
Azevedo et al. 1965	Sao Paolo, Brazil	122	21	3422	566	1.0603	0.0586	0.0556	17.9727	1.0530	0.0617
Covarrubias et al. 1965	Pedregoso Valley, Chile	58	1	25	1	0.4359	−0.8303	1.0554	0.9495	−0.7867	0.6533
DeLuca & Cramarossa 1965	Frosinone, Italy	81	25	364	87	1.3034	0.2650	0.0648	15.4416	4.0915	1.0841
Mendez de Araujo et al. 1972 (A)	Porto Alegre, Brazil	53	10	150	42	0.6950	−0.3638	0.1393	7.1785	−2.6119	0.9503
Mendez de Araujo et al. 1972 (B)	Porto Alegre, Brazil	15	2	48	12	0.3755	−0.9795	0.4932	2.0277	−1.9861	1.9454
Facchini et al. 1990	Bologna, Italy	61	14	255	56	1.0662	0.0641	0.1042	9.5927	0.6148	0.0394
								Totals	111.9944	−4.4014	12.3929

A, Caucasoids, B, Negroids.

Weighted mean value of $y = Y = \frac{\Sigma wy}{\Sigma w} = -0.0393$; SE $(Y) = \sqrt{\frac{1}{\Sigma w}} = 0.0945$.

Antilog of $Y = X$ = combined estimates of $x = 0.9610$.

The calculations have been carried out to six places of decimals but the figures have been rounded off to four places of decimals for presentation in this table.
Source: Method of Woolf (1954) as modified by Haldane (1955).

Table 32.12. *PTC non-tasting in athyreotic cretins*

Reference	Athyreotic cretins		Controls		Relative incidence
	Tasters	Non-tasters	Tasters	Non-tasters	
Fraser 1961	2	15	25[a]	12	21.1
Shepard 1961	9	18	104[b]	29	6.9

[a]Metabolic cretins, juvenile myxoedema and Pendred's syndrome (McKusick 26070).
[b]Healthy adults and children.
Relative incidence computed on the assumption that there is an association between PTC non-tasting and athyreotic cretinism by the method of Woolf (1954) as modified by Haldane (1955).

Table 32.13. *PTC tasting phenotypes in the relatives of athyreotic cretins*

Reference	Relation	Tasters	Non-tasters	% non-tasters
Fraser 1961	Parents	15	18	54.5
Shepard 1961	Fathers	15	12	44.4
	Mothers	15	15	50.0
	Siblings	11	18	62.1

Table 32.14. *Serum protein-bound iodine concentrations in tasters and non-tasters of PTC*

PBI concentration (γ per cent)	Numbers of persons	
	Tasters	Non-tasters
Low 1.0–3.9	3	12
Normal 4.0–7.9	288	150
High 8.0–15.0	46	10

$\chi_2^2 = 70.4$, $p < 0.001$.
From: Widström & Henschen 1963.

experimental subjects (presumably college students) who were taste-tested with propylthiouracil and quinine. It was found that 'tasters' disliked significantly more foods than non-tasters. Similar findings were obtained by Forrai & Bankovi (1981). However, the food preferences of 282 students – nearly all Caucasian – were investigated by Mattes & Labov (1989) and the foods were categorized according to their capacity to inhibit thyroid iodine uptake. No difference between the PTC taster phenotypes was found in any category.

In view of accounts like those of Greer & Astwood (1948) and Clements (1957), it is clear that a huge number of bitter-tasting goitrogenous plants have not had their active principles defined and have not been investigated for their ability to detect the PTC tasting polymorphism.

Other conditions

A comprehensive table showing various conditions studied for their associations with PTC tasting phenotypes has been published by Mourant *et al.* (1978), and therefore Table 32.15 has been constructed mainly to show some observations made since that time.

The most striking entry in this table is that of Mourao & Salzano (1978), showing the association of tasters with tuberculosis. The association of non-tasters with glaucoma is also an observation which has been reported by more than one research group (e.g. Becker & Morton 1964 as well as Soodan *et al.* 1978).

As far as thyroid disorders other than polynodular goitre and athyreotic cretinism are concerned there is no hint of a positive association with either phenotype.

Table 32.15. *Studies of associations of PTC taste phenotypes with miscellaneous disorders and variables*

Reference	Condition	Conclusion
Kitchin *et al.* 1959 Mendez de Araujo *et al.* 1972 } Facchini *et al.* 1990	Single thyroid adenoma	No significant difference in phenotype frequency from controls
Mourao & Salzano 1978	Tuberculosis	Five series analysed by the method of Woolf (1954) for association of tasters with tuberculosis. Significance of deviation of X from unity $\chi_1^2 = 26.70$ ($p < 0.001$) Heterogeneity $\chi_4^2 = 15.67$ ($p < 0.01$)
Sriram *et al.* 1975	Diabetes mellitus	No association (agreeing with Harris *et al.* 1949)
Mascie-Taylor *et al.* 1983	Psychometric variables (personality and intelligence quotient test scores in university undergraduate students)	Non-tasters more placid (rather than apprehensive), relaxed (rather than tense) and practical (rather than imaginative) and scored higher on the more visuo-spatial component of an IQ test than their taster counterparts
Whittemore 1986	Depression rating (mainly in college students)	Tasters had higher depression scores ($p = 0.026$) and also higher mean scores on: – feeling like a failure – self hatred – somatization – boredom – guilt feelings as compared with non-tasters
Kimmel & Lester 1987	Psychoticism Extraversion Neuroticism History of thinking about suicide, threatening suicide, attempting suicide	No significant difference between tasters and non-tasters
Soodan *et al.* 1978	Glaucoma	Increased incidence of non-tasters which agrees with Becker & Morton (1964)
	Cataract	Slightly increased incidence of non-tasters
Gasset & Houde 1977	Keratoconus	No association
Stanchev *et al.* 1985	Duodenal ulcer	298 duodenal ulcer patients, 15% non-tasters 213 duodenal ulcer patients with a positive family history 10% non-tasters. 408 controls, 23% non-tasters Both comparisons significant $p < 0.01$
Frank & Korchmar 1985	Reaction times to various gustatory stimuli	The reaction times were swifter in PTC tasters for all tastes
Whissell-Buechy & Wills 1989[a]	Age of reaching 15 indices of physiological maturity in girls and 12 indices in boys	In girls PTC tasters achieved the indices earlier than non-tasters. In boys the reverse was true
Li *et al.* 1990	Duodenal ulcer Gastric ulcer	134 duodenal ulcer patients, 26% non-tasters 164 gastric ulcer patients, 15% non-tasters. 299 controls, 19% non tasters. Difference between duodenal ulcer series and control not significant

[a]Contains also data on 56 families.

EPILOGUE

The PTC tasting polymorphism was shown to be present in primates by Fisher *et al.* (1939) and Chiarelli (1963). Considerable differences between various strains of mouse in their consumption of PTC have been found by Whitney & Harder (1986) and Lush (1986), but there has been no clear demonstration in rodents of a tasting polymorphism.

The fact that the polymorphism has survived in the human race since the anthropoid and hominid stocks separated means that there is a stable equilibrium. The implication of this, as Fisher *et al.* (1939) pointed out, is that there must be according to the Darwinian view a selective advantage for the heterozygotes.

It has been suggested that the heterozygote advantage might be somehow related to either protection from excessive natural goitrogen ingestion or survival when dietary iodine was scarce. While the molecular basis of the polymorphism is unknown the nature of the selective advantage will probably remain a mystery.

Since it is suspected that the site of action in the thyroid gland of the $N-C\!\!=\!\!S$ containing antithyroid compounds is peroxidase, it is speculated that the PTC polymorphism may be concerned with this enzyme. As has been mentioned earlier, Fischer & Griffin (1964) started investigating salivary peroxidase in the two phenotypes and found an activity difference between them, but the subject was apparently not pursued.

It is interesting to note that in a discussion of the underlying mechanism of the PTC tasting polymorphism and the phenotyping methods available Mourant *et al.* (1978) state, 'Perhaps one day a test will be devised using living cells from tongue scrapings.' This vision of the future would now be a distinct possibility using the technique of polymerase chain reaction (Peake 1989; Vosberg 1989) if the structure of the relevant polymorphic DNA or RNA were known.

The author would like to express his gratitude to Emeritus Professor Sir Cyril A. Clarke, FRS, University of Liverpool, UK who made many helpful suggestions about the contents of this chapter.

Akcasu, A. & Özalp, E. (1977). Distribution of taste thresholds for phenylthiocarbamide among different age groups in Turkey. *Pahlavi Medical Journal*, **8**, 294–304.

Anonymous items (1931). *Science*, **73**, (Suppl 14).

Aquaron, R., Kamden, L., Menard, J.-Cl., Bridonneau, C. & Battaglini, P. F. (1984). Etudes séroanthropologiques des populations albinos et melanodermes Bamilekes (Cameroun); groupes erythrocytaires ABO et Rhesus hemoglobine S et sensibilité gustative à la phenylthiocarbamide. *Medicine Tropicale*, **44**, 311–18.

Astwood, E. B., Bissell, A. & Hughes, A. M. (1945). Further studies on the chemical nature of compounds which inhibit the function of the thyroid gland. *Endocrinology*, **37**, 456–81.

Azevedo, E., Kriger, H., Mi, M. P. & Morton, N. E. (1965). PTC taste sensitivity and endemic goiter in Brazil. *American Journal of Human Genetics*, **17**, 87–90.

Barnicot, N. A., Harris, H. & Kalmus, H. (1951). Taste thresholds of further eighteen compounds and their correlation with PTC thresholds. *Annals of Eugenics (London)*, **16**, 119–28.

Becker, B. & Morton, W. R. (1964). Phenylthiourea taste testing and glaucoma. *Archives of Ophthalmology*, **72**, 323–7.

Beidler, L. M. (1961). The chemical senses. *Annual Review of Psychology*, **12**, 363–88.

Ben-David Koblinski, I., Mikla, S., Hershkovitz, I. & Arensburg, B. (1983). Taste sensitivity to phenylthiocarbamide in Bedouin of South Sinai. *Harefuah*, **105**, 56–9.

Bhatia, S., Sharma, K. N., Tandon, O. P. & Singh, S. (1979). Relation of PTC responses and secretor status to blood groups. *Indian Journal of Physiology and Pharmacology*, **23**, 269–76.

Blakeslee, A. F. (1932). Genetics of sensory thresholds, taste for phenyl thiocarbamide. *Proceedings of the National Academy of Sciences (USA)*, **18**, 120–30.

Blakeslee, A. F. & Salmon, M. R. (1931). Odor and taste blindness. *Eugenical News*, **16**, 105–9.

Blakeslee, A. F. & Salmon, T. N. (1935). Genetics of sensory thresholds, individual taste reactions for different substances. *Proceedings of the National Academy of Sciences (USA)*, **21**, 84–98.

Boyce, A. J., Harrison, G. A., Platt, C. M. & Hornabrook, R. W. (1976). Association between PTC taster status and goitre in a Papua New Guinea population. *Human Biology*, **48**, 769–73.

Boyd, W. C. (1950a). *Genetics and the Races of Man.* Oxford: Blackwell. (Cited by Harris & Kalmus 1951.)

Boyd, W. C. (1950b). Taste reactions to antithyroid substances. *Science*, **117**, 153.

Brand, N. (1963). Taste sensitivity and endemic goiter in Israel. *Annals of Human Genetics (London)*, **26**, 321–4.

Chautard-Freire-Maia, E. A. (1974). Linkage relationships between 22 autosomal markers. *Annals of Human Genetics (London)*, **38**, 191–8.

Chiarella, B. (1963). Sensitivity to PTC (phenyl-thiocarbamide) in primates. *Folia Primatologica*, **1**, 88–94.

Clements, F. W. (1957). A goitrogenic factor in milk. *Medical Journal of Australia*, **44**, 645–6.

Clements, F. W. & Wishart, J. W. (1956). A thyroid-blocking agent in the etiology of endemic goiter. *Metabolism*, **5**, 623–39.

Cohen, J. & Ogdon, D. P. (1949). Taste blindness to PTC as a function of saliva. *Science*, **110**, 532–3.

Conneally, P. M., Dumont-Driscoll, M., Huntzinger, R. S., Nance, S. E. & Jackson, C. E. (1976). Linkage relations of the loci for Kell and phenylthiocarbamide taste sensitivity. *Human Heredity*, **26**, 267–71.

Covarrubias, E., Barzelatto, J., Stevenson, C., Bobadilla, E., Pardo, A. & Beckers, C. (1965). Taste sensitivity to phenylthiocarbamide and endemic goiter among Pewenche Indians. *Nature*, **205**, 1036.

Das, S. R. (1956). A contribution to the heredity of the PTC taste character based on a study of 845 sib pairs. *Annals of Eugenics (London)*, **20**, 334–43.

Das, S. R., (1966). Application of phenylthiocarbamide taste character in the study of racial variation. *Journal of the Indian Anthropology Society (Calcutta)*, **1**, 63–80.

Dawson, W., West, G. B. & Kalmus, H. (1967). Taste polymorphism to anetholtrithione and phenylthio-carbamate. *Annals of Human Genetics (London)*, **30**, 273–6.

De Luca, F. & Cramarossa, L. (1965). Phenylthiourea and endemic goiter. *Lancet*, **1**, 1399–400.

De Stefano, G. F. & Molieri, J. J. (1976). PTC tasting among three Indian groups of Nicaragua. *American Journal of Physical Anthropology*, **44**, 371–3.

De Villiers, H. (1976). Studies on the ability to taste phenylthiocarbamide; red-green colour blindness and the age at menarche in Johannesburg Chinese school children. *South African Journal of Medical Sciences*, **41**, 279–83.

Facchini, F., Abbati, A. & Campagnoni, S. (1990). Possible relations between sensitivity to phenylthiocarbamide and goiter. *Human Biology*, **62**, 545–52.

Fischer, R. & Griffin, F. (1960). Factors involved in the mechanism of taste-blindness. *Journal of Heredity*, **51**, 182–3.

Fischer, R. & Griffin, F. (1961). 'Taste-blindness' and variations in taste-threshold in relation to thyroid metabolism. *Journal of Neuropsychiatry*, **3**, 98–104.

Fischer, R. & Griffin, F. (1964). Pharmacogenetic aspects of gustation. *Drug Research (Arzneimittel-Forschung) (Aulendorf)*, **14**, 673–86.

Fischer, R., Griffin, F., England, S. & Pasamanick, B. (1961). Biochemical-genetic factors of taste-polymorphism and their relation to salivary thyroid metabolism in health and mental retardation. *Medicina Experimentalis*, **4**, 356–66.

Fischer, R., Griffin, F. & Mead, E. L. (1962). Two characteristic ranges of taste sensitivity. *Medicina Experimentalis*, **6**, 177–82.

Fischer, R., Griffin, F. & Pasamanick, B. (1965). The perception of taste, some psychophysiological pathophysiological pharmacological and clinical aspects. In *Psychopathology of Perception*, ed. P. Hoch & J. Zubin, pp. 129–64. New York, Grune & Stratton.

Fischer, R., Griffin, F. & Rockey, M. A. (1966). Gustatory chemoreception in man, multidisciplinary aspects and perspectives. *Perspectives in Biology and Medicine*, **9**, 549–77.

Fisher, R. A., Ford, E. B. & Huxley, J. (1939). Taste-testing the anthropoid apes. *Nature*, **144**, 750.

Forrai, G. & Bankovi, G. (1981). Geschmacksempfinding für Speisen und Schmeckvermögen für PTC bei ungarischen Schulkindern *Arztliche Jugendkunde (Leipzig)*, **72**, 246–51.

Fox, A. L. (1932). The relationship between chemical constitution and taste. *Proceedings of the National Academy of Sciences (USA)*, **18**, 115–20.

Frank, R. A. & Korchmar, D. L. (1985). Gustatory processing differences in PTC tasters and non-tasters, a reaction time analysis. *Physiology and Behaviour*, **35**, 239–42.

Fraser, G. R. (1961). Cretinism and taste sensitivity to phenylthiocarbamide. *Lancet*, **1**, 964–5.

Frisancho, A. R., Klayman, J. E., Schessler, T. & Way, A. B. (1977). Taste sensitivity to phenylthiourea (PTC), tongue rolling, and hand clasping among Peruvian and other native American populations. *Human Biology*, **49**, 155–63.

Gasset, A. R. & Houde, W. L. (1977). Pharmacogenetics in keratoconus. *Annals of Ophthalmology*, **9**, 57–8.

Goedde, H. W. & Ohligmacher, H. (1965). Zur problematik des polymorphisms des Bitterschmeckens: vergleichende Untersuchungen an Thioharnstoffderivaten und Anetholtrithion. *Humangenetik*, **1**, 423–36.

Greer, M. A. & Astwood, E. B. (1948). The antithyroid effect of certain foods in man as determined with radio-active iodine. *Endocrinology*, **43**, 105–19.

Griffin, F. & Fischer, R. (1960). Differential reactivity of saliva from 'tasters' and 'non-tasters' of 6-*n*-propyl-thiouracil. *Nature*, **187**, 417–19.

Haldane, J. B. S. (1955). The estimation and significance of the logarithm of a ratio of frequence. *Annals of Human Genetics (London)*, **20**, 309–11.

Harris, H. & Kalmus, H. (1949a). The measurement of taste sensitivity to phenylthiourea (PTC). *Annals of Eugenics (London)*, **15**, 24–31.

Harris, H. & Kalmus, H. (1949b). Chemical specificity in genetical differences of taste sensitivity. *Annals of Eugenics (London)*, **15**, 32–45.

Harris, H. & Kalmus, H. (1951). The distribution of taste thresholds for phenylthiourea of 384 sib pairs. *Annals of Eugenics (London)*, **16**, 226–30.

Harris, H., Kalmus, H. & Trotter, W. R. (1949). Taste sensitivity to phenylthiourea in goitre and diabetes. *Lancet*, **2**, 1038–9.

Henkin, R. I. & Kopin, I. J. (1964). Abnormalities of taste and smell thresholds in familial dysantonomia: improvement with methacholine. *Life Sciences*, **3** 1319–25.

Hollingsworth, D. R. (1963). Phenylthiourea taste testing in Hiroshima subjects with thyroid disease. *Journal of Clinical Endocrinology*, **23**, 961–3.

Hopkins, C. Y. (1938). A sulphur containing substance from the seed of *Conringia orientalis*. *Canadian Journal of Research B*, **16**, 341–4.

Hopkins, C. Y. (1942). Taste differences in compounds having the NCS linkage. *Canadian Journal of Research B*, **20**, 268–73.

Ibraimov, A. & Mirrakhimov, M. M. (1979). PTC-tasting ability in populations living in Kirghizia with special reference to hypersensitivity: its relation to age and sex. *Human Genetics (Annals of London)*, **46**, 97–105.

Kalmus, H. (1958). Improvements in the classification of the taster genotypes. *Annals of Human Genetics (London)*, **22**, 222–30.

Kalmus, H. (1959). A contribution to a discussion. In *Biochemistry and Human Genetics*, ed. G. E. W. Wolstenholme. & C. M. O'Connor. CIBA Foundation Symposium. London: Churchill. (Cited by Fischer & Griffin 1961.)

Kalmus, H. (1976). PTC testing of infants. *Annals of Human Genetics (London)*, **40**, 139–40.

Kalmus, H. & Farnsworth, D. (1959). Impairment and recovery of taste following irradiation of the oropharynx. *Journal of Laryngology and Otology*, **73**, 180–2.

Kalmus, H. & Smith, S. M. (1965). The antimode and lines of optimal separation in a genetically determined bimodal distribution, with particular reference to phenyl-thiocarbamide sensitivity. *Annals of Human Genetics (London)*, **29**, 127–38.

Kalmus, H. & Trotter, W. R. (1962). Direct assessment of the effect of age on PTC sensitivity. *Annals of Human Genetics (London)*, **26**, 145–9.

Kang, Y. S. & Cho, W. K. (1968). Genetic studies on the isolated populations in Korea on the frequency of color-blindness and tastability to PTC. *Proceedings of the International Seminar on Occupational Health in Developing Countries*. Lagos, Nigeria, April 1968, pp. 534–6.

Kaplan, A. R., Fischer, R., Karras, A., Griffin, F., Powell, W., Marsters, R. W. & Glanville, E. V. (1967). Taste thresholds in twins and siblings. *Acta Geneticae Medicae et Gemellologiae (Roma)*, **16**, 229–43.

Kaplan, A. R., Glanville, E. V. & Fischer, R. (1964). Taste thresholds for bitterness and cigarette smoking. *Nature*, **202**, 1366.

Kimmel, H. L. & Lester, D. (1987). Personalities of those who can taste phenylthiocarbamide. *Psychological Reports*, **61**, 586.

Kitchin, F. D., Howel-Evans, W., Clarke, C. A., McConnell, R. B. & Sheppard, P. M. (1959). PTC taste-response and thyroid disease. *British Medical Journal*, **1**, 1069–74.

Kusenov, K. U. (1984). Taste sensitivity to phenylthiocarbamide among the population of West Kazakhstan. *Genetika (Moskva)*, **20**, 702–4.

Lee, B. F. (1934). A genetic analysis of taste deficiency in the American negro. *Ohio Journal of Science*, **34**, 337–42.

Leguebe, A. (1960). Génétique et anthropologie de la sensibilité à la phenylthiocarbamide. 1. Fréquence du gène dans la population Belge. *Institut Royal des Sciences naturelles de Belgique*, **36**, 1–27.

Li, Z.-L., McIntosh, J. H., Byth, K., Stuckey, B., Stiel, D. & Piper, D. W. (1990). Phenylthiocarbamide taste sensitivity in chronic peptic ulcer. *Gastroenterology*, **99**, 66–70.

Lugg, J. W. H. (1966a). Extremely high acuities of taste for phenylthiocarbamide in human population groups. *Nature*, **212**, 841–2.

Lugg, J. W. H. (1966b). Taste thresholds for phenylthio-carbamide of some population groups III: The threshold of some groups living in Japan. *Annals of Human Genetics (London)*, **29**, 217–30.

Lugg, J. W. H. (1970). Unusually high taste acuity for phenylthiocarbamide in two Formosan aboriginal groups. *Nature*, **228**, 1103–4.

Lush, I. E. (1986). Differences between mouse strains in their consumption of phenylthiourea (PTC). *Heredity*, **57**, 319–23.

McKusick, V. A. (1992). *Mendelian Inheritance in Man*, 10th edition. Baltimore, Md: Johns Hopkins University Press.

Mascie-Taylor, C. G. N., McManus, I. C., MacLarnon, A. M. & Lanigan, P. M. (1983). The association between phenylthiocarbamide (PTC) tasting ability and psychometric variables. *Behaviour Genetics*, **13**, 191–6.

Mathur, V. D., Mathur, S. & Bahadur, B. (1983). Taste deficiency for phenylthiocarbamide in Mathur Kayasths community of Hyderabad AP. *Indian Journal of Physiology and Pharmacology*, **27**, 92–100.

Mattes, R. & Labov, J. (1989). Bitter taste responses to phenylthiocarbamide are not related to dietary goitrogen intake in human beings. *Journal of the American Diet Association*, **89**, 692–4.

Mendez de Araujo, H. M., Salzano, F. M. & Wolf, H. (1972). New data on the association between PTC and thyroid disease. *Humangenetik*, **15**, 136–44.

Merton, B. B. (1958). Taste sensitivity to PTC in 60 Norwegian families with 176 children. Confirmation of the hypothesis of single gene inheritance. *Acta Geneticae Medicae et Gemellologiae (Roma)*, **8**, 114–28.

Mitchell, R. J., Cook, R. M. & Sunderland, E. (1977). Phenylthiocarbamide (PTC) taste sensitivity in selected populations in the Isle of Man and Cumbria. *Annals of Human Biology*, **4**, 431–8.

Mohr, J. (1951). Taste sensitivity to phenylthiourea in Denmark. *Annals of Eugenics (London)*, **16**, 282–6.

Mourant, A. E., Kopec, A. C. & Domaniewska-Sobzak, K. (1976). Other biochemical polymorphisms. In *The Distribution of the Human Blood Groups and Other Polymorphisms*, pp. 44–6 & 786–98. Oxford: Oxford University Press.

Mourant, A. E., Kopec, A. C. & Domaniewska-Sobzak, K. (1978). The phenylthiocarbamide tasting system. In *Blood Groups and Diseases*, pp. 39–41 & 245–51. Oxford: Oxford University Press.

Mourao, L. A. C. B. & Salzano, F. M. (1978). New data on the association between PTC tasting and tuberculosis. *Revista Brasileira de Biologia*, **38**, 475–9.

Negoescu, I., Ciovirnache, M., Simescu, M. & Ghisa, D. (1980). Some aspects concerning taste sensitivity to PTC and dermatoglyphics in children from endemic goitre areas. *Endocrinologie*, **18**, 35–41.

Olson, J. M., Boehnke, M., Neiswanger, K., Roche, A. F. & Siervogel, R. M. (1989). Alternative genetic models for the inheritance of the phenylthiocarbamide taste deficiency. *Genetic Epidemiology*, **6**, 423–34.

Panayotou, T., Kritsikis, S. & Bartsocas, C. S. (1983). Taste sensitivity to phenyl thiocarbamide in the Salamis Island population (Greece). *Human Heredity*, **33**, 179–80.

Peake, I. (1989). The polymerase chain reaction. *Journal of Clinical Pathology*, **423**, 673–6.

Pentzos-Daponte, A. & Grefen-Peters, S. (1983). Über die verteilung einiger morphologischer Merkmale sowie der PTC-Schmeck fähigkeit in der nordgriechischen Bevölkerung. *Anthropologischer Anzeiger*, **41**, 21–31.

Rao, D. C. & Morton, N. E. (1977). Residual family resemblance for PTC taste sensitivity. *Human Genetics*, **36**, 317–20.

Rastogi, S. & Tyagi, D. (1975). Phenylthiocarbamide taste threshold distribution among the Rastogis of India. *Acta Geneticae Medicae et Gemellologiae (Roma)*, **24**, 167–8.

Reddy, B. M. & Rao, D. C. (1989). Phenylthiocarbamide taste sensitivity revisited: complete sorting test supports residual family resemblance. *Genetic Epidemiology*, **6**, 413–21.

Riddle, W. J. B. & Wybar, K. C. (1944). Taste of thiouracil and PTC. *Nature*, **154**, 669.

Rife, D. C. (1933). Genetic studies of monozygotic twins. *Journal of Heredity*, **24**, 339–45.

Rubin, T. R., Griffin, F. & Fischer, R. (1962). A physico-chemical treatment of taste thresholds. *Nature*, **195**, 362–4.

Scott-Emuakpor, A. B., Uviovo, J. E. & Warren, S. T.

(1975). Genetic variation in Nigeria I, The genetics of phenylthiourea tasting ability. *Human Heredity*, **25**, 360–9.

Setterfield, W., Schott, R. G. & Snyder, L. H. (1936). Studies in human inheritance XV. The bimodality of the threshold curve for the taste of phenyl-thio-carbamide. *Ohio Journal of Science*, **36**, 231–5.

Shamil, S. & Birch, G. G. (1990). A conceptual model of taste receptors. *Endeavour New Series*, **14**, 191–3.

Shepard, T. H., II (1961). Phenylthiocarbamide non-tasting among congenital athyrotic cretins: further studies in an attempt to explain the increased incidence. *Journal of Clinical Investigation*, **40**, 1751–7.

Shepard, T. H., II & Gartler, S. M. (1960). Increased incidence of non-tasters of phenylthiocarbamide among congenital athyreotic cretins. *Science*, **131**, 929.

Shepard, T. H., Lorincz, A. E. & Gartler, S. M. (1963). Desulfuration of thiourea by saliva. *Proceedings of the Society for Experimental Biology and Medicine*, **112**, 38–42.

Snyder, L. H. (1931). Inherited taste deficiency. *Science*, **74**, 151–2.

Snyder, L. H. (1932). Studies in human inheritance IX. The inheritance of taste deficiency in man. *Ohio Journal of Science*, **32**, 436–40.

Snyder, L. H. & Davidson, D. F. (1937). Studies in human inheritance XVIII. The inheritance of taste deficiency to diphenyl-guanidine. *Eugenical News*, **22**, 1–2.

Soodan, S. S., Gupta, S., Rahi, A. H. & Saiduzzaffar, H. (1978). Phenyl thiourea (PTC) taste sensitivity in ocular disorders. *Indian Journal of Ophthalmology*, **4**, 30–2.

Sriram, K., Balaraman, V. T. & Usha, J. (1975). The

association between taste sensitivity to phenylthio-carbamide and diabetes mellitus. *Indian Journal of Medical Research*, **63**, 390–5.

Stanchev, I., Tsonev, K. & Mincher, M. (1985). Duodenal ulcer: genetic analysis by the phenylthiocarbamide test. *Folia Medica*, **27**, 13–16.

Vosberg, H.-P. (1989). The polymerase chain reaction: an improved method for the analysis of nucleic acids. *Human Genetics*, **83**, 1–15.

Wheatcroft, P. E. J. & Thornburn, C. C. (1972). Toxicity of the taste testing compound phenylthiocarbamide. *Nature New Biology*, **235**, 93–4.

Whittemore, P. B. (1986). Phenylthiocarbamide (PTC) tasting and reported depression. *Journal of Clinical Psychology*, **42**, 260–3.

Whissell-Buechy, D. & Wills, C. (1989). Male and female correlations for taster (PTC) phenotypes and rate of adolescent development. *Annals of Human Biology*, **16**, 131–46.

Whitney, G. & Harder, D. B. (1986). Phenylthiocarbamide (PTC) preference among laboratory mice: understanding of a previously 'unreplicated' report. *Behaviour Genetics*, **16**, 605–10.

Widström, G. & Henschen, A. (1963). The relation between PTC taste response and protein-bound iodine in serum. *Scandinavian Journal of Clinical and Laboratory Investigation*, **15**, (Suppl. 69), 257–61.

Woolf, B. (1954). On estimating the relation between blood group and disease. *Annals of Human Genetics (London)*, **19**, 251–3.

33 Hereditary anticoagulant resistance

CLINICAL EXPERIENCE

IN 1964 O'Reilly *et al.* (1964) published the first recorded kindred of exceptional resistance to coumarin anticoagulant drugs. As with some other pharmacogenetic examples discussed in this book a striking clinical picture in a patient led to the discovery.

A 73 year old male oil prospector of English–Irish extraction had been quite well until he sustained a myocardial infarction. It was intended to treat him with warfarin (Fig. 33.1) but the drug was not given because his prothrombin time was found to show 55 to 65% of normal activity. The bleeding time (Duke method) was 1½ minutes, coagulation time (Lee–White method) 11 minutes and prothrombin complex activity 41%. The following specific blood-clotting factors were determined: factor II 74%, factor V 130%, factor VII 46%, factor IX 112% and factor X 85% of normal.

One month after his infarction long term treatment with oral anticoagulation was started. Warfarin at 20 mg daily had no significant effect on the prothrombin time, and therefore the patient was referred to a consultant for more extensive investigations.

Later O'Reilly (1970, 1972) outlined some of the possible mechanisms of resistance to oral anticoagulant drugs, as follows:

1 decreased gastrointestinal absorption of the drug;
2 increased metabolic transformation, excretion or volume of distribution of the drug;

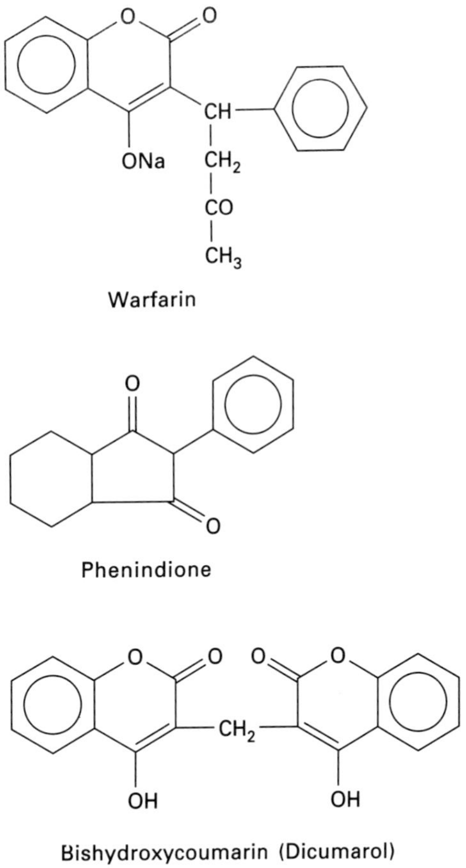

Fig. 33.1. Structural formulae of some anticoagulant drugs.

3 increased production of clotting factors dependent on vitamin K;
4 prolonged biologic half-life of clotting factors dependent on vitamin K;
5 presence of an alternate pathway for production of clotting factors, bypassing vitamin K;
6 increased activity or altered metabolism of vitamin K;
7 presence of an enzyme or receptor site with altered affinity or permeability for vitamin K or anticoagulant drug.

The above considerations were evaluated by the following observations made on the proband (O'Reilly *et al.* 1964), who was not taking any other medication.

1 Following a single oral dose of 1.5 mg warfarin per kg body weight (BW) the maximal plasma concentration was 12 mg/l in 9 hours and the plasma disappearance half-life was 36 hours, both being values within normal limits. The prothrombin time was only slightly prolonged.
2 An oral dose of 12 mg warfarin per kg BW (660 mg) gave a duration and magnitude of prothrombin response within the range of values given by normal persons after 1.5 mg/kg. The time curve of the prothrombin response was normal, but the warfarin concentration was 8 times higher than normal.
3 The dose–response curve was parallel to that obtained in normal persons but shifted to the right (Fig. 33.2).
4 The plasma elimination half-life and apparent volume of distribution of warfarin did not vary significantly with the size of the dose.
5 The degree of binding of warfarin to plasma proteins was normal.
6 The rates of disappearance of four vitamin K dependent clotting factors from the plasma following a single large intravenous dose of warfarin were normal.
7 A similar resistance to that encountered to warfarin was also observed using bishydroxycoumarin and phenindione (Fig. 33.1).
8 The response to heparin was normal.
9 The effect of vitamin K on the prothrombinopenic response to warfarin was much greater in the proband than in the normal.
10 On continued treatment with high doses of warfarin for therapeutic purposes to achieve a prothrombin activity of 20 to 35%, the liver function (as assessed by bromsulphthalein clearance) remained unimpaired, no bleeding tendency occurred and no evidence of a direct toxic vascular effect was observed.

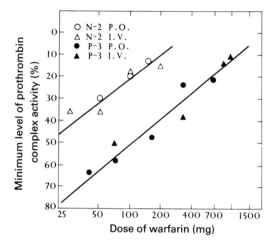

Fig. 33.2. Comparison of the dose–response relation in the propositus (P-3) and the normal subject (N-2). The response is expressed on a linear scale as the minimum level of prothrombin activity achieved after the dose administered and is plotted as a function of the log of the dose. Regression lines were fitted to the data by the method of least squares. (From O'Reilly *et al.* 1964.)

So the evidence pointed very definitely towards the seventh in the theoretical list of possibilities given above, namely an abnormal molecule concerned with vitamin K metabolism or action with a greatly lowered affinity for warfarin.

The family of the proband (including his twin brother) was investigated, and of the nine persons tested, seven exhibited anticoagulant resistance the same as the proband. The pattern of inheritance was suggestive of an autosomal dominant mode of transmission but X-linked autosomal dominance could not be excluded.

A second much larger family was studied by O'Reilly (1970). The proband was a 43 year old man of Scottish ancestry who had suffered from recurrent thrombophlebitis and pleurisy. The same tests were performed on him as on the initial proband, with the same results. Fifty-two of his fifty-nine living family members free of drug exposure and over the age of 2 years were investigated. The prothrombin-complex activity 48 hours following a single dose of 1.5 mg warfarin per kg BW gave two widely separate frequency distribution modes, allowing unequivocal phenotyping. The pedigree was consistent with inheritance as an autosomal dominant character (Fig. 33.3).

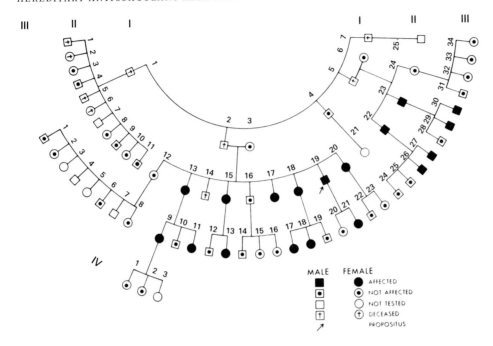

Fig. 33.3. Pedigree of family McC. (From O'Reilly 1970.)

VITAMIN K

As is made very clear in the review of Hathaway (1987), the vitamin K group of compounds exists in two major forms: (1) phylloquinone (Vitamin K_1) found in green plants, and (2) menaquinones (vitamin K_2) which are a group of compounds synthesized by intestinal bacteria and which have variable numbers of side chains. Vitamin K is an essential co-factor in the carboxylation of glutamic acid residues in clotting factor proteins II, VII, IX and X which confers on them calcium-binding properties. The carboxylation apparently occurs after formation of the primary gene product, after removal of the signal peptide, after disulphide bonding and after carbohydrate addition but before beta-aspartyl hydroxylation and sialylation (Suttie 1986). During this process the reduced vitamin K (hydroxy-

A third proband, a 57 year old black woman was described by Alving *et al.* (1985). She presented with weakness of the left arm 4 months after the insertion of a prosthetic mitral valve. The same tests as have been described above were carried out on this proband and her daughter and yielded the same results.

quinone) is oxidized to vitamin K 2,3-epoxide. The reduction of this intermediary compound back to hydroxyquinone constitutes a metabolic cycle and is the site of action of 4-hydroxycoumarins such as warfarin (Fig. 33.4). The principal site of mammalian clotting factor production is the liver.

HEREDITARY WARFARIN RESISTANCE IN RATS

Although it is not the purpose of this book to discuss pharmacogenetics in animals, it is, however, necessary to discuss hereditary warfarin resistance in rats at this point. The reason for this is that studies in rats have revealed the probable mechanisms responsible for hereditary warfarin resistance in humans.

Warfarin was introduced as a rodenticide in 1953. Genetically determined resistance was described from an area on the Scottish lowlands in 1958 (Boyle 1960) and from part of the Welsh/English border region in 1960 (Drummond 1966). Subsequently warfarin-resistant rats were reported to occur in Denmark (Lund 1964), the Netherlands (Ophof & Laneveld 1968) and the USA (Jackson & Kaukeinen 1972).

A monogenic basis was found in Scottish rats to

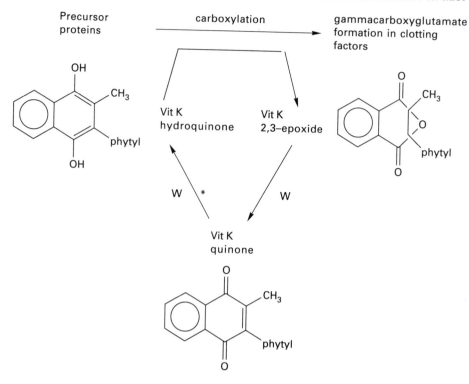

Fig. 33.4. The vitamin K cycle. W, Reactions inhibited by warfarin.* This reaction is mediated by an NADH-dependent reductase as well as by a dithiol-dependent reductase inhibited by warfarin.

Vit K: the type of vitamin K shown is phylloquinone.

phytyl is $-CH_2-CH=\overset{CH_3}{\underset{|}{C}}-\left[-CH_2-CH_2-CH_2-\overset{CH_3}{\underset{|}{CH}}-\right]-CH_3$

(Adapted from Suttie & Preusch 1986.)

explain the resistance as an autosomal dominant trait (Evans & Sheppard 1966).

The genetics of warfarin resistance in Welsh rats was investigated by Pool *et al.* (1968), who subjected the animals to 250 ppm in the drinking water with exposure for 48 hours and testing at 48 hours by measuring the prothrombin time. There was an excellent separation between the phenotypes. The breeding data indicated an autosomal dominant mode of transmission of warfarin resistance.

It was shown that the absorption, distribution and excretion of warfarin were normal in the resistant rats. Later it was discovered that the resistant rats had an abnormally high requirement for vitamin K. It was suggested that a protein involved in clotting factor synthesis, interacting with both vitamin K and with warfarin, might be altered in the resistant rats in such a way that its affinity for both vitamin K and warfarin might be reduced, the latter to a greater degree. This hypothesis formed the basis for possible heterozygote advantage. Rats heterozygous for resistance, having some of the altered protein, could synthesize clotting factors in the presence of high levels of warfarin which would account for resistance appearing as a dominant character. If, however, in the absence of warfarin there was enough vitamin K available to permit the synthesis of clotting factors only in the presence of the normal protein, the heterozygote would be at an advantage over the homozygote which has only the altered protein (Greaves & Ayres 1969). These proposed differential affinities were demonstrated experimentally by O'Reilly (1971), who showed that heterozygous resistant rats needed 25 times more warfarin than normal rats to achieve a comparable hypoprothrombinaemia yet required 10 times less vitamin K_1 to retard the prothrombin response.

A possible counterpart to this observation in the wild was provided by Lund (1967) in that the resistant rats in Denmark were less viable: on removal of the selective pressure imposed by the anticoagulant rodenticide the proportion of resistant mutants in the population decreased substantially in 4 years.

Progress was then made in identifying the enzymic basis of the warfarin resistance. Bell & Caldwell (1973), using radio labelled vitamin K_1 and its oxide, found that phylloquinone oxide stimulated prothrombin synthesis in resistant rats given warfarin but was ineffective in control normal Sprague–Dawley rats treated with the anticoagulant. In the latter 0.1 mg warfarin per 100 g body weight increased the oxide/K_1 ratio and decreased the concentration of vitamin K_1 in the liver, whereas in resistant animals the same dose of warfarin did not increase the oxide/K_1 ratio and had little effect on the amount of K_1 in the liver. In the Sprague–Dawley rats given [^{3}H]phylloquinone oxide, the same dose of warfarin almost completely blocked its conversion to vitamin K_1, but 5 mg warfarin per 100 g body weight was required to produce the same effect – as well as to inhibit prothrombin synthesis in resistant rats. Similar findings were also reported by Zimmermann & Matschiner (1974).

It was also pointed out by Bell & Caldwell (1973) that the vitamin K requirements of the resistant rats were much greater than for the normal rats. This finding was corroborated by Greaves et al. (1977), who also advanced the view that there is a balanced polymorphism in rat populations subjected to frequent warfarin poisoning – based on the reciprocal warfarin resistance/vitamin K requirement characteristics of the two homozygotes.

Vitamin K epoxide reductase converts vitamin K 2,3-epoxide to vitamin K quinone and is a membrane-bound microsomal enzyme (Fig 33.4). This enzyme was solubilized using detergents by Hildebrant et al. (1984) from both normal and warfarin-resistant liver microsomes. It seemed likely that an active-site disulphide was involved in the enzymatic reaction. The enzyme preparation from warfarin resistant rats had a significantly lower V_{max} (0.75 nmol/min/g liver) compared with that from sensitive rats (3 nmol/min/g liver), with a similar affinity for vitamin K epoxide. The authors suggested that the inability of the slower reductase of the resistant rat to recycle vitamin K epoxide might account for the greater vitamin K requirements.

There seems to be a wide measure of agreement that the epoxide reductase is the principal site of

action of warfarin to produce a lowering of prothrombin activity in sensitive individuals.

Most of the early work on warfarin-resistant rats was done on the Welsh variety, but later the enzymological characteristics of the Scottish variety were examined (Thijssen 1987; Vermeer et al. 1988). In the Welsh warfarin-sensitive rats warfarin was found to be bound irreversibly to vitamin K 2,3-epoxide reductase. In the Welsh resistant variety the enzyme had a reduced substrate affinity and reduced affinity for warfarin (and other 4-hydroxycoumarins). In the Scottish resistant variety the enzyme, though sensitive to 4 hydroxycoumarins, was not irreversibly inactivated by these compounds.

It seems that in Scottish resistant rats the dithiol-dependent vitamin K quinone reductase is sensitive to inhibition by warfarin but, like the epoxide reductase, the enzyme can be re-activated by an extensive washing procedure.

Also by investigating the pharmacokinetics of micro-doses of [^{14}C]warfarin, Thijssen & Baars (1987) demonstrated that the compound could be displaced from a 'deep' compartment by displacers such as acenocoumarol and other 4-hydroxycoumarins. Hepatic microsomes prepared from rats treated in this way showed that their [^{14}C]warfarin content was only a third of controls whereas the cytosol and plasma contained more. These data suggested that the microsomal enzyme, vitamin K 2,3-epoxide reductase was the hepatic binding site as well as the site of action for warfarin.

From these observations Vermeer et al. (1988) concluded that the mutation causing warfarin resistance differed between the Welsh and Scottish strains. The fact that two enzymic activities are affected in the Scottish strain indicated that the same enzyme might conduct both biotransformations.

The work of Trivedi et al. (1988) suggests the possibility that hydroxy-vitamin K can be formed directly from the 2,3-epoxide in both warfarin-sensitive and warfarin-resistant rats, but is of much greater importance in the latter.

RELEVANCE OF THE WORK IN RATS TO HUMAN HEREDITARY WARFARIN RESISTANCE

To find out the exact metabolic defect in the human with hereditary warfarin resistance is obviously a very difficult undertaking. So far, it is not known whether the human mutant resembles either of the two rat mutants.

The behaviour of humans under conditions of vitamin K deprivation was studied by O'Reilly (1971). He placed four normal individuals and one with hereditary anticoagulant resistance on a vitamin K-deficient diet and gave them neomycin or tetracycline to inhibit vitamin K production by intestinal bacteria. The prothrombin activity remained in the normal range for 32 days in the normal individuals, but fell markedly after 8 days in the individual with hereditary anticoagulant resistance. After this, whilst still on the experimental diet 80 μg vitamin K_1 daily by injection were required to normalize this subject's prothrombin activity.

An analogous behavior was shown by O'Reilly (1971) using the Welsh strain of resistant rats. They required less vitamin K than did normal rats to reverse warfarin anticoagulation (when it had been achieved with large doses), but in the absence of anticoagulants required much more vitamin K to maintain physiological prothrombin activity.

Shearer et al. (1977) investigated the relationship between increasing doses of warfarin in man and the metabolism of phylloquinone. Increasing amounts of phylloquinone epoxide were found to accumulate in the plasma. In the urine the normal phylloquinone aglycones diminished and abnormal aglycones increased as the dose of warfarin increased. The study of inter-individual variability was not the objective of this study and the point of mentioning it here is that it indicated that the manner of action of oral anticoagulants in man was to inhibit the cyclic interconversion of vitamin K and vitamin K epoxide, thus agreeing with the work on rats discussed above.

On the strength of the evidence available it is tempting to suggest that humans who have hereditary oral anticoagulant resistance may have a mutation in vitamin K 2,3-epoxide reductase similar to that seen in one of the strains of resistant rats.

VARIATION IN THE RESPONSE TO ORAL ANTICOAGULANTS IN NON-EXTRAORDINARY SUBJECTS

Abnormal responses of patients to oral anticoagulants are not uncommon clinical events and

schemes to elucidate the basis in a given individual have been published (Bentley et al. 1986).

The anticoagulant-resistant human subjects and rats described in the foregoing sections can be regarded as exceptional individuals representing a rare phenotype with an abnormal pharmacodynamic response.

In ordinary individuals there is a very substantial variability in the prothrombin time response to anticoagulants such as warfarin. The factors which might be responsible for such a variation were thoroughly reviewed by O'Reilly & Aggeler (1970). They include intestinal absorption of the drug, its plasma albumin binding and rate of biotransformation (which is heavily influenced by 'inducing' drugs). On the response side there is the degree of repletion with vitamin K, the rate of synthesis of clotting factors and their rate of decay.

The possibility that there might be genetic control over some of these components has been investigated. Vesell & Page (1968) demonstrated, using monozygous and dizygous twins that there was a considerable genetic influence on the disposition of dicoumarol as shown by its half-life with a heritability estimate of 0.97. The same problem was approached by Motulsky et al. (1964) with a family study whose result was disappointing because no significant parent–child or mid-parent–mean-offspring correlations (to provide an estimate of heritability) could be demonstrated. Wilding et al. (1977) showed, again using twins, that the association constants of warfarin binding to albumin and the number of warfarin binding sites per albumin molecule were more similar within monozygotic than among dizygous twinships. Heritability estimates of 0.89 and 0.85, respectively, were obtained for these two measurements.

The activities of 11 cytochromes P450 expressed individually in Hep-G2 cells were investigated with warfarin enantiomers by Rettie et al. (1992). Only cytochrome P450 2C9 was able to form 7-hydroxy-S-warfarin. The variations known to exist in the constitutive, induced and inhibited activities of cytohromes P450 may account for some of the clinical variability in response to warfarin.

The variation in the response of individuals to vitamin K was investigated by Zieve & Solomon (1969), who made observations on healthy volunteers. Vitamin K was given before, simultaneously with, and after a large dose of warfarin. Their experiments indicated the presence of considerable variation in the normal population in response to vitamin K, independent of the variability in warfarin plasma level. The authors mentioned differences in rate of metabolism or excretion of the vitamin, differences in the affinity of the receptor sites in the liver for the vitamin, differences in efficacy of the vitamin at these sites and differences in the rates of synthesis of vitamin K-dependent clotting factors as being possible explanations.

The advent of assays for vitamin K 2,3-epoxide in the plasma made it possible more precisely to examine the *in vivo* behaviour of the reductase. Choonara *et al.* (1988) gave seven healthy volunteers a daily small dose of warfarin to bring them into steady state. Then a single intravenous injection of vitamin K_1 was given. Plasma warfarin concentrations, prothrombin activity, vitamin K_1 (the biologically active *trans*-isomer) and vitamin K_1 2,3-epoxide were all assayed. There was a correlation between the concentration of the epoxide and the concentration of warfarin, but there was, in addition, considerable inter-individual variation in the level of the epoxide independent of the warfarin concentration. This raises the possibility that there may be minor alleles responsible for a background variation in the activity of vitamin K 2,3-epoxide reductase in the population.

Alving, B. M., Strickler, M. P., Knight, R. D., Barr, C. F., Berenberg, J. L. & Peck, C. C. (1985). Hereditary warfarin resistance. *Archives of Internal Medicine*, **145**, 499–501.

Bell, R. G. & Caldwell, P. T. (1973). Mechanism of warfarin resistance. Warfarin and the metabolism of vitamin K_1. *Biochemistry*, **12**, 1759–62.

Bentley, D. P., Backhouse, G., Hutchings, A., Haddon, R. L., Spragg, B. & Routledge, P. A. (1986). Investigation of patients with abnormal response to warfarin. *British Journal of Clinical Pharmacology*, **22**, 37–41.

Boyle, C. M. (1960). Case of apparent resistance of *Rattus norvegicus* Berkenhout to anticoagulant poisons. *Nature*, **188**, 517.

Choonara, I. A., Malia, R. G., Haynes, B. P., Hay, C. R., Cholerton, S., Breckenridge, A. M., Preston, F. E. & Park, B. K. (1988). The relationship between inhibition of vitamin K_1 2,3-epoxide reductase and reduction of clotting factor activity with warfarin. *British Journal of Clinical Pharmacology*, **25**, 1–7.

Drummond, D. (1966). Rats resistant to warfarin. *New Scientist*, **30**, 771–2.

Evans, D. A. P. & Sheppard, P. M. (1966). Some preliminary data on the genetics of resistance to anticoagulants in the Norway rat. *WHO Seminar on Rodents and Rodent Ectoparasites Vector control*, **66**, 5.4, 1–6.

Greaves, J. H. & Ayres, P. (1969). Linkages between genes for coat colour and resistance to warfarin in *Rattus norvegicus*. *Nature*, **224**, 284–5.

Greaves, J. H., Redfern, R., Ayres, P. B. & Gill, J. E. (1977). Warfarin resistance: a balanced polymorphism in the Norway rat. *Genetical Research (Cambridge)*, **30**, 257–63.

Hathaway, W. E. (1987). New insights on vitamin K. *Haematology/Oncology Clinics of North America*, **1**, 367–79.

Hildebrandt, E. F., Preusch, P. C., Patterson, J. L. & Suttie, J. W. (1984). Solubilization and characterization of vitamin K epoxide reductase from normal and warfarin-resistant rat liver microsomes. *Archives of Biochemistry and Biophysics*, **228**, 480–92.

Jackson, W. B. & Kaukeinen, D. (1972). Resistance of wild Norway rats in North Carolina to warfarin rodenticide. *Science*, **176**, 1343–4.

Lund, M. (1964). Resistance to warfarin in the common rat. *Nature*, **203**, 778.

Lund, M. (1967). Resistance of rodents to rodenticides. *World Review of Pest Control*, **6**, 131–8.

Motulsky, A. G. (1964). Pharmacogenetics. In *Progress in Medical Genetics*, Vol. 3, Chapter 2, ed. A. G. Steinberg & A. G. Bearn. New York: Grune & Stratton.

Ophof, A. J. & Laneveld, D. W. (1968). Warfarin resistance in the Netherlands. *WHO Vector Biology and Control*, **68**(109), 1. (Cited by O'Reilly 1972.)

O'Reilly, R. A. (1970). The second reported kindred with hereditary resistance to oral anticoagulant drugs. *New England Journal of Medicine*, **282**, 1448–51.

O'Reilly, R. A. (1971). Vitamin K in hereditary resistance to oral anticoagulant drugs. *American Journal of Physiology*, **221**, 1327–30.

O'Reilly, R. A. (1972). Genetic factors in the response to oral anticoagulant drugs. *Proceedings of the IV International Congress of Human Genetics. Excerpta Medica*, pp. 428–42.

O'Reilly, R. A. & Aggeler, P. M. (1970). Determinants of the response to oral anticoagulant drugs in man. *Pharmacological Reviews*, **22**, 35–96.

O'Reilly, R. A., Aggeler, P. M., Hoag, M. S., Leong, L. S. & Kropatkin, M. L. (1964). Hereditary transmission of exceptional resistance to coumarin anticoagulant drugs. *New England Journal of Medicine*, **271**, 809–15.

Pool, J. G., O'Reilly, R. A., Schneiderman, L. J. & Alexander, M. (1968). Warfarin resistance in the rat. *American Journal of Physiology*, **215**, 627–31.

Rettie, A. E., Korzekwa, K. R., Kunze, K. L., Lawrence, R. F., Eddy, A. C., Aoyama, T., Gelboin, H. V., Gonzalez, F. J. & Trager, W. F. (1992) Hydroxylation of warfarin by human cDNA-expressed cytochrome P-450: a role for P-450 2C9 in the aetiology of (S)-warfarin–drug interactions. *Chemical Research in Toxicology*, **5**, 54–9.

Shearer, M. J., McBurney, A., Breckenridge, A. M., Barkhan, P. (1977). Effect of warfarin on the metabolism of phylloquinone (vitamin K_1): dose–response relationships in man. *Clinical Science and Molecular Medicine*, **52**, 621–30.

Suttie, J. W. (1986). Report of workshop on expression of vitamin-K dependent proteins in bacterial and mammalian cells, Madison, Wisconsin, USA, April 1986. *Thrombosis Research*, **44**, 129–34.

Suttie, J. W. & Preusch, P. C. (1986). Studies of the vitamin K-dependent carboxylase and vitamin K epoxide reductase in rat liver. *Haemostasis*, **16**, 193–215.

Thijssen, H. H. W. (1987). Warfarin resistance. Vitamin K epoxide reductase of Scottish resistance genes is not irreversibly blocked by warfarin. *Biochemical Pharmacology*, **36**, 2753–7.

Thijssen, H. H. W. & Baars, L. G. M. (1987). Hepatic uptake and storage of warfarin. The relation with the target enzyme vitamin K 2,3-epoxide reductase. *Journal of Pharmacology and Experimental Therapeutics*, **243**, 1082–8.

Trivedi, L. S., Rhee, M., Galivan, J. H. & Fasco, M. J. (1988). Normal and warfarin-resistant rat hepatocyte metabolism of vitamin K 2,3-epoxide: evidence for multiple pathways of hydroxy vitamin K formation. *Archives of Biochemistry and Biophysics*, **264**, 67–73.

Vermeer, C., Soute, B. A. M., Aalten, M., Knapen, M. H. J. & Thijssen, H. H. W. (1988). Vitamin K reductases in normal and in warfarin-resistant rats. *Biochemical Pharmacology*, **37**, 2876–8.

Vesell, E. S., Page, J. G. (1968). Genetic control of dicoumarol levels in man. *Journal of Clinical Investigation*, **47**, 2657–63.

Wilding, G., Paigen, B. & Vesell, E. S. (1977). Genetic control of interindividual variations in racemic warfarin binding to plasma and albumin of twins. *Clinical Pharmacology and Therapeutics*, **22**, 831–42.

Zieve, P. D. & Solomon, H. M. (1969). Variation in the response of human beings to vitamin K. *Journal of Laboratory and Clinical Medicine*, **73**, 103–10.

Zimmermann, A. & Matschiner, J. T. (1974). Biochemical basis of hereditary resistance to warfarin in the rat. *Biochemical Pharmacology*, **23**, 1033–40.

34 NADH-cytochrome *b*5 reductase

THE PURPOSE of including a chapter on this topic is to bring out the fact that sometimes the administration of a standard dose of a therapeutic drug to an adult patient causes methaemoglobin-aemia. This event occurs because the person concerned is heterozygous for an inadequate variant form of NADH-cytochrome *b*5 reductase (EC 1.6.2.2: formerly known as methaemoglobin reductase and NADH diaphorase).

THE NATURE OF METHAEMOGLOBIN

Methaemoglobin is correctly defined as an oxidation product of haemoglobin in which the sixth co-ordination position of ferric haem is bound to a water molecule in the acid form, or a hydroxyl group in the alkaline form. In the former case the colour is brown (absorption maxima 631 and 500 nm) and in the latter case the colour is dark red (absorption maxima 575 and 540 nm). Methaemoglobin lacks an electron in comparison with deoxyhaemoglobin. The sixth coordination position in the latter molecule is thought to be vacant and available to bind oxygen reversibly (Jaffe 1981).

Since haemoglobin is a tetramer only some of the four haem groups may be oxidized. This has the effect on the remaining non-oxidized haem groups of increasing their affinity for oxygen, with the consequence that the oxygen is given up to the tissues less readily (Schwartz *et al.* 1983). The oxygenation curve of a 2,3-DPG-free haemolysate of methaemoglobin is shifted to the left as compared with normal haemoglobin (Park & Nagel 1984).

Methaemoglobin is not only inferior as an oxygen carrier: it is also prone to further oxidative damage and to bind to other molecules, factors which lead to its being denatured within the erythrocyte. However, this is probably not the route by which haemoglobin is customarily degraded (Jaffe 1981).

THE FORMATION OF METHAEMOGLOBIN

About 3% of haemoglobin is converted to methaemoglobin every day. This figure was computed from the reappearance of methaemoglobin after its complete reduction in patients lacking the normal mechanism for performing this biotransformation (Mansouri 1985). The formation of methaemoglobin is thought to occur in the following way. When oxyhaemoglobin is formed there is a partial transfer of an electron from the iron atom to oxygen to form super-oxo-ferri-haem ($Fe^{3+}O_2$). When this molecule dissociates to give up its oxygen the electron moves back to the iron. A failure of this process will result in the formation of methaemoglobin and the superoxide anion $O_2^{\bullet-}$ (Mansouri 1985).

PHYSIOLOGIC MECHANISMS FOR REDUCTION OF METHAEMOGLOBIN

Since only about 1% of the total haemoglobin is in the form of methaemoglobin there is obviously a dynamic equilibrium between factors responsible for methaemoglobin production and factors responsible for its reduction.

It was found that a substrate such as glucose or triose phosphate or lactate was required for the reduction of methaemoglobin in normal cells. Gibson (1948) showed that this reaction did not occur in the blood of persons with idiopathic methaemoglobinaemia and suggested that there was a deficiency of a methaemoglobin reducing enzyme. The first direct evidence for the existence of such an enzyme was provided by Scott & Griffith (1959). These authors used NADH to reduce 2,6-dichlorobenzenone-indophenol (DCBI) and observed that normal red cell haemolysates speeded the reaction while red cells from native Alaskans with hereditary methaemoglobinaemia slowed the reaction. They called the responsible enzyme 'diaphorase'.

Sodium nitrite converts haemoglobin to methaemoglobin by mechanisms which are not fully understood. Normal erythrocytes treated with nitrite and supplied with glucose were used by Jaffe *et al.* (1966) to study the regeneration of haemoglobin and this model was subsequently used to study the effect on the process of adding various substances. NADH enhanced the rate of the reaction and so also did cytochrome $b5$. NADH-cytochrome $b5$ reductase was isolated from human erythrocytes and characterized by Passon & Hultquist (1972), who clarified the electron transport chain from NADH to methaemoglobin as it is now understood. It was reasoned that absence of cytochrome $b5$ reductase or of cytochrome $b5$ itself could be responsible for idiopathic methaemoglobinaemia. In fact one individual has been described with deficiency of cytochrome $b5$ in the erythrocytes (Hegesh *et al.* 1986), who proved to have methaemoglobinaemia, which demonstrates the importance of this cytochrome in the reduction of methaemoglobin *in vivo*. No information was given by the authors regarding any features other than methaemoglobinaemia in this 27 year old woman, so it is not clear whether cytochrome $b5$ mediated functions were normal or not in cells other than erythrocytes.

The different enzymic activities previously known as NADH-dehydrogenase, NADH-methaemoglobin-ferrocyanide reductase, and NADH-cytochrome $b5$ reductase were shown to be mediated by a single protein obtained from a calibrated column of Sephadex gel (Jaffe 1981).

Ancillary mechanisms thought to be involved are those required to destroy superoxide, namely superoxide dismutase; and hydrogen peroxide (formed from superoxide), namely glutathione peroxidase and catalase. It would seem, however, that they are not of great importance because persons with hereditary deficiency of either one of the latter two enzymes are not methaemoglobinaemic (Schwartz *et al.* 1983).

As was recognized by Gibson (1948), there are other systems in the erythrocyte dependent on NADPH dehydrogenases which are capable of reducing methaemoglobin. These were found not to be of importance in the natural state, but on the addition of methylene blue they took part in bringing about a great acceleration of methaemoglobin reduction.

Other compounds which act in a similar manner to methylene blue (MB) are ascorbic acid (AA), riboflavin (R) and glutathione. It is known, however, that methaemoglobinaemia is not a feature of scurvy, riboflavine deficiency, glutathione synthase deficiency, NADPH dehydrogenase deficiency and G6PD deficiency (Jaffe 1981). However, it is important to note that AA and R can be effective when given therapeutically to reduce methaemoglobin, and the use of MB can sometimes be life-saving.

A simplified scheme of the pathways for methaemoglobin reduction is shown in Fig. 34.1 and more details of the main physiological process are shown in Fig. 34.2.

ORIGIN AND DEVELOPMENT OF ERYTHROCYTIC NADH-CYTOCHROME *b*5 REDUCTASE

The enzyme NADH-cytochrome $b5$ reductase is plentiful in the endoplasmic reticulum of many cells in the body and has been extensively studied in, for example, the liver. Similarly the enzyme, and the cytochrome $b5$ (a haem-containing flavoprotein), are present in the endoplasmic reticulum of the nucleated cells which are the precursors of erythrocytes in the marrow.

During the course of erythrocytic maturation the enzyme and the cytochrome both appear in a soluble form. This transformation from being membrane-bound to being soluble is thought to occur by proteolytic digestion by the lysosomes of the immature erythrocyte.

The ability of the erythrocytes of infants to reduce methaemoglobin is very much less than that of adults, as demonstrated by Lee *et al.* (1967) and

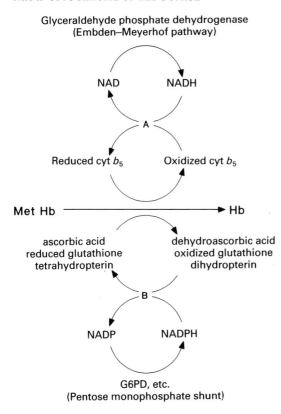

Fig. 34.1. The principal mechanisms by which methae-moglobin is reduced to haemoglobin. A, NADH cytochrome (cyt) b5 reductase (previously called methaemoglobin reductase). The NADH mechanism is the powerful mechanism occurring naturally *in vivo* which ensures that less than 1% of haemoglobin is in the methaemoglobin form. B, Specific reductases operate at this point, e.g. glutathione reductase and de-hydroascorbic acid reductase.

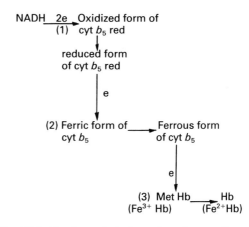

Fig. 34.2. The flow of electrons to reduce methaemo-globin to haemoglobin. cyt, cytochrome; Met Hb, methaemoglobin; (1), (2), (3), a complex is formed by binding at these points, and electrons are transferred.

Hegesh *et al.* (1986). This is ascribed to immaturity of cytochrome b5 reductase. This is of very great clinical importance and will be discussed later.

The ability of red cell haemolysates to reduce methaemoglobin was shown by Feig *et al.* (1972) to wane with red cell age.

GENETIC VARIATION OF NADH-CYTOCHROME *b*5 REDUCTASE

Information on genetic variability in this enzyme has come mainly from two sources, first, the study of individuals with hereditary methaemoglobin-aemia and secondly, population surveys using elec-trophoretic techniques.

It was pointed out by Schwarz *et al.* (1983) that congenital cyanosis without obvious cardiac or pul-monary disease was reported by Francois (1845) and familial clusters of idiopathic congenital cyan-osis were described by Hitzenberger (1932).

Since those early observations it has become clear that it is necessary to differentiate sulphaemoglobin-aemia (which is excessively rare) from methaemo-globinaemia (which is done spectroscopically), and to differentiate methaemoglobinaemia due to haemo-globin variants (M haemoglobins) from that due to enzymic variants.

Recessive methaemoglobinaemia was described in Alaskan Eskimos and Indians by Scott & Hoskins (1958) in whom the condition seemed to be com-moner (15 per 20 000) than in Caucasian type populations. They found that the degree of met-haemoglobinaemia varied, probably being reduced by ascorbic acid, the intake of which was seasonal. Extending these studies, Scott (1960) showed that the frequency distribution of the rate of DCBI reduc-tion was trimodal in 318 subjects, and that these modes represented the three genotypes due to two autosomal alleles.

Since then many patients with congenital defi-ciency of cytochrome b5 reductase have been described in different populations. Some authors have collected impressive series from certain ethnic groups. For example, in Yakutsk, Siberia, hetero-

Table 34.1. *Results of enzyme activity measurement and starch gel electrophoresis of the cytochrome* b5 *reductase of erythrocyte haemolysates in congenital methaemoglobinaemia*

Patient number	% of normal enzyme activity	Result on SGE in patient	Result on SGE in relative
1	10	No band visible	–
2	10	Weak band with normal mobility	–
3	25	Absence of normal band. Weak faster band present	Daughter had two bands, one with normal and one with faster mobility. Her % of normal enzyme activity was 55

SGE, starch gel electrophoresis.   *Data from:* Kaplan & Beutler 1967.

zygotes constituted 7% of the population (Jaffe 1981). Three Puerto Rican women with congenital methaemoglobinaemia were described by Hsieh & Jaffe (1971) and Schwartz *et al.* (1972). Various Mediterranean populations contributed eight such patients to the study of Kaplan *et al.* (1979). Similarly, Balsamo *et al.* (1964) described three patients in Navajo Indians. It is possible that some of these series merely represent bias of ascertainment. It is strange that there are apparently no reports of increased frequency of the disorder in Asian populations in which consanguinity is very prevalent.

An important step forward was made by Kaplan & Beutler (1967), who devised a way of visualizing cytochrome *b*5 reductase on starch gel, and used it to examine the red cells of three patients with congenital methaemoglobinaemia. The results, shown in Table 34.1, revealed that there was genetic heterogeneity in this phenotype; they called the electrophoretically fast variant the 'California variant'.

Similarly, other electrophoretic variants were found in patients with congenital methaemoglobinaemia by other authors, e.g. West *et al.* (1967); Bloom & Zarkowsky (1969). The latter authors also described a patient with NADPH dehydrogenase deficiency but who did not have methaemoglobinaemia.

Five different electrophoretic variants were discovered by Hsieh & Jaffe (1971) in congenital methaemoglobinaemia patients from different racial groups. One of these variants, occurring in Puerto Ricans, was shown to be an unstable cytochrome *b*5 reductase molecule. Its activity in red cells fell from 37% of normal mean activity in young erythrocytes to 1% in old cells. The K_m^{NADH} was raised and thermal stability moderately reduced (see also Schwartz *et al.* 1972).

In a population survey involving nearly 3000 unrelated people Hopkinson *et al.* (1970) found 29 individuals with five different abnormal electrophoretic phenotypes of cytochrome *b*5 reductase. One sort of abnormal phenotype or another occurred in about every 100 individuals amongst Europeans, Indians, Negroes and Greek Cypriots. The variants were shown to be constant on retesting and in 16 cases family studies were performed which revealed that the variants were genetic. No individuals with methaemoglobinaemia were discovered during this survey. Since the variant 'Dia 6-1 pattern' had an electrophoretic band faster than normal and so resembled the California variant of Kaplan & Beutler (1967), it was suggested by Hopkinson *et al.* (1971) that they might be the same. Two persons possessing this band were found amongst 1975 Europeans.

Subsequently many variants with different activities and electrophoretic mobilities were discovered in congenital methaemoglobinaemia patients in various ethnic groups. A table of 25 such variants was provided by Schwartz & Jaffe (1978), together with five examples of the disease where no electrophoretic variant was found.

DIFFERENT CLINICAL TYPES OF CONGENITAL METHAEMOGLOBINAEMIA

After understanding had been gained of the basic enzymology of the condition, more patients with congenital methaemoglobinaemia were studied. It was perceived by Worster-Drought *et al.* (1953), Fialkow *et al.* (1965) and later others such as Jaffe *et al.* (1966), Beauvais & Kaplan (1978) and Takeshita *et al.* (1982) that in some families the congenital methaemoglobinaemia was accompanied by mental retardation. This was termed Type II to differentiate it from Type I in which there was no abnormality outside the erythrocytes. It was shown by Leroux *et al.* (1975) that there was a gross deficiency of soluble NADH-cytochrome *b5* reductase activity in erythrocytes and of membrane-bound NADH-cytochrome *b5* reductase in leucocytes, muscle and liver in Type II probands.

These two types of disorder were presumed to be due to two different mutations, one involving the soluble form of the enzyme and the other the microsomal form. It is understandable that the latter might cause grave neurological and mental effects because cytochrome *b5* is involved in desaturation of fatty acids, an important process in lipid metabolism in nervous tissue.

A complicating turn to the story has occurred with the discovery of Type III congenital methaemoglobinaemia (Tanishima *et al.* 1985, 1987). In this variety cytochrome *b5* reductase is absent in erythrocytes, leucocytes and platelets. Yet the patients concerned were neurologically and mentally normal, and the enzymic activity was present in hair root cells and buccal mucosal cells.

The enzymological explanation for Type III is at present obscure.

STRUCTURES AND MOLECULAR GENETICS OF NADH-CYTOCHROME *b5* REDUCTASE AND CYTOCHROME *b5*

The membrane-bound type of the flavoprotein cytochrome *b5* reductase is 300 amino acids long, having both membrane binding and catalytic domains. The soluble (erythrocytic) enzyme has only 275 of these amino acids, namely the catalytic domain. Both enzymes by virtue of their structures must be controlled by a single gene (Kobayashi *et al.* 1990).

Examination of the organization and complete nucleotide sequence of the NADH-cytochrome *b5* reductase (*b5*R) shows the gene to be about 31 kb

long, containing nine exons and eight introns (Tomatsu *et al.* 1989).

The exact defects for all three Japanese types of congenital methaemoglobinaemia have now been elucidated by determining the structures of the genes in affected individuals (Table 34.2). These defects were present in homozygous form in the affected individuals. The same defect was present in all three Type II individuals in one family. Other mutant forms of *b5*R may well be found in non-Japanese populations.

In order to examine the functional consequences Yubisui *et al.* (1991) created variant enzymes by site-directed mutagenesis at codon 127. Serine was thus replaced by proline and by alanine. The enzymes were produced by *E. coli* and purified. The mutant enzymes were demonstrated to be less thermostable and to have a very inferior affinity for NADH using cytochrome *b5* as an electron receptor as compared with the normal (wild type) enzyme. So it was concluded that amino acid 127 is in the NADH binding portion of the *b5*R enzyme and present in both the membrane-bound and soluble forms of the enzyme.

Exactly how these different amino acid substitutions give rise to the phenotypic features of the three types of congenital methaemoglobinaemia (CM) is unknown. It is possible that examination of more patients with CM may reveal other variant forms of *b5*R.

Cytochrome *b5* is a flavoprotein which contains a haem group. The erythrocytic form is derived from a membrane-bound form, by proteolysis during cell development, and contains 97 amino acids.

CHROMOSOMAL LOCALIZATION

The gene for cytochrome *b5* reductase has been localized to chromosome 22. Fisher *et al.* (1977) showed complete concordance between the presence of the enzyme and the possession of chromosome 22 in somatic cell hybrids. The same conclusion was obtained in a similar way by Junien *et al.* (1978).

ACQUIRED METHAEMOGLOBINAEMIA

Methaemoglobinaemia can be congenital or acquired. The congenital form can be due to either an abnormal haemoglobin or an enzyme deficiency.

Table 34.2. *Mutant forms of NADH-cytochrome b5 reductase (b5R) in congenital methaemoglobinaemias*

Reference	Type of congenital methaemoglobinaemia	Name of variant	Codon number[a]	Base change	Amino acid change
Katsube *et al.* 1991	I	Toyoake	57	CGG → CAG	arginine → glutamine
Kobayashi *et al.* 1990	II	Hiroshima	127	TCT → CCT	serine → proline
Katsube *et al.* 1991	III	Kurobe	148	CTG → CCG	leucine → proline

[a]The number shown here is that for the complete membrane-bound enzyme. For the soluble erythrocyte type the number would be 25 less.

The latter has been discussed in some detail, as this is how the biochemical mechanisms involved were elucidated. Acquired methaemoglobinaemia may be commoner than the congenital variety and to some degree it is preventable; it is also treatable.

It is pointed out by Jaffe & Hultquist (1989) that many different drugs have the propensity to change haemoglobin to methaemoglobin. Oxidant drugs such as menadione, doxorubicin and methylene blue can produce free radicals by reaction with haemoglobin; these free radicals can produce superoxide $O_2^{\bullet-}$ from oxygen. Reducing drugs can reduce oxygen to produce the same results and examples in this category are nitrites and hydrazines. Many drug compounds are metabolized to produce oxidants or reductants, and examples are primaquin, sulphanilamide, dapsone, phenacetin, acetanilide, benzocaine and phenazopyridine.

The acquired form has a different basis in infants and in adults so they will be discussed separately.

In infants the enzyme cytochrome $b5$ reductase is not properly developed, and this renders them liable to develop methaemoglobinaemia from seemingly trivial exposure to certain chemicals. Perhaps the most sinister occurs when infant feeds are made up with well water which is contaminated by nitrates. This condition was described by Comly (1945) when he was a paediatric resident (Lukens 1987). The nitrate (which gets into wells after having been applied as fertilizer to nearby fields) is converted to nitrite either prior to ingestion or after ingestion by intestinal organisms, and the nitrite after absorption converts the haemoglobin to methaemoglobin. The same unfortunate toxicological event continues even now to occur in infants (e.g. Miller, 1971), sometimes with fatal consequences (e.g. Johnson *et*

al. 1987), but the nitrate content of processed infant foods has been exonerated (Filer *et al.* 1970). (Well water used for home peritoneal dialysis has also caused methaemoglobinaemia in an adult: Carlson & Shapiro 1970.) Other agents causing methaemoglobinaemia in babies include prilocaine (Menahem 1988), prilocaine/lidocaine cream (Nilsson *et al.* 1990), metoclopramide (Kearns & Fiser 1988), glycerited asafoetida (Kelly *et al.* 1984) and aniline-based diaper marking dyes absorbed percutaneously.

Children of 1 to 6 years of age were shown by Frayling *et al.* (1990) to develop 0.85% methaemoglobin 12 hours after 5 g of prilocaine cream had been applied to the arm before surgery. Obviously this was in itself only a minor abnormality, but if another oxidant drug was simultaneously administered then clinically relevant methaemoglobinaemia might be produced, as happened in the patient described by Jakobson & Nilsson (1985), who received trimethoprim-sulphamethoxazole with prilocaine-lidocaine cream.

In adults the development of methaemoglobinaemia either signifies the administration of a larger than usual dose of the causative agent, or the inability of the red cell to cope with a modest oxidative stress. Obviously poisoning with monolinuron (a constituent of 'Gramanol', which also contains paraquat: Ng *et al.* 1982; Proudfoot 1982) belongs to the former category. Sometimes two oxidizing drugs administered together may result in methaemoglobinaemia, as described by Kaplan *et al.* (1985) in a patient receiving oral phenazopyridium and intravenous nitroglycerin.

Other recently published examples in adults include dapsone in association with an anaesthetic

Table 34.3. *Drug therapy and enzymic phenotypes in patients who developed methaemoglobinaemia*

Reference	Number of patients and ethnic group	Drug and dose	% met	Result of erythrocytic cytochrome b5 reductase assay
Robicsek 1985	1	Nitroglycerin 90 µg/min[a]	16.5	Normal
Gibson et al. 1982	1	Nitroglycerin 6 µg/kg/min	9.6	Normal
Kaplan et al. 1985	1	Nitroglycerin 4.1 µg/kg/min[b]	12.0	Normal
Cohen et al. 1968	6 white	Malaria chemoprophylaxis[c]	2.5 to 23.6	All heterozygous
Daly et al. 1983	1 white	Phenazopyridine 200 mg PO QID	53.5	Patient, brother, father and aunt heterozygous
Horne et al. 1979	1	Butyl nitrite[d]	18.0	Patient and father heterozygous
Collins 1990	1 Aleut	Benzocaine[e]	74.7	Patient heterozygous

met, methaemoglobin.
[a]Patient's weight not provided.
[b]Also receiving phenazopyridine.
[c]Various standard dosages of chloroquine, primaquine and dapsone.
[d]Dose not quantifiable.
[e]3 to 4 sprays of 20% benzocaine repeated after 30 minutes.

(Mayo et al. 1987) and given to treat *Pneumocystis carinii* pneumonia in a patient with AIDS (Reiter & Cimoch 1987), sulphamethoxazole and trimethoprim therapy (Damergis et al. 1983) and pickled pork treated with an excessively high concentration of nitrite (Walley & Flanagan 1987), nitroglycerin (Husum et al. 1982; Bojar et al. 1987), benzocaine (Ferraro et al. 1988; Kotler et al. 1989), amyl nitrite (Laaban et al. 1985; Pierce & Nielsen 1989), butyl nitrite (Shesser et al. 1980), and isobutyl nitrite (Wason et al. 1980). However, in only a few examples have measurements been made of both the methaemoglobin level and the erythrocytic b5 reductase activity. These examples are shown in Table 34.3. Obviously the nitroglycerine doses were fairly large and the patients had a normal enzyme activity. Saxon & Silverman (1985) investigated 15 patients with myocardial infarction and found that intravenous nitroglycerin infusions of up to 2.12 µg/min/kg produced no significant methaemoglobinaemia. In the lower part of the table are examples where methaemoglobinaemia developed with customary doses of drugs and where the persons involved were shown to be heterozygotes.

The methaemoglobin production which occurs in persons given antimalarial drugs depends on first the drug load, secondly the enzymic phenotype and thirdly the presence or absence of malaria. Cowan & Evans (1964) showed in 59 healthy Caucasians

taking 15 mg primaquine base daily for 14 days that the highest methaemoglobinaemia was 0.72 g%. Greaves et al. (1980) showed, in 30 healthy Caucasians taking chloroquine 450 mg base for 3 days, concurrently with 15 mg primaquine base daily, continued for a total of 14 days, that the highest methaemoglobinaemia was 1.6 g%. It is thought that the presence of malaria adds further oxidative stress within the erythrocyte (Jones et al. 1953) but it is obviously the enzymic phenotype that really makes the difference. One combination chloroquine–primaquine tablet given by Cohen et al. (1968) to a heterozygote produced a methaemoglobin level of 23.6%. In another heterozygote two doses of dapsone on consecutive days gave a level of 9.0%.

Phenacetin is a drug known to be capable of causing methaemoglobinaemia, and formerly when it was widely used by patients with rheumatoid arthritis it was not uncommon to see otherwise unexplained cyanosis in such patients (personal observation). When the use of phenacetin was discontinued this phenomenon disappeared.

GENE FREQUENCY OF NADH-CYTOCHROME b5 DEFICIENCY IN CAUCASIANS

A very rough idea of the allele frequency can be gleaned from the observation of Hansen et al. (1954)

Table 34.4. *Methaemoglobinaemia-producing variants of haemoglobin (Hb M)*

Place after which Hb M is named	Amino acid substitution
Adult	
Boston	α58 His → Tyr
Saskatoon	β63 His → Tyr
Milwaukee-1	β67 Val → Glu
Iwate	α87 His → Tyr
Hyde Park	β92 His → Tyr
Fetal	
Osaka	γ63 His → Tyr

Compiled from information in: Weatherall *et al.* 1989.

that one soldier in 3000 developed methaemo-globinaemia on antimalarial therapy, suggesting $2pq$ might be $1/3000 = 0.00033$. Since $p =$ approximately 1, $q = 1/6000$, i.e. 0.00017; hence $q^2 = 0.000000028$. This figure would indicate that one person with congenital methaemoglobinaemia is present in every 36 million Caucasians, which is probably an underestimate.

METHAEMOGLOBINAEMIA DUE TO HAEMOGLOBIN VARIANTS

It is not the purpose of this chapter to discuss these variants and they are mentioned here only because they should be considered in the diagnosis of congenital methaemoglobinaemia. This brief summary is adapted from that given by Weatherall *et al.* (1989).

Five adult forms and one fetal form of haemoglobin M are known. Hb M indicates a form of haemoglobin which circulates as methaemoglobin. The different forms are shown in Table 34.4. Most are explained by the substitution of tyrosine for histidine. The phenolic group of the abnormal tyrosine forms a covalent link with the haem iron. These amino acid substitutions stabilize the haem group in the oxidized form. Once oxidized it cannot be reduced.

The forms with α chain substitutions exist from birth, whereas those with β chain substitutions arise

a few months after birth when these chains start being manufactured.

The person with this form of methaemoglobin-taemia is an asymptomatic Mendelian dominant heterozygote. Normal haemoglobin is made under the control of his normal genes. The homozygous Hb M individual is presumed to be lethal.

In this context it is of interest to note that Tassi-opoulos *et al.* (1985) provided evidence that patients with homozygous thalassaemia β, particularly when they have been subjected to splenectomy, have a raised Met Hb concentration (0.61 g/dl). They also have twice the normal activity of the reductase. (Similar findings were also reported by Perry & Anderson 1991.) It is not clear whether they have a greater or lesser propensity than normal to develop clinical methaemoglobinaemia when treated with the relevant drugs.

On the other hand, sickle cells had relatively less methaemoglobin reductase than normal bearing in mind their low average age (Zerez *et al.* 1990). The clinical significance of this finding is at present uncertain.

DIAGNOSIS

On a clinical level in a patient with cyanosis there are four points of importance:

1 the length of time the cyanosis has been present;
2 the family history;
3 the drug history;
4 evidence of a disorder of the heart or lungs.

These points are shown in a flow chart in Fig. 34.3.

In congenital methaemoglobinaemia concentrations of 10 to 20% are tolerated without apparent ill effects but levels of 30 to 40% may be associated with mild exertional dyspnoea and headaches (Jaffe 1981). In methaemoglobinaemias acquired due to drugs and chemicals, levels of 40 to 60% give rise to headache, lethargy, confusion, dyspnoea and chest pain whilst levels above 70% cause coma and are fatal unless treated.

A simple bedside diagnostic test in toxic methaemoglobinaemia is to observe that the blood does not become bright red when shaken with air; it remains a dark brownish-red.

For the laboratory diagnosis of NADH-cytochrome $b5$ reductase deficiency a number of methods are available, as shown in Table 34.5.

Table 34.5. *Methods of assessing NADH-cytochrome* b5 *reductase activity in erythrocytes*

Reference	Method
Scott & Griffith 1959	Reduction of 2,6-dichlorobenzanone-indophenol (DCBI) by haemolysate of nitrite-treated cells supplied with NADH
Jaffe *et al.* 1966	Nitrite-treated washed cells incubated with glucose and reduction of methaemoglobin observed in comparison with cells from a normal subject
Kaplan *et al.* 1970	Depends on the fact that NADH fluoresces in ultraviolet light. Nitrite-treated whole blood is added to a mixture containing a haemolysing agent, NADH and DCBI. In the presence of the reductase the dye DCBI is reduced and NADH becomes NAD which does not fluoresce (spot screening test)
Passon & Hulquist 1972	Change in absorbance of cytochrome *b*5 measured directly, or coupled with cytochrome *c*, in presence of NADH and the reductase either in crude haemolysate or purified by column chromatography on DEAE cellulose, etc.
Board 1981	Simple method based on NADH-ferricyanide reductase activity, using haemolysates directly and follows oxidation of NADH by change of OD at 340 nm
Hegesh *et al.* 1986	Ferrihaemoglobin made from reductase-free haemoglobin with potassium ferricyanide. NADH supplied and reduction indicated by change in optical density
Borgese *et al.* 1987	Quantitative radio-immuno-blotting method using affinity-purified polyclonal antibodies against rat liver microsomal NADH-cytochrome *b*5 reductase as a probe

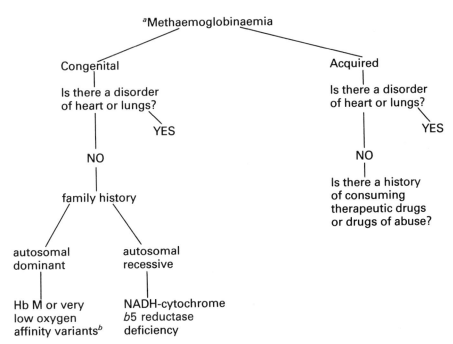

Fig. 34.3. Clinical diagnostic steps in methaemoglobinaemia. [a] Sulphaemoglobinaemia can be differentiated by the following properties: (1) the absorption peak at about 620 nm does not disappear quickly on adding potassium cyanide (which is the case with methaemoglobin); (2) the absorption peak at about 620 nm increases in height on adding carbon monoxide (which does not occur with methaemaoglobin or haemoglobin M); (3) different properties on isoelectric focusing (Park & Nagel 1984). [b] Haemoglobins such as Hammersmith, Kansas, Beth Israel and St Mande.

TREATMENT

The treatment for congenital methaemoglobinaemia Type I is cosmetic only since the condition does not usually give rise to any symptoms (these patients have been described as 'more blue than sick'). The level of methaemoglobin can be reduced by methylene blue (MB), ascorbic acid (AA) and riboflavin. There are disadvantages with MB such as bladder irritation, the passage of blue or green urine and haemolysis in the presence of glucose-6-phosphate dehydrogenase deficiency. High doses of AA for a long time are known to cause oxalate stones. So riboflavin is the most innocuous of the three compounds (Jaffe 1981).

The treatment of Type II congenital methaemoglobinaemia can reduce the level of methaemoglobinaemia but does not influence the neurological features.

The first thing in the treatment of acquired methaemoglobinaemia, as in any poisoning, is to eliminate the cause. Further treatment depends on the degree of methaemoglobinaemia. Below about 40% methaemoglobinaemia the natural process of reduction will usually suffice. For higher levels the administration of a specific therapeutic agent is indicated. Intravenous MB at a dose of 1 to 2 mg per kg body weight usually produces a dramatic improvement. This drug is, however, not devoid of peril, particularly in adults with glucose-6-phosphate dehydrogenase deficiency (Harvey & Keitt 1983) and in infants even when this condition is absent (Menahem 1988). This is because MB depends for its action on an adequate supply of NADPH. When this supply is not adequate MB can worsen the methaemoglobinaemia and cause haemolysis (Mansouri 1985).

Haemodialysis to remove the causative chemicals and red blood cell transfusions to improve the oxygen carrying capacity are indicated in patients with severe toxic methaemoglobinaemia (Schwartz et al. 1983).

Balsamo, P., Hardy, W. R. & Scott, E. M. (1964). Hereditary methemoglobinemia due to diaphorase deficiency in Navajo Indians. *Journal of Pediatrics*, **65**, 928–31.

Beauvais, P. & Kaplan, J. C. (1978). La méthémoglobinémie congénitale récessive: étude de huit cas avec encéphalopathie. Nouvelle conception nosologique. *Journal Parisiennes Pédiatrie*, 145–57.

Bloom, G. E. & Zarkowsky, H. S. (1969). Heterogeneity of the enzymatic defect in congenital methemoglobinemia. *New England Journal of Medicine*, **281**, 919–22.

Board, P. G. (1981). NADH-ferricyanide reductase, a convenient approach to the evaluation of NADH-methaemoglobin reductase in human erythrocytes. *Clinica Chimica Acta*, **109**, 233–7.

Bojar, R. M., Rastegar, H., Payne, D. D., Harkness, S. H., England, M. R., Stetz, J. J., Weiner, B. & Cleveland, R. J. (1987). Methemoglobinemia from intravenous nitroglycerine: a word of caution. *Annals of Thoracic Surgery*, **43**, 332–4.

Borgese, N., Pietrini, G. & Gaetani S. (1987). Concentration of NADH-cytochrome b5 reductase in erythrocytes of normal and methemoglobinemic individuals measured with a quantitative radio-immuno-blotting assay. *Journal of Clinical Investigation*, **80**, 1296–302.

Carlson, D. J. & Shapiro, F. L. (1970). Methemoglobinemia from well water nitrates. A complication of home dialysis. *Annals of Internal Medicine*, **73**, 757–9.

Cohen, R. J., Sachs, J. R., Wicker, D. J. & Conrad, M. E. (1968). Methemoglobinemia provoked by malarial chemoprophylaxis in Vietnam. *New England Journal of Medicine*, **279**, 1127–31.

Collins, J. F. (1990). Methemoglobinemia as a complication of 20% benzocaine spray for endoscopy. *Gastroenterology*, **98**, 211–13.

Comly, H. H. (1945). Cyanosis in infants caused by nitrates in well water. *Journal of the American Medical Association*, **129**, 112–16.

Cowan, W. K. & Evans, D. A. P. (1964). Primaquine and methemoglobin. *Clinical Pharmacology and Therapeutics*, **5**, 307–9.

Daly, J. S., Hultquist, D. E. & Rucknagel, D. L. (1983). Phenazopyridine induced methemoglobinemia associated with decreased activity of erythrocyte cytochrome b5 reductase. *Journal of Medical Genetics*, **20**, 307–9.

Damergis, J. A., Stoker, J. M. & Abadie, J.-L. (1983). Methemoglobinemia after sulfamethoxazole and trimethoprim therapy. *Journal of the American Medical Association*, **249**, 590–1.

Feig, S. A., Nathan, D. G., Gerald, P. S. & Zarkowski, H. S. (1972). Congenital methemoglobinaemia: the result of age-dependent decay of methemoglobin reductase. *Blood*, **39**, 407–14.

Ferraro, L., Zeichner, S., Greenblott, G. & Groeger, J. S. (1988). Cetacaine-induced acute methemoglobinemia. *Anesthesiology*, **69**, 614–15.

Fialkow, P. J., Browder, J. A., Sparkes, R. S. & Motulsky, A. G. (1965). Mental retardation in methemoglobinemia due to diaphorase deficiency. *New England Journal of Medicine*, **273**, 840–5.

Filer, Ll. J., Lowe, C. U., Barness, L. A., Goldbloom, R. B., Heald, F. P., Holliday, M. A., Miller, R. W., O'Brien, D., Owen, G. M., Pearson, H. A., Scriver, C. R., Weil, W. B., Kine, O. L., Cravioto, J. & Whitten, C. (1970). Committee on Nutrition: Infant methemoglobinemia: the role of dietary nitrate. *Pediatrics*, **46**, 475–8.

Fisher, R. A., Povey, S., Bobrow, M., Solomon, E., Boyd,

Y. & Carritt, B. (1977). Assignment of the DIA₁ locus to chromosome 22. *Annals of Human Genetics (London)*, **41**, 151–5.

Francois. (1845). Cas de cyanose congénitale sans cause apparente. *Bulletin de l'Académie Royale de Médécine de Belgique*, **4**, 498. (Cited by Schwartz *et al.* 1983.)

Frayling, I. M., Addison, G. M., Chattergee, K. & Meakin, G. (1990). Methaemoglobinaemia in children treated with prilocaine-lignocaine cream. *British Medical Journal*, **301**, 153–4.

Gibson, Q. H. (1948). The reduction of methaemoglobin in red blood cells and studies on the cause of idiopathic methaemoglobinaemia. *Biochemical Journal*, **42**, 13–23.

Gibson, G. R., Hunter, J. B., Raabe, Jr. D. S., Manjoney, D. L. & Ittleman, F. P. (1982). Methemoglobinemia produced by high-dose nitroglycerin. *Annals of Internal Medicine*, **96**, 615–16.

Greaves, J., Evans, D. A. P. & Fletcher, K. A. (1980). Urinary primaquine excretion and red cell methaemoglobin levels in man following a primaquine-chloroquine regime. *British Journal of Clinical Pharmacology*, **10**, 293–5.

Hansen, J. E., Cleve, E. A. & Pruitt, F. W. (1954). Relapse of vivax malaria treated with primaquine and report of one case of cyanosis (methemoglobinemia) due to primaquine. *American Journal of Medical Science*, **227**, 9–12.

Harvey, J. W. & Keitt, A. S. (1983). Studies of the efficacy and potential hazards of methylene blue therapy in aniline-induced methemoglobinemia. *British Journal of Haematology*, **54**, 29–41.

Hegesh, E., Calmanovici, N. & Avron, M. (1968). New method for determining ferrihemoglobin reductase (NADH-methemoglobin reductase) in erythrocytes. *Journal of Laboratory and Clinical Medicine*, **72**, 339–44.

Hegesh, E., Hegesh, J. & Kaftory, A. (1986). Congenital methemoglobinemia with a deficiency of cytochrome b5. *New England Journal of Medicine*, **314**, 757–61.

Hitzenberger, K. (1932). Autotoxische cyanose (intra-globuläre methämoglobinamie). *Wiener Archiv für Innere Medizin und Deren Grenzgebeite* **23**, 85. (Cited by Schwartz *et al.* 1983.)

Hopkinson, D. A., Corney, G., Cook, P. J. L., Robson, E. B. & Harris, H. (1970). Genetically determined electrophoretic variants of human red cell NADH diaphorase. *Annals of Human Genetics (London)*, **34**, 1–10.

Horne, M. K., Waterman, M. R., Simon, L. McE., Garriott, J. C. & Foerster, M. S. (1979). Methemoglobinemia from sniffing butyl nitrite. *Annals of Internal Medicine*, **91**, 417–18.

Hsieh, H.-S. & Jaffe, E. R. (1971). Electrophoretic and functional variants of NADH-methemoglobin reductase in hereditary methemoglobinemia. *Journal of Clinical Investigation*, **50**, 196–202.

Husum, B., Lindeburg, T. & Jacobsen, F. (1982). Methemoglobin formation after nitroglycerine infusion. *British Journal of Anaesthesia*, **54**, 571.

Jaffe, E. R. (1981). Methaemoglobinaemia. *Clinics in Haematology*, **10**, 99–122.

Jaffe, E. R. & Hultquist, D. E. (1989). Cytochrome b5 reductase deficiency and enzymopenic hereditary methemoglobinemia. In *The Metabolic Basis of Inherited Disease*, 6th edn, ed. C. R. Scriver, A. L. Beaudet, W. S.

Sly & D. Vale, Ch. 92, pp. 2267–80. New York: McGraw-Hill.

Jaffe, E. R., Neumann, G., Rothberg, H., Wilson, F. T., Webster, R. M. & Wolff, J. A. (1966). Hereditary methemoglobinemia with and without mental retardation. A study of three families. *American Journal of Medicine*, **41**, 42–55.

Jakobson, B. & Nilsson, A. (1985). Methemoglobinemia associated with a prilocaine-lidocaine cream and trimethoxazole. A case report. *Acta Anaesthesiologica Scandinavica*, **29**, 453–5.

Johnson, C. J., Bonrud, P. A., Dosch, T. L., Kilness, A. W., Senger, K. A., Busch, D. C. & Meyer, M. R. (1987). Fatal outcome of methemoglobinemia in an infant. *Journal of the American Medical Association*, **257**, 2796–7.

Jones, R., Jackson, L. S., DiLorenzo, A., Marx, R. L., Levy, B. L., Kenny, E. C., Gilbert, M., Johnston, M. N. & Alving, A. S. (1953). Korean vivax malaria III curative effect and toxicity of primaquine in doses of 10 to 30 mg daily. *American Journal of Tropical Medicine*, **2**, 977–82.

Junien, C., Vibert, M., Weil, D., Van-Cong, N. & Kaplan, J.-C. (1978). Assignment of NADH-cytochrome b5 reductase (DIA₁ locus) to human chromosome 22. *Human Genetics*, **42**, 233–9.

Kaplan, J.-C., Leroux, A. & Beauvais, P. (1979). Formes cliniques et biologiques du deficit en cytochrome *b5* reductase. *Comptes rendus des séances de la Société de Biologie*, 1979; **173**, 368–379.

Kaplan, J.-C. & Beutler, E. (1967). Electrophoresis of red cell NADH-and NADPH-diaphorases in normal subjects and patients with congenital methemoglobinemia. *Biochemical and Biophysical Research Communications*, **29**, 605–10.

Kaplan, J.-C., Nicolas, A. M., Hanzlickova-Leroux, A., Beutler, E. (1970). A simple spot screening test for fast detection of red cell NADH-diaphorase deficiency. *Blood*, **36**, 330–3.

Kaplan, K. J., Taber, M., Teagarden, J. R., Parker, M. & Davison, R. (1985). Association of methemoglobinemia and nitroglycerin administration. *American Journal of Cardiology*, **55**, 181–3.

Katsube, T., Sakamoto, N., Kobayashi, Y., Seki, R., Hirano, M., Tanishima, K., Tomoda, A., Takazakura, E., Yubisui, T., Takeshita, M., Sakaki, Y. & Fukumaki, Y. (1991). Exonic point mutations in NADH-cytochrome b5 reductase genes of homozygotes for hereditary methemoglobinemia Types I and III: putative mechanisms of tissue-dependent enzyme deficiency. *American Journal of Human Genetics*, **48**, 799–808.

Kearns, G. L. & Fiser, D. H. (1988). Metoclopramide-induced methemoglobinemia. *Pediatrics*, **82**, 364–6.

Kelly, K. J., Neu, J., Camitta, B. M. & Honig, G. R. (1984). Methemoglobinemia in an infant treated with the folk remedy glycerited asafoetida. *Pediatrics*, **73**, 717–19.

Kobayashi, Y., Fukumaki, Y., Yubisui, T., Inoue, J. & Sakaki, Y. (1990). Serine–proline replacement at residue 127 of NADH-cytochrome b5 reductase causes hereditary methemoglobinemia, generalized type. *Blood*, **75**, 1408–13.

Kotler, R. L., Hansen-Flaschen, J. & Casey, M. P. (1989). Severe methaemoglobinaemia after flexible bronchoscopy. *Thorax*, **44**, 234–5.

Laaban, J. P., Bodenan, P. & Rochemaure, J. (1985). Amyl nitrite poppers and methaemoglobinaemia. *Annals of Internal Medicine*, **103**, 804.

Lee, W. M., Bragg, F. E. & Jaffe, E. R. (1967). Reduction of methemoglobin in human adult and cord blood erythrocytes incubated with glucose or inosine. *Proceedings of the Society for Experimental Biology and Medicine*, **124**, 214–16.

Leroux, A., Junien, C. & Kaplan, J.-C. (1975). Generalized deficiency of cytochrome *b*5 reductase in congenital methaemoglobinaemia with mental retardation. *Nature*, **258**, 619–20.

Lukens, J. N. (1987). The legacy of well-water methemoglobinemia. *Journal of the American Medical Association*, **257**, 2793–5.

Mansouri, A. (1985). Review: Methemoglobinemia. *American Journal of Medical Sciences*, **289**, 200–9.

Mayo, W., Leighton, K., Robertson, B. & Ruedy, J. (1987). Intraoperative cyanosis: a case of dapsone-induced methemoglobinemia. *Canadian Journal of Anaesthesia*, **34**, 79–82.

Menahem, S. (1988). Neonatal cyanosis, methaemo-globinaemia and haemolytic anaemia. *Acta Paediatrica Scandinavica*, **77**, 755–6.

Miller, L. W. (1971). Methemoglobinemia associated with well water. *Journal of the American Medical Association*, **216**, 1642–3.

Ng, L. L., Naik, R. B. & Polak, H. (1982). Paraquat ingestion with methaemoglobinaemia treated with methylene blue. *British Medical Journal*, **284**, 1445–6.

Nilsson, A., Engberg, G., Henneberg, S., Danielson, K. & deVerdier, C.-H. (1990). Inverse relationship between age-dependent erythrocyte activity of methaemoglobin reductase and prilocaine-induced methaemoglobinaemia during infancy. *British Journal of Anaesthesia*, **64**, 72–6.

Park, C. M. & Nagel, R. L. (1984). Sulfhemoglobinemia. *New England Journal of Medicine*, **310**, 1579–84.

Passon, P. G. & Hultquist, D. E. (1972). Soluble cytochrome b5 reductase from human erythrocytes. *Biochimica et Biophysica Acta*, **275**, 62–73.

Perry, G. M. & Anderson, B. B. (1991). Utilization of red cell FAD by methemoglobin reductases at the expense of glutathione reductase in heterozygous β-thalassaemia. *European Journal of Haematology*, **46**, 290–5.

Pierce, J. M. T. & Nielsen, M. S. (1989). Acute acquired methemoglobinaemia after amyl nitrite poisoning. *British Medical Journal*, **298**, 1566.

Proudfoot, A. T. (1982). Methaemoglobinaemia due to monolinuron – not paraquat. *British Medical Journal*, **285**, 812.

Reiter, W. M. & Cimoch, P. J. (1987). Dapsone-induced methemoglobinemia in a patient with *P. Carinii* pneumonia and AIDS. *New England Journal of Medicine*, **317**, 1740–1.

Robicsek, F. (1985). Acute methemoglobinemia during cardiopulmonary bypass caused by intravenous nitroglycerin infusion. *Journal of Thoracic and Cardiovascular Surgery*, **90**, 931–4.

Saxon, S. A. & Silverman, M. E. (1985). Effects of continuous infusion of intravenous nitroglycerin on methemoglobin levels. *American Journal of Cardiology*, **56**, 461–4.

Schwartz, J. M. & Jaffe, E. R. (1978). Hereditary methemoglobinemia with deficiency of NADH dehydrogenase. In *Metabolic Basis of Inherited Disease*, 4th edn, ed. J. B. Stanbury, J. B. Wyngaarden & D. S. Fredrickson, Ch. 61, pp. 1452–64. New York: McGraw-Hill.

Schwartz, J. M., Paress, P. S., Ross, J. M., DiPillo, F. & Rizek, R. (1972). Unstable variant of NADH methemoglobin reductase in Puerto Ricans with hereditary methemoglobinemia. *Journal of Clinical Investigation*, **51**, 1594–1601.

Schwartz, J. M., Reiss, A. L. & Jaffe, E. R. (1983). Hereditary methemoglobinemia with deficiency of NADH cytochrome b5 reductase. In *Metabolic Basis of Inherited Disease*. 5th edn, ed. J. B. Stanbury, J. B. Wyngaarden, D. S. Fredrickson, J. L. Goldstein & M. S. Brown, Ch. 75, pp. 1654–65. New York: McGraw-Hill.

Scott, E. M. (1960). The relationship of diaphorase of human erythrocytes to inheritance of methemoglobinemia. *Journal of Clinical Investigation*, 1960; 1176–9.

Scott E. M. & Griffith I. V. (1959). The enzymic defect of hereditary methemogloinaemia: diaphorase. *Biochimica et Biophysica Acta*, **34**, 584–586.

Scott E. M. & Hoskins D. D. (1958). Hereditary methemoglobinemia in Alaskan Eskimos and Indians. *Blood*, **13**, 795–802.

Shesser, R., Dixon, D., Allen, Y., Mitchell, J. & Edelstein, S. (1980). Fatal methemoglobinemia from butyl nitrite ingestion. *Annals of Internal Medicine*, **92**, 131–2.

Takeshita, M., Matsuki, T., Tanishima, K., Yubisui, T., Yoneyama, Y., Kurata, K., Hara, N. & Igarashi, T. (1982). Alteration of NADH-diaphorase and cytochrome b5 reductase activities of erythrocytes, platelets and leucocytes in hereditary methaemoglobinaemia with and without mental retardation. *Journal of Medical Genetics*, **19**, 204–9.

Tanishima, K., Tanimoto, K., Tomoda, A., Mawatari, K., Matsukawa, S., Yoneyama, Y., Ohkuwa, H. & Takazakura, E. (1985). Hereditary methemoglobinemia due to cytochrome b5 reductase deficiency in blood cells without associated neurologic and mental disorders. *Blood*, **66**, 1288–91.

Tanishima, K., Tomoda, A., Yoneyama, Y. & Ohkuwa, H. (1987). Three types of hereditary methemoglobinemia due to NADH-cytochrome b5 reductase deficiency. *Advances in Clinical Enzymology*, **5**, 81–6.

Tassiopoulos, Th., Fessas, Ph., Rombos, J. & Loukopoulos, D. (1985). Observations on oxygen delivery, methemo-globinemia and arterial oxygenation in patients with β-thalassemia. *Annals of the New York Academy of Sciences*, **445**, 135–47.

Tomatsu, S., Kobayashi, Y., Fukumaki, Y., Yubisui, T., Orii, T. & Sakaki, Y. (1989). The organization and the complete nucleotide sequence of the human NADH-cytochrome b5 reductase gene. *Gene*, **80**, 353–61.

Walley, T. & Flanagan, M. (1987). Nitrite-induced methemoglobinemia. *Postgraduate Medical Journal*, **63**, 643–4.

Wason, S., Detsky, A. S., Plat, O. S. & Lovejoy, F. H. (1980). Isobutyl nitrite toxicity by ingestion. *Annals of Internal Medicine*, **92**, 637–8.

Weatherall, D. J., Clegg, J. B., Higgs, D. R. & Wood, W. G. (1989). The hemoglobinopathies. In *The Metabolic Basis of*

Inherited Disease, 6th edn, ed. C. R. Scriver, A. L. Beaudet, W. S. Sly & D. Vale, Ch. 93, pp. 2281–339. New York: McGraw-Hill.

West, C. A., Gomperts, B. D., Huehns, E. R., Kessel, I. & Ashby, J. R. (1967). Demonstration of an enzyme variant in a case of congenital methaemoglobinaemia. *British Medical Journal*, **4**, 212–14.

Worster-Drought, C., White, J. C. & Sargent, F. (1953). Familial idiopathic methaemoglobinaemia associated with mental deficiency and neurological abnormalities. *British Medical Journal*, **2**, 114–18.

Yubisui, T., Shirabe, K., Takeshita, M., Kobayashi, Y., Fukumaki, Y., Sakaki, Y. & Takano, T. (1991). Structural role of serine-127 in the NADH- binding site of human NADH-cytochrome-b5 reductase. *Journal of Biological Chemistry*, **266**, 66–70.

Zerez, C. R., Lachant, N. A. & Tanaka, K. R. (1990). Impaired erythrocyte methemoglobin reduction in sickle cell disease: dependence of methemoglobin reduction on reduced nicotinamide adenine dinucleotide content. *Blood*, **76**, 1008–14.

35 Catalase

A CLINICAL OBSERVATION

THE INTEREST in the enzyme catalase in human pharmacogenetics started when Professor Shigeo Takahara, a Japanese otorhinolaryngologist, was performing an operation. His account of the event was as follows:

In 1946 I encountered an 11 year old girl with high fever and complaining of very severe ulcers in her mouth at our Ear, Nose and Throat Clinic. Extremely foul smelling granulation in her nose and a peculiar type of gangrene starting around the neck of a back tooth of upper jaw and encroaching upon the maxillary sinus and nasal cavity were noticed. In this case the infected part was radically excised and hydrogen peroxide was poured on the wound for sterilization. To my surprise, the blood that came in contact with the hydrogen peroxide, immediately turned brownish-black and the usual bubbles did not appear. At that time I suspected that the nurse might have handed me silver nitrate by mistake, but a fresh bottle of peroxide gave the same result. Thus I came to believe that there was some abnormality in the blood of this patient. In this family there are seven siblings and four of them had mouth gangrene of various degrees and their blood all reacted in the same manner just described. The other three had no oral lesions and their blood reacted in the normal fashion with peroxide. Thus I concluded that there was some close relationship between the blackening of blood and the mouth disease, and decided to study this disease more closely. Through exhaustive qualitative and quantitative analysis of the blood from these patients it was confirmed that catalase was completely absent in the blood. *(Takahara 1961)*

Subsequently Takahara (1952) published five more patients aged 8 to 18 years with progressive oral gangrene and no catalase activity in the blood or tissues adjacent to the disease site. Four of these five patients were siblings. In addition to these five persons with serious disease two with a milder form of the condition were found amongst four siblings in another family. All three families involved exhibited consanguinity.

ORAL GANGRENE (TAKAHARA'S DISEASE)

In the Japanese patients discovered by Takahara a rare and characteristic form of oral gangrene occurred. Ulcerations of the gums occurred at a young age and they were located around the necks of the teeth. Sometimes these lesions healed, but sometimes they progressed to damage the dental alveoli. When the teeth became loose and fell out, or were extracted, healing very often followed. In some instances there was a spreading gangrene damaging both soft and bony tissues and, for example, penetrating the maxillary sinuses and even involving the tongue or tonsil. Extensive surgery including bone grafting was required for the more seriously affected patients. After all the teeth had been removed and the mouth lesions were healed these patients were in general perfectly well but were left with scarring and deformity which caused difficulty in opening the mouth.

A lot more is known about the metabolism of

oxygen and allied chemical species in tissues than was the case in the late 1940s, and consequently a fairly convincing picture can be built up of the mechanisms causing Takahara's disease.

Some pathogenic organisms produce hydrogen peroxide. This topic is referred to also in Chapter 25, on glucose-6-phosphate dehydrogenase, but there the patient was at risk from organisms which did *not* produce hydrogen peroxide. In the present context it was organisms which did produce hydrogen peroxide which were the cause of the trouble. Examples of such organisms are haemolytic streptococci, *Streptococcus pneumoniae*, *S. faecalis* and *Bacillus acidophilus*, which not only produce hydrogen peroxide but also do not produce catalase. The first two were the organisms most commonly cultured by Takahara from the oral lesions of his patients.

Presumably organisms of this kind could invade the tissues via an abrasion on the gums. In the acatalasic subject the hydrogen peroxide formed would not be destroyed and would therefore be a cellular toxin. Haemoglobin would be oxidized to methaemoglobin so the tissues would be devitalized by anoxia. Also, as Matsunaga *et al.* (1985) showed, the acatalasic polymorphonuclear leucocytes do not function normally. Their migration, phagocytosis, membrane potential, and O_2^- production were all defective as compared with normal after exposure to peroxide.

With these defective defence mechanisms it was not surprising that progressive necrosis and infection occurred, sometimes to the extent of destroying adjacent bone. There is an obvious resemblance between Takahara's disease and two other conditions whose bases are quite different, namely the lazy-leucocyte syndrome (Miller *et al.* 1971) and chronic granulomatous disease (Johnston & Newman 1977).

The surprising thing, however, is that Professor Takahara, who saw dramatic patients between 1946 and 1950, did not see such severe disease in later years. He ascribed this change as possibly being due to two factors: first, the development, availability and liberal use of antibiotics, and secondly, the improvement in the grossly deficient nutritional and hygienic conditions which prevailed in Japan in the years immediately following World War II. The incidence rates of Takahara's disease in Japanese acatalasemic subjects born from 1876 to 1935 ($n =$

22), 1936 to 1945 ($n = 29$) and 1946 to 1965 ($n = 12$) were 0.46, 0.35 and 0.25, respectively (Ogata 1991). However similar patients with Takahara's disease have subsequently been described in Germany (Polster *et al.* 1968; Gross *et al.* 1977) and in Peruvian Mestizos (Delgado & Calderon 1979).

Mechanisms other than catalase which protect tissues against the noxious effects of hydrogen peroxide include (1) the presence of vitamin E, (2) degradation by glutathione peroxidase, (3) deviation into the myeloperoxidase–halide system for bacterial killing (Matsunaga *et al.* 1985). It is obvious that these processes could be depressed in states of malnutrition, just as catalase activity itself can be depressed in otherwise normal people by the existence of iron deficiency (Balcerzak *et al.* 1966).

CATALASE IN CELLS AND TISSUES OTHER THAN ERYTHROCYTES

Takahara (1952) had showed that tissue around the oral ulcers, and of the ethmoidal sinus, and nasal polyps from acatalasic subjects were devoid of catalase. Similarly, in Japanese acatalasics Kaziro *et al.* (1952) demonstrated that catalase was also absent from liver, muscle and bone marrow. The absence has also been shown in white blood cells, lymphoepithelial tissue, uterus, placenta and cultures of fibroblasts from skin biopsies. More modern techniques have shown that the catalase activity in the leucocytes of Swiss acatalasics is 28.5% of normal, whereas the activity in Japanese acatalasics is 2.4% of normal. Swiss acatalasic fibroblasts have 5% of the catalase activity of normal fibroblasts whereas in Japanese acatalasics no catalase activity can be detected in fibroblasts (Ogata 1991).

GENETICS OF ACATALASIA

Takahara had realized early on that acatalasia was a genetic disorder. Definitive information on the inheritance of the condition was obtained by Nishimura *et al.* (1959). They measured blood catalase activity in 206 randomly selected normal Japanese persons, and also in members of five acatalasemia families. The latter fell into three phenotypic categories, as shown in Fig. 35.1. The disposition of these phenotypes in pedigrees was in keeping with

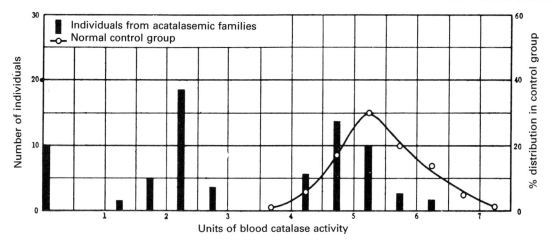

Fig. 35.1. Distribution of catalase values for members of the 5 acatalasemia families and comparison with a percentage distribution curve of values from a normal control group. (From Nishimura et al. 1959.)

the view that blood catalase activity was controlled by two autosomal co-dominant alleles.

In 1961 Aebi et al. published the finding of two Swiss males with acatalasia who were found as a result of screening 18 459 blood samples in the Army Blood Group Laboratory of the Swiss Red Cross Blood Transfusion Service. These individuals were healthy and it is to be noted that they possessed about ½% of the normal blood catalase activity, as compared with the total absence in most Japanese acatalasics. The estimated frequency of heterozygotes in Switzerland was 2%, compared with estimates of 0.09 and 1.4% in Japanese (Hamilton et al. 1961).

The inheritance pattern in the pedigrees of Swiss acatalasia individuals was consistent with control by two autosomal alleles, the same as with the Japanese. An unexplained exception was individual V37 in Fig. 2 of Aebi et al. (1963), who had a value of >2600 perborate units characteristic of a normal homozygote; this individual should have been a heterozygote because her mother was acatalasic.

CHROMOSOMAL LOCALIZATION OF THE CATALASE GENE

Wieacker et al. (1980) used the fact that mouse and human catalases have different electrophoretic mobilities. In hybrid mouse/human cells they found that the human enzyme co-segregated with chromosome 11. Subsequently using a human fibroblast cDNA probe the catalase gene was localized to 11p1305–11p1306 (Narahara et al. 1984; Schroeder & Saunders 1987). Deletions of this region of chromosome 11 may be associated with Wilms tumour, aniridia, genito-urinary abnormalities and mental retardation (Turleau et al. 1984).

MOLECULAR GENETICS

The isolation and sequencing of partial cDNA clones coding for human catalase were reported by Korneluk et al. (1984). These clones had been recovered from a human fibroblast cDNA library using oligonucleotide probes deduced from the amino acid structure of human erythrocyte catalase. The deduced amino acid sequence of the isolated cDNA showed a near perfect match to the known protein sequence. A 462 bp insertion was thought to be an intron. The gene was subsequently shown to have 13 exons, and to be 34 kb long (Quan et al. 1986). Human catalase has 526 amino acids.

In acatalasic fibroblasts Wen et al. (1988) probed the RNA using a part of human catalase cDNA (which was isolated from a human gene library using rat catalase cDNA). Catalase was not detectable in the fibroblast cultures and mRNA of normal size was deficient. However, genomic DNA showed no difference from normal in size. It was thought therefore that there was no large deletion, insertion or rearrangement of DNA.

The mutant gene was cloned from leucocytes of a Japanese acatalasic individual, and sequenced. Seven base differences were found, as compared with the normal gene. A guanine → adenine substitution at the fifth position of intron 4 (a splice site mutation) was responsible for the defective synthesis of catalase because of the alternative splicing of the precursor mRNA. Splicing in the mutant occurred between the 5' donor site of the preceding intron and the 3' acceptor site of the intron containing the substitution, so that one entire exon sequence was omitted (Ogata 1991). This same defect was found in four members of three Japanese acatalasic families by Kishimoto *et al.* (1992). The other base changes were polymorphic.

Rat cDNA has been isolated and its open reading frame encodes 527 amino acids (Furuta *et al.* 1985). An acatalasemic mouse strain has been investigated by Shaffer & Preston (1990). The molecular basis was a single nucleotide change (G → T), giving a change of amino acid 11 from glutamine (CAG) to histidine (CAT).

STRUCTURE OF CATALASE

Catalase (EC 1.11.1.6) has been extensively studied in many different types of organisms. Beef liver catalase has been crystallized and its three-dimensional structure determined (Fita & Rossmann 1985.) It is likely that all mammalian catalase molecules are built to a similar overall design. The enzyme is a tetramer with a molecular weight of 230 000. In each of the four subunits there is one protoporphyrin IX moiety containing a Fe^{3+} atom (see Chapter 26, on the hepatic porphyrias, for more information on this porphyrin). This haem group is deeply buried within the subunit molecule and is connected to the surface by a funnel shaped main channel and a subsidiary narrower channel. The major channel is probably the entrance for peroxide substrates whereby they can interact with the iron atom. As with other enzymes the amino acids forming the substrate channel are responsible for the proper functioning of the molecule. In the case of catalase a histidine and an asparagine seem to be of great importance in the formation of a presumed enzyme–substrate intermediary compound (Fita & Rossman 1985).

FUNCTION OF CATALASE

The prime function of catalase is to catalyse the rapid decomposition of hydrogen peroxide to water and oxygen (Ohmori *et al.* 1991). By this means it prevents cell constituents being damaged through oxidation (Easton 1991). When paracetamol is oxidized hydrogen peroxide is formed and cultured hepatocytes can be protected from damage by the presence of catalase (Kyle *et al.* 1987). The enzyme also has the ability to oxidize substrates, e.g. ethanol, by a peroxidase activity.

GENETIC VARIANTS OF ACATALASIA

It has already been pointed out that early studies showed that Swiss 'acatalasics' had a small amount of catalase activity, which suggested that they had a variant unlike the Japanese type. This view was supported by the fact that the heterozygotes, which were grouped quite separately from the normals in Japanese (Fig. 35.1), overlapped with the normals in the Swiss variety in frequency distribution histograms (Aebi *et al.* 1963). However, one Japanese family differed from the others in that the heterozygotes had catalase activity values which were almost normal.

Evidence for heterogeneity has also been found in other ways, and most effort has been spent in investigating the Japanese and Swiss varieties. The results are condensed in Table 35.1, with the presumed explanation. It has been suggested by Aebi & Wyss (1978) that in the Swiss acatalasics the unstable enzyme has almost completely disappeared from erythrocytes because they have a long half-life, and that the tissues generally may possess relatively more enzyme because the half-lives of their cells are shorter.

The prevailing ideas are as follows. Swiss acatalasia is probably due to a mutation causing a change in the structural gene, leading to an amino acid substitution either in the catalytic domain or disturbing the conformation of the enzyme causing it to have low stability (Crawford *et al.* 1988). The common Japanese type acatalasia has been explained above.

Other variants may well exist; for example, Baur (1963) found a Caucasian catalase variant with increased electrophoretic mobility but with the same activity and stability as a normal catalase.

Table 35.1. *Properties of catalase from Japanese and Swiss acatalasics*

Property	Japanese acatalasic	Swiss acatalasic
Red cell catalase activity (% of normal)	0.16%	0.5 to 2%
White cell catalase activity (% of normal)	2.40%	9 to 20%[a]
mRNA	Nil[b,c]	Normal amounts[b]
Catalase protein by immunoblot analysis	Nil[c]	Present
Heat stability	Normal[d]	Decreased[e]
Stability against concentrated urea	–	Decreased[e]
Electrophoretic mobility	Normal[f]	Increased[g,h]
Antigenic properties	–	Identity with the normal enzyme[i]
Isoelectric focusing followed by immunofixation	A normal person shows proteins at pI 5.3 and 5.9. The latter was absent[j]	–
Presumed explanation	Variant with normal stability but low specific activity[h]	Variant with low stability but approximately normal specific activity[h]

[a]Wyss & Aebi 1975.
[b]Crawford *et al.* 1988.
[c]Wen *et al.* 1988.
[d]Ogata *et al.* 1987.
[e]Shapira *et al.* 1974.

[f]Ogata 1991.
[g]Scherz *et al.* 1976.
[h]Aebi & Wyss 1978.
[i]Aebi *et al.* 1974.
[j]Ogata & Mizugaki 1982.

On the basis of the criteria described above, Aebi & Wyss (1978) proposed the existence of seven different variants. It is obvious, however, that the matter can be put on a firm basis only as a result of genomic analysis accompanied by genotype/phenotype correlations for each variant.

ETHNIC DISTRIBUTION OF ACATALASIA

Evidence for the presence of acatalasia or hypocatalasia (heterozygous carriers) has also been found in ethnic groups other than Japanese and Swiss. They have been described in Koreans (Hamilton *et al.* 1961), Swedes (Engstedt & Paul 1965), Mexicans (Saldivar *et al.* 1974), Peruvians (Delgado & Calderon 1979; Wilson & Rosa 1979), Israelis of Persian origin (Szeinberg *et al.* 1963), white and black Americans (Baur 1963; Taylor & Haut 1967) and Germans (Gross *et al.* 1977; Polster *et al.* 1968).

A SPECULATION

It seems strange that so few experiments have been conducted to study the interactions of xenobiotics (other than hydrogen peroxide for wound sterilization) with acatalasic red blood cells and white blood cells. There is a possibility that such experiments might be informative.

Aebi, H., Heiniger, J. P., Bütler, R. & Hässig, A. (1961). Two cases of acatalasia in Switzerland. *Experientia*, **17**, 466.

Aebi, H., Jeunet, F., Richterich, R., Suter, H., Bütler, R., Frei, J. & Marti, H. R. (1963). Observations in two Swiss families with acatalasia. *Enzymologia Biologica Clinica*, **2**, 1–22.

Aebi, H. E. & Wyss, S. R. (1978). Acatalasemia. In: *The Metabolic Basis of Inherited Disease*, 4th edn., ed. J. B. Stanbury, J. B. Wyngaarden & D. S. Fredrickson, Ch. 78; pp. 1792–1807. New York: McGraw-Hill.

Aebi, H. E., Wyss, S. R., Scherz, B. & Skvaril, F. (1974). Heterogeneity of erythrocyte catalase II. Isolation and characterization of normal and variant erythrocyte catalase into their subunits. *European Journal of Biochemistry*, **48**, 137–45.

Balcerzak, S. P., Vester, J. W. & Doyle, A. P. (1966). Effect of iron deficiency and red cell age on human erythrocyte catalase. *Journal of Laboratory and Clinical Medicine*, **67**, 742–56.

Baur, E. W. (1963). Catalase abnormality in a Caucasian family in the United States. *Science*, **140**, 816–17.

Crawford, D. R., Mirault, M. E., Moret, R., Zbinden, I. & Cerutti, P. A. (1988). Molecular defect in human acatalasia fibroblasts. *Biochemical and Biophysical Research Communications*, **153**, 59–66.

Delgado, W. & Calderon, R. (1979). Acatalasia in two Peruvian siblings. *Journal of Oral Pathology and Medicine*, **8**, 358–68.

Eaton, J. W. (1991). Catalases and peroxidases and glutathione and hydrogen peroxide: Mysteries of the bestiary. *Journal of Laboratory and Clinical Medicine*, **118**, 3–4.

Engstedt, L. & Paul, K. G. (1965). Nonhereditary hypocatalasia. *Scandinavian Journal of Clinical and Laboratory Investigation*, **17**, 295–6.

Fita, I. & Rossmann, M. G. (1985). The active center of catalase. *Journal of Molecular Biology*, **185**, 21–37.

Furuta, S., Hayashi, H., Hijikata, M., Miyazawa, S., Osumi, T. & Hashimoto, T. (1986). Complete nucleotide sequence of cDNA and deduced amino acid sequence of rat liver catalase. *Proceedings of the National Academy of Sciences (USA)*, **83**, 313–17.

Gross, J., Scherz, B., Wyss, S. R., Künzel, W., Maiwald, H. J., Hartwig, A. & Polster, H. (1977). Charakterisierung der Katalase roter Blutzellen eines Patienten mit den Symptomen einer TakaharaKrankheit. *Kinderärtzliche Praxis*, **36**, 793–5.

Hamilton, H. B., Neel, J. V., Kobara, T. Y. & Ozaki, K. (1961). The frequency in Japan of carriers of the rare 'recessive' gene causing acatalasemia. *Journal of Clinical Investigation*, **40**, 2199–208.

Johnston, R. B. & Newman, S. L. (1977). Chronic granulomatous disease. *Pediatric Clinics of North America*, **24**, 365–676.

Kaziro, K., Kikuchi, G., Nakamura, H. & Yoshiya, M. (1952). Die Frage nach der physiologischen Funktion der Katalase im menschlichen Organismus. Notiz über die Entdeckung einer Konstitutionsanomalie 'Anenzymia catalasea'. *Chemische Berichte*, **85**, 886. (Cited by Wyngaarden, J. B. & Howell, R. R.). (1960). Acatalasia. In: *The Metabolic Basis of Inherited Disease*, ed. J. B. Stanbury, J. B. Wyngaarden & D. S. Frederickson, Ch. 46, pp. 1398–414. New York: McGraw-Hill.

Kishimoto, Y., Murakami, Y., Hayashi, K., Takahara, S., Sugimura, T. & Sekiya, T. (1992). Detection of a common mutation of the catalase gene in Japanese acatalasemic patients. *Human Genetics*, **88**, 487–90.

Korneluk, R. G., Quan, F., Lewis, W. H., Guise, K. S., Willard, H. F., Holmes, M. T. & Gravel, R. A. (1984). Isolation of human fibroblast catalase cDNA clones. *Journal of Biological Chemistry*, **259**, 13819–23.

Kyle, M. E., Miccadei, S., Nakae, D. & Farber, J. L. (1987). Superoxide dismutase and catalase protect cultured hepatocytes from the cytotoxicity of acetaminophen. *Biochemical and Biophysical Research Communications*, **149**, 889–96.

Matsunaga, T., Seger, R., Höger, P., Tiefenauer, L. & Hitzig, W. H. (1985). Congenital acatalasemia: a study of neutrophil functions after provocation with hydrogen peroxide. *Pediatric Research*, **19**, 1187–90.

Miller, M. E., Oski, F. A. & Harris, M. B. (1971). Lazy leucocyte syndrome. A new disorder of neutrophil function. *Lancet*, **1**, 665–9.

Narahara, K., Kikkawa, K., Kimira, S., Kimoto, H., Ogata, M., Kasai, R., Hamawaki, M. & Matsuoka, K. (1984). Regional mapping of catalase and Wilms' tumor aniridia, genitourinary abnormalities, and mental retardation triad loci to the chromosome segment 11p1305-p1306. *Human Genetics*, **66**, 181–5.

Nishimura, E. T., Hamilton, H. B., Kobara, T. Y., Takahara, S., Ogura, Y. & Doi, K. (1959). Carrier state in human acatalasemia. *Science*, **130**, 333–4.

Ogata, M. (1991). Acatalasemia. *Human Genetics*, **86**, 331–40.

Ogata, M., Fujii, Y., Meguro, T., Kira, S., Matsuda, A., Izushi, F., Kimoto, T. & Takahara, S. (1987). The level and stability of residual catalase in cultured acatalasemic skin fibroblasts. *Acta Medica Okayama*, **41**, 201–4.

Ogata, M. & Mizugaki, J. (1982). Heterogeneity of erythrocyte catalase in Japanesetype acatalasemia by electrofocussing. *Biochemical Genetics*, **20**, 265–9.

Ohmori, T., Takamoto, K. & Ogata, M. (1991). The role of catalase in protecting erythrocytes against methemoglobin formation. *Acta Medica Okayama*, **45**, 321–4.

Polster, H., Beyreiss, K. & Nostilz, H. J. (1968). Akatalasie bei einem vierjährigen Jungen. *Kinderaeräztliche Praxis*, **36**, 367–70.

Quan, F., Korneluk, R. G., Tropak, M. B. & Gravel, R. A. (1986). Isolation and characterization of the human catalase gene. *Nucleic Acids Research*, **14**, 5321–35.

Saldivar, A. A., Carrasco, R. M. D. & Reyes, G. R. (1974). Deficiencia de catalasa entrocitica en la civdad de Peubla. *Revista de Investigacion Clinica (Mex)*, **26**, 47–52.

Scherz, B., Kuchinskas, E. J., Wyss, S. R. & Aebi, H. (1976). Heterogeneity of erythrocyte catalase. Dissociation of recombination and hybridization of human erythrocyte catalases. *European Journal of Biochemistry*, **69**, 603–13.

Schroeder, W. T. & Saunders, G. F. (1987). Localization of the human catalase and apolipoprotein AI genes to chromosome 11. *Cytogenetics and Cell Genetics*, **44**, 231–3.

Shaffer, J. B. & Preston, K. E. (1990). Molecular analysis of an acatalasemic mouse mutant. *Biochemical and Biophysical Research Communications*, **173**, 1043–50.

Shapira, E., BenYoseph, Y. & Aebi, H. (1974). Nature of residual erythrocyte catalase activity in Swiss-style acatalasemia. *Enzyme*, **17**, 307–18.

Szeinberg, A., de Vries, A., Pinkhas, J., Djaldetti, M. & Ezra, R. (1963). A dual hereditary red blood cell defect in one family: hypocatalasemia and glucose-6-phosphate dehydrogenase deficiency. *Acta Geneticae Medicae et Gemellologiae*, **12**, 247–55.

Takahara, S. (1952). Progressive oral gangrene probably due to lack of catalase in the blood (acatalasemia) – report of nine cases. *Lancet*, **2**, 1101–4.

Takahara, S. (1961). *Acatalasemia*. Address at the Second Congress of Human Genetics, Rome, 1961.

Taylor, E. H. & Haut, A. (1967). Hypocatalasia in two American men. *Clinical Research*, **15**, 289–91.

Turleau, C., de Grouchy, J., Tournade, M.-F., Gagnadoux, M.-F. & Junien, C. (1884). Del 11p/aniridia complex. Report of three patients and review of 37 observations from the literature. *Clinical Genetics*, **26**, 356–62.

Wen, J.-K., Osumi, T., Hashimoto, T. &, Ogata M. (1988). Diminished synthesis of catalase due to the decrease in catalase mRNA in Japanese type acatalasemia. *Physiological Chemistry and Physics and Medical NMR* **20**, 171–6.

Wieacker, P., Mueller, C. R., Mayerova, A., Grzeschik, K. H. & Ropers, H. H. (1980). Assignment of the gene coding for human catalase to the short arm of chromosome 11. *Annales de Génétique*, **23**, 73–7.

Wilson, D. A. & Rosa, C. (1979). Acatalasia in two Peruvian siblings. *Journal of Oral Pathology and Medicine*, **8**, 358–68.

Wyss, S. R. & Aebi, H. (1975). Properties of leukocyte catalase in Swiss type acatalasemia: A comparative study of normals, heterozygotes and homozygotes. *Enzyme*, **20**, 257–68.

36 Antibiotic-induced deafness, chloramphenicol toxicity and other topics

ANTIBIOTIC-INDUCED DEAFNESS

IT is well known that aminoglycoside antibiotics (streptomycin, kanamycin, gentamicin, tobramycin, neomycin) can lead to hearing loss. Following isolated reports of familial aggregation a systematic survey of the problem was undertaken in Shanghai by Hu *et al.* (1991). They ascertained 763 deaf mutes and amongst them found 167 caused by aminoglycosides. These led to 36 informative pedigrees which were found to contain 108 cases of aminoglycoside antibiotic-induced deafness (AAID) (including the probands).

In 22 pedigrees the manner of transmission could be ascertained. Even though there was an approximately equal sex frequency of AAID, transmission always seemed to be through females. Affected males did not transmit the character to their offspring. The maternal transmission could be explained by mitochondrial inheritance. As Hu *et al.* (1991) point out most mitochondrially inherited disorders in man are rare. Antibiotic induced deafness is rare. Since not everybody in the pedigrees had been treated with the relevant antibiotics the actual prevalence of persons with susceptibility to AAID would be higher than indicated by the affected cases.

Aminoglycoside antibiotic therapy should be avoided in patients with a family history of ototoxic side effects from the drug (especially in the maternal relatives).

FLUOROURACIL AND FAMILIAL PYRIDINAEMIA

The pyrimidine analogue 5-fluorouracil (FU) (Fig. 36.1) was established as an anti-tumour drug by Heidelberger *et al.* (1957) and exerts some of its effects, as predicted, by blocking the synthesis of thymidylic acid. Blockade of the thymidylate synthase reaction inhibits DNA synthesis (Cohen *et al.* 1958). Thymidylate synthase (EC 2.1.1.45) catalyses the transfer of a methyl group to deoxyuridine-5'-monophosphate to form thymidine-5'-monophosphate. It is important for the *de novo* production of the latter compound for DNA synthesis.

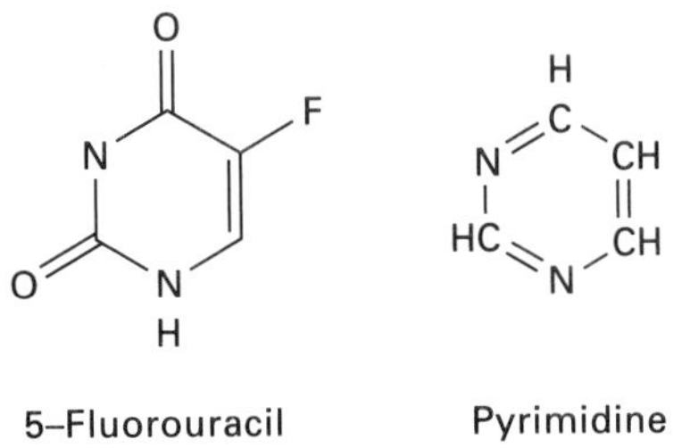

5–Fluorouracil   Pyrimidine

Fig. 36.1. The molecular structures of pyrimidine and 5-fluorouracil.

The drug FU is used as an antimetabolite in the treatment of a variety of solid tumours such as cancers of the breast, ovary, gastrointestinal tract and liver.

Toxicity has long been known to be unpredictable (see, for example, Calabresi & Parks 1975) and consists of

1 gastrointestinal symptoms (eg vomiting, diarrhoea, stomatitis, etc.);
2 myelouppression: especially leucopenia which reaches a nadir at the ninth to 14th day;
3 hair and nail changes;
4 neurological manifestations such as a cerebellar disturbance.

Fluorouracil toxicity was established as a pharmacogenetic entity by Tuchman *et al.* (1985), who described a 27 year old woman who had undergone a left modified radical mastectomy for an infiltrating duct carcinoma. After conventional dosages of cyclophosphamide methotrexate and FU the patient developed leucopenia and gastrointestinal symptoms. Three weeks after the second course of treatment she developed sluggish speech and cerebellar ataxia followed by confusion and semicoma. These features started to improve after 5 weeks.

High levels of uracil and thymine were found in her plasma and urine, abnormalities which continued for a long time after the last dose of FU. Her plasma uric acid was not raised, indicating that there was no extraordinarily extensive nucleotide breakdown. Similar high levels of uracil and thymine were not seen in other patients with the same disease treated in the same way. Family investigations revealed that the patient's mother had values not significantly different from 17 normal controls. No dihydrouracil or dihydrothymine were detected in the urine or blood of the patient or the affected brother. The thymidine kinase activity of the patient's white cells was found to be normal.

The evidence thus indicated strongly that this patient and her brother had a genetic abnormality in pyrimidine metabolism which rendered her liable to severe toxic effects when treated with FU.

Dietary explanations having been discounted, three metabolic processes dealing with pyrimidine metabolism were considered as possible locations for the metabolic abnormality. These were production, salvage and degradation. The absence of orotic aciduria eliminated the first suggestion. The second explanation seemed unlikely because of the finding of a normal leucocyte thymidine kinase activity. The third possibility (Fig. 36.2) specifically involving the

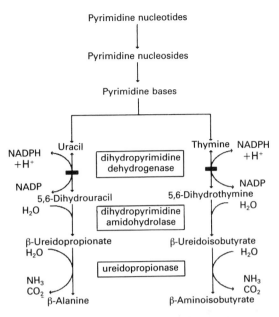

Fig. 36.2. The degradation pathway of pyrimidine nucleotides. The rate-limiting enzyme for degradation of the pyrimidine bases uracil and thymine is dihydropyrimidine dehydrogenase (DPD). NADPH = reduced nicotinamide adenine dinucleotide. (From Tuchman *et al.* 1985.)

enzyme dihydropyrimidine dehydrogenase (DPD; EC 1.3.1.2) seemed to be the most attractive because:

1 there is a known increase in endogenous pyrimidine production during cancer therapy;
2 both uracil and thymine were present in increased amounts in the patient's body fluids;
3 there was no increase in dihydrouracil and dihydrothymine;
4 DPD is the rate-limiting enzyme in the metabolism of FU, so if it was defective more FU would be available for incorporation into RNA and to bind to thymidylate synthase;
5 thymidine, which prolongs the plasma half-life of FU, is converted to thymine which may compete with the binding of FU to DPD.

A second patient, who was the product of a pedigree positive for consanguinity and who also presented with an infiltrating ductal breast carcinoma, was described by Diasio *et al.* (1988). The patient was treated with cyclophosphamide, methotrexate and FU, and developed neutropenia and later

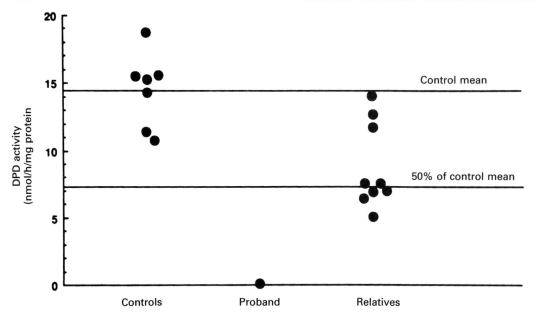

Fig. 36.3. Relative activity of DPD in peripheral blood mononuclear cells obtained from the proband, nine of her family members, and seven healthy volunteers (controls). DPD activity is expressed as nanomoles of catabolite formed/h/mg protein. (From Harris *et al.* 1991.)

paralysis from which she eventually recovered. Her serum and urine contained high concentrations of uracil and thymine. A small test dose of [6-³H]-FU was given to this proband and revealed an elimination half-life from the plasma of 159 minutes whereas control cancer patients gave a vale of 13 ± 7 minutes. Minimal catabolite production was demonstrated in that 89.7% of the dose was recovered unchanged in the urine over 24 hours whereas in control patients the corresponding figure was 9.8% and substantial catabolite formation was evident 2 hours after dosing. Peripheral blood monocyte DPD activities were zero in the proband, reduced in her father and children and normal in one brother, findings consistent with her being an autosomal recessive character. Presumably this finding in the blood monocytes reflected the metabolic capacity of the liver but this presumption has never been proven.

A third patient reported by Harris *et al.* (1991) also had an extensive invasive ductal breast carcinoma without metastases. Following treatment with cyclophosphamide methotrexate and FU she sustained neutropenia and mild neurological toxicity (difficulty with balance and spelling simple words).

This patient, her family and control subjects were investigated in the manner described above. It is not clear why the controls in this study gave blood monocyte DPD activities 20 times lower than those in the paper of Diasio *et al.* (1988). The pedigree of this proband indicated that she had a recessive character consisting of absent DPD activity (Figs 36.3 and 36.4).

The fact that all three probands were suffering from an infiltrating ductal breast carcinoma may have had nothing to do with the toxicity of FU. The fact that they were given the FU in combination with cyclophosphamide and methotrexate could (as discussed by Harris *et al.* 1991) have had some influence on the metabolism of FU.

It seems likely that the marrow and nervous system toxicities exhibited by the probands were due to high concentrations of FU in the plasma and cerebrospinal liquid, respectively. Catabolite production was either extremely small or absent. Why the neurological adverse effects should follow the haematological adverse effects after a time lag is unclear.

What relationship if any this classic pharmacogenetic condition has to paediatric syndromes with

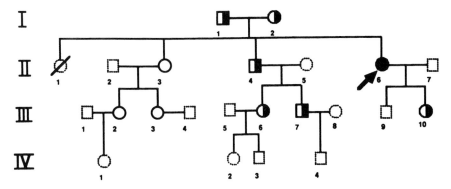

Fig. 36.4. Pedigree of the proband and family members showing the inheritance of a defect in DPD activity. The proband is indicated by an arrow, deceased family members are indicated by a diagonal line through the symbol, and family members who were alive but not examined are indicated by a dashed symbol. Non-shaded symbols indicate control levels of DPD activity, half-shaded symbols indicate partial deficiency of DPD activity (i.e. approximately 50% of controls), and fully shaded symbols indicate complete deficiency of DPD activity. (From Harris et al. 1991.)

neurologic dysfunction, mental retardation and developmental abnormalities (MIM 274270) remains to be determined.

As mentioned by Harris et al. (1991), whilst the homozygote for DPD deficiency may suffer severely, the heterozygote may also be somewhat more prone than normal individuals to suffer side effects on FU administration.

The gene frequency of DPD deficiency in the population is unknown. This might be a point of some importance in order to decide whether the screening of patients for DPD deficiency prior to FU therapy is a practical and cost-effective possibility.

CHLORAMPHENICOL-INDUCED MARROW DEPRESSION

Three instances have been recorded of bone marrow depression following the therapeutic use of chloramphenicol.

Aplastic anaemia in one identical twin with a possibly related thrombocytopenia in the other were described by Fernbach & Trentin (1960), as mentioned by Best (1967).

Secondly, a 36 year old white male developed pancytopenia following the use of chloramphenicol eyedrops. Recovery following the cessation of the medication was followed by relapse when they were

recommenced. Two years previously a 5 year old niece, daughter of the patient's sister, died of aplastic anaemia following ingestion of chloramphenicol (Rosenthal & Blackman 1965).

Thirdly, white male twins born to non-consanguineous parents were treated for a fever at the age of 6 months with chloramphenicol and both developed marrow toxicity. Studies for Fanconi's anaemia and paroxysmal nocturnal haemoglobinuria were negative, there was no evidence of associated hepatitis and the humoral and cellular immunity was intact.

The authors, Nagao & Mauer (1969), pointed out that estimates of the frequency of aplastic anaemia following chloramphenicol exposure were 1/200 000 and 1/60 000, and so the simultaneous appearance of the disease in twins was very unlikely to be due to chance.

Bone marrow cells from persons who had recovered from chloramphenicol toxicity were found by Howell et al. (1975) to be less sensitive than cells from normal controls to the toxic effects of chloramphenicol in vitro. It has been suggested by Fine (1978) that possibly chloramphenicol sensitivity is determined by mitochondrial inheritance and that in the episode of toxicity there is selection for cells carrying mitochondria bearing genes conferring resistance.

NAIL PIGMENTATION FOLLOWING CANCER CHEMOTHERAPY

The formation of pigmentary bands of melanin in the nails of patients undergoing chemotherapy was observed among close relatives in Sardinia by Sulis & Flores (1980). Both transverse and longitudinal bands were seen, and either a few or all the nails could be affected. The phenomenon was concomitantly observed in a brother and sister treated with adriamycin for carcinoma, and in a mother treated with cyclophosphamide for breast carcinoma and her daughter treated with cyclophosphamide for resistant rheumatoid arthritis. The incidence of the ungual pigmentation in Sardinian cancer patients treated with chemotherapy was reported to be 8%, and so the occurrence in close relatives was unlikely to be due to chance and there may be a genetic basis for the phenomenon.

HEREDITARY PREDISPOSITION IN DRUG-INDUCED PARKINSONISM

Phenothiazine drugs are known to produce a mimic of Parkinson's disease, and the susceptibility of different patients to develop this complication varies greatly. The idea that the susceptibility to develop this complication is related to the aetiology of 'idiopathic' Parkinsonism was explored by Myrianthopoulos et al. (1962). Patients who had been treated for schizophrenia and other psychiatric illnesses with phenothiazines were divided into two groups: 59 who developed Parkinsonian signs (propositi) and 67 who did not do so after similar dosages of the same drugs (controls). Details of 728 relatives of the propositi and 777 relatives of the controls were examined. Thirteen cases of Parkinson's disease were found in the former and three in the latter group.

This study suggests the possibility that the occurrence of phenothiazine induced extra-pyramidal signs mimicking Parkinsonism may indicate the presence of genes conferring a liability to develop the naturally occurring variety of the disease.

MINOCYCLINIC INDUCED POTASSIUM LOSS FROM ERYTHROCYTES

Minocycline induces potassium loss from all human erythrocytes, an effect which is inhibited by calcium. During studies to investigate this phenomenon Kornguth & Calvin (1978) discovered a 39 year old healthy male laboratory technician whose red cells under the influence of minocycline lost 3.5 times more potassium than those of other volunteers. The

red cells of the propositus contained normal amounts of potassium when not under the influence of minocycline. The relatives of the propositus were then investigated. The pedigree strongly suggested an autosomal dominant mode of inheritance of the trait of increased potassium loss under the influence of minocycline. The pedigree study also revealed that the red cells of affected individuals leaked a little more potassium than normal when they were not under the influence of minocycline, so that the antibiotic was amplifying a property which was present under basal conditions. It was speculated that the minocycline effect might reflect a difference in membrane lipids or an alteration in a membrane protein directly involved in the control of ion permeability. The red blood cell membranes, osmotic fragility, and Ca^{2+}-dependent and ouabain-sensitive $(Na^+ K^+)$-dependent adenosine triphosphatase activity were normal in the affected subjects.

This 'minocycline effect' was investigated by Lannigan & Evans (1982). A population of 86 randomly selected healthy volunteers showed a wide variation. The repeatability was 0.70. In 30 families there was no correlation between parents and the 'heritability' was 0.63. Eleven persons who had suffered vestibular side effects following minocycline administration had a distribution of the minocycline effect not significantly different from the healthy family members. It would seem probable, therefore, that the minocycline effect is controlled in a polygenic fashion and that Kornguth & Calvin (1978) had found an unusual allele which conferred a magnified effect.

TUMOUR RESISTANCE TO MULTIPLE CHEMOTHERAPEUTIC AGENTS

There are many possible reasons why a malignant tumour can be resistant to chemotherapy. Hochhauser & Harris (1991) mention pharmacokinetic factors which might impair bioavailability and might vary from poor absorption to a poor blood supply to the tumour. A more subtle reason is the development of multidrug resistance (MDR) which is the phenomenon whereby exposure to one drug induces cross-resistance to a variety of chemical classes to which the cell has never been exposed;

typically these are adriamycin, vinca alkaloids and mitomycin C.

Multidrug resistance occurs because of the over-expression of the *MDR* genes. This property can be conferred upon sensitive cells by transfection with this gene. The over-expression can arise by means of induction and by means of gene amplification in tumours. The two genes *MDR1* and *MDR2* are located at 7q21.1; more is known about the former than the latter. They probably belong to an *MDR* gene family.

In the case of *MDR1* the mechanism responsible is a 170 kDa P-glycoprotein ('P' for permeability) which is an ATP-energized membrane transporter. The glycoprotein has the ability to eject the cytotoxic drug from the cell; consequently the intracellular concentration of the anti-cancer drug does not become effective.

It is suggested that the molecules have a physiological function as a cytoplasmic detoxifier possibly eliminating carcinogens. The amount of MDR in normal tissue has been assessed by observations of the relevant mRNA and histochemically, and appears to be very variable. Restriction fragment length polymorphisms have been described in both *MDR1* and *MDR2* (Pauly *et al.* 1992). The suggestion has been made (Weinstein *et al.* 1990) that there may be different sub-populations of people who are either high or low expressors of *MDR*. Also, expression of different isoforms may be genetically determined (Weinstein *et al.* 1990). However there is no solid proof to support this idea.

LITHIUM

Lithium has been used for over 40 years in the treatment of manic-depressive psychosis. It is well known that there are inter-individual differences in blood levels, therapeutic response and toxicity following lithium administration.

The idea that the distribution of lithium ions may be genetically determined was investigated by Dorus *et al.* (1974). They measured the 24 hour erythrocytic uptake of lithium *in vitro* in 10 monozygotic and seven dizygotic twin pairs. The heritability was about 0.8. The intra-erythrocytic lithium concentration is always lower than in the plasma but the ratio is very variable. It was pointed out by Jenner & Lee (1976) that the red cell lithium/plasma lithium

concentration ratio (y) should be studied at different plasma lithium concentrations (x) in each person. This recommendation was made because the relationship between y and x was very variable between individuals.

The ratio y was found by Rybakowski (1977) to have a unimodal frequency distribution in a population of 60 patients. The inter-individual variability of y was shown by Greil *et al.* (1977) to be due to variations in the efficiency of the Na^+-dependent Li^+ counter-transport system (Na–Li CNT).

In a large and meticulous study of 238 unrelated individuals, and of 245 individuals in 50 pedigrees from the population, Boerwinkle *et al.* (1986) found a bimodal distribution of Na–Li CNT. Various sophisticated analyses showed that there was a large measure of genetic control, and that environmental influences were not responsible for the bimodality observed. However, the family data did not fit a simple Mendelian model. In a similar type of study Rebbeck *et al.* (1991) reached the conclusion that there must be at least two different explanations for the mixture of distributions of Na–Li CNT in the general population.

The suggestion was made that persons who responded favourably to psychiatric lithium treatment had higher values of ratio y than those with poor responses (Mendels & Frazer 1973). This suggestion was subsequently both confirmed (Casper *et al.* 1976) and refuted (Rybakowski & Strzyzewski 1976). Firmer evidence was in favour of red blood cell lithium levels (like plasma levels) being higher in patients experiencing side effects (Hewick & Murray 1976).

It was claimed by Rybakowski (1977) that there was a higher incidence of affective illness in first-degree relatives of patients with a high value of y. This, it was claimed, might indicate a possible link between y and genetic factors in manic-depressive psychosis.

The Na–Li CNT has been one of a number of red cell sodium transport mechanisms examined in relation to hypertension. A total of 434 persons in 10 hypertensive families was studied by Dadone *et al.* (1984). There was no spouse–spouse correlation, which if present would indicate an environmental influence. The mid-parent–offspring correlation was 0.44 and pedigree analysis indicated that polygenic inheritance was most likely. High mean levels of

Na–Li CNT have been found consistently in hypertensive compared with normotensive groups in both clinical and experimental studies (Trevisan & Laurenzi 1991). Unfortunately the explanation for this association remains a mystery.

BLACK THYROID ASSOCIATED WITH MINOCYCLINE THERAPY

A pathological curiosity is the finding at surgical biopsy or post-mortem of a black discoloration of the thyroid gland. This occurs in patients who have been taking the antibiotic minocycline, usually for long periods such as one year for acne or for chronic respiratory infections.

Although pigmentation in other anatomical sites (skin, bones and teeth) has been recorded, it is not mentioned in accounts of the black thyroids studied at autopsies.

The black colour of the thyroid was found to be due to small round brown/black granules of pigment present in the apical cytoplasm of the follicular cells. The pigment was thought to be related to lipofuscin, but it has also been suggested that minocycline itself had been converted into a black pigment (Medeiros et al. 1984). Because the same electron-dense material is sometimes found within lysosomal bodies it has been proposed that the abnormality may be the result of incomplete lysosomal degradation of pigment.

There was no evidence of thyroid hypofunction in most of the patients described, but Medeiros et al. (1984) mention a 32 year old man with the black thyroid after minocycline whose thyroid function test results 'were low normal', and Alexander et al. (1985) document a 30 year old man with low T4 and raised TSH levels with a black thyroid found at open biopsy.

It is quite unclear whether the occurrence of this phenomenon is universal after prolonged minocycline therapy or whether it afflicts only certain people. Presumably autopsies must have been performed on many people who died of respiratory disease who had received long term minocycline. Possibly the striking nature of the black thyroid caused these exceptional cases to be reported, whereas the occurrence of non-pigmented thyroids in such patients aroused no comment. It can be speculated that the propensity to develop the black thyroid may be due to a genetic variant of minocycline metabolism or of tissue response to this drug (see Reid 1983; Attwood 1983; Medeiros et al. 1984; Delprado & Carter 1984; Alexander et al. 1985; Ohaki et al. 1986).

A GREEN MAN AFTER INDOMETHACIN

A unique patient who suffered from rheumatoid arthritis which was treated with indomethacin was described by Fenech et al. (1967). This 46 year old man was treated with 75 mg a day of the compound and after 3 weeks his skin, urine and serum turned green. This was due to biliverdin, and was accompanied by a general disturbance of liver function tests. Over a period of 3 months all the abnormalities gradually disappeared.

A pharmacogenetic perspective leads to a suggested explanation which was hinted at by the authors, namely that this man had a rare genetic variant of biliverdin reductase which was inhibited by indomethacin. Unfortunately no family studies were performed.

DRUG BINDING TO PLASMA PROTEINS

The degree to which a drug is bound to the plasma proteins affects the rate of elimination as well as the apparent volume of distribution. Increased binding gives less glomerular filtration and a larger apparent volume of distribution.

Some examples exist to show that the binding of drugs to plasma proteins is under both genetic and environmental control. Seven monozygotic (MZ) and 10 dizygotic (MZ) same sex twin pairs were studied by Alexanderson & Borga (1972). The binding of nortriptyline (NT) to plasma proteins was determined by a plasma/plasma equilibrium dialysis method. These twins had previously had their steady state plasma concentrations of NT determined after 8 days on a dosage of 0.2 mg NT per kg body weight. The variation of the plasma protein binding ratio was significantly greater in the DZ than in the MZ twinships. Interestingly, the interindividual differences in NT-binding to plasma proteins could not be correlated with steady-state plasma concentrations.

The binding of racemic warfarin to plasma was investigated by Wilding et al. (1977), again using equilibrium dialysis, in 10 MZ and 10 DZ twins. The heritability of the association constant K_a and the number of warfarin binding sites per molecule were computed by different methods to lie between 0.70 and 0.87. Similar results were obtained using purified albumin. This overcame the objection (levelled at the study of Alexanderson & Borga 1972) that greater dietary similarities between MZ twins could have led to exogenous molecules occupying the binding sites in a more similar manner in them than in DZ twins, thus giving a falsely inflated impression of the genetic control.

A microfiltration technique was used by Alvan *et al.* (1983) to measure the binding of propanolol to plasma proteins in 432 individuals of 132 nuclear families. Path analysis showed a rather small estimate of 0.21 for the heritability of the unbound fraction of propanolol.

So the conclusion from these examples is that the binding of drugs to plasma proteins is variable between persons and that variability is in part accounted for by genetic factors. However, it seems that this variability in binding is much less in degree than the variability in biotransformation which is known for many drugs and which is heavily influenced by genetic factors.

CHLOROQUINE-INDUCED PRURITIS

The adverse effect of itching produced by chloroquine was investigated by Ajayi et al (1989). They considered itching to be a significant drawback in the tolerability and possibly in the compliance with drug treatment in areas of hyperendemic malaria. It has also been suggested that it may result in inadequate chemosuppression and so contribute to the emergence of resistant strains of plasmodia. Pruritis may be a commoner side effect of chloroquine in Africans than in Europeans.

A survey conducted by means of a questionnaire found that 810 of 1100 respondents living on a university campus in Nigeria reported itching on antimalarial treatment. There was no sex predilection. Amongst the 810 'reactors' 61% described itching on chloroquine alone, and the frequency appeared to increase with age. The peak intensity of the pruritis occurred 6 to 24 hours after dosing, which is the time when the plasma concentrations of chloroquine and its metabolites are highest.

Evidence indicating that the phenomenon might be genetically determined was as follows. Of the 810 'reactors' 345 had an affected full sibling compared with 66 of 290 'non-reactors'. However among 16 pairs of monozygotic twins (both 'reactors' and 'non-reactors') the concordance rate was 75%, whereas in 25 pairs of dizygotic twins the concordance was 72%. The concordance between spouses was 60%.

An experimental investigation was conducted by Ogunranti *et al.* (1992), who gave either four tablets of chloroquine phosphate 250 mg each or four multivitamin tablets to 176 subjects in a cross-over blind trial. None of the subjects complained of pruritis after the multivitamin tablets. Sixty per cent of subjects were 'reactors'. The sickle haemoglobin status of the subjects was recorded as either AA or AS and 66% with AA were 'reactors', compared with 45% of AS individuals ($p < 0.01$). The explanation of this association is unknown.

Intradermal chloroquine injection gives a larger flare response in 'reactors' than in 'non-reactors' but this is not thought to be mediated by histamine. However, it would be interesting to determine the *N*-methyltransferase status of these two apparent phenotypes (see Chapter 20, p. 341).

A well conducted family study is required in order properly to clarify the genetics of this interesting polymorphism.

Ajayi, A. A., Oluokun, A., Sofowora, O., Akinleye, A. & Ajayi, A. T. (1989). Epidemiology of anti-malarial pruritis in Africans. *European Journal of Clinical Pharmacology*, **37**, 539–40.

Alexander, C. B., Herrera, G. A., Jaffe, K. & Yu, H. (1985). Black thyroid: clinical manifestations, ultrastructural findings and possible mechanisms. *Human Pathology*, **16**, 72–8.

Alexanderson, B. & Borgå, O. (1972). Interindividual differences in plasma protein binding of nortriptyline in man. A twin study. *European Journal of Clinical Pharmacology*, **4**, 196–200.

Alvan, G., Bergström, K., Borgå, O, Iselius, L. & Pedersen N. (1983). Family study of genetic and environmental factors determining the protein binding of propanolol. *European Journal of Clinical Pharmacology*, **25**, 437–41.

Attwood, H. D. (1983). A black thyroid and minocycline therapy. *Medical Journal of Australia*, **11**, 549.

Best, W. R. (1967). Chloramphenicol-associated dyscrasias: review of cases submitted to American Medical Association Registry. *Journal of the American Medical Association*, **201**, 181–8.

Boerwinkle, E., Turner, S. T., Weinshilboum, R., Johnson, M., Richelson, E. & Sing C. F. (1986). Analysis of the distribution of erythrocyte sodium lithium countertransport in a sample representative of the general population. *Genetic Epidemiology*, **3**, 365–78.

Calabresi, P. & Parks, R. E. Jr (1975). Alkylating agents, antimetabolites, hormones, and other antiproliferative agents. In *The Pharmacological Basis of Therapeutics*, 5th edn, ed. S. Goodman & A. Gilman, pp. 1274–7. New York: Macmillan.

Casper, R. C., Pandey, G., Gosenfeld, L. & Davis, J. M. (1976). Intracellular lithium and clinical response. *Lancet*, **2**, 418–19.

Cohen, S. S., Flaks, J. G., Barner, H. D., Loeb, M. R. & Lichtenstein, J. (1958). The mode of action of 5-fluorouracil and its derivatives. *Proceedings of the National Academy of Sciences (USA)*, **44**, 1004–12.

Dadone, M. M., Hastedt, S. J., Hunt, S. C., Smith, J. B., Ash, K. O. & Williams, R. R. (1984). Genetic analysis of sodium–lithium countertransport in 10 hypertension-prone kindreds. *American Journal of Medical Genetics*, **17**, 565–77.

Delprado, W. J. & Carter, J. J. (1984). Minocycline hydrochloride and thyroid pigmentation, a case report with histological and ultrastructural study. *Pathology*, **16**, 339–41.

Diasio, R. B., Beavers, T. L. & Carpenter, J. T. (1988). Familial deficiency of dihydropyrimidine dehydrogenase: biochemical basis for familial pyrimidinuria and severe 5-fluorouracil-induced toxicity. *Journal of Clinical Investigation*, **81**, 47–51.

Dorus, E., Pandey, G. N., Frazer, A. & Mendels, J. (1974). Genetic determinant of lithium ion distribution. *Archives of General Psychiatry*, **31**, 463–5.

Fenech, F. F., Bannister, W. H. & Grech, J. L. (1967). Hepatitis with biliverdinaemia in association with indomethacin therapy. *British Medical Journal*, **2**, 155–6.

Fernbach, D. J. & Trentin, J. J. (1962). Isologous bone marrow transplantation in identical twin with aplastic anaemia. In *Proceedings of the VIIIth International Congress of Haematology*, Vol. I, *Nucleonics and Leukaemia*, pp. 150–5. Tokyo, 4–10 September 1960. Organized by International Society of Haematology and Science Council of Japan. Tokyo: Pan-Pacific Press.

Fine, P. E. M. (1978). Mitochondrial inheritance and disease. *Lancet*, **2**, 659–62.

Greil, W., Eisenfried, F., Becker, B. F. & Duhm, J. (1977). Interindividual differences in the Na$^+$-dependent Li$^+$-countertransport system and in the Li$^+$ distribution ratio across the red cell membrane among Li$^+$-treated patients. *Psychopharmacology*, **53**, 19–26.

Harris, B. E., Carpenter, J. T. & Diasio, R. B. (1991). Severe 5-fluorouracil toxicity secondary to dihydropyrimidine dehydrogenase deficiency. *Cancer*, **68**, 499–501.

Heidelberger, C., Chaudhuri, N. K., Danneberg, P., Duchinsky, R., Schnitzer, R. J., Pleven, E. & Scheiner, J. (1957). Fluorinated pyrimidines; a new class of tumour-inhibitory compounds. *Nature*, **179**, 663–6.

Hewick, D. S. & Murray, N. (1976). Red blood cell levels and lithium toxicity. *Lancet*, **2**, 473.

Hochhauser, D. & Harris, A. L. (1991). Drug resistance. *British Medical Bulletin*, **47**, 178–96.

Howell, A., Andrews, T. M. & Watts, R. W. E. (1975). Bone-marrow cells resistant to chloramphenicol-induced aplastic anaemia (letter). *Lancet*, **2**, 81–2.

Hu, D.-N., Qiu, W.-Q., Wu, B.-T., Fang, L.-Z., Zhou, F., Gu, Y.-P., Zhang, Q.-H., Yan, J.-H., Ding, Y.-Q. & Wong, H.

(1991). Genetic aspects of antibiotic-induced deafness: mitochondrial inheritance. *Journal of Medical Genetics*, **28**, 79–83.

Jenner, F. A. & Lee, C. R. (1976). Intracellular lithium and clinical response. *Lancet*, **2**, 641–2.

Kornguth, M. L. & Kunin, C. M. (1978). Minocycline-induced loss of potassium from erythrocytes, identification of a family with an augmented response. *The Journal of Infectious Diseases*, **138**, 455–62.

Lannigan, B. G. & Evans, D. A. P. (1982). The effect of minocycline on potassium leakage from red cells: a study of the genetics and relationship to vestibular adverse reactions. *Journal of Medical Genetics*, **19**, 354–9.

Medeiros, L. F., Federman, M., Silverman, M. L. & Balogh, K. (1984). Black thyroid associated with minocycline therapy. *Archives of Pathology and Laboratory Medicine*, **108**, 268–9.

Mendels, J. & Frazer, A. (1973). Intracellular lithium concentration and clinical response: towards a membrane theory of depression. *Journal of Psychiatric Research*, **10**, 9–18.

Myrianthopoulos, N. C., Kurland, A. A. & Kurland, L. T. (1962). Hereditary predisposition in drug-induced Parkinsonism. *Archives of Neurology*, **6**, 5–9.

Nagao, T. & Mauer, A. M. (1969). Concordance for drug-induced aplastic anaemia in identical twins. *New England Journal of Medicine*, **281**, 7–11.

Ogunranti, J. O., Aguiyi, J. C., Roma, S. & Onwukeme, K. E. (1992). Chloroquine-induced puritis and sickle cell gene trait in Africans: possible pharmacogenetic relationship. *European Journal of Clinical Pharmacology*, **43**, 323–4.

Ohaki, Y., Misugi, K. & Hasegawa, H. (1986). 'Black thyroid' associated with minocycline therapy – a report of an autopsy case and review of the literature. *Acta Pathologica Japonica*, **36**, 1367–76.

Pauly, M., Ries, F. & Dicato, M. (1992). The genetic basis of multidrug resistance. *Pathology Research and Practice*, **188**, 804–7.

Rebbeck, T. R., Turner, S. T., Michels, V. V. & Moll, P. P. (1991). Genetic and environmental explanations for the distribution of sodium–lithium countertransport in pedigrees from Rochester MN. *American Journal of Human Genetics*, **48**, 1092–104.

Reid, J. D. (1983). The black thyroid associated with minocycline therapy. A local manifestation of a drug-induced lysosome/substrate disorder. *American Journal of Clinical Pathology*, **79**, 738–46.

Rosenthal, R. I. & Blackman, I. (1965). Bone marrow hypoplasia following use of chloramphenicol eye drops. *Journal of the American Medical Association*, **191**, 136–7.

Rybakowski, J. (1977). Pharmacogenetic aspect of red blood cell lithium index in manic-depressive psychosis. *Biological Psychiatry*, **12**, 425–9.

Rybakowski, J. & Strzyzewski, W. (1976). Red blood cell lithium index and long-term maintenance treatment. *Lancet*, **1**, 1408–9.

Sulis, E. & Floris, C. (1980). Nail pigmentation following cancer chemotherapy. A new genetic entity? *European Journal of Cancer*, **16**, 1517–19.

Trevisan, M. & Laurenzi, M. (1991). Correlates of sodium–lithium countertransport. Findings from the Gubbio epidemiological study. *Circulation*, **84**, 2011–19.

Tuchman, M., Stoeckeler, J. S., Kiang, D. T., O'Dea, R. F., Ramnaraine, M. L. & Mirkin, B. L. (1985). Familial pyrimidinemia with pyrimidinuria associated with severe fluorouracil toxicity. *New England Journal of Medicine*, **313**, 245–9.

Weinstein, R. S., Kuszak, J. R., Kluskens, L. F. & Coon, J. S. (1990). P-glycoproteins in pathology. The multidrug resistance gene family in humans. *Human Pathology*, **21**, 34–49.

Wilding, G., Paigen, B & Vesell, E. S. (1977). Genetic control of interindividual variations in racemic warfarin binding to plasma and albumin in twins. *Clinical Pharmacology and Therapeutics*, **22**, 831–42.

PART XI   Polygenic effects in pharmacogenetics

37   Polygenic effects in pharmacogenetics

INTRODUCTION

THE TECHNIQUES of quantitative (or biometric) genetics have been greatly neglected in medicine, which is a pity since they offer a way of measuring genetic influences on common phenomena. Consider, for example, the variability in normal blood pressure. There are no well defined alleles at a single locus which control it. Yet successful attempts have been made to quantify the contribution made by heredity to the variability.

The analogy between blood pressure and drugs is worth developing one step further. Blood pressure is prone to short-term variability depending on the physical activity and mental state of the individual. Since these will at a given moment vary between individuals they will add to the variance of the population. They are largely non-genetic and so will contribute mostly to the environmental component of the population variance.

The situation is similar with regard to many examples in drug metabolism. The majority of drugs are metabolized by microsomal oxidases, and these enzyme systems are frequently subjected to increase (induction) or decrease (repression) of their activities by environmental influences. Since these environmental influences will vary in nature and degree of effect between individuals they will increase the inter-individual variances and so render the genetic influences less obvious.

It will be apparent from the foregoing that the primary aim of quantitative genetics is to establish what proportion of the population variance can be ascribed to genetic factors (and so it also offers a way of ascribing a proportion of the population variance to environmental factors).

Three main methodologies have been applied in the pharmacogenetic field: first, the study of twins, secondly, the study of two-generation family units and thirdly, the study of distributions within generations of families. All these approaches are derived from classical genetic antecedents. The first two were originally devised by Sir Francis Galton though the interpretations are more modern. The third was derived from classical botanical genetic experiments of the early years of this century. The point of including this chapter is as follows. Adverse reactions to a drug can be caused, for example, by a high plasma concentration, and lack of efficacy by a low concentration. In some instances it has clearly been shown that a substantial proportion of the total variance is due to genetic factors. This is even though the biochemical mechanisms controlling the plasma concentration may not be understood and the effects of single alleles not recognized. Yet in practice, this type of variation – without fully understanding the origin or mechanisms involved – can be managed by attention to clinical end points and in some cases by plasma drug level estimations. This situation can be contrasted with monogenic systems where a phenotyping test can be performed on an individual and the frequencies of different phenotypes determined in a population.

NORTRIPTYLINE

This drug is a particularly good example to illustrate the foregoing. High drug levels have been well correlated with adverse reactions (Åsberg *et al.*, 1970). The antidepressive effect has been shown to occur in a restricted concentration range (Åsberg *et al.* 1971a). A twin study has shown a substantial genetic influence on drug plasma concentration (Alexanderson *et al.* 1969). A family study was based on propositi who had been studied because they suffered side effects on conventional dosages and had been found to have high plasma concentrations. The variance of the nortriptyline plasma concentrations in the relatives of the high-level propositi was shown to be greater than in random subjects (Åsberg *et al.* 1971b) (Fig. 37.1).

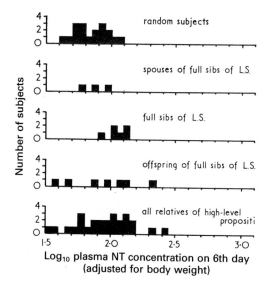

Fig. 37.1. Distributions of $\log_{10}$ plasma nortriptyline on the 6th day, adjusted for body weight, for various categories of subjects. L.S. was a patient who developed adverse reactions on conventional doses of nortriptyline and was discovered to have very high plasma concentrations. (From Åsberg *et al.* 1971b.)

The classical experiment of East (1916) was carried out with the plant *Nicotiana*. Two pure lines, which had long and short flowers, were crossed. The first filial generation (F1) had flowers of intermediate length. The second filial generation (obtained by cross-fertilisation of F1) had a mean similar to F1 but a considerably greater variance.

This is exactly the result expected if alleles at a number of loci controlled flower length. It is, of course, impossible to do this type of experiment in man, but the observation on the relatives of propositi showing high plasma nortriptyline concentrations is, broadly speaking, analogous.

More recently, following the discovery of the debrisoquine/sparteine polymorphism, further light has been shed on the genetic control of nortriptyline metabolism in man.

A correlation has been found between the metabolic clearance of nortriptyline by 10-hydroxylation in the E position (not in the Z position) with the 'metabolic ratio' of debrisoquine (q.v.) (Mellstrom *et al.* 1981). This has been confirmed in Swedes and Ghanaians (Woolhouse *et al.* 1984). There is competitive inhibition of sparteine oxidation by human liver *in vitro* by nortriptyline (Otton *et al.* 1983). Correlations have been found *in vivo* and *in vitro* (using liver microsomal preparations) of the metabolism of nortriptyline by 10-hydroxylation and debrisoquine hydroxylation (von Bahr *et al.* 1983).

So, one of the sources of the overall genetic variability in the metabolism of nortriptyline is its control by the alleles responsible for the debrisoquine/sparteine polymorphism which govern cytochrome P450 2D6. What proportion of the total variability is accounted for by the effect of this polymorphism has not been measured.

PHENYLBUTAZONE

Phenylbutazone is a drug which was in use for over 30 years as an anti-inflammatory agent particularly in rheumatic disorders. It produced a wide range of adverse reactions (Davies 1977) many of which were likely to occur more frequently the higher the plasma concentration.

A twin study revealed that the half-life of the drug in the plasma was largely under genetic control, since the intrasibship variability was much greater for dizygotic twins than for monozygotic twins (Vesell & Page 1968a) (Table 37.1).

If a parameter is under polygenic control then a correlation should be demonstrable between the mean value for the offspring and the mean value for the parents. Sir Francis Galton (also of fingerprint fame) demonstrated this phenomenon for human stature. Such data are often represented as a scattergram in which each family yields one point. Fisher,

Table 37.1. *Half-lives of phenylbutazone in plasma of twins. The difference between monozygotic and dizygotic twins in intrapair variance is significant at the 0.01 level with A.M. excluded (F, 7.5; n_1, 6; n_2, 7) or at the 0.001 level with A.M. included (F, 79.5; $n_1 = n_2 = 7$)*

Twin	Age, sex	Half-life (days)
Identical twins		
J.G.	22, M	2.8
P.G.	22, M	2.8
D.H.	26, F	2.6
D.W.	26, F	2.6
D.T.	43, F	2.8
U.W.	43, F	2.9
Ja.T.	44, M	4.0
Jo.T.	44, M	4.0
Ge.L.	45, M	3.9
Gu.L.	45, M	4.1
He.M.	48, M	1.9
Ho.M.	48, M	2.1
C.J.	56, F	3.2
F.J.	56, F	2.9
Fraternal twins		
A.M.	21, F	7.3
S.M.	21, M	3.6
L.D.	21, F	2.9
L.W.	21, F	3.0
Ja.H.	24, F	2.6
Je.H.	24, F	2.3
E.K.	31, F	1.9
R.K.	31, M	2.1
S.A.	33, F	2.1
F.M.	33, F	1.2
D.L.	36, F	2.3
D.S.	36, F	3.3
F.D.	48, M	2.8
P.D.	48, M	3.5

From: Vesell & Page 1968a.

in a classic paper, showed that the slope of the calculated regression line of mean-offspring values on mean-parent values gives an estimate of 'heritability' (Fisher 1918) which is that component of variance which can be ascribed to the additive effects of the (unknown) alleles concerned.

A family study of phenylbutazone using two-generation family units yielded interesting results.

When the family members had their single-dose plasma phenylbutazone half-lives determined in an unpremedicated state such a correlation was found but was deemed to be due to environmental influences since there was a highly significant correlation between spouses. However, when all the family members were tested again immediately after consuming a short course of phenobarbitone, a highly significant mean-offspring/mean-parent correlation was observed. Since there was then no correlation between spouses it could be assumed that the slope of the regression of mean-offspring values on mean-parent values gave an estimate of the heritability which was 0.65 ± 0.21 (approximately) (Figs 37.2 and 37.3). In other words, 65% of the variability of phenyl butazone half-lives in this population under the circumstances of this experiment (Whittaker & Evans 1970) was due to the additive effects of genes. It is not surprising that this compound's overall pharmacokinetics exhibits a multifactorial (or polygenic) pattern because it is known to be oxidized at two different sites, one aliphatic giving an (ω-1) oxidation product of the butyl side chain and the other aromatic giving parahydroxylphenyl butazone (Williams 1959).

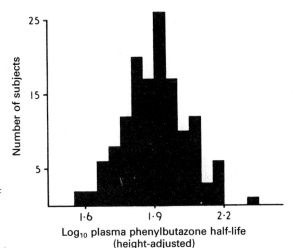

Fig. 37.2. Frequency distribution of $\log_{10}$ post-phenobarbitone plasma phenylbutazone half-lives adjusted to a standard height. (From Whittaker & Evans 1970.)

A correlation was demonstrated between the plasma clearance of phenylbutazone and the plasma clearance of acetanilide (Cunningham *et al.* 1974). Using the latter as a probe drug in eight individuals with hypoplastic anaemia following phenylbutazone therapy revealed a diminished clearance as

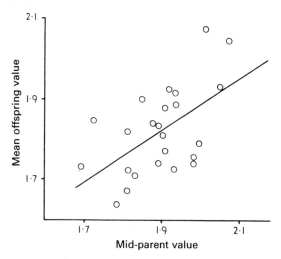

Fig. 37.3. Regression of mean offspring $\log_{10}$ post-phenobarbitone plasma phenylbutazone half-lives on mid-parent values. These results have been adjusted to a standard height. (From Whittaker & Evans 1970.)

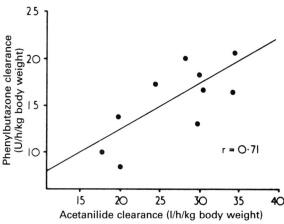

Fig. 37.5. Acetanilide clearance and phenylbutazone clearance in 10 volunteer subjects. Slope of regression line is significantly different from zero ($p < 0.05$). (From Cunningham *et al.* 1974.)

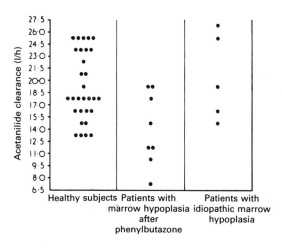

Fig. 37.4. Acetanilide clearance in three groups of subjects studied. (From Cunningham *et al.* 1974.)

compared with healthy volunteers. (Figs 37.4 and 37.5) It was thought likely that this result indicated that persons with low plasma clearance capability – a largely genetically determined property – would be more than usually liable to develop marrow damage from phenylbutazone.

DICUMAROL

A twin study revealed a considerable measure of genetic control over dicumarol plasma concentration half-lives (Vesell & Page 1968b).

An earlier family study (Motulsky 1964), however, showed the presence of an unimodal distribution of plasma dicumarol half-lives with considerable variation (25.2 ± 11 hours). There was a significant sib–sib correlation of 0.347 ± 0.091 but no significant mean-offspring/mean-parent regression. It is likely that environmental factors were responsible for the sib–sib correlation. Possibly having the family members in varying degrees of induction (due to environmental influences) had overwhelmed the genetic component so that its existence was no longer demonstrable.

Clearly, there is a disparity which is unresolved between the twin and family studies.

Even though the dosage of the drug is in practice determined by the response of the prothrombin time, it would still be of interest to have a better understanding of the relative roles of genetic and environmental factors on the blood level.

ANTIPYRINE

There is a vast literature on the metabolism of antipyrine. It has been studied in detail by such a large number of experimenters because it has been pro-

Table 37.2. *Half-life of antipyrine in plasma. The difference between monozygotic and dizygotic twins in intrapair variance is significant: p < 0.001 (F = 64.5, $n_1 = n_2 = 9$)*

Twin	Age, sex	Half-life (h)
Identical twins		
JG	22,M	11.5
PG	22,M	11.5
DH	26,F	11.0
DW	26,F	11.0
JaD	29,M	11.0
JoD	29,M	12.0
SD	34,F	11.1
ML	34,F	11.5
DT	43,F	10.3
UW	43,F	9.6
JaT	44,M	14.9
JoT	44,M	14.9
GeL	45,M	12.3
GuL	45,M	12.8
HeM	48,M	11.3
HoM	48,M	11.3
CJ	56,F	6.9
FJ	56,F	7.1
Fraternal twins		
AM	21,F	15.1
SM	21,M	6.3
LD	21,F	8.2
LW	21,F	6.9
JaH	24,F	12.0
JeH	24,F	6.0
EK	31,F	7.7
RK	31,M	7.3
SA	33,F	5.1
FM	33,F	12.5
DL	36,F	7.2
DS	36,F	15.0
NM	39,F	16.7
JR	39,F	13.4
LL	44,F	12.0
LR	44,F	16.7
FD	48,M	14.7
PD	48,M	9.3

From: Vesell & Page 1968c.

posed as a 'probe drug' of oxidation mechanisms in man.

An early twin study (Vesell & Page 1968c) yielded results indicating that genetic factors were predominantly responsible for the variability in antipyrine metabolism in man as revealed by the half-life of the plasma concentration (Table 37.2).

One family study (Blain *et al.* 1982) used anti-pyrine clearance as an indicator of metabolism. Significant correlations were found between siblings (r = 0.59) and spouses (r = 0.32) but not between parents and their offspring. Hence the conclusion from this study was that environmental factors accounted for most of the inter-individual variance in antipyrine clearance.

Examples of environmental factors which have been shown to influence antipyrine pharmacokinetics are:

1 living in the Sudan was accompanied by a lower clearance in Sudanese, compared with living in England (Branch *et al.* 1978);
2 cimetidine co-administration decreased the metabolic clearance rate of antipyrine but only in slow acetylators (Gachalyi *et al.* 1987);
3 the antipyrine clearance per volume of liver was significantly higher in smokers than in non-smokers (Spoelstra *et al.* 1986), even though the excreted amounts of three metabolites were not significantly different between the two groups.

A further family study then appeared (Penno & Vesell 1983) in which 13 two-generation family units were carefully selected for absence of inducing agents such as smoking and ethanol. The elimination rate constant for the unchanged drug and the rate constants of formation of 4-hydroxy-antipyrine, 3-hydroxymethyl- antipyrine and N-demethylantipyrine were determined in all subjects.

In addition to the 13 families a population sample of 83 unrelated individuals was also studied in the same way. The results were claimed to reveal trimodal distributions for all four parameters. The three metabolite-production rate constants appeared to be inherited as independent genetic polymorphic characters with different allele frequencies. In all cases the allele controlling the high rate constant had a frequency of 0.20 or less.

This important work will require corroboration. Other workers will probably take up the suggestion of the authors that several other drugs should be examined in a similar fashion.

It is clear that none of the three biotransformations of antipyrine are controlled by the debrisoquine/sparteine polymorphism (Danhof *et al.* 1981; Eichelbaum *et al.* 1983).

THEOPHYLLINE

A similar situation to that of antipyrine prevails with the drug theophylline (1,3-dimethylxanthine), which is in widespread clinical use. Plasma concentrations are known to vary widely between healthy people and between patients following standard doses. The prevailing state of knowledge was neatly summarized by Jenne (1982) who pointed out that:

1 clearance was accelerated by cigarette smoking (the same as with antipyrine),
  protein food shortened the plasma half-life;
2 there were elevated plasma levels, increased half-lives, reduced clearance, and reduced production of the metabolites 3-methylxanthine and 1,3-dimethyl uric acid on erythromycin,
  marked reduction in clearance on troleandomycin, cimetidine prolonged the half-life,
  carbohydrate foods prolonged the half-life,
  plasma levels were increased by various events which might cause interferon production (e.g. fever, BCG, influenza vaccines).

The genetic aspects of the inter-individual variability in theophylline metabolism were investigated by Miller *et al.* (1984) in 13 monozygotic twin pairs and 11 dizygotic twin pairs. The pharmacokinetics of the unchanged drug and the urinary excretion of the three major metabolites 1-methyluric acid, 3-methylxanthine and 1,3-dimethyluric acid were studied. Some of the studied individuals smoked. The heritabilities of the pharmacokinetic parameters (half-life elimination rate constant, etc.) of the unchanged drug and the individual metabolite productions were low.

A study of 79 unrelated adults, six sets of monozygous twins, six sets of dizygous twins and six two-generation families was published by Miller *et al.* (1985). They made similar measurements to those described above and carefully screened their subjects for absence of smoking, alcohol drinking, drug consumption and chemical exposure. Significant heritabilities were demonstrated for the production rate constants of each of the three metabolites. On the basis of the population and family studies the authors suggested that there were genetic polymorphisms of these biotransformations and that they might be related for those described above for antipyrine. These suggestions have not been independently corroborated.

Now it is known that theophylline is metabolized by cytochrome P450 1A2 which is induced by polycyclic aromatic compounds, 3-methylcholanthrene and omeprazole (see the general chapter (Ch. 4) on cytochromes P450). The formation of 3-methyl-xanthine and 1-methylxanthine with microsomes from 22 different human livers correlated best with an immunoreactive protein representing cytochrome P450 1A2 (Sarkar *et al.* 1992).

The properties of inducibility by erythromycin and inhibition by cimetidine are characteristic of cytochrome P450 3A4. It remains to be seen whether this cytochrome mediates biotransformation of theophylline.

The whole subject may well be considerably clarified by observing the biotransformation of theophylline *in vitro* by individual cytochromes P450 expressed in, for example, yeasts and tissue culture cells (see Chapter 5, page 19).

CONCLUSION

The metabolism of drugs and the effects of drugs on receptors in cells may be controlled by a number of genes which are allelic at different loci. Since the individual genetic systems are usually unknown the genetic influence can be demonstrated only by the mass effect of the heredity. In some examples there is clear evidence of an interplay between environmental and inherited factors. The information can be used in a meaningful way in clinical management either by paying attention to physiological end points or by monitoring of drug plasma concentrations. It seems probable that the newer methods of DNA analysis may be applied to find the allelic genes which contribute to the overall genetic variability.

On a mathematical level, very few attempts have been made to explore how a single relevant polymorphism contributes to a multifactorial (polygenic) system. An attempt to approach this type of problem in a non-pharmacogenetic example was made by Eze *et al.* (1974), who studied human red cell acid phosphatase. They were able to say that about 60% of the phenotypic variability was due to the electrophoretic polymorphism which thus made a large contribution to the heritability of $0.82 \pm \text{SE } 0.11$. It would be interesting to approach this type of problem again using pharmacogenetic systems.

Alexanderson, B., Evans, D. A. P. & Sjöqvist, F. (1969). Steady-state plasma levels of Nortriptyline in twins: influence of genetic factors and drug therapy. *British Medical Journal*, **4**, 764–8.

Åsberg, M., Cronholm, B., Sjöqvist, F. & Tuck, D. (1970). The correlation of subjective side-effects with plasma concentrations of nortriptyline. *British Medical Journal*, **4**, 18–21.

Åsberg, M., Cronholm, B., Sjöqvist, F. & Tuck, D. (1971a). Relationship between plasma level and therapeutic effect of nortriptyline. *British Medical Journal*, **3**, 331–4.

Åsberg, M., Evans, D. A. P. & Sjöqvist, F. (1971b). Genetic control of nortriptyline kinetics in man – a study of relatives of proposita with high plasma concentrations. *Journal of Medical Genetics*, **8**, 129–35.

Blain, P. G., Mucklow, J. C., Wood, P., Roberts, D. F. & Rawlins, M. D. (1982). Family study of antipyrine clearance. *British Medical Journal*, **284**, 150–2.

Branch, R. A., Salih, S. Y. & Homeida, M. (1978). Racial differences in drug metabolizing activity. A study with antipyrine in the Sudan. *Clinical Pharmacology and Therapeutics*, **24**, 283–6.

Cunningham, J. L., Leyland, M. J., Delamore, I. W. & Evans, D. A. P. (1974). Acetanilide oxidation in phenylbutazone-associated hypoplastic anaemia. *British Medical Journal*, **3**, 313–17.

Danhof, M., Idle, J. R., Tennissen, M. W. E., Sloan, T. P., Breimer, D. D. & Smith, R. L. (1981). Influence of the genetically controlled deficiency in debrisoquine hydroxylation on antipyrine metabolite formation. *Pharmacology*, **22**, 349–58.

Davies, D. M. (1977). *Textbook of Adverse Drug Reactions*. Oxford: Oxford University Press.

East, E. M. (1916). Studies on size inheritance in *Nicotiana*. *Genetics*, **1**, 164–76.

Eichelbaum, M., Bertilsson, L. & Sawe, J. (1983). Antipyrine metabolism in relation to polymorphic oxidations of sparteine and debrisoquine. *British Journal of Clinical Pharmacology*, **15**, 317–21.

Eze, L. C., Tweedie, M. C. K., Bullen, M. F., Wren, P. J. J. & Evans, D. A. P. (1974). Quantitative genetics of human red cell acid phosphatase. *Annals of Human Genetics (London)*, **37**, 333–40.

Fisher, R. A. (1918). The correlation between relatives on the supposition of Mendelian inheritance. *Transactions of the Royal Society (Edinburgh)*, **52**, 399–433.

Gachalyi, B., Vas, A., Csillag, K., Nagy, B., Kocsis, F. & Kaldor, A. (1987). Pharmacogenetic differences in the inhibitory effect of cimetidine on the metabolism of antipyrine. *European Journal of Clinical Pharmacology*, **31**, 613–15.

Jenne, J. W. (1982). Theophylline – a remarkable window to the hepatic microsomal oxidases. *Chest*, **81**, 529–30.

Mellstrom, B., Bertilsson, L., Sawe, J., Schulz, H. U. & Sjöqvist F. (1981). E- and Z-10-hydroxylation of nortriptyline; relationship to polymorphic debrisoquine hydroxylation. *Clinical Pharmacology and Therapeutics*, **30**, 189–93.

Miller, C. A., Slusher, L. B. & Vesell, E. S. (1985). Polymorphism of theophylline metabolism in man. *Journal of Clinical Investigation*, **75**, 1415–25.

Miller, M., Opheim, K. E., Raisys, V. A. & Motulsky, A. G. (1984). Theophylline metabolism: variation and genetics. *Clinical Pharmacology and Therapeutics*, **35**, 170–82.

Motulsky, A. G. (1964). Pharmacogenetics. In *Progress in Medical Genetics 3*, ed. A. G. Steinberg & A. G. Bearn, Ch. 2. New York: Grune & Stratton.

Otton, S. V., Inaba, T. & Kalow, W. (1983). Inhibition of sparteine oxidation in human liver by tricyclic anti-depressants and other drugs. *Life Sciences*, **32**, 795-800.

Penno, M. B. & Vesell, E. S. (1983). Monogenic control of variations in antipyrine metabolite formation. *Journal of Clinical Investigation*, **71**, 1698-1709.

Sarkar, M. A., Hunt, C., Guzelian, P. S. & Karnes, H. T. (1992). Characterizaton of human liver cytochromes P-450 involved in theophylline metabolism. *Drug Metabolism and Disposition*, **20**, 31–7.

Spoelstra, P., Teunissen, M. W. E., Janssens, A. R., Weeda, B., Van Duijn, W., Koch, C. W. & Breimer, D. D. (1986). Antipyrine clearance and metabolite formation: the influence of liver volume and smoking. *European Journal of Clinical Investigation*, **16**, 321–7.

Vesell, E. S. & Page, J. G. (1968a). Genetic control of drug levels in man: phenylbutazone. *Science*, **159**, 1479–80.

Vesell, E. S. & Page, J. G. (1968b). Genetic control of dicumarol levels in man. *Journal of Clinical Investigation*, **47**, 2657–63.

Vesell, E. S. & Page, J. G. (1968c). Genetic control of drug levels in man: Antipyrine. *Science*, **161**, 72–3.

von Bahr, C., Birgersson, C., Blanck, A., Goransson, M., Mellstrom, B. & Nilsell, K. (1983). Correlation between nortriptyline and debrisoquine hydroxylation in the human liver. *Life Sciences*, **33**, 631–6.

Whittaker, J. A. & Evans, D. A. P. (1970). Genetic control of phenyl-butazone metabolism in man. *British Medical Journal*, **4**, 323–8.

Williams, R. T. (1959). *Detoxication Mechanisms*, p. 576. London: Chapman & Hall.

Woolhouse, N. M., Adjepon-Yamoah, K. K., Mellstrom, B., Hedman, A., Bertillson, L. & Sjöqvist, F. (1984). Nortriptyline and debrisoquine hydroxylations in Ghanaian and Swedish subjects. *Clinical Pharmacology and Therapeutics*, **36**, 374–8.

PART XII   Common themes

38   Common themes

INTRODUCTION

THE PURPOSE of this chapter is to gather together some themes which are common to a number of previous sections in this book in order to view them with a cohesive perspective. It seems an opportune time to examine these topics because the present rapid advance of molecular genetics makes it possible to achieve a much more satisfactory understanding of the problems involved than was previously possible.

Many of the laboratory techniques deployed to work out the molecular genetic basis of pharmacogenetic variability are standard and are mentioned repeatedly in different chapters. Similar molecular mechanisms have been found to account for pharmacogenetic variability in a number of examples. These molecular mechanisms at the DNA level include base substitution, base insertion, base deletion, which can result in a change in an amino acid in the relevant protein or in the creation of a premature stop codon, or incorrect splicing. These rearrangements give rise to an enzyme with greatly changed catalytic properties, or one with grossly deformed structure which is non-functional.

The consequences of these changes are manifested in phenotypes in terms of a changed ability to metabolize a drug substrate at the usual rate. Most often this is an inability, but sometimes (as in the rare Cynthiana variant of cholinesterase) it is a super-ability. Receptor molecules are presumably subject to similar changes but there are insufficient well-explored pharmacogenetic examples at present to discern common themes in this area.

Throughout the preceding chapters it has been pointed out that pharmacogenetic variability can affect the efficacy of drug treatment and the occurrence of adverse effects. Pharmacogenetic genes can also have an influence on the occurrence of non-iatrogenic disorders. Common themes can also be discerned in this area.

Inter-ethnic variability either in the frequency or the nature of pharmacogenetic phenomena has been described in almost all examples and this constitutes another common theme.

OCCUPATIONAL MEDICINE

The idea that individuals with a particular phenotype within a polymorphism might not be appropriate for particular occupations came into being after a railway accident at Lagerlunda in Sweden. In order to detect persons who were unable properly to read red and green coloured signals, Holmgren devised a suitable test in 1876 (Hunter 1978).

However, when one moves to consider chemical exposure at work the situation is much more complicated. The degree of exposure may vary. More than one chemical may be involved and their effects may interact. Acute over-exposure may give different effects to chronic exposure of moderate degree. The habits, life-style or domicile of the individual may determine the outcome: for example, the effects of asbestos are more deleterious in smokers.

Table 38.1. *Pharmacogenetic polymorphisms as determinants of the sequelae of industrial exposure*

Reference	Polymorphism	Nature of exposure	Outcome
Cartwright 1984	*N*-acetyltransferase	Benzidine in dye manufacture	Slow acetylators prone to develop bladder cancer
Dewan *et al.* 1986	*N*-acetyltransferase	Benzidine in dye manufacture	Urinary non-conjugated benzidine excretion higher in slow acetylators
Le Walter & Korallus 1985	*N*-acetyltransferase	Aniline	Slow acetylators form more methaemoglobin with low rates of exposure. After an accidentally high exposure a slow acetylator had 45% methaemoglobin whereas a rapid acetylator had 7%
Harris *et al.* 1986		China dolls made of clay containing iron. Exposed to sulphur containing compounds in the poor sulphoxidizer operative's sweat	Black speckling presumably due to iron sulphides.
Prody *et al.* 1989	Cholinesterase	Parathion	Gene amplification in a heavily exposed individual with the 'silent' phenotype. Clinical sequelae unclear but resembles disturbances found in some tumours
Denborough *et al.* 1988	Malignant hyperthermia	Bromochlorodifluoromethane	Malaise, stiffness and weakness of forearms and hands at the end of the working week in the father of a malignant hyperthermia proposita
Anonymous 1931; Fox 1932	PTC tasting	Airborne PTC powder at work	The polymorphism was discovered because Dr Fox was a non-taster and his co-worker Dr C. R. Noller was a taster
Dean 1963	Porphyria variegata	Sunlight exposure on the dorsal surfaces of the hands of farmers	'Van Rooyen's skin' scarred skin due to blisters produced by photosensitivity
Doss *et al.* 1984	Plumboporphyria	Usual lead exposure in a painter	Developed abdominal colic and paraesthesia. He was heterozygous for a variant form of PBG-S
Föst *et al.* 1991	Erythrocytic glutathione-S-transferase	Exposure to ethylene oxide at work	Increased sister-chromatid exchanges in 'non-conjugators' only, which correlates with the finding of chromosomal aberrations and abortions in exposed workers

PBG-S, porphobilinogen synthetase (previously known as δ-aminolevulinate dehydratase).

Nevertheless, now that quite a lot is known about the role of genetic factors in the way individuals metabolize and respond to exogenous chemicals, there is a growing awareness that some of this knowledge may well be applicable to occupational disorders. A book devoted to the topic (Omenn & Gelboin 1984) explored many of the possibilities. The general principles on which the relevant considerations are based were expertly expounded by Vesell (1987).

Despite all this, concrete examples where a defined phenotype within a polymorphism is more susceptible than another to an adverse effect are few and they are shown in Table 38.1. It must be admitted that some are tenuous and others facetious, but they serve to illustrate the general principle.

One can speculate about other possibilities. Pythagoras is thought to have been glucose-6-phosphate dehydrogenase (G6PD) deficient because he is said to have been killed by his pursuers as he paused at the edge of a bean-field (Beutler 1990). It would be interesting to know, in areas where beans are grown and where G6PD deficiency is common, whether the affected men-folk work in bean fields.

Persons with high serum paraoxonase activity should be better able to survive parathion poisoning than the persons with low activity – an idea put forward by Taylor et al. (1965), Flugel et al. (1978) and Geldmacher v-Mallinckrodt (1978) and reiterated in the discussions of the papers of Ortigoza-Ferado et al. (1984) and La Du & Eckerson (1984). Despite this no convincing survey has been reported. Geldmacher v-Mallinckrodt (1978) commented

If a man is working in a factory which is producing paraoxon, he is better protected. He will have more paranitrophenol in his urine and his cholinesterase will be better if he has high paraoxonase activity. If he does not have much paranitrophenol in the urine, his cholinesterase is low and it would be better for him to work in another factory.

There has been a tremendous growth in the knowledge of P450 enzymes, some of which deal with both drugs and carcinogenic compounds to which workers are exposed. The Ah receptor in mice occurs in two forms, high-affinity and low-affinity. These two forms result in huge differences in cyp 1A1 inducibility. Similar differences are believed to exist in man though an actual genetic polymorphism has not yet been demonstrated. Nebert (1988) has put forward the idea that pre-employment screening and disallowing genetically susceptible individuals to become exposed to industrial carcinogens such as polycyclic hydrocarbons might be feasible.

There is little doubt that such a proposition might give rise to serious political issues. Despite this, with the advent of easier phenotyping methods and the discovery of more genetic systems, pre-placement assessments for some jobs may in the future include pharmacogenetic (or ecogenetic) phenotyping.

It is surprising that a recent book devoted to occupational health did not address this problem (Landrigan & Selikoff 1989).

TOXICOLOGICAL IMPLICATIONS

Toxicology is defined as the study of harmful interactions between chemicals and biological systems (Timbrell 1989). A look at the table of contents of a textbook of toxicology reveals that it deals with harmful substances from a wide variety of sources. Examples are industrial processes, food additives, pesticides, environmental pollutants, and natural products (plant, fungal and bacterial). Also included in the list are drug compounds which, although designed to be beneficial, nevertheless sometimes become toxins. Generally drugs become toxic either because their concentrations in the body reach too high a level or because they are biotransformed into toxic metabolites, or because target cells or organs have an unusual susceptibility.

It has been shown in this book that variability in drug effects is due in considerable measure to variability in the genetic constitutions of the patients and that in some examples toxic effects arise because of ineffective biotransformation of the parent compound and/or of a toxic metabolite. In many instances these genetic factors are now becoming understood at a molecular level.

The same ideas can be applied to phenomena caused by non-drug chemicals. The implications in occupational disorders have been discussed in another section. The number of well-worked-out examples where genetic factors have been shown to be responsible for the different effects of toxins encountered in everyday life are few. However, the following (which are dealt with in full in the appropriate sections) can be mentioned. Favism due to eating the broad bean Vicia faba is a haemolytic anaemia in glucose-6-phosphate dehydrogenase deficient individuals. The ingestion of naphthalene mothballs can have the same effect. Modest doses of lead are particularly deleterious to people with variant enzymes involved in the synthesis of porphyrins (especially porphobilinogen synthase).

Many of the vast numbers of organic chemicals produced by modern industries for various purposes and which get into the human body must be biotransformed in the body by the enzymic mechanisms discussed in this book. Since a growing number of these enzymes are being shown to be polymorphic it therefore follows that the toxic effects of environmental chemicals (particularly at low levels of exposure) can be expected to display considerable variability between individuals because of their different genetic constitutions. This rather obvious perspective should be taken into account when investigating suspected environmental pollution events.

CANCER

The idea that a particular pharmacogenetic phenotype within an enzymic polymorphism may be more prone than another to develop cancer is an intriguing one. It is believed that drug metabolism enzymes have come into being during evolution, to deal with naturally occurring exogenous compounds. Man-made therapeutic substances happen to have molecular structures which form appropriate substrates for some of these enzymes. The fact that an enzyme exhibits a balanced polymorphism may indicate that one or other phenotype has a survival advantage in particular situations. It is clear that many different exogenous chemicals, both natural and man-made, have the ability to cause cancer and it is, therefore, supposed that individuals with different attributes to deal with these chemicals may vary in their liability to develop the relevant malignant neoplasm.

Seven pharmacogenetic polymorphic enzyme systems have been studied in relation to cancer incidence and they are listed in Table 38.2. Six are directly concerned with the metabolism of foreign compounds whilst glucose-6-phosphate dehydrogenase is in a separate category.

The evidence in favour of and against the associations between cancers and pharmacogenetic phenotypes has been presented in detail in the relevant chapters.

It is to be noted that there are important criteria to be met in any studies seeking an association between a disease and a genetically determined phenotype and these are detailed in the chapter on *N*-acetyltransferase. Some other points are given in the review of Caporaso *et al.* (1991), as follows.

1 See whether the disease and the phenotype show an association within families. This is the approach originally suggested by L. S. Penrose for the study of ABO blood groups and duodenal ulcer (see Clarke *et al.* 1956). It is undoubtedly the ideal approach, but difficult to apply to cancer because this comes on mainly in older age groups, which makes the appropriate family studies difficult to carry out.
2 Prospective studies: namely, phenotype a large healthy population and in the fullness of time, see which ones have developed cancer.
3 Ascertain the phenotype when the tumour is present, and also after it has been removed.
4 Find out if the frequencies of metabolic phenotypes alter during the course of the disease.

Bronchial carcinoma, because it is so common and because it is strongly associated with the inhalation of carcinogenic chemicals in cigarette smoke, has been the disorder investigated in many experiments to find associations with pharmacogenetic phenotypes. There is a difficulty about such studies, which arises from the fact that bronchial carcinoma is well known to have profound and diverse effects on many different metabolic processes in the body. So any apparent association with a metabolic phenotype might simply be an epiphenomenon – a result of the presence of the neoplasm and not a factor involved in its causation.

However, there is now the promise that there will be available more direct and satisfactory ways of resolving the difficulty. The techniques of molecular biology allow direct genotyping of the DNA of the leucocytes of the individual patient, as well as the expression of individual genes, e.g. recombinant cytochrome P450 cDNA clones in mammalian or yeast cells (Gonzalez 1990).

At the time of writing, 11 studies have been published illustrating this new approach (see Table 38.2).

Three studies have been made to elucidate *CYP 2D6* in bronchial cancer patients. Gough *et al.* (1990) give insufficient details for their results on 140 lung cancer patients to be evaluated. Sugimura *et al.* (1990) obtained both *Xba*I and *Eco*RI restriction fragments. Their results in 45 lung cancer patients did not show a significant association of any particular fragment with the disorder. However, it must be observed that they did not differentiate between the different types of the *Xba*I 29 kb fragments. Wolf *et al.* (1992) found that the genotype frequencies were not significantly different in 361 lung cancer patients compared with 720 controls.

The results of Kawajiri *et al.* (1990) are more indicative of the shape of things to come. As has been explained in a preceding chapter the matter of *CYP 1A1* in humans has been a difficult one. There

Table 38.2. *Summary of studies to assess associations between phenotypes within pharmacogenetic polymorphisms and neoplastic disorders*

Polymorphism	Neoplasm investigated	Number of studies	Phenotype associated with the disorder
P450 2E1	Bronchial cancer	1	NS[a]
P450 1A1	Bronchial cancer	>10	[b]
	Bronchial cancer *Msp*I RFLP	2	Type C homozygote in Japanese. No association in Europeans
	Bronchial cancer Ile/Val polymorphism	1	Increased frequency of Val genotypes
	Gastric cancer	1	NS
	Colorectal cancer	1	NS
	Breast cancer	1	NS
P450 2C18 (mephenytoin)	Bladder cancer	1	NS
P450 2D6 (debrisoquine/ sparteine)	Bronchial cancer	9	Extensive metabolism
	Bronchial cancer RFLP	3	1 study genotyping not predictive 1 study genotype frequencies not different to controls 1 study insufficient detail given
	Breast cancer	4	NS
	Liver cancer	1	Extensive metabolism
	Bladder cancer	5	Extensive metabolism
	Bladder cancer	1	Insufficient detail given
	Bladder cancer RFLP	1	Increase in frequency of heterozygotes
	Colorectal cancer	2	NS
	Prostate	1	NS
	Malignant melanoma	1	NS
	Leukaemia	1	Apparent increased frequency of poor metabolizers
N-acetyltransferase	Bladder cancer	16	Slow acetylation
	Breast cancer	7	NS
	Bronchial cancer	4	NS
	Colorectal cancer	4	NS
	Gastric cancer	1	Slow acetylation
	Lymphoma	2	NS
	Laryngeal cancer	2	Contradictory 1 slow acetylation and 1 NS
Glutathione-S-transferase (*trans*-stilbene oxide conjugation)	Bronchial cancer	5[c]	Deficient conjugation according to 2 studies but the other 3 disagree
Glucose-6-phosphate dehydrogenase deficiency	Various, mainly haematological	4	NS

[a]The present author disagrees with the statistical deduction of Uematsu *et al.* 1991.
[b]The results suggest that high P450 IA1 activity is associated with bronchial cancer but there was no clearly defined separate susceptible phenotype.
[c](4 molecular).
RFLP, restriction fragment length polymorphism; NS, nil significant.

have been strong background reasons for thinking that variability in the activity of the products of this gene might explain differential susceptibility to bronchial carcinoma amongst smokers. There has, despite much effort, been no success in delineating a polymorphism with defined phenotypes. Knowledge of an *Msp*I polymorphism of *CYP 1A1* was applied to the lung cancer problem by Kawajiri *et* *al.*, using a probe obtained as a result of *Xba*I–*Eco*RI digestion of the gene. Three fragment patterns were found: 2.7, 2.3, –, 0.8 (homozygote A); 2.7, 2.3, 1.9, 0.8 (heterozygote B); 2.7, –, 1.9, 0.8 (homozygote C). Sixteen persons had the last genotype amongst 68 lung cancer patients, compared with 11 out of 104 healthy control persons (all Japanese). Unfortunately, Tefre *et al.* (1991) found almost exactly the same distribution of genotypes amongst 221 lung cancer patients and 212 controls (all Norwegian). Why there should be this disparity in the results of these two series which were apparently conducted most carefully and in an identical manner is not clear. Possibly some unidentified racial factor may account for the difference.

Studying a new polymorphism in the *CYP 1A1* gene, Hayashi *et al.* (1992) found a significant association of one genotype with smoking-related bronchial cancers in Japanese.

A similar type of study was undertaken by Uematsu *et al.* (1991). They studied an intronic RFLP of *CYP 2E1* detected with *Dra*I, which showed three genotypes. Amongst 56 controls six persons of type CC were found whereas there were none amongst 47 patients with lung cancer. The present author does not agree with Uematsu *et al.* (1991) that these figures denote significantly different distributions in the diseased and healthy populations.

With regard to the polymorphism of the mu type of glutathione-S-transferase there is also dispute. Zhong *et al.* (1991), Brockmoller *et al.* (1992) and Heckbert *et al.* (1992) did not find convincing evidence of an association of the null genotype with smoking-associated bronchial cancer. On the other hand, Seidegård *et al.* (1990), using an enzymic phenotyping method and Hayashi *et al.* (1992), using a polymerase chain reaction technique in 116 Japanese patients of this type, did find such an association.

It is as yet early days in the study of these types of investigations. Modern techniques of genotyping give much more precise information than has been available in the past and it is possible, relatively easily, to survey large numbers of persons. There seems little doubt that it is worth pursuing the study of associations of genotypes with disease processes.

INTER-ETHNIC VARIABILITY

The subject of inter-ethnic variability in the response to drugs dates back to the observations of Chen & Poth (1929) of the Johns Hopkins Hospital on the effects of mydriatics. They investigated the effects of L-ephedrine, DL-ephedrine, D-pseudoephedrine, cocaine and euphthalamine in Caucasian, Chinese and Negro subjects with normal eyes. The pupil-dilating effect was compared under standardized conditions with accurate measurements. It was found to be greatest in Caucasians and least in Negroes, with the Chinese being intermediate, for all five compounds. It was speculated that this effect might be due to the pigment in the iris. The interesting suggestion was made that albinos of all three races might be investigated. As far as the present author is aware this idea was never taken up.

More recently the topic of inter-ethnic differences in reactions to drugs and xenobiotics has attracted a great deal of attention and has been the subject of an entire monograph (Kalow *et al.* 1986) as well as a number of reviews (Kalow 1982, 1991).

It is quite apparent that there are considerable differences between ethnic groups with regard to many biological characteristics. Facial appearances, body build and skin pigmentation are obvious examples which must be controlled by a number of genes as well as by environmental influences.

So it is to be expected that mechanisms which control drug metabolism and drug effects, e.g. amount of drug metabolizing enzymes, structures of drug-metabolizing enzymes, and the numbers and structures of drug receptors, may well each be subjected to a particular selective pressure, the former by virtue of the substrates with which they deal naturally. In this regard pharmacologic mechanisms would be expected to show inter-ethnic differences analogous to those already known for blood group antigens (Mourant *et al.* 1976), haemoglobin types (Weatherall *et al.* 1989), enzyme polymorphisms (Harris 1970) and HLA (Bodmer *et al.* 1987).

Single gene (major gene) phenomena

The inter-ethnic variability of pharmacogenetic phenomena controlled by single genes has received a lot of attention in the last 30 years, and individual examples have been discussed in preceding chapters (Table 38.3).

Recent advances in pharmacogenetics have revealed some previously unexpected difficulties in the area of inter-ethnic comparisons. It is not as easy to compare pharmacokinetics and pharmacodynamics between races as it is, for example, to

Table 38.3. *Single gene (or major gene) pharmacogenetic phenomena which exhibit inter-ethnic variability*

The debrisoquine/sparteine polymorphism
The mephenytoin hydroxylation polymorphism
N-acetyltransferase
Plasma paraoxonase
Cholinesterase
Glucose-6-phosphate dehydrogenase
Acetaldehyde dehydrogenase
Phenylthiocarbamide tasting

---

compare the ABO blood groups. This is particularly true where the test is carried out *in vivo*, i.e. by administering the drug to test subjects (which is true in most examples at present).

Where a polymorphism is represented by means of a bimodal frequency distribution curve the antimodal point by which phenotypes are defined may be different in different racial groups, e.g. debrisoquine in the Venda (Sommers *et al.* 1989) and in Ngawbé Guaymi Amerindians of Panama (Arias & Jorge 1989). The antimode may be obscured in some racial groups when they are assessed by means of a particular test (eg Africans and Chinese in the paraoxonase study of Playfer *et al.* 1976). Phenotypes which have seemed to be similar may eventually be discovered to be different. For example, Yue *et al.* (1989) found Chinese extensive hydroxylators of debrisoquine with *Xba*I RFLP pattern 44 kb/44 kb which would predict a poor hydroxylator in Europeans, but Mura *et al.* (1991) by using different electrophoresis conditions found the Chinese fragment to be one of 40 kb not 44 kb, thus differentiating it from the European fragment. Phenotypes which seemed to be different may on closer examination prove to be the same, e.g. glucose-6-phosphate dehydrogenase variants Mediterranean, Sassari and Cagliari (De Vita *et al.* 1989). Many drugs undergo biotransformation at more than one site in the molecule. These biotransformations can be controlled by the products of different genes whose frequencies vary independently between ethnic groups (e.g. propanolol, which is metabolized by cytochromes P450 2D6 and P450 2C18).

The perils of blindly extrapolating the effects of a genetic polymorphism from one ethnic group to another are illustrated by the following example.

Diazepam (DZ) is metabolized by *N*-demethylation in the endoplasmic reticulum of the liver to demethyldiazepam (DMDZ), which is similarly biologically active. In turn the DMDZ is hydroxylated at the C3 position to form oxazepam. It was shown by Bertilsson *et al.* (1989) that poor Caucasian hydroxylators of mephenytoin were relatively unable to perform both these biotransformations, leading to low clearances and long half-lives. This study was followed by a similar one in Chinese subjects (Zhang *et al.* 1990), and it was discovered that there was no difference in the metabolism of DZ in them between the two mephenytoin phenotypes. They all resembled Caucasian poor metabolizers. There was, however, a difference between the Chinese mephenytoin phenotypes with regard to the oxidation of DMDZ. These findings may be the metabolic basis for medical practitioners prescribing lower doses of diazepam for Chinese patients than those commonly used in Caucasians (Bertilsson *et al.* 1990).

Another disparity between ethnic groups has already been referred to in Chapter 7 (Debrisoquine polymorphism). In Caucasians slow hydroxylators of debrisoquine are also slow hydroxylators of sparteine, but this appears not to be the case in Ghanaians or apparently in the South African Venda. To sort out anomalies like the two above it will be necessary directly to elucidate the relevant gene structures.

Not only genetic factors but also environmental influences operate to produce differences in drug metabolism and responses to drugs between populations. Environmental influences in drug metabolism have been emphasized by Vesell (1977, 1986) and include disease, exercise, occupational exposure, drugs, circadian and seasonal variations, stress, alcohol intake and smoking. The particular mechanism stimulated by environmental influences which is best understood is enzyme induction. Environmental influences may operate differentially on individual phenotypes within some polymorphic systems. When the polymorphism is portrayed as a bimodal frequency distribution histogram, enhanced environmental influences have the effect of increasing the variance in each mode. All these factors may make phenotype definition difficult. Now, however, the situation is changing. With the advent of allele-specific DNA probes and the use of RFLPs the confounding influence of environmental factors can be set aside. Nevertheless to be of practical value it will still be necessary to examine the pharmacokinetics and pharmacodynamics of a new drug in each phenotype in the different major ethnic groups.

Quantitative, multifactorial or polygenic systems

The same environmental influences referred to above also operate on the multifactorial systems which are expressed as a single frequency distribution curve. The greater the variability of the environmental influences the greater the variance which is observed. It is undoubtedly a large effect of this type that caused the intra-group variability to be as great as the inter-group variability in the study of Fotherby *et al.* (1981) in Table 38.4.

It is in relatively few apparent quantitative multifactorial or polygenic systems that any of the individual responsible genes have been identified. By comparing ethnic groups with regard to their drug metabolism or drug effect, one is observing the mass effect of several genetic systems which may be varying between the ethnic groups accompanied by a variable environmental background.

Some recent examples of this type of work are condensed in Table 38.4.

The study of Zhou *et al.* (1989a) merits comment. These workers studied the biotransformation and pharmacokinetics of and pharmacodynamic responses to propanolol in both Caucasian and Chinese. They found that the Chinese metabolized the drug faster and produced lower plasma concentrations. However, in relation to a given plasma concentration the response of the Chinese in terms of hypotensive effect and slowing of heart rate was much greater. The resultant of these two opposing trends was the fact previously established on clinical grounds, namely that the dose of propanolol required per kilogram to treat a Chinese patient is less than that required to treat a Caucasian. It is suspected that the basis for this difference is polygenic. The contributions of the two known polymorphisms to the inter-ethnic difference in biotransformation were unlikely to have been important. As regards cytochrome P450 2D6 (debrisoquine polymorphism), if q^2 for Caucasians was 0.05 then $2pq$ would be 0.35, so about a third of the sample would be expected to be heterozygous (the one Caucasian poor metabolizer of debrisoquine found was excluded from the analysis). For the Chinese the corresponding figures would be 0.01 and 0.18. It is possible that this polymorphism may have influenced the biotransformation to 4-hydroxy-propanolol to some degree but would not influence the pharmacodynamic result significantly because 4- hydroxypropanolol is a much weaker β-blocking drug than propanolol itself. As regards cytochrome P450 2C18 (mephenytoin polymorphism), 0.35 of Caucasians and about 0.49 of Chinese would be expected to be heterozygous. This polymorphism controls the biotransformation of propanolol to naphthaoxylactic acid but the genotypic distributions are not sufficiently different to account for the large pharmacodynamic inter-ethnic difference.

So the presumption was that some unknown genes, with an environmental component, were probably responsible for the inter-ethnic differences observed in pharmacokinetics and pharmacodynamics of propanolol.

Because of the coexistence of white and black Americans and the frequency of cardiovascular disorders (particularly hypertension) in both groups, inter-ethnic comparisons of cardiovascular drugs have received more attention than any other class.

The effects of antihypertensive therapy in black and white patients have been compared by Freis (1986), Seedat (1989) and Weinberger (1990) and are summarized in Table 38.5. Drugs are given to produce some sort of effect on the patient and in the cardiovascular system the effect can be fairly simply measured. The variation in this effect (pharmacodynamics) may be heavily influenced by the biotransformation of the drug molecule and the pharmacokinetics of it and of its metabolites. Hence a really analytical study should examine both aspects. Only few examples exist (see Table 38.4) (Olatunde & Evans 1982; Vincent *et al.* 1986; Zhou *et al.* 1989a).

The deduction that there are genetic differences between racial groups because they respond differently to standard drug dosages may well be correct but is difficult to prove because of the effects of environmental influences.

A PUBLIC HEALTH PERSPECTIVE

Some governments have insisted that new drugs should be tested on their own populations before being released for general use. In other words they were unwilling to accept that results usually obtained in American and European laboratories and trials would be generally applicable. Though there was sometimes a suspicion that their motives were political and chauvinistic rather than altruistic

Table 38.4. *Some inter-ethnic comparisons of drug metabolism and drug effects*

Reference	Subjects investigated	Drug(s) investigated	Pharmacokinetic observations	Pharmacodynamic observations	Comment(s)
Zeigler & Biggs 1977	13 black Americans 22 white Americans depressed patients	Amitriptyline as clinically indicated	*Plasma levels of amitriptyline, nortriptyline and total tricyclic antidepressants not different between the 2 groups	–	–
	13 black Americans 17 white Americans depressed patients	Nortriptyline as clinically indicated	*Plasma levels of nortriptyline higher in blacks *(Plasma levels corrected for individual dosages so that the plasma level was based on a 1 mg/kg/day dose)	–	Possibly accounts for more rapid improvement of blacks on tricyclic anti-depressants
Branch *et al.* 1978	11 Sudanese in Sudan 9 Sudanese in England 19 English in England	Single dose of 1200 mg antipyrine	No significant difference between Sudanese living in England and the English. Sudanese in Sudan had significantly lower mean clearance	–	An environmental effect was demonstrated
Spector *et al.* 1980	10 Oriental 10 Caucasian	Diphenhydramine orally and intravenously	Plasma levels lower in Orientals. V_D and clearance about 70% larger in Orientals	Significantly less sedation and deterioration in psychomotor performance in Orientals	–
Fotherby *et al.* 1981	Up to 7 women in each of 14 centres in 13 countries	One 50 μg dose of ethynyl-oestradiol	Intra-centre variability for a range of pharmacokinetic parameters as great as variability between centres	–	–

Table 38.4. (*cont.*)

Reference	Subjects investigated	Drug(s) investigated	Pharmacokinetic observations	Pharmacodynamic observations	Comment(s)
Olatunde & Evans 1982	7 white British (4M 3F) 7 Nigerians (5M 2F)	Single 400 mg oral dose of quinidine	Plasma (P) and intra-erythrocytic (I) quinidine concentra-tions tend to be higher in Nigerians. The I/P ratio was not different in the 2 groups	ΔQT_c (i.e. change in QT_c from control value) was greater in relation to both P and I in the British than in the Nigerians	The differentiation between genetic and environmental influences unclear because the British were studied in Liverpool and the Nigerians in Ibadan
Vincent et al. 1986	6 Caucasians 6 Nigerians all residing in Glasgow	Three procedures: – 100 mg i.v. trimazosin – 200 mg oral trimazosin – i.v. 0.9% NaCl (placebo) on different occasions	Overall pharmaco-kinetic profile similar in the 2 groups. The volume of distribution was greater in Caucasians but Nigerians excreted more 1-hydroxy-trimazosin	No significant differences in blood pressure responses between the two groups	Suggests similar peripheral α_1-adrenoceptor mechanisms in the two ethnic groups
Critchley et al. 1986	111 Scottish Caucasians 67 Ghanaians 20 Kenyans	1.5 g single oral dose of paracetamol	Ghanaians and Kenyans excreted a little more glucuronide than Caucasians but the latter excreted as much mercapturic acid and cysteine conjugate	–	–
Sommers et al. 1987	20 rural Venda 20 westernized Venda 20 Caucasians	1 g single oral dose of paracetamol	No significant differences between the three groups as regards formation rate constants and percentage of dose eliminated as sulphate and glucuronide	–	–

Reference	Subjects	Intervention	Results	Comments
Alam et al. 1988	Asymptomatic healthy normal volunteers not exposed to any drugs: I 95 white Americans 5 black Americans in New York city II 32 white Americans in Dhaka, Bangladesh III 100 Bangladeshis in Dhaka IV 95 Bangladeshis in New York City	A single dose of 0.25 mg digoxin orally	Cardio-inactive reduced metabolites of digoxin were produced by bowel micro-organisms. Both the metabolism of digoxin and the prevalence of the responsible micro-organisms were greater in white Americans than in Bangladeshis. Hence this ethnic difference was considered environmental	Differences in drug metabolism between ethnic groups may not be due to enzymic differences in the tissues of the persons
Rutledge et al. 1989	8 black Americans 8 white Americans	Isoproterenol injection i.v. Initial dose of 0.1 μg increased stepwise until heart beat 30 to 45 beats/min above baseline	–	Greater change in heart rate in blacks than in whites Could be due to differences in β-receptor responses but withdrawal of vagal tone is an alternative possible explanation
Zhou et al. 1989a	10 Chinese (in the USA) 10 white Americans	Increasing oral doses of propanolol	Propanolol clearance (mainly due to 4-hydroxypropanolol formation) was twice as high in Chinese and propanolol plasma levels lower	Dose–response curves: (1) Reduction in heart rate with rise in plasma propanolol concentration (2) fall in blood pressure with rise in plasma propanolol concentration both lay more to the left in Chinese These data (1) were not due to stereoselective metabolism (Zhou et al. 1989b) (2) could explain why the doses of propanolol prescribed in China are much lower than those prescribed in USA and Europe
Joubert & Brandt 1990	8 black 8 white non-smokers not taking any medications with diastolic blood pressures (BP) below 75 and systolic blood pressures below 130 mm Hg	Angiotensin I infusion	–	Fall in diastolic BP with rising dose was greater in blacks than in whites (average 1.8 μg/min in blacks and 3.9 μg/min in whites for diastolic to reach 95 mm Hg). Systolic BP and decrease in heart rate were similar in the 2 groups Some of the apparent increased sensitivity of blacks to angiotensin I could be due to a higher sodium intake

Table 38.4. (*cont.*)

Reference	Subjects investigated	Drug(s) investigated	Pharmacokinetic observations	Pharmacodynamic observations	Comment(s)
Zhou *et al.* 1990	8 Chinese (in USA) 8 Caucasian	Acidic: warfarin diazepam salicylic acid	*In vitro* study. >90% of the drugs bound to albumin in both groups	–	–
		Basic: diphenhydramine propanolol disopyramide	*In vitro* study. These drugs are bound to both albumin and α_1-acid glycoprotein (AGP). Total binding less in Chinese due to lower AGP concentration	–	Lower binding leads to a larger volume of distribution and in the case of a poorly bound drug to increased systemic clearance (as has been shown with diphenhydramine in Chinese)
Johnson & Burlew 1992	13 black and 13 white subjects	Propanolol 80 mg 3 times daily	Area under the concentration-time curve less and apparent oral clearance greater in black than in white subjects	–	May provide an explanation why propanolol is less effective at e.g. lowering blood pressure in blacks than in whites

Table 38.5. *Comparison of efficacy of antihypertensive treatments in black and white patients*

Drug	Effect on raised blood pressure
Thiazide and other diuretics (e.g. chlorthalidone, hydrochlorothiazide, butizide, clopamide)	Produce a greater fall in blacks than in whites, probably because blacks have an expanded intracellular volume and low plasma renin activity
α_1-blockers (e.g. prazosin)	Equally effective in both groups
β-blockers (e.g. atenolol, propanolol, metopranolol, pindolol, oxprenolol)	Effective in whites but no more effective than placebos in blacks. Have hypotensive action when combined with diuretics
α_1, β_1, and α_2-adrenergic receptor blocker (e.g. labetalol)	Effective in lowering BP in both groups
Angiotensin converting enzyme inhibitors (e.g. captopril, enalapril, lisinopril)	Response in blacks is poor when used alone but equal to that in whites when combined with a diuretic
Calcium channel blockers (e.g. verapamil, nifedipine, diltiazem)	Response is about the same in both groups
Cerebrally acting anti-sympathetic agents (e.g. reserpine[a], methyldopa, clonidine)	Equal responses in both groups
Ganglion blocking drugs (e.g. guanethidine[a])	No data as to inter-ethnic comparisons
Direct acting vasodilators (e.g. hydralazine)	No data as to inter-ethnic comparisons

[a]Obsolete   *Data derived from:* Seedat (1989) and Weinberger (1990).

and scientific, it seems that their stance was to some extent justified because inter-ethnic variability has turned out to be greater than was formerly suspected.

Nevertheless, to test every new drug on every population would be very time-consuming and expensive. It is possible that some of this labour could be curtailed by using cells in culture which contain expression vectors for the main polymorphic enzymes (Kalow 1990; Meyer 1990; Meyer *et al.* 1990). Such a system might quickly give an indication of the biotransformation characteristics of a drug. This might lead to simplified forms of clinical trials.

MOLECULAR MODELLING

The modern era in therapeutics was initiated by Paul Ehrlich who in 1909, in a discussion of chemotherapy, stated 'we must learn to aim and to aim in a chemical sense' (Holmstedt & Liljestrand 1963). This statement was made in connection with the development of arsenicals for use in trypanosomiasis. The same idea was used in the outstandingly successful development of salvarsan as a treatment for syphilis. At this time the analogy was enunciated of a drug fitting into its biological receptor in the same way as a key fits into a lock.

Rational drug design thereafter consisted of making modifications to a compound proven to

have the desired biological activity, and then testing these to see if an enhancement had been obtained (and/or toxicity diminished).

For many years it has been a main activity of pharmaceutical scientists, particularly those in the pharmaceutical industry, to introduce modifications into the molecular structures of drugs under development. Systematic studies of structure–activity relationships have produced drugs with much improved therapeutic properties; examples are sulphonamides, penicillins and cephalosporins. An example of a similar activity in pharmacogenetics has been the investigation of congeners of phenylthiocarbamide (PTC), an activity which hitherto, however, has not led to a clear view of the essential structure required to detect the PTC-tasting polymorphism.

This way of proceeding proved increasingly expensive and was also slow (Gund *et al.* 1980). Meantime, computer graphics technology became available and it is now possible to portray the three-dimensional molecular structure of a drug, either in 'ball and stick' or in a space-filling format. Drug molecules are often sterically strained or contain rings, and computer programs can produce strain-minimized geometry. Also, rigid rotation is possible around various bonds and conformational studies can be conducted by means of molecular orbital calculations (Gund *et al.* 1980).

A recent application of this modern approach was

that of Lipkowitz & McCracken (1991), who studied triclabendazole (TCZ), a potent orally active benzimidazole anthelmintic active only against *Fasciola* species. Their studies indicated that the broad-spectrum anthelmintic benzimidazoles have L-shaped molecules, whereas TCZ has a U-shaped molecule.

Using these new approaches it proved possible to make deductions about the conformation of the 'lock' by the study of the 'keys', and so to predict the shape of the 'key' which will provide an even better fit.

Turning now to consider the 'lock', precise three-dimensional structures of proteins were determined from crystallographic data and in some instances physical models were subsequently built, which greatly advanced understanding. Examples were DNA, haemoglobin and some enzymes such as carbonic anhydrase (Kannan 1980).

The X-ray crystallographic approach has been invaluable but is expensive. For compounds of molecular weight <12 000, NMR and computer methodology can now be used to determine structures. The two techniques are complementary because it may be difficult to obtain suitable heavy atoms for X-ray crystallography and since NMR looks at the molecule in solution it represents its functional state. Hence small proteins or the important sections of proteins can usefully be examined in this new way (Wüthrich 1990).

Because of these recent developments there are now computer-based attempts to understand how the drug molecule interacts in a three-dimensional manner with the enzyme or receptor which it influences. Thorough understanding of this process has enabled more rational design of new therapeutic drugs. The *Journal of Computer-aided Molecular Design* publishes articles devoted to this activity. Examples are described by Martin (1991) of designing nicotinic agonists, a potential D2 dopaminergic agent and a novel potent inhibitor of HIV protease. She explains how the 3-D structure of a protein can be predicted from its amino acid sequence and, further, how the shape and charges of the receptor site can be displayed. This information can then be utilized by the computer to sift through a very large number of 3-D structures of compounds (54 296 in one example) which would interact with the macromolecule.

A note of caution was, however, sounded in an editorial in *Science* (R.S. 1992), which emphasized that computer-based drug design must go hand in hand with investigations of biological potency.

The existence of genetically determined variants with different activities in enzymes and receptors may, on the one hand, make the task of understanding the interaction with drugs more complex. However, on the other hand, once the molecular basis of the variability has been determined, it may provide clues for the more rational design of inhibiting or enhancing compounds.

With molecular biological methods it is possible to go one step further than nature. New genes can be created and the properties of their products examined *in vitro*. Examples of this process which have been mentioned in this volume include the following.

1   The work of Imai *et al.* (1989) in which by site-directed mutagenesis the amino acid at position 253 in cytochrome $P450_{cam}$ was replaced by others. This led to the conclusion that an amino acid bearing a hydroxyl group is essential at this point in the molecule for enzymic function.

2   The construction of chimeric alleles of human *N*-acetyltransferases (NAT2) by Blum *et al.* (1991) showed that both nucleotide substitutions in mutant M1 were required to cause the diminished production of a less stable protein, presumably by defective translation. However, in the M2 mutant the amino acid change 197 Arg → Gln alone was responsible for the production of a less stable protein than the 'wild type' enzyme.

3   Chimeric *CYP 2D6* genes were constructed by Kagimoto *et al.* (1990) each containing a 5'-end, a middle portion and a 3'-end derived variously from the wild type and 29B mutant of *CYP 2D6* alleles. These chimeric genes were expressed in COS-1 cells in culture. Mutations in exon 1 resulted in a functionally deficient protein and the mutation at intron 3/exon 4 splice site in an absent protein. Mutations in exons 2 and 9 were of no consequence for function. This work not only emphasised the functional significance of the 2D6(B) mutations, but also indicated which parts of the P450 molecule were of greatest importance for activity and stability.

4   About 5% of the approximately 220 amino acid residues are conserved in the cytosolic glutathione *S*-transferases (GST), which have been characterised. The technique of site-directed mutagenesis has been used to create new genes, which were expressed in *E. coli* JM103. The wild type and mutant enzymes

were purified by affinity chromatography. The results obtained indicated, first, that arginine residues may be involved in binding the co-factor glutathione and secondly, that when Tyr[8] was mutated to Phe in human alpha class GST the specific activity to three substrates was lowered to 2 to 8% of that of the wild type enzyme. It seems likely that the hydroxyl group of the tyrosine activates the sulphydryl groups of glutathione. Detailed understanding of the chemical mechanism of GST will require further studies of the relationship between structure and function (Stenberg *et al.* 1991).

5 A whole range of man-made variations for the cytochrome P450 molecule was described by Johnson (1992), who emphasized a new concept. Instead of finding out which genomic base changes cause amino acid changes leading to *loss* of enzymic activity the converse strategy can be studied, namely how to *confer* new enzymic activity on a given cytochrome P450 molecule. By introducing mutations into cytochrome P450 2C4 to change three amino acids the K_m for progesterone 21-hydroxylation was lowered from >25 µM to *c.* 2 µM which is indistinguishable from P450 2C5. Yet in the natural way these two enzymes differ at 24 of 490 amino acids. Consequently, site-directed mutagenesis has identified the three amino acids which account for the large difference in enzymic activity between two cytochromes.

Although the P450 cytochromes are the best studied examples it is to be noted that nearly all of our information about the three-dimensional structure of these enzymes comes at present from the soluble bacterial P450$_{cam}$, which has only a 10 to 20% sequence identity with mammalian forms (Porter & Coon 1991). It is necessary to know more about the endoplasmic varieties (Poulos 1988). Also, the diversity of structures of the different classes of human P450 cytochromes and their genetic variants, and the manner in which they react with their substrates in three dimensions, need to be studied.

It is clear that despite being able to produce variants in the structure of the enzymic substrates (especially drugs) and being able to study variants in the structure of the enzymes (both naturally occurring mutants and those produced by site-directed mutagenesis), there is a long way to go in understanding how they interact (Martin 1991). Nevertheless, the potential rewards of the investment required to achieve this understanding are very large, namely, being able more rationally to design therapeutic compounds with predictable properties for specific purposes. Knowledge of genetic diversity and the application of genetic techniques make important contributions.

IMPLICATIONS OF PHARMACOGENETIC POLYMORPHISMS FOR DRUG DEVELOPMENT AND REGULATION

It seems amazing in retrospect that up to the 1950s much of the pharmaceutical industry thought mainly in terms of means and did not consider variances in measurements of drug biotransformation and pharmacological effect. Furthermore, some quite major (and successful) companies employed only chemists (i.e. no biochemists, pharmacologists or statisticians). With growing knowledge of drug metabolism this situation began to change – a process which was greatly boosted by the thalidomide disaster. It was clear by 1965 (Evans 1965) that polymorphisms should be kept in mind when investigating the human pharmacology of new drugs, in the investigation of cases of drug toxicity and in the design of drug trials.

Pharmacogenetic considerations have achieved much greater prominence in the thinking of both industry and regulatory bodies since the discovery of the cytochrome P450 2D6 (debrisoquine/sparteine) polymorphism, because such a large number and variety of commonly used drugs are involved (Clarke 1987).

As pointed out by Idle *et al.* (1983), who based their remarks mainly on the debrisoquine model, the differences between the two phenotypes place the poor metabolizer greatly at risk because (1) high plasma levels of an unchanged pharmacologically active drug can occur due to a very small first pass effect, giving an exaggerated response; (2) where elimination depends on metabolite formation there may be toxic accumulation of the parent compound; (3) where the metabolite is the therapeutically active entity there may be a lack of efficacy; (4) if the usual major metabolic pathway handles only relatively few molecules in the poor metabolizer then an alternative, usually minor pathway may handle many more molecules and form a toxic metabolite. The potential clinical importance of a poly-

Table 38.6. *Hypothetical drug development scheme based on the supposition that there is a genetic polymorphism of biotransformation*

---

1 The chemical configuration of a new compound may suggest the most probable main route(s) of metabolism
2 Investigation *in vitro* with:-
    (a) microsomal liver preparations of known phenotypes
    (b) hepatocytes (cultured or fresh) of known phenotypes (Beaune & Guengerich 1988, Vesell 1989)
    (c) cells carrying expression vectors incorporating known genes, e.g. COS-1 (Meyer 1990), yeasts (Ellis *et al.* 1992)
    (d) as (c) with inhibitors such as quinidine or previously recognized polymorphic substrates
    (e) as (c) with antibodies to specific known polymorphic enzymes
3 Animal studies (in more than one species) indicate the main route(s) of metabolism and toxicological aspects
4 Investigation in a few humans *in vivo* to confirm the results of animal studies
5 If the existence of a biotransformation polymorphism substantiated: test on typed panels of healthy individuals of different major ethnic groups, who represent the different phenotypes of the main polymorphisms
6 If polymorphism confirmed: investigate single dose and multiple dose kinetics in relation to the pharmacological effect:
    (a) in phenotyped healthy individuals, of different major ethnic groups (Festing 1987, Guttendorf & Wedlund 1992)
    (b) in phenotyped patients suffering from the condition(s) for which the drug is being developed
7 Formulate appropriate policies and procedures, e.g.
    • information about the polymorphism and its implications, incorporated in the official data sheet
    • advocate phenotyping (or direct DNA genotyping) before starting treatment
    • and/or therapeutic drug monitoring of plasma levels as seems appropriate

---

morphism is much greater when the difference in metabolic performance between the phenotypes is large.

It is now possible (and desirable) to consider the existence of polymorphism of biotransformation or of polymorphism of pharmacologic effect at an early stage in the development of a new drug (Lennard *et al.* 1983). In the former case the polymorphism may be already known or may be a hitherto undiscovered system.

A hypothetical scheme can be considered as portrayed in Table 38.6. Not all steps need necessarily be undertaken for each drug and the exact choice of procedures would depend on the nature of the drug and the circumstances. An interactive manner of proceeding is required so that the plan developed for any given compound may be unique. Taking the cytochrome P450 2D6 polymorphism, which has been the main impetus to the development of such a scheme as an example, the *in vitro* tests in Section 2 of Table 38.6 are now feasible and would enable the presence of polymorphic biotransformation to be established quickly and relatively cheaply.

In the case of a new drug undergoing a number of different biotransformations (such as paracetamol) it would be possible in the future to have banks of preparations representing different polymorphisms with which the drug could be tested. The successful introduction of *CYP 2D6* into yeast

by Ellis *et al.* (1992) is likely to be an important step because a great deal is already known about yeast genetics and about the practical aspects of keeping large yeast cultures functioning indefinitely.

The detection of an hitherto unknown and unsuspected polymorphism is altogether a different matter. Up to the present, such a finding has generally emerged from either testing a large number of individuals in a standard manner or by observing some unusual pharmacological response (e.g. hypotension on a small dose of debrisoquine). It is difficult to plan in such a way as to have a high probability of observing such an event. The only thing that can be said is that a new drug should be tested on a much larger number of healthy volunteers (and/or liver preparations) than has been customary in the past. In addition, the major ethnic groups of mankind should also be surveyed.

Similar considerations apply to variability in pharmacodynamic response.

Even if a polymorphism is not found (or demonstrated not to be of any clinical importance) it is still desirable to know the range of variability in biotransformation and pharmacological response and so this is also an argument in favour of surveying sizeable populations. Decisions about the desirability of phenotyping before starting treatment and/or therapeutic drug monitoring can follow.

Many drugs are metabolized by more than one

route, so the contribution of a polymorphism to the overall metabolism of a compound needs to be evaluated in quantitative terms (Balant *et al.* 1989).

Opinions vary as to the proper course of action to take when a polymorphism is shown to have an important influence on the metabolism of a new drug.

An interesting point was made by Eichelbaum & Gross (1990), who stated that the

occurrence of a genetic polymorphism in the metabolism of a drug has been considered a disadvantage since therapeutic use of such drugs is no doubt complex. However, it should not be overlooked that other drugs which are not subject to polymorphic metabolism also exhibit substantial interindividual variation in their disposition, which, in addition, can be affected to a much greater extent by environmental factors such as inducing agents.

Lennard *et al.* (1983), Idle *et al.* (1983) and Idle & Smith (1984), discussing polymorphism, were of the opinion that 'drugs without this undesirable property are to be preferred'. Balant *et al.* (1989), however, state, 'The fact that the metabolism of a new drug is under substantial polymorphic control, resulting in considerable pharmacokinetic variability should not be an *a priori* reason for stopping its development.' They also remark that following a policy of stopping the development of new drugs whose metabolism is polymorphic would have prevented many valuable drugs being marketed.

Whilst animal studies have their usefulness for indicating likely routes of metabolism in man, the validity of extrapolations made from them is always suspect. Furthermore, animal studies are very unlikely to give a clue to the existence of human polymorphisms (Smith 1986; Balant *et al.* 1989).

In the matter of drug design it would probably be advantageous to incorporate features in the molecule so that it would be metabolized by a number of different enzyme systems and hence would not be too dependent on one biotransformation which might turn out to be polymorphic (G. T. Tucker, personal communication, 1992).

Another idea which has re-emerged is to combine a compound ('B') with the active compound 'A' so as to prolong the time course of the latter. Probenecid was used to eke out scarce penicillin in this way many years ago. The new interest has been generated by the effect of quinidine on the cytochrome P450 2D6 polymorphism, which makes an exten-

sive metabolizer resemble a poor metabolizer. Hence mixing quinidine with a drug which is a substrate for this polymorphism would in theory reduce the variability in the population. However, the price to be paid for this advantage would be to run the risk of hypersensitivity-type reactions to quinidine (e.g. asthma and thrombocytopenia) and these might occur in the 7% of the population who would not stand to benefit.

PHARMACOGENETIC APPROACHES TO THE STUDY OF THE AETIOLOGY OF COMMON DISORDERS

Despite a tremendous amount of effort in the last 50 years the exact causation of most common disorders remains a mystery. Nevertheless, it is obvious that many of them represent the outcome of interaction between environmental and genetic factors. The discovery of environmental factors has properly been the function of epidemiologic research, but with the realization of the importance of genetic predisposition or resistance in the production of common disorders a new field of study, namely genetic epidemiology, has come into being and now there is a monograph (Morton 1982) and a journal bearing that title. Pharmacogenetics makes a contribution to this area of activity. Studies of pharmacogenetics specifically carried out in relation to various types of cancer are discussed in another subsection. Here we discuss a general point in relation to the strategy of how to gain more knowledge about the causation of common disorders using pharmacogenetic polymorphisms.

The appeal of the pharmacogenetic alleles in this type of research is that they control enzymes (or receptors) which handle known chemical structures. Therefore, if a statistical association is discovered between a given common disorder and a particular pharmacogenetic phenotype within a polymorphism it constitutes a clue to the involvement of a particular type of chemical grouping in the causation. Conversely, if no association is demonstrable then it is most unlikely that the relevant chemical grouping has any part to play in the production of the disorder being studied.

Examples of the first kind are shown and discussed in the subsection on cancer, to which can be added alcoholism in Japanese, a disorder to which

Table 38.7. *Studies of associations of pharmacogenetic phenotypes with Parkinson's disease*

Pharmacogenetic system	Number of studies	Conclusion
Paracetamol 3-hydroxylation (cytochrome P450 2E1)	1	No significant difference between the activity in normals and PD patients
Mephenytoin hydroxylase (cytochrome P450 2C18)	1	No association found between either phenotype and PD
Debrisoquine/sparteine hydroxylase (cytochrome P450 2D6)	8 (Two direct genotyping)	The largest study (which involved direct genotyping) showed an increased frequency of PM in PD
Phenytoin hydroxylase	1	There was no proof of the hypothesis that slow DPH parahydroxylation is associated with PD
N-acetyltransferase	1	No association between either phenotype and PD
Thiolmethyltransferase (TMT)	1	Erythrocyte TMT activity lower in PD
Sulphoxidation	1	Poor sulphoxidation associated with PD

PD, Parkinson's disease; PM, poor metabolizer.

aldehyde non-dehydrogenase deficient individuals are particularly prone. Examples of the second kind include the lack of association of either of the acetylator phenotypes with systemic lupus erythematosus and coronary artery disease, indicating that hydrazine and primary aromatic amine compounds are most unlikely to play any part in pathogenesis. This aspect of genetic epidemiology can thus be used to eliminate as well as to point towards causative environmental agents.

Looking to the future, it is explained in another subsection, that establishing the pharmacogenetic genotypes of individuals and populations is going to be a lot easier with direct DNA genotyping methods, than phenotyping by the administration of drugs.

Consequently it is to be expected that applying knowledge of pharmacogenetic alleles will form an important contribution to elucidating the nature of some common disorders.

An example where seven different systems have been investigated is Parkinson's disease (Table 38.7). Many of the studies involved rather small numbers of patients and controls. The largest study was of the debrisoquine/sparteine polymorphism (*CYP 2D6*) using modern molecular genetic techniques on large numbers of patients. This study yielded a positive association whereas previous studies failed to do so. It must be re-emphasized that in such studies the phenotype definition (or genotype definition), the clinical diagnosis and the epidemiological plan must all be of the highest scientific standard.

It has been customary in the past to consider many common disorders in terms of the addition of variances. Components of variance are considered to be contributed by both environmental and hereditary factors. The disorder is presumed to occur when an arbitrary threshold value is exceeded (Fig. 38.1). Typical examples are hypertension and diabetes mellitus (Emery 1976; Emery & Mueller 1988).

The introduction of a single gene system (i.e. a major polymorphism) into the model can have the effect of removing a substantial component of variance represented by the difference between the means of the two phenotypes (Fig. 38.1), and also of being able to discuss phenomena in terms of frequencies. Applying knowledge of a pharmacogenetic polymorphism in this way may make it possible to identify relevant aetiological chemical substances and eliminate them from the environment.

The mathematical aspect of the contribution of a genetic polymorphism to the overall heritability in a biometrical (polygenic, multifactorial) system has been relatively little explored (see p. 590). However, the contributions of individual phenotypes within polymorphisms to total population variances have been assessed. A non-pharmacological example was the study of plasma cholesterol concentrations by Tikkanen *et al.* (1990), in which the phenotype E_4/E_4 contributed about 9.7% of the total variance when the population was on baseline diet. After 6 to 12 weeks on a low fat, low cholesterol diet the mean

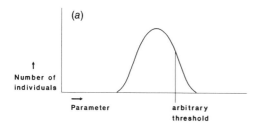

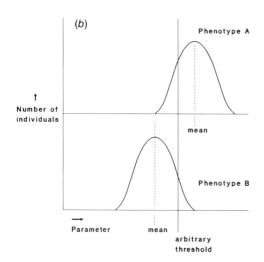

Fig. 38.1.(a) A model for the development of a multi-factorial disorder which occurs when a parameter exceeds an arbitrary threshold. (b) The different liabilities of two phenotypes within a genetic polymorphism to develop the disorder.

value for the E_4/E_4 phenotype plasma cholesterol concentration had fallen by 24% (more than the other phenotypes) and the attributable proportion of the total variance to about 6.3%. A return to the original diet was accompanied by a return of the plasma cholesterol concentrations to resemble those at baseline. Hence dietary changes produced differential effects dependent on genetically determined phenotypes.

The complicated theoretical considerations required properly to plan an epidemiological study of a polymorphic genetic marker in relation to a common disorder are spelled out in detail in the paper of Khoury et al. (1987).

The nature of the interaction between environmental and genetic factors may be expected to differ between ethnic groups, and so will need to be examined at least in the major racial groups of mankind.

Since there appears only to be a relatively limited number of pharmacogenetic polymorphic systems dealing with xenobiotics, it will shortly be possible to test all of them that may be relevant in common disorders whose aetiologies are not understood.

Alam, A. N., Saha, J. R., Dobkin, J. F. & Lindenbaum, J. (1988). Inter-ethnic variation in the metabolic inactivation of digoxin by the gut flora. Gastroenterology, 95, 117–23.

Anonymous. (1931). Science Supplement, 73, Suppl. 14.

Arias, T. D. & Jorge, L. F. (1989). An observation on the ethnic uniqueness of the debrisoquine and sparteine antimodes: a study in the Ngawbé Guaymi Amerindians of Panamá. British Journal of Clinical Pharmacology, 28, 493–4.

Balant, L. P., Gundert-Remy, U., Boobis, A. R. & von Bahr, Chr. (1989). Relevance of genetic polymorphism in drug metabolism in the development of new drugs. European Journal of Clinical Pharmacology, 36, 551–4.

Beaune, P. H. & Guengerich, F. P. (1988). Human drug metabolism in vitro. Pharmacology and Therapeutics, 37, 193–211.

Bertilsson, L., Baillie, T. A. & Reviriego, J. (1990). Factors influencing the metabolism of diazepam. Pharmacology and Therapeutics, 45, 85–91.

Bertilsson, L., Henthorn, T. K., Sanz, E., Tybring, G., Sawe, J. & Villen, T. (1989). Importance of genetic factors in the regulation of diazepam metabolism: Relationship to S-mephenytoin but not debrisoquine hydroxylation phenotype. Clinical Pharmacology and Therapeutics, 45, 348–55.

Beutler, E. (1990). The genetics of glucose-6-phosphate dehydrogenase deficiency. Seminars in Hematology, 27, 137–64.

Blum, M., Demierre, A., Grant, D. M., Heim, M. & Meyer, U. A. (1991). Molecular mechanism of slow acetylation of drugs and carcinogens in humans. Proceedings of the National Academy of Sciences (USA), 88, 5237–41.

Bodmer, J. G., Kennedy, L. J., Lindsay, J. & Wasik, A. M. (1987). Applications of serology and the ethnic distribution of three locus HLA haplotypes. British Medical Bulletin, 43, 94–121.

Branch, R. A., Salih, S. Y. & Homeida, M. (1978). Racial differences in drug metabolizing ability: a study with antipyrine in the Sudan. Clinical Pharmacology and Therapeutics, 24, 283–6.

Brockmöller, J., Gross, D., Kerb, R., Drakoulis, N. & Roots, I. (1992). Correlation between trans-stilbene oxide-glutathione conjugation activity and the deletion mutation in the glutathione-S-transferase class Mu gene detected by polymerase chain reaction. Biochemical Pharmacology, 43, 647–50.

Caporaso, N., Landi, M. T. & Vineis, P. (1991). Relevance of metabolic polymorphisms to human carcinogenesis: Evaluation of epidemiologic evidence. Pharmacogenetics, 1, 4–19.

Cartwright, R. A. (1984). Epidemiological studies on N-acetylation and C-center ring oxidation in neoplasia. In Genetic Variability in Responses to Chemical Exposure, ed. G. S. Omenn & H. V. Gelboin, pp. 359–68. Banbury Report 16, Cold Spring Harbor Laboratory.

Chen, K. K. & Poth, E. J. (1929). Racial differences as illustrated by the mydriatic action of cocaine, euphthalamine and ephedrine. *Journal of Pharmacology and Experimental Therapeutics*, **36**, 429–45.

Clarke, C. A., Wyn Edwards, J., Haddock, D. R. W., Howel-Evans, A. W., McConnell, R. B. & Sheppard, P. M. (1956). ABO blood groups and secretor character in duodenal ulcer. Population and sibship studies. *British Medical Journal*, **2**, 725–31.

Clarke, D. W. J. (1987). Genetic polymorphisms in drug oxidation: implications for drug therapy. *ISI Atlas of Science: Pharmacology*, pp. 274–9.

Critchley, J. A. J. H., Nimmo, G. R., Gregson, C. A., Woolhouse, N. W. & Prescott, L. F. (1986). Inter-subject and ethnic differences in paracetamol metabolism. *British Journal of Clinical Pharmacology*, **22**, 649–57.

De Vita, G., Alcalay, M., Sampietro, M., Cappelini, D., Fiorelli, G. & Toniolo, D. (1989). Two point mutations are responsible for G6PD polymorphism in Sardinia. *American Journal of Human Genetics*, **44**, 233–40.

Dean, G. (1963). *The Porphyrias: A Story of Inheritance and Environment*. London: Pitman Medical.

Denborough, M. A., Hopkinson, K. C. & Banney, D. G. (1988). Firefighting and malignant hyperthermia. *British Medical Journal*, **296**, 1442–3.

Dewan, A., Jani, J. P., Shah, K. S. & Kashyap, S. K. (1986). Urinary excretion of benzidine in relation to the acetylator status of occupationally exposed subjects. *Human Toxicology*, **5**, 95–7.

Doss, M., Laubenthal, F. & Stoeppler, M. (1984). Lead poisoning in inherited δ-aminolevulinic acid dehydratase deficiency. *International Archives of Occupational and Environmental Health*, **54**, 55–63.

Eichelbaum, M. & Gross, A. S. (1990). The genetic polymorphism of debrisoquine/sparteine metabolism – clinical aspects. *Pharmacology and Therapeutics*, **46**, 377–94.

Ellis, S. W., Ching, M. S., Watson, P. F., Henderson, C. J., Simula, A. P., Lennard, M. S., Tucker, G. T. & Woods, H. F. (1992). Catalytic activities of human debrisoquine 4-hydroxylase cytochrome P450 (CYP2D6) expressed in yeast. *Biochemical Pharmacology*, **44**, 617–20.

Emery, A. E. H. (1976). *Methodology in Medical Genetics*, pp. 51–62. Edinburgh: Churchill Livingstone.

Emery, A. E. H. & Mueller, R. F. (1988) *Elements of Medical Genetics*, 7th edn, pp. 200–1. Edinburgh: Churchill Livingstone.

Evans, D. A. P. (1965). Individual variations of drug metabolism. *Annals of the New York Academy of Sciences*, **123**, 178–87.

Festing, M. F. W. (1987). Genetic factors in toxicology: Implications for toxicological screening. *CRC Critical Reviews in Toxicology*, **18**, 1–26.

Flugel, M. & Geldmacher-v Mallinckrodt, M. (1978). Zur Kinetik des paraoxonspaltenden Enzyms in menschlichen Serum (EC 3,1,1,2). *Klinische Wochenschrift*, **56**, 911–16.

Föst, U., Hallier, E., Ottenwalder, H., Bolt, H. M. & Peter, H. (1991). Distribution of ethylene oxide in human blood and its implications for biomonitoring. *Human Experimental Toxicology*, **10**, 25–31.

Fotherby, K., Akpoviroro, J., Abdel-Rahman, H. A., Toppozada, H. K., de Souza, J. C., Coutinho, E. M.,

Koetsawang, S., Nukulkarn, P., Sheth, U. K., Mapa, M. K., Gopalan, S., Plunkett, E. R., Brenner, P. F., Hickey, M. V., Grech, E. S., Lichtenberg, R., Gual, C., Molina, R., Gomez-Rogers, C., Kwon, E., Kim, S. W., Chan, T., Ratnam, S. S., Landgren, B. M., Shearman, R. P., Goldzieher, J. W. & Dozier, T. S. (1981). Pharmacokinetics of ethynyloestradiol in women from different populations. *Contraception*, **23**, 487–96.

Fox, A. L. (1932). The relationship between chemical constitution and taste. *Proceedings of the National Academy of Sciences (USA)*, **18**, 115–20.

Freis, E. D. (1986). Antihypertensive agents. In *Ethnic Differences in Reactions to Drugs and Xenobiotics*, ed. W. Kalow, H. W. Goedde & D. P. Agarwal. *Progress in Clinical and Biological Research*, **214**, 313–22. New York: Alan R. Liss.

Geldmacher v-Mallinckrodt, M. (1978). Polymorphism of human serum paraoxonase. *Human Genetics*, Suppl. 1, 65–8.

Gonzalez, F. J. (1990). Molecular genetics of the P-450 Superfamily. *Pharmacology and Therapeutics*, **45**, 1–38.

Gough, A. C., Miles, J. S., Spurr, N. K., Moss, J. E., Gaedigk, A., Eichelbaum, M. & Wolf, C. R. (1990). Identification of the primary gene defect at the cytochrome P-450 *CYP2D* locus. *Nature*, **347**, 733–6.

Gund, P., Andose, J. D., Rhodes, J. B. & Smith, G. M. (1980). Three-dimensional molecular modelling and drug design. *Science*, **208**, 1425–31.

Guttendorf, R. J. & Wedlund, P. J. (1992). Genetic aspects of drug disposition and therapeutics. *Journal of Clinical Pharmacology*, **32**, 107–17.

Harris, H. (1970). Enzyme and protein diversity in human populations. In *The Principles of Human Biochemical Genetics*, ed. H. Harris. *North-Holland Research Monographs Frontiers of Biology*, **19**, 211–42. Amsterdam: North-Holland.

Harris, C. M., Waring, R. H., Mitchell, S. C. & Hendry, G. L. (1986). The case of the black-speckled dolls: an occupational hazard of unusual sulphur metabolism. *Lancet*, **1**, 492–3.

Hayashi, S.-I., Watanabe, J. & Kawajiri, K. (1992). High susceptibility to lung cancer analyzed in terms of combined genotypes of P450 IA1 and Mu-class glutathione S-transferase genes. *Japanese Journal of Cancer Research*, **83**, 866–70.

Heckbert, S. R., Weiss, N. S., Hornung, S., Eaton, D. L. & Motulsky, A. G. (1992). Glutathione S-transferase and epoxide hydrolase activity in human leukocytes in relation to risk of lung cancer and other smoking-related cancers. *Journal of the National Cancer Institute*, **84**, 414–22.

Holmstedt, B. & Liljestrand, G. (1963). *Readings in Pharmacology*, p. 286. New York: Macmillan.

Hunter, D. (1978). *Diseases of Occupations*, 6th edn, p. 80. London: Hodder & Stoughton.

Idle, J. R., Oates, N. S., Shah, R. R. & Smith, R. L. (1983). Protecting poor metabolisers: a group at high risk of adverse drug reactions. *Lancet*, **1**, 1388.

Idle, J. R. & Smith, R. L. (1984). The debrisoquine hydroxylation gene: a gene of multiple consequence. In *Proceedings of the Second World Conference on Clinical Pharmacology and Therapeutics*, ed. L. Lemberger & M. M. Reidenberg. pp. 148–64. Bethesda, M. D. American Society of Pharmacology and Experimental Therapeutics.

Imai, M., Shimada, H., Watauabe, Y., Matsushima-Hibiya,

Y., Makino, R., Koga, H., Horiuchi, T. & Ishimura, Y. (1989). Uncoupling of the cytochrome P450$_{cam}$ mono-oxygenase reaction by a single mutation, threonine-252 to alanine or valine: A possible role of the hydroxy amino acid in oxygen activation. *Proceedings of the National Academy of Sciences (USA)*, **86**, 7823–7.

Johnson, E. F. (1992). Mapping determinants of the substrate selectivities of P450 enzymes by site-directed mutagenesis. *Trends in Pharmaceutical Sciences*, **13**, 122–6.

Johnson, J. A. & Burlew, B. S. (1992). Racial differences in propanolol pharmacokinetics. *Clinical Pharmacology and Therapeutics*, **51**, 495–500.

Joubert, P. H. & Brandt, H. D. (1990). Apparent racial difference in response to angiotensin I infusion. *European Journal of Clinical Pharmacology*, **39**, 183–5.

Kagimoto, M., Heim, M., Kagimoto, K., Zeugin, T. & Meyer, U. A. (1990). Multiple mutations of the human cytochrome P450 II D6 gene (CYP2D6) in poor metabolisers of debrisoquine *Journal of Biological Chemistry*, **265**, 17209–14.

Kalow, W. (1982). Ethnic differences in drug metabolism. *Clinical Pharmacokinetics*, **7**, 373–400.

Kalow, W. (1990). Pharmacogenetics: past and future. *Life Sciences*, **47**, 1385–97.

Kalow, W. (1991). Interethnic variation of drug metabolism. *Trends in Pharmacological Sciences*, **12**, 102–7.

Kalow, W., Goedde, H. W. & Agarwal, D. P. (ed). (1986). Ethnic differences in reactions to drugs and xenobiotics. *Progress in Clinical and Biological Research*, Vol. 214. New York: Alan R. Liss.

Kannan, K. K. (1980). Crystal structure of carbonic anhydrase. In *Biophysics and Physiology of Carbon Dioxide*, ed. C. Bauer, G. Gros & H. Bartels, pp. 184–205. Berlin: Springer-Verlag.

Kawajiri, K., Nakachi, K., Imai, K., Yoshi, A., Shinoda, N. & Watanabe, J. (1990). Identification of genetically high risk individuals to lung cancer by DNA polymorphisms of the cytochrome P-450 I A1 gene. *FEBS Letters*, **263**, 131–3.

Khoury, M. J., Stewart, W. & Beaty, T. H. (1987). The effect of genetic susceptibility on causal inference in epidemiologic studies. *American Journal of Epidemiology*, **126**, 561–7.

La Du, B. N. & Eckerson, H. W. (1984). Could human paraoxonase polymorphism account for different responses to certain environmental chemicals? In *Genetic Variability in Responses to Chemical Exposure*, ed. G. S. Omenn & H. V. Gelboin. Banbury Report 16, Cold Spring Harbor Laboratory.

Landrigan, P. J., Selikoff, I. J. (eds) (1989). Occupational health in the 1990s – developing a platform for disease prevention. *Annals of the New York Academy of Sciences*, **572**, 1–295.

Lennard, M. S., Ramsay, L. E., Silas, J. H., Tucker, G. T. & Woods, H. F. (1983). Protecting the poor metabolizer: clinical consequences of genetic polymorphism of drug oxidation. *Pharmacy International*, **4**, 53–7.

Le Walter, J. & Korallus, U. (1985). Blood protein conjugates and acetylation of aromatic amines. New findings on biological monitoring. *International Archives of Occupational and Environmental Health*, **56**, 179–96.

Lipkowitz, K. B. & McCracken, R. O. (1991). A molecular modeling approach to *in vivo* efficacy of triclabendazole *Journal of Parasitology*, **77**, 998–1005.

Martin, Y. C. (1991). Computer-assisted rational drug design. In *Molecular Design and Modeling – concepts and applications, Part B*, ed. J. J. Langone. *Methods of Enzymology*, **203**, 587–612. San Diego: Academic Press.

Meyer, U. A. (1990). Molecular genetics and the future of pharmacogenetics. *Pharmacology and Therapeutics*, **46**, 349–55.

Meyer, U. A., Zanger, U. M., Grant, D. & Blum, M. (1990). Genetic polymorphisms of drug metabolism. In *Advances in Drug Research*, Vol. 19, ed. B. Testa, pp. 197–241. Orlando, FL: Academic Press.

Morton, N. E. (1982). *The Outline of Genetic Epidemiology*. Basel: Karger.

Mourant, A. E., Kopec, A. C. & Domaniewska-Sobezak, K. (1976) *The Distribution of the Human Blood Groups and Other Polymorphisms*, 2nd edn. London: Oxford University Press.

Mura, C., Broyard, J. P., Jacqz-Aigrain, E. & Krishnamoorthy, R. (1991). Distinct phenotypes and genotypes of debrisoquine hydroxylation among Europeans and Chinese. *British Journal of Clinical Pharmacology*, **32**, 135–6.

Nebert, D. W. (1988). Genes encoding drug-metabolizing enzymes: possible role in human disease. In *Phenotypic Variation in Populations*, ed. A. D. Woodhead, M. A. Bender & R. C. Leonard, pp. 45–64. New York: Plenum.

Olatunde, E. & Evans, D. A. P. (1982). Blood quinidine levels and cardiac effects in white British and Nigerian subjects. *British Journal of Clinical Pharmacology*, **14**, 513–18.

Omenn, G. S. & Gelboin, H. V (ed.) (1984). *Genetic Variability in Responses to Chemical Exposure*. Banbury Report 16, Cold Spring Harbor Laboratory.

Ortigoza-Ferado, J., Richter, R., Furlong, C. & Motulsky, A. G. (1984). Biochemical genetics of paraoxonase. In *Genetic Variability in Responses to Chemical Exposure*, ed. G. S. Omenn & H. V. Gelboin. Banbury Report 16, pp. 177–88. Cold Spring Harbor Laboratory.

Playfer, J. R., Eze, L. C., Bullen, M. F. & Evans, D. A. P. (1976). Genetic polymorphism and inter-ethnic variability of plasma paroxonase activity. *Journal of Medical Genetics*, **13**, 337–42.

Porter, T. D. & Coon, M. J. (1991). Cytochrome P450. Multiplicity of isoforms substrates and catalytic and regulatory mechanisms. *Journal of Biological Chemistry*, **266**, 13469–72.

Poulos, T. L. (1988). Cytochrome P450: Molecular architecture, mechanism and prospects for rational inhibitor design. *Pharmaceutical Research*, **5**, 67–75.

Prody, C. A., Dreyfus, P., Zamir, R., Zakut, H. & Soreq, H. (1989). *De novo* amplification within a 'silent' human cholinesterase gene in a family subjected to prolonged exposure to organophosphorus insecticides. *Proceedings of the National Academy of Sciences (USA)*, **86**, 690–4.

R. S. (1992). Computerized drug design: Still promising, not yet here. *Science*, **256**, 441.

Rutledge, D. R., Cardozo, L. & Steinberg, J. D. (1989). Racial differences in drug response: isoproterenol effects on heart rate in healthy males. *Pharmaceutical Research*, **6**, 182–5.

Seedat, Y. K. (1989). Varying responses to hypotensive agents in different racial groups: black versus white differences. *Journal of Hypertension*, **7**, 515–18.

Smith, R. L. (1986). Polymorphism in drug metabolism – implications for drug toxicity. *Archives of Toxicology*, Suppl. 9, 138–46.

Sommers, De.K., Moncrieff, J. & Avenant, J. C. (1987). Paracetamol conjugation: an interethnic and dietary study. *Human Toxicology*, **6**, 407–9.

Sommers, De.K., Moncrieff, J. & Avenant, J. (1989). Non-correlation between debrisoquine and metoprolol polymorphisms in the Venda. *Human Toxicology*, **8**, 365–8.

Spector, R., Choudhury, A. K., Chiang, C.-K., Goldberg, M. J. & Ghoneim, M. M. (1980). Diphenhydramine in Orientals and Caucasians. *Clinical Pharmacology and Therapeutics*, **28**, 229–34.

Stenberg, G., Board, P. G. & Mannervik, B. (1991). Mutation of an evolutionarily conserved tyrosine residue in the active site of a human class Alpha glutathione transferase. *FEBS Letters*, **293**, 153–5.

Sugimura, H., Caporaso, N. E., Shaw, G. L., Modali, R. V., Gonzalez, F. J., Hoover, R. N., Resau, J. H., Trump, B. F., Weston, A. & Harris, C. C. (1990). Human debrisoquine hydroxylase gene polymorphisms in cancer patients and controls. *Carcinogenesis*, **11**, 1527–30.

Taylor, W. J. R., Kalow, W. & Sellers, E. A. (1965). Poisoning with organo-phosphorus insecticides. *Canadian Medical Association Journal*, **93**, 966–70.

Tefre, T., Ryberg, D., Haugen, A., Nebert, D. W., Skaug, V., Brogger, A. & Børresen, A.-L. (1991). Human CYP1A1 (cytochrome P_1450) gene: lack of association between MspI restriction fragment length polymorhism and incidence of lung cancer in Norwegian population. *Pharmacogenetics*, **1**, 20–5.

Tikkanen, M. J., Huttunen, J. K., Ehnholm, C. & Pietinen, P. (1990). Apolipoproetin E_4 homozygosity predisposes to serum cholesterol elevation during high fat diet. *Arteriosclerosis*, **10**, 285–8.

Timbrell, J. A. (1989). *Introduction to Toxicology*. London: Taylor & Francis.

Uematsu, F., Kikuchi, H., Motomiya, M., Abe, T., Sagami, I., Ohmachi, T., Wakui, A., Kanamuaru, R. & Watanabe, M. (1991). Association between restriction fragment length polymorphism of the human cytochrome P450 II E1 gene and susceptibility to lung cancer. *Japanese Journal of Cancer Research*, **82**, 254–6.

Vesell, E. S. (1977). Genetic and environmental factors affecting drug disposition in man. *Clinical Pharmacology and Therapeutics*, **22**, 659–79.

Vesell, E. S. (1986) Dynamic interactions among host factors that influence antipyrine metabolism: implications for the design and interpretation of studies on ethnic pharmacokinetic variations. In *Ethnic Differences in Reactions to Drugs and Xenobiotics*, ed. W. Kalow, H. W. S. Goedde & D. P. Agarwal. *Progress in Clinical and Biological Research*, **214**, 425–51. New York: Alan R. Liss.

Vesell, E. S. (1987). Pharmacogenetic perspectives on susceptibility to toxic industrial chemicals. *British Journal of Industrial Medicine*, **44**, 505–9.

Vesell, E. S. (1989). Pharmacogenetic perspectives gained from twin and family studies. *Pharmacology and Therapeutics*, **41**, 535–52.

Vincent, J., Elliott, H. L., Meredith, P. A. & Reid, J. L. (1986). Racial differences in drug responses – a comparative study of trimazosin and α_1-adrenoceptor responses in normotensive Caucasians and West Africans. *British Journal of Clinical Pharmacology*, **21**, 401–8.

Weatherall, D. J., Clegg, J. B., Higgs, D. R. & Wood, W. G. (1989). The hemoglobinopathies. In *The Metabolic Basis of Inherited Disease*, 6th edn, ed. C. R. Scriver, A. L. Beaudet, W. S. Sly & D. Vale, Chapter 93, pp. 2281–339. New York: McGraw-Hill.

Weinberger, M. H. (1990). Racial differences in antihypertensive therapy: evidence and implications. *Cardiovascular Drugs and Therapy*, **4**, 379–82.

Wolf, C. R., Smith, C. A. D., Gough, A. C., Moss, J. E., Vallis, K. A., Howard, G., Carey, F. J., Mills, K., McNee, W., Carmichael, J. & Spurr, N. K. (1992). Relationship between the debrisoquine hydroxylase polymorphism and cancer susceptibility. *Carcinogenesis*, **13**, 1035–8.

Wüthrich, K. (1990). Protein structure determination in solution by NMR spectroscopy. *Journal of Biological Chemistry*, **265**, 22059–62.

Yue, Q. Y., Bertilsson, L., Dahl-Puustinen, M. L., Säwe, J., Sjöqvist, F., Johansson, I. & Ingelman-Sundberg, M. (1989). Disassociation between debrisoquine hydroxylation phenotype and genotype among Chinese. *Lancet*, **2**, 870.

Zhang, Y., Reviriego, J., Lou, Y.-Q., Sjöqvist, F. & Bertilsson, L. (1990). Diazepam metabolism in native Chinese poor and extensive hydroxylators of S-mephenytoin: Inter-ethnic differences in comparison with white subjects. *Clinical Pharmacology and Therapeutics*, **48**, 496–502.

Zhong, S., Howie, A. F., Ketterer, B., Taylor, J., Hayes, J. D., Beckett, G. J., Wathen, C. G., Wolf, C. R. & Spurr, N. K. (1991). Glutathione S-transferase Mu locus: use of genotyping and phenotyping assays to assess association with lung cancer susceptibility. *Carcinogenesis*, **12**, 1533–7.

Zhou, H.-H., Adedoyin, A. & Wilkinson, G. R. (1990). Differences in plasma binding of drugs between Caucasians and Chinese subjects. *Clinical Pharmacology and Therapeutics*, **48**, 10–17.

Zhou, H.-H., Koshakji, R. P., Silberstein, D. J., Wilkinson, G. R. & Wood, A. J. J. (1989a). Racial differences in drug response – altered sensitivity to and clearance of propanolol in men of Chinese descent as compared with American whites. *New England Journal of Medicine*, **320**, 565–70.

Zhou, H.-H., Silberstein, D. J., Wilkinson, G. R. & Wood, A. J. J. (1989b). Racial differences in drug response. *New England Journal of Medicine*, **321**, 259.

Ziegler, V. E. & Biggs, J. T. (1977). Tricyclic plasma levels. *Journal of the American Medical Association*, **238**, 2167–9.

PART XIII   Conclusions

39   Conclusions

THERE are implications from the contents of this book on both practical and theoretical levels. Even though modern therapeutics is outstandingly successful and a great monument to human intellectual endeavour, every perspicacious doctor realizes after he has been practising medicine for a few years that when he gives a drug to a patient it is an act which has many similarities to an experiment. The outcome of prescribing a drug is never a hundred per cent certain. The desired beneficial effect may be observed or there may be unexpected adverse effects or there may be a failure of treatment. There may be a number of reasons for such variable sequelae. The examples given in this book make it clear that genetic factors are frequently responsible.

An attempt has been made to demonstrate the manner of operation of pharmacogenetic principles by giving known examples. Genetic factors are very likely to be of importance in the metabolism of, and response to, many more drugs. Consequently genetic factors are worth considering when any unexpected clinical event such as an adverse reaction (particularly of a non-hypersensitivity type) is observed.

Adverse reactions may be determined by genetic factors operating in a variety of ways, e.g. excess substrate due to low rate of biotransformation, toxic metabolite production through the activity of an alternative pathway or undue susceptibility because of a variant form of the tissue or enzyme receptor. More than one genetic mechanism may be involved in the production of clinical phenomena from one drug (e.g. phenytoin).

Discontinuous variability observed during the course of clinical pharmacological surveys may indicate the existence of a previously unknown polymorphism. Family studies are required to demonstrate that a polymorphism is genetic, and they also reveal the manner of inheritance.

The elicitation of an appropriate family history from a patient can frequently be very revealing in Mendelian dominant conditions and may sometimes be of value in recessive characters. Very striking instances have occurred of patients warning medical attendants that fatal porphyria and fatal malignant hyperthermia had occurred in close relatives, and these warnings have been disregarded with fatal consequences to the patient. Predictive tests are worth considering when indicated either by the family history and clinical examination or by the prospect of long-continued treatment with a drug known to have polymorphic metabolism or effect.

Where a genetic influence has been demonstrated but the individual alleles concerned have not been identified, monitoring procedures may be instituted during drug therapy. Plasma concentration determinations are standard practice with many drugs. Tonometry should be carried out at regular intervals in patients on long-term therapy with corticosteroids.

In a genetic polymorphism some benefits and disadvantages in different clinical situations may be associated with each phenotype. For example, slow acetylators of isoniazid are more prone to neuropathy on conventional doses. On the other hand, rapid acetylators have an unsatisfactory response of their tuberculosis to once-weekly dosage schedules. This differential liability of phenotypes has some similarity to Darwinian selection.

When the genetic basis of an adverse reaction is understood it may not be necessary to discard a useful drug. For example, perhexilene was considered a useful drug for angina pectoris. About 5% of the population could not metabolize it properly and they were particularly prone to develop peripheral neuropathy. Because of this the drug was withdrawn. Consequently 95% of the population who could have used it with only minimal risk of neuropathy were denied the possible benefits of the drug. It would in theory have been more logical to have introduced a phenotyping test.

A new adverse reaction may reveal a new allele. Knowledge gained by applying genetic methodology to pharmacological phenomena may reveal important mechanisms or even a factor in the aetiology of the disorder being treated. A change of attitude is needed, therefore, to regard adverse reactions as being Nature's way of revealing secrets, rather than simply being events to inconvenience patient and doctor.

Hitherto the pattern of development of any individual pharmacogenetic system has followed a conventional path starting with phenotypic recognition followed by unravelling of the pharmacologic and/or biochemical mechanism leading to purification of an enzyme or receptor finally yielding identification of the gene. It seems likely that the new techniques of reverse genetics may enable future discoveries to be made in different ways.

Metabolic accounting should be the norm for all new drugs. Well-established methods make it feasible to know the fate of all ingested drug molecules, and the structures of metabolites should be identified. In the past these exercises have been carried out on small numbers of people. It is necessary to examine larger numbers of persons in order to assess the inter-individual variability. With these approaches the influences of pharmacogenetic polymorphisms on new drugs may be either predicted or detected early.

Epidemiologic studies will be made much easier to carry out by using allele-specific probes in association with the polymerase chain reaction. Examples where this technology is immediately available for application include the following: aldehyde dehydrogenase, porphyrin pathway enzymes, glucose-6-phosphate dehydrogenase variants, pseudocholinesterase variants, the acetylation polymorphism and the debrisoquine/sparteine polymorphism. This approach should enable better progress to be made in the study of the role of pharmacogenetic factors in both drug-induced and spontaneous disorders.

Clinical trials of a normally structured type should contain adequate numbers of persons, so that an unrepresentative genetic constitution of control and experimental groups does not arise by chance.

Sometimes industrial processes use compounds which have a similarity to drugs. Therefore when a genetic polymorphism has been defined in relation to the metabolism or effect of a drug it may find application in the prevention of occupational disorders, e.g. by restricting certain jobs to individuals of a particular phenotype.

The development of a reproducible biochemical or physiological phenotyping test has clarified the doubt and vagueness associated with a purely clinical description. Examples are acute intermittent porphyria and malignant hyperthermia where the genetic basis of an adverse reaction became clear when the relevant test was introduced. It is expected that genotyping with specific probes will be even more definitive.

Despite the fact that animal work is not emphasized in this book, it is nevertheless clear that a new use for animal tissues has arisen recently. An animal DNA for a particular enzyme may resemble the human DNA closely enough that it can be used as a specific probe with which to study the human genome.

The development of biotinylated probes (as developed, for example, for the pseudocholinesterase variants) should lessen the use of radioactivity in biomedical laboratories.

It will be observed that some of the pharmacogenetic systems described have been very thoroughly studied down to gene level. Their influence on clinical phenomena has also been extensively explored. Other systems are a long way from this state of development and possess only phenotypic descriptions, e.g. phenylthiocarbamide (PTC) tasting, mephenytoin hydroxylation, chlorpropamide – alcohol flushing, anticoagulant resistance, and the effects of glucocorticoids on intraocular pressure. It is anticipated that these topics should also be elucidated at a molecular level in the future.

Many modern drugs are complex molecules and

liable to more than one biotransformation. Consequently their metabolism may be influenced by the products of different genes, each of which may have alleles with differing properties. Examples are propanolol and imipramine whose metabolisms are controlled by both the debrisoquine/sparteine (CYP 2D6) and the mephenytoin (CYP 2C18) polymorphisms. Presumably, therefore, the total variability in their metabolism and action in the population is a composite with contributions from different components. No one has yet actually demonstrated this phenomenon. It is likely that the variability in phenylbutazone metabolism (shown to be 'polygenic') may be of this composite nature because the molecule is known to be oxidized at two positions, aromatic and aliphatic, which are biotransformations most likely catalysed by different gene products.

Determining the genetic constitution of an individual using specific gene probes circumvents the difficulties in pharmacogenetic studies caused by induction phenomena. Therefore by direct examination of the genome it will be easier to make comparisons of genetic make-up between patients with different disorders (e.g. cancer) and on different drug treatments.

A different pattern of adverse reactions may occur when a drug is used in a new ethnic population. There may be a different incidence of a known reaction or the occurrence of new reactions. If such a different pattern of adverse reactions is observed, then an attempt should be made to correlate them with the metabolic fate of the compound. However, inter-ethnic comparisons have proven difficult to make particularly when the parameter being examined is inducible. The availability of allele-specific probes and the other techniques of molecular genetics will allow genotypes to be compared directly. The effects of environmental variables as well as genetic effects should consequently become more measurable.

The intellectual appeal of the 'common' genetic polymorphisms in medicine is that they allow phenomena to be analysed in terms of frequencies of phenotypes. Another attraction of pharmacogenetic polymorphisms as objects for research is that they deal with well defined substrates, which must have a close similarity to the natural substrates of the relevant enzymes. The drug substrates were created in the first place because they had an action on some mechanism which was important in relation to a disease process. Because of this, the investigation of a pharmacogenetic polymorphism may result in the identification or elimination of a particular class of candidate substances in the causation or pathogenesis of a disorder which (like most) is due to the interplay of environmental and genetic factors.

Recently it has become possible to introduce individual pharmacogenetic alleles using expression vectors into bacteria, yeasts and tissue culture cells. These techniques allow the relevant enzyme activities to be studied in isolation and hence with greater definition. This ability may well prove advantageous where there are overlapping specificities between enzymes as, for example, with cytochrome P450 activities, glucuronyltransferases and glutathione-S-transferases.

In order properly to understand the nature of many pharmacogenetic phenomena it will be necessary to have knowledge of the three-dimensional structures of the macromolecules involved. Nuclear magnetic resonance spectroscopy and computer techniques make it possible that in the immediate future information of this type will be more easily obtainable than it was with X-ray crystallography.

The laboratory scientific aspects of pharmacogenetics have raced ahead in the last few years. The need at present is for clinical surveys to make use of this knowledge, and these should be much better planned than has been the case in the past, with more rigorous definition of phenotypes.

Even with the startling new advances in molecular biology it is still necessary to correlate phenotype with genotype. On a practical level it is with the phenotype that the physician has to contend, but knowledge of genetic factors in drug therapy may enable him to make a better job of looking after his patients.

PART XIV Appendices

Appendix I Computing the degree of dominance for a Mendelian character exhibiting a bimodal population frequency distribution

LET us suppose that a given measured character is stable in the individual (i.e. very similar results are obtained on repeated testing) and bimodally distributed in the population. Then pedigree studies may reveal that the character is inherited in a Mendelian manner, and that one mode consists of homozygous recessives and the other of dominants. Within the latter mode there are two types of individuals – heterozygotes and homozygotes. It is of interest to know what are the distributions of these genotypes within the observed phenotypic mode. There follows an explanation of how this information can be obtained using simple arithmetic (Evans *et al.* 1980).

It must be remembered that dominance is a variable character and a property of the phenotype, not of the genotype. When the mean heterozygote value is equal to the mid-point between the means of the two homozygotes on a linear scale of values, then dominance is zero. When the mean heterozygote value is the same as the mean homozygote value, then dominance is 100%.

An approximate estimate of the mean value of homozygous dominants can be made by the following procedure.

1 Identify homozygous recessives (poor metabolizers) from population phenotyping data.
2 Obtain the mean value for recessives.
3 Identify obligate heterozygotes from pedigrees.
4 Obtain the mean value for heterozygotes.
5 Compute the number of heterozygotes in the population sample using the Hardy–Weinberg equilibrium.
6 Compute the number of homozygous dominants in the population sample.
7 Use the values obtained in the following equations:

| Sum of observed values for all dominants in population sample. | − | Product of estimated number of heterozygotes in population sample multiplied by mean value for obligate hetero zygotes in family study. | = | Sum of values for the homozygous dominants in the population sample. |

| Computed sum of values for the homozygous dominants in the population sample. | ÷ | number of homozygous dominants estimated in population sample. | = | mean value for homozygous dominants. |

619

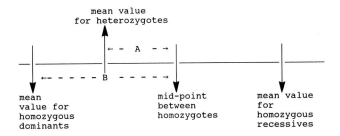

Fig. A.1. Diagrammatic representation of the concept of dominance. Percentage dominance is given by A/B%. Complete dominance (100%) is where A = B. Zero dominance (0) is where A = 0.

When this information has been obtained then the information can be used for a computation of dominance as shown in Fig. A.1.

Evans, D. A. P., Mahgoub, A., Sloan, T. P., Idle, J.R. & Smith, R. L. (1980). A family and population study of the genetic polymorphism of debrisoquine oxidation in a British white population. *Journal of Medical Genetics*, **17**, 102–5.

Appendix II   Exponential decay

THE PURPOSE of this appendix is to explain the relationship between plasma concentration and time which for most drugs is exponential or a first-order process after the distribution phase has come to an end.

The relationship between half-life and elimination rate constant will also be shown.

The elimination of most drugs from the body is by a first-order process. The rate of fall of the plasma concentration is dependent on the concentration so that when the latter is high the former is large. This is known an an exponential function so that

$$C = C_0 . e^{-kt} \tag{1}$$

where C = concentration at a given time; C_0 = estimated concentration at zero time; e = the mathematical constant 2.7183; k = the elimination rate constant (sometimes known as the first-order rate constant); t = the time which has elapsed from zero. Equation 1 can be conveniently restated as

$$\log_e C = \log_e C_0^{-kt} \tag{2}$$

which has the same format as the formula for a straight line graph

$$y = a - kt \tag{3}$$

where y = ordinate value, t = abscissa value, a = ordinate, i.e. value of y when $t = 0$, k = slope, i.e. increment in value of y for each unit increment in the value of t.

It is conventional to refer to the time that it takes for the value of the plasma concentration C to fall by half (plasma concentration half-life $t_{1/2}$). This half life has the same value whether C is large or small. Since the half-life is the time taken to reduce C_0 to half its value, equation 1 can be re-written

$$0.5 = e^{-kt_{1/2}} \tag{4}$$

$$\text{or } 2 = e^{kt_{1/2}} \tag{5}$$

Taking natural logarithms

$$\log_e 2 = 0.69315 = k \cdot t_{1/2} \tag{6}$$

$$\text{or } t_{1/2} = \frac{0.69315}{k} \tag{7}$$

It is often preferred to use equation 2 in the form of common logarithms and since

$$\log_e X = \text{approximately } 2.3 \log_{10} X$$

$$\log_{10} C = \log_{10} C_0 - 0.434 \, kt$$

When $\log_{10} C$ is halved its value falls by 0.3010 (i.e. $\log_{10} 2$) and the time taken for this to occur is the half-life.

Other natural phenomena, such as the decay of a radioactive isotope, Hook's law of the spring and Newton's law of cooling can be represented mathematically the same way.

The alternative to a first-order process in pharmacokinetics is a zero-order process where the rate of fall in plasma concentration is independent of the plasma concentration. This is very unusual but does apply to ethyl alcohol.

The author would like to express his gratitude to Dr Ken Leach, Department of Medical Physics, Riyadh Armed Forces Hospital, Saudi Arabia who made many helpful suggestions about the contents of this Appendix.

621

Appendix III   The disentanglement of overlapping frequency distribution curves

IN some of the early examples of pharmacogenetics, e.g. G6PD deficiency and pseudocholinesterase variants, the modes were well separated by the phenotyping methods so that there was no confusion about the assignment of an individual. When 'isoniazid inactivator' phenotyping came along there was a small difficulty.

The problems of interpretation were extensively discussed by Murphy (1964), who by showing the results of sampling experiments and citing examples from the literature (including famous Platt–Pickering hypertension controversy) made clear the pitfalls which await the unwary.

Since then the same type of problem has recurred again and again. Table A.1 gives some of the main pharmacogenetic authors who have attempted various solutions.

A classical pharmacologic approach to the problem has been strongly advocated by Kalow (see, for example, Kalow 1982). This is the use of probit plots. The probit y is defined as the normal equivalent deviate $x - \mu/\sigma$ increased by 5 where x is the log of each data point and μ and σ are the mean and standard deviation respectively of the population so that

$$y = 5 + x - \mu/\sigma$$

Regression lines are formed when probits are plotted against a pharmacokinetic parameter (often they are depicted above the frequency distribution histogram). For a single normal distribution curve the probit plot gives a straight line whose slope is determined by the standard deviation and centre by the mean. Where one such line meets another the inflection point on the probit plot indicates the position of the antimode. This technique is discussed by Jackson *et al.* (1986a) who concluded that the probit plot is of only limited use in the detection of polymorphisms of drug metabolism

and that the presence of a sharp discontinuity in the probit plot is a sufficient but not a necessary criterion for the presence of a polymorphism.

However, despite all the effort put into these mathematical aspects it needs to be pointed out that their use is subservient to sound biological and chemical techniques. For example, Lee (1988), discussing debrisoquine phenotyping states 'It is recommended . . . that the antimode discriminating extensive and poor metabolizers be redefined with each study'. This is obviously wiser than using an antimodal value derived from some different population to define phenotypes.

Sometimes independent external reference information can be obtained to indicate groups making up compound distribution curves. One classic example concerns red cell acid phosphatase where electrophoretically determined genotypes were shown to make individual contributions to the frequency distribution curve of enzyme activities (Harris 1966).

Another example concerns the identification of heterozygotes from pedigrees and then seeing what contribution they make to the frequency distribution curve of a pharmacokinetic variable for dominants (e.g. Evans *et al.* 1960, 1980, 1983). See Appendix I.

The same mathematical considerations occur in many other branches of science. An example related to laboratory techniques used in pharmacology is the existence of overlapping distribution curves (which are very often approximately normal) in chromatography. A method of calculating the areas of such overlapping curves was given by Smith & Bartlet (1961).

A graphical method of analysis of polymodal frequency distributions was described in 1949 by J. P. Harding (*J. Mar. Biol. Ass. UK*, **28**, 141–53). This method, although laborious and requiring large numbers for analysis, illustrates the basis on which later

Table A.1. *Mathematical techniques to disentangle overlapping frequency distribution curves*

Reference	Summary of method
Smith & Bartlet 1961	Computation from the classical mathematics of normal probability curves
Kalmus & Maynard Smith 1965	Computations of the antimode on the assumptions that equal proportions of both frequency distribution curves and equal numbers of individuals are misclassified
Murphy & Bolling 1967	Maximum likelihood
Bliss, 1967	Iterative programme
McClean *et al.* 1976	Removal of skewness in analysis of commingled distributions
Scott & Poffenbarger 1979	Computer-based non-linear curve fitting
Geldmacher-v Mallinckrodt *et al.* 1979	Iterative technique representing a cluster-analytical approach
Spielman & Weinshilboum 1981	Assumptions that the three distributions of the genotypes in a two-allele system are normal with no dominance. Maximum likelihood computer method (Kaplan & Elston 1972) used to find the combination of parameter values which maximizes the likelihood of the entire sample
Kalow 1982	Probit plots
Evans *et al.*, 1983	Normal distributions estimated with maximum likelihood with unequivocal observations and antimode computed at point of equal density. Maximum likelihood also used to resolve genotypes from dominant phenotype distribution
Jack 1983	Rosin-Rammler Sperling Weibull distribution
Schmid *et al.* 1985	Intersection point of two density functions equals the antimode in a discontinuous frequency distribution histogram
Jackson *et al.* 1986b	Insertion of parameter values into a pharmacokinetic model, description of clearance via the polymorphic pathway using the Hardy–Weinberg Law and the generation of frequency distributions using a computer stimulation. Experimentally observed data compared with computer predictions
Iyun *et al.* 1986	Kernel density estimates to investigate multimodality
Henthorne *et al.* 1989	A likelihood ratio χ^2 statistic was computed to test whether there was an improvement of fit with a mixture of distributions over a single one

computer analyses were designed, the latest and most effective of which is that due, in 1975, to Yong and Skillman of the South-West Fisheries Centre, Honolulu Laboratory, National Marine Fisheries Service, NOAA, Honolulu HI 96812, USA. This program accepts a list of values of the chosen parameter, e.g. whole blood cholinesterase, arranges them in order of magnitude as a cumulative frequency distribution, converts from percentage probabilities to probits and then finds the polynomial function which best fits the probit data. The second derivative of this polynomial is then tested for inflection points, the roots of the polynomial are calculated, and the means, standard deviations and percentage of each subpopulation are estimated. The predicted frequencies of values, taking all populations together, are then calculated and tested for correspondence with the original data using the Chi-squared test. (Personal communication, Dr D. V. Roberts, Department of Physiology, University of Liverpool, 18 November 1981.)

Bliss, C. L. (1967). *Statistics in Biology*. Vol. 1, pp. 156–165. New York: McGraw-Hill. (Cited by Messeri, G., Tozz, P., Boddi, V. & Ciatto, S. (1985). Glucose-6-phosphate dehydrogenase activity and estrogen receptors in breast cancer. *Journal of Steroid Biochemistry*, **19**, 1647–50.)

Evans, D. A. P., Harmer, D., Downham, D. Y., Whibley, E. J., Idle, J. R., Rithie, J. & Smith, R. L. (1983). The genetic control of sparteine and debrisoquine metabolism in man with new methods of analysing bimodal distributions. *Journal of Medical Genetics*, **20**, 321–9.

Evans, D. A. P., Mahgoub, A., Sloan, T. P., Idle, J. R. & Smith, R. L. (1980). A family and population study of the genetic polymorphism of debrisoquine oxidation in a white British population. *Journal of Medical Genetics*, **17**, 102–5.

Evans, D. A. P., Manley, K. A. & McKusick, K. A. (1960). Genetic control of isoniazid metabolism in man. *British Medical Journal*, **2**, 485–91.

Geldmacher-v Mallinckrodt, M., Hommel, G. & Dumbach, J. (1979). On the genetics of the human serum paraoxonase (EC 3.1.1.2). *Human Genetics*, **50**, 313–26.

Harris, H. (1966). Enzyme polymorphisms in man. *Proceedings of the Royal Society of London, Ser. B*, **164**, 298–310.

Henthorn, T. K., Benitez, J., Avram, M. J., Martinez, C.,

Llerena, A., Cobaleda, J., Krejcie, T. C. & Gibbons, R. D. (1989). Assessment of the debrisoquine and dextromethorphan phenotyping tests by gaussian mixture distributions analysis. *Clinical Pharmacology and Therapeutics*, **45**, 328–33.

Iyun, A. O., Lennard, M. S., Tucker, G. T. & Woods, H. F. (1986). Meroprolol and debrisoquine metabolism in Nigerians; Lack of evidence for polymorphic oxidation. *Clinical Pharmacology and Therapeutics*, **40**, 387–94.

Jack, D. B. (1983). Statistical analysis of polymorphic drug metabolism data using the Rosin Rammler Sperling Weibull distribution. *European Journal of Clinical Pharmacology*, **25**, 443–8.

Jackson, P. R., Lennard, M. S. A., Tucker, G. T. & Woods, H. F. (1986a). Is the probit plot of use to detect polymorphism of drug metabolism? *Acta Pharmacologica et Toxicologica*, **59** (Suppl. 5), 215.

Jackson, P. R., Tucker, G. T., Lennard, M. S. & Woods, H. F. (1986b). Polymorphic drug oxidation; pharmacokinetic basis and comparison of experimental indices. *British Journal of Clinical Pharmacology*, **22**, 541–50.

Kalmus, H. & Maynard-Smith, S. (1965). The antimode and lines of optimal separation in a genetically determined bimodal distribution with particular reference to phenylthiocarbamide sensitivity. *Annals of Human Genetics (London)*, **29**, 127–38.

Kalow, W. (1982). Ethnic differences in drug metabolism. *Clinical Pharmacokinetics*, **7**, 373–400.

Kaplan, E. B. & Elston, R. C. (1972). A subroutine package for maximum likelihood estimation (MAXLIK). *UNC of Statistics Mimeo Series No. 823*. Chapel Hill: University of North Carolina.

Lee, E. J. D. (1988). Diurnal effects on debrisoquine hydroxylation phenotyping. *European Journal of Clinical Pharmacology*, **35**, 441–2.

MacLean, C. J., Morton, N. E., Elston, R. C. & Yee, S. (1976). Skewness in commingled distributions. *Biometrics*, **32**, 695–9.

Murphy, E. A. (1964). One cause? Many causes? The argument from the bimodal distributions. *Journal of Chronic Diseases*, **17**, 301–24.

Murphy, E. A. & Bolling, D. R. (1967). Testing single locus hypotheses where there is incomplete separation of the phenotypes. *American Journal of Human Genetics*, **19**, 322–34.

Schmid, B., Bircher, J., Preisig, R. & Kufer, A. (1985). Polymorphic dextromethorphan metabolism: co-segregation of oxidative O-demethylation with debrisoquine hydroxylation. *Clinical Pharmacology and Therapeutics*, **38**, 618–24.

Scott, J. & Poffenbarger, P. L. (1979). Pharmacogenetics of tolbutamide metabolism in humans. *Diabetes*, **28**, 41–51.

Smith, D. M. & Bartlet, J. C. (1961). Calculation of the areas of isolated or overlapping normal probability curves. *Nature*, **191**, 688–9.

Spielman, R. S. & Weinshilboum, R. M. (1981). Genetics of red cell COMT activity analysis of thermal stability and family data. *American Journal of Medical Genetics*, **10**, 279–90.

Appendix IV   Chromosomal locations of genes referred to in the text

Abstracted with permission from McKusick, V.A. (1992) *Mendelian Inheritance in Man*, 10th edition. Baltimore, MD: John Hopkins University Press (ISBN 0-8018-4411-8).

Location	Symbol	Title	Mɪᴍ No.	Status
1pter–q12	ARNT	Aryl hydrocarbon receptor nuclear translocator	126110	P
1p34	UROD	Uroporphyrinogen decarboxylase	176100	C
1p34–p12	CYP 4B1	Cytochrome P450 Subfamily 4B member 1	124075	P
1p31	GST 1	Glutathione-S-transferase 1	138350	C
1p11 – qter	EPHX, EPOX	Epoxide hydroxylase, microsomal (epoxide hydrolase)	132810	P
1q21–q23	GNT2	Bilirubin UDP-glucuronosyltransferase (Crigler–Najjar)	218800	P
2q33–q35	CHE2	Cholinesterase, serum 2 (C5 component)	177500	P
2	UGT1 GNT 1	UDP-glucuronosyltransferase Family 1 (phenols & bilirubin)	191740	P
3p21	ALAS 1	Delta-aminolevulinate synthase	125290	C
3q26.1–q26.2	BCHE, CHE 1	Cholinesterase 1	177400	C
3	GST 1-L, GSTM	Glutathione-S-transferase-like (mu-like)	138270	P
4q21 – q25	ADH 5, ADHX	Alcohol dehydrogenase class III	103710	C
4q22	ADH C1	Alcohol dehydrogenase class I cluster		
	ADH 1	Alcohol dehydrogenase alphapolypeptide	103700	C
	ADH 2	Alcohol dehydrogenase betapolypeptide	103720	C
	ADH 3	Alcohol dehydrogenase gammapolypeptide	103730	C
	ADH 4	Alcohol dehydrogenase Class I. pi-polypeptide	103740	P
6p21.3	CYP 21	Cytochrome P450 Subfamily 21; steroid 21-hydroxylase	201910	C
6p12.2	GST 2	Glutathione-S-transferase 2	138360	C
7p14–cen	BLVR	Biliveridin reductase	109750	C
7q	PTC	Phenylthiocarbamide tasting	171200	P
7q11.2	POR	Cytochrome P450 reductase	124015	P
7q21.1	PGY 1, MDR 1	P-glycoprotein-1 (multidrug resistance)	171050	C
7q21.1	PGY 3, MDR 3	P-glycoprotein-3 (multidrug resistance-3)	171060	P
7q21.3–q22.1	CYP3	Cytochrome P450 Sub-family 3 nifedipine oxidase	124010	C
7q22	PON, ESA	Paraoxonase	168820	C P
8pter–q11	AAC 1	Arylamine-*N*-acetyltransferase-1	108345	P
8pter–q11	AAC 2	Arylamine-*N*-acetyltransferase-2	243400	
8q21	CYP 11 B1	Cytochrome P450 Subfamily 11 B, 11 beta-hydroxylas	202010	P
9q21	ALDH 1	Aldehyde dehydrogenase-1	100640	P
9q34	ALAD	Delta-aminolevulinate dehydratase	125270	C
9	ALDH 5	Aldehyde dehydrogenase-5	100670	P
9	CPRR, CPO	Coproporphyrinogen oxidase	121300	P

Appendix IV. (*cont.*)

Location	Symbol	Title	Mɪᴍ No.	Status
10q24.1–q24.3	CYP2C	Cytochrome P450 Subfamily 2C (mephenytoin 4'-hydroxylase)	124020	C
10q24.3	CYP 17	Cytochrome P450 Subfamily 17; steroid 17-alpha-hydroxylase	202110	P
10q25.2–q26.3	UROS	Uroporphyrinogen III synthase	263700	P
10	CYP2E	Cytochrome P450 Subfamily 2E (ethanol inducible)	124040	P
11p13	CAT	Catalase	115500	C
11q	PORC	Porphyria, Chester type	176010	P
11q13	GST P1, GST 3	Glutathione-S-transferase-P1	138370	C
11q23	DRD 2	Dopamine receptor 2	126450	P
11q24.1–q24.2	PBGD, UPS	Porphobilinogen deaminase (uroporphyrinogen I synthase)	176000	C
12q24.2	ALDH 2	Aldehyde dehydrogenase, mitochondrial	100650	C
12	GST 12	Glutathione-S-transferase 12 (microsomal)	138330	P
13q34	DJS	Dubin–Johnson syndrome	237500	L
14q32	VP, PPOX	Protoporphyrinogen oxidase	176200	P
15q21.1	CYP 19, ARO	Cytochrome P450 Subfamily 19 (aromatization of androgens)	107910	C
15q22–qter	CYP 1A1, CYP 1	Cytochrome P450 Sub-family I (aromatic compound inducible) member 1	108330	P
15q22–qter	CYP 1A2	Cytochrome P450 Sub-family I (aromatic compound inducible) member 2	124060	P
15	CYP 11A	Cytochrome P450 Subfamily 11A (cholesterol side chain cleavage)	118485	P
17q23.1–q25.3	SCN 4A	Sodium channel, voltage-gated type 4, alpha polypeptide	170500	C
17	ALDH 3	Aldehyde dehydrogenase 3	100660	P
17	G6PDL	Glucose-6-phosphate dehydrogenase-like	138110	P
18q21.3–q22	FECH	Ferrochetalase	177000	C
18	CYB5	Cytochrome *b*5	250790	P
19q12–q13.2	CCO, CCD	Central core disease of muscle	117000	C
19q13.1	RYR, RYDR	Ryanodine receptor (sarcoplasmic reticulum calcium release channel)	180901	C
19q13.1–q13.3	CYP 2A	Cytochrome P450 Subfamily 2A (phenobarbital inducible)	123960	C
19q13.1–q13.3	CYP 2B	Cytochrome P450 Subfamily 2B (phenobarbital inducible)	123930	C
19q13.1–q13.3	CYP 2F	Cytochrome P450 Subfamily 2F	124070	P
22q11.2	COMT	Catechol-*O*-methyltransferase	116790	P
22q11.2–q12.2	CYP2D	Cytochrome P450 Subfamily 2D (debrisoquine/sparteine hydroxylase)	124030	C
22q13.31–qter	DIA 1	NADH-diaphorase 1 (cytochrome *b*5 reductase)	250800	C
Xp21.1	CYBB CGD	Chronic granulomatous disease	306400	C
Xq28	G6PD	Glucose-6-phosphate dehydrogenase	305900	C

Mitochondrial genes: Aminoglycoside antibiotic induced deafness; chloramphenicol sensitivity and resistance.
MIM, McKusick, V.A., *Mendelian Inheritance in Man*, Baltimore, Johns Hopkins University Press.
C, Confirmed; P, Provisional; L, 'in limbo', inconsistent evidence.

Appendix V   General bibliography

Aldrete, J. A. & Britt, B. A. (ed.) (1978). *Malignant Hyperthermia*. New York: Grune & Stratton.

Dutton, G. J. (1980). *Glucuronidation of Drugs and Other Compounds*. Boca Raton: CRC Press.

Goedde, H. W. & Agarwal, D. P (ed.) (1987). *Genetics and Alcoholism. Progress in Clinical Biological Research 241*. New York: Alan R. Liss.

Goedde, H. W., Doenicke, A. & Altland, K. (1967). *Pseudocholinesterasen – pharmakogenetik, Biochemie, Kinik*. Berlin: Springer-Verlag (in German).

Ingleman-Sundberg, M., Gustafsson, J. A. & Oppenius, S. (ed.) (1990). *Drug Metabolizing Enzymes: Genetics, Regulation and Toxicology*. Stockholm: Karolinska Institute.

Kalow, W. (1962). *Pharmacogenetics. Heredity and the Response to Drugs*. Philadelphia: Saunders.

Kalow, W. (ed.) (1992). *International Encyclopedia of Pharmacology and Therapeutics. Pharmacogenetics of Drug Metabolism*. Oxford: Pergamon Press.

Kalow, W., Goedde, H. W. & Agarwal, D. P. (ed.) (1986). *Ethnic Differences in Reactions to Drugs and Xenobiotics. Progress in Clinical and Biological Research 214*. New York: Alan R. Liss.

Kiese, M. (1974). *Methemoglobinaemia: A Comprehensive Treatise*. Cleveland: CRC Press.

Mantle, T. J. & Pickept, C. B. (ed.) (1990). *Glutathione S-Transferases and Drug Resistance*. London: Taylor & Francis.

Meier, H. (1963). *Experimental Pharmacogenetics*. New York: Academic Press. (Deals mainly with animal work.)

Moore, M. R. (ed.) (1990). *A Century of Porphyria*. London: Pergamon Press.

Moore, M. R., McColl, K. E. L., Rimington, C. & Goldberg, A. (1987). *Disorders of Porphyrin Metabolism*. New York: Plenum Press.

Omenn, G. S. & Belboin, H. V. (ed.) (1984). *Genetic Variability in Responses to Chemical Exposure*. Banbury Report 16. Cold Spring Harbor Laboratory.

Sies, H. & Ketterer, B. (ed.) (1988). *Glutathione Conjugation*. London: Academic Press.

Siest, G., Magdalou, J. & Burchell, B. (1988). *Cellular and Molecular Aspects of Glucuronidation*. Colloque INSERUM, Vol. 173. John Libbey Eurotext Ltd.

Szórady, I. (1973). *Pharmacogenetics. Principles and Paediatric Aspects*. Budapest: Akadémiai Kiado.

Testa, B. & Jenner, P. (1976). *Drug Metabolism: Chemical and Biochemical Aspects*. New York: Dekker.

Weber, W. W. (1987). *The Acetylator Genes and Drug Response*. New York: Oxford University Press.

Whittaker, M. (1986). *Cholinesterase* In *Monographs in Human Genetics*, Vol. II, ed. L. Beckman. Basel: Karger.

Index